Third Edition

The Complete Guide to Aromatherapy

Volume I – Foundations & Materia Medica

Salvatore Battaglia

Black Pepper Creative
Brisbane

First published in 1995 by
Perfect Potion
7 Guardhouse Road
Banyo QLD 4014
Australia
ISBN 0 646 20670 2
Reprinted 1997, 1998, 1999, 2000, 2001, 2002

Second edition published in 2003 by
The International Centre of Holistic Aromatherapy
PO Box 273
Zillmere QLD 4034
Australia
Reprinted 2003, 2004, 2005, 2007, 2008, 2009, 2011, 2012, 2014, 2015, 2017

Third edition published in 2018 by
Black Pepper Creative Pty Ltd
PO Box 273
Zillmere QLD 4034
Australia
ISBN 978-0-6482606-0-8
Reprinted 2018, 2020

Note to the reader
Knowledge in this field is constantly changing. As new research and experience become available, changes in research methods, professional practices or medical treatment may be necessary. The author and the publisher have, as far as possible, taken care to ensure that the information given herein is accurate and up to date. Practitioners and researchers must rely on their own experience and knowledge in evaluating and using any information, methods or remedies described herein. In using such information they should be mindful of their own safety and the safety of others, including parties for whom they have professional responsibility. Readers are strongly advised to confirm that the information complies with the latest legislation and standards of practice.

To the fullest extent of the law, neither the author nor the publisher, contributor or editor assumes any liability for any injury and/or damage to persons or property as a matter of product liability, negligence or otherwise, or from any use or operation of any methods, products, instructions or ideas contained in this book.

National Library of Australia Cataloguing-in-Publication data:
Battaglia, Salvatore
The complete guide to aromatherapy, volume I – foundations and materia medica.
Bibliography.
Includes index.
ISBN 978-0-6482606-0-8
1. Aromatherapy. 2. Essences and essential oils – therapeutic use. 3. Oils Volatile – therapeutic use. 4. Alternative Medicine.

Edited by Kyoko Mizoguchi
Proofreading by Gail Cartwright
Cover design by Joanna Cristy
Text design by Bill Adrisurya
Typeset in Palatino by Watson Ferguson and Company, Brisbane.
Printed and bound in China by Everbest Printing Investment Ltd

Cover images - ylang ylang flower provided by © pittapitta at dreamstime.com; chamomile flower provided by © Lucian Milasan at dreamstime.com.

FSC
www.fsc.org
100%
Paper from well-managed forests
FSC® C124385

Contents

Acknowledgements

I wish to acknowledge all those individuals who have contributed to promoting aromatherapy and the use of essential oils in a holistic and professional manner. I am grateful for all the sources of information referenced throughout the book.

I wish to express my gratitude to all the therapists and individuals who have provided me with feedback over the years.

I gratefully acknowledge the professional associations that have endorsed *The Complete Guide to Aromatherapy* as a textbook. I acknowledge the contributions that many of my colleagues, educators, researchers, therapists and clinicians have made to aromatherapy.

I am indebted to all my teachers and people who have inspired me to pursue my career in traditional Chinese medicine, natural therapies and aromatherapy. I am grateful to have had the opportunity to train with Madame Micheline Arcier, a person whose dedication and commitment to aromatherapy taught me humility and respect. She has always been a major source of my inspiration.

I wish to thank all my past, present and future students who are responsible for providing me with the inspiration I needed to write this book.

I am indebted to Kyoko Mizoguchi, who has done an outstanding job editing this book. I would like to also acknowledge Dan Kelly and the team at Watson Ferguson and Company for the typesetting, design and layout of this book.

A special thank you goes to the wonderful team at Perfect Potion for being so patient while I spent many hours away from the business writing this book.

The photograph on page 51 has been reproduced with the kind permission of Inkata Press, the publisher of the book *Eucalyptus Leaf Oils: Use, Chemistry, Distillation and Marketing*, 1991, edited by DJ Boland, JJ Brophy and APN House, ACIAR / CSIRO, Canberra.

Last, but not least, I am sincerely grateful and indebted to my wife Carolyn Stubbin for her constant support, patience and encouragement.

I almost forgot a very special furry companion, Charlie, my pet beagle who always waits patiently by my side for her daily walk while I would say: 'Just a few more minutes, as soon as I finish this sentence we will go for a walk.' A few minutes often became an hour later.

Salvatore Battaglia

2018

Preface to Third Edition

When I first wrote the first edition of *The Complete Guide to Aromatherapy* in 1996, aromatherapy was still in its infancy. I did not ever imagine that aromatherapy would become as popular as it is today.

While aromatherapy continues to blossom as one of the most popular forms of health care, it is still the least understood and often the most vulnerable to commercial exploitation. Many of the issues raised in the first and second edition of the book remain unresolved.

Aromatherapy as a health care profession is at a very challenging cross road. More than ever before, aromatherapists need to stand united. Aromatherapy has the opportunity to make a significant contribution to the way conventional health care is provided, but for this to happen we must establish a framework that allows aromatherapy to develop into a profession. There are some who suggest aromatherapy is not a profession, and that it will be difficult for aromatherapy to ever become a profession. I would like to prove them wrong.

We must also convince health regulators to understand the unique holistic principles of aromatherapy, and to find other ways of measuring health care outcomes that are not solely reliant on the pharmacological model. Essential oils are one of the very few natural remedies that can be used in a holistic way to balance the body, mind and spirit.

One area of aromatherapy that has often been criticised is the lack of scientific evidence. It is exciting to see the enormous growth in clinical evidence and scientific research on essential oils. These studies are beginning to confirm many of the traditional actions that had been assigned to essential oils.

The third edition of *The Complete Guide to Aromatherapy* has undergone a major transformation. It has become necessary to publish the book as two volumes. *Volume I – Foundations and Materia Medica* and *Volume II – Science and Therapeutics*. Volume II will be available in the near future.

Much of the information in the second edition has been updated and revised. The essential oil monographs have undergone considerable transformation, with new subsections on adulteration, pharmacopoeias and standards, and a very detailed section summarising the pharmacological and clinical studies. I have expanded the section on subtle aromatherapy, the personality profiling and the energetics of essential oils. There is also a new section on blending for aromatherapy and perfumery purposes.

Many of the actions traditionally assigned to essential oils have been appropriated from old herbals. We know that the properties often attributed to essential oils are not necessarily going to be the same as the herbs. This is why I have expanded the monographs to include the use of the plant in herbal medicine, and where necessary, I have clearly explained that it may be more appropriate to use the herb rather than the essential oil.

In the second edition I often referred to the 'typical chemical composition' of the oil. We now know that there is no such thing as a typical essential oil composition. Most of the essential oil monographs have had the section on chemical composition updated. We also now know so much more about the botanical origins of essential oils, and how so many ecological variables can influence the chemistry of the essential oils. As a result, there is now a new section dedicated to the role of botany and understanding the botanical factors that influence the quality of essential oils.

In looking to the future, we sometimes need to understand the past. I am very excited to have expanded the history of aromatherapy, to take into account the spiritual and cultural context in which scent has been used.

I challenge all aromatherapists and health care professionals passionate about aromatherapy to embrace the diversity of aromatherapy and develop strategies to ensure that aromatherapy can flourish within an integrative medicine framework.

I hope that you enjoy the third edition of *The Complete Guide to Aromatherapy* and that aromatherapy becomes an important part of your health practice or health care regime.

Salvatore Battaglia

2018

Preface to Second Edition

Eight years have passed since the publication of the first edition. During this period aromatherapy has blossomed into one of the most popular complementary health care modalities.

Through my own training, new research and feedback from other educators in aromatherapy, students and aromatherapists, I have been able to expand on many of the existing chapters and added five new chapters.

The essential oil profiles have been extensively updated. I have included new categories on pharmacological and clinical studies, the energetics of essential oils, the subtle effects of essential oils and the personality profile of essential oils.

There is now a considerable amount of research, which has scientifically validated much of what we know of the essential oils. For this, I am indebted to Bob Harris, who has provided us with the most comprehensive database on scientific research dedicated to aromatherapy.

I have included a section on the energetics of essential oils. As an acupuncturist, I have always utilised the essential oils according to the principles of traditional Chinese medicine (TCM). I must acknowledge the work of Gabriel Mojay and Peter Holmes, who have made the principles of TCM accessible to aromatherapists.

I have included a category on the subtle effects of each essential oil – that is how the essential oils may influence our subtle bodies, chakras and spiritual wellbeing. For this, I am indebted to Patricia Davis and Valerie Ann Worwood, who have nurtured, promoted and created awareness of this wonderful facet of aromatherapy.

In each essential oil monograph, I have included a section on method of administration. This provides the reader with clear advice on the most appropriate methods of use. In some cases, I have played the devil's advocate in suggesting internal ingestion. I do not teach internal ingestion and I certainly do not expect you to start recommending ingestion – especially without the appropriate medical and clinical training. I have cited The German Commission E Monographs, which recommend the ingestion of some essential oils.

I believe it is important for us to be aware that many doctors and phytotherapists have been successfully using essential oils by ingestion. This gives us an opportunity to broaden our knowledge and skills base. However, we should exercise some caution, and ensure that any move to promote ingestion of essential oils is backed up by comprehensive and authoritative training relevant to ingestion, and that relevant government legislation regarding the prescribing of therapeutic substances is not breached.

While it is important to have excellent skills and knowledge, to be a successful aromatherapist it is also important to have sound business skills. I have therefore included information necessary to develop these business skills in the chapter, *Requirements for Professional Practice*.

The safe use of essential oils in aromatherapy has created some controversy in the last five years or so. While it is better to err on the safe side – especially when it comes to our client's safety – I believe that this has led to dogma within our industry. Therefore, in some cases, I may sound ambiguous when I cite opposing views regarding safety and don't necessarily 'take sides'. This is done intentionally – I hope that this encourages healthy debate and discussion, which will ultimately benefit aromatherapy.

I am also excited to have introduced five new exciting chapters. The main reason I became involved in complementary medicine in the first place was because of my fascination with the subtle anatomy – it is therefore with great pleasure that I introduce a chapter on subtle aromatherapy.

I can now confidently say that this book is 'complete'. While much research has been conducted into the chemistry and pharmacology of essential oils, I believe it is the subtle vibrational effects of essential oils that will make aromatherapy the holistic medicine of the 21st century.

Aromatherapy has become an integral part of mainstream healthcare in many hospitals and nursing homes. It is therefore appropriate that the role of aromatherapy in mainstream healthcare be addressed in the chapter on *Aromatherapy for the Health Professional*.

A criticism of many books on aromatherapy has been the lack of information in developing skills to blend essential oils. This has been addressed in this edition with an entire chapter dedicated to blending of essential oils.

Many aromatherapists hunger for new and exciting essential oils to use in aromatherapy. I have introduced a new chapter on essential oils that may not necessarily be new or novel, but are not typically part of mainstream aromatherapy. Adventurous aromatherapists will find the chapter on *Exotic Essential Oils* very exciting.

The role of aromatherapy in skin care is as old as the origins of aromatherapy itself; however an exciting new phenomena in the last eight years has been the rise of the day spa industry. Aromatherapy has played a critical role in the success of the spa industry. For individuals wishing to know more about the spa industry and how aromatherapy can complement it, the chapter on *Aromatherapy and Day Spas* is a must.

I hope that you find this new edition provides you with a very strong platform on which you can confidently practise aromatherapy.

Salvatore Battaglia
2003

Preface to First Edition

The booksellers' shelves are crammed with aromatherapy books. Much of the information is usually recycled from earlier English or French texts. While books such as *The Art of Aromatherapy* by Robert Tisserand and Tricia Davis's book *Aromatherapy: An A-Z* have become classics, and are useful reference books, the majority of books on aromatherapy are not as useful as one would wish. They often provide an entertaining series of recipes and often misguided information, sometimes making unsubstantiated claims.

This makes it difficult for the modern holistic aromatherapist who needs to be multidisciplined practitioner with training in remedial therapies, counselling, chemistry, botany, pharmacology, anatomy, physiology and pathophysiology.

The Complete Guide to Aromatherapy addresses all the topics listed above. This is the first time a book on aromatherapy has been aimed specifically at people with a serious interest in aromatherapy and the health professional working in the field of aromatherapy.

While this book addresses in detail both the theoretical and practical aspects of aromatherapy, I have ensured that it remains true to the main principles of holistic healing which embraces three basic principles:

- a holistic approach to health which treats the patient as an individual
- the wisdom of the past and the validity of traditional empirical knowledge;
- the analytical back-up provided by modern pharmacology and chemistry.

I believe that the future of aromatherapy as a powerful, safe and effective form of natural healing is embodied in the issues that I have raised in this book, and I hope that this book contributes to the achievement of that future.

Salvatore Battaglia
1995

Organisation of this book

Volume I – Foundations and Materia Medica

Unit 1 – Foundations

Unit 1 provides you with the knowledge required to develop a holistic framework for the practice of aromatherapy. This is achieved by:

- examining the holistic role of aromatherapy in promoting health and wellbeing
- tracing the history of aromatherapy
- defining the botanical origins of essential oils and explaining the methods of extraction
- examining the need for establishing standards for the quality of essential oils for aromatherapy use
- developing parameters for the safe practice of aromatherapy
- describing the methods on how to use essential oils in aromatherapy.

Unit 2 – Materia Medica

Unit 2 provides you with an extensively updated materia medica with detailed monographs of over 110 essential oils. The essential oils monographs are divided into six sections as follows:

Identification – includes information on the botany and origins, method of extraction, detailed organoleptic profile of the oil, chemical profile, risk of adulteration, and pharmacopoeias and standards that exist for the essential oils.

History and traditional uses – includes information on the history of the plant and essential oil, the role of the plant in herbal and traditional medicine, and examines other uses of the essential oil.

Therapeutics – examines pharmacological and clinical studies that have been conducted for each essential oil, along with the range of actions that are commonly assigned to the essential oil.

Aromatherapy uses – explains the therapeutic application of essential oils in clinical aromatherapy, and the role of the essential oil in energetics, subtle aromatherapy and personality profiling.

Dosage and administration – includes information on aromatherapy blending and perfumery blending, along with recommended methods of use.

Safety profile – provides information to ensure essential oils are used safely by identifying and examining contraindications and toxicity of the oil, as well as identifying the regulatory status relevant for the safe use of the essential oil.

Volume II – Science and Therapeutics

(coming soon)

Unit 3 – Science

Unit 3 will provide you with the knowledge required to understand how aromatherapy works. This is achieved by:

- outlining the chemistry and pharmacology of essential oils
- reviewing the latest research and clinical trials in aromatherapy
- outlining the pharmacokinetics of essential oils
- reviewing the mechanisms of olfaction.

Unit 4 – Holistic frameworks

Unit 4 will help you develop a holistic integrative approach to using essential oils. This will be achieved by:

- integrating the principles of traditional Chinese (TCM) medicine with your aromatherapy knowledge and skills
- examining the subtle effects of essential oils
- examining the relationship between essential oils and personalities
- examining the role of nutrition and healthy lifestyle interventions in the prevention of illnesses and promotion of wellbeing.

Unit 5 – Practical matters

Unit 5 will provide you with the knowledge and skills required for the practice of aromatherapy. This is achieved by:

- establishing an optimal healing environment
- establishing a holistic healing encounter
- developing skills for blending essential oils
- outlining a step-by-step description of the Micheline Arcier aromatherapy massage
- examining the role of aromatherapy within professional health care environment
- examining the role of aromatherapy within skincare and day spa environment.

Unit 6 – Therapeutics

Unit 6 will provide you with an up-to-date, clear and detailed guide to the treatment of a wide range of conditions. Each condition is grouped according the specific body system involved.

A detailed description of the aetiology, the symptoms, a holistic treatment strategy, the need for referral along with detailed treatments that include aromatherapy, diet, herbs, acupressure and other holistic therapies is provided for a range of conditions.

UNIT

1

Foundations

1. **Framework**
   In which we develop a holistic framework for the practice of aromatherapy
2. **History**
   In which we trace the history of essential oils and aromatherapy
3. **Botany**
   In which we explain the botanical origins of essential oils
4. **Production**
   In which we describe the production methods of essential oils
5. **Quality**
   In which we establish standards for the quality of essential oils used in aromatherapy
6. **Safety**
   In which we develop parameters for the safe use of essential oils
7. **Use**
   In which we explain how to use essential oils in aromatherapy

Framework

CHAPTER

1

Contents

Introduction

Why are people drawn to aromatherapy?

The following comments by prominent aromatherapists provide us with some clues:

> *Getting to know these heavenly scents is something like falling in love. They will touch your heart, make you keenly aware of the beauty surrounding you, and open the door to your soul. Suddenly, every facet of your life will be touched by magic.*[1]

Fischer-Rizzi suggests that essential oils have the ability to cast a magical spell upon us and that they can have profound influence on our spiritual wellbeing:

> *... essential oils invite one to appreciate the beauty and wonders of creation, providing us inner contentment. As a gate to our soul, essential oils give us the impetus to search for meaning in our lives.* [1]

Tisserand assigns life-like and ethereal qualities to the essential oils:

> *Essences are like the blood of a person. They are not the whole plant, but are whole, organic substances in themselves. Like blood they will die (lose their lifeforce) if they are not properly preserved. Like blood they incorporate the characteristics of the body (plant) from which they came. They are like the personality, or spirit, of the plant. The essence is the most ethereal and subtle part of the plant, and its therapeutic action takes place on a higher, more subtle level than that of the whole, organic plant, or its extract, having in general a much more pronounced effect on the mind and emotions than herbal medicine.*[2]

Schnaubelt points out that aromatherapy contributes to the realisation of health that no science can – it accepts and integrates the phenomenon of the soul. He explains that essential oils are intricately involved with the chemistry of life. Essential oils can play an important role in the psychosomatic networks, and through olfaction they interact with our emotions, and create a powerful imprint on our consciousness.[3]

Schnaubelt suggests that the willingness to embrace aromatherapy may also be a response to humanity's deep desire to reconnect with nature.[3]

A desire to reconnect with nature

Fischer-Rizzi explains that people want to assume more responsibility for their wellbeing, and to concentrate on preventing illness in the first place. She states that we are drawn to a holistic approach towards healing.[1] We now understand that many illnesses originate in the mind and that a holistic approach for healing involves balancing the body, mind and soul.

She states that the discontent growing within our society has reconnected us with plants and herbs:

> *The number of unhappy people in our society has grown steadily. While in some parts of the world we have been able to satisfy many of our needs for food, protection, property, and security, we have lost our spiritual richness. We know that inner emptiness cannot be filled by external prosperity or diversion. And maybe that's why we are 'ready'*

> *now for those long-neglected healing methods – the pure essential oils – the concentrated fragrant components of plants and herbs that may benefit everyone.*[1]

Schnaubelt also expresses discontent with modern society:

> *Society is not only distinguished by high mobility, flexibility, freedom and an abundance of ideas and innovative concepts, but also by a high degree of inequality, hyper-materialism, crime, violence, a constant rise in psychological disorders, and a drug subculture out of control.*[3]

He explains that quiet connection to nature, holistic health and happiness and many other factors contributing to wellbeing are in short supply; however, aromatherapy provides us with great potential for physical healing and psychological regeneration.[3]

Tisserand suggests that aromatherapy returns us to a time when there was no distinction between science and art and we were in tune with nature:

> *The herbalists of previous centuries had a deep love of nature and respect for plants, and in some ways seemed to understand them. They knew where to find their plants growing naturally. They knew in which season and at what time of the day to pick them; which planets ruled them, and how this affected their properties. They knew virtually nothing of the chemical constituents of the herbs, or why they had certain properties. But they knew a little about disease, and knew which herbs were good for certain ailments. This knowledge was based on no kind of science, except that of trial and error, added to the experience of their predecessors and perhaps more significantly, their intuition.*[2]

However, Lau is critical of this romantic New Age notion that suggests those whose knowledge predated 'science' somehow had an instinctive understanding of nature and a spiritual relationship with the environment.[4]

The popularity of aromatherapy

Throughout the world, there has been a dramatic rise in aromatherapy's popularity. Many factors have contributed to aromatherapy's popularity:

- the ease with which essential oils can be incorporated into so many different products, whether they be products to scent the home, skin care products or bath products just to name a few
- essential oils are readily available to the general public
- aromatherapy is very much associated with a feel-good therapy
- the aesthetic appeal of aromatherapy, which involves two senses that are often neglected in today's society – touch and smell
- essential oils have potent proven therapeutic properties.

In recent years, multi-level marketing (MLM) companies have hijacked aromatherapy and undermined the role of the professional aromatherapist. Many professionally trained aromatherapists are concerned with incorrect information and the unsafe practices being disseminated. There is a concern that if someone reads a bit about essential oils or if they belong to an MLM company, they think they are then qualified to tell others how to use essential oils. This situation undermines the qualifications and experience of professionally trained aromatherapists, and also puts the public at risk of unsafe usage recommendations.

I am pleased that more people than ever are being introduced to aromatherapy; however, it is imperative that aromatherapy is promoted with integrity. Essential oils must not be promoted as a quick fix cure, and consumers should not be misled by fraudulent claims inferring that essential oils such as frankincense have potential anticarcinogenic properties.

Tisserand states that there has not been one peer-reviewed journal article in which frankincense essential oil was successfully used to treat any kind of cancer.[5]

I also agree with Tisserand when he expresses his concerns that consumers with no understanding of aromatherapy are encouraged to use high doses of undiluted essential oils topically, especially when they have been told that any skin redness they experience is a natural, healing reaction and not an adverse reaction, and especially when the recipient is a baby or a pregnant woman. He states that it is possible that harm is going much deeper than a skin reaction.[6]

For aromatherapy to develop as a professional holistic health care modality, several important issues need to be addressed. These include:

- clearly defining the term aromatherapy
- the role of aromatherapy in an integrative medicine framework
- developing guidelines for research into aromatherapy
- improving education standards for the training of professional aromatherapists
- developing standards and regulations for the quality of essential oils.

What is Aromatherapy?

Defining aromatherapy

Aromatherapy has been defined as a branch of phytomedicine that uses essential oils as its principal therapeutic tools. However, there are quite stark divergences in training, emphasis and style between aromatherapy and phytomedicine.[7]

The English word 'aromatherapy' is derived from the French word 'aromatherapie', which was first coined by French chemist Gattefossé in the 1930s. Whilst I do not agree with Buchbauer's semantic objection to the term aromatherapy, I do agree that the term often implies the therapeutic use of fragrances by inhalation only. Buchbauer suggests that, since aromatherapists predominant use essential oils by other means, more suitable names could be 'essence therapy' or 'essential oil therapy'.[8]

Kusmirek suggests the word aromatherapy has a nice sound, it flows and fits the essence of the ideas it is representing. He defines aromatherapy as:

> *The use of pure essential oils to seek to influence, to change or modify, mind, body or spirit; physiology or mood.*[9]

Unfortunately, this statement also encompasses the use of essential oils in perfumery, cosmetics, medicine, both orthodox and alternative, and psychotherapy.

It has been the failure to clearly define aromatherapy that has led to a misunderstanding and abuse of the term. There is no doubt that the use of the term has given commercial advantage, as the therapeutic implication of aromatherapy has been used to provide credibility for frivolous products. We see, for example, skin and hair care products, to name a few, all promising to introduce the user to the benefits of aromatherapy. The fact that these products contain essential oils does not mean they will have the efficacy of essential oils used by a professional aromatherapist.

Schnaubelt states that aromatherapy is deeply rooted in the Western, industrialised and science-based societies of our time. He refers to Gattefossé's theories which place aromatherapy within the modern scientific paradigm:

> *Gattefossé's aromatherapy was biased toward the concept of active ingredients. Not surprisingly, aromatherapy according to Gattefossé was used to treat a symptom or disease the same way conventional medicine did. In Gattefossé's approach there really was no division between medicine and aromatherapy; in fact he considered aromatherapy to be an integral part of medicine.*[3]

Tisserand lists five fields in which aromatherapy is practised – medical, nursing, holistic, psychotherapeutic and aesthetic.[10]

Sheen states that aromatherapists include those who focus on the use of essential oil in massage and those who use essential oils orally as aromatic medicine. At the same time, Sheen explains that there are many other health care professionals who have a background in Ayurveda, traditional Chinese medicine, nursing, beauty therapy or kinesiology who incorporate aromatherapy into their practice.[11]

Whatever our concept or method of practice is, we need to realise the complexity of aromatherapy. While we can remain true to our own concept of aromatherapy, we should also be exploring other aspects of aromatherapy and respect our colleagues who may have a different approach.

Anglo-Saxon aromatherapy

Harris explains that 'Anglo-Saxon aromatherapy', as practised in the UK and taught in many countries around the world, originates from French Biochemist Madame Maury who wrote *The Secret of Life and Youth*. This style of aromatherapy was promoted as an external therapy and closely associated with massage and beauty therapy. Anglo-Saxon aromatherapy is commonly perceived as a 'soft therapy' that lacks a scientific basis, and hence is limited in its contribution to health care.[12]

Jenkins states that some therapists in Britain realise the potential of the French style of aromatherapy treatment, whilst still maintaining the holistic philosophy which the Anglo-Saxon style aromatherapy was originally based on.[13]

However, she claims that the link to beauty therapy can be a two-edged sword. The therapy is seen as gentle and non-invasive, offering little risk of harm, and providing a soothing and relaxing massage with pleasantly scented oils. Jenkins claims that this view has prevented aromatherapy from being taken seriously.[13]

As more aromatherapists are exposed to the French approach of 'aromatic medicine' in which essential oils are often used at higher concentrations or internally, Jenkins states that the level of training needs to improve. Most aromatherapy educators focus on the holistic, topical and energetic methods of treatment. However, aromatherapists who wish to incorporate 'aromatic medicine' into their practice must be required to do more training in 'aromatic medicine', which involves the internal use of essential oils. Jenkins advocates the need for more integrated training and training to a higher level. It is important that the aromatherapist be well grounded in anatomy and physiology, pathology, chemistry and pharmacology, and be able to evaluate research findings and able to think and reason for themselves to practise safely and effectively.[13]

Jenkins cites Mojay, who suggests that aromatherapy may benefit from a single professional body, and recommends adopting a multi-level platform for practitioners such as novice, competent and expert. She states that this is already in place for nursing.[13]

Aromatic medicine/medical aromatherapy

While there is no approved definition for the term 'medical aromatherapy', for the purpose of this book, I will refer to medical aromatherapy as the style of aromatherapy as practised by doctors in France. French doctors have pioneered the clinical treatment of infectious diseases using essential oils.

Asked to comment on the internal use of essential oils, Dr Lapraz, a French doctor who uses essential oils and phytotherapy extensively in the treatment of cancer, states:

> *Our position with regards to the internal use of aromatherapy is very clear. As essential oils are extremely active agents having some demonstrable effects on the different organs of the body, they need to be administered under medical supervision.*[14]

Dr Pénoël, a prominent French doctor who uses aromatherapy, suggests that in the case of serious infections, the only way that aromatherapy can help is an internal, massive and repetitive aromatic treatment involving strong antimicrobial essential oils taken by oral ingestion every 20 minutes. He suggests that within three days the infection can be completely eliminated by such a treatment.[15]

However, Dr Pénoël points out that the French patient in a stressful situation cannot easily make an appointment to receive an aromatherapy treatment 'in the English way', which he claims to be a delightful and highly efficacious treatment. The French doctor trained in aromatherapy is also not likely to include lifestyle changes, which are necessary as part of a holistic aromatherapy treatment.[15]

Holistic aromatherapy

A holistic practitioner of any particular therapy has a deep respect for the individual's inherent capacity for self-healing. This, claims Hoffmann, facilities a relationship of active partnership in the healing process, as opposed to an unequal dynamic between expert healer and passive healer.[16]

Hoffmann states that the mere use of herbal medicines does not make a treatment holistic. In fact, using a herbal remedy as a natural alternative to a prescription medication relegates the herb to the status of an organic drug delivery system. What makes herbs part of an holistic treatment is the context within which the herbs are prescribed and used.[16] I agree with Hoffmann and suggest that the same principles apply to the use of essential oils.

A holistic aromatherapy treatment aims at treating the whole person. A holistic approach may include identification and treatment of the disease, but it does not focus exclusively on symptoms. It should focus on the development of wellbeing and enjoyment of life in a system of self-responsibility.

Holistic aromatherapy often incorporates the pharmacological, the psychotherapeutic and the metaphysical activities of the essential oils.

Aromatherapy is part of complementary and alternative medicine (CAM). CAM is defined as a group of diverse medical and health care practices, and products that are not currently considered to be part of conventional medicine.

Kotsirilos et al. cite the National Center for Complementary and Alternative Medicine that classifies natural, complementary and alternative medicines into five categories or domains:[17]

- **alternative medical systems** – complete systems of theory and practice such as homoeopathic and naturopathic medicine, traditional Chinese medicine (TCM) and Ayurveda
- **mind-body interventions** – these interventions include patient support groups, meditation and mindfulness, prayer, spiritual healing, and therapies that use creative outlets such as art, music or dance
- **biological-based therapies** – these therapies include herbs, food and nutritional supplements
- **manipulative and body-based therapies** – these methods include chiropractors, osteopaths and massage therapists
- **energy therapies** – involve the use of energy fields such as qi gong, chakras, therapeutic touch and use of electromagnetic fields.

So which category does aromatherapy fit into?

I am sure you will agree with me that aromatherapy can easily be classified into any of the five categories.

Integrative Medicine

What is integrative medicine?

> *Integrative medicine is about changing the focus of medicine to one of healing rather than disease. This involves an understanding of the influences of mind, spirit and community as well as of the body. It entails developing insight into the patient's culture, beliefs and lifestyle that will help the provider understand how best to trigger the necessary changes in behaviour that will result in improved health. This cannot be done without a sound commitment in the therapist-patient relationship.*[17]

Kotsirilos et al. describe integrative medicine as the practice of medicine in a way that relates to complete patient care. They state that it should not reject conventional therapies nor uncritically accept alternative / complementary ones.[17]

Rakel states that an integrative medicine approach to health care should:[18]

- emphasise relationship-centred care
- develop an understanding of the patient's culture and beliefs to help facilitate the healing response
- focus on the unique characteristics of the individual person based on the interaction of mind, body, spirit and community
- focus on prevention and maintenance of health with attention to lifestyle choices, including nutrition, exercise, stress management and emotional wellbeing
- require providers to act as educators, role models and mentors to their patients
- use an evidence-based approach from multiple sources of information to integrate the best therapy for the patient, be it conventional or complementary
- regard the patient as an active partner who takes personal responsibility for health
- integrate conventional and complementary methods for treatment and prevention
- activate the body's innate healing response
- search for and remove barriers that may be blocking the body's innate healing response
- see compassion as always helpful, even when other therapies are not
- use natural, less invasive interventions before costly, invasive ones where possible
- maintain that healing is always possible, even when curing is not.

Rakel suggests that any therapy used in integrative medicine should be based on an understanding of the physical, emotional, psychological and spiritual aspects of the individual.[18]

He explains that there should be more emphasis on 'healing' rather than 'curing'. Cure refers to doing something to alleviate a troublesome condition or disease. Healing is a dynamic process of recovery, repair, reintegration and renewal that increases resilience, coherence and wholeness.[18]

Healing is a transformative process of the whole person – physical, mental, emotional, social, spiritual and environmental. It is a unique, personal and communal process and experience that may or may not involve curing.[18]

For example, it is easy for a doctor to 'cure' hypertension with a pharmaceutical without ever healing the patient. Healing requires improved diet, promotion of exercise, reduction in stress and an increase in the person's sense of community. In doing this, we help improve the balance of health of the body that may result in the ability to discontinue a pharmaceutical drug and thereby reduce the need for the cure and reduce the cost of the health care intervention.

The National Center for Complementary and Integrative Health states that there are many definitions of 'integrative' health care, but all involve bringing conventional and complementary approaches together in a coordinated way. Most complementary health approaches fall into one of two subgroups – natural products or mind and body practices.[19]

- **Natural products** – This group includes a variety of products, such as herbs, vitamins and minerals. They are widely marketed, readily available to consumers and often sold as dietary supplements. It is claimed that researchers have done large, rigorous studies on a few natural products, but the results do not always support the claims.
- **Mind and body practices** – Mind and body practices include a large and diverse group of procedures or techniques administered or taught by a trained practitioner or teacher. Yoga, chiropractic and osteopathic manipulation, meditation and massage therapy are among the most popular mind and body practices used. Other mind and body practices include acupuncture, relaxation techniques (such as breathing exercises, guided imagery and progressive muscle relaxation), tai chi, qi gong, healing touch, hypnotherapy and movement therapies (such as Feldenkrais method, Alexander technique, Pilates, Rolfing Structural Integration and Trager psychophysical integration).
- **Other complementary health approaches** – The two broad areas outlined above – natural products and mind and body practices – capture most complementary health approaches. However, some approaches may not neatly fit into either of these categories. For example, Ayurvedic medicine, TCM, homoeopathy and naturopathy.

The Australasian Integrative Medicine Association (AIMA) states that integrative medicine refers to the blending of conventional and natural/ complementary medicines and therapies along with lifestyle interventions and a holistic approach – taking into account the physical, psychological, social and spiritual wellbeing of a person – with the aim of using the most appropriate, safe and evidence-based modalities available.[20]

Aromatherapy and complementary & alternative medicine (CAM)

Buckle states that, of all the complementary

therapies, aromatherapy is the most misunderstood. She explains that it is misaligned, misrepresented and can be very confusing. She explains that while aromatherapy has been ridiculed by some, a growing number of health care practitioners believe that aromatherapy has a valid place in integrative medicine.[21]

Rakel suggests that the deterioration of the patient-provider relationship, the overuse of technology and the inability of the medical system to treat chronic disease adequately have contributed to the interest in CAM.[18]

Buckle states that the popularity and growth of CAM has led to a power struggle between the supporters of Western medicine and the supporters of CAM. She explains that both appear to be entrenched in their philosophies, but share the idea that if one is correct, the other is wrong.[21]

Buckle states that the rationale behind CAM, including aromatherapy, is multidimensional and not aimed at one specific body system. CAM therapists are interested in the individuality of the patient and what has led the patient to his or her particular disease process or set of symptoms.[21]

CAM therapists feel that when a patient is balanced, homoeostasis can return and the disease will be unable to survive. Emphasis is placed on teaching the patient preventative medicine to avoid a relapse, and on providing support during the healing process. The patient is often encouraged to rest while the healing process is in progress.[21]

More and more people find natural therapies to be more aligned with their own values, beliefs and physical orientations towards health and life. Sheen surveyed nurses about the role of aromatherapy and the general feeling was that aromatherapy complements their profession. Nurses felt that it often provides a safer option than pharmacological medicines and could reduce the costs and pressure on the health care system. They mentioned the increased effectiveness, increased family involvement, positive public relations and staff benefits.[11]

Harris cites a report stating that the increasing public use of CAM is due to:[12]

- a degree of public dissatisfaction with orthodox medicine
- perceived limitations of modern medicine, especially with regard to chronic, degenerative or stress-related diseases, mental health or addiction
- recognition of the need for a more humane approach to health
- a desire to take more responsibility for self-care
- increased publicity and positive reporting in the media.

Harris states that the top five conditions reported as being helped by aromatherapy as a result of surveying UK aromatherapy associations included:[12]

- stress / anxiety
- headaches / migraine
- insomnia
- musculoskeletal problems
- hormonal problems.

On the other hand, a survey of the members of the public found that the main reasons for choosing aromatherapy included:[12]

- stress relief
- relaxation
- as a 'pick me up'
- aches and pains
- loss of mobility / injury.

Harris concludes that most people choose aromatherapy to help with chronic problems, especially of a musculoskeletal or stress nature. The majority of clients have already sought conventional treatment for the same problem with limited success and are thus not going to an aromatherapist for a diagnosis.[12]

Aromatherapy and nursing

Despite the lack of statutory regulation, aromatherapy is increasingly being integrated into some areas of orthodox medicine. Aromatherapy is one of the most popular complementary therapies practised by nurses.[12]

Harris states that the main uses for incorporating aromatherapy within a clinical practice for nurses include:[12]

- relaxation
- stress reduction
- pain relief
- insomnia
- palliative care
- minor problems in pregnancy.

Many examples where aromatherapy has been successfully integrated into orthodox medicine include oncology, hospice care, pain management, intensive care, midwifery and aged care.[12]

A study in Norway examining why a growing number of nurses were choosing to offer CAM identified four main reasons:[22]

- a desire to perform holistic nursing
- a tendency to value self-realisation
- a wish to experience meaning to their work and develop a stronger professional identity
- a freedom to mix care and cure.

Johannessen states that in order to understand why nurses choose to offer CAM, it is useful to look at the general trends in nursing. She claims nursing, as a practical profession and as a scientific discipline, has developed in different directions over recent years. Nursing science is a young science with a strong influence from the United States, where most of the nursing and caring theories are developed. However, practical nursing is governed by other theories such as medical, economic and organisational theories. This gap between theoretical and practical nursing has created a debate among nurses.[22]

Johannessen states that one of the concerns is the management approach which focuses mainly on productivity, output and profits. She claims that this kills the professional discretion and the holistic approach, which is essential to nursing care. In theoretical nursing, care of the whole person is emphasised; however, in practice, nurses of today have a feeling of coming up short, and there are very few opportunities for them to realise their ideals.[22]

Johannessen states that nurses often leave the profession because they are frustrated and burned out when they are not able to be the nurses they would like to be.[22]

Rizzo Gnatta et al. explain that aromatherapy should be part of nursing practice. They use several theories of nursing practice that align with the philosophy of different CAM therapies and aromatherapy.[23]

For example, a correlation is made with the model of Florence Nightingale nurse care, which is grounded in attention to the aspect of the environment. They state that Nightingale indicated the use of lavender essential oil in the frontal regions of wounded soldiers with the intention of providing comfort and relief, which would allow for an environment that facilitates the natural healing and restoration of the patient.[23]

Jean Watson's theory suggests that healing is facilitated by transpersonal care. In this respect, aromatherapy can be offered in conjunction with touch, massage and the gentle application directly to the skin. The healing process is not only understood as a cure, but as a restorative non-invasive process. For Watson, health was conceptualised as an integral harmony in the interrelationship between the person and the environment. Therefore, aromatherapy can create a sense of harmony with the environment and the body.[23]

According to Martha Rogers, nursing is considered a humanistic and humanitarian science, focused on the description and explanation of the human being as a whole. The principle of Roger's theory is based on integrality and resonance, and addresses the concepts of energy fields in constant exchange. Each essential oil may be seen as a pattern of unique vibrational frequencies, in the same way that each person is considered a unique pattern of energy frequencies.[23]

Rizzo Gnatta et al. state that the relationship between aromatherapy and the nursing theories contributes to a better understanding of the role of aromatherapy in nursing practice:

> *Humanistic and holistic principles, guided in interpersonal relationships and in the integral approach of the human being as discussed in the current context of nursing, find accordance with complementary practices such as aromatherapy, contributing to the expansion of care towards offering an approach that reaches not only the physical, but mental, emotional and spiritual wellbeing of the patients.*[23]

It is, therefore, not surprising that Sheen suggests that the practice of aromatherapy should be integrated into nursing practice:

> *... the most likely pathway for the practice of aromatherapy to develop within the Australian health care system is by integration into nursing practice. This is because of a philosophical match between aromatherapy and nursing practice.*[11]

Developing Guidelines for Research

The need for evidence

Harris acknowledges the diversity of aromatherapy, and that many therapists use essential oils in association within their practice with great success. He states that the fact that aromatherapy is effective outside the scientific paradigm is advantageous to practitioners and clients.[24]

However, aromatherapy is often the target of ridicule and criticism by those involved in conventional science. Harris suggests that, as an emerging profession, if we wish to be taken seriously, that is, if we wish for aromatherapy to be accepted as an effective therapeutic intervention, we need to place more value on the scientific aspects of aromatherapy. He warns us that in many countries, impending draconian legislation may tighten control on the use of essential oils if we do not provide a scientific paradigm proving that aromatherapy works.[24]

If aromatherapy is to fit within the integrative medicine framework, then it is often expected to conform to the conventions of the biomedical framework. For example, in discussing the role of aromatherapy in the management of depression, Kotsirilos et al. state:

The antidepressant properties of essential oils such as bergamot and geranium were summarized in a report offering clinical and neuropharmacological perspectives of aromatherapy in managing psychiatric disorders. Although some studies demonstrated an association between aromatherapy and improvement in mood in healthy adults, there was a notable lack of methodologically useful trials in clinical depressed populations, hence no conclusions could be drawn regarding the efficacy of aromatherapy in treating depression until controlled trials are conducted.[17]

This mantra 'hence no conclusions could be drawn regarding the efficacy of aromatherapy in treating such and such condition until controlled trials are conducted' appeared time and time again under every single subsection for aromatherapy. This means that aromatherapy is often not included as a recognised therapy within the integrative medicine framework because of the lack of controlled clinical trials.

Rakel states that short-term, but not persistent benefits were found for aromatherapy massage with citrus oils in patients with cancer who were dealing with depression. Rakel concludes that aromatherapy may be promising as a gentle adjunctive therapy, but larger, well-designed trials are necessary before conclusions can be reached.[18]

I most certainly endorse the need for larger controlled studies. However, I ask: 'Why is it necessary for aromatherapy to comply with the biomedical framework?'

The problem with pharmacology

Holmes states that, whether we are trying to describe how an essential oil works on the body or soul, or whether we are trying to explain why a particular blend has such miraculous effect on a certain client, we are usually attempting to validate aromatherapy in terms of chemistry or pharmacology, yet aromatherapy is essentially an *energy medicine*.[25]

Pharmacology does play an important role in understanding aromatherapy, but it concerns me that government legislators around the world are fixated on the pharmacology model to understand the therapeutic action of natural remedies such as essential oils.

We may be tempted to think of drugs or essential oils as magic bullets that can cure our ailments; however, a more integrative approach is to understand the complex relationship between the illness and the patient.

It is not surprising that some doctors are now interested in a more integrative health care system. Dr Agus, a world-renowned oncologist, states:

We've had a hard time moving past the germ theory of disease, which has dominated and in many ways defined, medicine in the 20th century. According to this theory, if you can figure out what species of germ you are infected with, then your problem is solved because this tells you how you should treat this disease. This became the general paradigm of medicine. Doctors would perform laboratory test to determine what the infectious agent was, then apply a treatment that was specific for that agent. The treatment only cared about the invading organism … it did not care to define or understand the host (the human being) or even where the infection was happening in the host. That is why we use the same drug in every patient with a particular infectious disease.[26]

He points out that the scientific approach to medicine is relatively new. He goes on to state:

Historically doctors had theories that resembled the traditional Hindu system of Ayurveda medicine, with its emphasis on balance between the various forces in the body … the idea was to try to restore the order of the various forces that were controlling the body. Unfortunately, this approach to medicine of honoring the body as a whole was all but abandoned in the early 20th century. [26]

Dr Agus is especially critical of the attitude of Western medicine towards cancer. Cancer is not as straightforward as infectious diseases. Diagnosing, categorising and treating may make a lot of sense for infectious diseases because organisms causing infections can be treated as invaders.[26]

Mills describes conventional pharmacology as being entirely pragmatic, and an unprincipled science because it suppresses inflammation, kills pathogens, blocks pathological deteriorations and potentially damages physiological responses.[27]

In pharmacology, nature is effectively disintegrated so that the actions of isolated chemicals on isolated pieces or functions of the body can be observed as precisely as possible in a variable world. These observations are then stuck together to make a jigsaw picture of the effect of that substance on the body. On that basis drugs are given to real people.

Most pharmacological research has focused on finding the 'active' principle or constituent. The trace constituents are often seen as a problem that have to be removed. This is the case with eucalyptus oil. Eucalyptus oil is commonly redistilled or rectified.

The so-called 'active' principle in eucalyptus oil is 1,8-cineole. 1,8-cineole has excellent expectorant properties. However, Dr Pénoël says that the residue left behind in the redistillation of eucalyptus oil contains precious molecules such as the rare phenol, australol. Even though the amount of australol is low, it works in synergy with the main components and should not be removed if we wish to utilise the essential oil's full healing potential.[28]

Mills suggests that any pharmacology suited to aromatherapy must be different. At no time must the view of the whole be lost. Traditional pharmacology's role is to draw from human experience and the effects of the mind and body to enable the aromatherapist to better predict the action of each essential oil in the infinitely variable circumstances that will be encountered in practice.[27]

Schnaubelt best summarises the role of science in aromatherapy:

> *Subordinating aromatherapy to what can be proven scientifically is either folly or execution of a hostile agenda. The role of science in aromatherapy is clear: it can help us to understand some of the more complex mechanisms in which oils can be used to treat symptoms of diseases, but science is not equipped to explain the miracles of life to which the interaction with essential oils and plants open a glimpse.*[3]

The need for new sciences

Science has helped us to make some remarkable discoveries. Science is important for the advancement of humankind; however, a purely scientific approach to health care is an extremely alienating paradigm. Within an aromatherapy context, science has helped us to understand the chemical nature of the essential oils and how the essential oils work at a pharmacological level. However, you might be surprised to know that we still do not fully understand the mechanisms of olfaction or the intricate relationship between smell, the limbic brain and our emotions.

Schnaubelt states that the current scientific method is unable to make meaningful statements regarding the role of scent and emotions. He suggests the need for new sciences that would allow us to understand the existence of psychosomatic networks.[3]

For example, the currently accepted model of olfaction is based on shape theory – that scent is recognised by the molecular shape of the aroma molecules. However, in 1996, a biophysicist and chemist Luca Turin challenged this olfactory theory. Turin suggests that olfactory villa detect smell by molecular vibration rather than molecular shape.[29]

How interesting!

Yes, you heard right – vibrations. Vibrations which are frequencies are the basis of subtle energy medicine and energy healing. Perhaps one day in the near future subtle anatomy will become part of mainstream medicine.

Smith explains how all energy medicines such as homoeopathy, acupuncture and healing are all linked through the commonality of frequencies. He provides us with a sound scientific framework for understanding how frequencies affect our health and wellbeing.[30]

There are people doing some excellent scientific research into vibrational and energy medicine. Konstantin Korotkov, professor of physics at St Petersburg State Technical University in Russia, has developed the Gas Discharge Visualisation technique (GDV) to study the human energy field. He has also conducted studies examining the subtle energetic influences of essential oils on our subtle body.[31] Wisneski & Anderson provide us with a detailed scientific investigation of subtle energy therapies in their book *The Scientific Basis of Integrative Medicine*.[32]

Unfortunately, much of this work does not fit well with the current scientific framework supported by the pharmaceutical industry.

We will examine the subtle energy of essential oils in far more detail in volume II of *The Complete Guide to Aromatherapy* in the chapter on *Subtle Aromatherapy*.

We will also examine the ongoing debate between those who suggest that olfaction is molecular shape-based and those who suggest that it is molecular vibrational based in volume II of *The Complete Guide to Aromatherapy* in the chapter on *Olfaction*.

There is no need for me to remind you how limiting it is to think of essential oils as only having a pharmacological effect that must be measured by double-blind, controlled clinical trials.

Bone & Mills also explain the drawbacks of conventional science and state the need for a new physiology to study the complex dynamic living organism.[33]

Improving Education Standards

Aromatherapy as a health care profession

Sheen's PhD thesis – *The professionalisation of aromatherapy: a case study of the professionalisation of complementary and alternative medicine in the Australian health care system* – argues that aromatherapy, as it is currently practised, fails to meet the criteria for being considered a profession in the 'true' sense. Sheen proposes that one of the most likely pathways for the development of aromatherapy in the Australian health care system is within nursing practice.[11]

Nurses are increasingly using aromatherapy.

Sheen explains that one of the main reasons that nurses are drawn to aromatherapy is the similar underlying philosophical principles such as giving people control of their own health, taking a vitalistic approach and moving away from the more technical curative aspects of modern medicine.[11]

Another option is that the medical profession could take on the oral and medicinal use of essential oils in their practice.[11] While this practice has been adopted in other countries such as Japan and Korea, there is very little evidence of interest by the Australian medical profession to take on this role.

Another option is that naturopathy or Western medical herbalists could consider this role.[11] These roles are distinctly different from the nursing approach, whose emphasis is on nurturing and self-care aspects of aromatherapy practice compared to the naturopathy or medical profession's distinctly task and pharmacological orientated approach.

The need for regulations?

Many practitioners of aromatherapy do not have conventional medical qualifications. Typically, an aromatherapist will undergo one year or less of training at a private school to become registered with a suitable professional organisation after qualifying.

There is no single governing body for all practitioners of complementary medicine, in fact, there are often several governing bodies for each therapy. Practitioners can train in a number of different schools. Each school offers qualifications that vary in the length and intensity of the course offered and the approach of the teaching.

There are those who argue that the future of all complementary medicines would appear to lie in statutory self-regulation of the therapies on a therapy-by-therapy basis. In the UK, osteopathy and chiropractic are the only two groups of CAM practitioners that have succeeded in gaining statutory recognition (including protection against the use of the title 'osteopath' or 'chiropractor' by unqualified practitioners) in Acts which were passed in 1993 and 1994 respectively.[34]

Back in 1996, Vickers stated that it is unlikely that massage or aromatherapy will ever become subject to statute in the near future. Vickers argued that complementary therapies are not a unified professional discipline; rather, it is a term of convenience to group together a disparate collection of different therapies. He states that the lack of philosophical and practical cohesion of the complementary therapies limits generalisations about 'complementary medicine' as a whole. This is reflected in the practice and organisation of complementary medicine, in which a number of different governing bodies compete for recognition and status.[34]

Others argue that the lack of regulations leads to concerns about patient safety. Smith states that there are two approaches that should be considered to the regulation of CAM – statutory and voluntary.[35]

Statutory regulations require the therapist to join a register otherwise it would be unlawful for them to practise. However, a voluntary body does not have any statutory status. A practitioner does not need to join a voluntary organisation to practise or need to participate in continuing professional development.[35]

Smith states that the disparity of regulations across CAM therapies has led to confusion for clinical nurses wishing to recommend CAM therapies for their patients, or to train to deliver a particular CAM therapy. It has become problematic for clinical nurses to distinguish between a well-trained CAM therapist and someone who has only undertaken a short course.[35]

Smith is also concerned with the continuing fragmentation between CAM representative bodies and statutory registered practitioners such as clinical nurses. In the UK, acupuncturists, medical herbalists and non-medically qualified homoeopaths are currently regulated by voluntary bodies. Other CAM therapies such as aromatherapy, massage, yoga therapy and reiki are working towards voluntary self-regulation.[35]

Smith states that the principal purpose of regulation of any health-related profession is to protect the public from unqualified or inadequately trained practitioners. However, many of the issues associated with the regulation of CAM remain to be resolved.[35]

Sheen points out that aromatherapy is promoted to be a relatively safe practice. This is detrimental to aromatherapy ever becoming a profession with statutory regulation:

> *A further critical issue is that to become a true profession, with statutory regulation, a significant 'risk' must be demonstrated requiring the state to act in order to protect the public. As aromatherapy practice is promoted to be and accepted as a relatively safe practice this criterion is not fulfilled. Aromatherapy practice as a true profession is a very unlikely outcome.*[11]

Cultural Dimensions of Aromatherapy

The commodification of aromatherapy

Barcan states that aromatherapy thrives in a consumer culture, where the beauty industry and the New Age have provided vehicles for the translation of its folk medical and herbalist principles into a receptive popular culture. She goes on to state that aromatherapy is one of the most amenable CAM therapies to commodification and most easily picked up by amateurs and hobbyists.[36]

While Schnaubelt is critical of the exploitation and commercialisation of esoteric aromatherapy, he explains that it has helped to create an awareness of the connection between aroma, consciousness and the spiritual dimension.[3]

Lau states that New Age capitalism has transformed aromatherapy practices into a collection of products that fragment the body into a series of parts and separate the mind and soul into various states of being, each 'treatable' with different aromatherapy products. She is also critical of books written by aromatherapists who provide a 'therapeutic index' for determining the best essential oil for specific conditions. This she claims is contrary to the holistic practice of aromatherapy.[4]

Lau also questions the way in which New Age capitalism has hijacked the environmental movement. She states that aromatherapy benefits from the association of organically grown botanicals; however, she asks:

> *The exact ways in which aromatherapy protects the planet from demise, however, are unclear. Everyone from aromatherapists to essential oil suppliers and aroma researchers praises the earth-friendly nature of aromatherapy, but no one articulates the precise nature of its environmentalism.*[4]

Lau explains that aromatherapy has jumped on the bandwagon of the 'save the earth' green movement and that the association seems as simple as plants = green = earth friendly. In fact, 'green consumerism' has inspired a worldwide increase in essential oil production and created even more markets for aromatherapy products.[4]

Rashkow states that the New Age movement contributed to the demise of the sandalwood industry and tree in India.[37] As a result, the sandalwood tree in India is now listed as a threatened and endangered species.[38]

The plants for producing essential oils are usually harvested by either 'wild harvesting' them in nature or from cultivated plants. We examine the challenges of sourcing of essential oil-bearing plants in *Chapter 3 – Botany*.

I believe that those aromatic plants that have been cultivated using certified organic practices, or those aromatic ingredients that have been sustainably harvested using traditional indigenous practices, are both environmentally and socially sustainable.

The feminisation of aromatherapy

Barcan explains that aromatherapy is a feminised practice because the majority of its clients and practitioners are women. She states that this female centredness holds for both aesthetic and therapeutic aromatherapy – where clients, usually women, enjoy an aromatherapy treatment from a beauty therapist or massage therapist. Aromatherapy massage is considered a practice of intimate care.[7]

Aromatherapy's different styles and explanatory paradigms are bound up in attitudes towards science, rationality and the esoteric in which gender plays a significant role. Barcan explains that, aromatherapy revalues culturally trivialised sensory practices, bringing to the centre both fragrances and the sense of smell. In doing so, she claims that aromatherapy reunites the separated realms of sensuality, spirituality and medicine, reviving religious meanings and uses of scents, but also places them within a consumerist context in which healing and pampering are not mutually exclusive.[7]

Lau is not surprised that women are the primary targets for and consumers of aromatherapy products. She states that women have long been linked with perfume and fragrance, with flowers and nature, with cosmetics and beauty. She claims that aromatherapy sells more than essential oils and the promise of holistic health – it also sells the dominant ideologies of beauty and romance, and it is these gendered ideals that in turn compel women to aromatherapy.[4]

Barcan explains that the feminisation of aromatherapy is an ambiguous blessing for aromatherapy, which sometimes struggles to assert its legitimacy against the 'hard' sciences. Aromatherapy is both valued and maligned for its connections to smell and the feminine, and is professionally divided between a quest for scientific validation and a more radical inclusive holism.[7]

Johannessen states that there is an imbalance in Western medicine, with a preponderance of masculine values at the expense of feminine values.[34] She states that this is seen as a power/powerless relationship:

> *A holistic approach is perceived to be based on feminine values and feminine energy. Given the human capacity for self-healing, informants will provide treatments they call holistic. These treatments appeal to women, especially nurses.*[22]

On the other hand, Schnaubelt acknowledges and embraces the fact that aromatherapy is essentially a female modality that emphasises female qualities and cooperative approaches. He suggests that aromatherapy returns the power of healing back to the individual, especially the individual woman. He also claims that women generally have a better sense of smell than men, and are better equipped to be creative in the interface of rational and intuitive conclusions for those in need of healing.[3]

The role of myths

Barcan states that the broader cultural dimensions to the variability of olfactory experiences means that, the sense of smell involves a physical encounter with myths. These may be marketing myths or broader cultural stories. She explains that, in the Western context, both the mythology and the language of aromatherapy represent history, luxury and the exotic.[36]

Barcan uses a description of jasmine by Fischer-Rizzi to critique orientalism, however, she also explains that these cultural myths; however politically dubious or historically feeble, are a genuine part of the aromatherapy experience for those consumers who literally buy into them.[36]

> *In India the jasmine plant is called 'queen of the night' or 'moonshine in the gardens'. This plant with blossoms the color of moonlight generously emits, especially at night, a magical fragrance. Like the waters of a sweet river, this fragrance penetrates the deepest layer of our souls, opening the doors to our emotions … In a secret way queen of the night excites sensuality. As if touched by a silvery wand, men and women under its influence opens up to sensual love. Naturally sensuality grows from a state of wholeness, which requires that we trust ourselves and others. Jasmine helps set the stage for experiencing warm love, total abandon, trust and relaxed physical awareness. It envelops people with a mantle of mystery and magic. In India people have known about the power of the jasmine plant for centuries. Many portrayals of lovers bathed in moonlight near a garden or lake include the jasmine plant, which mirrors the mysterious moonlight in its blossoms.*[1]

The strong role of culture, experience, expectations and learning in the actual sensory perception of smells, even to the point where perception can be 'inconsistent with the actual sensory output', means that these cultural resonances are part of the phenomenological experience of an aromatherapy treatment.[36]

Schnaubelt states that throughout most previous cultures, plant aromatics were intimately involved in defining human identity, influencing our physical, emotional and spiritual being:

> *At the dawn of recorded history, aromatic substances already were the substances of choice for ritual and magic. Medicinal and religious applications were identical and cultures knew how to use and respect them. Difficult as it may be for Western man (and perhaps less so for Western women) to return to a belief system where the unified use of aromatic plants is the norm.*[3]

He suggests that it is self-deceptive to believe that plants stopped working right around the time the pharmaceutical industry took control of healing.[3]

Barcan states that aromatherapy's aesthetics of smell is multilayered – weaving together the scientific, the mythological and the therapeutic. She uses Fischer-Rizzi's description of neroli oil to explain how the odour, the pharmacological properties, the effects and the associated metaphors and symbols, though they can be separated for analytical purposes, are understood to be entirely interwoven functionally and even ontologically.[36]

> *For people who have become thin-skinned, neroli can strengthen their inner being and build a protective shield … neroli has been assigned to the diamond. Both provide light that reduces inner emptiness and anxiety. Neroli offers the gift of strength and courage that helps us see life's beauty. Neroli helps treat psychosomatic illness, used in the aroma lamp, the bath, a compress or a massage oil …*[1]

The role of olfaction

Schnaubelt states that our sense of smell was once a vital and essential tool for survival; however, it has been claimed that it now has lost most of its significance. It is likely, he claims, that losing our appreciation for natural fragrances we may have also lost our faculties inherent in a natural lifestyle.[3]

Smell is linked to memory because the olfactory neurons go directly to the limbic region of the brain. The olfactory bulb connects to the hippocampus which plays an important role in learning and memory. When we smell an odour, it triggers the emotions associated with earlier experiences of it. Smelling, therefore, involves a complex interplay of experience and pharmacology.

Barcan states that the psychophysiological responses to smell are an interesting blend of objective pharmacological properties, personal experiences and the larger cultural contexts in which smells are experienced.[36]

Reinarz states that many Western philosophers considered the sense of smell as less developed, feeble and atrophied, and the least productive of our senses.[39]

Nietzsche was one of the few Western philosophers to value smell and its connection to our animal instincts. Nietzsche linked smell to intuitive awareness, claiming for it the ability to read people's hearts and souls and to sniff out falsity and illusion.[40]

Conclusion

Sheen states that the philosophy of a healing practice is very important both personally and professionally, as it gives 'spirit and integrity' to the practice and plays a critical role in underpinning the art and practice of healing.[11]

However, Sheen states that aromatherapy lacks its own philosophy of health and disease, theory of aetiology, system of disease classification and coherent diagnostic framework:

> *As a practice aromatherapy relies on theories of health, illness and diagnosis from other health care frameworks.*[11]

Schnaubelt is concerned that a tendency for aromatherapy to move from one paradigm to another in an attempt to gain acceptance from conventional medicine is counterproductive.[3]

However, I suggest: Why not accept components from other health care frameworks on which aromatherapy can be practised? This I believe would embody the true meaning of integrative health care.

Hoffmann is wary of any attempt to bridge and integrate the various herbal traditions of the world. I agree with him that it can be problematic and needs a high level of critical thinking. He uses the term *intellectual imperialism,* an assumption in the Western mindset that we can spontaneously understand the concepts and visions of another culture. Hoffmann states that there is a wealth of knowledge and experience in TCM, but not all herbalists who use these insights have the necessary training in the principles of TCM.[16]

Hoffmann explains that a key insight for practitioners is to understand the limits of both their therapies and themselves. He states that we take for granted that well-qualified practitioners will be skilled in their chosen healing art, but a true holistic healer will think beyond their training to focus on the overall needs of the patient. This raises questions about the educational standards.[16]

I agree with Hoffmann that we need to review educational standards. However, if we take the time to learn healing traditions such as Ayurveda or TCM, it will provide us with an opportunity to understand aromatherapy within a holistic framework.

Perhaps one of Sheen's other proposals should also be considered – that aromatherapy develops as a tool within other occupations:

> *The development of aromatherapy practice in other modalities involves the development of specialist knowledge for each occupation for example – nursing, midwifery, psychological practices, naturopathy or TCM. Consequently, this approach still requires the development of an appropriate knowledge base however its development may be supported by those within the individual fields relating the essential oil use to the specific practice. This pathway for the development of aromatherapy is within healthcare modalities rather than as a unique health care modality.*[11]

Schnaubelt suggests that aromatherapy acknowledges the phenomena of the soul and is far more effective in treating real problems of our times than conventional medicine. He argues that it is futile for aromatherapy to gain acceptance by the conventional system:

> *Trying to gain acceptance for aromatherapy by the conventional system, that is, hoping that doctors would start to implement it if there only was more scientific documentation, is counterproductive. It ignores the fact that scientific procedures have long lost their independence and serve mainly to perpetuate the economic status quo.*[3]

He claims that fragrance has always transcended the material planes of consciousness and communicated directly with those of the soul. Aromatherapy does not mandate a spiritual belief system, but it does have a spiritual element that many indigenous people have always recognised in plants.[3]

References

1. Fischer-Rizzi S. *Complete aromatherapy handbook*. Sterling Publishing, New York, 1990.
2. Tisserand R. *The art of aromatherapy*. C.W Daniel Company, Saffron Walden, 1977.
3. Schnaubelt K. *Medical aromatherapy*. Frog, Berkeley, 1999.
4. Lau KJ. *New age capitalism*. University of Pennsylvania Press, Philadelphia, 2000.
5. Tisserand R. *Frankincense oil and cancer in perspective*. Retrieved March 3, 2016, from http://tisserandinstitute.org/frankincense-oil-and-cancer-in-perspective/
6. Tisserand R. *Multi-level marketing and aromatherapy*. Aromatherapy Today, 48; 2010; 32-33.
7. Barcan R. *Aromatherapy and the mixed blessing of feminization*. The Senses and Society, 2014; 9(1): 31-54.
8. Buchbauer G. *The biology of essential oils and fragrance compounds*. In AROMA'95 Conference Proceedings, Aromatherapy Publications, Sussex, 1995.
9. Kusmirek J. *Perspectives in aromatherapy*. In Van Toller S, Dodds GH eds. *Fragrance: the psychology and biology of perfume*. Elsevier Applied Science, UK, 1992: 277-285.

10. Tisserand R. *Aromatherapy today – part II*. The International Journal of Aromatherapy, 1993; 5(4): 3-5.
11. Sheen JG. *The professionalisation of aromatherapy: a case study of the professionalisation of complementary and alternative medicine in the Australian health care system*. PhD thesis, Southern Cross University, Lismore, 2006.
12. Harris R. *Anglo-Saxon aromatherapy: its evolution and current situation*. International Journal of Aromatherapy, 2003; 13(1): 9-17.
13. Jenkins S. *Modern British aromatherapy – the way forward: education and regulation*. The International Journal of Aromatherapy, 2006; 16(2): 85-88.
14. Lapraz J. *In profile*. International Journal of Aromatherapy, 1991; 3(4): 12-14.
15. Pénoël D. *This is also aromatherapy*. The International Journal of Aromatherapy, 1991; 3(3): 14-16.
16. Hoffmann D. *Medical herbalism – the science and practice of herbal medicine*. Healing Arts Press, Rochester, 2003.
17. Kotsirilos V, Vitetta L, Sali A. *A guide to evidence-based integrative and complementary medicine*. Churchill Livingstone, Sydney, 2011.
18. Rakel D. *Integrative medicine*. 3rd edn. Elsevier Saunders, Philadelphia, 2012.
19. National Center for Complementary and Integrative Health. *Complementary, alternative, or integrative health: what's in a name?* Retrieved Dec 28, 2017, from https://nccih.nih.gov/health/integrative-health#cvsa
20. Australasian Integrative Medicine Association. *What is integrative medicine?* Retrieved Dec 28, 2017, from https://www.aima.net.au/what-is-integrative-medicine/
21. Buckle J. *Clinical aromatherapy – essential oils in practice*. 2nd edn. Churchill Livingstone, Edinburgh, 2003.
22. Johannessen B. *Why do registered nurses choose to offer complementary and alternative medicine?* Tang Humanitas Medicine, 2012; 2(1): 1-4. doi: 10.5667/tang.2011.0021.
23. Rizzo Gnatta J et al. *Aromatherapy and nursing; historical and theoretical conception*. Journal of School of Nursing USP, 2016; 50(1): 127-133.
24. Harris B. *Editorial comment*. The International Journal of Aromatherapy, 2002; 12(1): 1.
25. Holmes P. *Energy medicine*. The International Journal of Aromatherapy, 1998/1999; 9(2): 53-56.
26. Agus BA. *The end of illness*. Simon & Schuster, London, 2012.
27. Mills S. *The essential book of herbal medicine*. Arkana Penguin Books, England, 1991.
28. Pénoël D. *Winter shield*. The International Journal of Aromatherapy, 1992; 4(4): 10-12.
29. Burr R. *The emperor of scent*. Random House, New York, 2002.
30. Smith CW. *Energy medicine united*. Complementary Therapies in Nursing & Midwifery, 2003; 9(4): 169-175.
31. Korotkov KG. *Human energy field – study with GDV bioelectrography*. SPIFMO, St Petersburg, 2000.
32. Wisneski LA, Anderson L. *The scientific basis of integrative medicine*. 2nd edn. CRC Press, Boca Raton, 2009.
33. Bone K, Mills S. *Principles and practice of phytotherapy*. 2nd edn. Elsevier, Edinburgh, 2013.
34. Vickers A. *Massage and aromatherapy – a guide for health professionals*. Springer-Science+Business Media, London, 1996.
35. Smith GD. *Editorial: regulation in complementary and alternative medicine: is it time for statutory regulation of CAM in the UK?* Journal of Clinical Nursing, 2010; 19(7/8): 901-903. doi: 10.1111/j.1365-2702.2010.03221.x.
36. Barcan R. *Aromatherapy oils – commodities, material, essences*. Cultural Studies Review, 2014; 20(2): 141-171.
37. Rashkow E. *Perfumed the axe that laid it low: the endangerment of sandalwood in southern India*. Indian Economic & Social History Review, 2014; 51(1): 41-70. doi: 10.1177/0019464613515553.
38. Asian Regional Workshop (Conversation & Sustainable Management of Trees, Vietnam, August 1996). *Santalum album, sandalwood*. The IUCN Red List of Threatened Species 1998: eT31852A9665066. doi: 10.2305/IUCN.UK.1998.RLTS.T31852A9665066.
39. Reinarz J. *Past scents – historical perspectives on smell*. University of Illinois Press, Urbana, 2014.
40. Le Guérer A. *Olfaction and cognition: a philosophical and psychoanalytic view*. In Rouby C et al. eds. *Olfaction, taste, and cognition*. Cambridge University Press, Cambridge, 2002: 3-15.

History

CHAPTER

2

Contents

Introduction

While the term aromatherapy was only coined in the 1930s, aromatic plants have been used since antiquity. In order to trace the history of aromatherapy we need to examine the role of essential oils and aromatic plants throughout the history of humanity. Understanding the relationship our ancestors had with aromatic plants, essential oils and scent will help us to appreciate the framework in which contemporary aromatherapy has developed.

In the past, essential oils had always been an integral part of perfumery and herbal medicine, therefore in many ways the history of aromatherapy is the history of perfumery and herbal medicine.

The Role of Scent in Culture

Classen, Howes and Synnot, authors of *Aroma – the cultural history of smell* provide us with a comprehensive exploration of the cultural role of scent throughout history. They explain that, while smell is often considered one of the most undervalued senses of the modern West, many traditional and ancient cultures considered scent very important. They argue that smell is simply not a biological and psychological phenomenon – it is cultural, hence a social and historical phenomenon. They suggest that many odours represented cultural values and were used as a means of interacting with the world.[1]

According to Hippocrates, the sense of smell bridged the gap between the body and the soul. Reinarz states that smells were generally understood to be tactile in orientation, their detection involving some form of direct contact between the object being smelled and the subject.[2] Galen considered smell to be a superior sense because he believed that the nostrils were a direct link to the brain, allowing the scent vapors to reach the brain and be processed without the need of an intervening sensory nerve.[3] He observed what we all now know of aromatherapy – that smells appear to have a direct and discernible impact on the way we feel.

The devaluation of smell in the contemporary West dates back to the eighteenth and nineteenth centuries. Scholars of this period decided that sight was the sense of reason and smell was the sense of savagery. Darwin, Freud and others argued that the sense of smell had been left behind and that sight was more important.[2]

However, some intellectuals of the time stressed the importance of the senses in the acquisition of knowledge. Jean-Jacques Rousseau (1712-1778) held the senses in high regard, as the mind could only develop when it worked in unison with the body.[2]

German philosopher Immanuel Kant (1724-1804) declared that smell was the least productive of all the senses. He explained that smell revealed very little about the true nature of external objects, although he explained that smell could be useful in distinguishing those items that humans wished to avoid.[2]

Friedrich Nietzsche (1844-1900) claimed that religion taught Christians to be ignorant of their body and to restrain their animal instincts. However, the prevailing belief of the time was that the 'sense of science' was sight, while smell, which was so hard to measure, name or recreate, was not suited to the rigours of science.[2]

Sigmund Freud (1856-1939) stated that the repression of the senses was part of an evolutionary process and a defining feature of civilized man. In 1930, Freud associated the decline in the perceptive powers of the sense of smell with the rise of modern civilization and the transformation of humans.[2]

Reinarz argues that neither Freud nor others disseminating such arguments for the decline in the sense of smell in humans corroborated their theories by referencing scientific research available at the time. For example, he states that in the early 1800s, Ludwig Jacobson found that the vomeronasal organ, located in the nose of adult humans, is able to detect pheromones and is also common to mammals. However, some argued that the vomeronasal organ is a useless and functionless organ that stops developing after the first months of fetal life. This they claimed was linked to the evolutionary passage from animality to humanity. Smell was consequently abandoned to the animal kingdom and has been treated dismissively by many other psychologists since Freud.[2]

Classen suggests that contemporary society demands that we distance ourselves from emotions, that social structures and divisions be seen more objectively and not emotionally, and that personal boundaries be respected.[1]

In 1875, a report by WS Watson appeared in *The Medical Press and Circular*, where Watson stressed the exhilarating effects of odours on the mentally ill.[2]

The psychology of fragrance as an academic field of research in its own right began its development at the end of the 1970s. The psychology of fragrance has been helpful in the development of perfumes and personal care products containing perfume, environmental fragrances and aromatherapy products. It encompasses behavioural effects of a product on the user in respect of others' perceptions of appearance, personality, projected image of the user, and self-perception issues such as self-image, mood, self-esteem, confidence and attitudes. It also examines the relationship of fragrances to different situations and lifestyles, links individual fragrances with personality types, and assesses therapeutic effects at a mental and emotional level.[3]

Sacred Scents

The spiritual interpretation of scents

In many traditional cultures, pleasant aromas were often associated with good food and health or virtuous people, tied to concepts of immortality, and even announced divine presence, whereas bad smells carried negative connotations, represented illness, disorder, decay, divine disapproval, destruction and ultimately death. Religious ceremonies and rituals used odours to clean, purify, heal, ward off or initiate communion with the divine.[2]

In ancient Egyptian culture, it was believed that scents had divine origins, having sprung from deities' bones, or even their eyes in the case of Ra. The Greek gods were also associated with fragrant scents, and it is not surprising that the scent representing Buddha has always been associated with sandalwood.[2]

According to early Christian beliefs, heaven was reputed to be a place of beautiful sights and distinctive scents. These smells were considered divine in contrast to the stenches encountered on earth, which reminded people of their sinful nature.[2]

According to early Christian beliefs, the physical consequences of immortality, including sickness, bodily decay and disintegration, were also regularly interrupted as the direct result of sin. To be mortal was to reek of sin, therefore life on earth stinks, while heavenly scents only come after death.[4]

In Mesopotamian mythology, the descent of Ishtar into the underworld was described as the absence of pleasant odours in the realm of the dead.[2]

German abbess Saint Hildegard von Bingen described hell as 'a long and wide marsh filled with filth and vermin of many types and emitting the worst stink'.[2]

An another example where stench or foul odours were associated with evil:

> *The jinn in Muslim culture also inflict harm through evil odors and were believed to inhabit dung heaps, while Buddhists' flesh-eating demons were equally described as foul-smelling.*[2]

The role of scent in early Christianity

Professor Susan Ashbrook Harvey, author of

Scenting salvation, explores the role of bodily sensory experience in early Christianity. Her book examines the ancient understanding of smell and how it came to influence Christian religious practices.[4]

Ashbrook Harvey explains that at first, the Christian leaders forbade the use of aromatics in religious ceremonies as pagan practice was not to be copied. However, after Constantine's edict of Milan in 313 AD which legitimised Christianity, the use of incense was only allowed with sacred rituals. Until that time, Christian liturgists associated fragrance with polytheistic rituals, particularly emperor worship, and condemned its use. As Christianity evolved into a state cult, it integrated incense into the liturgy as a way to compete with its various pagan counterparts.[4]

By the eighth century, every aspect of Christian practice became 'drenched' in the fragrance of incense. Incense was used in every Christian home, shrine, tomb, church, pilgrimage site and monastic cell, and transformed these terrestrial spaces into ceremonial places.[5]

Sacrificial scents

Scent was a very important part of sacrificial practices which were very common in all ancient cultures. Religious sacrifice helped establish and maintain the relationship that bound communal order and identity, and connected communities of believers to the divine presence.[5]

In Christian and Judaic traditions, a properly performed sacrifice soothed the god's anger, removed collective guilt and sin and guaranteed divine deliverance. Holy oils and holy incense were often offered as aromatic sacrifices. Holy oils used by early Christians included myrrh, cinnamon, aromatic cane, cassia and olive oil. Holy incense was composed of sweet spices and aromatics such as stacte, onycha, galbanum, frankincense and salt. In Jewish literature, balsam and myrrh were deemed as the most important aromatics. In Roman tradition, fragrant offerings were often accompanied by garlands and floral crowns which were said to please the gods and goddesses of love who not only were sweetly scented, but delighted in floral scents.[2]

While the act of burning incense is a destructive process, it was considered to be a metamorphic process. The scent released was able to transform an ordinary space to a ceremonial space. The smoke of the burning aromatics travelled heavenward with the worshipper's prayers and the lingering aromas attuned the mind to devotion and adoration, both before and after the performance of the religious rite.[2]

Reinarz states that the ritual of baptism is rich in olfactory meaning. By anointing the forehead, ears and nostrils with baptismal oil, the individual being baptised is being granted new senses that open and become attuned to the divine.[2]

The decadence of perfume

By the first millennium, if scent was not used for sacred purposes it was considered to lead to temptation and sin. Some Christian writers expressed strong suspicion of perfume, suggesting that it has the potential to stimulate impure desires. While cleanliness was considered godly and fitting for a chosen people, scent also caused skepticism that only increased with the proliferation of manufactured scents. When scents were used as perfumes, it was interpreted as a sign of inner filthiness and worthy of confession. Sweet scents were denounced when used as aphrodisiacs.[2]

The smell of health and disease

Mary Thurlkill, associate professor of Religious Studies at the University of Mississippi and author of *Sacred scents in early Christianity and Islam*, states that early Christians contextualised illness and suffering in a different way to their pagan and Jewish counterparts. While physical suffering could be punishment from God, it was also accepted as a unique path to salvation. Suffering was redemptive. It linked the Christian to the body of Christ, who had suffered unimaginable pains and torments. The illness and suffering became sweet. They purged the body of sin and transformed the suffering into salvation.[5]

Thurlkill explains that Greek scholar and early Christian theologian Origen (185-254 AD) recognised God as the supreme healer who mercifully provided medical knowledge to human beings. Origen introduced a dichotomy that continued into early Middle Ages – that very pious Christians relied upon only God as the healer while interpreting their illness as a punishment or simply God's will.[5]

This is in contrast to Islamic tradition that acknowledged that both the disease and the healing come only from God. Unbelievers see the plague as divine punishment while Muslims rejoice in it as God's will. One Islamic tradition noted that 'there is no disease that Allah has created, except that He also has created its treatment.'[5]

Thurlkill compares the development of physicians in early Christianity and in the Islamic world:

> *The paradigm of spiritual healing, either directly through Allah or more 'magical' forms, did not proliferate as aggressively as it did in early Christianity. This may be because, in the West,*

medical knowledge and (eventually) hospital care came to reside in monasteries, churches or ecclesiastical schools. Christian theology largely directed medical theory and practices. Physicians in the Islamic world – certainly working within a religious context, ultimately attributing all healing to Allah – experienced a more secular divide.[5]

Many plants have become ingrained in our psyche for their healing properties and their use in spiritual practice. Dorothy Abram, author of *Seven scents – healing and the aromatic imagination,* provides us with an in-depth study of seven plants and the role they have played in healing and spiritual practices throughout the history of humankind. The seven plants that she explores are sandalwood (*Santalum album*), lotus (*Nymphaea caerulea*), neem (*Azadirachta indica*), terebinth (*Pistacia terebinthus*), tulsi (*Ocimum sanctum*), spikenard (*Nardostachys jatamansi*) and jasmine (*Jasminum officinale*).[6]

The History of Aromatics

Most of the information about aromatic plants in the ancient world comes from the writers of Greece and Rome. However, Classen explains that in many respects the cultures of the ancient Middle East such as Egypt and Persia had more developed and refined olfactory traditions than those developed by the Greeks and Romans.[2]

The Egyptians

Egypt was the cradle of the sciences, including medicine, perfumery and cosmetology. Throughout the ancient world, Egypt was famous for the use of aromatic substances. In their religious cults, the Egyptians consumed great quantities of *Boswellia papyrifera*, frankincense, and *Commiphora erythraea*, myrrh resin.

This was not the same frankincense and myrrh presented at the birth of Christ or burned in great abundance by the Romans. That was from another species not yet known to the Egyptians which was found in Arabia. The Egyptians sourced frankincense and myrrh from the land called Punt, which is believed to be in the region of Somalia.

Incense was always burned before the opening of a shrine, at the coronation of the pharaoh, and for national celebrations. The souls of the dead were thought to ascend above as a cloud of smoke, and incense was burned to avert baneful spirits from the bodies of the deceased.

The Egyptians believed in the transmigration of souls. They believed that the soul, after leaving the body, entered the body of some other animal, and, having successively passed through all the creatures of the earth, water and air, it again assumed a human shape. The journey was to be accomplished in 3000 years. This belief accounted for the great care they took in embalming the bodies of their dead, so that after the long journey, the souls might find their original body in a tolerable state of preservation.

The embalming process involved eviscerating the dead body, which was then washed with natron (sodium nitrate salts) from the Wadi El Natrum, and stuffed the cavities with myrrh, pine resin and oakmoss.

As distillation had not yet been discovered, the main method of extracting the essential oils was by enfleurage and maceration. This was done by steeping the resins, flowers or splinters of wood in oil. The materials were placed in a cloth which was wrung until every last drop of fragrance had been retrieved.

Alternatively, maceration involved boiling of the aromatic substances in the oil. The oils most commonly used were moringa, balanos, castor oil, linseed, sesame, safflower, olive and sweet almond.

The human body also became an object of esteem to be anointed with perfumed oils. Cosmetics used included aromatic substances such as frankincense, myrrh, lilies, pine, cedar of Lebanon, gum mastic, mints and other herbs.[7]

One of the best-known perfumes was kyphi. Kyphi was burnt in the temples. A recipe for making kyphi was as follows:[8]

- Take 270 g each of: Acorus calamus, mastic, cassia, cinnamon. Grind and sieve. Only the powder is to be used.
- Take 270 g each of juniper berries; an unidentified plant; *Cyperus slongus*. Grind. Add to this 2,250 g of wine. Leave until the next morning. Half the wine will be absorbed by the herbs. The rest will be discarded.
- Take 1,800 g raisins and 2,250 g oasis wine. Grind together well. Remove the rind and pips of the raisins. Place the rest in a pot with the herbs. Leave for five days.
- Mix 1,200 g frankincense and 3,000 g honey in a vessel. Boil gently until it thickens and reduce by 1/5. Mix the other ingredients and leave for five days.
- Add to this 1,143 g of finely ground myrrh and you have kyphi.

According to Greek historian Plutarch, kyphi had the ability to relieve anxiety, brighten dreams and heal the soul.[1]

One of the ingredients of kyphi was calamus, which Tisserand describes as having potent narcotic and sedative properties. Calamus contains up to 80% asarone, a toxic phenol, which is a precursor of

TMA-2, a phenylethylamine capable of powerful narcotic effects.[9]

The Ebers Papyrus, a comprehensive document that dates back to about 1550 BC, was discovered in 1874 by German Egyptologist Georg Ebers, and contains extensive information about surgery and internal medicine. It also lists some 800 medicinal and aromatic plants that are still used today such as aniseed, caraway, cassia, coriander, fennel, cardamom, onions, garlic, thyme, mustard, sesame, fenugreek, saffron and poppy seed. The Egyptians used these herbs and spices in medicine, cosmetics, perfumes, aromatic oils, cooking, fumigation and embalming.[10]

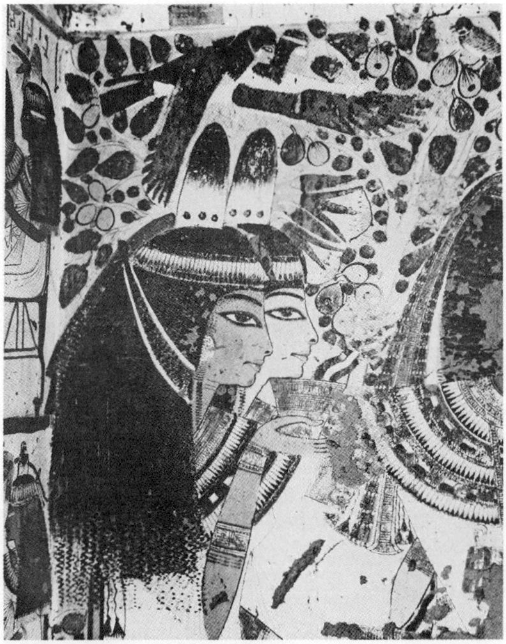

Egypt, wigs with cones of unguent, tomb of Userhat, Thebes. Courtesy of Wellcome Collection.

As myrrh was not from Egypt, in 1485 BC, Queen Hatshepsut sent an expedition of five sailing vessels from Thebes to travel down the Nile to the Delta, through a channel into the Red Sea, then south along the East African coast until they reached Punt. When the ships returned, they were reported to be heavily laden with precious commodities such as ivory, gold, silver, cinnamon and large quantities of myrrh resin.[10]

Throughout the ancient world, the Egyptians were famous for their scents and perfumes. Theophrastus explained that the secret to the Egyptian perfume makers was knowing at which precise moment to add the various aromatic ingredients, and at which temperature. One of the most famous Egyptian perfumes was made in the city of Mendes in the Delta region of the Nile. It consisted of balanos oil, myrrh and other resins. The perfume was known as 'The Egyptian'. It was known to have a very long shelf life, and once applied to the skin it lasted well.[8]

Metopion, another Egyptian ointment, was based on galbanum. It consisted of oil from bitter almonds and unripe olives, scented with cardamom, sweet rush, sweet flag, honey, wine, myrrh, seed of balsamum, galbanum and turpentine resin. According to Dioscorides, the best *Metopion* should smell more like cardamom and myrrh than galbanum. Medicinally it was soothing, heat and sweat producing, and was used to 'open the vessels, to purge ulcers and to treat injuries'.[8]

Greeks and Romans, like Dioscorides and Pliny, documented all the skills that had been developed by the Egyptians for using aromatics as pharmaceuticals and perfumes.[7]

The incense and spice trade routes

For more than a millennium, incense and other luxury goods were traded from the southern coast of Arabia to the insatiable markets in the Mediterranean region and Mesopotamia. Historians are not sure of the dates of the earliest incense trade. It has been suggested that the original interest in the trade of incense gums dates back to Egypt in 3000 BC.[11]

The Egyptians were not the only users of incense. Herodotus reports that a substantial trade of incense existed between Arabia and Greece by 500 BC. Theophrastus wrote the first eye witness account of incense trees and the harvesting of incense from the reports of reconnaissance ships sent out by Alexandria the Great. Pliny the Elder, near the end of the first century AD, provides us with details of the trade route from its sources in southern Arabia and its processing in the north.[11]

Cinnamon and cassia were among the earliest spices used. They were considered to be among the most precious aromatic ingredients in ancient Greece and Rome. There are indications that, as early as the second millennium BC, cassia and cinnamon from China and South East Asia might have been brought from Indonesia to Madagascar in primitive canoes, along a 'cinnamon route' which might have existed at the time. The aromatic barks were then transported northward along the east coast of Africa to the Nile valley, and from there to the land of 'Punt'.[11]

It has been suggested that the founders of the spice trade between India and the rest of the world were either the Phoenicians or the Arabs. The Phoenicians were accomplished sailors and may have been responsible for transporting spices from the east to the west.[11]

In Ezekiel, Chapter 27, high praises are given to the richness of Tyre, the capital of the Phoenicians under the emperor Hiram. There are also references to the Arab merchants carrying spices. It is very likely that the Phoenicians were the first to carry spices such as cinnamon and cassia to Greece.[11]

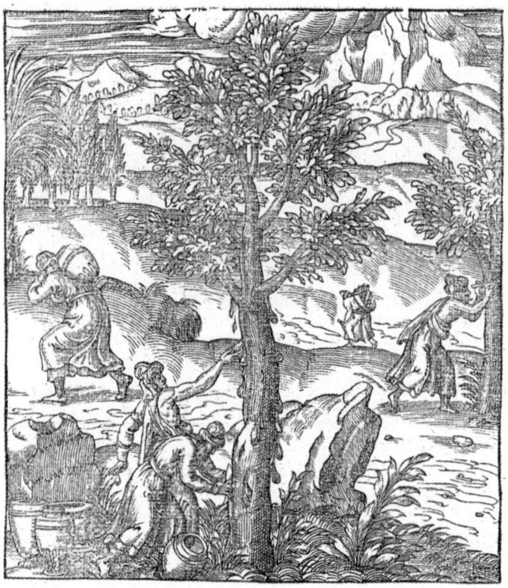

Indigenous people collecting resin or incense. Courtesy of Wellcome Collection.

In ancient times, the southern Arabian region was occupied by a nomadic race, the Sabians, who were skilled at sailing and sea trading. Their main merchandise was spices. It is likely that they traded with the ancient Egyptians. While there is insufficient evidence to come to any conclusion on the relative role played by the Arabians and the Phoenicians, it is most likely that the people of the south Arabian region held a monopoly on the spice trade for a very long time.[11]

Herodotus and Theophratus recorded mythical stories perpetuated by the Sabians about the source of cinnamon and cassia. Theophrastus describes south-west Arabia as the land of myrrh, frankincense, cinnamon and cassia. The Sabian traders were very successful at shrouding the source of cinnamon in mystery. One such story was:

> *Far away in a distant land, said Arab traders to spice buyers from Europe, there is a great lake. It is surrounded by deep and fragrant woods and high cliffs. On those cliffs nest a great dragon-like bird with a scimitar-sharp beak and talons like Saladin's sword. The nest of this bird is made only of one material: the bark of a rare tree. And when it has made its nest, it does not lay eggs in it. Oh no. It does not need to. It flaps its wings so fast that the bark catches fire and then the bird sits in the middle of its blazing pyre. And then, lo and behold, it emerges from the flames refreshed, renewed, rejuvenated. The name of the bird is Phoenix. And the name of the bark? Ah! It is cinnamon. And that is why, that is exactly why, cinnamon is so expensive.*[11]

The Arabs not only were able to enhance the value of cinnamon, but they kept its origins a mystery for many centuries. It would only be in the fifteenth century, when Europeans started sailing around the world in search of pepper, that they discovered cinnamon and cassia grew relatively easily in South East Asia.[11]

The Arab control of the spice trade was broken by the Romans around AD 40. Mariner Hippalus discovered the trade winds system in the Indian Ocean that had only been known to the Arabs. It is believed that Hippalus travelled to India and back around AD 40, opening direct trade between Rome and the west coast of India. By the end of the first century, the use of spices in Rome had grown enormously.[11]

By the end of the third century AD, the Arabs had established trade relationships with China, mostly for the trading of cassia.[11]

With the collapse of the Roman empire, the Arabs once again became the masters and controlled the spice trade. This lasted until the fifteenth century, when the sea route to India was discovered and Vasco da Gama landed on the west coast of India in 1498.[11]

The Greeks

The ancient Greeks further advanced the use of aromatics. The first treatise on scent was the study *Concerning odours* by Theophrastus. Not only did he take an elaborate inventory of Greek and imported aromatics, but he discussed ways in which they could be used. Theophrastus commented on the therapeutic nature of perfumes, saying:

> *It is to be expected that perfumes should have medicinal properties in view of the virtues of their spices. The effect of plasters and of what some may call poultices prove these virtues, since they disperse tumours and abscesses and produce a distinct effect on the body and its interior parts.*[7]

He was referred to as the father of botany. He observed one of the fundamentals of holistic aromatherapy, that essential oils applied externally affect the internal organs and tissues.

Theophratus even provides us with blending

instructions to enhance the tenacity of a perfume blend by taking into consideration the odour intensity of various aromatic ingredients:

> *Now the composition and preparation of perfumes aim entirely, one may say, at making odours last. That is why men make oil the vehicle of them, since it keeps a very long line and also is most convenient for use.*
>
> *They use spices in the making of all perfumes; some to thicken the oil, some in order to impart their odour. The less powerful spices are used for the thickening, and then at a later stage they put the one whose odour they wish to secure. For that which is put in last always dominates even if it is in small quantity; thus if a pound of myrrh is put into a half-pint of oil, and at a later stage a third of an ounce of cinnamon is added, this small amount dominates.*[12]

However, Socrates declined to use scent as he felt it was only for women. The Spartans often drove the perfume merchants from the state for wasting precious edible oils as solvents for perfumes.[12]

While Hippocrates is referred to as the father of modern medicine, it would be more fitting to dub him the father of holistic medicine. He promoted the benefits of massage:

> *The physician must be experienced in many things, but assuredly in rubbing … for rubbing can bind a joint that is too loose, and loosen a joint that is too rigid.*[13]

Greek medicine as developed by Hippocrates was based on the four elements – Air, Earth, Fire and Water, and the four humours corresponding to the chief fluids in the body – choleric (yellow bile), sanguine (blood), phlegmatic (phlegm) and melancholic (black bile). The properties of the herbs corresponded to one or more of the four elements. The cornerstone of Greek medicine was the concept of mental, emotional and physical balance. Disease was a disturbance of this balance, and it was the duty of the physician to restore and assist the patient's own natural healing powers. Hippocratic teaching emphasised that a healthy body was one in which the four elements were equally balanced.[14]

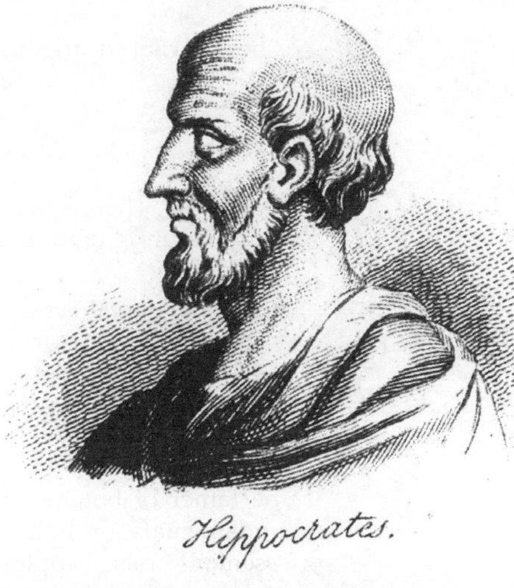

Hippocrates. Line engraving. Courtesy of Wellcome Collection.

Four centuries later, Galen adopted the Hippocratic teachings of the four elements and made it the cornerstone of an elaborate and rigid system of medicine which would remain unchallenged for the next 1,500 years.[14]

Pedanius Dioscorides, of Anazarba in Asia Minor, wrote a treatise on herbal medicine during the first century AD. His book remained the medical reference work in Western medicine for over 1,000 years after his death, and much of our present knowledge of medicinal herbs originates from Dioscorides.[13]

His book contains five sections, one of which deals with aromatics. Many of the remedies he discusses are still used today in aromatherapy:[13]

- *Myrrh* – strengthens the teeth and gums and is soporiferous.
- *Juniper* – is described as a diuretic.
- *Marjoram* – is described as soporific.
- *Cypress* – the lux of the belly (diarrhoea). It doth also stanch the blood.
- *Costus* – provokes venerie.

Aromatherapists are aware of the sedative properties of marjoram, that juniper is a diuretic, and that the astringent properties of cypress are beneficial in cases of diarrhoea. Costus, traditionally used as an aphrodisiac, is now wisely avoided, since it can cause allergic reactions.[13]

Dioscorides attributes the following properties to cinnamon:

> *Cinnamon provoked urine, it cleared the eyes and made the breath sweet. An extract of cinnamon would bring down the menses and would counteract the stings and bites of venomous beasts, reduce inflammation of the intestines and kidneys, comfort the stomach, break wind, would aid digestion and when mixed with honey would remove spots from the face that was anointed there with.*[11]

Some 300 years after Hippocrates, Asclepiades, a Greek physician who was closer to our concept of an aromatherapist than Hippocrates or Dioscorides, was a great believer in massage. He practised in Greece and Rome, believed in curing his patients with as little discomfort as possible for them, and was against the excessive use of purgatives and emetics, which were then so much an integral part of medicine. Instead, he advocated the use of massage, music and perfume as soothing and healing agents.[13]

The Romans

The Roman armies helped spread the knowledge of Mediterranean healing plants around Europe. The Romans took good care of their armies, especially when they were posted in distant countries. The legions travelled with their own doctors and surgeons, and when good local doctors could be found, they too were consulted and often enlisted.[14]

In the case of wounds, a lotion of wine and myrrh was prescribed for burns and for relieving inflammations. Roman physician Pliny suggested rue infused in vinegar for comatose patients, to be used as a kind of smelling salts, while the scent of pennyroyal was used to protect from cold or heat and to lessen thirst.[1]

Galen believed that it was not the nose which perceived smell, but the brain. Proof of this, he held, lay in the way in which different odours were known to affect the brain.[14]

Rome had an insatiable appetite for incense. Nero is said to have burnt more incense than Arabia could produce in a year at his wife Poppeae's funeral. Rome was said to have consumed 3,000 tons of frankincense and 600 tons of myrrh from southern Arabia. Pliny was critical of the abuse of aromatics by his contemporaries.[1]

Of all the aromatic substances, Romans loved rose the most. They adorned themselves with it at banquets, decorated their homes with it, and on occasions of a victory, strew roses through the street. At one of Nero's feasts, guests were asphyxiated by showers of roses.[7]

It was the Romans who developed bathing to such an extent that baths in public buildings became like modern social clubs. Butler describes the most likely scenario:

> *The bather undressed, was anointed with perfumed oil by a slave, then after a period of violent exercise went into a steam room. It was probably here that the body was scraped with a strigil, a curved metal instrument used to remove accumulated oil, dirt and perspiration. The bather then went to the warm room and thence the cold one where there was often a swimming pool.*[12]

Scents were absorbed directly into the body so they were often regarded as having important healing qualities. The best recipe for health, wrote the poet Alexis, 'is to apply sweet scents unto the brain.' Anointing the head with perfume when drinking wine, for example, was believed to counteract the intoxicating effect of wine, anointing the breasts with perfume, in turn, was thought to be beneficial for the heart. Philonides, the physician, recommended a rose garland to alleviate a headache, whereas a myrtle garland would act as a stimulant and counteract drunkenness.[12]

The scholars of the day documented the medicinal virtues of aromatic ingredients. Pliny the Elder (23-79 AD) wrote on chemistry and botany, including the use of aromatics and perfumes, while Dioscorides, in a Materia Medica, documented all known animal, vegetable and mineral substances used. In the second century AD, Galen wrote about the many branches of medicine, including hygiene and pharmacy.[15] He also formulated *Ceratum refrigerans*, a cooling wax or balm. He added as much water as could be incorporated into a mixture of 1:4 of beeswax and olive oil in which rose petals had been steeped.[12]

The influence of Galen persisted in the medical world for many centuries. Many of his treatments were based on medicinal herbs.[15] In many ways, Galen established a framework for using herbs that is still very relevant today. Before using a remedy, he suggested that the following eight conditions must be considered:[16]

- The drug must be of good unadulterated quality.
- The illness must be simple, not complex.
- The illness must be appropriate to the action of the drug.
- The drug must be more powerful than the illness.
- One should make careful note of the course of illness and treatment.
- One must ensure that the effect of the drug is the

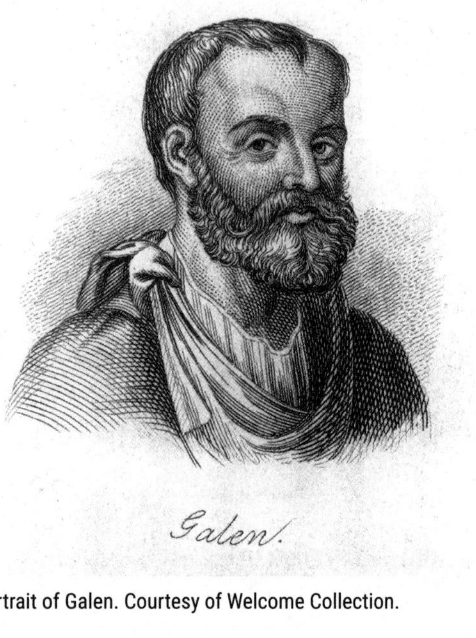

Portrait of Galen. Courtesy of Welcome Collection.

same for everyone at every time.

- One must see that the effect of the drug is specific for human beings (in an animal it can have another effect).
- One must distinguish the effect of drugs (working by their qualities) from food (working by their substance).

One of Galen's most important approaches to health was diet. He believed in regulating food and drink to both cure and maintain good health. He strongly recommended prescribing food and herbs according to the humoral theory. Galen stated that a healthy diet was one filled with diverse foods that complemented each other with their humoral qualities. He also believed that moderate and balanced food choices signalled wisdom and self-discipline, while he suggested that anything less led to one's enslavement to gluttony and desire.[5]

After the fall of the Roman Empire, the active development of medicine ceased in the West. Early Christianity believed that diseases were divine punishment for their sins and that their cure was a matter for heaven and not for mankind to tamper with.[15]

The Jews and the Bible

The earliest mention in the Bible of aromatic substances being used is in Genesis 2:12 in reference to the land of Havilah, 'and the gold of the land is good; there is bdellium, and the onyx stone.' Bdellium refers to the fragrant gum resin obtained from *Commiphora mukul*, which grew in the arid regions of western India. Bdellium was often sold as a less expensive substitute for myrrh.[17]

The ancient Jews used incense and aromatic plants for religious ceremonies. According to Butler, the first reference to trade in aromatics is about 1730 BC in the Bible, when the Ishmaelites came from Gilead with their camels bearing 'spices and balm and myrrh'. In Exodus, the Lord commanded Moses to build an alter to burn incense upon. Instructions were given for a holy anointing oil of myrrh, cinnamon, sweet calamus and cassia in olive oil, and another for a sweet incense which included sweet spices, stacte, onycha, galbanum and frankincense. According to Pliny, stacte may have been the gum extract from myrrh, while others say it is storax. Onycha may have been labdanum.[12]

The Assyrians and the Babylonians burned incense and aromatic gums to honour their gods. While the Assyrians produced vast quantities of frankincense, they also had to import a thousand talents of frankincense a year from Arabia. Saffron, cinnamon and fenugreek were other aromatics that would have been used and traded.[12]

Myrrh was commonly used in Assyria as an incense to exorcise the demons from the body of a sick person. It was believed to have purifying and medicinal properties, and it was ordained by Jewish Law in the purification of women.[12]

The Queen of Sheba brought spices to the court of Solomon. The region of Sabaea or Sheba was the spice centre of Arabia. The Sabians not only produced most of the myrrh and frankincense of the Middle Eastern countries, but were on the trade route for the spices and aromatic gums from India and the Far East. This would have included sandalwood, incense, vetiver, musk, henna, jasmine, lotus and rose.[12]

References to cinnamon and cassia exist in the old testament of the Bible. In Exodus, the lord spoke to Moses on the top of Mount Sinai and gave instructions that the children of Israel should build a tabernacle, so that he might dwell among them; and gave further instructions for the preparation of an anointing oil for the tabernacle containing aromatic ingredients such as myrrh, calamus, cinnamon and cassia.[11]

> *The Lord spoke unto Moses. Take thou also unto thee principle spices, of pure myrrh five hundred shekels, and of cinnamon half so much, two hundred and fifty shekels, and of sweet calamus two hubdred and fifty shekels. and of cassia five hundred shekels, after the shekel of the sanctuary, and of oil olive and hin: and thou shalt make it an oil of holy anointment, an ointment compound after the art of the apothecary: it shall be an holy anointing oil. And thou shall anoint the tabernacle of the congregation therewith and ask of testimony.*[18]
>
> Exodus 30:23-26 (King James Version)

The Bible is saturated with images of scent in the Song of Solomon:

> *Thou hast ravished my heart, my sister, my spouse; thou hast ravished my heart with one of thine eyes; with one chain of thy neck. How fair is thy love, my sister, my spouse! How much better is thy love than wine! And the smell of thine ointments than all spices! Thy lips, O my spouse, drop as the honeycomb: honey and milk are under thy tongue; and the smell of thy garments is like the smell of Lebanon. A garden inclosed is my sister, my spouse; a spring shut up, a fountain sealed. Thy plants are an orchard of pomegranates, with pleasant fruits; camphire, with spikenard, spikenard and saffron; calamus and cinnamon, with all trees of frankincense; myrrh and aloes, with all the chief spices: a fountain of gardens, a well of living waters, and streams from Lebanon. Awake, O north wind, and come, thou south; blow*

upon my garden, that the spices thereof may flow out. Let my beloved come into his garden, and eat his pleasant fruits.[18]

Song of Solomon 4:9-16 (King James Version)

Morris explains that this dialogue between two lovers intoxicated by the scent of each other's bodies, by their perfumes, and by the setting of a garden blooming with lilies and hyacinths is also a complicated allegory between the soul and the divine, Israel and Yahweh. Morris explains that perfume is used throughout the poem as an invisible but unescapable attractant.[7]

During biblical times, spikenard would have come from India along with other spices mentioned in the Bible, such as cassia and cinnamon. Spikenard was then used in incense and expensive perfumes.[7]

It was therefore not surprising that when Mary Magdalene used spikenard to perfume the feet of Christ, she was rebuked by those around her, but not by Christ:

Then took Mary a pound of ointment of spikenard, very costly and anointed the feet of Jesus, and wiped his feet with her hair; and the house was filled with the odour of the ointment.[18]

John 12:3 (King James Version)

The scent of spikenard was associated with royalty:

While my king sitteth at his table, my spikenard sendeth forth the smell thereof.[18]

Song of Solomon 1:12 (King James Version)

Duke's handbook of medicinal plants of the Bible provides us with the most detailed and comprehensive description of the medicinal and sacred plants referenced in the Bible, along with quotes from various translations of the Bible.

Duke states that frankincense is mentioned 22 times in the bible, 16 times as an item of worship, three times as a product in the garden of Solomon, twice as a tribute of honor and only once as an item of merchandise.[19]

And the lord said unto Moses, take unto thee sweet spices, stacte and onycha, and galbanum; these sweet spices with pure frankincense: of each shall there be a like weight.[18]

Exodus 30:34 (King James Version)

And when they came into the house, they saw the young child with Mary his mother, and fell down, and worshipped him: and when they had opened their treasures, they presented unto him gifts; gold, and frankincense, and myrrh.[18]

Matthew 2:11 (King James Version)

Duke states that myrrh shows up in the bible at least a dozen times. He explains that we will never know exactly which species it is referring to, as *Commiphora* is a complicated genus. However, many scholars equate *C. molmol* to the biblical myrrh.[19]

The origins of alchemy

Morris states that from the first century AD through to the fourth, we find a religious revival that focused on personal salvation. The origins of alchemy began when Christianity and Gnosticism attempted to find a release from the limitations of the world. Alchemists were convinced that the spark of divinity could be discovered by submitting botanical and mineral substances to heating in water baths and stills. The alchemists hoped to extract the divine, external spirit.[7]

Morris claims that records of the alchemists indicate that the first true still was the invention of Maria the Jewess, of whom we know very little.[7]

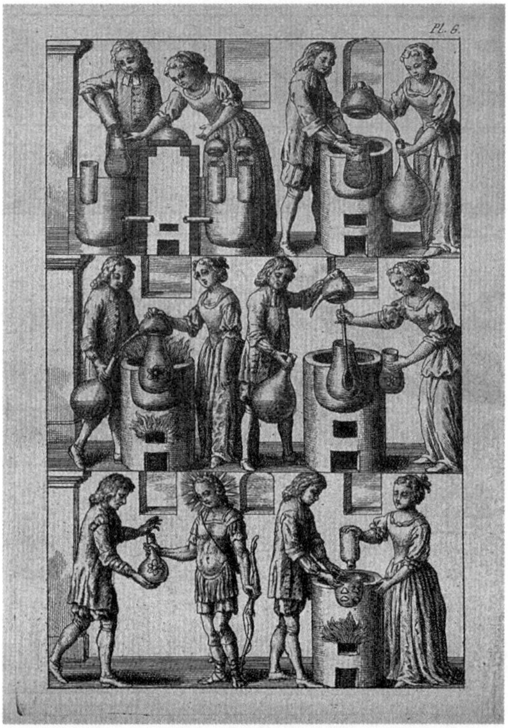

A man and a woman demonstrating the process of fermentation and distillation in alchemy. Etching, ca 17th century. Courtesy of Wellcome Collection.

The philosophy of the alchemists was 'to sublimate that which was bodily and to embody that which was spirit'. Morris explains that, in Alexandria, a long line of alchemists continued to explore the utilisation of distillation throughout the late Roman, Christian and Byzantine periods. Among them we find Hermes Trimegistus, Ostanes of Persia, Cleopatra (not the Queen), Isis, Zosimus and his consort Theosebeia, Christianus, and Theodorus, author of *Corpus hermeticum*, the repository of the writings of these alchemists. This work was prepared after Alexandria had passed to the Arabs in the seventh century. Islam did not extinguish the scientific spirit which it encountered.[7]

The Middle East

The writings of Dioscorides, Galen, Pliny and Zosimus, which were translated into Arabic, gave birth to a purely Islamic body of knowledge.

Westerners are accustomed to the belief that when Europe went through the Dark Ages, the rest of the world did so as well. Islamic culture is so often disregarded in Western culture, yet it is during this period that the use of aromatics flourished in the Middle East, and indeed gave rise to many of the skills and techniques which are still used today.[7]

Arabs used scent domestically in much the same ways as Romans. They regularly fumigated their homes with a mixture of frankincense and thyme. Ninth century Islamic scholar Ali b. Sahl Rabban al-Tabari referred to a common practice of crushing musk and ambergris, then dusting it inside pockets and sleeves for a pleasant personal odour.[5]

The prophet Muhammad stressed the importance of sweet-smelling breath and encouraged the use of aloeswood soaked in rosewater as toothbrushes. Early Islamic perfume texts describe the various perfumes that could be used for the clothing and body; however, there was much more information about perfumes for men than women. Women were permitted to wear perfumes, but its appreciation should only be for the husband.[5]

Islamic expectations of modesty and sexuality meant that a woman's fragrance should be reserved for her spouse. If the scent could be detected by other men, it called into question her chastity. A perfume mixing vessel, a *madaf,* was an important possession for a woman so that she could mix scents to please her husband.[5]

Islamic religious leaders had no concerns celebrating sexuality within religiously sanctioned unions. Arabs understood that sweet smells on the body and within sleeping quarters enhanced sexual pleasure.[5]

We would assume that the Arabs had a great love of frankincense and myrrh, but Harvey cites tenth century poet al-Sari al-Raffa, who compiled an anthology of popular poetic references to lovers and beloveds, scents and drinking in which he discusses musk, ambergris, camphor and aloeswood, but never mentions frankincense or myrrh.[5]

It is the Persians who are credited with having perfected the art of distillation. Ibn-Sina (980-1037), known in the West as Avicenna, was known as the 'Prince of Physicians', whose book *Canon of medicine* would later provide the basis of medical schools in Europe.[7]

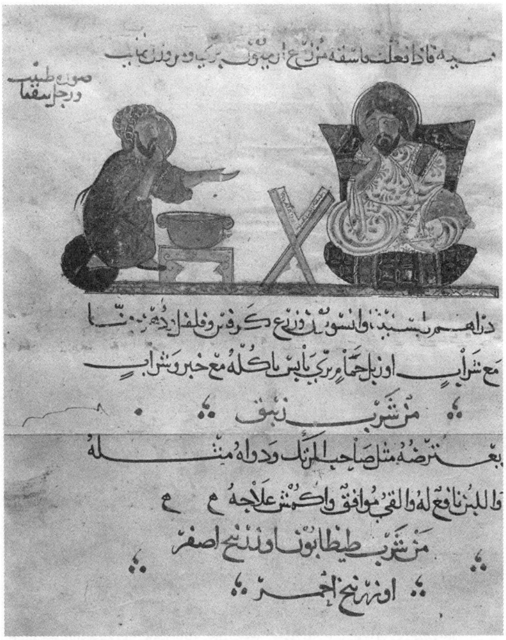

Arab physician and patient. 13th century. Courtesy of Wellcome Collection.

Both Roman and Arab physicians agreed that spices and other aromatics affected the body. The same assumption held true for the influence of scent on the mind and spirit. Blends of aloeswood, myrtle, violet, jasmine and marjoram inspired pride, generosity and nobility. Rose, narcissus and wallflower promoted pleasure, yearning and desire. Al-Kindi also labelled blends as masculine or feminine.[5]

Scent played an important role in Arab medical manuals. Ibn Masawaih compiled a pharmacology devoted solely to the healing properties of aromatics. Ibn Masawaih served various caliphs as personal physican, trained numerous young doctors and wrote 44 books. One text, entitled *Kitab jawahir al-tib almufrada* (Simple aromatic substances), discusses the five primary scents as musk, ambergris, aloe, camphor and saffron. He then refers to 24 secondary aromatics, including nard, clove, pepper, cardamom and nutmeg.[5]

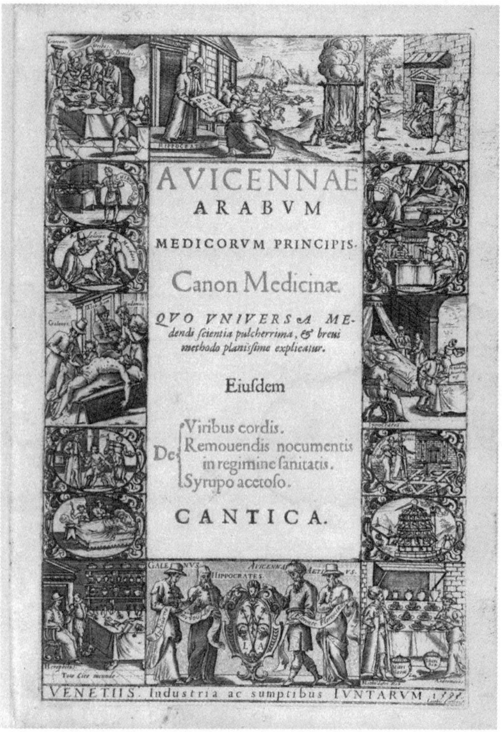
AVICENNAE
ARABVM
MEDICORVM PRINCIPIS.
Canon Medicinæ.
QVO VNIVERSA MEdendi ſcientia pulcherrima, & breui methodo planiſſime explicatur.
Eiuſdem
De { Viribus cordis. Remouendis nocumentis in regimine ſanitatis. Syrupo acetoſo.
CANTICA.
VENETIIS. Industria ac sumptibus IVNTARVM.

Avicenna, Canon Medicinae. Courtesy of Wellcome collection.

Ibn Masawaih explains that musk benefits the heart and stops bleeding; ambergris balances the humors of the aged; aloe treats the nerves, liver and stomach; camphor keeps wounds from stretching and saffron addresses all the humors. Along with healing properties, Ibn Musawaih discusses popular cooking combinations such as clove and nutmeg, as well as applications in perfumery and incense. Thurlkill states that this confirms that Arabs valued a large variety of scents for many different purposes.[5]

Ibn el Beithar (1197-1248), a famous Arab doctor, wrote an extensive book on medicinal plants in which he describes the medical practices of Diosocrides and Galen. He listed the names of the remedies in alphabetical order and specified the names of the remedies in various languages.[15]

It was in the Middle East that glassware was perfected, including pieces that could withstand the heat of distilling. Unlike Christianity, Islam was relatively relaxed as far as the comforts of life were concerned. Muhammed is said to have loved perfumes above all else.[7]

Of all the aromatics in the Arabic treasury, pride must be given to the attar of rose. Legend also holds that when Muhammad rose to heaven, his sweat fell to earth, and he said, 'whoever would smell my scent would smell the rose'.[7]

Islamic culture not only forged a solid bridge between the ancient world and medieval Europe, but it also laid great foundations upon which plant-based holistic medicine could flourish.

Aromatics of the East

Morris explains that the great importance of the role of Islam was that it placed the West in contact with two very rich cultures – India and China. He states that the cultural and technical sophistication of these two countries helped to create modern Europe.[7]

India

No other region in the world possessed such a wealth of aromatic plants. The religion of the Jains, the Buddhists and the Brahmins all encouraged frequent baths, ritual washings and the use of fragrant oils, powders and pastes to be applied to the body after these cleansings.[7]

One Sanskrit author described the pleasures which the ritual necessity of the daily bath could give to the ruler, followed by a massage with an oil in a base of sesame seed oil perfumed with jasmine, coriander, cardamom, basil, costus, pandanus, agarwood, pine, saffron, champaka and clove. Once this rub down was complete, the king would be dressed in a clean cotton garment and, fully refreshed, emerged to face the day.[7]

Just as Greece had a zone of influence beyond her borders, known as Magna Graecia, the term greater India refers to those countries to the south and east – Sri Lanki, Thailand, Cambodia, Burma, Sumatra, Java and Malaysia. Indian culture percolated down to these areas through numerous traders from India who came in search of materials not found at home.[7]

The perfume dealer in India was the *gandhika.* Treatises dating between 500 and 1000 AD provided the *gandhika* with practical advice on the choice of materials. Gangadhara, author of one such text, the *Gandhasara,* gave the following advice:

> *The science of cosmetics and perfumery is helpful in the worship of gods; which requires the use of auspicious perfumes and incense; it contributes to the pleasures of men; it leads to the attainment of the three ends of human life (viz, religious merit, worldly prosperity and sensual enjoyment); it removes one's poverty; it contributes to the pleasures of kings and it gives highest delight to the minds of accomplished ladies.*[7]

McHugh, a Sanskrit scholar and author of *Sandalwood and carrion,* describes in great detail the art of perfumery that developed in India.

Perfumery played a very important role in every aspect of Indian life.[20]

The greatest contribution from India must be sandalwood, whose soft scent was said to induce the calm sought by all the spiritualities of India. Another well-known essential oil whose origin is from India is patchouli. Patchouli is a tropical member of the mint family. It was initially used to ward off moths from carpets and fine woven goods such as shawls and jackets. The leaves and stems, which turn brown upon drying, were chopped up and sprinkled among the fabrics.[7]

Cardamom was first mentioned in the Ayurvedic texts of the fourth century BC. Another highly prized Indian aromatic is tulsi, the herb sacred to Krishna. Exquisite floral aromatics such as jasmine, champaka (a close relative of our garden magnolias) and lotus are believed to have originated from India.[7]

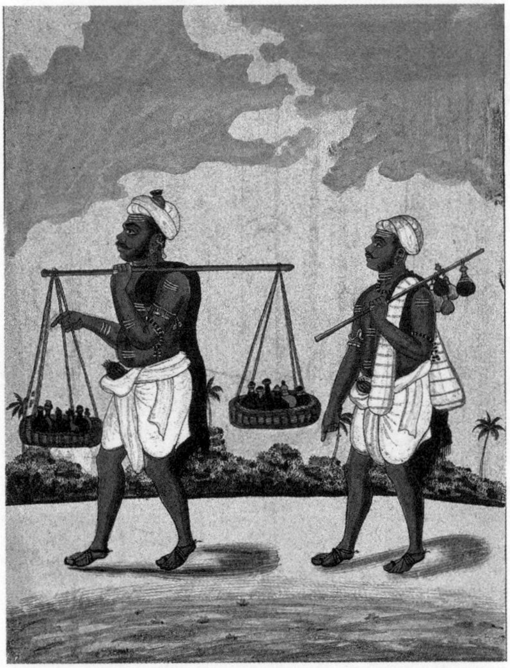

Indian perfume sellers. Gouache drawing. Courtesy of Welcome Collection.

The lotus is considered the sacred symbol of India. The scent is described as sweet and fruity, with a hint of anise. Buddhism adopted the flower as a symbol of its dharma because the roots are in the mud, while it blooms pure and clear above the waters.[7]

Apart from the lotus flower, tulsi, also known as sacred basil, was considered to be the most important holy plant in the Indian repertoire. It promoted cognitive clarity and union with the divine. It was considered the herb of transcendence.[6]

Another important aromatic oil from India is vetiver, which in Sanskrit literature is referred to as *reshira* or *sugandhimula*. It is cultivated in the south of India, and wild plants can be found on the Himalayan foothills. Spikenard was exported to the West in Roman times, and was considered a very precious aromatic ingredient. Ginger and galangal, two very important aromatic ingredients used for flavor and fragrance, originate from India.[7]

China

From the sixth to the thirteenth century, China was considered the world's greatest power and Chinese culture was considered the world's greatest splendour. Science and technology were much more advanced than in Europe at the time.[12]

China's most important contribution to aromatherapy was the citrus species. Almost all the citrus species are believed to have originated from China. *Citrus aurantium,* originating in China, first reached the Mediterranean world in the tenth century (through the Arabs). It is hard to imagine that all of these common fruits were completely unknown to the Greeks and Romans.[7]

The camphor tree was also a very important part of Chinese civilisation. It was extensively used in perfumery, medical and building applications.[7]

The ninth century text of al-Kindi describes camphor distillation in the Arabic world. It is likely that the Chinese who supplied the camphor were also distilling it. Morris states that an independent tradition of distillation occurred among Chinese alchemists, coming slightly later than the distillation apparatus developed in the West.[7]

The Chinese contributed to many improvements in distillation techniques. They isolated the step that extracted the ethyl alcohol from wine. This was the cooling of the condenser by means of cold water.[7]

Aromatics formed an important part of the compendiums of Chinese medicine, the *Great Herbal of Li Shih-Chen* and the *Pen Ts'au Kang Mu* of 1578. The carminative properties of essential oil-bearing plants were well known.[7]

The Middle Ages

The decline of the Roman Empire was considered the general decline in the level of civilisation in Europe, and most of the knowledge on aromatics was lost for some time. Personal use of fragrances was considered a frivolous luxury, tending towards debauchery, by church leaders. Many early Christians even ceased washing themselves, and were proud to reek of 'honest' dirt and sweat.[1]

It was a time of great superstition. The plagues had become an unavoidable part of life in medieval Europe. While science now recognises that the plague had been spread primarily by rat fleas carrying the plague germs, at the time, more dramatic agents were put forward as being responsible for the deadly sin.

One of the most popular beliefs of the time was that foul odour was considered one of the most common causes of many diseases. Classen describes a typical European city:

> *European cities were then the most filthy places. Food remains, human and animal waste, blood and entrails of slaughtered animals, dead cats and dogs – to name some. Even blood let from patients by barber-surgeons would be cast into the street as often as not.*[1]

It is not surprising that people generally tended to the strongly aromatic herbs and oils to mask the foul odours which were believed to be the cause of most diseases.[1]

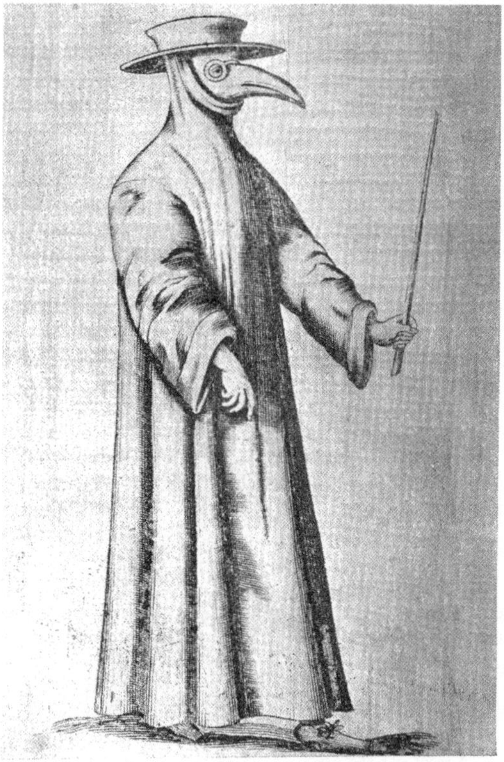

Plague doctor: ein Kieydung under den Todt. Courtesy of Wellcome Collection.

Aromatics were considered not only useful for preventing disease, but for curing it. Medical theory of the time suggested that the nose gave direct access to the brain, and that any medication inhaled through the nose would act directly on the brain, hence the spirit. It was also imagined that the spirit, or the life force, was similar in nature to odour, hence making smell the best means of correcting its disorders.[1]

It was here that we find that measures against the plague were directed in controlling and combating corrupt air. Municipal authorities lit bonfires of aromatic woods in the streets to purify the atmosphere. A popular device of the time was a pomander: an orange stuck full of cloves. Physicians recommended that the sickrooms have herbs at the window, an aromatic fire burning in the fireplace, and rosewater and vinegar sprinkled on the floor. Doctors often wore a nose-bag as shown in the picture opposite. The use of such smells was not without medical value as the essential oils used are now known to be considered powerful germicides.[1]

However, the Crusades once again introduced the spices and perfumes of the East, that had previously so fascinated the Greeks and Romans, to medieval Europe.

Spiritual and curative powers were often attributed to scent by early Christendom. For example, aromatic ingredients played an important role during the periods of the plague, when the battle of disease was essentially a war between fragrant and foul scents.[1]

In medieval Europe, Paracelsus, a Swiss fifteenth century doctor, developed the 'Doctrine of Signatures'. He believed that plants were created to serve humankind and that they had been given their shape and colour by the Divine Creator as a sign, in accordance with the objective that they were to serve. For example, heart-shaped leaves and flowers were believed to heal the heart; kidney-shaped fruits were used to treat the kidneys, red flowers and plants were considered excellent tonics for the blood, while yellow plants were used for curing jaundice.[15]

During the Middle Ages, we see the formation of the guilds that became the precursors to the professional associations we have nowadays. Butler provides us with a very detailed account of the formation of the various guilds, which more than likely contributed to the way medicine and healing has become fragmented today:

> *An apothecary in the Middle Ages, by definition, was a warehouseman, but by application the term became restricted to those who prepared and sold drugs. In England by the sixteenth century apothecaries were granted the right to issue licenses to practice medicine. The dealers in drugs were included in the Guild of Pepperers formed in*

1190. This in turn was merged with the Spicers in 1345 to form the Fraternity of St Anthony. In 1373 the name of grocer first appears in the records, so that by 1500 the Guild of Grocers had full control of drugs sold by apothecaries. By the fifteenth century England was dependent on spices from the East.[12]

Gattefossé explains the origins of the 'four thieves vinegar', which was considered to be a prophylactic more than a remedy for the pneumonic plague. It is believed that the formula was developed in 1720-21 by four thieves who robbed the bodies of a plague victim, without the fear of disease.[21] When the thieves were arrested, their lives were to be spared on the condition that they disclose their formula. The formula was follows:

Take three pints of strong white wine vinegar, add a handful each of wormwood, meadowwood, wild marjoram and sage, fifty cloves, two ounces of angelica, rosemary, and horehound and three large measures of camphor. Place the mixture in a container for fifteen days, strain and express, then bottle. Use by rubbing it on the hands, ears and temples from time to time when approaching a plague victim.[21]

There is another version of the origins of the four thieves vinegar which dates back to the great plague of 1413. However, in this case, the four thieves were condemned to be burnt alive, but to lighten their sentence, they disclosed their formula and were hanged instead. Gattefossé states that whatever the origins of the story, the plants used in the four thieves vinegar are rich in essential oils which have strong antimicrobial properties.[21]

The Age of Discovery

During the Middle Ages the spices that started reaching Europe were considered the finest gifts to royalty and the privileged.[11]

By the thirteenth century, Java had become the main trading centre for nutmeg, mace and cloves that came from the Moluccas Islands, and the Arabs controlled the trade of spices from Java to Europe. However, by the sixteenth century, the East Indies had attracted merchants from Western Europe.[11]

The Western European countries had to establish a sea route to the eastern spice lands such as India and the East Indies after the fall of Constantinople to the Ottoman Turks in 1453. At the end of the fifteenth century, the Portuguese started direct trading in spices with the Malabar Coast. This was the end of the Arab supremacy over the spice trade. Very soon the Portuguese established a monopoly in the spice trade, not only with India, but also with Sri Lanka and the spice islands of the East Indies.[11]

The Portuguese forced the Sinhala kings to supply over 11,000 kg of cinnamon bark, which led to the cinnamon forests being ruthlessly over-harvested. The rising price of spices in Europe because of the Portuguese monopoly caused resentment amongst other Europeans. Dutch navigator Cornelius Van Hortman reached the East Indies (Indonesia) in 1596, and established trade relations with some of the islands in spite of resistance from the Portuguese. Gradually the Dutch took control of all the important spice-producing islands of the East Indies, putting an end to the Portuguese monopoly.[11]

The Dutch now had a virtual monopoly of the trade of nutmeg and cloves. They concentrated their cultivation of nutmeg trees on the islands of Banda and Amboina, and cloves on Amboina. In 1651 they devised a scheme to uproot all nutmeg and clove trees on the remaining islands to protect their monopoly. By 1681, approximately 75% of all the wild nutmeg and clove trees on the Moluccas had been destroyed, thus creating an artificial scarcity of these spices in Europe and driving the prices up for the benefit of the Dutch East India Company.[17]

In 1658, the Dutch took control of the Portuguese establishments in Ceylon, and in 1663, they also conquered Cochin and Cannanore off the Malabar Coast. The Dutch then held a very strict and tightly controlled monopoly on the trade of spices from Asia to Europe.[11]

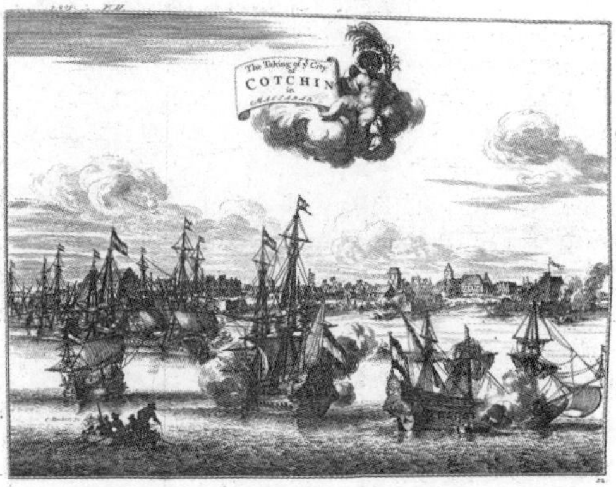

Scene showing the taking of Cochin in Malabar by the Dutch East India Company. Courtesy of Wellcome Collection.

Between 1770 and 1772, Pierre Poive, the French administrator of the island of Mauritius, managed to smuggle clove, nutmeg and cinnamon plants out of the Dutch-controlled spice islands. New spice plantations were established in Réunion, the

Seychelles and other French colonies.[17]

However, in 1799, the Dutch East India Company went bankrupt and Holland's greatest period of trading affluence came to an end. The Dutch ports of India's Malabar coast were taken over by England as Holland lost its leadership in European commerce. In 1795, the British planted clove trees in Penang, an island near the west coast of the Malay Peninsula. By 1796, England had taken over all Dutch possessions in the East Indies except for Java.[17]

The Rise of Modern Perfumery

Morris, author of *Fragrance – the story of perfume from Cleopatra to Chanel,* provides us with a detailed account of the unfolding of perfumery in the West from the end of the Dark Ages in Europe through to the perfume industry we know today.

He explains that there were several factors that significantly contributed to the development of the modern perfumery industry:[7]

- the discovery of alcohol around 1200
- an extensive range of studies appeared in the Renaissance on all topics related to perfumery such as distillation, botany, chemistry and glass making
- the bypassing of the old Arab trade network to the spice producing countries of Asia.

There was a fourth factor that contributed to the growth of perfumery that Morris refers to as the 'new humanism', that was ushered in by the Renaissance:

> *Adorning the body and celebrating the glory of man were no longer unusual concepts. The nobility of the human condition, which had been preached by the Neoplatonists of the Academy of the Medici at Florence, was taken up by thinkers throughout Italy and then absorbed by the French.*[7]

The growing capitalism of the Renaissance also assured the ability to buy whatever could be had from the rich sources of supplies made available by the new trade routes.[7]

After the fall of the Roman Empire, the knowledge of aromatics was preserved by the monks in cloistered gardens from the sixth through to the eleventh centuries. Monks and nuns grew classical herbs such as bay laurel, basil, sage, lavender, dill, thyme, rosemary, valerian, chamomile, pennyroyal, spearmint and peppermint. Most of these herbs were reserved for healing. Two early texts on the uses of these herbs were the work of Odo, Abbot of Beauprai, called *De viribus herbarum* (On the powers of herbs), and the *Causae et Curae* (Cause of illness and cures) by St Hildegarde, Abess of Bingen (1098-1179). Her highest praise went to lavender.[7]

Morris explains that the Dark Ages came to an end with the Crusades. He claims that, thanks to the Crusades, Europeans received an invaluable schooling in medicine, pharmacy, chemistry, commerce and perfumery. Platearius made many translations of Arab pharmacological works around 1150, Gerard of Cremona translated ar-Razi, and at the end of the twelfth century, Alfred of Sarshel translated Ibn-Sina, the pharmacist known as Avicenna.[7]

Reinarz explains that, in the early days of perfume making, rose water and orange flower water were often used as bases for perfumes. The perfumer's main competitors were the apothecaries and distillers who produced alcoholic extracts of herbs which were often sold as medical elixirs. One perfume that became very popular during the eigtheenth century was originally used as a medical remedy to treat constipation, fever and the plague. This perfume was *Eau de Cologne*.[2]

It was originally created by Renato Bianco, the perfumer of the Florentine and queen consort of France. The recipe then travelled to Cologne with an Italian perfumer, Giovanni Femini, who renamed it *Acqua di cologne*. It was commercialised by Italian expatriate, Johann Maria Farina. The scent initially comprised rosemary and citrus essences dissolved in grape spirit.[2]

Reinarz explains that by the eighteenth century the luxury goods market in France was vibrant. According to historians, the French drenched themselves with eau de Cologne. During this period, scents were also applied to fabrics that the user was wearing, including gloves, handkerchiefs and dresses. Perfumes for scenting gloves was a necessity to help counteract the putrid smells required in the process of tanning leather.[2]

Two cities in southern France led the production of alcohol-based perfumes – Montpellier and Grasse. Montpellier was well connected through its port to foreign supplies of aromatic ingredients, and its local apothecaries manufactured medicines and perfumes. During this period, the apothecaries separated from the spice and drug merchants, as well as the glove makers and perfumer-distillers. The perfume trade became the preserve of the *gantier-parfumeurs,* and was protected by a guild. Membership required a seven-year apprenticeship, after the successful completion of which the title of master perfumer was earned. By the mid-eighteenth century there were 250 master perfumers in all of France.[2]

Although Montpellier was long known as the centre for perfume, it slowly and gradually lost ground to Grasse, the economic capital of Western

Provence, which soon became the nation's perfume capital after its two dozen manufacturers of scented leathers were granted separate status in 1729. The climate in Provence was better suited to the cultivation of the aromatic plants required by perfumers.[2]

However, as the tanning trade began to wane, its perfumers would split from the tanner's guild and apply their skills to other sectors. Over time, perfumers broke free from the ancillary trades, including those of the apothecary, distiller and grocer, but success in the eighteenth century only came to those who collaborated with the coiffeurs, soap makers and other emerging beauty trades.[2]

The Breakthrough of Distillation

When alcohol was first extracted is not clear. Albert the Great (1193-1280), a scholar and saint, gave instructions for making a new substance:

> *When wine is sublimed like rosewater, a light, inflammable liquid is obtained.*[7]

Alcohol was referred to as *admirable water, burning water, water of wine, water of life, spirit of wine, subtle spirit* and the *soul of heaven*. It was considered the *quintessence*, the fifth essence that complemented Water, Fire, Air and Earth.[7]

The trick to making alcohol was an efficient water-cooling system. The 'Moor's head' cooling cap for the still had been modified into a bucket filled with constantly running cold water into which the tube from the still had been fitted by coiling it.[7]

Alcohol was a success from the very beginning. Cardinal Vitalis de Furno declared it to be a 'panacea' for all ills. Very soon, every pharmaceutical school began busily distilling alcohol. All the herbs inherited from the classical world could be steeped into this solution to produce numerous liqueurs, which were initially used for medicinal purposes only.[7]

Improvements to distillation also helped in the extraction of essential oils. Large plantations of lavender, rose and sage were set up in Burgundy in the fourteenth century, and by 1370, perfumes as we know them today began to appear. A combination of rosemary and lavender essential oils with alcohol, known as *Hungary water*, was named after Queen Elizabeth of Hungary.[7]

A second perfume, *eau de Carmes*, was compounded in 1379 by the nuns of Abbaye St Juste for Charles V of France. This blend, known as Carmelite water, was a blend of melissa, angelica and other herbal extracts.[7]

Many books on distillation were written during the sixteenth century, especially in Germany, which seems to have been the centre of this aromatherapy renaissance. The books also referred to alchemical practices.

Alchemy was very popular at this time, and the distillation of all kinds of substances was one of the alchemists' favourite pastimes in their pursuit of the *quintessence* of matter.

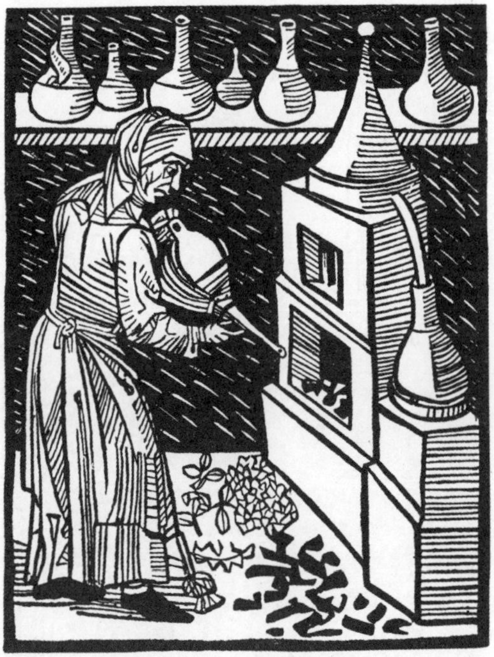

Distillation in 1475, Von den Gebrannten Wassern. Courtesy of Wellcome Collection.

Distillation was still unperfected, but in the early fifteenth century, the *Libellus de distallatione philosophia* noted that tinctures of herbs in alcohol were impervious to decay, and it gave the advice that herbs should not be distilled in vessels of lead.[13]

In Germany, Hieronymus Braunschweig, often referred to as Jerome of Brunswick, who was a physician, wrote several books on distillation. His last great work, the new *Vollkomen Distillierbuch*, was published in 1597. It includes reference to 25 essential oils, including rosemary, lavender, clove, cinnamon, myrrh and nutmeg. Braunschweig's books on distillation went through 680 editions, appearing in every European language.[13]

Other contributions to the development of aromatherapy were made by Conrad Gesner, and by Ryff, a Strasburg physician, who published *Neu Gross Destillierbuch* in 1545. In *The treasure of Euonymus*, published in 1559, Conrad Gesner writes of essential oils having the power to conserve all strengths and to prolong life. His findings on the properties of rosemary oil are remarkably perceptive:

> *It strengtheneth the harte, the braine, the sinews [muscles] and the hoole bodye ... members [limbs] sick of the palsy it heateth them for moste parte, and healeth them sometimes. Fistulaes and Cancars that give not place to other medicines, it healeth them throughlye.*[13]

Many of these comments, especially the properties ascribed to rosemary oil, would be regarded as valid by aromatherapists today.

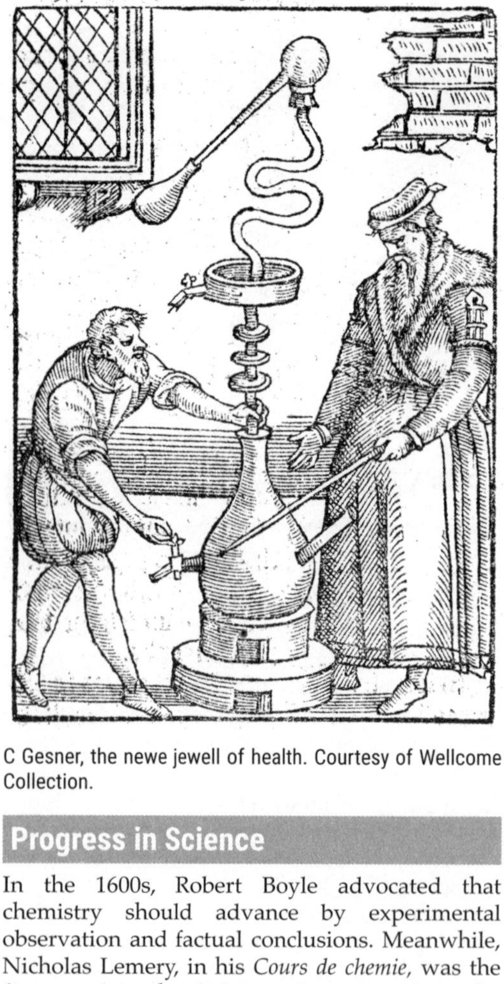

C Gesner, the newe jewell of health. Courtesy of Wellcome Collection.

Progress in Science

In the 1600s, Robert Boyle advocated that chemistry should advance by experimental observation and factual conclusions. Meanwhile, Nicholas Lemery, in his *Cours de chemie,* was the first to adopt the division of compounds in the animal and vegetable world as organic and those in the mineral world as inorganic.[12]

By the late eighteenth century, many scholars followed Boyle's precept of a century before, discarding abstract theory and turning to careful observation of laboratory experiments. By the early 1800s, John Dalton put forward the Atomic Theory of Matter. It was at this point that we begin to see chemistry diverging from medicine, which was still concerned with herbs and resins.[12]

The 'vital force' theory was shattered in 1828, when Wohler created an organic compound – urea – in the lab from two inorganic compounds – cyanic acid and ammonia. In the first half of the nineteenth century, we also see Berzelius, Gay-Lussac, Dalton and Avogadro provide us with a better understanding of the distinction between atoms and molecules. In 1805, Gay-Lussac and Humboldt found that water consisted of hydrogen and oxygen in the ratio of 2:1.[12]

By the second half of the nineteenth century, commercial production of aromatic chemicals such as linalool, linalyl acetate and coumarin began.[12]

By 1900, the introduction of solvent extraction using hydrocarbon such as ether or benzene allowed concretes to be made from which a range of absolute florals became available. The perfumer at the turn of the century had more natural oils, absolutes and isolates, together with synthetic aromatic chemicals, than ever before to create new perfumes.[12]

In 1913, Gildemeister wrote a comprehensive text describing essential oils. This book clearly established a scientific framework for the manufacture and understanding of essential oils. It provided chemical tests for identifying inferior or adulterated oils. Gildemeister also provided a detailed historical account of many of the essential oils that we use nowadays.[22]

Holmes explains that, in the first half of the twentieth century, the perfume industry had long abandoned the principles of natural perfumery and the use of essential oils and turned to isolates, chemically altered oils and synthetic fragrances.[24]

Between the wars, chemical and physical examination and olfactory assessment were all qualitative testing techniques used to test the purity of essential oils. This included tests such as specific gravity, optical rotation, refractive index and solubility in alcohol, just to name a few. However, in 1959, Langenau and Rogers reported the instrumental analysis of essential oils. By the 1980s, the development of gas-liquid chromatography to high resolution mass spectrometry allowed the identity and purity of the constituents of essential oils to be determined much more quickly and accurately.[12]

The Rise of Modern Medicine

Philippus Theophrastus Bombastus von Hohenheim (1493-1541) (commonly known as Paracelsus) was credited with revolutionising medicine. He lay the foundations of both modern and alternative medicine. However, modern medicine would become more interested in active constituents and chemicals rather than the entire plant.[14]

He castigated those in the medical profession who merely followed the texts of ancient Greek and Roman herbalists and would not test their materials and processes by experiences.[14]

The Medical Act of 1511 saw the formalisation of training for physicians. The Royal College of Physicians was given the power to fine unauthorised practitioners. In 1540, barbers and surgeons were given similar powers, when the king had approved their company. Without hesitation, the barber-surgeons began a rampage of prosecuting 'unauthorised practitioners'. These 'quacks' were healers who relied on traditional knowledge of herbs and healing. Most were poor and served the poor.[14]

So ruthless was the persecution that, within two years, there were insufficient healers. So in 1542, King Henry enacted the Quacks Charter, which exempted many unauthorised practitioners from the 1511 Act. The medical elite were outraged, so their target then shifted from the 'quacks' to women, when the king passed the first penal law against witches. Witches had become a convenient scapegoat for the medical establishment.[14]

Hygiene and sanitation in larger European cities was not very advanced. It is not surprising that these conditions contributed to the plague epidemics in the seventeenth century. Most houses did not have bathrooms, but wooden tubs that were bought into the bedrooms by servants, along with the hot and cold water, so the task of keeping clean was often very tedious. The Law of Gallantry in 1640 recommended that the entire body be bathed occasionally, that the hands be washed at least every day, the face almost as often, and the head from time to time.[12]

Butler states that, even a large dwelling, in which 60 servants might be employed, had no proper lavatory, only a stinking 'house of easement'. Houses had no gutters, and rain and traffic made gunnels in the narrow streets. Into these went all kitchen waste and other garbage, to be washed away by the next downpour of rain. It is not surprising that disease was common.[12]

After the Restoration, perfumes had become popular, mainly to cover obnoxious smells. The courtiers held perfumed handkerchiefs to the nose and the ladies had posies of flowers. Pomanders were carried to ward off infections and aromatic gums were sucked to cover bad breath. During the great plague, cinnamon, juniper berry, lavender, cassia and cardamom were burned in the streets and houses in the belief that the infection was airborne.[12]

The seventeenth century was known as the 'golden age' of English herbalists, notably Nicholas Culpeper, John Parkinson and John Gerardes. Essential oils had become a regular part of the herbalist's repertoire.[5] For instance, Culpeper says of rosemary:

> *The chemical drawn from the leaves and flowers is a sovereign help … to touch the temples and nostrils with two or three drops for all diseases of the head and brain spoken of before, as also to take one drop, two or three, as the case requires, for inward diseases; yet it must be done with discretion, for it is very quick and piercing.*[23]

Of lavender, Culpeper states:

> *It is of especial use for pains in the head and brain, following cold, apoplexy, falling-sickness, the dropsy or sluggish malady, cramps, convulsions, palsies and faintings. It provokes women's courses, and expels the dead child and afterbirth.*[23]

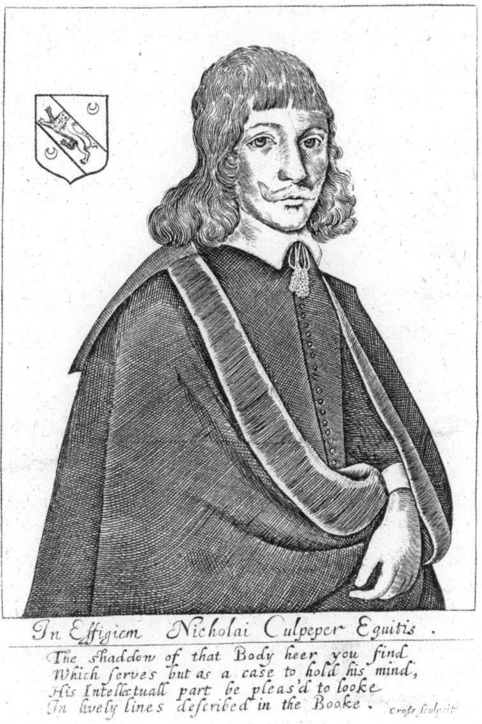

Portrait of N Culpeper by Cross. Courtesy of Wellcome Collection.

It is apparent that essential oils were successfully being used for a variety of internal and external problems. Both doctors and herbalists used them, a trend that would continue until the end of the nineteenth century. By this stage, dosages had been established and the need for dilution and suitable vehicles for internal use had become clear.

A gradual division between the physicians who used chemical drugs and those that remained faithful to herbs occurred. Over time, the medical establishment became obsessed with science and chemistry, and plant-based therapies began to fall out of favour, especially when it was believed that the 'active constituents' could be extracted from the plant, or even better, synthetically derived.

For example, willow (*Salix alba*) is used in herbal medicine for the relief of aches, fevers and rheumatic pain. However, in 1852, salicylic acid, the active constituent in willow, was synthetically derived. The laboratory was now replacing the herb garden as a source of principal materia medica.

Holmes explains that the development of chemistry-based pharmacognosy, pharmacy and medicine saw a profound transformation throughout the nineteenth century. Doctors began to value the simple empirical, sensory evidence of clinical experience, but Western medicine began to abandon the science-based research that had been previously conducted on essential oils, and the material reductionism reigning in allopathic medicine reached a tipping point in favour of pharmacy. Holmes claims that, incapacitated by the political imperatives of the drug industry, medical practitioners were no longer able to prescribe essential oils as clinical remedies.[24]

The Pioneers of Modern Aromatherapy

Aromatherapy in France

In the 1860s, Antoine Béchamp and later Louis Pasteur confirmed the existence of microbes and that they were the cause of disease. However, Holmes points out that Béchamp was adamant that microbes were not necessarily the cause of infectious disease, but the individual's tissue terrain with healthy commensal microbes was fundamental in the balance of health and sickness.[24]

Somebody drew attention to the low incidence of tuberculosis in the flower-growing districts of France, especially in the south. Tuberculosis was a very common illness at the time; however, it was noted that most of the workers who processed the flowers and herbs remained free of respiratory diseases. The most likely cause of this was believed to have been the essential oils contained in these plants. This led, in 1887, to the first recorded laboratory test on the antibacterial properties of the essential oils.[13]

In the 1880s, Chamberland, Cadeac and Meunier published similar studies that showed that the micro-organisms of glandular and yellow fever were easily killed by essential oils. They noted the active properties of oregano, Chinese cinnamon, angelica and geranium.[13]

In July 1910, Rene-Maurice Gattefossé discovered the healing properties of lavender oil after severely burning his hands in a laboratory explosion. While he was not the first person to use essential oils therapeutically, he has been given credit for having coined the term *aromatherapie* in 1937.

Gattefossé used essential oils for the treatment of soldiers in military hospitals during the First World War. Some of his observations included:

> *Wounds to the scalp: healed in 10 days*
> *Firearm wounds: healed in 15 days*
> *Crushing of the thigh, open leg fracture; varices becoming ulcerated; delayed healing of an amputation stump of the thigh: healed in 21 days after failing with all other medications.*[21]

He concluded by stating:

> *It must be conceded that, while the antiseptic power of essences is of enormous interest, especially since it is not attended by any of the disadvantages found to such a large degree with all the other antiseptics used hitherto, greater attention needs to be devoted to the power they have of revitalising tissue.*[21]

Gattefossé cites many case studies involving the work of Dr Marchand, who regularly used lavender oil to treat infected ulcerated lesions. One of the case studies was reported as follows:

> *Infected ulcerated lesion of the lower third of the leg. 24th December, first application of lavender. 31st December: improvement, the purulent suppurating base was granulating and pink. By 16th January, the sore was half the original size. By 10th February, it had healed completely.*[21]

Gattefossé is to be commended for having the insight to see that the therapeutic application of essential oils constituted a discipline in its own right. He was a chemist, so while he did not have much to do with the holistic approach to aromatherapy, he knew the importance of the chemical understanding of the essential oils, and as a perfumer he recognised the psychotherapeutic benefits of the fragrance of the essential oils.[21]

Although Gattefossé deserves full credit for his vision of aromatherapy, he was not the only person at the time to recognise the benefits of essential oils. In 1939, another Frenchman, Albert Couvreur, published a book on the medicinal properties of the essential oils.[13]

Dr Jean Valnet is also credited with the further development of aromatherapy. As an army surgeon, he began to use, with great success, essential oils as antiseptics in the treatment of war wounds during the Indochina war from 1948-1959.

After the war, he continued using essential oils in his capacity as a doctor, and in 1964 published a comprehensive text entitled *Aromatherapie* (also available in English), which has since earned him global recognition.[14]

While Valnet understood the powerful antimicrobial activity of essential oils, he also understood that the role of the microbe is far less important than the site. He suggests that infection does not automatically follow the penetration of an organism by a microbe. The germ has to find a suitable breeding ground.[25]

Valnet describes the benefits of using essential oils:

> *Essential oils are especially valuable as antiseptics because of their aggression towards microbial germs and their harmlessness to tissue – one of the chief defects of chemical antiseptics is that they are likely to be as harmful to the cells of the organisms as to the cause of the disease.*[25]

Valnet was keen to understand the chemistry of the essential oil in order to understand the therapeutic activity of the oil, but he also emphasised the importance of using the natural essential oil rather than adulterated oils or synthetic oils. He cites the work of Cuthbert Hall who, in 1904, demonstrated that the antimicrobial properties of eucalyptus were much more powerful than the principal constituent eucalyptol, also known as 1,8-cineole.[25]

Valnet cites a study conducted in 1958 that confirmed that the vapours of essential oils had antiseptic activity which inhibited certain *staphylococci* and *coliform bacilli*. He cites the work of Dr Girault, a gynaecologist and obstetrics surgeon, who was convinced of the frequent harmful effects of regularly prescribed hormones, synthetic corticoids and antibiotics, which were regularly being dispensed far too freely and in exceedingly high doses. Dr Girault suggested that plant extracts and essential oils not only had anti-infective properties, but were considered general physiological restoratives for the circulation, endocrine glands and nervous systems.[25]

Herbs, essential oils and careful attention to diet formed an integral approach of Dr Valnet's therapeutic strategy. The prescription his patients were likely to take with them usually combined a mixture of herbs and essential oils in an alcohol base, to be taken in a glass of lukewarm water before meals.[14]

However, for most French doctors of the time, plants were yesterday's medicine. Scientifically, clinically tested synthetic drugs had become the norm of the day. In 1972, three doctors, Lapraz, Duraffourd and Belaiche, gathered around Valnet to form the nucleus of a new organisation devoted to the study and promotion of phytotherapy.[14]

While they realised that Valnet's empiric approach was effective, to give aromatherapy credibility, they had to work within the framework of modern medicine, not outside it. Belaiche developed a scientifically based medical application of essential oils based on scientific research.[14]

However, the very success of phytotherapy was its own undoing:

> *There were obvious dangers in much of this self-medication by legions of largely amateur herbal enthusiasts, but the herbs and essential oils available for over-the-counter sale were severely limited by French law. Far more of a threat to the public health were the growing legions of doctors armed with a prescription pad, and just enough of a sketchy training to allow them to impress patients with their mastery of phytotherapy.*[14]

Grigg cites Valnet, who was horrified with the irresponsible prescribing of essential oils:

> *On one occasion, a pharmacist rang to ask his opinion of prescription: it consisted of a mix of essential oils and tinctures in capsule form, a cream, an ointment and a liquid preparation, in total, thirty essential oils – including hyssop, sage and rosemary – and seventeen plant tinctures.*[14]

It was the over-commercialisation and charlatanism rampant in the French herbal world that led to its downfall. The cost of essential oils dispensed by pharmacists was reimbursed by the French National Health Scheme. However, with a drug budget already escalating out of control, in 1989, the French Ministry of Health ceased to reimburse herbal prescriptions. Doctors whose consulting rooms had been crammed with patients eager for the new plant medicines saw them empty dramatically once patients knew that they would have to foot the prescription bill themselves.[14]

The origins of holistic aromatherapy

It was Marguerite Maury, a French biochemist and beautician, who is often given much credit in the development of holistic aromatherapy as it is practised today. While her book (now published in English) *The secret of life and youth*, does not give much practical information on the essential oils, she understood the impact of our emotions on our physical wellbeing and at a cellular level:

> *Whether it be hatred or love, envy or anger which come to light in the course of an analysis, the material and physical life of the patient is always in danger. All these emotions have immediate repercussions on the different functions. Every physiologist knows the inhibition and disturbances of digestive or renal function, the excessive production of acid in the stomach*

as a result of worries and upsets. It is common knowledge.[26]

She emphasised the importance of the essential oils, not only in massage, but also as psychotherapeutic substances capable of bringing about changes in one's mood:

The greatest interest is the effect of fragrance on the psyche and mental state of the individual. Powers of perception become clearer and more accurate and there is a feeling of having, to a certain extent, outstripped events. They are seen more objectively, and therefore in truer perspective.[26]

She explained that scents may not be able to entirely transform an individual, but she explained that it may awaken latent faculties and thoughts which slumber in the lowest depths of the memory. She explained that the inner brakes which have been damaged by traumas can be made to function. She also suggested that scent:

... procures us a state of relaxation that makes it easy to dispel traumas. Our problems appear under another light and with greater clarity.[26]

She was adamant that aromatherapy should not be compared with perfumery. She explained that perfumes were typically presented in an alcoholic base, making them very diffusive. According to Maury, when we wear a perfume:

We do it to externalize certain qualities, to please and to attract. In other words, we do it to influence our entourage whereas the use of essential oils concerns only ourselves.[26]

However, she was grateful to the perfume industry for providing us with so many essential oils.[26]

Maury emphasised the importance of applying the essential oils externally, diluted in vegetable oil, in combination with massage:

Massage of the conjunctive, neuro-muscular or soft tissues pave the way admirably for the penetration of odoriferous substances, and the resultant rejuvenation ... It is therefore clear that preparations with a basis of essential oils with vegetable oils used as carriers, will be of great assistance.[26]

Maury also understood how essential oils could be used to enhance many of the spa treatments available at the time. However, she also explained that immediately after a steam bath, the skin is in a state of elimination for several hours, and this makes it impossible for anything such as essential oils to be absorbed.[26]

It is at this point that we see a clear shift in the original meaning of the French word *aromatherapie*. Maury, who became Chairperson for CIDESCO (Pour le Comite International D'esthetique et de Cosmetologie), forged a link between aromatherapy and the beauty industry. As a result, beauty therapists, who were already working in the context of wellbeing, were able to introduce additional benefits, such as massage and the essential oils, to their treatment.

While it may be tempting to suggest that Maury focused purely on the aesthetic or anti-aging uses of essential oils, she understood that nervous exhaustion and stress and a lack of sleep are responsible for preventing the body's natural healing process.[26]

Maury was familiar with the principles of the Ayurveda and TCM, and incorporated these principles in the way she practised aromatherapy and her concept of the individual mixture or individual prescription:

The individual mixture is designed to reflect the weaknesses and violence of an individual; it has to compensate for the deficiencies and reduces the excesses. It serves above all to normalize the rhythm of the functions.[26]

At a beauty therapy conference in 1959, Micheline Arcier met Marguerite Maury. This led to Micheline Arcier's lifelong devotion to aromatherapy. She trained with both Marguerite Maury and Dr Jean Valnet.[27] Micheline Arcier has developed some of the most effective aromatherapy techniques being used today.

Robert Tisserand is also attributed with the development of holistic aromatherapy. Tisserand's book *The art of aromatherapy*, published in 1977, was the first to leave the purely medical approach of aromatherapy, combining medical applications with a more holistic and esoteric view of essential oils.[28]

It is at this point that aromatherapy became a semi-medical modality, which allowed the lay person to attempt self-therapy for many common ailments. Many other interpretations of aromatherapy began to develop. Some of these interpretations were esoteric, while others began to focus on the fragrance aspect.[28]

Schnaubelt explains that the development of aromatherapy after 1980 diversified into four basic strands:

- medical aromatherapy
- popular and esoteric aromatherapy
- holistic aromatherapy
- and the scientific study of fragrance.[28]

Aromatherapy Today

Aromatherapy as a health profession

In many countries, it is still difficult or impossible to practise aromatherapy because of very strict government control. Why is this so, considering that aromatherapy continues to be one of the most popular forms of natural therapies amongst the public?

In 1999, Schnaubelt made the following comment:

> *At the end of the twentieth century, the practice of aromatherapy appears to consist of whatever the particular practitioner or user of essential oils might make it to be. Disjointed and scattered it is a practice without a theory. Whatever definitions exist are massively colored by commercial interests.*[29]

Unfortunately, Schnaubelt's comment is more relevant today than it ever was.[29]

In some countries, doctors think they should be the only ones to practise aromatherapy. In other countries, doctors think aromatherapy is a load of quackery. Often nurses think they are best suited to practice aromatherapy, beauty therapists also think they should be aromatherapists, even people who make soaps and cosmetics say that they are aromatherapists.

Why can we not just have one professional association that represents all health care practitioners of aromatherapy – irrespective of how aromatherapy is practised? We simply need to establish different categories of membership for doctors, nurses, massage therapists, natural therapists and beauty therapists.

Meanwhile, multi-level marketing (MLM) aromatherapy companies have taken advantage of the lack of a globally united aromatherapy profession. A market report for the sales of essential oils states that direct sales channels now dominate the distribution of over 60% of the aromatherapy market. The United States is the largest market, valued at over $4 billion in 2017-2018.[30]

While this renewed interest in essential oils is welcomed, we must be sure that it is done responsibly and with integrity. Many professionally trained aromatherapists are concerned with several issues regarding information being disseminated throughout the internet and within essential oil MLM companies.[31]

Klipse is concerned that if someone reads a bit about essential oils, or if they belong to an MLM company, they are then qualified to tell others how to use them. This situation undermines the qualifications and experience of professionally trained aromatherapists, and also puts the public at risk of unsafe usage recommendations.[31]

For example, Watt has expressed his concern at claims made promoting frankincense oil as a treatment for cancer.[32] Tisserand explains that almost all the research on frankincense and cancer is on the gum, which contains boswellic acid. However, there is no boswellic acid in the essential oil. Frankincense extracts contain about 50% boswellic acid, and there has been extensive research on the antitumoral activity of boswellic acid, but this does not apply to the essential oil.[33]

Tisserand states boswellic acid is much too heavy a molecule to be volatile so it is impossible to find it in the essential oil. Boswellic acid has a molecular weight in the range of 450-500. However, volatile molecules all have molecular weight below 300.[33]

Therefore, to suggest that frankincense essential oil has boswellic acid and to promote it as a cancer treatment is misleading and irresponsible.

It is not surprising that aromatherapy was the topic of Janelle Sheen's PhD thesis:

> *The Professionalization of Aromatherapy – a case study of the professionalization of complementary and alternative medicine in the Australian health care system.*[34]

Sheen claims that aromatherapy has an identity crisis. She claims that aromatherapy lacks a theoretical framework, and that aromatherapy still lacks scientific research. Sheen argues that aromatherapy was never a profession. While the definition of 'what is a profession' varies within literature, Sheen has identified some core characteristics that define a profession:

> *a recognised body of knowledge requiring degree level training; an emphasis on service to society within a service ideal; and autonomy via monopolistic control.*[34]

Sheen argues that, according to this definition of a profession, the practice of aromatherapy does not meet the criteria and therefore should not be considered a profession.[34]

We could spend all day arguing if aromatherapy is a profession or not within mainstream health care, but the fact is that aromatherapy does have many challenges that have undermined its professional status:

- the lack of commonality in ideology for the practice of aromatherapy
- the lack of regulations regarding the quality of essential oils
- there is little scientific evidence to validate aromatherapy
- there is no holistic framework for the practice of aromatherapy
- the hijacking of the term 'aromatherapy' for the purposes of marketing MLM, cosmetics and toiletry products
- no unity or agreement amongst aromatherapy practitioners of different backgrounds
- still too many charlatans promoting 'quick fixes'

- compared to other natural therapies very little training required to become aromatherapist.

In Australia, the popularity of aromatherapy within conventional health care such as nursing homes and hospitals remains strong. Indeed, it is most interesting that Sheen proposes that aromatherapy should be integrated into nursing practice:

> *It is presented that the most likely pathway for the practice of aromatherapy to develop within the Australian healthcare system is by integration into nursing practice. This is because of a philosophical match between aromatherapy and nursing practice, nursing interest and nursing's available resources to develop aromatherapy practice.*[34]

This makes a lot of sense. I agree that integrating aromatherapy into nursing practice is a very exciting direction that aromatherapy can take and is taking. However, if Sheen is proposing that one should become a nurse to become an aromatherapy practitioner, that is where I disagree.

Sheen states that aromatherapy has been used as a tool to enhance other practices. This is true. She notes that beauty therapists take up aromatherapy without the comprehensive skills of a medical herbalist. She states that generally aromatherapy is allied to other theories or philosophies and is often integrated into any other health care modality emphasising its versatility. As a practice, she says that it relies on theories of health, illness and diagnosis from other healthcare frameworks.[34]

This is exactly what 'integrative aromatherapy' should be.

Aromatherapy in Australia

Natural therapies such as aromatherapy have become an integral part of Australia's health care system. More than 70% of Australians have used natural therapy as a regular part of their overall health care.[35]

The Australian public is encouraged to take out private health insurance, which also includes health care cover for many complementary therapies including aromatherapy.

Currently, the Australian Government provides a private health insurance rebate to individuals and families to encourage the uptake and maintenance of private health insurance. Most people are eligible for a 30% rebate on their health insurance costs. This typically includes the cost of optional extras such as natural therapies.[35]

However, a review of the Australian Government rebate on private health insurance for natural therapies was announced in the 2012–13 budget to ensure private health insurance covers clinically proven treatments. The health department reviewed 'natural therapies' to identify services that could not be underpinned by a robust evidence base and for which the private health insurance rebate should be withdrawn.[36]

The review found that no such evidence was available and recommended the withdrawal of health insurance rebates for many natural therapies, including aromatherapy.[36]

I believe, like many others, that this review ignored good quality, evidence-based research which shows complementary medicine is effective.

Based on this review, in 2017 the Australian Government made an announcement that it will be cutting off government rebates to a range of natural therapies, including aromatherapy and herbalism. The government spokesperson said that private health insurers can still cover natural therapies, but they will no longer be eligible for Commonwealth subsidies. The government claimed that the crackdown on natural therapies was the 'right move' based on the advice from the Chief Medical Officer.[37]

The review also ignored the recommendations provided in the WHO guidelines for methodologies on research and evaluation of traditional medicines. While the WHO document supports the need for scientific research to provide evidence of safety and efficacy, it also acknowledged that the theories and concepts of the individual traditional practices must be taken into account.[38]

The WHO document recommends a grading system for the requirements for proof of efficacy, and that the documentation required to support the therapeutic claims should depend on the nature and level of the indications. The evidence should correspond to the nature of the illness to be treated.[38]

The review also appears to be in direct conflict with the Therapeutic Goods Administration (TGA) position of regulating all medicines and medical devices. The TGA appears to have adopted the WHO recommendations by grading the level of evidence required according to the nature of the illness or condition being treated.

The TGA acknowledges that there are two types of evidence which may be used to support claims. These are:

- Evidence based on traditional use of a substance or product; and
- scientific evidence.[39]

The TGA states that traditional therapies are considered to include TCM, traditional Ayurvedic medicine, traditional Western herbal medicine, traditional homoeopathic medicine, aromatherapy and other indigenous medicines.[39]

The Australian Natural Therapists Association (ANTA) submission to the Chief Medical Officer stated that there is strong scientific evidence supporting many natural therapies. It also highlighted that the educational standards in Australia for all complementary medicines are among the highest in the world. All educational standards are set by the Australian Qualification Framework, and approved packages of training for health practitioners require qualifications from universities, tertiary colleges and registered private providers for bachelor degrees, advanced diplomas or diplomas.[40]

The practice of aromatherapy in Australia has been defined by the Government National Health Training Package HLT51407, introduced in 2002.

The ANTA submission also reported that the level of complaints received by the Australian Health Practitioner Regulation Agency, the Health Care Complaints Commission (NSW) and the ANTA Complaints Register show that the level of consumer satisfaction is high and the risk factor is very low.[40]

It was also mentioned that natural therapies have a positive impact on cost effectiveness, both in the short and long term. This is because they provide relief to a currently already overburdened health care system through:

- reducing the number of visits to GPs for minor ailments
- reducing the consumption of drugs and their undesirable side effects
- reducing the number of claims made on the health system
- contributing to the prevention and treatment of conditions that may otherwise lead to the need for hospital care.[40]

The future of aromatherapy

It has been said that there is no consensus on the ultimate direction of aromatherapy. There are those who suggest that if the aromatherapy profession wants to be respected and acknowledged by conventional Western medicine, then whether we like it or not, we have to show substantial and replicable clinical evidence of our claims.[29]

While scientific research may help us to identify and validate the active constituents, aromatherapy is inherently a vitalistic modality, and the current scientific approach may not be the most appropriate platform for aromatherapy to develop in the future.[29]

Schnaubelt states that what is needed for the future is a framework that provides a platform that will allow aromatherapy to develop as a viable, holistic and confident therapy. This can be achieved by clarification of the relationship aromatherapy has with science. The scientific exploration of essential oil constituents contributes to the knowledge about the pharmacology of essential oils and their quasi-medicinal application, but it does not explain the living nature of essential oils from plants.[29]

We also need to understand the role of olfaction and fragrance and its inherent problems. How does one account for the hedonistic qualities of odour?

Schnaubelt asks – How can liking or disliking a fragrance be eliminated? It is not surprising that scientific methods run into problems when dealing with the interconnected phenomena such as fragrance, feelings and culture. He states that science will be unable to make meaningful statements in this field as long as it is dependent on measuring the changes of only one variable.[29]

It is also important to recognise that the interaction of aromatherapy with humans cannot be reduced to a single variable experiment. Essential oils are made up of hundreds of different chemical constituents, which initiate different processes all happening simultaneously. Essential oils can elicit complex responses from the psychosomatic networks of any one person.[29]

Finally, there is also a need for new sciences that understand and allow the existence of psychosomatic networks of the mind and body. Schnaubelt says that these new sciences will give us an insight into the interaction of highly effective sesquiterpene compounds found in essential oils and receptor systems.[29]

A holistic approach acknowledges that aromatherapy connects to the phenomena of life much more closely and intimately than conventional medicine. Schnaubelt beautifully describes the role of essential oils:

> *Essential oils reawaken odour awareness and the connection to individuality, and greater independence improves the ability to take responsibility for one's own health. Self-confidence and wellbeing are influenced, providing an improved flow of biological information through the psychosomatic network of body and mind.*[29]

I believe that the future for aromatherapy is a very promising one, in which essential oils are integrated into all aspects of life.

References

1. Classen C, Howes D, Synnott A. *Aroma – the cultural history of smell.* Routledge, London, 1994.

2. Reinarz J. *Past scents – historical perspectives on smell.* University of Illinois Press, Urbano, 2014.
3. Graham JA. *Chapter 25: The psychology of fragrance and aromatherapy.* From *Poucher's perfumes, cosmetics and soaps.* Edited by Hilda Butler, 10th ed, Kluwer Academic Publishers, 2000.
4. Ashbrook Harvey S. *Scenting salvation – ancient Christianity and the olfactory imagination.* University of California Press, Berkeley, 2006.
5. Thurlkill M. *Sacred scents in early Christianity and Islam.* Lexington Books, Lanham, 2016.
6. Abram D. *Seven scents – healing and the aromatic imagination.* Singing Dragon, London, 2017.
7. Morris E. *Fragrance: the story of perfume from Cleopatra to Chanel.* Product of Nature and of Art, New York, 1984.
8. Manniche L. *An ancient Egyptian herbal.* British Museum Press, London, 1993.
9. Tisserand R. *Essential oils as psychotherapeutic agents.* In *Proceedings of perfumery: The psychology and biology of fragrance.* Chapman & Hall, UK, 1987.
10. Rosengarten F. *The book of spices.* Jove Publishing, New York, 1969.
11. Ravindran PN, Nirmal Babu K. *Chapter 1 – introduction.* From *Cinnamon and cassia – the genus Cinnamomum.* Edited by Ravindran PN, Nirmal Babu K. CRC Press, Boca Raton, 2004.
12. Butler H. *Cosmetics through the ages.* From *Poucher's perfumes, cosmetics and soaps.* Edited by Hilda Butler, 10th ed, Kluwer Academic Publishers, 2000.
13. Tisserand R. *Aromatherapy for everyone.* Penguin Books, UK, 1988.
14. Griggs B. *Green pharmacy.* 2nd edn. Healing Arts Press, Rochester, 1997.
15. Yaniv Z. *Introduction: medicinal plants of ancient traditions.* From *Medicinal and aromatic plants of the Middle-East.* Eds Yaniv Z, Dudai N, Springer Science+Business Media, Dordrecht, 2014.
16. Bone K, Mills S. *Principles and practices of phytotherapy.* 2nd edn, Churchill Livingstone, Edinburgh, 2013.
17. Rosengarten F. *The book of spices.* Jove Publishing, New York, 1969.
18. https://www.kingjamesbibleonline.org
19. Duke J. *Duke's handbook of medicinal plants of the Bible.* CRC Press, Boca Raton, 2008.
20. McHugh J. *Sandalwood and carrion – smell in Indian religion and culture.* Oxford University Press, New York, 2012.
21. Gattefossé R. *Gattefossé's aromatherapy.* C.W. Daniel, Saffron Walden, 1993.
22. Gildemeister E. *The volatile oils – first volume.* 2nd edn, John Wiley and Sons, 1913.
23. Potterton D. *Culpeper's colour herbal.* W Foulsham & Company, UK, 1983.
24. Holmes P. *Aromatica – a clinical guide to essential oils therapeutics.* Singing Dragon, London, 2016.
25. Valnet J. *The practice of aromatherapy.* C.W. Daniel Company, Great Britain, England, 1980.
26. Maury M. *Marguerite Maury's guide to aromatherapy: The Secret of Life and Youth.* C.W. Daniel Company, Saffron Walden, 1964.
27. Arcier M. *Aromatherapy.* The Hamlyn Publishing Group Ltd, London, 1990.
28. Schnaubelt K. *Essential oils – Viable wholistic pharmaceutical for the future.* In Proceedings of the 13th International Congress of Flavours, Fragrances and Essential Oils. Istanbul, 1995; 269-279.
29. Schnaubelt K. *Medial aromatherapy.* Frog, Berkeley, 1999.
30. Rico H. *Direct selling dominates the aromatherapy and essential oil market.* Retrieved on Nov 4, 2017 from https://globanewswire.com/news-release/2016/02/03/807472/0/en/Direct-Selling-Dominates-the-Aromatherapy-and-Essential-Oils-Market.html
31. Klispie J. *A path to aromatherapy credentialing: General evaluation of the Aromatherapy Registration Council (ARC).* Retrieved on Nov 4, 2017 from https://ijpha.wordpress.com/2017/08/14/a-path-to-aromatherapy-credentialing-general-evaluation-of-the-aromatherapy-registration-council-arc/
32. Watt M. *Frankincense essential oil and claims for its cancer curing activity made by distributors of Young Living and DoTerra.* Retrieved on Nov 4, 2017 from http://www.aromamedical.org/pdf/frankincense_oil_for_cancer.pdf
33. Tisserand R. *Frankincense oil and cancer in perspective.* Retrieved on Nov 4, 2017 from http:tisserandinstitute.org/frankincense-oil-and-cancer-in-perspective/
34. Sheen J. *The professionalisation of aromatherapy: A case study of the professionalisation of complementary and alternative medicine in the Australian health care system.* PhD thesis, Southern Cross University, Lismore, 2006.
35. Staindl P, Grace S, Khoury R. *Australian Traditional Medicine Society Ltd submission to Chief Medical Officer: Natural therapies – review of private health insurance rebate.* ATMS, Meadowbank, 2013.
36. Baggoley C. *Review of the Australian Government rebate on natural therapies for private health insurance.* Australian Government Department of Health, Canberra, 2015.
37. Elton-Pym J. *Yoga out, mental health in: sweeping reforms to private health insurance revealed.* Retrieved on Nov 4, 2017 from http://www.sbs.au/news/article/2017/10/13/yoga-out-mental-health-under-sweeping-reforms-private-health-insurance

38. *General guidelines for methodologies on research and evaluation of traditional medicine.* World Health Organization, Geneva, 2000.
39. *Guidelines for levels and kinds of evidence to support indications and claims for non-registerable medicines, including complementary medicines, and other listable medicines.* Australian Government, Therapeutic Goods Administration, Version 1.1, April 2011.
40. *Australian Natural Therapists Association – Submission to the private health insurance rebate review, Chief Medical Officer, Department of Health and Aging*. GRS Communications, 2013.

Botany

CHAPTER

3

Contents

Introduction

Knowledge of the basic principles of botany will help us to understand:

- the importance of taxonomy of plants to help us to identify essential oils according to the botanical name of their plant source
- how the plants make essential oils
- the biological role of essential oils within the plant
- the biological factors that influence the chemical composition of essential oils.

Defining an Essential Oil

Before we begin our discussion on botany, it is beneficial for us to examine the descriptions commonly assigned to essential oils. An essential oil is described as a volatile material derived by a physical process from an odorous plant material of a single botanical form and species.[1]

The ISO (International Organization for Standardization) defines an essential oil in terms of its extraction process:

> *An essential oil is a product obtained from natural raw material, either by distillation with water or steam, or from the epicarp of citrus fruits by mechanical processing, or by dry distillation. The essential oil is subsequently separated from the aqueous phase by physical means.*[2]

While this description describes how essential oils are extracted, it does not provide us with an explanation of their origins or purpose. Drs Franchomme and Pénëol describe an essential oil in terms of the photosynthesis process:

> *Plant essences, in the physiological meaning of the term are most certainly true life essences, elaborated by the secretory cells of the plants that have tapped the photo-electro-magnetic energy of the sun and have converted it, with the intervention of enzymes, into biochemical energy under the form of highly diversified aromatic molecules.*[3]

Franz & Novak describe essential oils in terms of the biosynthesis pathways within the plant:

> *Essential oils are complex mixtures of volatile compounds produced by living organisms and isolated by physical means only (pressing and distillation) from a whole plant or plant part of known taxonomic origin. The respective main compounds are mainly derived from three biosynthetic pathways only, the mevalonate pathway leading to sesquiterpenes, the methyl-erithrytol pathway leading to mono- and diterpenes, and the shikimic acid pathway en route to phenylpropenes.*[4]

Price & Price describe essential oils in terms of their biological, commercial and therapeutic significance:

> *… of these secondary metabolites the essential oils have the greatest commercial significance … whatever else they may do, they give the plant its*

aroma and flavour and often have a significant physiological effect on people.[5]

Jean Rose's description of an essential oil gives us an insight into the physiological role of an essential oil in a plant:

> *... what is this elusive essence of plant material called essential oil? It is the heart and soul of the plant. It is the essence that deters bugs from eating the plant. It is the fragrant aromatic heart of the plant that attracts bees and pollinating insects. It is the chemical component contained in the tiny plant cells that are liberated during the extraction process.*[6]

Lavabre adopts a more esoteric approach in describing essential oils:

> *Essential oils are the fragrant principle of the plant. They are the chemical components that give a plant its characteristic fragrance. In the spiritual approach to aromatherapy, essential oils are considered the life force, the energy of the plant. Alchemists regard them as the quintessence, the soul, the spirit of the plant.*[7]

Sadgrove & Jones explain that, while essential oils may be considered significantly important for the survival of the plant, the term 'essential oil' did not originate from this function. It is a common misconception that essential oils are called 'essential' to highlight their importance in the biological survival of the plant. The term 'essential' has its origin from the term *quinta essentia* (quintessence). This term was coined by Swiss medical pioneer, Bombastus Paracelsus von Hohenheim (1493-1541). His theory was that the essential oil was the most pure and concentrated form of the medicinal principal of any plant.[8]

The term 'quintessence' referred to the fifth element of the Aristolean paradigm which described matter as being composed of five elements – earth, fire, water, air and spirit. Quintessence was regarded as the spirit or life force of the plant, which could be removed and contained by the distillation process.[8]

Other names that have been assigned to 'essential oil' include essence, fragrant oil, volatile oil, aetheroleum or aromatic oil.[8]

Plant Taxonomy

Essential oils should be traded under the botanical name assigned to their plant sources. While Hoffmann is referring to herbs the following comment is also valid for essential oils:

> *There is at least one vitally important reason for phytotherapists to be concerned with understanding how plants are named. When using plants in medicine, it is essential to know exactly which herb is being prescribed. Botanical names are exact and internationally recognized, and each Latin binomial refers to one plant and one plant only. Common names, on the other hand, vary from place to place, and much confusion can result when several plants are called by the same common name.*[9]

The coining of botanical names occurs in the field of taxonomy, a branch of science dedicated to the arrangement of living organisms into categories based on natural similarities such as structure, development, biochemical or physiological function, and evolutionary history.[9]

The botanical naming of all plant species takes place according to the International Rules of Botanical Nomenclature Convention. This provides botanists with the guiding principles to ensure a precise system of nomenclature, which is used by botanists around the world. The scientific names of all groups are usually taken from Latin or Greek.[10]

Carolus Linnaeus, a Swedish botanist, introduced the modern system of classification in 1753. The basic unit in the Linnaean system is the species – a group of organisms that resemble each other more closely than those of any other group and are capable of mating with one another to produce fertile offspring.[1]

Species are arranged into higher groupings that are progressively more inclusive. Species that are closely related are grouped together into a genus. Genera with similar characteristics and origins are grouped into families. Families in turn are grouped into orders and orders into classes. Classes are then grouped into divisions (if plants) or phyla (if animals). Finally, related phyla or divisions are placed together into kingdoms.[9]

These are the main units used in plant nomenclature, using lavender as an example:[11]

Kingdom – Plantae (plant kingdom)

Subkingdom – Tracheobionta (vascular plants)

Superdivision – Spermatophyta (seed plants)

Division – Magnoliophyta (flowering plants)

Class – Magnoliopsida (dicotyledons)

Subclass – Asteridae

Order – Lamiales

Family – Lamiaceae (a large group of aromatic annuals or perennial herbs)

Genus – *Lavandula*

Species – *Lavandula angustifolia* Mill. (English lavender); *Lavandula* x *intermedia* Emeric ex Loisel. (lavandin); *Lavandula latifolia* Medikus (spike lavender); *Lavandula stoechas* L. (French lavender).

The botanical name is expressed as a Latin binomial, or two-part name. The first part of the name identifies the genus, which is a group of species more closely related to one another than any other group. The second part of the name identifies the species. The botanical name is normally written in italics, with only the genus name having a capital letter.[9]

An example of a genus name is *Thymus*, which is used for every species of *Thymus*. The common English word 'thyme' is traditionally used to name both the genus and its most commercially used species. Some of the species commercially used in the production of thyme oil include:

- *Thymus vulgaris* – common thyme
- *Thymus zygis* – Spanish thyme
- *Thymus serpyllum* – creeping thyme
- *Thymus citriodorus* – lemon thyme.

There are 215 reported species for the *Thymus* genus.[12]

Several explanations exist regarding the origin of the name *Thymus*. Some authors state that the Latin name *Thymus* comes from the Greek word *thyo* (perfume), while another interpretation of its etymology considers the Greek word *thymos* (courage, strength).[12]

The abbreviations sp. and spp. are used to indicate one specie or several species of a particular genus, respectively. For example, *Thymus* spp. suggests that we are talking about a number of species in the *Thymus* genus.

Species are sometimes divided into subspecies, which refers to minor variation of a species. This may include difference in colour or structure of a plant part.[13] For example, *Lavandula angustifolia* ssp. *angustifolia* differentiates this subspecies of lavender from *Lavandula angustifolia* ssp. *pyrenaica*.[1]

Some plants are hybrids of two other plants of the same genus. This is indicated by an 'x' between the genus name and the species name, as in *Mentha* x *piperita* L.

Another addition to the botanical name that is often used to identify essential oils is the chemotype (ct.). Some plants from anatomically identical species may produce essential oils of different odour and chemical composition. The chemotype name is usually in reference to the predominant chemical constituent in the oil. For example, *Rosmarinus officinalis* ct. 1,8-cineole means that 1,8-cineole is the predominant compound in this rosemary oil.

Bowles states that, in an ideal world, all essential oils used for aromatherapy should be from one species or one chemotype of a species and from one geographic location; however, often only those suppliers who are sourcing their oils directly from the grower can provide this stringent quality assurance.[13]

Many species have a capital 'L.' following their names. This indicates that it was Linnaeus who first classified them. As new species are discovered, or old ones reclassified, the name of the botanist who most recently created a name gets added in abbreviated form.[13]

For example, the name *Eucalyptus smithii* F. Muell. ex R.T. Baker indicates that the name was ascribed to Baron Sir Ferdinand Jacob Heinrich von Mueller but was published by Richard Thomas Baker.

Knowledge of Latin helps us to understand how botanical names have been selected. William Stearn, author of *Botanical Latin*, provides us with the most detailed study on the origin of Latin names used in taxonomy.[14]

Latin names can be grouped into categories based upon their derivation. A few examples include:[9]

- names of mythical origins such as *Achillea* (genus name for yarrow), from the Greek Achilles, hero of Homer's Iliad, whose bleeding ankle was treated with yarrow
- names of a geographical origin such as *montana* (species name for winter savory) which means growing in mountainous places
- place names such as *sinensis* (species name for sweet orange) which means from China
- uses or properties such as *officinalis* (species name for many plants) which means once used in the official pharmacopoeia
- historical names such as Narcissus (genus name for Narcissus) which originates from the character of the same name in Greek mythology, who was renowned for his beauty
- anatomical names that highlight visible plant features such as *perforatum* (species name for St John's wort) which is characterised by small perforations along the leaf edges
- colour names such as *niger* (species name of black pepper) meaning black
- Aroma names such as *odorata* (species name of ylang ylang) meaning sweet-smelling.

Plant families

Plant families involving species that are commonly used for the production of essential oils include:

Plant family	Part of plant	Common name	Botanical name
Annonaceae	Flower	Ylang ylang	*Cananga odorata*
Apiaceae (also known as Umbelliferae)	Fruit or root	Angelica	*Angelica archangelica*
	Seed	Aniseed	*Pimpinella anisum*
	Seed	Sweet fennel	*Foeniculum vulgare* var. *dulce*
	Seed	Coriander	*Coriandrum sativum*
Asteraceae (also known as Compositae)	Flower	German chamomile	*Matricaria recutita*
	Flower	Everlasting	*Helichrysum angustifolium*
Burseraceae	Resin	Frankincense	*Boswellia carterii*
	Resin	Elemi	*Canarium luzonicum*
	Resin	Myrrh	*Commiphora myrrha*
Cupressaceae	Leaf	Cypress	*Cupressus sempervirens*
	Fruit	Juniper	*Juniperus communis*
Geraniaceae	Leaf	Geranium	*Pelargonium* spp.
Lamiaceae (also known as Labiatae)	Leaf	Basil	*Ocimum basilicum*
	Leaf & flower	Clary sage	*Salvia sclarea*
	Leaf & flower	Lavender	*Lavandula angustifolia*
	Leaf	Peppermint	*Mentha x piperita*
	Leaf	Rosemary	*Rosmarinus officinalis*
Lauraceae	Leaf	Bay laurel	*Laurus nobilis*
	Wood, bark or leaf	Camphor	*Cinnamomum camphora*
	Bark or leaf	Cinnamon	*Cinnamomum verum*
	Wood	Rosewood	*Aniba rosaeodora*
Myristicaceae	Seed	Nutmeg	*Myristica fragrans*
Myrtaceae	Leaf	Cajeput	*Melaleuca cajuputi*
	Leaf	Eucalyptus, Blue Mallee	*Eucalyptus polybractea*
	Leaf	Fragonia	*Agonis fragrans*
	Leaf	Tea tree	*Melaleuca alternifolia*
Oleaceae	Flower	Jasmine	*Jasminum grandiflorum*
Piperaceae	Seed	Black pepper	*Piper nigrum*
Poaceae (also known as Gramineae)	Leaf	Citronella	*Cymbopogon winterianus*
	Leaf	Lemongrass	*Cymbopogon flexuosus*
	Leaf	Palmarosa	*Cymbopogon martinii*
	Root	Vetiver	*Vetiveria zizanioides*
Rosaceae	Flower	Rose	*Rosa centifolia*
Rutaceae	Fruit	Bergamot	*Citrus bergamia*
	Fruit	Grapefruit	*Citrus paradisi*
	Fruit	Lemon	*Citrus* x *limon*
	Fruit	Lime	*Citrus* x *aurantifolia*
	Fruit	Orange	*Citrus sinensis*
	Flower	Neroli	*Citrus* x *aurantium*
	Leaf	Petitgrain	*Citrus* x *aurantium*
Santalaceae	Wood	Sandalwood	*Santalum album*
Styraceae	Resin	Benzoin	*Styrax benzoin*
Zingiberaceae	Rhizome	Ginger	*Zingiber officinale*
	Seed	Cardamom	*Elettaria cardamomum*

Lavabre states that the classification of essential oils by botanical families can tell us so much about their therapeutic activity. He explains that this approach is based on more classical systems of traditional herbal medicine in that there are some obvious similarities between the recommended uses of essential oils from plants in the same family.[7]

Plant Anatomy

In plant anatomy, we examine the anatomical features of plants such as the leaves, flowers, fruits, shape and size of the plants. Different anatomical features of plants form the basis for plant classification. The family of the plant is often determined by its different anatomical features such as shape, orientation and structure. Variations in leaf shapes and different flower colours often help to determine the genus of a plant.

Lavabre explains that we can learn from the part of the plant where its creativity is most developed – where its essential oil is produced. He refers to this as the plant's domain of creativity.[7]

Roots and rhizomes

The roots are the underground part of the plant, providing the plant with stability and anchorage. The roots also play a very important role in keeping the soil together and preventing erosion. The rhizomes are the underground stems that grow horizontally. Rhizomes are also referred to as creeping root stalks. The role of rhizomes is food storage and vegetative propagation.

The roots are the first part of the plant that appears when the seed germinates. The roots push down into the soil, in search of nutrients and water. The roots become the foundation of the plant.

Lavabre explains that essential oils from roots tend to have a very grounding energy and food-like qualities. They usually have a strong tonic effect on our vital functions.[7]

Stems

Plants do not always have stems; however, they often do have a structure that supports the flowers and the leaves. The stems, trunk or main branches form the main structural element of a plant. The branching structure can be extensive and intricate or just made up of a number of upright stems. When identifying a plant, botanists consider whether the stem is woody or herbaceous. Stems that are woody are usually self-supporting.

Lavabre explains that essential oils from wood tend to be centring and balancing. He explains that the creative process is drawn to the heart of the wood. He states that these oils have the power to expand our consciousness to higher spheres without making us lose control. This is why they have been used in spiritual practices around the world for millennia.[7]

Leaves

Leaves come in so many different shapes, textures, colours and smells. Typically leaves are flat and thin. The shape and structure of leaves is determined by the climate, available light, available nutrients and ecological competition from other plants. Botanists have developed an extensive range of terms to describe the characteristics of a leaf such as the shape and texture of the leaf.

Leaves have a determinate growth. This means that they grow to a specific pattern and shape and then stop. Other parts of the plant have a non-determinant growth and usually continue to grow as long as the resources are available. Plants, through their leaves, breathe in carbon dioxide, and during photosynthesis, they break down the carbon dioxide molecule into carbon and oxygen.

Leaves are responsible for photosynthesis. Leaves are the primary organs responsible for transpiration. The leaves can also store nutrients and water. Leaves are generally very rich in proteins, minerals and sugars. This assists in the photosynthesis process. Hence leaves are a very important source of nutrients for many animals, including humans.

The upper surface of the leaf processes energy from the sun while the underside is involved in gas exchange through tiny openings called stomata. As Buhner explains, plants breathe just like us. Stomata are like lungs:

> *When an individual stoma is full, the opening closes and carbon dioxide and any other usable molecules are separated from the air. What remains, along with the oxygen generated from the breakdown of carbon dioxide, is released back to the atmosphere as the stoma opens again and breathes out. This cycle is powered by sunlight; at nights the plants rest, photosynthesis stops, the stoma are closed.*[15]

According to Lavabre, essential oils from leaves tend to correspond to the vital body and have a strong affinity with our *Qi* or *Prana* energy. They have a strong affinity with the respiratory system and tonify the vital body.[7]

Flowers

Flowers are the plant's reproductive structures. Plants bearing flowers are classified as angiosperms. Flowers are usually both male and female. The biological function of flowers is reproduction.

Flowers have a male part called stamens that

produce a sticky powder called pollen. Flowers also have a female part called the pistil. The top of the pistil is called the stigma. It is usually sticky. The seeds are created at the base of the pistil, in the ovule. To be pollinated, pollen must be moved from the stamen to the stigma. When pollen from the plant's stamen is transferred to the same plant's stigma, it is called self-pollination. When pollen from the plant's stamen is transferred to a different plant's stamen, it is called cross-pollination. Cross-pollination produces stronger plants.

Plants that rely on pollination by animals are often brightly coloured and have a stronger scent to attract animal pollinators. Plants that are pollinated by the wind often have a long stamen and pistil. Since they do not need to attract animal pollinators, they often lack colour and are not scented, and often have small or no petals since no insect needs to land on them.

Lavabre states that essential oils from flowers tend to be the most spiritually evolved fragrances. He explains that this indicates a sign of strong astral activity. They tend to be very refined and are often very difficult to extract.[7]

Fruits and seeds

Fruits can be fleshy or dry. Dry fruits can be dehiscent, meaning they split open to release their seeds (such as a bean pod), or indehiscent (remaining closed, such as a hazelnut). Fleshy fruits can be simple, such as a tomato or rosehip, or multiple such as a mulberry. A berry is a fleshy fruit that contains many seeds, an apple is referred to as a pome, an orange is a hesperidium and a peach is a drupe. While we would consider a drupe as a type of fleshy fruit, it is actually an indehiscent dry fruit surrounded by an outer fleshy layer. Other examples of drupes are plums, olives and cherries.[16]

Fruits are the means by which seeds are disseminated. Fleshy fruits tend to be eaten by animals, allowing the seeds to spread by the animal droppings. Dry seeds are either eaten, carried by the wind or water, or they attach themselves to passing animals.[16]

Like leaves and flowers, many terms exist to describe seeds by their shape. Seeds can be rounded, square, oblong, ovate, lenticular (lentil-shaped) or reniform (kidney-shaped). Seeds can also be distinctively coloured, patterned or textured.[16]

Lavabre states that essential oils from seeds tend to be less sophisticated, more humble and straightforward. The oils from fruits and seeds are invigorating and fortifying and have a strong affinity with the digestive system.[7]

Plant Physiology

Plant physiology is the science that studies plant functions, such as the dynamic processes of growth, metabolism and reproduction in living plants. An understanding of the basic principles of plant physiology helps us understand the biosynthesis of essential oils and the biological functions of essential oils. Plant physiology can also help explain some of the important processes of plant biochemistry and metabolism such as photosynthesis.

Photosynthesis

The photosynthesis process involves chloroplasts of plants capturing light from the sun and converting it to chemical energy, which is then stored in the bonds of sugar and other organic molecules made from water and carbon dioxide.

Cells cannot create their own energy, but as open systems, they are able to absorb energy from their surroundings. Photosynthetic cells acquire their energy in the form of light, which they use to make the organic compounds that provide energy to other cells. Hence photosynthesis nourishes almost all the living world directly or indirectly.

The energy collecting cells of plants are called chloroplasts, but the leaves are the major sites of photosynthesis in most plants. The colour of the leaf is due to a green substance known as chlorophyll.

Photosynthesis can be summarised with this chemical equation:[17]

$$6\ CO_2 + 12\ H_2O + \text{light energy} = C_6H_{12}O_6 + 6\ O_2 + 6\ H_2O$$

The carbohydrate $C_6H_{12}O_6$ is glucose, a major product of photosynthesis. The free energy from the sun has, therefore, been stored in the form of a complex molecule, glucose.

Secondary metabolites

All the chemical reactions that take place in the plant are called metabolism. Most of the carbon, nitrogen and energy ends up in molecules that are common to all cells and are required for the proper functioning of cells and organisms. These molecules such as lipids, proteins, nucleic acids and carbohydrates are called primary metabolites. Unlike animals, most plants divert a significant proportion of assimilated carbon and energy to the synthesis of organic molecules that may have no obvious role in cell function. These molecules are known as secondary metabolites.[18]

At a biosynthetic level, primary and secondary metabolites share many of the same intermediates and are derived from the same core metabolic pathways. Secondary metabolites often occur in relatively low quantities, and their production may be widespread or restricted to particular plant families, genera or even species. They are often of significant economic and medicinal value to humans.[18]

Essential oils are referred to as secondary products. While they are not necessary for primary cellular function, they do have important biological tasks such as providing the plant with protection against predators, pollination, supporting wound healing, or protecting the plant against trauma and offering defense against excessive perspiration.[4]

Bowles states that the secondary plant chemicals found in essential oils include:[13]

- **Terpenoid molecules** – These are the most common essential oil molecules and are used by plants to repel predators and prevent bacterial and fungal infections. Terpenoid compounds found in flowers are also used as insect pollinators.
- **Phenolic and phenylpropanoid molecules** – A few phenolic compounds are found in essential oils. These are likely to be used by the plant to repel predators.
- **Non-terpenoid aliphatic molecules** – These are often found in citrus peels and are likely to be used to repel predators.
- **Heterocyclic molecules** – These are found only in a few oils and include molecules containing atoms other than carbon in closed rings. This includes nitrogen-containing molecules such as indole and methyl anthranilate.

Other secondary compounds found in plants include alkaloids, flavonoids and saponins. Bowles explains that many of these compounds have notable pharmacological effects on humans. One example is caffeine, the alkaloid found in tea and coffee. However, these compounds are not extracted into essential oils by steam distillation.[13]

Essential oil storage structures

Franz & Novak explain that all plants possess the ability to produce essential oils; however, quite often only trace amounts. They refer to 'essential oil plants' as those plant species that provide us with essential oils of commercial interest.[4]

A plant is referred to as an essential oil plant if it meets one of the following conditions:[4]

- Some flowers, such as rose, jasmine sambac or tuberose, produce and immediately emit the essential oils from the epidermal cells of their petals. The yield in an intensive smelling flower is usually very low, and specialised extraction techniques are required to recover the essential oil.
- In other plants, the secretion and accumulation of volatiles are stored in specialised anatomical structures. This often leads to a higher concentration of the essential oil in the plant. These structures are secretory idioblasts (secretory cells), cavities/ducts or glandular trichomes.

Ragusa explains that it is possible to distinguish two types of secretory tissues:[19]

- those that excrete substances secreted out of the plant or even, in the interior of it, in the intercellular spaces after they had thus been secreted extracellularly
- those that eliminate substances secreted in the vacuoles and then store them in the interior of the cells (intracellular secretion).

The type of structure is generally plant family or species specific. Some examples are described below.

Secretory cavities and ducts

Cavities or ducts consist of extracellular space that originates from schizogeny (created by the dissolution of the middle lamella between the duct initials and formation of an intercellular space) or by lysogeny (programmed death and disintegration of cells). In both cases, peripheral cells become epithelial cells that are highly active in the synthesis and secretion of their product into the extracellular cavities. Schizogenic oil ducts can be found in plants from the Apiaceae family or the Pinaceae family. Lysogenic cavities can be found in plants belonging to the Rutaceae and Myrtaceae plant families.[4]

Glandular trichomes

These are modified epidermal hairs and can be found covering leaves, stems and parts of flowers in many plants from the Lamiaceae family or the *Pelargonium* species.[20] Glandular trichomes are either peltate or capitate trichomes. Peltate glands are made up of a basal epidermal cell, a neck-stalk cell and a secreting head of four to 16 cells, with a large subcuticular space on the apex in which

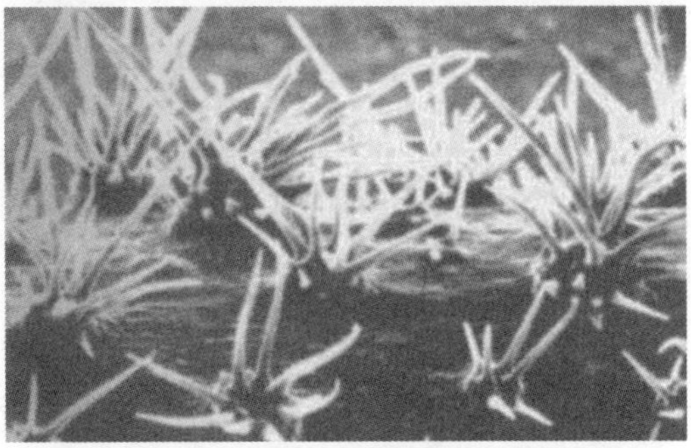

A scanning electron micrograph of the leaf surface of a eucalyptus leaf showing the stellate hairs associated with the oil glands. (Picture courtesy of the Australian Centre for International Agricultural Research)

the secretion product is accumulated. Capitate trichomes possess only 1-4 secreting cells with a small subcuticular space.[4]

Epidermal cells

Essential oils obtained from flowers such as rose and jasmine are not usually secreted by glandular hairs, but diffuse through the cytoplasm and cell walls of the plant to the outside. The yield of essential oil obtained from these plants is usually very low.[20]

Oil cells

These are cells that occur within the plant tissue and differ from the cells adjacent to them, both in their content and size. They can be found in plants from Lauraceae, Magnoliaceae, Piperaceae, Valerianaceae and Gramineae plant families.[21]

Biosynthesis of Essential Oils

Basic biosynthesis pathways

Sell explains that all chemicals produced in nature can be classified as primary metabolites or secondary metabolites. The primary metabolites are those that are considered the basic building blocks of life – proteins, carbohydrates, nucleic acids and lipids. These primary metabolites do not directly contribute to the formation of essential oils; however, some essential oil components are a degradation of lipids.[22]

On the other hand, secondary metabolites are components that are present in some species but not others. They are usually classified as terpenoids, shikimates, polyketides and alkaloids. The most important secondary metabolites for the formation of essential oils are the terpenoids and shikimates. A small number of polyketides and very few alkaloids are also involved.[22]

Photosynthesis allows green plants to convert carbon dioxide and water into glucose. Cleavage of glucose produces phosphoenolpyruvate, which is the key building block for both the shikimic acid and acetyl coenzyme-A.[22]

This is critical for the synthesis of secondary metabolites and some primary metabolites such as lipids. Those metabolites along the acetyl coenzyme-A path include lipids, polyketides and terpenes, whilst those along the shikimic acid path include coumarins, flavonoids and lignin. Lignin is a complex monomer of aromatic alcohols called monolignols, an integral part of the secondary cell wall of plants. The lipids also include free fatty acids that appear in fixed oil and sometimes essential oils.[8]

Where the path splits at acetyl coenzyme-A, on one side mevalonic acid is produced, made from three molecules of acetyl coenzyme-A. This is a precursor to the isoprenes which are the building blocks of terpenes. On the other side we have the carboxylation of acetyl coenzyme-A to give us malonyl coenzyme-A. This combines with acetic acid then decarboxylates to give us a β-ketoester. If this process is repeated, a molecule will form with a carbonyl group on every alternating alcohol, which is then eliminated with the corresponding carbon hydrogenated, providing us with the beginning of a fatty acid.[8]

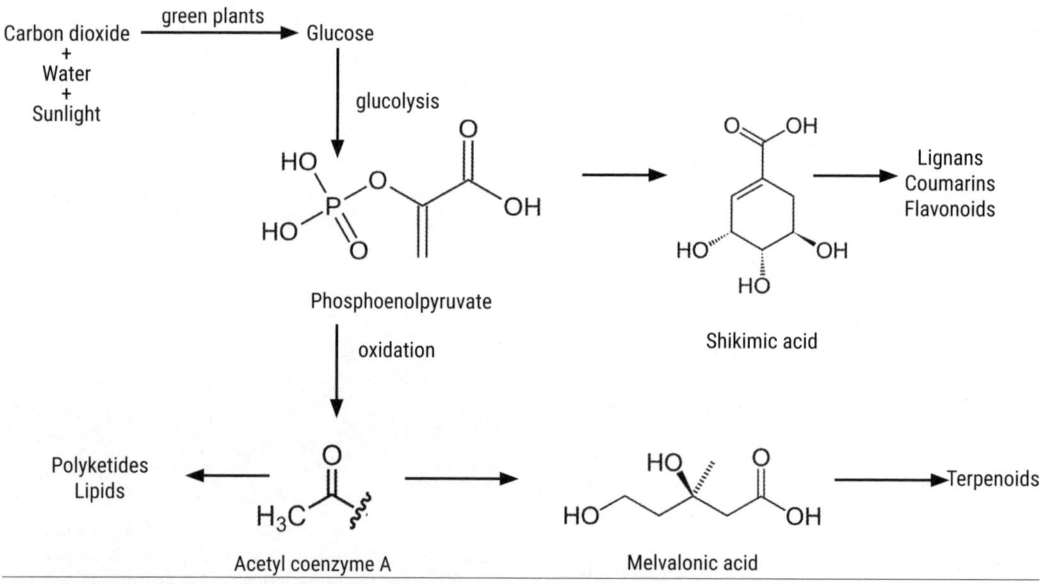

General pattern of biosynthesis of secondary metabolites

The biosynthesis of shikimates is from the shikimic acid pathway. The biosynthesis of shikimic acid itself starts with phosphoenolpyruvate and erythrose-4 phosphate, which is a precursor to carbohydrates. This means that the biosynthesis of shikimates diverges from the carbohydrate pathway.[8]

Terpenoid essential oils are biosynthesised from the mevalonate pathway. Isoprene units combine to create terpenes, involving repeated carbon chains in multiples of five.[8]

Terpenoids are by far the most important group of molecules for the formation of essential oils. They are defined as substances composed of isoprene (2-methylbutadiene) units. Isoprene is not found in essential oils, but the isoprene skeleton is easily discernible in terpenoids. The terpenoids are classified according to the number of carbon atoms they contain (multiples of 5). The first group containing molecules with 10 carbon atoms are called monoterpenes, those containing molecules with 15 carbon atoms are called sesquiterpenes, those with 20 carbon atoms diterpenoids and so on.[23]

In general, only monoterpenoids and sesquiterpenoids are sufficiently volatile to be components of essential oils.

There are more than 30,000 known terpenoids, isolated from plants, microorganisms and animals, many of which occur in essential oils. These terpenes are classified into groups according to their size and structural composition. The monoterpenes are known to comprise 25 different classes of terpenoids, 147 classes exist for sesquiterpenes and 118 classes exist for diterpenes.[8]

The term terpene was coined by Kekule in 1880 because terpenes were first discovered in turpentine oil. Terpenes are the most common essential oil components, followed by the non-terpenoid group – the phenylpropanoids.[8]

The role of endophytes

Microbial endophytes can also play an important role in the biosynthesis of essential oils. Sadgrove & Jones state that, while we still do not fully understand how endophytes are involved, it is now clear that endophytes may be involved in the final chemical alteration before the essential oil becomes the end product. Such microbial reactions are referred to as biotransformations.[8]

It is known that bacterial endophytes influence the plant's physiology, nutrient uptake and growth vigour via the biosynthesis of phytohormones such as ethylene, indol-3-acetic acid, acetoin and 2,3-butanediol. Bacterial endophytes from *Lavandula angustifolia* Mill were isolated and demonstrated to secrete metabolites that were inhibitory to human pathogens.[8]

Due to the similarity of inhibition demonstrated between the endophytes and the essential oil, it was suggested that the endophytes may be involved in the synthesis of the essential oil. In another study involving fungal endophytes of *Mentha piperita* L., it was demonstrated that the fungal organism was biosynthesising all the essential oil components in the rhizosphere of the plant, although the composition of the components was regulated by a plant interaction.[8]

Biological Role of Essential Oils

Essential oils are biologically regarded as metabolites of secondary importance to the plant because, in contrast to primary metabolites, they are not found in all plants nor do they constitute any of the basic building blocks of life.

It is known that the plant will not reabsorb the essential oils that have formed in a leaf before shedding it in winter. Sugar and starches, however, are returned to the main body of the plant prior to the shedding of the leaf. It was not surprising that many botanists concluded that essential oils were merely 'waste products' of the plant's metabolism.[24]

While secondary metabolites are generally regarded as metabolic by-products, they may provide an evolutionary advantage to the plant such as protection against graziers such as fungi, insects or herbivores. There is now evidence that essential oils play an important biological and ecological role within the plant such as:[8,25]

- attracting pollinators
- defense mechanism against insect and animals
- providing plants with antimicrobial protection
- allopathic interactions
- attracting herbivores for seed dispersal
- improving drought tolerance.

Attracting pollinators

There are three main attractants: odour (produced by the volatile essential oil), colour and morphology. Many of the compounds found in the odour glands of insects are also found in flower fragrances and plant volatiles.[25]

Odour is important for night flying insects and other animals where visual stimulus is practically absent. Bat-pollinated flowers, for example, may have a fruity or cabbage-like scent, while moth-pollinated flowers are generally very strongly and sweetly scented. Bird-pollinating flowers generally have no scent, as birds do not respond to scent.[25]

Insects are very sensitive to small concentrations of volatile chemicals. This means that flowers which do not have a strong odour to human senses may still produce enough odour to attract insects.[25]

The maximum scent production coincides with the time when the pollen is ripe and the flower is ready for pollination. Scent is also generally at its peak at the time of the day when the pollinator is around.

Defense mechanisms

The terpenoid compounds have a wide range of functions in plant interactions with insects and animals. Studies confirm the role of terpenes in the defence of the plant against herbivores and microbial pathogens. There is evidence that indicates that terpenes can be toxic or repulsive to mammals.[18]

The goats that scourge the forest around the Mediterranean normally spare many of the pungent herbs such as wild thyme and wild marjoram. Citronella and camphor oils repel certain insects and sandalwood is impervious to termites. Sage, wormwood, tansy and thuja all contain thujone, which is so powerful against parasites that it has been used as a vermifuge in traditional medicine.

Antimicrobial compounds

Some terpenoid compounds produced by plants have been identified as having antimicrobial activity. These compounds protect the plant from fungal attacks and other microbes.[25]

Allelopathy

Monoterpenes, the most abundant class of terpenoid compounds found in essential oils, are known to be cytotoxic to plant tissues, impairing respiration and photosynthesis and decreasing cell membrane permeability. These compounds prevent the growth of competing vegetation near established plants by inhibiting germination.[25]

Improving drought intolerance

The essential oils found on the surface of a leaf have been found to reduce the rate of water loss through transpiration.[25]

Sourcing Essential Oil Plants

The plants for producing essential oils are usually harvested either by 'wild harvesting' them in nature or from cultivated plants.

Wild harvesting and sustainability

The increasing demand for standardisation and a homogeneous raw material has led to many wild species being domesticated and systematically cultivated. However, many plant species used for essential oil production are still harvested from the wild because:[4]

- many plants and plant products are used for the subsistence of rural populations
- small quantities of the respective species are required for the essential oil industry, which is making the cost of cultivation prohibitive
- some species are difficult to cultivate because of slow growth rate or the requirement of a special microclimate
- market uncertainties or political circumstances do not allow investment in long-term cultivation
- the market desire for 'wildcrafted' material.

Franz & Novak state that less than two decades ago, almost all oregano worldwide came from wild harvested plants.[4]

It is imperative that the harvesting of wild plants for commercial purposes is regulated to ensure long-term sustainability – to prevent overharvesting or loss of habitat. International organisations such as IUCN (International Union for Conservation of Nature), WWF/TRAFFIC and World Health Organization (WHO) have launched together the Convention on Biological Diversity, the Global Strategy for Plant Conservation and the Guidelines for the Sustainable Use of Biodiversity. These guidelines provide the herbal and essential oil industry with specific guidelines to ensure sustainable sourcing practices.[4]

Unfortunately, a number of essential oil-bearing plants such as Atlas cedarwood, spikenard, sandalwood and rosewood are now listed as endangered or as vulnerable species due to overharvesting or poor sustainability practices.

Cultivation

Cultivation of essential oil-bearing plants offers a number of advantages over wild harvest for the production of essential oils:[4]

- avoidance of admixtures and adulterations by reliable botanical identification
- better control of harvesting volumes
- ability to select genotypes with desirable traits, especially quality
- controlled influence of the plant material and of postharvest handling.

However, it also requires the availability of arable land, a strategy for screening the most suitable chemotypes, developing the most appropriate propagation methods, being aware of potential pests and diseases, and developing the appropriate cultivation methods for the plant being cultivated.[4]

Williams explains that, in its natural habitat, the *Melaleuca alternifolia* tree grew in remote swampy locations that were significant obstacles to the collection of the leaf for the production of the essential oil.[26]

The development of a reliable source of supply was the only way to overcome these challenges. In the late 1970s, cultivation of the tree was undertaken by Thursday Plantation. This subsequent development of sophisticated oil extraction processes and reliable chemotypes of the plant were essential to developing a successful industry. Tea tree oil has progressively gained a remarkable level of support from good pharmacological and clinical research. This was the stimulus that was to eventually lead to its outstanding success in the local and international marketplace.[26]

One of the most exciting recent developments in cultivation of an essential oil crops has been *Santalum album* in Australia. Excessive harvesting of sandalwood tree from the wild without a strategy for replanting has substantially reduced the availability of sandalwood in India. This has resulted in global shortages and soaring market prices of *Santalum album.* As a result of the declining levels of *Santalum album* in the wild, the tree was given vulnerable status by the International Union for Conservation of Nature and Natural Resources (IUCN) in 1998.[27]

All early attempts to cultivate sandalwood proved to be complete failures. Before the first quarter of the twentieth century, European foresters could not work out how to grow sandalwood effectively. The main reason is that sandalwood is a hemiparasite. John Scott, curator of the Royal Botanical Garden in Calcutta, discovered this back in 1871; however, it was never taken seriously.[28]

Experimental growing of Indian sandalwood first occurred in Kununurra in 1983 by FPC and the former Department of Conservation and Land Management. The Australian Centre for International Agricultural Research (ACIAR) funded the sandalwood research with the then WA Department of Conservation and Land Management (CALM) from 1987 to 1995 in Indonesia and Australia. This helped develop reliable nursery techniques for mass production of high-quality seedlings, and for identifying and assessing the practicality and value of second-stage and third-stage host plants.[29]

The first harvest *of S. album* in Australia occurred in September 2013. The first harvest consisted of 144 hectares of sandalwood trees that were planted in 1999 and 2000.[30,31] As global supplies of *S. album* oil from India dwindle, Australia is set to become the world leader in the growth and sustainable supply of *S. album.*

Genetic variation and plant breeding

Plant breeding not only helps to improve essential oil content and composition, but it also helps the plant develop resistance to pests and diseases as well as abiotic stress. It can lower the nutritional requirements to save production costs, and improve homogeneity and suitability for technological processes at harvest and post-harvest, especially in preparation for distillation.[4]

Bhatt explains that, while the composition of the essential oil varies with the plant's genetic make-up, stage of growth and environmental factors, the presence or absence of a particular chemical constituent at any stage of growth is determined exclusively by the genes.[32]

Bhatt states that considerable progress has been made in recent years to understand the role of genes in controlling the biosynthetic pathways responsible for the production of essential oil in the plant. For example, new cultivars of lavender, peppermint and melissa have been developed to provide desirable oil composition and higher yields.[32]

Propagation from seed or clones

Plants can be grown from seed or propagated asexually by cloning.[33]

Lavender that has been raised from seed is kept for one year in pots before transplanting it into the field. It then takes another three years before the plantation yields enough flowers for commercial harvesting and distillation. The plants that have been grown from seed always exhibit wide genetic variations among the progeny. Improvement of the crop can be achieved by selective breeding of those genotypes that yield the most desirable oil, but is is often a very slow process requiring years to accomplish.[33]

Cloning is the preferred method for replication of plants having desirable commercial qualities. Clones are obtained from the buds or cuttings of the same plant. One advantage of clones is that commercial harvest may be possible after a shorted time compared with plantations grown from seed. However, Schmidt states that one big risk exists – if the mother plant is diseased, all clones will be affected and the plantation would have to be destroyed.[33]

Selection by exploiting natural variability

Franz & Novak state that many essential oil-bearing plants species are in transitional phase from wild plants to systemic cultivation.

When individual plants showing the desired phenotype are identified, they are selected to be either generatively or vegetatively propagated. Selection is considered the most common method of genetic improvement for the majority of varieties and cultivars of essential oil crops. The vegetative propagation of selected high performance individual plants has been used in the development of many plants including peppermint (*Mentha* x *piperita*) and lavandin (*Lavandula* x *hybrida*).[4]

Schmidt explains that Denny, who established the Tasmanian lavender industry in 1921, selected within 11 years 487 genotypes from a source of 2,500 genotypes of *L. angustifolia* for closer examination, narrowing them down to just 13 strains exhibiting larger yields of a superior oil. Finally, four of these genotypes were grown on a large scale and mixed together in what is called *comunelles*. The quality of the oil produced was fairly consistent from year to year, both in terms of the chemistry and aroma.[33]

Fragonia oil from *Agonis fragrans* is another example where chemotype variations of the plant were investigated across its natural range to identify which chemotype would be most suitable for commercial development.[34]

Genetic modification

It can be a common practice to directly manipulate the genes of plants in the laboratory to improve the plant's tolerance to insects, disease, drought, salinity and temperature. Franz & Novak quote research involving spike lavender, in which an additional copy of the 1-deoxy-d-xylulose-5-phosphate synthase gene, the first step in the methylerythritol phosphate (MEP) pathway leading to the precursors of monoterpenes, from the *Arabidopsis thaliana,* was introduced and led to an increase of the essential oil of the leaves of up to 360% and an increase of the essential oil in the flowers of up to 74%.[4]

The essential oil composition of peppermint oil has also been modified using genetic manipulation of the genes involved in monoterpene biosynthesis.[4]

Organic farming

There has been an increasing awareness and concern worldwide over environmental issues such as pollution of the land, air and water, loss of biodiversity and damage to ecosystems resulting from intensive, chemical-based agricultural activities and unrestrained use of non-renewable resources. There has also been an increased recognition of the potential risks from pesticides and chemical residues in the food and water. This has led to a shift in world agriculture away from intensive farming systems towards organic farming practices based on environmentally sound principles and practices.[32]

The FAO/WHO Codex Alimentarius Commission defines organic agriculture as a holistic production management system, which promotes and enhances agroecosystem health, including biodiversity, biological cycles and soil biological activity. It emphasises the use of management practices in preference to the use of off-farm inputs, taking into account that regional conditions require locally adapted systems. This is accomplished, where possible, by agronomic, biological and mechanical methods as opposed to using synthetic materials to fulfil any specific function within the system.[35]

Since 1972, IFOAM – Organics International has established itself as the only international umbrella organisation of organic certifiers around the world.

IFOAM has defined organic agriculture as follows:

> *Organic agriculture is a production system that sustains the health of soils, ecosystems and people. It relies on ecological processes, biodiversity and cycles adapted to local conditions, rather than the use of inputs with adverse effects. Organic agriculture combines tradition, innovation and science to benefit the shared environment and promote fair relationships and a good quality of life for all involved.*[36]

IFOAM – Organics International states that organic agriculture must be based on:[37]

- The principle of health – organic agriculture should sustain and enhance the health of the soil, plant, animal, human and planet as one and indivisible.
- The principle of ecology – organic agriculture should be based on living ecological systems and cycles, work with them, emulate them and help sustain them.
- The principle of fairness – organic agriculture should build relationships that ensure fairness with regards to the common environment and life opportunities.
- The principle of care – organic agriculture should be managed in a precautionary and responsible manner to protect the health and well-being of current and future generations and the environment.

These principles of organic agriculture serve to inspire the organic movement in its full diversity.

The Australian Certified Organic (ACO) lists many reasons why certified organic practices should be supported:[38]

- reduce chemical runoff and residues into our drinking water, waterways and coastal areas

- restore soils for productive cropland and secure the future of Australian agriculture
- increase the resilience of farms during drought
- increase biodiversity and save disappearing native animal habitats
- safeguard the integrity of our food
- capture CO_2 into the soil in the form of humus
- reduce greenhouse gas emissions by eliminating synthetic nitrogen fertilisers.

In the second edition of *The Complete Guide to Aromatherapy* (2003), I stated that certified organic essential oils were rare and expensive. I am pleased to say that part of this original statement is now no longer true. An increased demand for certified organic products means that more essential oil suppliers with integrity are producing certified organic essential oils. However, in most cases, they are still considerably more expensive than the non-organic essential oils. The higher price reflects the true and fair price to produce the certified organic oil. The price is also high because the demand for certified organic oils often exceeds the rate of supply.

Factors Influencing the Composition of Essential Oils

The biosynthesis of essential oils in plants is particularly sensitive to many factors.[8] Some of the many factors that influence the production and quality of the essential oil include:

- polymorphism
- ecological variables
- insect stress and microorganisms
- harvesting time
- biomass used.

Polymorphism

The formation of essential oil depends on the tissues and the ontogenetic phase of the plant. The knowledge of these facts is important in harvesting the correct part of the plant at the right time.[4]

The composition of an essential oil often changes between different parts of the plant. Franz & Novak refer to this as phytochemical polymorphism.[4]

For example, the chemistry of cinnamon bark essential oil differs significantly from that of cinnamon leaf oil. The bark oil contains up to 70% cinnamaldehyde, whereas the leaf produces an essential oil that is predominant made up of eugenol.[4]

On the other hand, eugenol is the main compound found in clove, stem, leaf and bud essential oils. It was recently confirmed that the eugenol acetate was found in the bud oil up to 8%, whereas in the leaf oil only trace amounts are found.[4]

Even the height of the plant may play a role. Schmidt uses *Pinus pinaster* as an example. The essential oil obtained from the gum of the trunk at a height of 2 m will contain mainly pinenes with a significant amount of car-3-ene, while the oil obtained from the gum collected at a height of 4 m will contain very little or no car-3-ene. Schmidt explains that the reason for this may be to protect the bark from deer in the winter months.[33]

Franz & Novak state that in *Origanum vulgare* ssp. *hirtum,* a polymorphism could be detected on a much lower level between different oil glands of a leaf. This type of polymorphism may simply be related to the age of the oil glands. Polymorphisms can also be found when comparing the essential oil composition of individual plants of a distinct species and based on the plant's genetic background.[4]

The difference in the composition of two essential oils from the one plant species may often be difficult to assign to a specific chemotype, or to differences arising in the response of the plant to specific environmental conditions or different locations. It is suggested that the variation due to genetic differences is much bigger than the different environmental conditions.[4]

Ecological variables

The most important ecological variables include temperature, the hours of sunshine and the amount of precipitation. For example, Schmidt explains that one year the lavender yield from Provence decreased by one-third. This was because it was too cold at the beginning of the growth, then it was followed by very hot weather and a lack of water.[33]

Schmidt also explains that high humidity with elevated temperatures can produce conditions favourable for the proliferation of insects and microorganisms, which may have a devastating effect on essential oil yields.[33]

Essential oil formation in the plants is highly dependent on the length of the day, temperature and water supply.[4]

For example, peppermint is typically a long day plant. That means it prefers more hours of sunlight. A study found that peppermint cultivated in Germany had a higher menthol and menthyl acetate content than the oil extracted from the same plant cultivated in Turkey. The day length in Munich was 16 h 45 min, whereas in Izmir it was only 14 h 50 m.[4]

Herbs and spices usually require lots of sunshine. The duration of sunshine in the regions along the

Mediterranean Sea usually exceeds eight hours per day, making it highly desirable growing conditions for many herbs. In India, Indonesia and parts of China, the amount of sunshine is even higher, making it possible to have two or even three crops per year.[33]

Some plants such as lavender, thyme, oregano and clary sage require meagre but lime-rich soils. For example, the Jura Chalk of the Haute Provence produces an excellent quality lavender with an interesting top note compared to lavender oil of Bulgarian origin, which is growing on, a different soil type. Soil pH also significantly influences the oil yield and quality. Important elements necessary for some plants are less soluble in alkaline soils because they precipitate as hydroxides at high pH values.[33]

Mild and moderate water stress increases *Ocimum basilicum*'s essential oil content and alters the oil composition. Linalool and methyl chavicol increase as water stress increases, while the relative proportion of sesquiterpenes decreases.[39]

Experiments conducted to study the response pattern of *Pelargonium graveolens* to fertilisers and the variation of essential oil constituents under varied agroclimatic regions found that the essential oil yields were greater at lower altitudes than at higher altitudes. The oil produced at higher altitude locations was richer in menthone, citronellol, nerol and geraniol, while the oil produced from plants grown at lower altitude locations was richer in isomenthone, linalool and citronellyl formate. The variations in these growing conditions bring about a change in the quantity and quality of the essential oil produced.[40]

The effect of mineral fertilisers was evaluated on the basis of the fresh plant and essential oil yields. A study involving *Salvia officinalis* found that the concentrations of various chemical constituents were significantly affected by the various concentrations of fertilisers. An increase in fertilisers caused a reduction in the ratio of oxygenated components to hydrocarbons.[41]

It was found that higher nitrogen increased the biomass of peppermint and increased the essential oil yield, but it did not improve the quality of the oil. The oil had a lower menthol and higher menthone content. On the other hand, higher potassium forced the maturity of the plant and decreased the essential oil yield; however, the oil had higher menthol content.[4]

Insect stress and microorganisms

Plants are capable of interacting with neighbouring plants and warn them of any incipient danger from insect attack. These warning signals are the result of rapid changes occurring in their essential oil composition, which is then transferred to neighbouring plants. In this way the insect will come into contact with a chemically modified plant, which may not suit its feeding habits. Microorganisms can also significantly change the essential oil composition.[33]

Harvesting time

The timing of the harvest can be one of the most important factors affecting the quality of the essential oil. Often it can be a matter of days during which the quality of the essential oil reaches its optimum.[33]

Many studies have been conducted to determine the optimum time for harvesting. The conclusions are:[42]

- The volatile oil content of the leaf increases with time, and also with leaf size.
- The maximum leaf yield was measured at the same time for most species – late summer – but the maximum oil yield varied from species to species. Thus, it is important to know at what time in the plant's cycle the plant matter has been harvested.

It has been determined that the ester value in lavender is at its maximum value when about two-thirds of the lavender flowers are open. This is when harvesting should commence, as the ester value of lavender is one of the key indicators of a high-quality lavender oil.[33]

Oil yield can also be influenced by the time of the day in which the plant is harvested. For example, rose petals should be collected in the morning between 6 am and 9 am. As soon as the day temperature rises, the essential oil yield will diminish.[33]

The best time to harvest fennel seeds is the phase of full ripeness as the anethole content increases from <50% in unripe seeds to over 80% in full maturity.[4]

Investigations into the chemical profile of *Matricaria recutita* found that several extrinsic factors such as amount of daylight, temperature, air and soil humidity, sowing and harvesting times all affected the quantity and quality of the essential oil produced. It was found that the essential oil content was significantly higher if it were sown in spring rather than autumn.[43]

Another example is *Salvia officinalis*, which contains varying amounts of α-thujone depending on when it is harvested. It contains more after it has flowered, so it is better harvested before it flowers as the α-thujone is one of the more toxic constituents found in the oil.[41]

Considerable compositional differences could be found between older and younger leaves of sage

(*Salvia officinalis*). The younger leaves were rich in β-pinene, bornyl acetate and sesquiterpenes, while the mature leaves contained three times more camphor and camphene.[44]

It was found that *Ocimum basilicum* oil distilled from the whole plant gave an oil with a higher percentage of methyl chavicol, whereas the flower spikes produced an oil richer in linalool. For aromatherapy purposes, it is better to use basil with the least amount of methyl chavicol, as this constituent is considered a skin irritant and has possible carcinogenic effects.[45]

There was a marked difference in the menthol/ menthone and pulegone ratio of peppermint oil according to the harvesting time. It was concluded that the harvesting of peppermint before flowering yielded an oil rich in menthone and pulegone, two undesirable constituents, while harvesting the peppermint after flowering yielded an oil richer in menthol.[46]

Biomass used

The most economical way to extract an essential oil is to transport the harvested biomass directly to the distillery. For example, *Melissa officinalis* is very prone to quickly drying out, which results in significant loss oil.[33]

Schmidt explains that, as soon as the plant is cut, its life-sustaining processes slow down and finally stop altogether. The production of enzymes stops and autoxidative processes begin, including bacterial activity that will lead to rotting and molding. As a consequence of this, unless controlled drying or preparation are acceptable options, extraction of the essential oil from the biomass has to be prompt.[33]

In the case of peppermint, it was noted that drying leaves before distillation did not affect the chemical composition of the essential oil, and it was commercially more viable as it allowed larger amounts of plant material to be distilled.[47]

Some plants may require special treatment of the biomass before the essential oil is extracted. Certain harvested plants will need to be broken into smaller fragments and ground down, sometimes drying of the biomass may be beneficial. For example, until the 1980s, cut lavender and lavandin were dried in the field, a process taking about three days. The oil from this lavender exhibited the typical fine, floral aroma of lavender; however, the oil yield was low compared with the yield obtained from fresh material. However, the quality of essential oil from freshly cut lavender is often greener and harsher, requiring some time to harmonise.[33]

Clary sage is another good example in which there is a significant chemical difference between the essential oil distilled from dried plant and fresh plant.[33]

Constituent	Fresh – 'Vert Broyee'	Dried – 'traditional'
myrcene	0.9-1.0%	0.9-1.1%
limonene	0.2-0.4%	0.3-0.5%
cis-ocimene	0.3-0.5%	0.4-0.6%
trans-ocimene	0.5-0.7%	0.8-1.0%
α-copaene	0.5-0.7%	1.4-1.6%
linalool	13.0-24.0%	6.5-13.5%
linalyl acetate	56-70.5%	62.0-78.0%
β-caryophyllene	1.5-1.8%	2.5-3.0%
α-terpineol	1.0-5.0%	<2.1%
neryl acetate	0.6-0.8%	0.7-1.0%
δ-germacrene	1.1-7.5%	1.5-12.0%
geranyl acetate	1.4-1.7%	2.2-2.5%
geraniol	1.4-1.7%	1.2-1.5%
sclareol	0.4-1.8%	0.6-2.8%

Differences in the composition of clary sage essential oil, distilled from fresh or dried herb.[4]

Chemotypes

A typical essential oil consists of a small number of major chemical constituents, which make up the bulk of the essential oil; however, a large number of minor constituents are also present in smaller but significant proportions. Regardless of their relative amounts, every chemical component present contributes to the unique odour profile of the oil.[32]

In natural populations of many species of essential oil-bearing plants, large differences may occur in the chemical composition of the essential oil extracted from morphologically similar plants growing in different locations, or between individual plants growing on the same site. Depending on the major constituents of the oil, different chemotypes have been identified in the wild populations of many species.[32]

As previously stated, the composition of the essential oil may vary with the plant's genetic make-up, stage of growth and environmental factors; however, the absence or presence of a particular chemical constituent at any stage of growth is determined by the genes, whereas its concentration is governed by both genetic and environmental factors.[32]

Plants belonging to the Lamiaceae family are prone to hybridisation, which makes defining species and subspecies a difficult task. Hybridisation is when two different species cross-pollinate and the offspring is usually sterile.[48]

Of particular interest is thyme. There are over 150 subspecies of the genus *Thymus*. A subspecies occurs when a particular plant produces others like itself, usually with some marked differences between it and the parent species.[49]

Some of the different *Thymus* species investigated include the following:[49]

Thymus species	Main constituents
Thymus vulgaris	thymol, carvacrol, p-cymene, linalool
Thymus zygis	thymol, carvacrol
Thymus capitatus	carvacrol, thymol
Thymus satureoides	borneol, camphene, g-terpineol
Thymus mastichina	linalool, 1,8-cineole

This phenomenon – that chemical differences exist in morphologically identical species – is widespread among the Lamiaceae family. Two examples in which chemotypes exist are thyme and rosemary. There are six chemotypes of *Thymus vulgaris*:[50]

- thymol
- carvacrol
- linalool
- geraniol
- α-terpinyl acetate
- thuyan-4-ol.

It was found that there was a correlation between chemotype, sexual polymorphism and the environment. It was noticed that the phenol-containing species of thyme often showed two chemotypes, a thymol type, and a carvacrol type. Their common precursor *p*-cymene leads to either thymol or carvacrol, even though both substances can be found in many phenol-containing species, usually with one dominating.[49]

Rosemary essential oil from *Rosmarinus officinalis* has three main chemotypes:[50]

- camphor
- 1,8-cineole
- verbenone.

When purchasing certain essential oils it is important to know which chemotype you are buying, as the differences in the composition of the oil will affect the therapeutic properties of the oil. It is useful to know the geographic and ecological origin of the essential oil, as this will give you information about its chemotype.

When such a difference occurs, it has become a standard practice to identify the oil by the Latin name of the plant followed by the predominant chemical component:

Rosmarinus officinalis ct. *camphor*

Conclusion

In this chapter we have found that there are many factors that influence the chemistry of the essential oil. The essential oil industry and aromatherapists would benefit from more carefully controlled studies aimed at pinpointing the key factors influencing the production and chemistry of essential oils.

References

1. Arctander S. *Perfume and flavor materials of natural origin.* Allured Publishing, Carol Stream, 1994.
2. Brud W. *Blending and compounding.* AROMA'93 Conference Proceedings. Aromatherapy Publications, Sussex, 1993: 44-54.
3. Franchomme P. *Phytoguide no.1: aromatherapy, advanced therapy for infectious illnesses.* International Phytomedical Foundation, La Coutete, 1985.
4. Franz C, Novak J. *Sources of essential oils.* In Baser KHC, Buchbauer G. eds. *Handbook of essential oils – science, technology and applications.* 2nd edn. CRC Press, Boca Raton, 2016: 43-86.
5. Price S, Price L. *Aromatherapy for health professionals.* Churchill Livingstone, Edinburgh, 1995.
6. Rose J. *The aromatherapy book.* Herbal Studies Course, California, 1992.
7. Lavabre M. *Aromatherapy workbook.* Healing Arts Press, Rochester, 1997.
8. Sadgrove N, Jones G. *A contemporary introduction to essential oils: chemistry, bioactivity and prospects for Australian agriculture.* Agriculture, 2015; 5(1): 48-102. doi: 10.3390/agriculture5010048.
9. Hoffmann D. *Medical herbalism – the science and practice of herbal medicine.* Healing Arts Press, Rochester, 2003.
10. *International rules of botanical nomenclature adopted by the fifth international botanical congress, Cambridge, 1930.* Taylor and Francis, London, 1934.
11. US Department of Agriculture. *Classification for kingdom plantae down to genus Lavandula L.* Retrieved Dec 29, 2017, from https://plants.usda.gov/classification.html
12. Morales R. *The history, botany and taxonomy of the genus Thymus.* In Stahl-Biskup E, Sáez F. eds. *Thyme – the genus thymus.* CRC Press, Boca Raton, 2002: 1-43.
13. Bowles J. *The chemistry of aromatherapeutic oils.* 3rd edn. Allen & Unwin, Crows Nest, 2003.
14. Stearn WT. *Botanical Latin.* 4th edn. Timber Press, Portland, 1992.
15. Buhner SH. *The lost language of plants.* Chelsea Green Publishing, White River Junction, 2002.
16. Bayton R, Maughan S. *Genealogy for gardeners.* Allen & Unwin, Crows Nest, 2017.

17. Bettelheim FA, March J. *Introduction to general, organic and biochemistry*. Saunders College Publishing, Philadelphia, 1984.
18. Ördög V, Molnár Z. *Plant physiology*. Retrieved January 5, 2018, from http:www.tankonyvtar.hu/en/tartalom/tamop425/0010_1A_Book_angol_01_novenyelettan/index.html
19. Ragusa S. *Physiology, taxonomy and morphology of aromatic plants*. In Bagetta G, Cosentino M, Sakurada T. eds. *Aromatherapy – basic mechanisms and evidence based clinical use*. CRC Press, Boca Raton, 2016: 43-58.
20. Svoboda K, Hampson J, Hunter T. *Secretory tissues*. The International Journal of Aromatherapy. 1998/1999; 9(3): 124-131.
21. Svoboda K. *The biology of fragrance*. Aromatherapy Quarterly, 1996; 49: 25-28.
22. Sell C. *Chemistry of essential oils*. In Baser KHC, Buchbauer G. eds. *Handbook of essential oils – science, technology and applications*. 2nd edn. CRC Press, Boca Raton, 2016: 165-194.
23. Statti G. *Phytochemical components of aromatic plants and factors influencing their variability*. In Bagetta G, Cosentino M, Sakurada T. eds. *Aromatherapy – basic mechanisms and evidence based clinical use*. CRC Press, Boca Raton, 2016: 59-83.
24. Boland DJ, Brophy JJ, House APN. *Eucalyptus leaf oils: use, chemistry, distillation and marketing*. Inkata Press, Canberra, 1991.
25. Shawe K. *Essential oils and their biological roles*. Aromatherapy Quarterly, 1996; 50: 23-28.
26. Williams C. *Medicinal plants in Australia – Vol. 2. Gums, resins, tannins and essential oil*. Rosenburg Publishing, Dural, 2011.
27. Asian Regional Workshop (Conversation & Sustainable Management of Trees, Vietnam, August 1996). *Santalum album, sandalwood*. The IUCN Red List of Threatened Species 1998: eT31852A9665066. doi: 10.2305/IUCN.UK.1998.RLTS.T31852A9665066.
28. Rashkow ED. *Perfumed the axe that laid it low: the endangerment of sandalwood in southern India*. Indian Economic & Social History Review, 2014; (51)1: 41-70. doi: 10.1177/0019464613515553.
29. Henderson W. *Sweet scent of success – sandalwood in Australia*. Retrieved May 2, 2017, from http://aciarblog.blogspot.com.au/2014/05/sweet-scent-of-success-sandalwood-in.html
30. McConnon T. *Sandalwood company happy despite low harvest*. (Sept 20, 2013) In ABC Rural. Retrieved May 2, 2017, from http://www.abc.net.au/news/rural/2013-09-20/tfs-happy-with-sandalwood-harvest/4970344
31. *TFS begins Indian sandalwood harvest*. Retrieved May 2, 2017, from http:www.perfumerflavorist.com.networking/news/company/TFS-Corp-begins-indian-sandalwood-Harvest-222169511.html
32. Bhat KKS. *Agrotechnology of aromatic plants*. In Tuley De Silva K. ed. *A manual on the essential oil industry*. United Nations Industrial Development Organization, Vienna, 1995.
33. Schmidt E. *Production of essential oils*. In Baser KHC, Buchbauer G. eds. *Handbook of essential oils – science, technology and applications*. 2nd edn. CRC Press, Boca Raton, 2016: 127-164.
34. Robinson C. *A new essential oil, Agonis fragrans: chemotype selection and evaluation*. Rural Industries Research and Development Corporation, RIRDC Publication No 06/090, Kingston, 2006.
35. Food and Agriculture Organization. *Organic agriculture: what is organic agriculture?* Retrieved Oct 18, 2017, from http://www.fao.org/organicag/oa-faq/oa-faq1/en/
36. IFOAM – Organics International. *Definition of organic agriculture*. Retrieved Oct 18, 2017, from https://www.ifoam.bio/en/organic-landmarks/definition-organic-agriculture
37. IFOAM – Organics International. *Principles of organic agriculture*. Retrieved Oct 18, 2017, from https//www.ifoam.bio/sites/default/files/poa_english_web.pdf
38. Australian Organic Ltd. *Australian organic guide to: what is organic?* Retrieved Oct 18, 2017, from http://www.austorganic.com/wp-content/uploads/2013/09/Consumer_Standards_Final_21.pdf
39. Simon J et al. *Water stress-induced alterations in essential oil content and composition of sweet basil*. The Journal of Essential Oil Research, 1992; 4(1): 71-75.
40. Bhaskaruni R. *Variations in yields and quality of geranium under varied climatic and fertility conditions*. The Journal of Essential Oil Research, 1990; 2(2): 73-79.
41. Piccaglia R. *Effect of mineral fertilisers on the composition of Salvia officinalis oil*. The Journal of Essential Oil Research, 1995; 7(2): 73.
42. Basker D, Putievsky E. *Seasonal variation in the yields of leaf and essential oil in some Labiatae species*. Journal of Horticultural Science, 1978; 53(3): 179-183.
43. Gasic O. *The influence of sowing and harvesting time on the essential oils of Chamomilla recutita*. The Journal of Essential Oil Research, 1991; 3(5): 295-302.
44. Németh-Zámboriné E. *Natural variability of essential oils components*. In Baser KHC, Buchbauer G. eds. *Handbook of essential oils – science, technology and applications*. 2nd edn. CRC Press, Boca Raton, 2016: 87-125.
45. Bonnardeaux J. *The effect of different harvesting methods on the yield and quality of basil oil in the Ord river irrigation area*. The Journal of Essential Oil Research, 1992; 4(1): 65-69.
46. Chalchat JC. *Variation of the composition of essential oil of Mentha piperita L. during the growing time*. The Journal of Essential Oil Research, 1997; 9(4): 463-465.

47. Perrin A, Colson M. *Timing of the harvest date for Mentha piperita based on observations of the floral development*. The Journal of Essential Oil Research, 1991; 3(1): 17-25.
48. Stahl-Biskup E. *The chemical composition of Thymus oils*. The Journal of Essential Oil Research, 1991; 3(2): 61-82.
49. Soulier J. *The Thymus genus*. Aromatherapy Records, 1995; 1: 38-49.
50. Lawrence BM. *Essential oils 1981-1987*. Allured Publishing, Wheaton, 1989.

Production

CHAPTER 4

Contents

Extraction Methods

While distillation is the most common method of essential oil extraction, special oils and absolutes may require more advanced equipment. The basic methods of extraction are:

- **Expression processes**
  - compression – sponge
  - écuelle à piquer
  - machine abrasion
- **Distillation processes**
  - water
  - water and steam
  - hydro-diffusion
- **Extraction with solvents**
  - solvent
  - enfleurage
  - hypercritical CO_2.

History of Essential Oil Production

The historical origins of essential oil production are not clear. According to some, China was the cradle of distillation while others suggest that it was first developed by the Indus culture. Some historians credit the Arabs as having developed distillation. It has been commonly stated that the earliest practical apparatus for water distillation has been dated from the Indus culture some 5,000 years ago; however, Schmidt believes that there are no written records to support these claims.[1]

The earliest documented records of a method and apparatus that appears to be a distillation apparatus dates back to Mesopotamia. The archaeological museum of Taxila in Pakistan has on exhibit an object made out of burnt clay that looks like a distillation apparatus, but it has been suggested that it is more likely to have been used for the purification of water. Schmidt explains that the Mesopotamian art of distillation was revived in ancient Egypt, as well as being expanded by the expression of citrus oils. The ancient Egyptians improved the processes for extracting natural aromatics so that they could be used for embalming.[1]

The thirteenth-century Arab writer Ad-Dimaschki described the process for the production of distilled rose water as well as improved cooling systems. Schmidt reminds us that the products produced at this time were not essential oils but fragrant distilled water extracts.[1]

The practice of distillation was introduced to Europe by the Crusades of the Middle Ages. Hieronymus Brunschwig describes 25 essential oils produced at the time in his treatise, *The True Art to Distil*.[1]

Schmidt explains that it is most likely that these extracts were fragrant alcohols or aromatic waters. The first evidence of the capability to extract genuine essential oils was provided in the sixteenth century. Our knowledge of the science of essential oils did not increase during the seventeenth century, and by the eighteenth century minor progress had been made to the design of the distillation equipment. However, in the nineteenth century, progresses in the understanding of the chemistry of essential oils led to the advancement of distillation methods. The 'Alambique Vial Gattefosse' was the first transportable distillation unit that was easy to transport and to be placed near the fields. The early stills had a capacity of about 50-100 kg of plant material; later their capacity increased to 1000-1200 kg.[1]

Schmidt states that the final chapter in the history of distillation was the introduction of a double-walled distillation plant. This method improved the speed of the distillation as well as the quality of the top notes of the essential oils produced.[1]

Expression

Expression or cold pressing is confined to the extraction of citrus oils. It involves the physical process in which the essential oil glands in the peel are crushed or broken to release the essential oil.[2]

The reason that citrus oils are extracted from the fruit rind by mechanical methods is the relative thermal instability of the aldehydes contained in them. Aldehydes such as heptanal, octanal, nonanal, decanal and dodecanal are readily oxidised by atmospheric oxygen, which gives rise to the formation of malodorous carboxylic acids. Likewise, the terpenoid aldehydes such as neral, geranial, citronellal and perilla aldehyde are sensitive to oxidation.[1]

The essential oil cells of citrus fruit are situated just under the epicarp, called the flavedo, in the coloured part of the fruit. Essential oils are also present in the juice cells; however, the amount of oil present in the juice cells is much smaller than the amount present in the flavedo and the composition is quite different.[1]

Until the beginning of the twentieth century, industrial production of cold-pressed citrus oils was very labour intensive. One method that was practised many years ago, particularly in Sicily, was the *spugna*, sponge method.[1]

The sponge method was one of the original methods used to obtain citrus essential oils. It has been reported that essential oils produced by the sponge process are different to essential oils which have been mechanically extracted.[3]

The fruit is cut transversely into two halves, from which the pulp is then removed. The fruit is then soaked in warm water for a short time in order to allow the pith to absorb a proportion of the water, which softens it and renders it more elastic. The softening process is completed by exposing the peel to the air for several hours, after which it is ready for the removal of essential oil.[4]

The peel is everted by the sponge, so that the flavedo is now on the inside of the hemisphere and is laterally compressed. This causes the rupture of many of the oil cells and the consequent release of the oil, which is absorbed by the sponge. The sponge is periodically squeezed into a collecting vessel, from which the essential oil is decanted.[4]

Lawrence states that the oil produced by this method contained more of the fruit odour character than oil produced by any other method.[2]

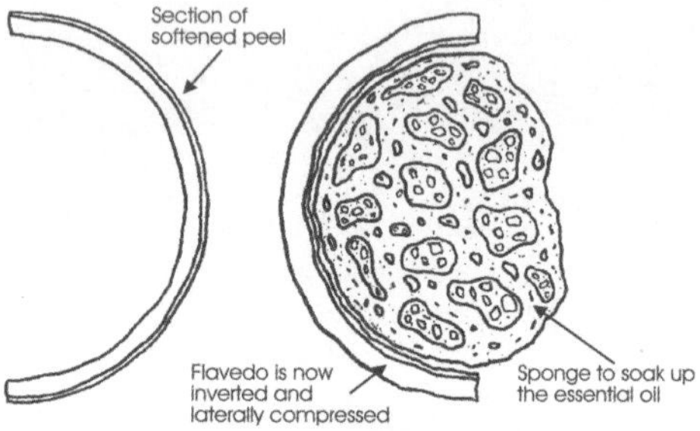

Eversion of fruit in sponge method

A second method is known as écuelle à piquer (or the scodella method). The whole fruit is rotated against the spikes around the rim in order to puncture the oil cells. These cells, contain not only essential oil, but also cell sap and protoplasm. The essential oil released is mixed with cell contents from these and surrounding cells, which are punctured in the process. The mixture of essential oil, other cell contents, including pigment, is then emptied into a collecting vessel, from which the oil is decanted after separation from the aqueous layer.[4]

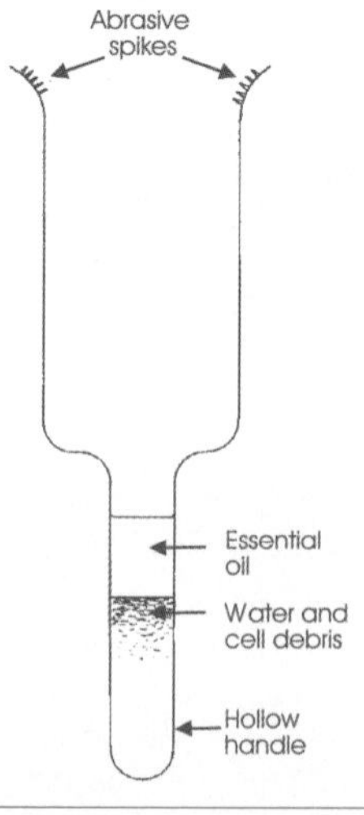

The équelle à piquer process

Lawrence states that these two methods are very labour intensive and impractical because they are very slow processes. On average, 1-2 kg of oil per day can be produced by a single person using one of these hand methods.[2]

As a result, a number of machines have been developed to either crush the peel of a citrus fruit or crush the whole fruit and then separate the oil from the juice. Nowadays there are four major processes that are used to extract citrus oils. These are pellatrice, sfumatrice, FMC extractor and the brown peel shaver. Expression extraction processes that are rarely used nowadays include the Pipkin roll press, screw press, Fraser brace excoriator and the AMC scarifier.[2]

Pellatrice process

The principle of the pellatrice process used for the production of citrus oils is no different from that of the écuelle à piquer process.

The whole fruits are fed from a hopper into a rotating drum with an abrasive shell. The fruit is rotated against the abrasive shell by a slow-moving Archimedian screw whose surface rasps the fruit surface causing some of the essential oil cavities on the peel to burst and release their oil. The screw further transports the fruit into a hopper in which the rollers covered with abrasive spikes burst the remaining oil cavities.[2]

As the fruit tumbles over the spikes, they are stripped of their outer peel, which in the form of a finely divided mixture of cell debris, essential oil and other cell contents, is washed away by running water into a centrifugal separator, which performs a very rapid separation of the essential oil from the aqueous matter.[3]

It should be noted, however, that in this process the essential oil is mixed with other cell contents so that the chance of alteration of the quality of the oil by enzyme action is higher.[4]

Sfumatrice process

The sfumatrice equipment consists of a metallic chain that is drawn by two horizontal ribbed rollers. The peels are conveyed through these rollers during which time they are pressed to release their oil. As in pellatrice process, the oil is washed away from the sfumatrice rollers by fine sprays of water. The oil is initially passed through a separator prior to being sent to two centrifuges in series, so that purified oil can be produced. At one time the sfumatrice process was the most popular process for production of citrus oils in Italy, however, the pellatrice method now appears to be more popular.[5]

The oil obtained by this method may also have to be 'wintered.' That is refrigerated in order to freeze out the peel waxes that can then be filtered off.[2]

FMC juice extractor

The most commonly used extractor is the Food Machinery Corporation (FMC) juice extractor. Schmidt states that more than 50% of extractors in the United States are of the FMC type. The advantage of this machine is that the fruit juice and the essential oil are produced in one step without the two coming into contact with each other.[1]

The processing requires the fruit to be graded according to size. Schmidt states that the technique is revolutionary in its concept. He explains how it works:

> *The fruit is carried to, and placed into, a fixed cup. Another cup, bearing a mirror image relationship to the fixed cup is positioned exactly above it. Both cups are built of intermeshing jaws. The movable cup is lowered towards the fixed cup thus enclosing the fruit. At the same time, a circular knife cuts a hole into the bottom of the fruit. When pressure is applied to the fruit the expressed juice will exit through the cut hole on to a mesh screen and be transported to the juice manifold while at the same time the oil is squeezed out of the surface of the peel. As before, the oil is collected using a jet of water. The oil-water emulsion is then separated by centrifugation.*[1]

Brown peel shaver

The brown peel shaver process is mainly used in the USA and South America, and less in Europe. It is similar to the Pellatrice method.[1]

Lawrence explains that the fruit is fed into the extractor where it settles between a pair of rollers. The fruit moves in a single layer across a bed of rollers covered with needle-like projections mounted in a shallow tank, all moving in the same direction. The rollers alternate between high and moderate speed. The entire surface of the fruit is punctured because the rollers not only rotate it vertically but also rotate it horizontally. The released oil-water emulsion is washed away from the fruit by water. After passing through a solids separator, the oil is removed from the water by centrifugal action.[2]

The advantages of expression processes

The benefit of the expression processes is that the essential oils are not subjected to heat. Heat may, under certain conditions, cause decomposition or damage the essential oil. This process is only available for the extraction of citrus oils.

Distillation

Distillation is the most popular and commonly used cost-effective method for producing essential oils throughout the world. Distillation of aromatic plants simply implies vaporising or liberating the essential oil from the plant cellular membranes in the presence of water or steam, by applying high temperature and then cooling the vapour mixture to separate the oil from the water on the basis that essential oils are immiscible in water.[6]

Principle of distillation

Distillation of aromatic plants involves three main physico-chemical processes:[5]

- hydro-diffusion
- hydrolysis
- decomposition by heat.

Hydro-diffusion

Diffusion of essential oils and hot water through the plant membrane is known as hydro-diffusion. In steam distillation the steam does not actually penetrate the plant cell membranes. Dry plant material can be exhausted with dry steam only when all the volatile oil has been released from the oil-bearing cells by thorough comminution of the plant material. When the plant material is soaked with water, exchange of vapors within the tissue takes place based on their permeability while in a swollen condition. The membranes of plant cells are almost impermeable to volatile oils. Therefore, at boiling water temperature, a part of the volatile oil dissolves in the water present within the glands, and this oil-water solution permeates, by osmosis, the swollen membranes and finally reaches the outer surface, where the oil is vaporised by passing steam.[5]

The speed of the oil vaporisation is not influenced by the volatility of the oil components but by the degree of solubility in water. Therefore, the higher-boiling and water-soluble constituents of the oil in the biomass distil before the lower-boiling and less water-soluble constituents. Since hydro-diffusion rates are slow, distillation of uncomminuted material takes longer time to distil than comminuted material.[5]

Often some of the essential oil constituents are not present in the plant but are artifacts of the extraction process. They can be products of enzymic splitting or chemical degradation occurring during distillation. Schmidt explains that many of the constituents found in rose otto such as citronellol, geraniol and nerol are products of fermentation that have taken place during the water distillation process.[1]

Hydrolysis

Hydrolysis refers to the chemical reactions that occur with certain constituents of the essential oil and water. In the presence of water, esters tend to react with water to form acids and alcohols.

If there is a large amount of water, the amount of alcohol and acid formed will be large, resulting in a decreased yield of essential oil. Furthermore, as it is a time-dependent reaction, the extent to which hydrolysis takes place depends on the contact time between the oil and water. This is considered one of the disadvantages of water distillation.[5]

Decomposition by heat

Almost all the essential oil constituents are unstable at high temperature. Therefore, to obtain the best quality oil, distillation should be done at low temperatures. The temperature in steam distillation is dependent on the operating pressure, whereas in water distillation and in water and steam distillation the operating pressure is usually atmospheric.[5]

Handa explains that all three factors – hydro-diffusion, hydrolysis and thermal decomposition – occur simultaneously and influence one another. The rate of diffusion usually increases with temperature as does the solubility of the essential oil in water. The same is true for the rate and extent of hydrolysis. In order to improve the yield and quality of the oil, it is important to:[5]

- maintain the temperature as low as possible
- use as little water as possible, in the case of steam distillation
- thoroughly comminute the plant material and pack it uniformly before distillation.

Methods of distillation

There are four types of hydro-distillation for extracting essential oils from plant materials:[6]

- water distillation
- water and steam distillation
- direct steam distillation
- distillation with cohobation.

The choice of a particular process for the distillation of an essential oil is generally dictated by the following considerations:[6]

- sensitivity of the essential oil to the action of heat and water
- volatility of the essential oil
- water solubility of the essential oil.

Water distillation

In water distillation, the plant material is completely covered with water. The still is brought to boil. If the air pressure in the still is reduced (e.g. by creating a vacuum), there will be a reduced crowding of molecules of the gases of air at the liquid surface, making it easier for molecules of the liquid to escape. By water distilling under a vacuum, it is possible to increase the speed of evaporation of any volatile liquid. Similarly, the boiling point of water or any other volatile liquid is reduced by reducing the pressure at its surface.[4]

Air pressure decreases with increased altitude, therefore water distillation conducted above sea level will ensue at temperatures below 100°C. A reduced distillation temperature can improve the quality of an essential oil.[4]

It is very important that, when the water is boiled by direct contact with a heat source, the water in the still must always be more than enough to last through the distillation, otherwise the plant matter can overheat and char. When this happens, off notes that are also referred to as still notes are formed.[2]

In order to ensure that the plant material can easily release the essential oil contained in the oil gland, hard fruits, seeds and woods are comminuted, that is, reduced to small pieces or powder, before distillation to render their essential oil cells accessible to the boiling water. Other materials such as patchouli are allowed to soak for a period before distillation, to allow fermentation to break down the cell walls to release the essential oil.[7]

Water distillation is a slow process that favours those essential oils which are not damaged by extensive contact with hot water. It is particularly aggressive towards essential oils containing a high percentage of esters, breaking them down to the corresponding alcohols and carboxylic acids. Because of this, many essential oils require the much faster process of steam distillation.[4,7]

Water distilled oils are typically darker in colour and have much stronger still notes than oils produced by other methods. Lawrence states that, if the oil contains high-boiling components such as phenols, ethers or sesquiterpenes, the distillation time is longer than those oils only containing monoterpene hydrocarbons and oxygenated constituents. It is usually not possible to have enough water in the still to last for the entire distillation cycle. To compensate for this a cohobation tube is placed in the side of the still and water is constantly returned to the distillation vessel.[2]

Lawrence states that water distillation tends to produce lower quality oil because:[2]

- The oil components such as esters are sensitive to hydrolysis, while other components such as acyclic monoterpene hydrocarbons and aldehydes are susceptible to polymerisation.
- Oxygenated components such as phenols have a tendency to partially dissolve in the still water, making it difficult to completely extract them.
- Most water distillations tend to be small so it takes a long time to accumulate much oil.
- Water distillation process is treated as an art by local distillers and few of them try to optimise the yield or quality.
- Water distillation is a slower process than either steam distillation or water and steam distillation, making it less energy efficient.

The one advantage of water distillation is that the cost of the equipment is low, the design of the stills, condensers and collection flasks is simple, and the requirement for electricity is not prohibitive.[2]

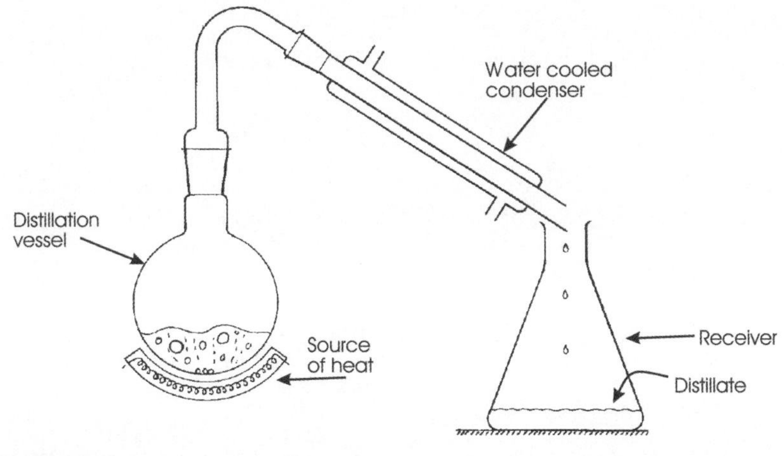

Simple water distillation process

Water and steam distillation

In the water and steam distillation process, live steam is generated in a separate apparatus and then led through the still, which is filled with plant material and water. This method is a compromise between water distillation and pure steam distillation.[4]

Like water distillation, water and steam distillation is commonly used in rural and remote areas. It does not require much more capital expenditure than water distillation. The equipment is usually similar to that of water distillation; however, the plant material is supported above the boiling water on a perforated grid. While this reduces the capacity of the still, it does improve the quality of the essential oil produced. If the amount of water is not sufficient to allow the completion of distillation, a cohobation tube is attached and condensate water added back to the still, thereby ensuring that the water, which is being used as the steam source, will never run out. This also controls the loss of dissolved oxygenated constituents in the condensate water because the re-used condensate water will once again become saturated with dissolved constituents after which more oil will dissolve in it.[5]

The advantages of water and steam distillation over water distillation are as follows:[5]

- higher essential oil yield
- oil constituents are less susceptible to hydrolysis and polymerisation
- the quality of the oil produced by water and steam distillation is more reproducible
- water and steam distillation is a faster extraction process than water distillation so it is more energy efficient.

The disadvantages of water and steam distillation are:[5]

- Due to the low pressure of the rising steam, oils of a high-boiling point range require a larger quantity of steam for vaporisation – hence longer hours of distillation.
- The plant material becomes wet, which slows down the distillation as the steam has to vaporise the water to allow it to condense further up the still

Cohobation

Cohobation is a procedure that can only be done for water distillation or water and steam distillation. It involves the practice of returning the distillate to the still after the oil has been separated from it so that it can be reboiled. The idea is to minimise the losses of oxygenated components which may dissolve in the distillate water. For most oils, this level of oil loss in the water is less than 0.2%; however, in phenol-rich oils, the amount of oil that may be dissolved in the water is between 0.2-0.7%.[5]

For example, rose otto contains phenylethyl alcohol, a colourless, rose-smelling constituent that is water- soluble. When rose is distilled, much of the phenylethyl alcohol is dissolved in the distilled water. In cohobation, the distilled water is collected and returned to the distillation vessel to be redistilled so that the phenylethyl alcohol can be recovered. The separated phenylethyl alcohol is then returned to the original distillate in the correct proportion to form rose otto oil.

Lawrence warns us that there is a higher risk of these water-soluble components becoming degraded as they are constantly being revaporised, condensed and revaporised again. It is, therefore, very important that the temperature to which the oxygenated constituents dissolved in the distillate are exposed is no higher than 100°C.[2]

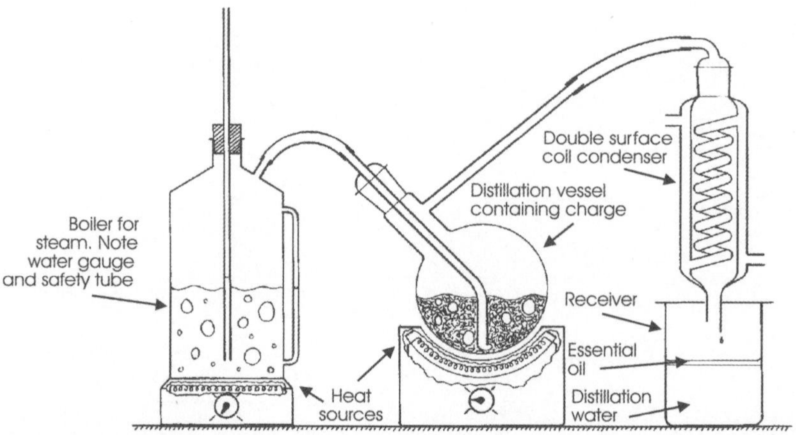

Water and steam distillation process

Steam distillation

In steam distillation, steam from a separate boiler is injected into the distillation vessel. The essential oil is extracted at a much faster rate than water distillation.

The steam is under greater pressure than that of the atmosphere, thus water from which it is produced is boiling at a temperature above 100°C. The object of steam distillation is to complete the process as quickly as possible, as certain essential oil components are thermolabile or heat sensitive. Therefore, damage to the essential oil through the effect of the steam is minimised.[4,7]

Constituents such as linalyl acetate found in lavender will decompose to linalool and acetic acid, and the matricin found in German chamomile will decompose into the intensely blue chamazulene.

The advantage of steam distillation over water distillation is that the essential oil is exposed to the risk of hydrolysis for a relatively shorter period.

Steam distillation is the most widely accepted process for the production of essential oils on a large scale and is considered superior to the other two processes.

The advantages of steam distillation include:[5]

- the amount of steam can be readily controlled
- no thermal decomposition of the essential oil constituents.

The main disadvantage is that steam distillation requires a much larger capital expenditure to build and set up.

Other distillation techniques

Fractional distillation

This process is conducted as per normal distillation; however, the essential oil is collected in batches as distillation proceeds, instead of being continuously collected. These batches of the essential oil are called fractions.

Ylang ylang essential oil is produced by fractional distillation. In this process, the distillation is stopped and restarted up to four times. The receiver is changed on each occasion. The first fraction is referred to as ylang ylang 'extra', and the subsequent fractions are referred to as 1st, 2nd and 3rd grade.[4]

The first fraction, ylang ylang extra, contains the most volatile constituents of the essential oil, along with a proportion of constituents of lower volatility. The second and third fractions contain larger quantities of less volatile constituents, while the final fraction is composed of the least volatile constituents of the oil.[4]

Dry distillation

Dry distillation involves heating in the absence of aerial oxygen, normally in a closed vessel, preventing combustion. The cells of the plant matter begin to char and brown smoky fumes are emitted, the density of which increases as the temperature rises. Eventually, a pale brown mobile liquid and a black, viscous tarry mass distil over and the 'smell of smoke' pervades the atmosphere. Birch tar and cade oil are both produced by this method.[4]

These two oils are no longer of any commercial importance as both oils contain carcinogenic phenols.[1]

Rectification

Some essential oils require rectification. This involves the redistillation of the crude oil in order to remove certain undesirable impurities, such as very small amounts of constituents of a very low volatility, carried over during the steam or water distillation, as well as a small amount of very volatile compounds that have an undesirable odour, thus affecting the top notes of the oils, such as dimethyl sulfide present in crude peppermint oil or isovaleric aldehyde present in *Eucalyptus globulus*.

In some cases, the purpose of rectification is done to enrich the essential oil with a preferred component, as is the case with eucalyptus oil and 1,8-cineole.[1]

The reason is that the standard for eucalyptus oil requires it to have a minimum of 70% cineole. If the distilled oil does not reach these high cineole levels, the essential oil will be redistilled so that so-called 'impurities' can be removed, hence increasing the cineole level.[8]

Hydro-diffusion

Hydro-diffusion was first described in 1983. Unlike traditional steam distillation, it works on the principle that steam is introduced at the top of the still and not at the base. The process uses the principle of osmotic pressure to diffuse oil from the oil glands.[6]

Condensation of the oil and steam mixture occurs inside the still directly below the grill or perforated tray supporting the material being processed. The yield of the oil is higher and the process is advantageous because of the reduced steam consumption, the shorter distillation time and an absence of hydrolysis, as the raw material does not come into contact with boiling water. However, because of the downward flow of steam and condensate, co-extraction of other non-volatile compounds such as lipids, chlorophyll, fatty acids and polar components make the

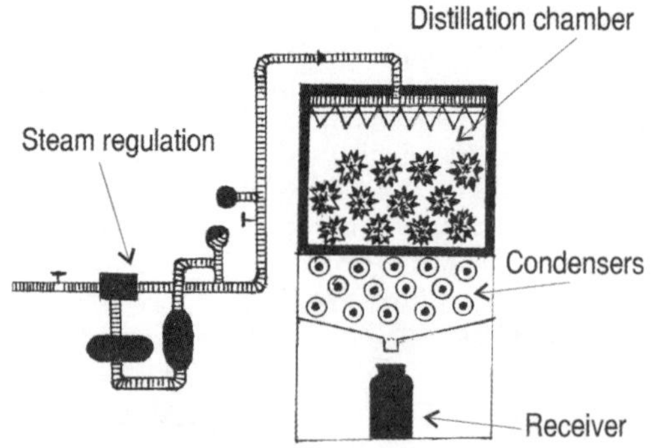

Hydro-diffusion process

process complicated. While hydro-diffusion is considered a better alternative to conventional distillation processes, the fact is that commercial operations based on hydro-diffusion have not been successful.[6]

Vacuum distillation

Vacuum distillation obtains oil from a still under a vacuum. This technique allows for very accurate control of the distillate since it can be adjusted according to the boiling points of the various essential oil constituents.[9]

Molecular distillation

This process is used to produce volatile essential oils from delicate materials containing some proportion of non-volatile matter often found in absolutes used in perfumery. The basic principle involves gentle evaporation of a thin film of material to be treated from a surface, over which the film is continuously replenished under vacuum conditions. Molecules of evaporating volatiles have only a short distance to travel before encountering a cooled surface on which to condense. The essential oil molecules can pass freely to this surface under vacuum conditions. Very little heat is used to cause the evaporation of the volatiles, and most molecules remain intact during the process.[4]

Parameters affecting yield and quality of essential oils during distillation

Tandon explains that the yield and quality of the essential oil from steam distillation can be affected by many processing parameters.

Mode of distillation

The distillation technique chosen should consider the boiling point of the essential oil and the characteristics of the plant, as the heat content and the temperature of the steam can alter the distillation characteristics. For example, woody oils such as sandalwood and cedarwood require a higher boiling point. Therefore, these oils should be extracted using boiler-operated steam distillation. The temperature of the steam depends on its pressure. Essential oils with higher-boiling point constituents normally require high-pressure steam. However, for rose and other florals, the plant material is immersed in water, as flowers tend to aggregate and form lumps which cannot be distilled using water and steam distillation or direct steam distillation.[6]

Material of fabrication of equipment

Essential oils can be very corrosive, so stills should be made of resistant materials such as aluminum, copper or stainless steel. Although copper was the most commonly used material for fabrication of distillation stills since ancient times, stainless steel is now the preferred material.[6]

Condition of raw material

Many raw materials need to be crushed, powdered or soaked in water to expose their oil cells.

Raw materials such as pepper, coriander seed, cardamom, celery seed, cumin, fennel seed and any other plant matter in the form of a hard grain need to be comminuted before water distillation. This is carried out in the presence of water, such as in a wet grinding turbine, and the water is used for the distillation. The stills will be equipped with blade stirrers to ensure that the biomass particles don't stick to the walls of the still, which could end up creating burnt notes. Dry grinding is likely to result in a significant loss of volatiles.[1]

Chopping the plant will also change the packing density of the plant material in the still. It is possible to pack up to 50% more plant material in the same still after comminution. Air drying and wilting of the herb prior to distillation can also have a considerable impact on the quality of the oil and the distillation process. If required, the drying of the herbs prior to distillation should be done in shaded areas and the dried material should not be stored in heaps.[6]

Time for distillation

The essential oil constituents are distilled according to their boiling points. The highest boiling point fractions will be the last to be extracted. If the distillation is terminated too soon, some of these higher boiling point constituents may be lost. In some plants such as vetiver, patchouli, sandalwood and agarwood, these high-boiling point fractions are very important due to the importance of their aroma. Therefore, the time of distillation must be chosen with care.[6]

Loading of raw material and steam distillation

Improper loading of the aromatic plant in the still may result in steam channelling causing incomplete distillation. The aromatic plant must be evenly and uniformly loaded in the tank without leaving voids. Excessive filling of the plant may also lead to 'rat holes', which may cause the steam to escape without vaporising any essential oil.[6]

Operating parameters

Proper control of injection rates and pressure in boiler-operating units is necessary to optimise the temperature of extraction for maximising yield.[6]

Problems of the distillation processes

It is important to remember that an essential oil produced by distillation will suffer some adulteration in its composition during the distillation process.

This occurs because of the hydrolysis of volatile esters and the hydrolysis of non-volatile constituents of the protoplasm known as glycosides. A glycoside that has undergone hydrolysis may be partially decomposed to form a sugar such as glucose, which is non-volatile, or it may form a compound called aglycone. The aglycones of certain glycosides present in essential oil-yielding plant matter are volatile, and end up forming part of the essential oil. Examples of such volatiles released during distillation include the rose alcohols, geraniol and citronellol.[7]

Williams suggests that it is inaccurate to refer to distilled essential oils as natural products, but more accurate to describe them as products prepared from their natural sources by distillation. Another reaction that takes place during distillation is the partial hydrolysis of protein forming the living matter of the cells. Weakly bonded fragments of the molecules split off to form highly odorous, sulphur-containing molecules, which distil over with the vapours of the essential oil, imparting an obnoxious odour, referred to as a 'still note'.[7]

Still notes present in essential oil can be eliminated by exposing the oil to air for several hours, or by blowing air into the oil for a short period. This promotes the evaporation of the responsible compounds.[7]

Solvent Extraction Processes

Not all odorous extracts of essential oil-bearing plants comply with the International Organization for Standardization (ISO) definition of an essential oil. Other types of volatile isolates that can be obtained commercially include concretes, absolutes, pomades, resinoids, oleoresins, extracts, infusions and tinctures:[2]

Concrete: An extract of fresh plant parts by the use of a hydrocarbon solvent. It is rich in hydrocarbon soluble material and devoid of water-soluble components. It is generally a waxy semi-solid dark coloured material free of the original solvent.

Absolute: A highly concentrated alcoholic extract of a concrete which contains only alcohol-soluble materials. It is primarily used for alcohol-based perfumes.

Pomade: The product of the enfleurage fat extraction of fresh flowers.

Resinoid: A solvent extract of a resin-rich exudate or dried plant material with a hydrocarbon solvent. Resinoids are generally viscous to semi-solid mixtures. They can be considered as concretes of dried materials.

Extract: A concentrate of a dried, less volatile aromatic plant part obtained by solvent extraction with a polar solvent.

Spice/herb oleoresin: A solvent extract of a dried spice or herb which is free from the solvent used in the extraction process. It is exclusively used by the food and pharmaceutical industries as a replacement for ground spices and spice tinctures.

Extract: An alcoholic extract of a pomade produced by enfleurage. It is a tincture of a pomade.

Balsam: A natural exudate obtained from a shrub or a tree. It is characterised by being rich in benzoic and cinnamic acids and their corresponding esters.

Gum resin: A natural exudate from a tree or plant. It is comprised of gums and resins. If the gum resin source also contains an essential oil, it is called an oleo-gum-resin.

Oleoresin: The natural tree trunk or bark exudate which is extremely rich in an essential oil.

These products are all obtained by solvent extraction methods; therefore they do not comply with the definition of an essential oil.

Solvent extraction is a very gentle process which tends to create less 'rearrangement' of the essential oil compounds compared to distillation methods. Compared with steam-distilled essential oils, solvent extracted oils have a richer fragrance. The disadvantage with this process is that not only the essential oil components of the plant, but also the non-volatile constituents such as waxes and plant dyes are extracted.

Solvent extraction is applied to those plants whose essential oils would be degraded by distillation. The methods of extraction with volatile solvents are:

- maceration
- extraction with volatile hydrocarbons
- enfleurage
- CO_2 extraction.

Maceration

Maceration is the simplest form of solvent extraction. Maceration in hot fat was one of the original processes of extracting the essential oils. This process is now almost obsolete. Maceration can be done using hot fat, alcohol, volatile solvents or cold fats. The process involving cold fats is referred to as enfleurage.

Scented flowers are immersed in highly purified, melted fat, or a mixture of fats, for a sufficient period of time so that the essential oil dissolves in the fat. Other constituents that would dissolve into the fat include natural waxes and plant pigments. The mixture is then strained to remove the exhausted flowers and other debris, and the process is then repeated several times using fresh flowers and the same fat.[4]

The end result is that you have a fatty extract solution that is highly fragrant. Once solidified, this product is referred to as the pomade. The essential oil may then be extracted from the pomade with alcohol by the procedure described for the extraction of concretes.[4]

Extraction with volatile hydrocarbons

Many flowers must be processed as soon as possible after they have been harvested because the odour of these flowers either changes or evaporates within a few hours of harvesting. Lawrence explains that the aromatic volatiles are glycosidically bound, and at a specific development stage and specific time in the 24-hour cycle of the flower, a controlled enzymatic degradation of the bound volatiles, along with other biosynthetic reactions, takes place resulting in the release of volatiles. Harvesting must be synchronised with the release of the volatiles to ensure the capture of the volatiles by the solvent used.[2]

Fresh flowers have a high water content (80-90%) compared with fresh leaves (60-80%). This means that if they were dried before extraction, a lot of volatiles would be lost during dehydration. Therefore, the solvent of choice must be non-water miscible, otherwise the water would dissolve in the solvent and change its polarity and its ability to dissolve the flower volatiles.[2]

The solvents used for the manufacture of concretes include butane, hexane, petroleum and toluene. About 30 years ago the solvent of choice used to be benzene; however, because of the toxicity associated with this solvent, it is no longer used.[2]

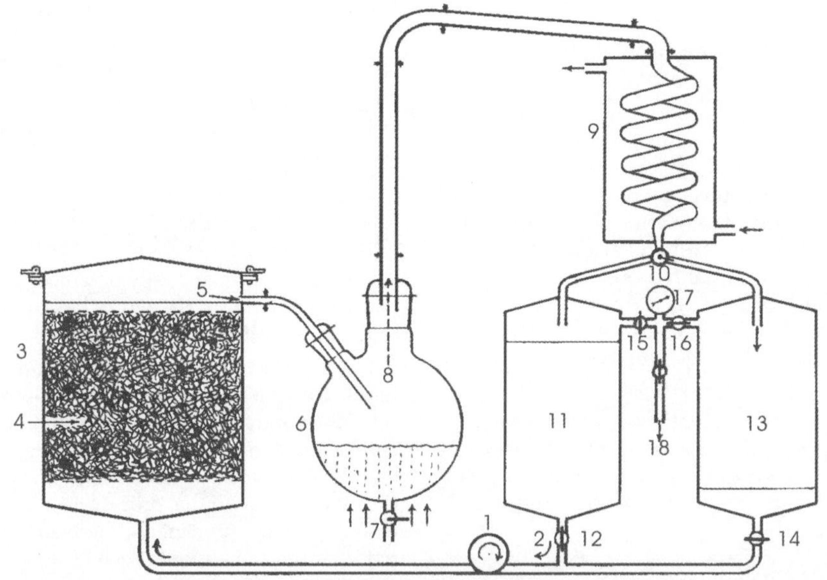

This diagram shows the basic equipment required for the extraction of essential oils with a volatile solvent, coupled with a vacuum still for recovery of the solvent after extraction.

1: Solvent pump; 2: Solvent to extraction vessel; 3 Extraction vessel; 4: Material for extraction; 5: Extract solution to distillation vessel; 6: Distillation vessel; 7: Drainage tap for recovery of concrete after extraction 8: Solvent vapour to condenser; 9: Water-cooler condenser; 10: Two-way tap; 11: Receiver containing recovered solvent being recirculated to extraction vessel; 12: Solvent outlet tap; 13: Receiver being filled with recovered solvent 14: Solvent outlet tap; 15 & 16: Vacuum taps; 17: Vacuum gauge; 18: To vacuum pump.

Concretes are produced in static extractors. These extractors are fitted with numerous perforated trays so that the flowers do not get compressed by their own weight. When stacking the flowers onto these trays, care must be taken to minimise bruising and damage of the flowers, because this can cause the release of enzymes in the flowers which would cause deterioration of the concrete. The basket stacked with flowers is immersed into the extraction vessel and the solvent of choice is introduced from the bottom into the extraction vessel until the plant material is completely immersed. Four to five washes are required until the material is exhausted.[2]

It is normal practice to circulate fresh solvent through a battery of extractors. At each cycle, the solvent becomes enriched with the flower volatiles until extraction is complete. Once the extraction is complete, the solvent, which is highly enriched with the flower extract, is pumped to a primary evaporator whose heat is maintained at the same temperature as the boiling point of the solvent. In this evaporator the solvent content is reduced to about one-tenth of the original volume. The recovered solvent is then re-used. The remaining solvent with the flower extract is pumped into a finishing evaporator where the solvent is removed more carefully under high vacuum. Again the solvent is recovered to be re-used. The resultant flower extract is referred to as the concrete. Usually it is a viscous to solid extract whose aroma is very similar to, but much stronger than the original material from which it was extracted.[2]

The concrete still contains many other hydrocarbon compounds such as waxes, diterpenes, fixed oil and free fatty acids. The approximate yield of concretes produced by various flowers is often less than 0.5%.[2]

The concrete is not very soluble in alcohol, so further conversion into an absolute is required if the material is to be used in perfumery. The concrete is mixed in pure ethanol and warmed to between 30° to 60°C and then strongly agitated to get everything into solution. It is then refrigerated to between -5 ° to -10°C so that the waxes can be removed by precipitation.[2]

The alcoholic solution is then chilled and this precipitates much of the poorly soluble, non-volatile matter. The alcoholic solution is then filtered and the alcohol is removed by distillation in a vacuum, still at the lowest possible temperature.

Concerns about using volatile hydrocarbons

Because the hydrocarbons used as solvents are highly volatile, they do present the risk of being highly flammable. The high volatility, however, means that they can be easily distilled off at relatively low temperatures under a vacuum.

While solvents such as benzene, used in the past, were considered to be extremely hazardous, solvents used today such as hexane are considered safer. The concern about the use of solvents has focused on several issues:

- solvent residues left in the oil
- the destruction of the life force.

Many of the solvent extracted products are used in food flavouring, and many countries have introduced strict regulations controlling the use and type of solvents.[9]

Holmes refers to the solvent extraction process as 'dry-cleaning' the plant. Solvent extraction produces a more complete plant extract. However, he says that contact with the solvent, which is usually a petroleum ether, may result in minute traces of solvent in the final absolute. He suggests that, from an energetic perspective, this may devitalise the essential oil through contact with a 'dead chemical substance'.[10]

The whole idea of solvent extraction is that it is done at relatively low temperature compared to traditional distillation techniques. I would suggest that the higher temperature of distillation is more likely to damage the lifeforce than the solvent extraction method.

In comparing rose absolute with rose otto, Wabner says that rose otto contains synthetic constituents that are not found in nature. A headspace analysis of a live rose was compared to the constituents of rose absolute of the same flower and rose otto of the same flower. While the chemical constituents of the rose absolute and live rose were similar, rose otto oil contained several constituents such as rose oxide and damascenone that were a by-product of distillation.[11]

Wabner also dispels the long-held belief that rose absolute should not be used in aromatherapy. To support his argument, he makes the following comments:[11]

- Water is not more alive than other chemicals.
- Absolutes can be prepared residue controlled and even residue free.

The most important thing is that you can lose up to 50% of the constituents found in the living flower. All the water-soluble components remain in the flower water.

Enfleurage

Jasmine season began at the end of July, August was for tuberoses. The perfume of these two flowers was both so exquisite and so fragile that not only did the blossoms have to be picked before sunrise, but they also demanded the most gentle and special handling. Warmth diminished their scent;

suddenly to plunge them into hot macerating oil would have completely destroyed it. The souls of these noblest of blossoms could not be simply ripped from them, they had to be methodically coaxed away. In a special impregnated room, the flowers were strewn on glass plates smeared with cool oil or wrapped in oil-soaked clothes, there they would die slowly in their sleep. It took three or four days for them to wither and exhale their scent into the adhering oil. Then they were carefully plucked off and new blossoms spread out.

This procedure was repeated a good, ten, twenty times, and it was September before the pomade had drunk its fill and the fragrant oil could be pressed from the clothes. The yield was considerably less than with maceration.

But in purity, it was unequalled, the jasmine oil radiated the sticky sweet, erotic scent of the blossoms with lifelike fidelity.[12]

Suskind has eloquently described the enfleurage extraction process in which the essential oil naturally released by fragrant flowers is absorbed by highly purified and odourless solid fat or oil.

Fresh blossoms, gathered in the early morning, are placed upon a thin layer of fat spread on a sheet of glass surrounded by a wooden frame known in French as a *chassis* or *corps*. Within a 24- to 48-hour period, depending on the nature of the flowers being processed, essential oil is transferred from the flowers to the fat, which absorbs it.

After a period of time, the flowers are removed from the chassis and are replaced by fresh, recently picked blossoms. This process is repeated until the enfleurage fat is saturated with the essential oil. This product is called an enfleurage pomade, and consists of the original fat and the absorbed essential oil.

The success of enfleurage depends to a large extent upon the quality of the fat used. It must be odourless and have a good consistency. If it is too hard, the blossoms will not have sufficient contact with the fat. On the other hand, if it is too soft, it will tend to engulf the flowers and the exhausted ones will adhere. When the flowers are removed they may retain adhering fat that will result in significant amount of the fat over the period of extraction. Many years of experience have confirmed that a mixture of one part of highly purified tallow and two parts of lard is the most suitable for enfleurage.[5]

Hypercritical carbon dioxide

This process produces essential oils of such a unique quality and purity that differ immensely from the essential oils produced by steam distillation. Lawrence states CO_2 extracts possess aroma profiles almost identical to the raw material from which they are extracted.[2]

The principle of CO_2 extraction is that any substance can exist in three different states – gas, liquid and solid – depending on its temperature and pressure. In addition, certain substances can be found in the hypercritical state. They are neither liquid nor gas, but rather they are both. The hypercritical fluids disperse as readily as gases and also have solvent properties.

Carbon dioxide is one gas that becomes hypercritical. Its hypercritical temperature is 33°C. Hypercritical carbon dioxide then becomes an excellent solvent of essential oils. The advantage is that the whole operation takes place at a low temperature, and therefore the essential oil is not affected by heat, as may occur in the distillation process.

The extraction process is almost instantaneous, and because the carbon dioxide is inert, there is no chemical reaction between carbon dioxide and the essential oil. Carbon dioxide can then be removed by simply releasing the pressure. The whole process takes place in a closed chamber.

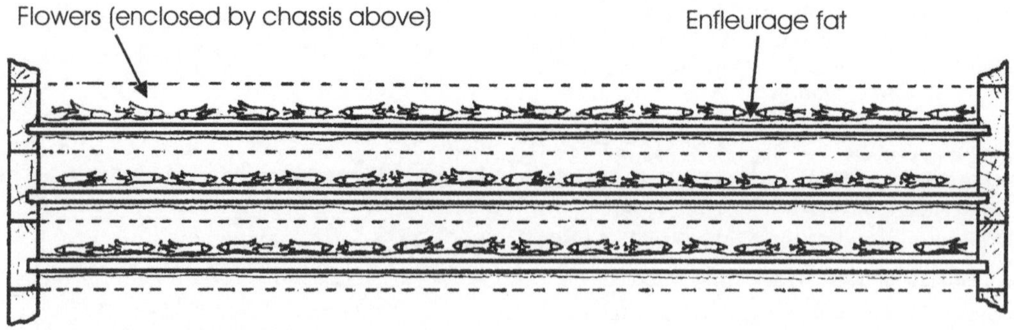

Enfleurage

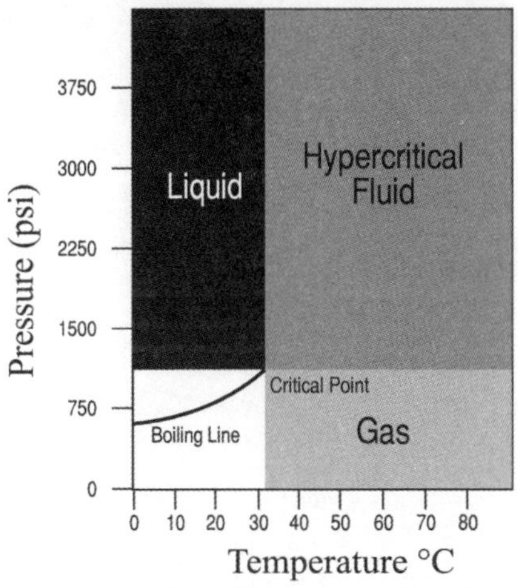

Physical states of carbon dioxide

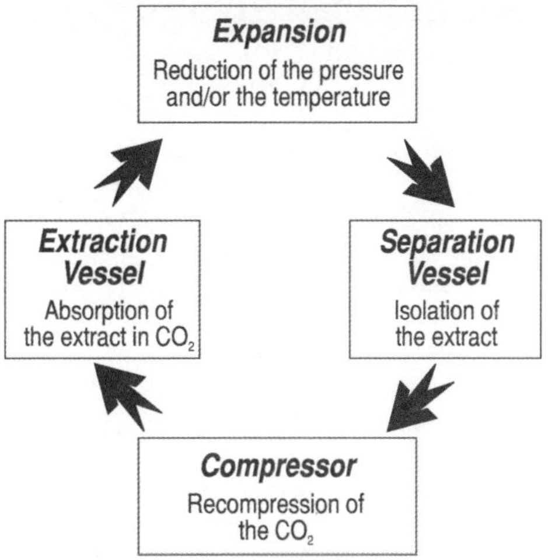

Hypercritical CO_2 extraction process

Carbon dioxide is a popular choice of solvent for hypercritical extraction because:[2]

- it is odourless, tasteless and non-toxic
- it is non-combustible
- it is inexpensive and readily available
- it is easily removed leaving no solvent residue
- low viscosity means it can easily penetrate comminuted dry plant material
- by varying the temperature and pressure, it can be used in a more selective manner.

Unfortunately, the hypercritical pressure for carbon dioxide is over 200 atmospheres. This is 200 times that of regular atmospheric pressure. As a result, the cost of the equipment is prohibitive except for large flavour, fragrance, beer or pharmaceutical manufacturers. Lawrence points out that almost all of the hop extracts used around the world are produced by CO_2 extraction.[2]

Liquid CO_2 is a good solvent for compounds whose molecular weight is below 250. This includes all the hydrocarbons and oxygenated monoterpene compounds found in essential oils. The solubility of compounds whose molecular weight is between 250 and 400 in liquid CO_2 is very poor, while compounds with molecular weights in excess of 400 are almost insoluble in liquid CO_2. This means that the CO_2 extracts will not contain the waxes, polyphenols, carbohydrates, carotenoids, chlorophylls etc.[2]

Some of the advantages of carbon dioxide extracts are as follows:[9]

- No organic solvents are employed.
- At low temperatures, thermally labile compounds are undamaged.
- There are no off notes, more top notes and more back notes.
- There is better solubility because no extra water-insoluble monoterpene hydrocarbons are generated during processing.
- No degradation products are formed and the true natural odour and flavour profile are obtained.

Steam-distilled ginger does not contain the non-volatile pungent principles for which ginger is highly esteemed. These constituents are found in the CO_2 extracted oil. This gives the CO_2 extract a more pungent and warming oil, which is said to contain up to 20% gingerol and 4% shogaol.[13]

Phytonics process

A new solvent based on hydrofluorocarbon-134a and a new technology to optimise its properties in the extraction of plant materials offers significant environmental and health and safety benefits over other traditional processes for the extraction of high quality natural essential oils and biological extracts.

Advanced Phytonics Limited has developed a patented technology termed 'phytonics process'. The properties of the new generation of fluorocarbon solvents have been applied to the extraction of plant materials. The solvent is hydrofluorocarbon-134a (HFC-134a). This solvent was developed to replace chlorofluorocarbons. The boiling point of HFC-134a is -25°C. It is not flammable or toxic and it does not contribute to the depletion of the ozone layer.[5]

There are many advantages to the phytonics process:[5]

- Unlike other processes that use high temperatures, the phytonics process is conducted at low temperature and is gentle, therefore its products are never damaged by exposure to temperatures in excess of ambient.

- No vacuum stripping is required, which often leads to the loss of precious volatiles.
- The process is carried out entirely at neutral pH and in the absence of oxygen; the products never suffer acid hydrolysis damage or oxidation.
- It requires a minimal amount of electrical energy.
- It releases no harmful emissions and the resultant waste products (spent biomass) are innocuous and pose no effluent disposal problems.
- The solvent used is not flammable, toxic or ozone depleting.
- The solvents are completely recycled within the system.

The phytonics process is being used for the extraction in biotechnologies such as the production of antibiotics, in the herbal drug industry, and in the food, essential oil and flavour industries.[5]

Modern Methods of Essential Oil Extraction

The traditional and more common methods of essential oil extraction have been examined in this chapter. These are the methods most commonly used on a commercial scale. However, new technologies have been developed which may not necessarily be used for the commercial production of essential oils, but may be useful for research and development purposes. These techniques include:[5]

- headspace trapping techniques such as static headspace technique, vacuum headspace technique and dynamic headspace technique
- solid phase micro-extraction (SPME)
- supercritical fluid extraction (SFE)
- phytosol (phytol) extraction
- protoplast technique
- simultaneous distillation extraction (SDE)
- microwave distillation
- controlled instantaneous decomposition (CID)
- microdistillation
- molecular spinning band distillation
- membrane extraction.

References

1. Schmidt E. *Production of essential oils.* In Baser KHC, Buchbauer G. eds. *Handbook of essential oils – science, technology and applications.* 2nd edn. CRC Press, Boca Raton, 2016: 127-164.
2. Lawrence BM. *The isolation of aromatic materials from natural plant products.* In Tuley De Silva K. ed. *A manual on the essential oil industry.* United Nations Industrial Development Organization, Vienna, 1995: 57-154.
3. Guenther E. *The essential oils – Vol. I.* Robert E Krieger Publishing, Malabar, 1948.
4. Diploma in Perfumery Correspondence Course Notes, Part 2: *Aromatic materials from natural sources.* Perfume Education Centre, London, 1980.
5. Handa SS. *An overview of extraction techniques for medicinal and aromatic plants.* In Handa SS et al. eds. *Extraction technologies for medicinal and aromatic plants.* United Nations Industrial Development Organization and the International Centre for Science and High Technology, Trieste, 2008: 22-54.
6. Tandon S. *Distillation technology for essential oils.* In Handa SS et al. eds. *Extraction technologies for medicinal and aromatic plants.* United Nations Industrial Development Organization and the International Centre for Science and High Technology, Trieste, 2008: 115-128.
7. Williams DG. *The chemistry of essential oils.* Micelle Press, Weymouth, 1996.
8. Boland DJ, Brophy JJ, House APN. *Eucalyptus leaf oils: use, chemistry, distillation and marketing.* Inkata Press, Canberra, 1991.
9. Weiss EA. *Essential oil crops.* CAB International, Wallingford, 1997.
10. Holmes P. *Rose – the water goddess.* The International Journal of Aromatherapy, 1994; 6(2): 8-11.
11. Wabner D. *A rose is a rose is a rose oil.* 2nd Australasian Aromatherapy Conference, Sydney, 1998.
12. Suskind P. *Perfume: the story of a murderer.* Penguin Books, London, 1986.
13. Arthur D. *Ginger.* The International Journal of Aromatherapy, 1996; 7(4): 20-23.

Quality

CHAPTER 5

Contents

Introduction

The need to define quality of essential oils

Whether for professional or home aromatherapy use, essential oils of the highest quality should be used. How do we define quality?

Holmes provides us with a good insight into the complexity of defining the quality of essential oils for use in aromatherapy when he asks the following question:

> *How do we know whether an essential oil is actually going to work in a therapeutic way?*[1]

In other words, he suggests defining the quality of an essential oil by its bioactivity.

The main challenge is that aromatherapists are not the only users of essential oils. Essential oils are extensively used in:

- food flavouring
- perfumery and fragrances
- pharmaceutical preparations
- chemical manufacturing.

Each of these industries has developed its own set of criteria for defining the quality of an essential oil.

Holmes suggests we must be cautious not to adopt industrial or scientific standards for essential oils used in aromatherapy:

> *Users of essential oils have unwittingly accepted from both the flavouring industry and pharmacognosy research an overly narrow focus on essential oil identity and purity at the expense of an equal striving for oil bioactivity. This one-sided concern has supplanted and confused the emergence of any true, authentic clinical definition.*[1]

Holmes suggests that the criteria for the quality of essential oils must come from the health-care practitioners rather than commercial enterprises and research science. He states that the definitions required should be specifically based on the criteria of therapeutics, and not ones designed to meet the biochemical standards set out in the pharmacopoeias, or perfume or food flavouring standards set out by international organisations such as ISO (International Organization for Standardization) or IFRA (International Fragrance Research Association).[1]

Defining quality

The term 'pure and natural' used by many suppliers of essential oils simply indicates that no synthetic materials are added. However, purity will not necessarily guarantee a high quality and bioactive essential oil. Holmes states that serious essential oil users have generally assumed a myopic analytical focus on essential oil constituents as a way to determine bioactivity.[1]

I agree with Holmes when he suggests that essential oil users often ignore the documented evidence provided by certificates of authenticity and of certified organic status, not to mention the evidence provided by simple analytical tests such as specific gravity, optical rotation and refractive index. He is concerned that even the most important sensory-based method of organoleptic examination has become marginalised.[1]

The terms 'genuine' and 'authentic' are often used to define the quality of essential oils for use in aromatherapy. In order for an essential oil to be genuine and authentic, I suggest that the following criteria must be used in defining the quality of essential oils:

- purity of essential oils
- role of standards and pharmacopoeias
- biological identification of essential oils
- integrity of the source plant and extraction process
- compliance with quality assurance and GMP standards
- quality control procedures for testing of essential oils.

However, Holmes states that the terms 'genuine' and 'authentic' only concern the essential oil's identity and purity that can be physically and scientifically substantiated. He suggests we should also consider the quality of the plant material used in the production of the essential oils and the extraction process.[1]

Purity of Essential Oils

The term purity is defined by the Macquarie Dictionary as 'the condition or quality of being pure; freedom from extraneous matter or anything that debases or contaminates; freedom from any admixture or modifying addition or freedom from foreign or inappropriate elements'.[2]

Purity is knowing that the essential oil in your small dispensing bottle is exactly the same oil that was originally distilled by the producer.[1]

The main concerns regarding purity of essential oils are:

- adulteration
- contamination
- degradation
- rectification and reconstitution.

Adulteration

Essential oils are often adulterated by:

- other essential oils and their constituents
- other essential oils of the same botanical origin
- its own main constituent
- a reconstituted oil
- a pure aroma chemical.

Brud states that the availability of true, natural steam-distilled oils that are not blended or treated is very scarce. Due to the high level of blending, mixing and adulteration, it is difficult to examine and differentiate a true product from a treated product.[3]

Adulteration is common with the most expensive essential oils such as jasmine, melissa, neroli, rose and sandalwood. Holmes states that most of the adulteration nowadays stems from the commercial need to produce a chemically standardised essential oil as opposed to an essential oil with minor seasonal and yearly variations in its aroma and constituents.[1]

Adulteration may also be done to simply increase the volume or the yield, which simply increases the profits. Schmidt & Wanner state that anyone who adulterates essential oils willfully and knowingly should be treated as a criminal:

> *It is a criminal act and never a wangle or minor offence. The target to cheat a customer by supplying an essential oil being not conform to any standard is a felony. There is no excuse for such unethical behaviour.*[4]

Terms such as cutting, stretching, blending, bouquetting or sophistication try to moderate this act.[4]

Adulteration can be done with other odorous substances including other essential oils that are less expensive, essential oil fractions or residues, synthetic aroma chemicals similar to those found in the essential oil, or aroma chemicals not found in the essential oils.[4]

Non-odorous adulterants, often called extenders, include ethanol, mineral oil, isopropyl myristate, glycols, phthalates and fixed oils. The most expensive oils and absolutes are subject to adulteration.[4]

Even common essential oils such as lavender are often subject to extensive adulteration. The most common additives or 'cutting' materials are acetylised lavandin oil, synthetic linalool and linalyl acetate, or fractions from the production of linalyl acetate from ho wood or rosewood.[5]

The only way to obtain true essential oils for aromatherapy purposes is to have reliable suppliers, either by having direct contact with the manufacturer of the oils, or by keeping in contact with a dealer who has enough contacts with producers to offer a full range of the best quality oils available.

Schmidt & Wanner state that, while a common nose may be fooled by adulteration, a professional well-trained perfumer is able to detect subtle changes to the organoleptic characteristics if an essential oil has been adulterated.[4]

While someone who is highly experienced in olfactory evaluation can detect essential oil adulteration, the best guarantee of purity is analysis by gas chromatography/mass spectrometry (GC/MS).[4]

Adulteration increases the risk of toxicity and reduces the therapeutic efficacy of the essential oil.

Contamination

Contamination of an essential oil may include pesticide or herbicide residues, while adulteration means that a substance has been added to modify the composition of the essential oil. Typically, the substance is a synthetic aroma chemical or an aroma chemical extracted from a less expensive essential oil.

Contaminants may potentiate the toxicity of an otherwise safe essential oil. It is believed that some of the allergic reactions to essential oils have been due to the pesticide or herbicide residue and not the essential oil.[6]

Biocides

Pesticides and herbicides are used in large-scale essential oil crop cultivation to control pests, diseases, parasites and weeds, and to raise harvest yields. It is known that biocides used in the cultivation of aromatic plants can be carried over during steam distillation. Solvent extracted essential oils and expressed oils are even more likely to retain biocides.[6]

Some of the pesticides are considered extremely persistent and there is a chance that, following extraction, pesticide residues will be found in the essential oil.[6]

According to Wabner, many biocide molecules contain chlorine or another halogen, which are readily soluble in oils and fats. If contaminated oils are applied to the skin during an aromatherapy treatment, these substances are likely to be transported into the nerve and fatty tissue of the body. While acute toxicity can be prevented by restricting the level of pesticide residue, there is very little research on the long-term accumulative effect of pesticides.[6]

Studies using propiconazole and mancozeb, two fungicides often used to control rust in peppermint and other essential oil crops, suggest that the poor solubility of these biocides and low volatility appear to preclude the co-distillation of residues in controlled laboratory conditions, even when contamination was found on the leaf; however, the authors of the study state that field-based stills may have a higher propensity for carryover of the biocides through the condenser at the point of breakthrough.[7]

It has been argued that the level of pesticide found in essential oils is usually not higher than levels found in food. Therefore, since essential oils are used in much smaller quantities and much less frequently than food products, this leads to the conclusion that aromatherapy is much safer than eating.[6]

However, biocides, by definition, are toxic, therefore they should not be welcome in either food or essential oils, even in trace amounts. The regulations state that only 0.1 to 0.5 ppb (parts per billion) of pesticide residue is allowable in drinking water, while the pesticide residue allowable in food is 0.5 to 1.0 ppm (parts per million).[6]

It is concerning that such levels of biocides are allowable in our food, certainly a tempting reason to grow your own vegetables or buy organic cultivated products.

Tisserand & Young cite Hotchkiss, who explains that biocides are poorly absorbed through the skin. They claim that the potential toxicity from biocides in essential oils is minimal.[8]

Wabner suggests that some reported allergic reactions to essential oils may be caused or enhanced by biocide residues and not by the essential oil themselves.[6]

Solvents

Tisserand & Young state that, while the use of benzene for the extraction of concretes has declined dramatically, it is still being used. It is a well-documented carcinogen. IFRA states that it should not exceed 1 ppm in fragrance products.[8]

Cyclohexane is now a commonly used replacement for benzene. It is not known to be genotoxic. Tisserand & Young state that the risk of solvent toxicity from the use of absolutes is negligible.[8]

Phthalates

Phthalates are often used intentionally as adulterants in essential oils to simply 'stretch' essential oils or to make unpourable resinoids more pourable.[8]

Phthalates are a group of chemicals used to make plastics more flexible and harder to break. They are used in vinyl flooring, adhesives, detergents, lubricating oils, automotive plastics and PVC plastics. Phthalates are used in plastic packaging film and sheets, garden hoses, inflatable toys, blood-storage containers, medical tubing and some children's toys. The Centers for Disease Control (CDC) cites a study examining the human exposure to environmental chemicals and states that CDC scientists measured 13 phthalate metabolites in urine of 2,636 participants aged six years and older who took part in the survey.

The report concluded that measurable levels of many phthalate metabolites occur in the general population. The CDC states that finding detectable levels of phthalates in urine does not imply adverse health effects.[9]

However, Tisserand & Young state that as a group, phthalates tend to be hepatotoxins, cause damage to the gastrointestinal tract, and may have a varying degree of reproductive toxicity and carcinogenicity.[8]

Diethyl phthalate (DEP) is commonly used to dilute essential oils. It is not toxic and has a good safety profile. The Research Institute of Fragrance Materials (RIFM) concludes that the level of dermal exposure from its use in fragrance is 0.73 mg/kg/day. The RIFM states that there is no significant risk to humans with regard to skin reactions, carcinogenicity, reproductive toxicity or oestrogenic activity. Phthalates other than DEP have been used to adulterate sandalwood oil.[8]

Contamination by phthalate esters of Sicilian and Calabrian citrus oils of lemon, orange and mandarin, produced in the crop years of 1994-1996, was believed to be from plastic materials used in the extraction process of the citrus oils.[10]

Tisserand & Young state that phthalate adulteration and contamination in essential oils is declining due to increased legislation and awareness of phthalate toxicity.[8] The addition of phthalates to essential oils is a big concern and should not be accepted.

Degradation

Chemical degradation is a process by which the quality of the essential oil is reduced over time. This usually occurs because of prolonged storage, or poor storage conditions. The main factors responsible for essential oil degradation are:

- oxygen
- heat
- light.

The effect of oxygen on essential oils is called oxidation and tends to occur in essential oils rich in monoterpene hydrocarbons such as citrus and pine oils. Oxidation is accelerated by both heat and light.

Expired essential oils may not only lose their therapeutic properties, but the chemical changes that an aged oil has undergone may make the oil more hazardous. An example is oxidised pine oil, which is more likely to cause dermal sensitisation than fresh pine oil.

Wabner cites research which found that oxidised tea tree oil was found to be the cause of severe dermatitis, whereas fresh tea tree oil on the same patients did not elicit the same negative reaction.[11]

Oxidised lemongrass oil was found to lose much of its antibacterial activity when compared to fresh un-oxidised lemongrass.[12]

To avoid degradation of essential oils, ensure that:

- The oils should be stored in dark glass bottles.
- Small amount of essential oils in large bottles should be transferred to smaller bottles to reduce the risk of oxidation.
- As with most organic products, essential oils have a limited shelf life. This should clearly be shown on the bottle as an expiry date.

Some essential oils undergo resinification. This is a process in which small molecules are joined together to form polymeric chains of two, three or more monomers. Resinification results in an increase in the oil's viscosity. It is often seen in old or poorly stored essential oils, and is commonly seen in essential oils such as angelica seed, myrrh, tagetes and tarragon.[8]

How to prevent oxidation

Oxidation of essential oils can be minimised by proper storage or the addition of antioxidants to susceptible essential oils. It is very important to keep essential oils in dark bottles and away from direct sunlight and sources of heat. The oils can be stored in a refrigerator, but do be aware that a few essential oils will become very viscous and will be difficult to pour until they are warmed to room temperature. The more air in the bottle, the higher the risk of oxidation. It is also preferable to store the oils under an inert gas such as nitrogen, but this is not practical for aromatherapists.[8]

Citrus oils and other oils that readily undergo oxidation should be stored in containers that have as little air space in them as possible. This will help reduce the risk of oxidation.

Tisserand & Young recommend using those essential oils that oxidise easily within 12 months. They also recommend the addition of an antioxidant such as BHT. Antioxidants are usually added at less than 0.1% However, they state that the addition of an antioxidant could be regarded as adulteration.[8]

Rectification and reconstitution

Rectification

Sometimes major or minor chemical constituents are removed from essential oils by a subsequent distillation to make the oil more acceptable or to comply with standards. These oils are referred to as rectified essential oils.

For example, the British Pharmacopoeia standard for eucalyptus requires a minimum of 70% 1,8-cineole content. As some eucalyptus oils have a cineole content less than this, the oil must be redistilled.

Pénoël best summarises the concerns of most aromatherapists:

> *Most of the products [eucalyptus oils] found on the usual aromatic market have been redistilled, rectified and refined. In reality, the residue left behind in the still from the rectification of the crude oils is rich in precious molecules (like the rare phenol australol). Even if their proportion seems low, they work in synergy with the main components and should be kept in order for the essential oil to express its full healing potential.*[13]

From a holistic aromatherapy perspective, it is recognised that the synergistic action of all the constituents of an essential oil is far superior to that of the redistilled oil.

Reconstitution

Reconstitution is a form of adulteration that often involves compounding or reconstituting an essential oil from essential oil fractions or synthetic aroma chemicals similar to those found in the essential oil. These oils are often used in perfumery to obtain an acceptable type of scent without incurring the high cost of using the pure essential oils. Melissa and lemon verbena are two essential oils that are commonly reconstituted as are many of the expensive floral absolutes.

The Role of Standards and Pharmacopoeias

Burfield & Kirkham state that over the decades a number of organisations have developed working standards for essential oils; however, most of them are geared towards the needs of the pharmaceutical, food and fragrance industries. Many of these standards are not suitable for establishing a quality framework for essential oils used in aromatherapy.[14]

Pharmacopoeias

Some essential oils are listed in pharmacopoeias such as the British Pharmacopoeia (BP). Price & Price explain that hospital pharmacies may require essential oils that comply with the BP standards. However, they explain that essential oils that are prepared to BP standards may not be suitable for aromatherapy.[15]

The BP standard specification is often very specific. This means that often only those essential oils that have been blended or rectified comply with the pharmacopoeia standard.

ISO standards

The main independent certifying body that publishes standards for individual essential oils is the ISO. However, the ISO standards are not designed or are not intended to define the efficacy or safety of an essential oil. The standard is only a guide to the essential oil composition. It helps us to know if an essential oil falls within the normal range as specified in the standard.

Harris states that an essential oil can still be very therapeutic and not fall within the ISO range.[16]

Sadgrove & Jones state that published standards sometimes take into consideration biological variables such as chemotypes. For example, the standard for tea tree oil (*Melaleuca alternifolia* Cheel) as specified by ISO specifies the chemotype being described as ISO 4730:2004 Oil of Melaleuca, Terpinene-4-ol Type (Tea Tree Oil).[17]

However, the ISO standard then goes on to define tea tree oil as:

> *Essential oil obtained by steam distillation of the foliage and terminal branchlets of Melaleuca alternifolia (Maiden et Betche) Cheel, Melaleuca linariifolia Smith, and Melaleuca dissitiflora F. Mueller, as well as other species of Melaleuca provided that the oil obtained conforms to the requirements given in this international Standard.*[17]

This is most interesting as the ISO standard clearly states that an essential oil can be labelled tea tree as long as it comes from the genus *Melaleuca* and complies with physical characteristics and chemical profile provided in the standard.[17]

For the purposes of use in aromatherapy, we should only accept and use those essential oils whose botanical origins are clearly known. This means that it is botanically pure and we know the botanical species used.

Standards are not enforced by law; however, the published standards are often used by manufacturers and essential oil traders as a reference to provide a guarantee of reproducibility and reliability of essential oil.[17]

Therapeutic grade oils

I can appreciate why some aromatherapy brands decided to use the term 'therapeutic grade'; however the truth is that there is no such thing as a 'therapeutic grade essential oil'. The term was only coined for the purposes of marketing essential oils in the aromatherapy industry. Burfield & Kirkham have clearly articulated that the term 'therapeutic grade' is misleading:

> *Let us be quite clear about this – there is no such thing as a 'therapeutic grade essential oil' and no standards for the authentication or performance of essential oils specifically exist within aromatherapy per se.*[14]

They suggest that it has been a failure of aromatherapy essential oil trading associations to issue guidelines for essential oil standards.[14]

Although Harris does not agree with the term 'therapeutic grade', he believes that if there was to be a definition, it should state that it would have to be a pure essential oil, preferably but not necessarily organically cultivated, that is supplied with a full chemical analysis of its constituents.[16]

The term 'certified pure therapeutic grade' has even been trademarked by a multi-level marketing company.

Biological Identification of Essential Oils

To identify a genuine essential oil the following information should be readily available:

- botanical name
- part of the plant used
- biological variability and chemotypes.

Botanical name

Price & Price state that it is often very difficult to procure essential oils that are considered genuine. They make a very valid point when they explain that the word natural does not mean that the essential oil is unadulterated or safe. They state that the essential oil trade often has a very limited knowledge of the botanical names. For example, the common name oregano applies to more than 43 species.[15]

The following examples highlight why referring to the oil by its common name or just the genus name will provide insufficient information about the oil. For a more detailed explanation, please refer to the individual essential oil monographs.

Chamomile

- *Matricaria recutita* – German chamomile
- *Anthemis nobilis* – Roman chamomile
- *Ormenis mixta* – Moroccan chamomile

An oil simply referred to as chamomile can refer to several different plants. All three species belong to the Asteraceae family and are similar in appearance; however, their chemical composition and organoleptic characteristics are distinctly different. German chamomile is also known as blue chamomile and is well known for its distinctive inky blue colour and strong herbaceous aroma. It is very high in sesquiterpene compounds, which are known to be anti-inflammatory, promote granulation and tissue regeneration. On the other hand, Roman chamomile is light in colour and has an almost sweet floral herbaceous aroma. It is very high in aliphatic esters, which are known to have spasmodic and sedative properties.[18,19]

Moroccan chamomile oil is not commonly used in aromatherapy. It has a fresh herbaceous and camphoraceous aroma. The chemical composition is distinctly different to that of German and Roman chamomile; however, the properties of *O. mixta* oil overlap those of German and Roman chamomile.[20,21]

Cedarwood

- *Cedrus atlantica* – Atlas cedarwood
- *Cedrus deodara* – Himalayan cedarwood
- *Juniperus virginiana* – Virginian cedarwood
- *Juniperus mexicana* – Texas cedarwood

There are many species of cedarwoods. Some belong to the Pinaceae family and others belong to the Cupressaceae family. Both families belong to the conifer class. The organoleptic characteristics and chemical composition of each species of cedarwood are unique.

Lavender

- *Lavandula angustifolia* – true lavender
- *Lavandula latifolia* – spike lavender
- *Lavandula* x *intermedia* – lavandin
- *Lavandula stoechas* – maritime lavender

The term 'lavender oil' is meaningless because there are so many species of lavender. The correctly defined botanical name of lavender provides us with the genus *Lavandula* in Latin, followed by a word which defines the species (e.g. *angustifolia, latifolia, stoechas, hybrida* etc). The organoleptic characteristics and chemical composition of each species of lavender are unique.

Spike lavender has a naturally higher camphor and 1,8-cineole content, making it useful as an inhalation for respiratory tract infections, for muscular aches and pains, and as an insect repellent.[21]

Marjoram

Origanum majorana – sweet marjoram

Thymus mastichina – Spanish marjoram

Thymus capitatus – Spanish oregano

Origanum majorana is the major botanical source of sweet marjoram oil. Sweet marjoram should not be confused with Spanish marjoram (*Thymus mastichina*) which belongs to the thyme species or Spanish oregano (*Thymus capitatus*) which is used to produce oregano oil.

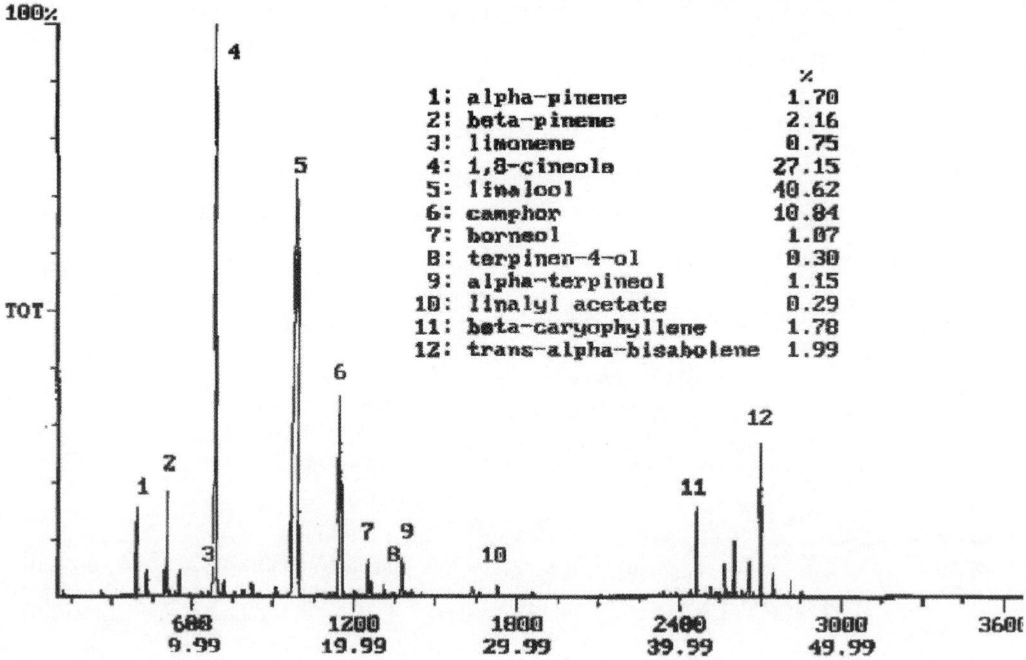

GC-MS analysis of spike lavender – *Lavandula latifolia*. Courtesy of John Fergeus from Australian Botanical Products

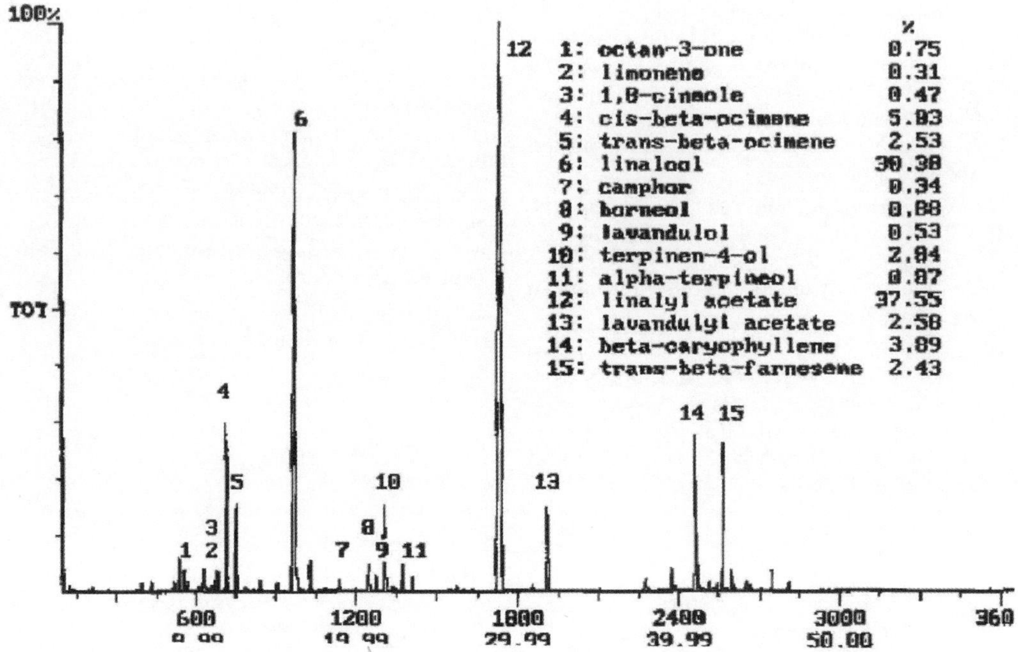

GC-MS analysis of lavender – *Lavandula angustifolia*. Courtesy of John Fergeus from Australian Botanical Products

Pine

- *Pinus mugo* var. *pumilio* – dwarf pine
- *Pinus palustris* – longleaf pine
- *Pinus sylvestris* – Scotch pine

There are numerous species of pine that yield an essential oil from their twigs and needles as well as their heartwood.

Sage

- *Salvia officinalis* – Dalmation sage
- *Salvia lavandulaefolia* – Spanish sage

There are several species and cultivars of sage such as Mexican sage (*S. azurea* var. *grandiflora*) and red sage (*S. colorata*), both of which are used medicinally. Essential oils can also be extracted from Spanish sage (*S. lavandulaefolia*) and clary sage (*S. sclarea*).[21]

Sandalwood

- *Santalum album* – True sandalwood
- *Santalum spicatum* – Australian sandalwood
- *Santalum lanceolatum* – Queensland sandalwood
- *Santalum austrocaledonicum* – Vanuatu sandalwood
- *Amyris balsamifera* – West Indian sandalwood, amyris

Four of the above sandalwood oils are produced from various species of the *Santalum* genus. The sandalwood oils that are most highly desirable are those with a higher santalol content. S. *album* has the highest percentage of naturally occurring santalols and is, therefore, the most sought after of the sandalwood oils. Sandalwood oil should be differentiated according to its botanical name and country of origin.

S. lanceolatum is a protected species by the Queensland government and is available in very limited quantities. *S. austrocaledonicum* is now being cultivated in Vanuatu. It is also available in limited quantities.

Amyris balsamifera bears no botanical relationship to the sandalwood oils from the *Santalum* genus. It grows on the Caribbean Islands and neighbouring countries of South America. Its aroma is reminiscent of guaiacwood and its chemical profile is totally different.

Thyme

- *Thymus vulgaris* – red thyme
- *Thymus zygis* – Spanish thyme
- *Thymus serpyllum* – wild thyme
- *Thymus capitatus* – Spanish oregano
- *Thymus mastichina* – Spanish marjoram

It is estimated that there are between 100 to 400 species of thyme. Most commercial thyme oils are commonly derived from *T. vulgaris* and *T. zygis*. Two types of thyme oil are produced: red thyme oil and white thyme oil. White thyme oil is obtained by rectifying red thyme oil.[22]

You can see from these few examples that we should always refer to an essential oil by its correct botanical name in order to avoid confusion.

Part of the plant used

Many essential oils are produced from the entire plant. However, for some oils, the part of the plant used must be specified, as the essential oil produced varies qualitatively according to the part of the plant used.

Bitter orange

Bitter orange is a classic example of a tree from which three essential oils are produced:

- neroli oil
- petitgrain oil
- bitter orange oil.

Neroli oil, water-distilled from the flowers, is a pale yellow mobile oil which tends to become darker and more viscous with age. It has a powerful, light and refreshing floral top note with very little tenacity.[5]

Petitgrain oil, steam-distilled from the leaves, is a pale yellow or amber coloured liquid of pleasant, fresh-floral, sweet odour, reminiscent of orange flowers, with a slightly woody-herbaceous undertone and very faint but sweet-floral dryout.[5]

Bitter orange oil, expressed from the fresh peel, is a dark yellow to olive-yellow liquid with a fresh citrus odour and a rich, sweet, bitter and dry undertone.

Therapeutically, petitgrain oil resembles neroli oil, though it is slightly less sedative. However, it would be misleading to assume that petitgrain as a substitute for neroli oil.[23]

Bitter orange oil and sweet orange oil exhibit similar pharmacological activities.[21,22]

Clove

- Clove leaf
- Clove stem
- Clove bud

Clove bud oil is a clear to yellow mobile liquid, becoming brown with a strong, sweet and spicy odour. Adulterants of clove bud oil are usually clove stem or leaf oil, or clove terpenes remaining after eugenol extraction.[24]

Clove leaf oil is a dark brown mobile liquid with a harsh, woody, phenolic, slightly sweet aroma. The leaf oil is often rectified and is usually a pale yellow colour with a sweeter, less harsh, dry woody odour closer to that of eugenol.[24]

Clove stem oil is a pale yellow to straw yellow coloured liquid of a strong spicy, somewhat woody, but quite a pleasant odour. The odour is similar to that of eugenol.[24]

The composition of the bud, stem and leaf oil can be differentiated as follows:[25]

Constituent	clove leaf	clove stem	clove bud
eugenol	85-90%	87-92%	80-85%
eugenyl acetate	0-10%	3-3.5%	8-12%
isoeugenol	-	trace	-
caryophyllene	10-15%	6-8%	6-10%
isocaryophyllene			0-2.0%

The stem and leaf oils are commonly used to adulterate the bud oil, which is considered to be of a superior quality.

Cinnamon

Cinnamon oil can be extracted from both the bark and the leaf. Cinnamon bark has a sweet, warm and spicy aroma with approximately 70% cinnamic aldehyde content. Cinnamon leaf oil is warm and spicy, but lacks the depth and body of cinnamon bark oil. It has a eugenol content of about 75%.

The chemical composition of cinnamon leaf and bark oil was reported as follows:

Leaf: eugenol (80-96%), eugenol acetate (1.0%), cinnamaldehyde (3%), benzyl benzoate (3%).[25]

Bark: cinnamaldehyde (40-50%), eugenol (4-10%), benzyl benzoate (1.0%), α-pinene (0.2%), 1,8-cineole (1.65%), linalool (2.3%), caryophyllene (1.35%).[25]

Cinnamaldehyde is considered the principal therapeutic constituent in cinnamon bark. Cinnamon leaf oil is primarily used as a source of eugenol and in perfumes and flavours.

Cinnamon bark is listed in the German Commission E for internal use for the treatment of gastrointestinal problems and for functional asthenia. However, it is not recommended for topical application because it is a dermal irritant and sensitisers.[26]

Biological variability and chemotypes

It is well known that essential oils produced from the same botanical species but grown in different countries can have a distinctly different chemical composition or chemotype, usually written as ct. or CT. Factors that may contribute to the various chemotypes include:

- prevailing climatic conditions
- soil type
- genetic factors.

Of particular importance are basil, the melaleucas, rosemary and thyme.

Basil

According to an extensive analysis of over 200 individual basil plants, five chemotypes of basil oil have been identified:

- linalool
- methyl chavicol
- methyl eugenol
- (*E*)-methyl cinnamate
- eugenol.[27]

The two most commonly available basil oils are:

- the true sweet basil oil, also known as European or sweet basil. This oil has a higher percentage of linalool. This oil is generally regarded as safe to use in aromatherapy[22]
- exotic or Réunion basil, which is distilled in the Comoro Islands, Malagasy Republic, Thailand and occasionally in the Seychelles. This oil has a higher percentage of methyl chavicol.[22]

The methyl chavicol chemotype basil is more pungent and is reputed to have an antispasmodic effect, whereas the linalool chemotype is reputed to be more sedating and relaxing due to the higher percentage of linalool.[28]

Methyl chavicol is mildly irritating and in high doses a possible carcinogen. It is recommended that basil oil with a methyl chavicol content of 5% or less is used in aromatherapy.[29] For this reason, it would be safer not to use methyl chavicol basil in aromatherapy.

Rosemary

Rosemary is another plant which has several chemotypes. Three principal chemotypes *of Rosmarinus officinalis* can be found growing in Europe:[30]

- camphor-borneol
- 1,8-cineole
- verbenone.

Due to their different compositions, these oils can be applied for different purposes to achieve maximum efficiency. Chemotypes with a high camphor content are more effective in cases of muscular aches and pain. The 1,8-cineole chemotype is best used for respiratory congestion, while the verbenone chemotype has excellent regenerative properties and is used in skincare preparations.[30]

Thyme

Tisserand & Young list seven chemotypes that exist for thyme oil:

- carvacrol
- thymol
- thymol/carvacrol
- borneol
- geraniol
- linalool
- thujanol.[8]

For example, *Thymus vulgaris* ct. *thymol* has potent antimicrobial activity; however, as it is high in phenols, it needs to be used with care in topical preparations as it may be irritating on the skin. On the other hand, *Thymus vulgaris* ct. *linalool* has less thymol and carvacrol. It is considered to be much more immunostimulant and less anti-infectious, and having less phenols, it is a safer choice for children.[31]

Integrity of the Source Plant and Extraction Process

Many of the factors influencing the composition of essential oils have been described in *Chapter 3 – Botany*.

Genetic variation and plant breeding

Due to the high chemical diversity found in some plants, the continuous selection of the desired chemotypes leads to a homogenous and reproducible population. When selecting plants, other factors that need to be considered apart from the essential oil content and composition include resistance to pests and disease, lower nutritional requirements and suitability for technological processes at harvest.

Ecological variables

Some of the most important ecological variables influencing the yield and chemistry of essential oils include altitude, climate, amount of precipitation and soil.[32]

Seasonal variations are common with many essential oils, causing significant chemical variability. For example, Tisserand & Young cite a study that shows the menthone content of French *Mentha* x *piperita* ranges from 6.1-8.1% in October to 48.8-54.5% in June. The thujone content of Italian *Salvia officinalis* ranges from 29.7% in April to 48.8% in October.[8]

Some plants such as lavender, thyme, oregano and clary sage prefer meagre but lime-rich soils.[32]

Mild to moderate water stress increases the linalool and methyl chavicol content, while the relative proportions of sesquiterpenes decreases.[33]

Time of harvesting

The time of harvesting can be one of the most important factors affecting the quality of essential oil.[32]

For example, the ester value of lavender is at its maximum value when about two-thirds of the lavender flowers are open. This is when the harvesting should commence, as the ester value of lavender is one of the key indicators of a high-quality lavender oil.[34]

The best time for harvesting fennel seeds is the phase of full ripeness as the anethole content increases from less than 50% in unripe seeds to over 80% in fully mature seeds.[34]

When the flowers of *Matricaria recutita* (German chamomile) are in full bloom, the chamazulene is at its highest level, whereas farnesene and α-bisabolol decrease from the beginning of flowering and the bisabolol oxides increase.[34]

Another example is *Salvia officinalis*, which contains varying amounts of α-thujone depending on when it is harvested. It contains more after it has flowered, so it is better harvested before it flowers as the α-thujone is one of the more toxic constituents found in the oil.[35]

Considerable compositional differences could be found between older and younger leaves of sage (*S. officinalis*). The younger leaves were rich in β-pinene, bornyl acetate and sesquiterpenes, while the mature leaves contained three times more camphor and camphene.[36]

Integrity of the biomass

Until the 1980s, cut lavender and lavandin was dried in the field, a process taking about three days. The oil from this lavender exhibited the typical fine, floral aroma of lavender; however, the essential oil yield was lower compared with the yield obtained from fresh material. The quality of essential oil from freshly cut lavender is often greener and harsher, requiring some time to harmonise.[32]

Clary sage is another good example in which there is a significant chemical difference between the essential oil distilled from dried plant and fresh plant. Clary sage oil from fresh clary sage has a much higher linalool content and lower sclareol content compared with oil produced from dried clary sage biomass.[34]

Extraction method

The following examples demonstrate the need to specify the method of extraction when using essential oils for aromatherapy.

Ginger

Ginger oil is produced by distillation of the dried, unpeeled, ground rhizomes of *Zingiber officinale*.

A CO_2 ginger extract produced by supercritical fluid extraction contains the aromatic and pungent principles from the ginger rhizomes. The CO_2 extract is considered near to the true ginger flavour and pungency.

Much of the scent of ginger is due to the essential oil. However, its sharp, pungent taste is from the gingerols and shogaol found only in the CO_2 extract. Most pharmacological studies state that the gingerols and shogaols are responsible for most of ginger's therapeutic properties. It is, therefore, unlikely that the distilled ginger oil has many of the actions commonly cited in aromatherapy.

Rose

Three main products are obtained from roses: an essential oil, a concrete and an absolute. The essential oil is obtained by steam distillation of the whole flowers, the concrete by solvent extraction of the leaves and flowers, and the absolute by further extracting the concrete.[24]

The three products vary from different cultivars or species, and also vary from the same cultivar or species grown in geographically separate areas.[24]

Rose otto, or otto of roses, is generally accepted to apply to the oil distilled from *Rosa damascena* and it is usually prefixed by the country of origin.[24]

Rose absolute is obtained by solvent extraction. Holmes refers to the solvent extraction process as 'dry-cleaning' the plant. Solvent extraction produces a more complete plant extract. However, Holmes suggests that contact with the solvent, which is usually a petroleum ether, may result in minute traces of solvent in the final absolute. He also states that, from an energetic perspective, this may devitalise the essential oil through contact with a 'dead chemical substance'.[37]

Wabner suggests that rose absolute produced by solvent extraction is superior to rose otto because rose otto actually contains synthetic constituents that are not found in nature.[38]

He did this by doing a headspace analysis of a live rose and comparing the constituents with that of rose absolute of the same flower and rose otto of the same flower. While the chemical constituents of the rose absolute and live rose were the same, the rose otto oil contained several constituents such as rose oxide and damascenone, by-products of distillation.[38]

He also dispels the long-held belief that rose absolute should not be used in aromatherapy. To support his argument, he makes the following comments:

- Water is not more alive than other chemicals.
- Absolutes can be prepared residue controlled and even residue free.

Up to 50% of the constituents found in the living flower can be lost during distillation. All the water-soluble components remain in the flower water.[38]

Rose absolute from *R. centifolia* is an orange-yellow to brown-orange viscous liquid with a sweet, deep-rosy, very tenacious odour. The spicy notes are usually less pronounced, while the honey-like notes are similar to that of *R. damascena*.[5]

Rose absolute from *R. damascena* is an orange-yellow to brown-orange viscous liquid with a rich, warm, spicy-floral and very deep rose odour and a pronounced honey undertone.[5]

Rose otto obtained from *R. damascena* from Bulgaria is a pale yellow or slightly olive-yellow liquid, which has a warm, deep-floral, slightly spicy odour, immensely rich with traces of honey.[24]

Rose otto obtained from *R. centifolia* is a colourless to pale yellow liquid, sometimes with a greenish tinge when fresh. It has a deep, sweet, warm, rich, but less spicy odour than Bulgarian or Turkish rose otto oils.[24]

Ylang ylang

The large flowers of ylang ylang are subjected to fractional steam distillation or fractional water and steam distillation, thus yielding in succession, ylang ylang extra; ylang ylang 1st grade, ylang ylang 2nd grade and ylang ylang 3rd grade. A complete essential oil is available by non-fractional steam distillation of the flowers or by combining the first three fractions.

In the production of ylang ylang, the first fraction of the distillate is collected over several hours and becomes the 'extra' fraction. It is rich in oxygenated constituents but is poor in the high-boiling point sesquiterpenes.

The operators of the stills producing ylang ylang oils grade the different qualities by specific gravity and by odour. Since there is no agreed standard, the quality of a given grade varies from one producer to another.

Passing from ylang ylang extra to ylang ylang 1st and 2nd and 3rd grade, the following observations may be made:

- There are decreases in specific gravity, volatility, floral odour character, proportion of oxygenated constituents and price.
- There are increases in sesquiterpene content and oiliness of odour character.

From a perfumer's aspect, ylang ylang extra is the best grade and the most highly valued of the four grades. The traditional use of ylang ylang in aromatherapy as a relaxant and antidepressant indicates that the extra or 1st grade would be more suitable than the 3rd grade, as esters are the chemical constituents which have such qualities.

Constituents	Extra	1st grade	2nd grade	3rd grade
linalool	13.6%	18.6%	2.8%	1.0%
geranyl acetate	5.3%	5.9%	4.1%	3.5%
caryophyllene	1.7%	6.0%	7.5%	9.0%
p-cresyl methyl ether	16.5%	7.6%	1.8%	0.5%
methyl benzoate	8.7%	6.4%	2.3%	1.0%
benzyl acetate	25.1%	17.4%	7.0%	3.7%
benzyl benzoate	2.2%	5.3%	4.7%	4.3%
other sesquiterpenes	7.4%	28.8%	54.5%	97%

The chemical composition of the various grades of ylang ylang.[39]

Quality Assurance and GMP Standards

QMS and GMP

Following a quality management system (QMS) and good manufacturing practice (GMP) standards is critical for pharmaceutical and cosmetics manufacturing. These standards are often enforced by government agencies.

All suppliers of essential oils should have in place a strict QMS and follow GMP procedures. GMP describes a set of principles and procedures that, when followed, will ensure that the goods are of high quality. The Therapeutic Goods Administration provides us with an excellent definition of the basic tenets of GMP:

- Quality cannot be tested into a batch of a product.
- Quality must be built into each batch of product during all stages of the manufacturing process.[40]

A quality system should ensure that the products being manufactured are fit for the intended use, and do not place the end users at risk due to inadequate safety, quality and efficacy. Achieving these quality objectives requires a comprehensively designed and correctly implemented quality system incorporating GMP and Quality Risk Management. The quality system should be fully documented and its effectiveness monitored.[41]

To build quality into a product, manufacturers must be disciplined to:[42]

- ensure all the staff receive thorough and continuous training in the requirements of GMP
- develop strict specifications for all starting materials and finished products
- ensure all batches of starting materials and finished products are sampled and tested for compliance with their specifications, using sampling and test procedures
- establish approved procedures and operating instructions for manufacturing all products
- ensure all products are manufactured in a controlled-environment laboratory designed and built to the strict GMP code
- maintain a detailed batch record system. The batch numbers ensure complete accountability and traceability of the starting material – an essential oil can be traced from the time the manufacturer receives it in its bulk container all the way to the final bottle of essential oil which reaches you, the end user
- monitor the product stability of both starting materials and finished products
- maintain an active self-inspection program to maintain compliance with GMP requirements
- create quality systems and follow set procedures.
- ensure that goods are produced according to protocols accepted for registration
- have high quality standards
- have a responsibility to the end user of the product.

Total Quality Management (TQM)

ISO 9000 series of international standards includes requirements for quality systems which can be used to achieve common interpretation, development, implementation and application of a quality management system. ISO 9000 quality system standards require the development and implementation of a documented quality system.[43]

Nowadays, more and more essential oil suppliers are striving for certification from a quality management system in order to prove that their company meets international standards ISO 9000 to 9004 and 1400.[43]

Suppliers who possess the ISO certification are considered as qualified suppliers and their products are more readily accepted by their clients.[43]

Baser states that the TQM system has surpassed the former quality concepts such as quality control, which only checks the quality of the final product, and quality management, which controls the quality of the product and the process. The TQM philosophy can be summarised as follows: customer orientation, process control and constant improvement of quality.[43]

Certified organic

Those suppliers providing certified organic essential oils are audited by the organic certifying body. In Australia, the Australian Certified Organic Standard (ACOS) outlines the requirements for selling produce as certified organic in Australia, and the associated use of the 'Australian Certified Organic' or 'ACO Certified Organic' logos.[44]

The ACOS covers the basic requirements outlined in the Standards Australia Standard for Organic and Biodynamic Products (AS6000-2009), as well as the National Standard for Organic and Bio-Dynamic Products, while also being a linking document to key international organic standards.[44]

In order to attain and maintain organic certification, the supplier must undergo regular independently accredited audits to ensure that they are complying with the standards. This can only be achieved if the supplier has comprehensive QMS and GMP procedures in place.

Quality Control of Essential Oils

According to d'Acampora Zellner et al., the need to establish systematic investigation of essential oils began in the first half of the nineteenth century when the production of essential oils became industrialised. It is interesting to point out that in 1908, very little was known about the composition of essential oils.[45]

To certify the authenticity of an essential oil, it must undergo a series of tests such as:

- nonanalytical physical tests such as organoleptic tests, specific gravity, refractive index, optical rotation
- analytical chemical tests such as acid value and determination of esters
- analytical physical tests such as GC/MS.

While odour evaluation is purely subjective, it can be a very effective test for someone with an experienced nose.

Various physical measures carried out on essential oils allow them to be compared with official standards. The density, refractive index and optical rotation are specific values of a pure essential oil that can be measured to establish consistency with a corresponding standard. However, adulterations are not easily detected with these physical tests, therefore it is necessary to turn to chemical analysis. Gas chromatography linked to mass spectrometry (GC/MS) remains the most thorough analysis technique available, as it is able to separate, measure and identify chemical constituents found in essential oils.

ISO standards are available for many of the analytical chemical tests and for individual essential oils. Where ISO standards exist for an essential oil they have been listed in the relevant essential oil monograph. A selected list of standards issued to describe test methods includes:

- ISO 279: Essential Oils – Determination of Relative Density at 20°C
- ISO 280: Essential Oils – Determination of Refractive Index
- ISO 592: Essential Oils – Determination of Optical Rotation
- ISO 709: Essential Oils – Determination of Ester Value
- ISO 1202: Essential oils – Determination of 1,8-cineole content
- ISO 1241: Essential oils – Determination of Ester Value after Acetylation and Evaluation of Free Alcohols and Total Alcohols Content
- ISO 1242: Essential oils – Determination of Acid Value.

A full list of standards for essential oils can be obtained from ISO.

Nonanalytical Physical Tests

Organoleptic testing

Smell is one of the two senses that respond to the presence of certain chemicals in a qualitative way, and for this reason is known as a chemical sense. The other chemical sense is that of taste, which, together with smell, contributes to the complex sensations we know as flavour.

The organoleptic 'odour' test is considered one of the most important control criteria for testing the quality of essential oils. While it is a very subjective test, it is possible to gain much information about the sensory properties and qualities of the essential oil. Careful smelling requires one to adopt and follow strict procedures, which yield the required information.

Sensory evaluation should be conducted by expert noses. This ability can be gained after many years of tedious and systemic olfactive training. To an experienced nose, the evaporation pattern of an essential oil on a smelling strip can reveal information about its source, age, main components and even its authenticity.[43]

Here are some guidelines for adopting the correct approach to smelling.

How to evaluate an essential oil?

Essential oils should be evaluated in terms of:

- odour quality — what are the notes present?
- odour intensity
- changes of odour on evaporation
- diffusiveness of odour.

A sample of the essential oil is absorbed to a depth of about 1 cm on a labelled smelling strip, and a sample of the standard is similarly taken at the same time. The strips are smelt for several minutes to compare top notes, again after 20 minutes to compare middle notes, and after several hours to compare base notes. At each stage, the aired sample is compared for odour with a fresh dip.

Odour description and classification

As there are no instruments where odour can be measured qualitatively to obtain a numerical value, odour description and classifications are matters of opinion based on human judgement, and as such may be subject to all the vagaries of human nature.

When an attempt is made to describe the qualities of an odour, the difficulty immediately arises that there is a lack of words in the English language which are set aside for the sole purpose of naming individual sensations of smell.

Other senses have their own vocabularies of descriptive terms, which are known and understood sufficiently well for the sensations to which they give rise to be put into words and communicated to the majority of people with fair accuracy. Odours alone are nameless and are usually described by reference to the name of their sources, and by the use of terms belonging to the vocabularies of other senses which have been adopted by the English language for the purposes of odour description.

For example, the odour of expressed lemon oil may be described as:

- *citrus* in reference to the nature of its source
- *refreshing* which is suggestive of an invigorating effect
- *sweet* which is truly descriptive of a sensation of taste but borrowed from usage to express a pleasing kind of odour
- *sharp* which is a term associated with the sour taste of lemon juice, but derived from reference to a finely tapering point or edge.[46]

If one was to define the odour of lemon oil as 'citrus' without reference to the other qualifiers, then this description has failed to distinguish the odour of lemon oil from those of sweet orange, grapefruit, lime and bergamot, each of which is 'citrus-like' but different from one another.[46]

Another possible way of describing the odour of lemon oil might be to say that it has the smell of 'lemons'. This expression associates odour-sensations with the names of the corresponding odour sources. This is not only stating the obvious, but it only has meaning for those people who are familiar with the odour in question and who associate it with the same source-name.[46]

Arctander acknowledges the challenge of organoleptic testing:

> *Part of the 'romance' or 'thrill' in perfumery work lies in the fact that, not only are all the materials different in odors but hardly ever will two perfumers give identical descriptions of the same material or the same perfume ... An odor is not 'woody' just because someone says so; it will always have a particular print in your mind. Unfortunately, you are more or less unable to translate this print verbally to fellow perfumers, let alone to laymen.*[5]

However, from the vast multitude of different essential oil odours present, a structure or system needs to be established for grouping together similar odours under appropriate class-names. For the purpose of odour description, there are certain terms, which are in common use throughout the essential oil industry, of which there is a fairly uniform agreement among users of essential oils. These terms fall into two categories:

- odour types
- odour characteristics.

Odour types

Some of the commonly used terms to describe odour types are described below.

Anisic

The word 'anisic' refers to the odour of the flavour of aniseed. Licorice confectionaries are still commonly flavoured with aniseed, and is there is a belief that aniseed 'tastes' or smells like licorice. Licorice rhizomes have only a slight, pleasant odour and licorice extract almost none at all when cold.[46] Essential oils with an anisic odour include aniseed, dill seed and sweet fennel.

Balsamic

A balsam is an oily or resinous material exuded by a plant either as a product of its natural life-processes or in response to injury of its tissues. A considerable variety of odours occur among balsams, they are usually typified as sweet, warm odours reminiscent of natural vanilla. Balsamic materials are soft and sweet and are usually fixatives and base notes.[46] Essential oils with a balsamic odour include balsam of Peru, balsam of tolu, benzoin and styrax.

Camphoraceous

Camphor is a colourless, crystalline solid having an odour frequently said to be characteristic of the odour of camphor.[46] Essential oils with a camphoraceous odour include cajeput, eucalyptus and rosemary.

Citrus

Citrus odours have the characteristic odour of citrus fruits. While the odour of citrus oils are uniquely different, they all partake of the quality of stimulating freshness which forms an essential part of the odour profile of the citrus type of note.[46] Essential oils with a citrus odour include bergamot, lemon and cold-pressed lime.

Conifer

The refreshing, evergreen tang of the pine forest is essentially invigorating.[46] Essential oils with a coniferous odour include fir, pine and spruce.

Earthy

An earthy scent can be best described as the smell that permeates the air whenever sun-baked soil receives the beneficence of rainfall. There is evidence that the clays present in the soil trap molecules of odorous vapours from the air and then release them when the soil is wet. Essential oils with an earthy odour include patchouli, oakmoss and vetiver.[46]

Floral

The word 'floral' signifies the fragrance of a single flower or of a bouquet of flowers. The term may be useful to describe an odour sensation recalling a flower or flowers.[46] Essential oils with a floral odour include jasmine, rose and ylang ylang.

Fruity

The class of fruity notes comprises odours of the kinds given by whole edible fruits in their natural condition, by crushed fruits and by fruit juices.[46] Among essential constituents, esters are usually classified as having a powerful fruity note. Citrus notes are usually also classified as fruity.

Green

A green scent is described as having the odour of crushed green leaves. These oils have a breathtakingly natural fragrance quality.[46] Essential oils with a green odour include galbanum and violet leaf absolute.

Herbaceous

The word 'herbaceous' refers to plants that wither away after flowering, while 'herbs' are understood to be those plants that are used in medicines or for culinary purposes. They are somewhat pungent, green and very slightly woody in character.[46] Essential oils with a herbaceous odour include lavender, marjoram, rosemary and red thyme.

Minty

Typically associated with the menthol odour of peppermint or spearmint.

Peppery

A peppery odour will have a characteristically warm dry and spicy odour. It displays a certain pleasant freshness, coupled with a woody note and an 'edge' or 'tingle', which makes it delightfully unique among essential oils.[46] Essential oils such as black pepper and elemi have a peppery odour.

Spicy

Spicy odours give the impression of 'warm', 'hot' or 'pungent'. Everyday experience shows the sensory properties of individual spices to be distinctively different from one another, and each also has its own, particular applications in the culinary art.[46] Essential oils with a spicy odour include clove bud, cinnamon and ginger.

Woody

Odours described as woody notes are those of woods such as sandalwood or cedarwood. They are usually unobtrusive and long lasting.[46]

Odour characteristics

Odour characteristics are terms which are used when the odour cannot be clearly defined by use of the odour names and so it is necessary, if further progress is to be made, to extend the scheme of classification to include descriptive terms representing sensations of odour which are recognisable, but which cannot be associated with any particular physical odour source. The terms are referred to as odour characteristics.

Balanced

A balanced fragrance or blend is one in which neither component overrides the other.[46]

Diffusive

An aromatic material is diffusive if, when exposed to the air, it rapidly permeates the surroundings with its odour. Oils such as geranium, ylang ylang and violet leaf absolute show this property to a certain degree.[46]

Dry

Odours that give the impression of dryness in association with objects or surroundings are physically dry. Patchouli essential oil has a 'dry' odour. A variation of a 'dry' note is a 'powdery' effect.[46]

Flat

A 'flat' odour impression is one which is featureless and without character.[46]

Fresh

The description of fresh is applied to a fragrance implying a stimulating and enlivening effect. Green and citrus notes are suggestive of freshness.[46]

Harsh

A harsh odour is one, which is crude, discordant and imbalanced – a rough and raucous smell. Citronella and red thyme are two classic examples.[46]

Heavy

Among odours considered heavy are jasmine absolute, ylang ylang and tuberose. In undiluted concentrations, they permeate the air with a heavy, sombre aroma, which is often regarded as oppressive.[46]

Light

Of all the fragrance qualities, lightness of effect is the most delicate with regard to aesthetic appeal. Lightness of odour suggests high volatility. Neroli and a good quality lavender have such a quality.[46]

Musty

The dry smell of old books and papers is typical of what is meant by a 'musty' note.[46] Essential oils such as patchouli and vetiver have a musty smell.

Rich

A rich odour is described as one which is able to flood the mind with sensation beyond the limit of aesthetic endurance. With rich odours the impression is one of concentration of odours.[46] Oils of rose, ylang ylang and clove bud are known for their richness.

Sharp

Sharpness of odour implies a penetrating effect similar to that found in an excellent quality lemon oil.[46]

Smooth

Smoothness of odour is typical of soft, sweet fragrances having a balsamic effect.[46] Wood oils such as sandalwood or rosewood would have this character.

Sweet

When an odour is described as 'sweet', this is the kind of sensation which describes an experience of pleasure, it may also denote such terms as 'soft', 'fragrant' and 'delicate'.[46] Examples may include rose or aniseed oil.

Warm

The term 'warm' is commonly used for many odours which produce an impression of warmth. It may apply to essential oils such as ginger or wintergreen, which have the association of warming liniments.[46] It may also be used to describe jasmine and rose absolute, which impart the qualities of 'life' and 'warmth'.

Specific gravity

The specific gravity of a substance is defined as the ratio of the mass of a given volume of the substance to the mass of an equal amount of water at a stated temperature.

$$\text{SG (at stated temperature)} = \frac{\text{Mass of a given volume of substance}}{\text{Mass of an equal volume of water}}$$

To measure specific gravity, a clean, dry specific gravity bottle of a nominal capacity is accurately weighed. Let us assume that the mass of the bottle and stopper is m1 g.

The bottle is then filled with freshly boiled and cooled distilled water (usually at 20°C). The bottle and contents are then accurately weighed (mass = m2 g).

The bottle is then emptied and thoroughly cleaned before it is filled with the test sample material at the same temperature and weighed with its content (mass = m3 g).

$$\text{Then SG} = \frac{m3 - m1}{m2 - m1}$$

Nowadays the specific gravity is measured by means of an electronic specific gravity meter.

The specific gravity of an essential oil is specified by an upper and lower limit as shown below:[47]

Essential oil	Specific gravity at 20°C
Bergamot oil	0.882 to 0.886
Clove bud oil	01.047 to 1.06
Lavender oil	0.883 to 0.895

The range allows for natural variations that may occur. If the specific gravity measured does not fall within the limits specified, then there is a reason for concern about the quality of the oil. It may indicate that the essential oil has been adulterated with an inexpensive chemical constituent.

Refractive index

When light passes from one medium to a denser medium, the light is partially refracted, but most of it takes a different path by changing direction at the interface and entering the denser medium at a smaller angle to the normal at the point of incidence than the angle of incidence.

The refractive index is defined as the ratio of the sine wave of the angle of incidence to the sine of the angle of refraction, when a ray of light of defined wavelength passes from air into the essential oil kept at a constant temperature.[48]

The refractive index of an essential oil is specified by an upper and lower limit as shown below:[47]

Essential oil	Refractive index at 20°C
Bergamot oil	1.464 to 1.467
Clove bud oil	1.528 to 1.537
Lavender oil	1.459 to 1.464

The refractive quality of an essential oil is very responsive to small changes in the composition of the oil, so an essential oil whose refractive index does not fall within the specified range may indicate possible adulteration or an oil of poor quality.

The refractive index is measured using a refractometer, an instrument looking much like a microscope.

Optical rotation

The optical rotation of an essential oil refers to the ability of an essential oil to rotate a plane of polarised light. Light waves are analogous to the waves produced when a rope, secured at one end, is flicked at the other end and creates a wave, which moves perpendicular to the surface to which the rope is secured. The wave generated is referred to as a transverse wave.[49]

Ordinary white light consists of transverse waves of different wavelengths, corresponding to the colours of the rainbow, together with the shorter and longer wavelengths. The waves comprise rays of ordinary light.[49]

A polarimeter is used to determine the optical activity of the essential oil. It comprises a filter, which is able to select light waves within a narrow range of wavelengths. To ensure that only light travelling in one plane is used, a 'polaroid lens' is used. This light is referred to as polarised light.

Certain substances (including natural essential oils) have the ability to rotate polarised light in either a clockwise or anti-clockwise direction. The polarimeter is able to determine the angle at which the essential oil rotates the polarised light.

Those substances which cause anti-clockwise rotation are laevorotatory and are symbolised *l-* , and those which cause clockwise rotation are dextrorotatory and are symbolised *d-*.

The optical rotation of an essential oil is specified by an upper and lower limit as shown below:[47]

Essential oil	Optical rotation at 20°C
Bergamot oil	+12° to +24°
Clove bud oil	-0° 20′ to -2° 30′
Lavender oil	-3° to -10°

Optical activity is conferred upon a substance by the presence in its molecule of a carbon atom, which is bonded to four different atoms or chemical groups. Such a carbon atom is said to be asymmetric.[47]

The optical rotation of an essential oil is the summation of the optical rotation of its constituents in relation to their proportion in the essential oil. Variations of the proportion of optically active constituents will give rise to a change in the optical rotation of the essential oil. Measurement of the optical rotation is an important aid in detecting synthetic adulterations to the essential oil.[49,50]

Analytical Chemical Tests

Williams explains that there are two types of analytical tests:

- qualitative tests – providing information on what is present in the essential oil
- quantitative – providing information on how much of a constituent is present in the essential oil.[47]

Analytical chemical tests involve chemical reactions to obtain qualitative characteristics about the essential oil. Chemical tests include the determination of aldehydes, acid value, ester value (for calculation of esters and combined alcohols), ester value after acetylation (for calculation of free alcohols), carbonyl value and phenol content.[43]

Acid value

As essential oils age, the content of free acid in many essential oils tends to increase. This increase results mainly from the oxidation of aldehydes and hydrolysis of esters to form equivalent quantities of organic acids, which in turn catalyse the further hydrolysis of esters.[47]

The acid value is a numerical value equivalent to the number of milligrams of potassium hydroxide required to neutralise the free acids present in 1 g of essential oil.[43]

Determination of esters

Essential oils such as lavender are highly valued for their natural ester content. An ester value lower than that indicated in the specification is often an indication of poor quality.[47]

However, there are no chemicals which react completely and quickly with esters. Potassium hydroxide reacts with acids, so to determine the amount of esters in an essential oil we need to understand that:

- water will hydrolyse esters to produce the equivalent amounts of free acids
- potassium hydroxide will catalyse hydrolysis and immediately neutralise the resulting free acids.[47]

Therefore, the ester value is the number of milligrams of potassium hydroxide required to neutralise the acids liberated by hydrolysis of the esters present in 1 g of essential oil.[43]

The ester value after acetylation is the numerical equivalent to the number of milligrams of potassium hydroxide required to neutralise the acids liberated by the hydrolysis of 1 g of the acetylated essential oil.[43]

Analytical Physical Tests

Instrumental techniques include chromatographic and spectroscopic techniques or their combinations.

Analytical physical tests of essential oil are able to:

- separate the constituents of the essential oil with absolute minimum of alteration to the composition of the molecular structure of the individual constituents. This usually involves gas-liquid chromatography and other forms of chromatography
- eucidate the molecular structure of the individual, separated constituents of essential oils. This usually involves mass spectrometry and infrared spectrophotometry.[47]

Baser lists the range of instrumental techniques often used for the analysis of essential oils.[43]

Chromatographic techniques

- Column chromatography (CC)
- Thin layered chromatography (TLC)
- Gas-liquid chromatography (GLC or GC)
- High pressure liquid chromatography (HPLC)
- Medium pressure liquid chromatography (MPLC)
- Supercritical fluid chromatography (SFE)
- Size exclusion chromatography (SEC)

Spectrophotometric techniques

- Ultraviolet and visible spectrophotometry (UV/ VIS)
- Infrared spectrophotometry (IR)

Spectroscopic techniques

- Mass spectrometry (MS)
- Nuclear magnetic resonance spectroscopy (NMR)

Combined techniques

- Gas chromatography/mass spectrometry (GC/MS)
- Liquid chromatography/mass spectrometry (LC/MS)
- Gas chromatography/fourier-transform infrared spectrophotometry (GC/FT-IR)
- Gas chromatography/fourier-transform infrared spectrophotometry/Mass spectrometry (GC/FT-IR/MS)
- Gas chromatography/atomic emission detector (GC/AED)
- Gas chromatography/isotope ratio mass spectrometry (GC/IRMS)
- Multidimensional gas chromatography (MDGC)

Thin layer chromatography

TLC was once commonly used for essential oil analysis; however, this technique is rarely used nowadays due to poor separation power of complex essential oils. Nevertheless, it can still be useful for the evaluation of simple mixtures.[43]

Gas-liquid chromatography (GLC)

GLC is the most important technique used nowadays for the separation of essential oil constituents. Baser states that, thanks to the advances in technology, there is now a wide range of column packing materials and detectors.[43]

In GLC, mixtures of gases and vapours are separated into their constituents. GLC equipment is able to ensure that every single molecule in the oil is vaporised, but not too quickly. A detector is then able to quantify the amount of constituent present and this is recorded on a graph, which is made up of a series of peaks. Each peak represents one component. The area under the peak is then used to help determine the percentage of the constituent making up the essential oil.[51]

While the GLC is extremely accurate, it has still not told us what each peak is. This is the job of either infra-red spectrophotometry or mass spectrometry.

Mass spectrometry

Mass spectrometry can determine the molecular mass of each molecule, thus identifying each constituent of the essential oil.[51]

GC/MS is a sophisticated technique whereby the MS detects the constituents that have been separated by a GC. The isolated compounds are illustrated in the form of a series of peaks in a total ion chromatogram (TIC). Modern GC/MS equipment has computerised libraries and advanced search systems. Mass spectrum of each component can be detected and then searched through thousands of mass spectra contained in the computerised library for identification. In the case of new compounds, analysis of fragmentation data gives a clue to its chemical structure.[43]

Infra-red spectrophotometry

The atoms in molecules are not rigidly bonded together, but tend to vibrate relative to one another in accordance with their mass, the distances apart, the proximity of other atoms and the flexibility of the bonds holding the atoms together.

Infra-red spectrophotometry involves measuring the frequencies at which the molecules vibrate in the presence of infra-red radiation. The infra-red spectrum of a material shows the frequencies at which its molecules absorb infra-red radiation. These are the frequencies at which the molecules are induced to resonate, and are therefore the characteristic frequencies of vibration of the different atoms and group of atoms in the molecules.[51]

Knowing these frequencies which are measured by a spectrophotometer, the analyst can:

- determine the chemical nature of the material under investigation
- determine the quality of the material relative to a standard sample.[51]

References

1. Holmes P. *Aromatica: a clinical guide to essential oil therapeutics – Vol. I.* Singing Dragon, London, 2016.
2. Delbridge A et al. *Macquarie dictionary.* 3rd edn. Macquarie Library, North Ryde, 1997.
3. Brud W. *Blending and compounding.* AROMA'93 Conference Proceedings. Aromatherapy Publications, 1993: 44-54.
4. Schmidt E, Wanner J. *Adulteration of essential oils.* In Baser KHC, Buchbauer G. eds. *Handbook of essential oils – science, technology and applications.* 2nd edn. CRC Press, Boca Raton, 2016: 707-745.
5. Arctander S. *Perfume and flavor materials of natural origin.* Allured Publishing, Carol Stream, 1994.
6. Wabner D. *Purity and pesticides.* The International Journal of Aromatherapy, 1993; 5(2): 27-29.
7. Garland SM, Menary RC, Oliver GS. *Determination of pesticide minimum residue limits in essential oils – report No 4.* Rural Industries Research and Development Corporation, Barton, 2004. RIRDC Publication No 04/104.
8. Tisserand R, Young R. *Essential oil safety.* 2nd edn. Churchill Livingstone, Edinburgh, 2014.
9. Centers for Disease Control and Prevention. *Phthalates.* Retrieved Nov 11, 2017, from https://www.cdc.gov/biomonitoring/phthalates_factsheet.html
10. Di Bella G et al. *Contamination of Italian citrus essential oils: presence of phthalate esters.* Journal of Agricultural and Food Chemistry, 1999; 47(3): 1009-1012. doi: 10.1021/jf980735b.
11. Wabner D. *The peroxide value – a new tool for the quality control of essential oils.* The International Journal of Aromatherapy, 2002; 12(3): 142-144.
12. Orafidiya LO. *The effect of autoxidation of lemon-grass oil on its antibacterial activity.* Phytotherapy Research, 1993; 7(3): 269-271.
13. Pénoël D. *Winter shield.* The International Journal of Aromatherapy, 1992; 4(4): 10-12.
14. Burfield T, Kirkham K. *The 'therapeutic grade' essential oil disinformation campaign.* Cropwatch Newsletter, August 2007. Retrieved from http://www.cropwatch.org.uk/newsletaug07.pdf
15. Price S, Price L. *Aromatherapy for health professionals.* 4th edn. Churchill Livingstone, Edinburgh, 2012.
16. Harris B. *Editorial.* International Journal of Aromatherapy, 2006; 16(2): 55.
17. Sadgrove N, Jones G. *A contemporary introduction to essential oils: chemistry, bioactivity and prospects for Australian agriculture.* Agriculture, 2015; 5(1): 48-102. doi: 10.3390/agriculture5010048.
18. Fleischner AM. *Plant extracts to accelerate healing and reduce inflammation.* Cosmetic Toiletries 1985; 100: 45-58.
19. Carle R et al. *The medicinal use of Matricaria flos.* British Journal of Phytotherapy, 1992; 2(4): 147-153.
20. Lavabre M. *Aromatherapy workbook.* Healing Arts Press, Rochester, 1997.
21. Lawless J. *The encyclopaedia of essential oils.* Element Books, Shaftesbury, 1992.
22. Khan I, Abourashed E. *Leung's encyclopedia of common natural ingredients used in food, drugs and cosmetics.* 3rd edn. John Wiley & Sons, New Jersey, 2010.
23. Davis P. *Aromatherapy: an A-Z.* 2nd edn. C.W. Daniel Company, Saffron Walden, 1999.
24. Weiss EA. *Essential oil crops.* CAB International, Wallingford, 1997.
25. Lawrence BM. *Essential oils 1976-1978.* Allured Publishing, Wheaton, 1979.
26. Blumenthal M et al. *The complete German commission E monographs: therapeutic guide to herbal medicine.* American Botanical Council, Austin, 1998.
27. Lawrence BM. *Essential oils: from agriculture to chemistry.* The World of Aromatherapy III Conference Proceedings, NAHA, 2000; 8-26.
28. Bowles J. *The chemistry of aromatherapeutic oils.* 3rd edn. Allen & Unwin, Crows Nest, 2003.
29. Tisserand R, Balacs T. *Essential oil safety.* Churchill Livingstone, Edinburgh, 1995.
30. Schnaubelt K. *Advanced aromatherapy.* Healing Arts Press, Rochester, 1995.
31. Soulier J. *Properties and indications: Thymus vulgaris.* Aromatherapy Records, 1995; 1: 50-53.
32. Schmidt E. *Production of essential oils.* In Baser KHC, Buchbauer G. eds. *Handbook of essential oils – science, technology and applications.* 2nd edn. CRC Press, Boca Raton, 2016: 127-164.
33. Simon J et al. *Water stress-induced alterations in essential oil content and composition of sweet basil.* The Journal of Essential Oil Research, 1992; 4(1): 71-75.
34. Franz C, Novak J. *Sources of essential oils.* In Baser KHC, Buchbauer G. eds. *Handbook of essential oils – science, technology and applications.* 2nd edn. CRC Press, Boca Raton, 2016: 43-86.
35. Piccaglia R. *Effect of mineral fertilisers on the composition of Salvia officinalis oil.* The Journal of Essential Oil Research, 1995; 7(2): 73.
36. Németh-Zámboriné E. *Natural variability of essential oils components.* In Baser KHC, Buchbauer G. eds. *Handbook of essential oils – science, technology and applications.* 2nd edn. CRC Press, Boca Raton, 2016: 87-125.

37. Holmes P. *Rose – the water goddess.* The International Journal of Aromatherapy, 1994; 6(2): 8-11.
38. Wabner D. *A rose is a rose is a rose oil.* 2nd Australasian Aromatherapy Conference, Sydney, 1998.
39. Lawrence BM. *Essential oils 1981-1987.* Allured Publishing, Wheaton, 1989.
40. Therapeutic Goods Administration. *Good manufacturing practice – an overview.* Retrieved Jan 4, 2018, from https://www.tga.gov.au/good-manufacturing-practice-overview
41. *Guide to good manufacturing practice for medicinal products – part I.* Pharmaceutical Inspection Co-operation Scheme, Geneva, 2017.
42. Battaglia S. *GMP, Quality control and quality assurance.* Aromatherapy Today, 1996; 3: 1-21.
43. Baser KHC. *Analysis and quality assessment of essential oils.* In Tuley De Silva K. ed. *A manual on the essential oil industry.* United Nations Industrial Development Organization, Vienna, 1995: 155-177.
44. *Australian certified organic standard 2016 v.4.* Australian Organic, Nundah, 2017.
45. d'Acampora Zellner B et al. *Analysis of essential oils.* In Baser KHC, Buchbauer G. eds. *Handbook of essential oils – science, technology and applications.* 2nd edn. CRC Press, Boca Raton, 2016: 195-228.
46. *Diploma perfumery correspondence course notes. Part 1: Odours and the sense of smell: odour description and classification.* Perfumery Education Centre, London, 1980.
47. Williams DG. *The chemistry of essential oils.* Micelle Press, Weymouth, 1996.
48. International Organization for Standardization. *Essential oils – Determination of refractive index.* (ISO 280-1976). 1976.
49. Clarke S. *Essential chemistry for safe aromatherapy.* Churchill Livingstone, London, 2002.
50. International Organization for Standardization. *Essential oils – Determination of optical rotation.* (ISO 592-1981). 1981.
51. *Diploma Perfumery Correspondence Course Notes. Part 9: Quality control and assurance.* Perfumery Education Centre, London, 1980.

Safety

CHAPTER 6

Contents

Introduction

This chapter establishes a framework for the safe use of essential oils within the practice of aromatherapy, and helps us make sense of the often-conflicting information and perceptions associated with the safety of essential oils.

Burfield states that perceptions of safety in aromatherapy fall into two categories:

- those who suggest that essential oils have very little or no risks or hazards
- those who adapt a more cautious approach where scientific data is not sufficient; for example, use of oils during pregnancy.[1]

Holmes suggests that we should consider essential oils as natural extracts from plants, and their safe use is the same as that for plants and foods from which they are extracted. We should free ourselves of the negatively biased approach of the aromatic chemical industry. He claims that much of the negative perception regarding the safe use of essential oils has been falsely exaggerated by the food, perfume and pharmaceutical industries. However, we need to have a good understanding of the safe use of essential oils grounded in science and facts.[2]

Guba states it is understandable that we err on the side of caution; however, exaggerated statements regarding essential oil safety have led to the common perception that the therapeutic use of essential oils is extremely risky.[3]

Holmes suggests that we should consider the following issues when considering essential oil safety:

- Essential oils are safe when selected and administered appropriately.
- Essential oils need to be administered with greater care than herbs or foods when used therapeutically as they are isolated plant extracts.
- Some essential oils need to be used with caution.[2]

I have used the 2nd edition of *Essential Oil Safety* by Robert Tisserand & Rodney Young as the benchmark for essential oil safety. This book is by far the most comprehensive resource available, providing us with an up-to-date and in-depth treatise on essential oil safety.

Some of the factors that need to be considered to ensure the safe use of essential oils include:

- quality of the essential oils being used
- packaging and labelling
- compliance with relevant legislative and regulatory bodies
- chemical composition of essential oils
- identifying essential oil hazards.

Quality of Essential Oils

The use of the highest quality essential oils is of the utmost importance in ensuring that aromatherapy is practised safely. Most of the essential oils produced are by the fragrance or flavouring industries. It is therefore important that essential oils that are used in aromatherapy meet the standards set by the aromatherapy industry, and not by other industries using essential oils.

To ensure that the highest quality essential oils are used in aromatherapy it is necessary to:

- use genuine essential oils
- avoid using essential oils that are subject to contamination and adulteration
- avoid using essential oils that have undergone degradation.

If these criteria are not satisfied, not only is the efficacy of the essential oil undermined, but there is also a higher risk that the essential oil may be hazardous or not safe to use. The key concerns regarding the quality of essential oils for use in aromatherapy are examined in *Chapter 5 – Quality*.

Packaging and Labelling

Packaging

Essential oil packaging should be such that it minimises the risks to the end user of essential oils. Accidental ingestion of essential oils by children is one of the biggest concerns. Therefore, it is imperative that the type of packaging used reduces such risks. Essential oils in open neck bottles probably represent the greatest risk of accidental ingestion in aromatherapy today. The use of the integral dropper-dispenser is very important in limiting the quantity of essential oil that a child could accidentally ingest. As many essential oils are sold undiluted, it is also important to consider the following:

- Do the essential oil bottles carry the appropriate warning and safety instructions?
- Are the essential oils packaged according to the current legislation of the country in which they are being sold or of any industry standard?
- What information should be on the label?

Labelling

Essential oil labels should contain the following information:

- proper identification of the essential oil such as botanical name, part of the plant and chemotype where applicable
- the amount of the essential oil in the bottle
- the concentration of the essential oil – normally expressed in mL/mL
- indication of useful shelf life of the essential oil
- storage conditions and precautions
- a unique batch number to ensure traceability to the original source of the essential oil
- clear instructions for the use of the essential oil
- first aid procedure if the essential oil is scheduled as a poison.

Regulatory Issues

The regulatory issues raised in this section are valid at the time of writing.

A recent review of the regulatory status of herbal drugs/products was conducted and it was found that there is a lack of harmonisation in the regulatory requirements of herbal products internationally.[4]

Food & Drug Administration

In the United States, herbal medicinal products can be prescription drugs or over-the-counter drugs. However, obtaining a licence to promote herbal products for medicinal use requires rigorous testing, including three distinct phases of clinical trials to ensure safety and efficacy, and very close scrutiny by the Food and Drug Administration (FDA).[4]

In August 2015, the FDA published a draft of the guidelines 'botanical drug development', which will replace the previous guideline of June 2004.[5] When herbal products are licensed as drugs, they must comply with the same strict regulated conditions as conventional pharmaceuticals.[6] The FDA considers most essential oils as being GRAS (generally recognized as safe) approved. GRAS is a term used by the FDA to define a substance that can be added to food and has been evaluated by experts.[6]

FDA regulates dietary supplements under the Dietary Supplement Health and Education Act of 1994. These do not require premarket approval, and it is the responsibility of the marketer to ensure the safety and labelling compliance of their products with the regulations. The claims must comply with the regulatory guidelines issued by the FDA.[4]

Therapeutic Goods Administration

In Australia, the Therapeutic Goods Administration (TGA) regulates herbal products under a category of complementary medicine.

Complementary medicines that do not require medical supervision are permitted, and need to be registered on the Australian Register for Therapeutic Goods (ARTG) before marketing. Low-risk medicines must be listed, while medicines for comparatively higher-risk therapeutic conditions require registration on the ARTG. Only evidence-based claims which are entered on the ARTG are permitted.[6]

Most essential oils fall under a low-risk or medium-risk claim. A low-risk claim would include health maintenance, relief of symptoms (not referring to a named disease or disorder) or claims for traditional syndromes and actions. Typically, the wording of a low-risk claim should be 'This (traditional) medicine has been traditionally used for (indication)'.[7]

The type of evidence required includes one of the four following sources that demonstrate adequate support for the indications claimed:[7]

- TGA approved pharmacopoeia
- TGA approved monograph
- three independent written histories of use in the classical or traditional medical literature
- availability through any country's government public dispensaries for the indication claimed.

A medium-risk claim would include health enhancement, reduction in frequency of a discrete event, reduction of risk of a disease, disorder or condition, aids or assists in the management of a named symptom, disease or disorder, relief of symptoms of a named disease, disorder or condition.[8]

Typically, the wording of a medium-risk claim should be 'This (traditional) medicine has been used for (indication)'.[7]

The type of evidence required includes two of the four following sources that demonstrate adequate support for the indications claimed:[6]

- TGA approved pharmacopoeia
- TGA approved monograph
- three independent written histories of use in the classical or traditional medical literature
- availability through any country's government public dispensaries for the indication claimed.

Essential oils that are supplied solely as starting material to practitioners are generally exempt from the requirement to be included in the ARTG before supply. This means that oils can be supplied only for the purposes of being subsequently dispensed or compounded for a particular person, for therapeutic application to that person.[8]

European Union

There are two ways of registering herbal medicinal products with the European Medicines Agency (EMA).

The first is a full market authorisation by submission of a dossier, which provides the information on quality, safety and efficacy of the medicinal product. This must include physico-chemical, biological or microbial tests, and pharmacological, toxicological and clinical trials data. This is under the directive 2001/83/EC.[4]

However, for traditional herbal products, which do not require medical supervision and where the evidence of long traditional use of the product exists, and adequate scientific literature to demonstrate a well-established medicinal use cannot be provided, a simplified procedure under directive 2004/24/EC exists.[4]

In the second way, the evidence of traditional use is accepted as evidence of efficacy of the product. However, authorities may still ask for evidence to support safety. Quality control requirements also require physico-chemical and microbiological tests to be included in the product specification. The product should comply with the quality standards in relevant pharmacopoeias of the member state or the European Pharmacopoeia. The bibliographic evidence should support that the product has been in medicinal use for at least 30 years, including at least 15 years within the EU. If the product has been in the EU for less than 15 years, the application for traditional use registration is referred to the Committee on Herbal Medicinal Products.[4]

The EMA has declared that essential oils are active substances in herbal medicinal products for both human and veterinary use, whereas in the United States, the FDA considers essential oils as either cosmetics or drugs, depending on their intended use. FDA decisions concerning the regulation of essential oils are made on a case-by-case basis according to the request of the applicant.[5]

National Poisons Scheduling Committee of Australia

Some essential oils must comply with the Standard for the Uniform Scheduling of Medicine and Poisons (SUSMP), and will require specific cautions and safety instructions. In Australia, the TGA is responsible for maintaining these standards. Some essential oils are classified in Schedule 5 or Schedule 6:

> *Schedule 5: Caution – Substance with a low potential to cause harm, the extent of which can be reduced through the use of distinctive packaging with simple warnings and safety directions on the label.*
>
> *Schedule 6: Poison – Substances with a moderate potential for causing harm, the extent of which can be reduced through the use of distinctive packaging with strong warnings and safety directions on the label.*[9]
>
> *It must be emphasised that an essential oil is not necessarily scheduled on the basis of toxicity. While toxicity is one of the factors considered,*

other factors include purpose of use, potential for abuse and the safety in use.

Any essential oil scheduled as a poison is required by Australian law to carry a label giving the appropriate first aid advice if poisoning occurs. This advice is as follows:

For advice, contact a Poisons Information Centre (Australia 131 126) or a doctor (at once).[9]

At the time of writing, the following essential oils require specific cautions, first aid instructions or are classified as poisons.

Schedule 5 essential oils

Anise oil, except when it is packaged in containers having a nominal capacity of 50 mL or less fitted with a restrictive flow insert; is labelled with the following warning: KEEP OUT OF REACH OF CHILDREN; and in preparations containing 50% or less of anise oil.[9]

Basil oil, except when it is packaged in containers having a nominal capacity of 25 mL or less fitted with a restrictive flow insert; is labelled with the following warning: KEEP OUT OF REACH OF CHILDREN; and in preparations containing 5% or less of methyl chavicol.[9]

Bergamot oil, except when it is steam distilled or rectified; in preparations for internal use; in preparations containing 0.4% or less of bergamot oil; in soaps or bath and shower gels that are washed off the skin; or when packed in containers with labels that state that application to the skin may increase sensitivity to sunlight.[9]

Camphor as a natural component in essential oils containing 10% or less camphor, except when it is in containers having a nominal capacity of 25mL or less fitted with a restrictive flow insert; is labelled with the following warning: KEEP OUT OF REACH OF CHILDREN and NOT TO BE TAKEN; in rosemary oil, sage oil (Spanish), or lavandin oils; or in preparations containing 2.5% or less of camphor.[9]

Cassia oil and **cinnamon bark oil,** except in food additives or in preparations containing 2% or less of these essential oils.[9]

Clove oil and **eugenol** for topical use in the mouth in a pack containing 5 mL or less of clove oil or eugenol, except in preparations containing 25% or less of clove oil or eugenol.[9]

Lemon oil, except when it is steam distilled or rectified; in preparations for internal use; in preparations containing 0.05% or less of lemon oil; in soaps or bath and shower gels that are washed off the skin; or when packed in containers with labels that state that application to the skin may increase sensitivity to sunlight.[9]

Lime oil, except when it is steam distilled or rectified; in preparations for internal use; in preparations containing 0.5% or less of lime oil; in soaps or bath and shower gels that are washed off the skin; or when packed in containers with labels that state that application to the skin may increase sensitivity to sunlight.[9]

Marjoram oil, except when it is packaged in containers having a nominal capacity of 50 mL or less fitted with a restrictive flow insert; is labelled with the following warning: KEEP OUT OF REACH OF CHILDREN; or in preparations containing 50% or less of marjoram oil.[9]

Methyl salicylate in preparations containing 25% or less of methyl salicylate.[9]

Nutmeg oil, except when it is packaged in containers having a nominal capacity of 25 mL or less fitted with a restrictive flow insert; is labelled with the following warning: KEEP OUT OF REACH OF CHILDREN; or in preparations containing 50% or less of nutmeg oil.[9]

Bitter orange oil, except when it is steam distilled or rectified; in preparations for internal use; in preparations containing 1.4% or less of bitter orange oil; in soaps or bath and shower gels that are washed off the skin; or when packed in containers with labels that state that application to the skin may increase sensitivity to sunlight.[9]

Thyme oil, except when it is packaged in containers having a nominal capacity of 25 mL or less fitted with a restrictive flow insert; is labelled with the following warning: KEEP OUT OF REACH OF CHILDREN or in preparations containing 50% or less of thyme oil.[9]

Schedule 6 essential oils

Bay oil, except when it is packaged in containers having a nominal capacity of 15 mL or less fitted with a restrictive flow insert; is labelled with the following warning: KEEP OUT OF REACH OF CHILDREN and NOT TO BE TAKEN; or in preparations containing 25% or less of bay oil.[9]

Cajeput oil, except when it is packaged in containers having a nominal capacity of 15 mL or less fitted with a restrictive flow insert; is labelled with the following warning: KEEP OUT OF REACH OF CHILDREN and NOT TO BE TAKEN; or in preparations containing 25% or less of cajeput oil.[9]

Cineole, except when it is packaged in containers having a nominal capacity of 15 mL or less fitted with a restrictive flow insert; is labelled with the following warning: KEEP OUT OF REACH OF CHILDREN and NOT TO BE TAKEN; or in preparations containing 25% or less of cineole; or in rosemary oil or white camphor oil.[9]

Cinnamon leaf oil, except when it is packaged

in containers having a nominal capacity of 15 mL or less fitted with a restrictive flow insert; is labelled with the following warning: KEEP OUT OF REACH OF CHILDREN and NOT TO BE TAKEN; or in preparations containing 25% or less of cinnamon leaf oil.[9]

Clove oil and **eugenol,** except when it is packaged in containers having a nominal capacity of 15 mL or less fitted with a restrictive flow insert; is labelled with the following warning: KEEP OUT OF REACH OF CHILDREN and NOT TO BE TAKEN; or in preparations containing 25% or less of clove oil or eugenol.[9]

Eucalyptus oil, except when it is packaged in containers having a nominal capacity of 15 mL or less fitted with a restrictive flow insert; is labelled with the following warning: KEEP OUT OF REACH OF CHILDREN and NOT TO BE TAKEN; or in preparations containing 25% or less of eucalyptus oil.[9]

Melaleuca oil (tea tree oil), except when it is packaged in containers having a nominal capacity of 15 mL or less fitted with a restrictive flow insert; is labelled with the following warning: KEEP OUT OF REACH OF CHILDREN and NOT TO BE TAKEN; or in preparations containing 25% or less of melaleuca oil.[9]

Pennyroyal oil, except when it is packaged in containers having a nominal capacity of 15 mL or less fitted with a restrictive flow insert; is labelled with the following warning: KEEP OUT OF REACH OF CHILDREN and NOT TO BE TAKEN; or in preparations containing 4% or less of *d*-pulegone.[9]

Sassafras oil or **safrole,** except for internal use; or in preparations containing 1% or less of safrole.[9]

Sage (Dalmatian) oil, except when it is packaged in containers having a nominal capacity of 15 mL or less fitted with a restrictive flow insert and child-resistant closure; is labelled with the following warning: KEEP OUT OF REACH OF CHILDREN and NOT TO BE TAKEN; or in preparations containing 4% or less of thujone.[9]

GRAS status

Most essential oils have GRAS status. This status has been granted by the Flavor and Extract Manufacturers Association (FEMA) and the FDA for food use. This was reviewed in 1996 after evaluation of the expert panel of the FEMA. The assessment was based on data of exposure. Lis-Balchin points out that most flavour ingredients are used at less than 100 ppm. Predictions regarding safety are assessed from data on their structurally related groups.[10]

Harris states that some essential oil suppliers are now promoting their essential oils as having GRAS status, implying that they are therapeutic quality and that they are safe to use internally.[11]

The fact is that almost all essential oils have GRAS status because they are commonly used in food flavouring. Lis-Balchin states that the concentrations used in food flavouring are extremely low; therefore, just because an essential oil has GRAS status, you should not infer that it is safe to use in aromatherapy and it definitely does not imply that it can be ingested.[10]

Material safety data sheet (MSDS)

Legislation around the world requires suppliers and manufacturers of essential oils to provide material safety data sheets. Material safety data sheets are required when the user intends to use that essential oil at work or if the substance is classified as dangerous. In most circumstances, the information on the label should suffice.

The National Occupational Health and Safety Commission (NOHSC) has published a national code of practice for the preparation of MSDSs. The MSDS includes information on the composition of the essential oil, analytical data, health hazards, first aid procedures, fire and explosive hazards, environmental implications, handling procedures and transportation, and labelling information.[12]

Burfield recommends that aromatherapists should have MSDS documentation on hand in their work setting (clinic) as it is a standard occupational health and safety requirement.[13]

A typical MSDS for an essential oil can be found in Appendix 4.

The role of RIFM and IFRA

The Research Institute for Fragrance Materials (RIFM) was established in 1966 by the American Fragrance Manufacturing Association. Its purpose is to gather and analyse scientific data, engage in testing and evaluation, distribute information, cooperate with official agencies and encourage uniform safety standards related to fragrance materials and essential oils.[14]

All of the RIFM's research is reviewed by an independent expert panel made up of dermatologists, toxicologists, environmental and respiratory scientists who have no commercial ties to the fragrance industry.[14]

Bickers et al. state that in the early years the expert panel was predominantly experts in the field of dermatology with expertise in skin toxicology. However, with a growing awareness of the potential for transdermal adsorption, inhalation and ingestion of fragrance materials which can contribute to systemic exposure and toxicity, it has become necessary to expand the panel's focus to include pharmacokinetics, toxicokinetics, toxicology, pathology and environmental science.[15]

The RIFM independent expert panel's conclusions form the basis for the standards set by the International Fragrance Association (IFRA). IFRA was founded in 1973 in Geneva to represent the collective interests of the fragrance industry. Its main purpose is to promote the safe enjoyment of fragrances worldwide. Many of those in the fragrance industry will adopt the recommendations of IFRA. IFRA maintains a database listing all essential oils that may be considered restricted materials based on their chemical composition. It also identifies the essential oil constituents that are responsible for the essential oil being considered a restricted material.[16]

Protocol for Conducting a Safety Assessment

Assessment of exposure

Bickers et al. explain that the safety assessment of a fragrance material is quite complex. Estimates of dermal exposure are crucial depending on the type of finished product being used. For example, is it a 'wash-off' or 'leave-on' product? Consideration is also given to how often the end consumer may be exposing themselves to the fragrance product. The total systemic exposure to a specific fragrance ingredient is usually expressed as mg/kg/body weight/day based on a 60 kg adult.[15]

Dermatological considerations

Dermatological studies often include evaluation of irritant dermatitis, allergic contact dermatitis, phototoxicity and photoallergy. It is essential that these evaluations be done on humans.[15]

Transdermal penetration and cutaneous metabolism

Many fragrance materials including essential oils may undergo significant percutaneous absorption into the systemic circulation. For example, the dermal absorption of some fragrance materials such as phenylethyl alcohol and coumarins is quite significant.[15]

Some fragrance materials are metabolised in the skin. Such metabolism may alter the biological activity of absorbed chemicals, particularly when compared to other routes of administration. It has been suggested that the dermal allergic responses linked to some fragrance materials may be related to their cutaneous transformation to bioactive metabolites capable of forming adducts with skin proteins able to function as allergens.[15]

Toxicological considerations

Toxicological evaluation of a fragrance material may include acute and chronic toxicity, mutagenicity, dermal irritation, skin sensitisation, photoirritation, photoallergy, developmental and reproductive toxicity, and carcinogenicity.[15]

Metabolism and toxicokinetic considerations

Knowledge of drug metabolism permits prediction of the likely metabolic fate of a fragrance or essential oil based on its chemistry. This is done by identifying the functional groups present in the fragrance and the metabolic options that these can present. For the majority of essential oil constituents such as esters, aldehydes and alcohols, it is possible to make reasonable predictions on their metabolic fate and detoxification process.[15]

Environmental consequences

Up to 60% of all fragrance materials used in soaps, fabric softeners, cleansers and detergents may end up in the environment by release into the water sewage system. There are two aspects of environmental concern that are addressed by the RIFM expert panel. The first is the potential ecological damage, with concerns for organisms in the water and soil, and emphasis on bioconcentration and biodegradation. The other concern is the unintended exposure of humans to fragrance materials from potential environmental contact. Modern analytical methodologies can assist in identification of fragrance materials in the environment, and it is important to determine whether there is any risk to human health from such exposure.[15]

Bickers et al. provide a detailed description of the approach used by the RIFM expert panel to examine all these factors in order to make a reliable determination of safe use under intended conditions.[15]

Chemical Composition

Essential oils may have 100 or more different essential oil constituents, which in combination give the essential oil its unique odour, therapeutic properties and, in some cases, its toxicity or potential hazards.

Aldehydes

Aldehydes can cause skin irritation and allergic reactions.[17,18]

Cinnamic aldehyde found in cinnamon bark oil is reported to be a dermal irritant and sensitiser. IFRA recommends that cinnamic aldehyde can be used at 0.05% maximum on the skin. Tisserand & Young recommend that the maximum percentage of cinnamon bark for dermal application should be 0.07%.[17]

Citral has been found to have an irritating effect on the skin. When essential oils such as may chang or lemongrass which are high in citral are blended in a 50:50 mix with essential oils such as lemon or sweet orange (both high in limonene, a monoterpene hydrocarbon), a quenching effect was observed. It has been suggested that the *d*-limonene is responsible for neutralising the irritancy effects of citral.[19]

Esters

Like alcohols, esters are considered non-hazardous, with the exception of sabinyl acetate found in savin and methyl salicylate found in wintergreen.[18]

Ketones

Ketones are considered the most common toxic constituents of all essential oil constituents. However, it is incorrect to assume all ketones are toxic. Ketones such as fenchone found in fennel, jasmone found in jasmine, italidione found in everlasting and carvone found in essential oils such as dill, caraway and spearmint essential oils are classified as non-toxic.[20]

Some ketones are known to be both toxic and neurotoxic. The most common toxic and neurotoxic ketones are camphor, pulegone, thujone and pinocamphone.[18]

Thujone is found in essential oils such as mugwort, sage, tansy, thuja and wormwood. While essential oils such as mugwort, tansy, thuja and wormwood should not be used in aromatherapy, sage essential oil needs to be considered more carefully.[18]

The thujone content of *Salvia officinalis* is anywhere from 35-60%. This alone would certainly render sage quite toxic. However, this contradicts most research on and experience with this oil, which clearly does not indicate the toxicity one would expect from such a thujone content.[20]

Schnaubelt states that the traditional use of sage in aromatherapy should not be considered hazardous. However, it would be wise to exercise extra care when using sage, and it should not be used by children or pregnant or nursing mothers.[20]

Another toxic ketone is pulegone. It is found (up to 85%) in pennyroyal essential oil.[21]

Pinocamphone is the primary constituent found in hyssop. Hyssop, according to the LD_{50} value, is distinctly more toxic than sage. Hyssop should always be used carefully in low doses, and should not be used by individuals with epilepsy or fever, during pregnancy, or by children under two years of age. It is preferable to use *Hyssopus officinalis* var. *decumbens*, as this oil is free of the potentially toxic ketones.[21]

Essential oil	Toxic ketone	Oral LD_{50} (g/kg)
Pennyroyal	pulegone	0.4
Sage	thujone	2.6
Tansy	thujone	1.15
Thuja	thujone	0.83
Wormwood	thujone	0.96
Hyssop	pinocamphone	1.40

Toxicity of essential oils with ketone constituents[21]

Phenols

While many essential oils that contain phenols are considered valuable in aromatherapy, they warrant a certain amount of caution. Essential oils such as thyme, oregano and savory are very useful essential oils in aromatherapy because of their antimicrobial activity. However, phenols are the most irritant of the constituents to the skin and mucous membranes, and cause contact dermatitis and sensitisation dermatitis.[18]

Phenyl methyl ethers

Many phenyl methyl ethers (also known as ethers) are considered psychotropic and carcinogenic.[18]

Myristicin and elemicin are two ethers found in nutmeg oil that are believed to be psychotropic.[18] Some of the more hazardous phenyl methyl ethers include methyl chavicol found in basil oil; safrole found in sassafras; and yellow or brown camphor essential oils. All are known to be liver carcinogens. Apiole found in parsley seed is reported to be an abortifacient, while asarone found in calamus is reported to be a neurotoxin and carcinogenic.[17]

Monoterpene hydrocarbons

Monoterpene hydrocarbons are the most commonly occurring essential oil constituents, and are generally considered to have very little risk associated with them. However, they are considered to be reactive (they tend to oxidise easily) and may cause skin irritations.[17,18]

Dangerous Practices

Aromatic perfusion

Aromatic perfusion involves using up to 20 mL of undiluted essential oil directly on the skin for specific conditions. Often essential oils such clove bud, red thyme or oregano are used. This treatment has the potential to cause severe burns and irritation to the skin.[10]

Ingestion

Price & Price state that the ingestion of essential oils should be left in the hands of a competent aromatologist or an aromatherapist working under the direction of a doctor.[19] I would also add that the doctor must have qualifications in medical aromatherapy.

Ingestion of essential oils is not recommended for pregnant women and very young children.[19]

Schnaubelt states that one or two drops of essential oil may deliver the full pharmacological effects; however, when essential oils are orally ingested, very little will actually reach the stomach or small intestines.[20]

Essential Oil Hazards

The hazards and risks associated with the use of essential oils include:

- toxicity
- skin reactions
- carcinogenesis
- neurotoxicity
- hepatotoxicity
- hazards during pregnancy.

Toxicity

Toxicity is what is commonly called 'poisoning', and at a certain level may become fatal. In aromatherapy, the degree of toxicity depends to a certain extent on the method of application. The toxicity of essential oils used in aromatherapy are usually classified as:

- oral toxicity
- dermal toxicity.

Oral toxicity is the degree of toxicity of a substance when it is ingested by swallowing. Dermal toxicity is the degree of toxicity of a substance when it is absorbed through the skin. Both types of toxicity are determined by lethal dose, which is the amount necessary to kill the organism.

The greatest hazard is associated with oral toxicity. In fact, the majority of incidents involving toxicity are from oral dosing. Toxicity is usually classified as acute or chronic.[21]

Acute toxicity is the result of the short-term use of an essential oil, usually involving a single dose, and may result in death. When the amount administered is less than a lethal dose, damage may occur to the liver or the kidneys.

Balacs cites a case in which a child who ingested clove oil almost died:

> *A two-year-old boy had drunk between 5-10 ml of clove oil from an open neck bottle. One hour after ingestion the boy was conscious but drowsy and distressed. Within three hours, the boy had fallen into a deep coma, had a very low blood glucose level and had a marked acidosis. Twenty-four hours after ingestion the boy was still in a coma and was showing signs of disseminated intravascular coagulopathy with concurrent liver failure.*
>
> *After three days of treatment with heparin, plasma, fibrinogen, antithrombin III, protein C and factor VII, the child began to recover. By the fifth day the boy's neurological state improved and he was fully conscious by the sixth. He made full recovery. It was suggested by the author that all essential oils should not be sold in open neck bottles (I fully concur) and that labelling should be more explicit.*[22]

Chronic toxicity is the result of often long-term use of small doses of essential oil. An example of chronic toxicity is cited by Lassak:

> *It appears that he had been in the habit, for about the past five years, of swallowing five to ten drops of eucalyptus oil to keep colds at bay and 'make him feel good'. Later during those five years he started to feel discomfort and even pain in the region of his liver. On entering hospital for a check-up, the matron apparently informed him that he suffered with cirrhosis of the liver and that, unless he stopped drinking immediately, his condition would further deteriorate. Now it so happened he was a tee-totaller and never so much as touched alcohol. The cause of his condition, as it turned out, was most likely the cineole he so regularly took to improve his health.*[23]

The result of chronic toxicity is usually organ tissue damage, most commonly degenerative changes in the liver and kidneys. Death may eventually result, but the problem here is one of slow tissue damage, rather than fatality. Chronic toxicity usually involves oral administration and it would be reasonable to assume the same applies to dermal administration.

Measuring toxicity

Animal testing

In the past for safety reasons and to comply with legal requirements, many substances used in food, medicine and cosmetics, including essential oils, were tested for toxicity on animals.[17]

Due to the pressure of public opinion and lobbying by animal rights groups, many countries have now banned animal testing of cosmetics. However, pharmaceutical drugs require more stringent testing than cosmetics.[17]

The most commonly used animals for toxicity studies are rats, mice, hamsters and guinea pigs. Rabbits are often used to assess dermal toxicity and eye irritation. Animal testing has also raised important concerns about its reliability and predictive value for human outcomes and for understanding human physiology. It has been suggested that animal experimentation often harms humans through misleading safety assessment.[24]

Determining LD_{50}

A common method of establishing a measure of toxicity is the LD_{50} experiment. LD_{50} is the dose of a specific substance that has been lethal for 50% in a group of test animals.[17]

This is usually not given as an absolute value but in grams of toxin per kilogram body weight. For example:

$$LD_{50} = 1\ [g/kg]$$

means that 1 g of essential oil per kg of body weight induces death in 50% of test animals. Using this value as a guide to toxicity in humans, it would mean, assuming the body weight to be 70 kg, that:

$$1\ [g/kg] \times 70\ [kg] = 70\ [g]$$

Therefore 70 g of essential oil would be a lethal dose in humans. LD_{50} values generally refer to oral toxicity. LD_{50} values are commonly accepted in establishing toxicity of a given substance in humans.

The LD_{50} value is not absolute. The LD_{50} value for the same substances frequently varies between the types of animals being used for testing, different laboratories, and methods of administration (e.g. oral, dermal or by injection).[21]

Clearly, the toxicity of the same substance in animals and humans can be quite different. The following table indicates the gross errors that are often assumed in using animal toxicity data to determine lethal doses of humans.

Essential oil	LD_{50} g/kg	Actual lethal dose for 70 kg person	Comment
Boldo	0.13	9.1g	Toxic
Hyssop	1.40	98.0g	Caution
Sage	2.52	176.0g	Safe
Chamomile	8.56	600.0g	Safe

LD_{50} values and corresponding lethal dose.[21]

Tisserand & Young state that LD_{50} is a crude measure of toxicity as it only uses an extreme end-point and does not tell us anything about the risks during pregnancy or carcinogenesis.[17]

The validity of animal testing

RIFM often conducts acute dermal toxicity studies on rabbits. It has, however, been clearly identified that human skin and rabbit skin do not absorb the same essential oils at the same rate. Hotchkiss, lecturer in biochemical toxicology at St Mary's Hospital Medical School, says that absorption is usually higher through animal skin, therefore existing information regarding dermal toxicity probably gives no useful indication of the toxicity of dermally applied essential oils.[25]

Tisserand says that it is a mistake to extrapolate LD_{50} values obtained from animal testing to determine oral toxicity in human beings.[26]

Apart from the ethical issues involved in testing to determine the LD_{50} value, clearly the toxicity of the same substance in animals and humans can be quite different.

The following table gives you an indication of the gross errors that may be assumed in using animal toxicity data to determine lethal doses for humans.[26]

Essential oil	Type of toxicity	Animal toxicity [g/kg]	Human toxicity [g/kg]
Eucalyptus	Acute oral	2.5	0.4-0.8
Wintergreen	Acute oral	1.2	0.23-0.37
Camphor	Acute oral	0.5-0.15	0.005-0.5
Pennyroyal	Acute oral	0.4	0.4

Alternatives to animal testing

Cosmetic testing on animals is considered controversial. It often involves general toxicity, eye and skin irritancy, phototoxicity and mutagenicity tests. As of March 11, 2013, the EU approved a complete ban on the sale of animal-tested cosmetics in Europe, even if the testing was done outside Europe.[27]

Several alternative methods to replace animal testing have been accepted worldwide. It appears that, while there is much support for minimising animal testing for biomedical research, the process of developing, realising, testing and validating an alternative method from idea to approval can be very tedious and time consuming. Various steps in designing valid alternatives to animal testing have been developed:[27]

Step 1: Define an alternative: The word alternative is used to describe any change in an animal test that achieves one or more of the '3Rs'. This is to replace animals, reduce the number of animals or refine the procedure to alleviate or minimise potential animal pain.

Step 2: Develop the alternative: New cell and tissue tests, computer models and other innovative methods can be used to replace existing animal tests. These alternatives are often more cost effective and more reliable than traditional animal experimentation.

Step 3: Validate the methods: The developed method needs to be scientifically validated in multiple laboratories to confirm that the results reliably predict outcomes in humans.

Step 4: Acceptance in scientific community: The International Cooperation on Alternative Test Methods (ICATM) was established in 2009 as a collaboration between validation bodies in Europe, US, Canada, Japan and Korea. Approximately 50 alternative methods and testing strategies have been developed, validated or accepted by the international regulatory authorities.

Often the topic of reducing the requirements of animal testing is perceived as a European regulatory issue; however, researchers are now recognising the benefits of using the 3Rs as a framework to improve science and reduce costs.[28]

New technologies and approaches are being developed in toxicological science to reduce the requirement for animal testing within the pharmaceutical industry.[28]

Some of the replacement techniques involve:[27]

- in vitro techniques which may involve organ culture, tissue slices, primary cell cultures, established cell lines or stem cells
- in silico methods which are often used to study diabetes, asthma and drug absorption. Virtual humans are constructed by creating mathematical models of known human reactions. This computer-based alternative is now being used in many countries
- the use of invertebrate animals – the most commonly used are *Drosophila melanogaster*, a fruit fly and *Caenorhabditis elegans*, a nematode worm.

Badyal & Desai state that, while a combination of newer in vivo and in vitro techniques provides a viable and cost-effective alternative to certain pharmacodynamic and pharmacokinetic evaluations of drugs, animal testing is still required for repeat dose toxicity, carcinogenicity of drugs and certain behavioural studies. They claim that animals are not entirely dispensable in research; however, the principles of the 3Rs must be adapted.[27]

Poisoning

Tisserand & Young state that all cases of poisoning from essential oils are a result of oral ingestion of much higher than normal therapeutic doses.[17]

The following oils have frequently appeared in cases of poisoning:

> *camphor, cinnamon, citronella, eucalyptus, hyssop, nutmeg, parsley, pennyroyal, sage, thuja, sassafras, wintergreen, wormwood, wormseed.*[21]

This does not mean that oils not appearing here are necessarily safe. It is very likely that any essential oil, ingested in sufficient quantities, may cause serious problems. In the unlikely event of accidental ingestion please refer to the first aid procedure in *General Safety Guidelines*.

The majority of cases involving poisoning involve children. Tisserand & Young cite an Australian report involving eucalyptus oil in which 78 of 109 children of five years or younger ingested solutions that were intended for vaporisation.[17]

Toxic essential oils

Tisserand & Young list the following essential oils as moderate oral toxins based on rodent LD_{50} values:

> *bitter almond (unrectified), boldo, calamus, Himalayan cedarwood, wormseed, white wormwood, and thuja.*[17]

They state that the following essential oils are moderate dermal toxins:

> *boldo, cassia, cinnamon bark, oregano, rose absolute, savory and wormseed.*[17]

Rose absolute is mentioned in this list because of the possible methyl eugenol content; however, in their profile for rose, Tisserand & Young state that the potential toxicity of rose absolute is not likely to cause any problems for use in aromatherapy.[17]

Adverse Skin Reactions

Skin reactions that often occur when using essential oils are:

- skin irritations
- sensitisation
- phototoxicity
- idiosyncratic reactions.

Compared with toxicity, skin reactions may vary considerably from one individual to another, and are therefore very difficult to predict.

Tisserand & Young state that some individuals will be more susceptible to adverse skin reactions than others. The health status of the individual, the level of psychological stress, age, gender, genetics and race can all influence the susceptibility to adverse skin reactions.[17]

Quenching

Price & Price state that quenching is an important aspect of synergy. Essential oils display a quenching effect whereby the potential unwanted side effects of one component are nullified by the presence of other components.[19]

A commonly cited example of quenching is the blending of sweet orange oil with lemongrass oil in a 50:50 mix. It is suggested that the monoterpenes found in sweet orange oil are able to quench the irritant properties of the aldehydes found in lemongrass.[19] Tisserand & Young state that quenching does not totally eliminate adverse reactions, but may significantly reduce their severity.[17]

Patch testing

Patch tests are conducted by dermatologists to determine the cause of dermatitis. Patients are often screened with the most likely allergens or suspected ingredients. Patch tests should be conducted by dermatologists or health care workers trained in the procedure.[17]

Tisserand & Young state that undiluted essential oils should not be used for patch testing. They also cite studies that suggest patch testing can sometimes induce positive reactions, which would not normally occur under everyday use conditions. Patch testing with essential oils and fragrance materials often suggests a much higher level of allergic contact dermatitis incidence than is apparent from consumer complaints or from the experience of most aromatherapists. The true incidence rates of the use of essential oils, whether in the general population or in dermatitis patients, should not be determined from patch tests.[17]

Procedure for dealing with an adverse skin reaction

If a reaction from a patch test, an accident or an aromatherapy treatment does occur, immediately wash the skin with a mild unperfumed soap to remove the oil from the surface of the skin. If necessary, apply an aloe vera gel to soothe the skin.

Irritation

An irritation is produced on the skin when the skin is exposed to a 'primary irritant', such as a corrosive chemical. Typically, a reaction occurs rapidly; the severity is dependent upon the concentration of the irritant.[21]

Essential oils that are known to be potential irritants are those that generally provoke dermal irritation at certain concentrations, although there is no guarantee that this will happen on a particular individual. At the same time, essential oils that are not considered to be irritants may occasionally cause irritation in someone with sensitive skin.[21]

Essential oils that are classified as dermal irritants

Essential oils such as horseradish, mustard and massoia at a dermal maximum of 0 to 0.1% are considered high risk dermal irritants.[17]

Essential oils such as immortelle absolute, wild mountain sage and garlic oil at a dermal maximum of 0.2 to 1.0% are considered moderate risk dermal irritants.[17]

Essential oils such as oregano, wild marjoram, Mexican oregano, winter savory, thyme ct. carvacrol, thyme ct. thymol, ajowan, summer savory, thyme ct. limonene, thyme ct. borneol, Siberian fir and dwarf pine at dermal maximum of 1.1 to 20% are considered low risk dermal irritants.[17]

Sensitisation

A dermal sensitisation reaction is sometimes referred to as an allergic urticaria. The skin normally reacts in the form of a rash, blotchy redness, often accompanied by irritation or slight blistering.

Sensitisation refers to an allergic reaction to a substance by an organism that involves the interaction of its immune system with a substance. Substances that are capable of inducing an immune response from an organism are called antigens. The antigens interact with the lymphocytes causing the formation of antibodies that will in turn react with the antigen, rendering it harmless. When an antigen induces an immune response at first exposure, the organism will experience altered body reactivity to subsequent exposure to the same or similar antigens. This may cause exaggerated reactions like sneezing and itching. This is defined as the allergic reaction.

Sensitisation is considered to be unpredictable, as some individuals will be sensitive to a potential allergen and some will not. Essential oil constituents such as cinnamic aldehyde found in cinnamon oil and cassia oil and the lactones found in costus and elecampane are known to be dermal sensitisers.[21]

If an essential oil causes an allergic reaction, its use should be discontinued immediately. What we do know about sensitisation is that once an individual has become sensitised to an essential oil, a severe inflammatory response may be evoked even with a small quantity of the sensitising essential oil.

Essential oils that are considered dermal sensitisers

Essential oils that are considered high risk dermal sensitisers at a dermal maximum of 0 to 0.1% include costus, elecampane, fig leaf absolute, massoia, saffron oil/absolute, lavandin or lavender absolute, cassia, cinnamon bark, oakmoss absolute and tree moss absolute.[17]

Essential oils that are considered moderate risk dermal sensitisers at a dermal maximum of 0.2 to 1.0% include tea leaf absolute, lemon verbena absolute, clary sage absolute, ginger lily absolute, Peru balsam, clove bud, cinnamon leaf, clove leaf, clove stem, opopanax, styrax, jasmine absolute, lemon myrtle, lemongrass, wild mountain sage, exotic basil, may chang, narcissus absolute, lemon-scented tea tree, ylang ylang oil/absolute, cananga, West Indian bay, melissa, honey myrtle, holy basil and lemon verbena.[17]

Essential oils that are considered low risk dermal sensitisers at a dermal maximum of 1.1 to 20.0% include lemon leaf, lemon basil, spearmint, East Indian sandalwood, benzoin resinoid, tolu balsam resinoid, basil ct. linalool, lemon-scented ironbark, lemon thyme, jasmine sambac absolute, palmarosa, tea tree, geranium, citronella, catnip and perilla.[17]

Occupational risk

There is an increased risk and higher prevalence of hand dermatitis in aromatherapists and massage therapists using essential oils.[17]

Many therapists are exposed to and in contact with essential oils every day for many hours. Other factors that may also contribute to increased risk of developing hand dermatitis include wet work, frequent hand washing and contact with latex.[29]

The results of a 12-month study of 350 therapists found that 15% of the therapists self-reported hand dermatitis. The locations of the skin symptoms for the self-reported cases were as follows: fingertips (36%), palms (33%), dorsum (49%), wrists (27%), and forearms (16%). 23% of the participants reported symptoms using a symptom-based method. The following symptoms were most commonly reported: erythema (70%), dryness with scale (77%), fissures (46%), pruritus (36%) and aching or pain (35%).[29]

The most commonly cited essential oils included tea tree, lavender, jasmine, rosewood, lemon, orange, citronella, cassia, ylang ylang and clove bud.[29]

Tisserand & Young suggest ways of reducing occupational hand dermatitis risks:

- using lower concentration of essential oils in massage
- avoidance of high risk and moderate risk essential oils
- avoidance of detergents for hand washing
- using hand cream after hand washing
- wearing thin plastic disposable gloves (not latex, as these can cause severe allergy)
- ensuring adequate ventilation.[17]

They also suggest that if a practitioner develops dermatitis it may be necessary to avoid the allergen. Wearing plastic gloves for some time may also be beneficial. They also state that individuals with a history of atopic dermatitis should be cautious of a career involving regular contact with essential oils.[17]

Photosensitisation

Photosensitisation is a skin reaction that occurs in the presence of ultraviolet light. It may be phototoxic or photoallergenic. Certain constituents of essential oils are capable of absorbing energy from ultraviolet light much more effectively than the skin. Essential oils listed as photosensitisers are hazardous only in this context. To simply apply these oils to the skin diluted or undiluted will not in itself produce a photosensitisation. It can only be achieved if the skin is covered in a photosensitising oil, and then exposed to the sun or any other source of ultraviolet light.

Photoallergenic

Tisserand & Young state that this is an uncommon type of skin reaction to UV light. It involves an allergic reaction to UV light. Photoallergens have been found to bind to proteins in the skin under the influence of UV light. The most common photoallergens are chemicals used in sunscreens, and three fragrance materials not found in essential oils such as musk ambrette, 6-methylcoumarin and 7-methoxycoumarin. These have all been banned by IFRA.[17]

While they report that there are no photoallergenic essential oils, they do cite one case study involving sandalwood oil and one using lavender oil. However, these are considered very rare cases; therefore, these oils should not be considered photoallergenic.[17]

Phototoxicity

The most common phototoxic agents are psoralens, otherwise known as furanocoumarins:

> *… these polycyclic molecules whose structure gives them the ability to absorb ultraviolet photons, store them for a while, and then release them in a burst on to the skin.*[21]

Citrus oils extracted by direct expression without distillation are the major group of phototoxic essential oils containing furanocoumarins. Bergamot and other expressed citrus oils contain small quantities of a furanocoumarin known as bergaptene or 5-methoxypsoralen or 5-MOP.[21]

As can be seen from the table below, the phototoxic potential of citrus oils is minimised when the furanocoumarin content is reduced to 0.0075%.

Essential oil	Furanocoumarin average content	Phototoxicity at 100%	Level when not phototoxic
Bergamot	0.44%	strong	1.0-2.0%
Lime	0.25%	strong	2.0-3.5%
Bitter orange	0.072%	moderate	3.5-7.0%

Essential oil *(continued)*	Furanocoumarin average content	Phototoxicity at 100%	Level when not phototoxic
Lemon	0.0032%	weak	5.0-10.0%
Grapefruit	0.0012%	weak	10.0-20.0%
Sweet orange	0.00005%	mild	No limit
Tangerine	0.00005%	mild	No limit
Mandarin	Trace	mild	No limit

Phototoxic potential of citrus oils.[30]

Essential oils that are phototoxic

Essential oils known to be phototoxic include angelica root, bergamot, cumin, fig leaf absolute, grapefruit, lemon, cold-pressed lime, mandarin leaf, bitter orange and rue oils.[17]

Essential oils that are possibly phototoxic include clementine, combava fruit, celery leaf, celery seed absolute, khella, lovage leaf and parsnip oils.[17]

The following essential oils are not phototoxic: distilled lemon oil, distilled lime oil, mandarin oil, sweet orange oil, satsuma oil, tangelo oil, tangerine oil and yuzu oil.[17]

Managing phototoxicity risk

There will be no risk of phototoxicity if the essential oils are used in a product that will be washed off the skin such as a soap, shampoo or bath product. There is also no risk if the skin is covered up with clothing fabric with a sun protection factor.

Tisserand & Young suggest that the risk of phototoxicity will remain for up to 12 to 18 hours following the topical application of any phototoxic essential oil.[17]

The best advice regarding the use of an essential oil that may cause a phototoxic reaction is to use less than 1% in a blend. Also advise your client not to go into the sun for at least 12 hours after a treatment, or to wear protective clothing and a sunscreen that will block out the UV light.

Idiosyncratic sensitisation

An idiosyncratic sensitisation is an allergic reaction to a substance that is generally not known to be an allergen. Like a food allergy, it is a phenomenon which can appear and disappear again with no apparent logic. The allergic reaction may be induced by dermal application, inhalation or by any other means. As with other types of sensitisation, the substances responsible can produce a severe reaction even in quite low dilutions, especially if the subject is already sensitised.

There is not much we can do in situations like this, except to ensure that when a person does have a history of allergic reactions to do a patch test first and to avoid the use of that oil in future.

Regulations to manage adverse skin reactions

The EU has adopted many of the IFRA guidelines and they have been enshrined into law in an attempt to reduce adverse reactions.[17]

In Europe, Directive 2003/15/EC amending the Cosmetics Directive 76/768/EEC (the 7th Amendment) lists 26 fragrance ingredients that are considered skin allergens. Of these, 16 occur in essential oils. The directive requires any cosmetic product sold in the EU member states and containing a listed material to declare it on the ingredients list if it occurs at more than 100 ppm (0.01%) in a wash off product or 10 ppm (0.001%) in a leave on product.

The essential oil constituents listed as allergens in the EU include:

> *d*-limonene, linalool, geraniol, eugenol, citral, benzyl benzoate, citronellol, farnesol, coumarin, benzyl alcohol, benzyl salicylate, isoeugenol, cinnamyl alcohol, benzyl cinnamate, anisyl alcohol.[31]

Tisserand & Young state the 7th Amendment has been criticised in its selection criteria. For example, one of the criteria states that positive patch test data from more than one patient in more than one independent centre would qualify the substance as a high-risk allergen.[17]

They also explain that no consideration has been given to the fact that many fragrance materials are probably low-risk allergens. They are also critical that no allowance was made for the fact that some constituents are more potent allergens than others. For example, they explain that it is very surprising that cinnamaldehyde and linalool are treated by the EU as if they have the same level of risk.[17]

They are also concerned because no consideration was given to the fact that limonene and linalool become allergenic once oxidation has set in, and that the addition of an appropriate antioxidant can significantly reduce the rate of oxidation.[17]

Carcinogenesis

This is defined as the stimulation of the formation and growth of cancerous cells in the body. Carcinogenesis involves at least three stages – initiation, promotion and progression – before the formation of a malignant neoplasm.[32]

Initiation involves the rapid, irreversible alteration in the cell's genetic material that primes the cell for the subsequent neoplastic development. The initiated cell may remain dormant until exposed to a tumour promoting agent that then allows the growth of clones from initiated cells, which will eventually produce a tumour.[32]

Promoting agents are chemicals that are not in themselves carcinogens, but when they are given repetitively, after a low dose of an initiating agent, they increase cancer incident. Progression is the development of a malignant tumour from a benign tumour.[32]

It has been suggested that at least 70 to 90% of all cancers are attributed to environmental chemical causes. Many substances such as benzene and asbestos have been identified as carcinogens. However, there may be many other unidentified carcinogens. Studies have shown that carcinogens require repeated application, usually several weeks or months, before any cancerous growth can be detected.[32]

Essential oils and constituents that are carcinogenesis

Tisserand & Young state that α-asarone, β-asarone, estragole, methyl eugenol and safrole are all carcinogenic in rodents. They explain that before they can produce malignant changes they must go through a two-stage process of enzyme-activated biotransformation. Therefore, the amount of carcinogen formed will be dependent on the activity of the relevant metabolic enzyme.[17]

While elemicin, *(E)*-anethole and eugenol may be carcinogenic at high doses in rodents, in low doses in humans there is negligible risk, because epoxidation is much less prevalent in humans and low doses are more easily detoxified.[17]

Tisserand & Young state that there are a few chemical carcinogens that are so powerful that even a single dose exposure to a dangerous level is likely to result in cancer. However, the studies reported for all the essential oil constituents below indicate that daily exposure to high oral doses over many months is required to induce cancer in rodents.[17]

Safrole

Safrole is considered to be a human carcinogen based on evidence of carcinogenicity from studies on experimental animals.[33]

It is a major component of sassafras essential oil and of both the yellow and brown fractions of camphor. Studies have also shown that safrole is a hepatocarcinogenic.[21,32]

Estragole

Estragole is also known as methyl chavicol. It is found in tarragon oil (70-87%) and in basil oil (5-87%). Methyl chavicol is a procarcinogen, becoming a carcinogen following metabolic activation. Studies on the toxicity of estragole conclude that estragole-containing essential oils should present no risk when used periodically at low doses.[34]

This conclusion is supported by the fact that rapid detoxification reactions occur immediately after estragole is metabolised into its carcinogenic form. It has also been determined that the level of estragole used in animal carcinogenicity studies is several hundred times higher than the estimated human daily intake.[34]

The EMA report states that estragole is a genotoxic carcinogen in rodents. There are currently no limits for estragole in medicinal products. The EMA report for products containing estragole states that the intake of 0.5 mg/person/day can be accepted for herbal medicinal products as short-term (maximum 14 days) intake.[35]

Tisserand & Young state that tarragon oil and basil oil are high in estragole and should not be taken orally.[17]

β-asarone

β-asarone is a potential hepatocarcinogenic constituent found in calamus oil.[34] Calamus essential oil should not be used in aromatherapy.[21]

β-asarone must first undergo metabolic hydroxylation in the liver before becoming toxic. Cytochrome P450 in the hepatocytes is responsible for secreting the hydrolysing enzymes that convert β-asarone into its genotoxic epoxide structure.[34]

Benzo[α]pyrene

Benzo[α]pyrene is a chemical constituent present in cade oil. It is considered a potential polynuclear hydrocarbon, which is well known as a carcinogen. Cade oil is obtained from the destructive distillation of the wood of *Juniperus oxycedrus*. It should not be used in aromatherapy.[21]

Role of glutathione

Tisserand & Young explain that cells have complex mechanisms of avoiding mutations, such as DNA repair enzymes and pathways that regulate cell growth or suppress oxidative stress.[17]

Glutathione is central for one of the most important detoxification enzyme systems. Studies have found that some essential oils can induce glutathione S-transferase which is responsible for the detoxification of electrophiles responsible for free radical damage to lipids and DNA. Some essential oils that have been found to induce glutathione S-transferase include caraway, cardamom, cumin, dill weed, sweet fennel, galangal rhizome, ginger, lemon, lemongrass, nutmeg, orange, sandalwood, tangerine and thyme.[17]

Depletion of glutathione has been associated with breast, stomach, colon, lung and prostate cancer. Glutathione depletion is also associated with chronic conditions such as emphysema, Alzheimer's disease, Crohn's disease, macular degeneration, Parkinson's and chronic fatigue syndrome. Depletion of glutathione is also associated with old age; hence older people will be more susceptible to chemical carcinogenesis.[17]

Massage and cancer

There is a common belief that massage will spread cancer cells from one part of the body to another by stimulating lymph flow. However, there is no clinical evidence that massage can spread cancer.[36]

It would be reasonable to assume that gentle massage would stimulate the lymph flow no more than gentle exercise or body movement. However, the following precautions should be observed before massaging a client with cancer:

- avoid deep massage of any kind, over or near the lymph glands
- avoid areas of the body that have been treated with radiation therapy, as the skin is usually very fragile
- massage should also be avoided over areas of skin cancer.

There are numerous clinical trials that report on the positive effects of massage on the wellbeing of patients with cancer. Any health professionals who decide to use massage should have a comprehensive understanding of both massage and cancer.

Neurotoxicity

Neurotoxicity is defined as an adverse effect in either the structure or function of the nervous system following exposure to a chemical agent. At a molecular level, a substance might interfere with protein synthesis, leading to reduced production of neurotransmitters and brain dysfunction.[32]

The potential adverse effects that essential oils can have on the central nervous system are:

- convulsant effects
- psychotropic effects.

A neurotoxic substance can cause temporary or permanent disruption to the structure or function of the nervous system.[17]

Convulsant effects

Convulsions and seizures are involuntary changes in behaviour which often involve movement, function, sensation and awareness. They can be sudden, violent muscle contractions, and may be accompanied by loss of consciousness, sensations of fear, visual disturbances or 'lost contact with the outside world' lasting for a few seconds.[17]

Ketones such as fenchone, pinocamphone, camphor and thujone have all been found to have convulsant activity at non-lethal doses in mice. Pulegone found in pennyroyal is also suspected to trigger convulsions at non-lethal doses in humans when ingested.[17]

Tisserand & Young state that essential oils containing significant amounts of these compounds may present a dose-dependent risk.[17]

Hyssop, camphor, mugwort, sage, wormwood and thuja essential oils have all been identified as having a convulsant effect.[21,37,38]

Pinocamphone

Tisserand & Young report that pinocamphone is a convulsant, and lethal in rats when administered by intraperitoneal injection above 0.05 mL/kg. The only essential oil that has more than 5% is the pinocamphone chemotype of hyssop. They suggest that there is a definite risk of seizures from ingesting hyssop oil, although they explain that the linalool chemotype which has only 0.5 to 1.0% pinocamphone is probably negligible, considering that linalool is an anticonvulsant.[17]

Thujone

α-thujone and β-thujone are both anticonvulsant and neurotoxic when administered by intraperitoneal injection in rats. Sage, thuja and wormwood all contain high percentages of thujones, and have been implicated in causing convulsions and seizures when ingested.[17]

Camphor

A review of national poison center data from 1990 through to 2003 in the US showed that there were approximately 10,000 ingestion exposures to camphor-containing products per annum.[39]

Tisserand & Young state that humans are more susceptible than rodents to camphor neurotoxicity. They also explain that camphor does not need to be ingested to trigger a convulsion. They cite a case where a 15-month-old child suffered loss of muscular coordination and seizures after crawling through camphorated oil spilled by his sibling. The child fully recovered.[17]

The mechanism by which camphor is toxic is not fully understood. Absorption from the gastrointestinal tract occurs rapidly, with detectable serum concentrations found within minutes of ingestion. Within five to 15 minutes, patients commonly complain of mucous membrane irritation, nausea, vomiting and abdominal pain. Generalised tonic-clonic convulsions are often the first sign of significant toxicity, and this can occur soon after ingestion. Central nervous system depression, headaches, dizziness, confusion, agitation, anxiety, hallucinations, myoclonus and hyperreflexia are also common.[39]

Manoguerra et al state that, even when applied to the skin in large quantities, camphor has only rarely been reported to cause systemic poisoning resembling the effects seen with acute ingestion exposures.[39]

Chronic oral administration of camphor has been reported to cause death, while chronic, low-dose, dermal exposure over many years was reported to cause granulomatous hepatitis in one case.[39]

Camphor appears to readily cross the placenta. Fetal deaths have been reported following camphor poisoning in the mother during the latter stages of pregnancy.[39]

Camphor presents a clear risk to humans and non-oral exposure of camphor to infants is considered a risk.[17]

Pulegone

Tisserand & Young state that the risk of seizures from pennyroyal is most likely limited to oral overdose.[17]

Rosemary oil

It has been recommended that rosemary oil not be used by individuals with epilepsy.[40,41] Valnet states that the essence of rosemary in excessive quantities has a strong tendency to induce epilepsy. However, he also suggests using rosemary oil in small internal doses to prevent seizures.[42]

A clinical study with animal experiments, in vivo, found that rosemary induced tonic-clonic convulsions. It was found that the oil inhibited oxygen consumption and the electrolyte gradients of sodium and potassium. It has been postulated that there may be a relationship between the metabolic effects of rosemary essential oil in vitro and convulsant activity in vivo.[43]

Tisserand & Balacs state that epileptics should exercise caution with rosemary, especially orally. The assumption being made here is that it is okay to use rosemary oil as long as you do not take it orally, even if you are prone to epileptic seizures.[21]

However, it is known that individuals who are prone to epilepsy may have idiosyncratic reactions to essential oils and odours in general.[21] It becomes almost impossible to predict the adverse effects. It is apparent that whether rosemary oil is taken orally, applied topically or inhaled, the potential exists to trigger a seizure. Therefore, since the effect of rosemary oil on seizures is unpredictable, I recommend that individuals with epilepsy use rosemary with caution.

Fennel

Fennel is also listed as being contraindicated for individuals with epilepsy, presumably for its fenchone content.[40,41] The fenchone content is usually higher in bitter fennel than sweet fennel.[44]

An epileptic seizure was reported in a 38-year-old woman known to be an epileptic patient, who was taking 300 mg per day of lamictal (an antiepileptic medication) to manage her epilepsy. She developed a typical generalised tonic-clonic seizure and remained unconscious for 45 minutes following the ingestion of a number of cakes containing an unknown quantity of fennel essential oil. It was suggested that the likely cause of the seizure was a pharmacodynamic mechanism involving the interaction between fennel oil and the antiepileptic medication.[45]

Tisserand & Young cite several studies that confirm that fennel essential oil is devoid of any convulsant activity; however they suggest that the likely cause of seizure in the above case is (*E*)-anethole, which significantly enhances the enzyme responsible for metabolising lamictal (an anti-epileptic medication). This could have had the effect of metabolising the drug and clearing it from the system too quickly, leaving the patient vulnerable to seizures.[17]

Eucalyptus

While Tisserand & Young list eucalyptus as a convulsant, they state that in the last 30 years there have not been any reported cases of eucalyptus oil causing convulsions. They explain that if eucalyptus oil was a convulsant, it would be natural to implicate 1,8-cineole. They cite several cases involving young children (less than five years in age) who accidentally ingested large amounts of eucalyptus oil (10 to 30 mL). They conclude that seizures linked to eucalyptus oil have only been reported in young children who ingest or inhale substantial quantities; therefore, it does not present a risk to older children or adults.[17]

Psychotropic effects

A psychotropic substance affects the brain in a way which causes changes in mood and behaviour. Reports of essential oils having psychotropic include:

- nutmeg
- thujone rich oils.

Some of the psychotropic effects reported after having used the above include hallucinogenic effects. These substances may also be classified as hallucinogens that are described as:

> *... chemicals which, in non-toxic doses, produce changes in perception, in thought, and in mood, but which seldom produce mental confusion,*

memory loss, or disorientation for person, place and time.[32]

Nutmeg

Most of the speculation regarding the psychotropic qualities of nutmeg oil focuses on two of the major constituents – myristicin and elemicin. Reports have shown that these two constituents are the principal psychotropic components. It has been suggested that a metabolic pathway converts the elemicin and myristicin to TMA (3,4,5-trimethoxyamphetamine) or MMDA (3-methoxy-4,5-methylenedioxyamphetamine), both known as hallucinogens.[21]

Myristicin has been shown to be an inhibitor of an enzyme important in eliminating monoamine oxidase. This may be the reason for nutmeg's euphoric properties. In animal tests, myristicin was found to increase levels of serotonin in rat brain. If this were also the case for humans, this would explain the psychotropic effect.[21]

However, closer investigation has revealed the following:[21]

Component	Psychotropic
Whole nutmeg	Highly active
Whole nutmeg less essential oil	Non active
Nutmeg oil	Weakly active
Myristicin	No activity

It appears that the psychotropic properties are due not only to the myristicin and elemicin, but to other constituents found in the whole nutmeg. While ground nutmeg is moderately to strongly psychotropic when taken in high doses, the effect of the essential oil is very weak, and it appears that non-oral doses will not have any effect at all.

Thujone-rich oils

It was suggested that thujone and δ-9-tetrahydrocannabinol, the most active ingredient in cannabis, interact with a common receptor in the CNS and so have similar psychotropic effects.[21]

However, Tisserand & Young state that thujone has a very low affinity to the cannabinoid receptors, therefore, the psychotropic activity of thujone will be much weaker than δ-9-tetrahydrocannabinol.[17]

Hepatotoxicity

The liver has a wider variety of functions than any other organ in the body. Apart from its major roles of carbohydrate and lipid metabolism, protein synthesis and secretion of bile, it is responsible for the detoxification of the blood. A substance is defined as a hepatotoxin if it causes damage to the liver cells.

It is unlikely that any essential oil is a hepatotoxic through dermal application; however, studies have shown that substances such as eugenol (clove and cinnamon leaf), cinnamaldehyde (cinnamon bark and cassia), and *trans*-anethole (aniseed) have caused depletion of glutathione in oral doses in laboratory experiments on rodents.[21]

Pulegone found in pennyroyal was also shown to be hepatotoxic similar to paracetamol toxicity. A toxic metabolite of pulegone, menthofuran, is produced in the liver's enzyme system and was found to produce acute liver and lung damage in rats.[21,34] The following table lists the essential oils and their corresponding constituents which are potentially hepatotoxic:[21]

Constituent	Essential oil
trans-anethole	Aniseed, fennel
cinnamaldehyde	Cassia, cinnamon bark
methyl chavicol	Basil (methyl chavicol), tarragon
eugenol	West Indian bay, cinnamon, clove
pulegone	Buchu, pennyroyal
safrole	Yellow and brown camphor

Glutathione depletion

Glutathione (GSH) is a very important antioxidant that assists the liver in detoxification of reactive molecules and free radicals before they damage DNA or protein.

Glutathione depletion occurs in the presence of large amounts of a reactive substance. This means that the reactive molecules are able to damage the liver and blood cells, before the glutathione is replaced.[17]

Tisserand & Young state that oral overdoses of essential oils could deplete hepatic glutathione; however, they explain that only a few oils present such a risk. They cite studies involving pennyroyal, cassia bark and essential oils with high doses of (*E*)-anethole that have been found to deplete glutathione. They recommend that it would be prudent for people taking drugs such as paracetamol, people with liver diseases such as cirrhosis and hepatitis, and people with alcoholism to avoid oral administration of essential oils such as pennyroyal and buchu.[17]

Hazards during Pregnancy

There is often a concern that some essential oils may not be safe to use during pregnancy. Some aromatherapists suggest that no essential oils should be used during pregnancy. This is being overcautious, as aromatherapy can be immensely beneficial in maintaining the general health of the expectant mother and in minimising the various discomforts of pregnancy. The main concerns during pregnancy in using some essential oils are that they:[21]

- may have a hormone-like activity, disturbing the normal, finely tuned balance of hormones
- may cause injury or malformation to the development of the foetus
- may cause abortion.

Essential oils with oestrogenic properties

Circulating levels of oestrogen and progesterone are much higher during pregnancy than at other times. The two most important female hormones are oestradiol, which is an oestrogen, and progesterone. Oestradiol controls the development and maintenance of the female sexual organs and gives a person her essentially feminine shape and physiology. Progesterone prepares the uterine lining for pregnancy each month.

Some essential oil constituents have hormone-like behaviour because their structure is similar to the hormones, so they interact with the same receptors that identify hormones. Oestrogenic activity has been found in essential oils of aniseed and fennel.[46]

Anethole, the main constituent in both these essential oils, is a methyl ether of oestradiol and is believed to be responsible for the oestrogenic activity of these oils. Essential oils with oestrogenic activity are known to influence menstrual cycle, lactation and secondary sexual characteristics. Balacs suggests that, until the absolute safety of anethole-rich oils such as aniseed and fennel is established, it would be prudent to avoid their use in pregnancy.[46]

Teratogenic effect of essential oils

Studying the effect of essential oils and drugs during pregnancy is highly problematic. Results of animal studies often correlate even more poorly with the human situation than in other fields of research. Interpreting the results obtained in animal toxicity studies to the human is very difficult indeed, if not totally inaccurate.

There are very few studies on the distribution and fate of drugs within the human embryo, because it is almost impossible to design safe clinical experiments. It is often assumed that drug or essential oil concentrations in the embryo would reach similar levels to that in the mother's serum. This may be inaccurate, and the truth is that we simply do not know whether foreign substances such as essential oils circulating in the mother's blood stream reach the developing child. As a rule of thumb, molecules which can cross the blood-brain barrier into the central nervous system are likely to reach the foetus. Essential oils would therefore be in this category.[21]

So can we safely use essential oils during pregnancy without harming the foetus? Tisserand & Balacs cite several studies involving rats which showed that 1,8-cineole does cross the placenta in sufficient quantities when given by subcutaneous injection to pregnant rats at a dose of 0.5 g/kg for four days.[21]

Tisserand & Balacs cite another study that involved a mother who ingested 2 ounces of camphorated oil, and had the first of three seizures 20 minutes later. She was admitted to hospital and gastric lavage was performed. The next morning, she had a spontaneous labour and the baby was born without complications, but smelling distinctly of camphor. The baby was closely monitored for several days and found to be okay. Another baby unfortunately died when the mother ingested the same amount of camphorated oil.[21]

In these cases, the amount of camphor ingested is approximately 12 mL. According to Tisserand & Balacs, this amount of camphor was more than the LD_{50} values given for camphor. They suggest that if the maximum concentration of essential oil for application by aromatherapy massage is 2%, then there is very little risk to the embryo and foetus. They are of the opinion:

> *... that the external use of camphor-rich oils such as rosemary are safe in pregnancy.*[21]

However, they state that:

> *... oral administration of camphor-rich essential oils should be avoided during pregnancy.*[21]

Other toxic oils discussed include safrole-rich oils such as sassafras, and thujone-rich oils such as wormwood and sage. These oils are obviously toxic and should be avoided altogether in aromatherapy.

Abortifacients

An abortifacient is an agent used to induce an abortion. There is no clear evidence that essential oils are abortifacients. Most essential oils that have been labelled as abortifacients are potentially toxic and are not recommended for used in aromatherapy.

All the 'abortifacient' oils are known to have a strong emmenagogue action. However, not all emmenagogues will induce abortion, and not all emmenagogue oils are toxic.

Many essential oils such as clary sage, cedarwood, cypress, sweet marjoram, peppermint, rosemary and rose are classified as contraindicated during pregnancy; however, they are not abortifacients. It has been suggested that these essential oils present no danger in pregnancy as long as they are not used orally.[21,34]

However, it would be prudent to avoid using these essential oils, as there is anecdotal evidence that indicates that they may be unsafe to use during pregnancy.

The following essential oils are known to have an abortifacient effect:

> *mugwort, parsley seed, pennyroyal, rue, sassafras, savin, thuja, tansy and wormwood.*

These oils are toxic and appear to be abortifacients in lethal dosages.[21]

Miscarriages are common, and women who use essential oils and then miscarry often suspect that the essential oils contributed or caused the miscarriage; however, in most cases there is no definite conclusion that the essential oils were actually responsible.

Essential oils to avoid during pregnancy

Tisserand & Young state that the following essential oils should be avoided by any route throughout pregnancy and lactation:[17]

> *aniseed, star anise, aniseed myrtle, sweet birch, buchu* ct. *diosphenol, buchu* ct. *pulegone, carrot seed, cassia, cinnamon bark, costus, blue cypress, dill seed (Indian), sweet fennel, bitter fennel, ho leaf* ct. *camphor, hyssop* ct. *pinocamphone, Spanish lavender, mugwort, myrrh, oregano, parsley leaf, parsley seed, pennyroyal, rue, Dalmatian sage, Spanish sage, savin, tansy, thuja, wintergreen, wormwood.*

Interactions between Essential Oils and Drugs

Tisserand & Young state that it is difficult to predict the probability of essential oil interactions with drugs.[14] They explain that:[17]

- there could be competition for binding sites in tissues or on plasma proteins
- there could be competition for specific cell surface or intracellular receptor sites
- there could be a change in the gut flora or gut motility
- metabolic enzymes may be induced or inhibited.

Topical application of essential oils that have high percentage of methyl salicylate such as sweet birch and wintergreen can potentiate the effects of warfarin, an anticoagulant used to inhibit platelet aggregation, and exacerbate blood thinning. This can cause internal heamorrhage.[17]

Some essential oils inhibit the cytochrome P450 enzymes (CYP1A2, CYP2C9, CYP2D6 and CYP3A4). These are drug metabolising enzymes, therefore interactions with drugs whose route of elimination is via cytochromes (especially CYP1A2) are possible.[19]

Some of the essential oils that have been implicated in studies to inhibit P450 enzymes include citronella, lemongrass, may chang, lemon myrtle and lemon-scented tea tree, melissa, palmarosa, German chamomile, yarrow and ho leaf ct camphor. It would appear that the essential oils would need to be taken in oral doses in order to potentiate drug action.[17]

Anyone who is taking aspirin, heparin and warfarin, which are all used as blood-thinning medication, should not take any of the following essential oils orally – aniseed, basil ct methyl chavicol, West Indian bay, cassia, cinnamon bark, clove bud, clove leaf, clove stem, corn mint, sweet or bitter fennel, lavandin, wild marjoram ct carvacrol, aniseed myrtle, oregano, savory, tarragon, thyme or wintergreen.[17]

General Safety Guidelines

Safety guidelines for the aromatherapist's wellbeing

When using essential oils please ensure that:

- the treatment room has good ventilation
- regular breaks are taken between clients
- hands are washed between appointments
- frequent hand washing with detergents may increase the risk of hand dermatitis, so their use should be minimised.

Safety guidelines for the general public

When recommending essential oils to the general public ensure that they:

- use less rather than more
- do not take essential oils internally, unless advice has been provided by an aromatic medicine practitioner
- do not purchase undiluted essential oils unless the bottles have a restrictive flow insert
- unless directed by an aromatherapist, do not use essential oils undiluted on the skin. The only exception is an emergency measure when a tiny amount of lavender or tea tree could be used on a sting, small burn or wound
- use no more than 1% concentration of essential oil, if there is a concern of possible skin reaction
- avoid essential oils that are poorly identified
- are aware of the safety issues concerning irritation, phototoxicity, pregnancy and other possible contraindications
- observe good personal hygiene and do not eat, drink or smoke whilst handling essential oils.

Safety guidelines for children

- Do not allow children to ingest essential oils.

- Keep essential oils out of reach of children.
- Purchase essential oils with a restrictive flow device or child resistant cap.
- Do not apply essential oils near a child's face.
- Do not apply essential oils into the nose of a child.

Waste disposal

- Essential oil waste may be a fire hazard.
- Spills should be wiped up with paper towel and placed in a closed metal waste container with a lid and a plastic liner.
- Waste containers should be emptied daily.

Safety guidelines for applications

Bath

It is preferable to add essential oils to a bath with a dispersing agent. Essential oils tend to clump together on the surface of the water, creating a higher risk of irritation to sensitive areas of the skin. A dispersant will ensure that the essential oil will be dispersed in the bath water. Follow the manufacturer's instructions when using a dispersant.

Use of undiluted oils

As a general rule, undiluted essential oils are neither used in massage nor applied to broken skin (cuts, wounds, surgery, sores etc.) and diseased skin. There may be some instances where the benefits of direct topical application may outweigh the risks. This might include instances such as insect bites and stings, burns, tinea, warts etc.

Inhalation

While asthma often responds well to the inhalation of essential oils, please be careful when recommending a steam inhalation, as it can be contraindicated for someone with asthma. Never leave a child unsupervised when using a steam inhalation.

Safety guidelines for the care of essential oils

To ensure the integrity of essential oils and the safe practice of aromatherapy, ensure the following:

- Essential oils have a use by date.
- Essential oils are stored in a dark glass bottle only (e.g. amber).
- Essential oils are stored below 30°C.
- Essential oils are kept in a cool place away from the sun.
- Small amounts of essential oil remaining in large bottles are transferred to smaller bottles, to reduce the risk of oxidation.

First aid procedures in case of an adverse reaction

If someone is suffering from a serious adverse reaction, seek medical help immediately. Contact a doctor, or call the Poisons Information Centre in your capital city for further advice. (In Australia, phone 13 11 26.)

Most of this information is adapted from the MSDS. A copy of an MSDS can be found in Appendix 5.

Procedure in case of essential oil ingested or swallowed

- Do not induce vomiting, unless advised to do so by a general practitioner.
- If the person is conscious and not convulsing, rinse mouth with water and call a hospital or poisons centre.
- If the person is convulsing or unconscious, do not give anything by mouth. Ensure that their airway is not obstructed and lay them on their side with the head lower than the body.
- Take the person to a hospital accident or emergency department and take the bottle with you.
- If the ingestion took place some time ago and the person is showing severe signs of poisoning such as loss of consciousness, telephone the ambulance emergency service.

Procedure in case of direct skin contact

- Remove contaminated clothing and wash the affected area.
- Seek medical attention if irritation persists.

Procedure in case of essential oils in the eyes

Flush the eyes with copious amounts of water for at least 15 minutes and seek medical attention if eye irritation persists.

References

1. Burfield T. *Safety of essential oils.* The International Journal of Aromatherapy, 2000; 10(1/2): 16-29.
2. Holmes P. *Aromatica: a clinical guide to essential oil therapeutics – Vol. I.* Singing Dragon, London, 2016.
3. Guba R. *Toxicity myths: the actual risks of essential oil use.* Aromatherapy Today, 1999; 11: 28-35.
4. Sharma S. *Current status of herbal product: regulatory overview.* Journal of Pharmacy & Bio-Allied Sciences, 2015; 7(4): 293-296. doi: 10.4103/0975-7406.168030.
5. US Food and Drug Administration/Center for Drug Evaluation and Research. *Botanical drug development – guidance for industry.,*

Silver Spring, 2016. Retrieved Nov 11, 2017, from http://www.fda.gov/Drugs/guidance ComplianceRegulatoryInformation/guidances/default.htm
6. Calapai G. *Regulatory issues in aromatherapy.* In Bagetta G, Cosentino M, Sakurada T. eds. *Aromatherapy – basic mechanisms and evidence based clinical use.* CRC Press, Boca Raton, 2016: 397-404.
7. Department of Health and Ageing/Therapeutic Goods Administration. *Guidelines for levels and kinds of evidence to support indications and claims for non-registerable medicines, including complementary medicines, and other listable medicines.* Version 1.1. Woden, 2011.
8. Department of Health/Therapeutic Goods Administration. *Australian regulatory guidelines for complementary medicines – part IV: general guidance.* Version 4.2. Woden, 2011.
9. Department of Health/Therapeutic Goods Administration. *Standard for the uniform scheduling of medicines and poisons. No.18 October 2017.* Woden, 2017.
10. Lis-Balchin M. *Aromatherapy science – a guide for healthcare professionals.* Pharmaceutical Press, London, 2006.
11. Harris B. *Editorial.* International Journal of Aromatherapy, 2006; 16(2): 55
12. *Planning occupational health & safety.* 5th edn. CCH Australia, North Ryde, 2000.
13. Burfield T. *Safety of essential oils: an overview of toxicology and safety testing.* Retrieved Apr 2, 2017, from http://www.users.gloalnet.co.uk/nodice/new/magazine/magsafetylecture.htm
14. Research Institute for Fragrance Ingredients. *About RIFM.* Retrieved Jan 18, 2018, from http://www.rifm.org/about.php#WI_9odGuaf0
15. Bickers DR et al. *The safety assessment of fragrance materials.* Regulatory Toxicology and Pharmacology, 2003; 37(2): 218-273.
16. International Fragrance Association. *What is IFRA?* Retrieved Jan 18, 2018, from http://www.ifraorg.org/en-us/about-ifra-text#.WI_gNGuaf0
17. Tisserand R, Young R. *Essential oil safety.* 2nd edn. Churchill Livingstone, Edinburgh, 2014.
18. Bowles EJ. *The chemistry of aromatherapeutic essential oils.* 3rd edn. Allen & Unwin, Crows Nest, 1991.
19. Price S, Price L. *Aromatherapy for health professionals.* 4th edn. Churchill Livingstone, Edinburgh, 2012.
20. Schnaubelt K. *Medical aromatherapy.* Frog, Berkeley, 1999.
21. Tisserand R, Balacs T. *Essential oil safety.* Churchill Livingstone, Edinburgh, 1995.
22. Balacs T. *Research reports.* The International Journal of Aromatherapy, 1994; 6(2): 33.
23. Lassak EV, McCarthy T. *Australian medicinal plants.* Methuen Australia, North Ryde, 1983.
24. Akhtar A. *The flaws and human harm of animal experimentation.* Cambridge Quarterly of Healthcare Ethics, 2015; 24(4): 407-419. doi: 10.1017/S0963180115000079.
25. Hotchkiss S. *How thin is your skin?* New Scientist, 29th Jan 1994: 24-27.
26. Tisserand R. *New perspectives on essential oil safety.* Aroma'95 Conference Proceedings, Aromatherapy Publications, England, 1995.
27. Badyal DK, Desai C. *Animal use in pharmacology education and research: the changing scenario.* Indian Journal of Pharmacology, 2014; 46(3): 257-265. doi: 10.4103/0253-7613.132153,
28. Chapman KL et al. *Pharmaceutical toxicology: designing studies to reduce animal use, while maximizing human translation.* Regulatory Toxicology and Pharmacology, 2013; 66(1): 88-103. doi: 10.1016/j.yrtph.2013.03.001.
29. Crawford GH et al. *Use of aromatherapy products and increased risk of hand dermatitis in massage therapists.* Archives of Dermatology, 2004; 140(8): 991-996.
30. *The IFRA's guidelines and recommendations on citrus oils.* Perfumer & Flavorist, 1980; 5(1): 1-17.
31. European Commission/Scientific Committee on Consumer Safety. *Perfume allergies.* Retrieved Jan 19, 2018, from http://ec.europa.eu/health/scientific_committees/opinions_layman/perfume-allergies/en/index.htm#1
32. Hodgson E, Levi P. A *textbook of modern toxicology.* 2nd edn. McGraw-Hill Higher Education, New York, 2000.
33. US Department of Health and Human Services/National Toxicology Program. *Safrole.* Retrieved Jan 19, 2018 from https://ntp.niehs.nih.gov/ntp/roc/content/profiles/safrole.pdf
34. McGuffin M et al. eds. *American herbal products association's botanical safety handbook.* CRC Press, Boca Raton, 1997.
35. Committee on Herbal Medicinal Products (HMPC). *Public statement on the use of herbal medicinal products containing estragole.* European Medicines Agency, London, 2014. Doc ref. EMA/HMPC/137212/2005 Rev 1.
36. Horrigan C. *Complementing cancer care.* International Journal of Aromatherapy, 1991; 3(4): 15-17.
37. Bruneton J. *Pharmacognosy.* 2nd edn. Lavoisier Publishing, Paris, 1999.
38. Blumenthal M et al. *The complete German commission E monographs: therapeutic guide to herbal medicine.* American Botanical Council, Austin, 1998.
39. Manoguerra AS et al. *Camphor poisoning: an evidence-based practice guideline for out-of-hospital management.* Clinical

Toxicology, 2006; 44(4): 357-370. doi: 10.1080/15563650600671696.
40. Davis P. *Aromatherapy: an A-Z*. 2nd edn. C.W. Daniel Company, Saffron Walden, 1999.
41. Lawless J. *The encyclopaedia of essential oils*. Element Books, Shaftesbury, 1992.
42. Valnet J. *The practice of aromatherapy*. C.W. Daniel Company, Saffron Walden, 1980.
43. Steinmetz MD et al. *Actions of essential oils of rosemary and certain of its constituents (eucalyptol and camphor) on the cerebral cortex of the rat in vitro*. Journal de Toxicologie Clinique et Expérimentale, 1987; 7(4): 259-271.
44. Khan I, Abourashed E. *Leung's encyclopedia of common natural ingredients used in food, drugs and cosmetics*. 3rd edn. John Wiley & Sons, New Jersey, 2010.
45. Skalli S, Bencheikh RS. *Epileptic seizure induced by fennel essential oil*. Epileptic Disorders, 2011; 13(3): 345-347.
46. Balacs T. *Hormones and health*. The International Journal of Aromatherapy, 1993; 5(1): 18-20.

Use

CHAPTER 7

Contents

Introduction

One of the advantages of aromatherapy is the ease with which essential oils can be administered in so many different ways:

- methods of percutaneous absorption such as massage, compresses, baths and skin care preparations
- inhalation
- internal use.

Using essential oils safely and correctly is important if the full benefits of their properties are to be realised.

Percutaneous Techniques

This means techniques that involve the application of the essential oil to the skin. Some of the commonly used methods are:

- massage
- topical application by the use of ointments, gels and creams
- bath
- compress.

Massage

Massage with essential oils is by far the most common method of using essential oils in holistic aromatherapy. Many studies have confirmed the importance of touch in the development of healthy human beings. Touch has been described as a basic human behavioural need, and its importance for both mental and physical health has been well researched.[1]

Therapeutic benefits of massage

The massage therapist may learn a variety of techniques that are designed to have a multitude of beneficial effects. The beneficial effects of massage include:

- inducing deep relaxation, relieving both mental and physical fatigue
- releasing chronic neck and shoulder tension and backache
- improving circulation to muscles, reducing inflammation and pain
- relieving neuralgic, arthritic and rheumatic conditions
- helping sprains, fractures, breaks and dislocations heal more readily
- promoting correct posture and helping improve mobility
- improving, directly or indirectly, the function of every internal organ
- improving digestion, assimilation and elimination
- increasing the ability of the kidneys to function efficiently
- stimulating the lymphatic system to eliminate toxins
- helping to disperse many types of headache
- helping to release suppressed feelings, which can be shared in a safe setting.[1]

Aromatherapy massage

Aromatherapy massage uses gentle, relaxing

techniques, and utilises the various energy systems of the body. The percussive techniques of Swedish massage or deep tissue massage are generally not suitable for aromatherapy massage because they are too intense and stimulating when used with essential oils.

Aromatherapists may utilise a range of massage techniques. This obviously depends on their training and background, and partly on their personal outlook and preference.

Davis says that it does not matter too much which technique is used, provided the therapist has been thoroughly trained in his or her chosen system and uses it with care and a nurturing attitude towards the client. It is far more important that the massage physically encompasses the whole body, and that the therapist takes into account the whole person – body, mind and spirit.[2]

I have been privileged to train with Madame Micheline Arcier, who developed a unique aromatherapy massage technique that will be described in Volume 2.

How to use essential oils in massage

For massage purposes, essential oils are usually diluted in a carrier oil. The standard carrier oils used are vegetable oils. The selection of the carrier oil is dependent on the benefits of the oil and the cost. For example, someone with dry skin would benefit from cold-pressed avocado oil, someone with mature skin would benefit from cold-pressed rosehip oil and wheatgerm oil, while someone with sensitive skin would benefit from cold-pressed jojoba or evening primrose oil being used as a base oil.

The recommended dilution rate used is a 1% to 3% dilution of the appropriate essential oil to the carrier oil.

A general rule of thumb is that 1 mL of essential oil is approximately 20 drops. This is only an estimate, as it will obviously depend on the size of the eye dropper or dripulator and the specific gravity of the essential oil.

If you are preparing a 3% dilution massage blend then:

- to 100 mL of carrier oil, you add 3 mL of essential oil, or 60 drops
- to 50 mL of carrier oil, you add 1.5 mL of essential oil, or 30 drops.

If you are using more than one essential oil to make your massage oil, it must be emphasised that the dilution refers to the total combination of essential oils.

When working with babies, children, pregnant women, the elderly and people with sensitive skin, you should only use 0.5% to 1.0% dilution.

If you are preparing a 1% dilution massage blend:

- to 100 mL of carrier oil, you add 1 mL of essential oil, or 20 drops
- to 50 mL of carrier oil, you add 0.5 mL of essential oil, or 10 drops.

Conditions that benefit from massage

Conditions that benefit from massage include circulatory problems, digestive problems, fluid retention, headaches, insomnia, menstrual problems, musculoskeletal disorders and nervous tension.

Contra-indications for massage

The aromatherapist must know when massage is recommended and when it should be avoided. The following conditions are generally contraindicated for massage:[3]

Abnormal body temperature – Massage is contraindicated when the client has a fever.

Acute infectious disease – Do not give a massage to an individual who is coming down with an acute viral infection such as a cold or flu. The massage will intensify the illness and also expose the therapist to the virus.

Inflammation – Where there is acute inflammation in a particular area of the body, massage is not advisable because it could further irritate the area or intensify the inflammation.

Osteoporosis – This condition leads to deterioration of bone. In advanced stages, bones become brittle, sometimes to the point that they are easily broken. Osteoporosis is usually prevalent in the elderly.

Varicose veins – Varicose veins are a condition in which the valves in the veins break down because of back pressure in the circulatory system. The veins bulge and may rupture, usually in the legs. The development of varicose veins is often the result of gravity or other obstructed venous flow, as the result of crossing the legs or other sitting postures that inhibit circulation to or from the legs.

However, essential oils such as cypress, lemon and geranium can be blended with calendula-infused oil to effectively treat varicose veins. Special care is needed in the execution of the massage, and only gentle, almost superficial, upward effleurage strokes should be used.

Oedema - Oedema is a circulatory problem that generally appears as puffiness in the extremities, but it can be more widespread. Specific massage techniques such as lymphatic drainage are considered beneficial for the treatment of oedema.

High blood pressure – Massage is often contraindicated for persons with high blood pressure. However, an aromatherapy massage that incorporates essential oils known to lower blood pressure, such as lavender, ylang ylang, sweet marjoram and may chang, will be beneficial.

Intoxication – Never massage a client who is intoxicated.

Other topical applications

These can be very useful mediums for the topical application of essential oils when a vegetable oil base is not suitable.

Balms and ointments

Balms and ointments are semi-solid and non-aqueous preparations that are not absorbed easily into the skin and are therefore used to provide a protective or remedial film over the skin. Being immiscible with water or skin secretions, ointments effectively form an occlusive layer over the skin, preventing evaporation.

The result is similar to an occlusive dressing. The skin becomes waterlogged (hydrated), permitting easier absorption of the essential oils in the ointment.

Balms and ointments have topical protective, healing, soothing, moistening and cooling properties, and provide a long-term effect when continuously applied. Some examples of the application of ointments are:

- For the treatment of boils, sores, infected cuts and fungal skin conditions, a soothing and antiseptic ointment can be made using tea tree oil and calendula-infused oil.
- The rubefacient and analgesic properties of arnica-infused oil, black pepper, ginger, hypericum-infused oil, cinnamon and peppermint can be used in an ointment to treat arthritis and sports injuries. Use before an event to keep the muscles warm and prevent injuries.
- To moisten, soothe and protect dry, irritated skin conditions such as eczema, dry chapped skin or lips, use calendula-infused oil, lavender, myrrh and German chamomile in an ointment.

Many recipes use lanolin, a wool fat, or petroleum jelly as a base. I prefer to use a vegetable derived ointment such as the base outlined below:

15 to 20 g beeswax or cocoa butter

80 to 85 mL vegetable oil

Alternatively, shea butter makes an excellent ointment base.

While the recommended dilution for essential oils in a massage oil or lotion is no more than 3% in an ointment or balm, the amount of essential oil used can be much higher. For example, a balm for wound care which incorporates essential oils such as lavender, everlasting and German chamomile could contain up to 20% or more essential oils. It is not uncommon to have an ointment for muscular aches and pain or for arthritis to be made with 40% or more essential oils. These ointments are usually applied to a localised area of the body only, and for a short period.

Gels

Gels are used to hydrate, soothe and cool the skin. Gels make an excellent base for essential oils when a vegetable oil base is not desired. Gels can be made from plants such as linseed, pectin from citrus peel, guar gum or xanthan gum. Gels can be used as:

- moisturisers
- masks
- treatments for skin problems such as acne and blemished skin.

A simple recipe for making a gel base is as follows:

2-5 g powdered pectin, guar or xanthan gum

100 mL purified water.

Sprinkle the pectin, guar or xanthan gum slowly into purified water that has been heated to 35-40° C. Use a whisk or electric hand mixer to ensure the powdered gum is evenly dispersed throughout the water. Strain the gel, and add more water if a thinner consistency is desired. Add up to 1% essential oil.

Liniments

A liniment is prepared by adding essential oils or herbal extracts to an alcohol solution. Liniments are typically used to relieve muscular aches and pains. Liniments should only be applied to unbroken skin. Liniments are very simple to make, as essential oils are soluble in alcohol and no preservatives are required.

Lotions and creams

Creams and lotions are examples of emulsions. They may be used to treat most skin conditions, or any condition where a massage oil is considered.

An emulsion is a stable system of two or more immiscible liquids in which the droplets of one liquid are held in suspension in the other by emulsifiers.[4]

An emulsifier is a chemical compound that is used to join oil and water to form a stable mixture called an emulsion. Each emulsifier molecule has the unique property of being able to attract both water and oil at the same time at different sites of its molecular structure.[5]

To create an emulsion, oil, water and an emulsifier must be mixed in a way to finely disperse the oil in water (or visa versa). Two types of emulsions can be made:

- oil in water emulsions

- water in oil emulsions.

The first disperses oil droplets in water and the second disperses water droplets in oil. If you are not too sure what kind of emulsion your favourite cream or lotion is made of, put some on your finger and let water run over it. If it washes off easily, it is an oil in water emulsion, if not, it is a water in oil emulsion. Sometimes it may be necessary to make a cream with more resistance to water, e.g. when making a sunscreen or for environmental and occupational protection.

The basic ingredients needed to make emulsions include:

- emulsifying waxes
- water
- emollients such as vegetable oils
- active ingredients such as essential oils or herbal extracts
- preservatives.

A simple recipe for making a cream is as follows:

Oil phase:

10 g emulsifying wax

30 mL sweet almond oil

Water phase:

5 mL vegetable glycerin

90 mL purified water

2 mL natural preservative

In one bowl, melt the wax in a bain-marie and stir in the vegetable oil. Bring the water and glycerin to the same temperature in a separate bowl. Remove both bowls from the heat and slowly stir the water phase into the oil phase. Continue beating until the mixture cools, add the citrus seed extract and then add 1-3% essential oil to the preparation and store in a jar.

Lotions and creams are often used for the preparation of skin care products or aromatherapy. They can be a suitable base for the treatment of inflammatory skin conditions.

Baths

Baths are an enjoyable method of using essential oils. Baths can be very effective because the essential oil can act in two ways: by absorption into the skin and by inhalation. Baths can also be an excellent way of using essential oils for client who cannot be massaged.

The main concern is that some aromatherapy books recommend adding the drops of essential oil directly to the water and then swishing it around to disperse the oil. Essential oils are not soluble in water, so I fail to understand how a swish is going to help disperse the essential oil. The main concern is that undiluted essential oils may come into contact with the skin and cause irritation to the skin.

Aromatherapy baths are generally safe provided that the essential oils are properly dispersed into the water. It is therefore recommended to use a dispersant whenever using essential oils in a bath.

Ensure that the dispersant is vegetable oil derived, as this will have an emollient effect on the skin. The warmth of the water aids absorption of the essential oil through the skin, and also causes the essential oil to vaporise so there is also the benefit via olfaction.

Essential oils can also be added to sea salt or magnesium sulphate. Bath salts can be used to promote detoxification, relax muscular tension and alleviate aches and pains. Aromatherapy bath salts can be made by adding up to 1 mL of essential oils to every 100 g of salt.

Foot and hand baths

For foot and hand baths, place five drops of an essential oil into a teaspoon of dispersant and add to a bowl of lukewarm water. After soaking the hands or feet for 10 to 15 minutes, wrap them in a dry towel.

Conditions that respond to hand and foot baths are arthritis, oedema, circulatory problems, dermatitis, rheumatism, varicose veins and dry skin.

Full bath

For a full bath, it is advisable to use a dispersant. Conditions that respond to a full bath include circulatory problems, fluid retention, headache, insomnia, menstrual problems, muscular disorders and nervous tension.

Be cautious when using essential oils that may readily oxidise, as these are likely to cause dermal irritation when used in a bath. This includes essential oils with a high percentage of monoterpene hydrocarbons such as lemon, grapefruit or sweet orange. If you experience an irritation while in the bath, you should immediately vacate the bath and wash the affected area in a shower with soapy water to reduce any irritation.

Essential oils that contain phenols and aldehydes are also very reactive and may cause dermal irritation when used in a bath. This includes essential oils such as cinnamon leaf, clove bud, oregano, savory, thyme, cinnamon bark, lemon-scented eucalyptus, lemongrass, lemon myrtle, may chang and melissa.

Sitz bath

Sitz baths are also known as hip baths. A bowl or normal bath may be used, filled with enough water to cover the hips up to the waist only. Add 5 drops of essential oil to a dispersant and add to the bath water. Sitz baths are very effective for treating urinary, genital and lower digestive conditions.

A hot hip bath is generally taken for 3 to 10 minutes at 40-46°C. It will stimulate, relax, warm and relieve pain, and is typically used for gynaecological conditions such as delayed or painful periods, and for lumbar pain, urinary ailments, gout, haemorrhoids and constipation.[6]

A neutral sitz bath is more appropriate for situations of acute inflammation, such as cystitis and pruritus of the anus or vulva. It is generally taken for 15 minutes at 33-35°C.[6]

A cold hip bath should only last for one to three minutes at a temperature of 13-24°C. It is stimulating, decongesting and is ideal for treating blood congestion. Cold hip baths are great for treating copious menstrual or inter-menstrual bleeding, and may also be used to prevent colds and flu and promote sound sleep.[6]

Douches

A douche is a vaginal wash using essential oils diluted in water. This method can be beneficial in the treatment of catarrhal or infectious conditions of the urinary tract, such as pruritus, cystitis or thrush.

Add 5 to 10 drops of essential oil to one litre of warm water and shake the mixture well. Add one tablespoon of cider vinegar to help maintain the pH balance. This mixture can be used in a sitz bath, bidet or in an enema or douche pot.[7]

The best position for applying a douche is lying on the back (to avoid spreading infection to the womb), and the douche should be retained for 10-20 minutes. Douches should be applied every day for up to a week when the symptoms are acute, and once a month for maintenance.[7]

It should be kept in mind that douching should not be done on a regular basis as it disrupts the normal, healthy bacterial balance.[2,7]

Compresses

Compresses are generally recommended when the affected area or condition is too painful to massage.

Compresses are a very effective way of using essential oils to relieve pain and swelling and reduce inflammation. Hot compresses are often used to reduce pain of a chronic nature, to draw out boils or splinters, and to relieve menstrual cramps. Cold compresses may be used to relieve tiredness due to overwork or stress, to alleviate acute pain, and as first aid for injuries such as sprains.

When preparing a compress, you should use a clean cloth, a face flannel or a clean handkerchief for a very small compress, and a folded hand towel for a larger one.

A hot compress should be replaced with a fresh one as soon as it has cooled to body heat.

To make a cold compress use some ice cubes. Davis says that a very large cold compress can be used to reduce a client's fever if it is dangerously high, but she says that this should only be done by therapists who are well trained in handling acute illness, and should never be applied to babies or elderly people, as their body heat control mechanisms are less efficient than those of adults and older children.[2]

Alternating warm and cold compresses may be used to help speed healing in pulled muscles, sprained ligaments and bruises.

The normal dilution of essential oils in a compress solution is 4 to 5 drops in 200 mL of water. Dip the cloth into the solution and wring it out so that it does not drip. Then cover the area being treated with the compress. Place a plastic wrap over the compress and then a towel or blanket on top. Leave the compress on for two to four hours. A cold compress should always be kept moist and renewed frequently to maintain the primary cold effect.

Inhalations

When essential oils are diffused into a room they have a multitude of effects. There is the obvious olfactory pleasure that is gained. Unpleasant odours can be replaced by the natural aromas of essential oils, thus stimulating our senses and imagination by the memories that they evoke.

Essential oils have specific therapeutic properties that affect the wellbeing of those who breathe them in. They have long been known for their airborne antiseptic properties, allowing them to disinfect and purify the air in the event of bacterial contamination. For example, Valnet states:

> *The essence of lemon is second to none in its antiseptic and bactericidal properties. The work of Morel and Rochaix has demonstrated that the vapours of lemon essence neutralize the meningococcus in 15 minutes, the typhus bacillus in less than an hour, pneumococcuss in 1-3 hours and staphylococcus aureus in 2 hours.*[8]

The use of essential oils as an inhalation for the treatment of respiratory conditions such as nasal congestion, coughs, colds and sore throat is a common and effective practice. Many essential oils can act as mucolytics and pulmonary decongestants.

Inhalation of essential oils works predominantly on the mind via the olfactory/limbic/hormonal/emotional response. Inhalations may therefore be effective in overcoming problems such as stress, depression or tiredness, and any other emotional dilemmas that may be encountered.

Buchbauer believes that the only effective way of administering essential oils is via inhalation:

> *Aromatherapy applied in the correct way by inhalation only (where the resultant plasma concentration of aroma compounds are 100 to 10,000 smaller) leads to the desired effect.*[9]

Maury describes the effect of fragrance on the psyche and mental state of the individual:

> *Powers of perception become clearer and more acute, and there is a feeling of having, to a certain extent, outstripped events. They are seen more objectively and therefore in truer perspective.*[10]

The use of essential oils as an inhalation for the treatment of respiratory conditions such as a congested nose, headache, sore throat and coughs is a common and effective practice. Bardeau found that essential oils that were vaporised were able to kill 90% of airborne microbes within three hours. The oils that were most effective when vaporised included clove, lavender, lemon, marjoram, mint, niaouli, pine, rosemary and thyme.[7]

Conditions that respond to inhalations include nervous tension, headaches, respiratory problems, colds, sore throat, blocked sinuses and coughs.

Methods of inhalation

Aroma mists

An aroma mist can be made by adding essential oils and an essential oil solubiliser to a bottle and then adding water to this mixture before shaking well. This can then be used as a body mist or a room spray. Avoid spraying directly into the face or the eyes. Aroma mists are usually made with an essential oil dilution of between 1 – 2%. Aroma mists can be very effective whenever we do not have access to an essential oil diffuser.

Direct inhalation

Apply 1 to 2 drops of neat essential oil, to a tissue or handkerchief, hold this near the nose for a few moments and inhale the vapours.

One of the simplest methods to inhale an essential oil is to add 3-4 drops of essential oil to a handkerchief and regularly inhale. Another possibility is to add 5-10 drops of essential oil to a bowl of steaming water and breathe the vapours emitted.

Steam inhalation

Add 5-10 drops of essential oil to a bowl of steaming water. Then place a towel over your head and the bowl and inhale the vapours for a few minutes. The eyes should be kept shut during inhalation. Steam inhalations are a traditional home remedy to ease congestion in the respiratory passage caused by colds, coughs and catarrh.

Nebulisers are considered safer, but many essential oils may be very corrosive to the plastic nebulisers, so care must be taken when using essential oils in nebulisers.

Vaporisation

The most effective method of using the essential oils as inhalations is by using an oil burner, vaporiser or diffuser.

To use a candle oil burner, place a small quantity of water in the small dish on top of the oil burner, then add 5-10 drops of essential oil. Light the candle and keep alight for approximately 15 to 30 minutes. Remember to never keep a burning object unattended, and never allow the oil and water in the oil burner to dry out. Keep the bowl clean by wiping it with a damp tissue or cleaning cloth.

Ultrasonic vaporisers are a very effective way to safely diffuse essential oils. The benefit of ultrasonic vaporisers is that they do not use heat to vaporise the oil. This reduces the risk of chemical alteration of the essential oil. When using an ultrasonic vaporiser, follow the instructions provided by the manufacturer, as each vaporiser is different.

Internal Use

Ingestion

The use of essential oils internally is the most controversial issue in aromatherapy today. We need to remember that internal use of essential oils is common practice in France. Dr Lapraz, a French doctor who uses essential oils, states:

> *Our position with regards to the internal use of aromatherapy is very clear. As essential oils are extremely active agents having some demonstrable effects on the different organs of the body, they need to be administered under medical supervision.*[11]

Pénöel suggests that in the case of serious infections, the only way that aromatherapy can help is an internal, massive and repetitive aromatic treatment involving strong antimicrobial essential oils taken by oral ingestion every 20 minutes. He suggests that within three days such an infection can be completely eliminated by such a treatment.[12]

However, as Pénöel points out, the French patient in a stressful situation cannot easily make an appointment to receive an aromatherapy treatment 'in the English way', which he claims to be a delightful and highly efficacious treatment. The French doctor trained in aromatherapy is also not likely to include lifestyle changes, which are necessary as part of a holistic aromatherapy treatment.[12]

Many professional aromatherapy associations do not endorse the internal ingestion of essential oils unless the aromatherapist has suitable training.

Oral ingestion of essential oils should only be recommended by suitably trained individuals such as doctors or medical herbalists who have an understanding of the pharmacological interaction of the essential oils, have an in-depth understanding of human physiology and pathology, and have extensive training in the French model of aromatherapy.

Oral administration does have some disadvantages:

- possibility of nausea and vomiting
- irritation of the gastrointestinal tract
- much of the essential oil will be metabolised by the liver
- destruction of the essential oil constituents by stomach acidity or enzymes in the intestines.[13]

The preferred method for administering essential oils internally is by adding the essential oil to a lipophilic medium such as a vegetable oil and adding this solution in a capsule. This will not only prevent gastric irritation but also helps to improve and slow down absorption.[14]

Price & Price suggest that, while oral ingestion is not harmful, continued ingestion for too long a period can eventually lead to toxic build-up in the liver. Therefore they recommend to have a rest from internal ingestion of essential oils after three weeks to allow the liver an opportunity to eliminate any accumulated toxins from essential oils.[15]

Gargles and mouthwashes

Gargles and mouthwashes can be prepared in water or in an alcohol-water solution. They are ideal for throat infections and to alleviate pain or inflammation of the mouth. They can be analgesic, antiseptic, anti-inflammatory or soothing. Honey can also be added to a gargle to soothe infection of the throat.

Price & Price recommend adding 2 to 3 drops in a quarter of a tumbler of water. For children, they recommend blending 1 drop of essential oil in a teaspoonful of honey before adding the water.[15]

Rectal

Suppositories are a common method of essential oil administration by French medical doctors. The advantages of using suppositories are:[16]

- The essential oils can be administered in higher doses than oral administration for the treatment of acute infectious conditions, especially lower respiratory tract conditions.
- There is the absence of the interaction between the essential oil and the gastrointestinal tract or the liver which possibly breaks down the essential oil.
- There is more rapid absorption of essential oil into the body.
- They reduce the possible hazardous effects on the liver, especially essential oils containing phenols. In order to excrete phenols the liver has to convert them into sulphonates which may cause damage to the liver by overworking it.
- Suppositories are easier to administer than oral ingestion.

It needs to be stressed that similar safety issues to those of oral administration need to be considered. Being lined with mucous membrane, the rectum is highly sensitive to irritation and there may be a risk of occasional irritation.

Benefits of internal use

Schnaubelt suggests that, to successfully deliver essential oils to the stomach or the intestines to treat conditions associated with the digestive system, the essential oils are best used internally.[17]

However, he does stress that oral ingestion will result in a fair degree of absorption in the mouth and esophagus. Only a very small amount of essential oil may make it to the intestines, as most of the ingested essential oil will be metabolised by the liver. He therefore recommends the use of suppositories.[17]

References

1. Price S, Price L. *Aromatherapy for health professionals*. 2nd edn, Churchill Livingstone, Edinburgh, 1999.
2. Davis P. *Aromatherapy an A-Z*. 2nd edn, C.W. Daniel Company, Saffron Walden, 1999.
3. Beck M. *Milady's theory and practice of therapeutic massage*. Milady Publishing, 1994.
4. Cowper A. *Manufacturing handbook for herbal medicines*. Allegro Printing Services, Australia, 1996.
5. Smeh N. *Creating your own cosmetics – naturally*. Alliance Publishing, USA, 1995.
6. Pizzorno J, Murray M. eds. *Textbook of natural medicine*. 2nd edn, Churchill Livingstone, Edinburgh, 1999.

7. Worwood V. *The fragrant pharmacy*. Bantam Books, 1991.
8. Valnet J. *The practice of aromatherapy*. C.W. Daniel Company, Saffron Walden, 1980.
9. Buchbauer G. *Molecular interactions*. International Journal of Aromatherapy, 1993; 5(1):11.
10. Maury M. *Marguerite Maury's guide to aromatherapy*. C.W. Daniel Company, Saffron Walden, 1994.
11. Lapraz J. *In profile*. International Journal of Aromatherapy 1991;3(4):12-14.
12. Pénoël D. *This is also aromatherapy*. The International Journal of Aromatherapy, 1991; 3(3):14-16.
13. Tisserand R. Balacs T. *Essential oil safety*. Churchill Livingstone, Edinburgh, 1995.
14. Tisserand R, Young R. *Essential oil safety*. 2nd edn, Elsevier, Edinburgh, 2014.
15. Price S, Price L. *Aromatherapy for health professionals*. 4th edn, Elsevier, Edinburgh, 2012.
16. Azemar J. *Galenic forms for aromatherapy – suppositories*. Aromatherapy Records, 1995; 1:86-89.
17. Schnaubelt K. *Advanced aromatherapy*. Healing Arts Press, Rochester, 1995.

UNIT

2

Materia Medica

How to use the Materia Medica

Essential Oil Monographs

- Amyris
- Angelica root
- Aniseed and Star Anise
- Aniseed myrtle
- Balsam, Peru
- Basil
- Bay laurel
- Bay, West Indian
- Benzoin
- Bergamot
- Birch, sweet
- Black pepper
- Boronia absolute
- Buchu
- Buddha wood
- Cabreuva
- Cajeput
- Camphor
- Caraway seed
- Cardamom
- Carrot seed
- Cassia
- Cedarwoods
- Celery seed
- Chamomile, German
- Chamomile, Roman
- Champaca absolute
- Cinnamon
- Cistus
- Citronella
- Clary sage
- Clove bud
- Coriander seed
- Cypress
- Cypress, blue
- Dill seed
- Elemi
- Eucalypts: 1,8-cineole rich
- Eucalyptus, broadleaf peppermint
- Eucalyptus, ironbark
- Eucalyptus, lemon-scented
- Everlasting
- Fennel, sweet
- Fir needle
- Fragonia
- Frankincense
- Galangal
- Galbanum
- Geranium
- Ginger
- Grapefruit
- Guaiacwood
- Ho leaf
- Hyssop
- Jasmine absolute
- Juniper berry

- Kanuka
- Kunzea
- Lavender
- Lavender, spike
- Lemon
- Lemongrass
- Lemon myrtle
- Lime
- Mandarin
- Manuka
- Marjoram, sweet
- May chang
- Melissa
- Myrrh
- Myrtle
- Neroli
- Niaouli
- Nutmeg
- Oakmoss absolute
- Opopanax
- Orange, sweet
- Oregano
- Palmarosa
- Parsley seed
- Patchouli
- Pennyroyal
- Peppermint
- Petitgrain
- Pine
- Ravintsara
- Rosalina
- Rose
- Rosemary
- Rosewood
- Sage
- Sandalwood
- Savory
- Spearmint
- Spikenard
- Spruce
- Tagetes
- Tangerine
- Tarragon
- Tea tree
- Tea tree, lemon-scented
- Thyme
- Tuberose absolute
- Turmeric
- Valerian
- Verbena
- Vetiver
- Violet leaf absolute
- Wintergreen
- Yarrow
- Ylang ylang

How to Use the Materia Medica

The monographs are headed and ordered according to the English common name of each essential oil. They have been designed to be as user-friendly as possible. This has been achieved by dividing the monographs into the following sections:

- identification
- history and traditional uses
- therapeutics
- aromatherapy uses
- dosage and administration
- safety profile.

Identification

Botanical name

This is the currently accepted botanical name of the plant from which the essential oil is extracted. When an essential oil is derived from more than one botanical source, I have attempted to include all the botanical species. I have used the website 'The Plant List' as a guide to confirm any disputed botanical names. The Plant List is a working list of all known plant species, and is a collaboration of the Royal Botanic Gardens, Kew and Missouri Botanical Garden. The Plant List provides the accepted Latin name along with all synonyms by which the species is known.[1]

Synonyms

Other English common names, alternative botanical names or names in other languages are listed.

Family

The name of the plant family is listed. The modern botanical nomenclature has been adopted. Where there is an alternative name for the plant family, this is given in the brackets.

Botany and origins

This section provides a brief description of the plant along with the origins of the plant.

Method of extraction

The typical method of extracting the essential oil is defined.

Characteristics

This section provides a detailed organoleptic description of the essential oil. In preparing this section, I am grateful to Steffen Arctander, author of *Perfume and Flavor Materials of Natural Origin*. This book is the most comprehensive reference providing us with the most detailed organoleptic description of essential oils.

Chemical composition

This section provides a chemical profile of the essential oil. The main chemical constituents and percentages of the constituents are provided.

We now know that there is no such thing as a typical chemical profile of an essential oil. The chemical variability of some essential oils can be significant. There are many factors that contribute to this such as country or region in which the plant is grown, seasonal variations or the time of harvesting. Many of these factors have been discussed in *Chapter 3 – Botany*.

In preparing this section, I am grateful to Brian M Lawrence for providing us with the most comprehensive database of essential oil chemical profiles that are published in the *Perfumer & Flavorist* magazine. Lawrence always indicates if the essential oil is a commercial sample, and identifies the country or region of origin along with chemotype where applicable.

In some instances where the essential oil is produced from plants grown in different countries or regions, I have provided more than one chemical profile. A comparative analysis is provided when there is a significant chemical variability.

Adulteration

We would expect, essential oils to be pure and natural substances. Unfortunately, adulteration is prolific in the essential oil industry and presents aromatherapy with a huge problem. It appears to be a commonly accepted practice for those who use essential oils for industrial purposes; however, in aromatherapy, it increases the risk of toxicity and undermines the therapeutic activity of the essential oil.

This section outlines the common practices of unscrupulous producers to fraudulently adulterate essential oils.

Pharmacopoeias and standards

This section lists any of the pharmacopoeias and standards in which essential oils appear. This may be of assistance to those involved in regulatory affairs. Some essential oils are listed in pharmacopoeias such as:

- ***German Commission E*** – The German Commission E was an expert committee of the German Federal Health Department set up in 1978. The committee reviewed the available scientific data and traditional information to assess the safety and efficacy of selected botanicals and essential oils. While the commission was discontinued in the early 1990s, much of the information remains valid.

- ***European Pharmacopoeia*** – The European Pharmacopoeia provides quality standards for the pharmaceutical industry in Europe to control medicines. It is a published collection of monographs which includes several essential oils.
- ***European Medicines Agency monographs*** – Many essential oils have been assessed by the European Medicines Agency Committee on Herbal Medicinal Products. The assessment reports and various documents associated with the botanicals are available from the European Medicines Agency website. [www.ema.europa.eu]
- ***WHO monographs*** – The WHO Monographs on Selected Medicinal Plants provide scientific information on safety, efficacy, quality control/ quality assurance of a wide range of medicinal herbs and essential oils. They have been developed to assist countries to develop their own monographs. The medicinal uses are categorised as those uses supported by clinical data, those uses described in other pharmacopoeia and in traditional systems of medicine, and those uses described in folk medicine, not yet supported by experimental or clinical data. Four volumes have been published.

Some of these monographs describe traditional systems of medicine; however, they tend to support only those claims that have been validated by clinical studies and pharmacological analysis.

ISO standards also exist for many essential oils. ISO standards are not designed or intended to define the efficacy or safety of an essential oil. The ISO standards are only a guide to the essential oil composition, and help us to know if an essential oil falls within the normal range as specified in the standard. As Harris states, an essential oil can still be very therapeutic and not fall within the ISO range.[2]

History and Traditional Uses

History

This section documents the history of the plant and the essential oil. This can often provide a valuable insight into the therapeutic uses of the essential oil.

Traditional medicine

This section discusses the role and use of the essential oil in traditional medicine such as Ayurveda, traditional Chinese medicine (TCM) and indigenous communities around the world.

Herbal

This section discusses the role of the herb from which the essential oil is extracted in herbal medicine.

Food, perfumery and flavouring

This section discusses the role of the essential oil in food flavouring and perfumery.

Other uses

This section identifies other uses of essential oils not covered by any the above categories.

Therapeutics

Pharmacology and clinical studies

This section lists a range of clinical studies and research which provide pharmacological or clinical evidence to support the actions assigned to the essential oils.

The studies are prepared in alphabetical order according to their activity. In selecting these studies, I have accessed various databases. The most important database is *The Essential Oil Bioactivity Research Database* dedicated to aromatherapy, which was established by Bob Harris of Quintessential Aromatics Ltd. The database is regularly updated and is composed of published, peer-reviewed research papers that investigate the bioactivity of many essential oils.

In some cases, I have cited in vitro studies. I am aware that most pharmaceutical regulatory guidelines state that in vitro studies have no relevance to clinical evidence. Many of the antimicrobial activity studies involving essential oils are in vitro studies. One of the main weaknesses of in vitro studies is that they fail to replicate the precise cellular conditions of the organism.[3]

An in vivo study involves whole, living organisms. Animal studies and clinical trials are two forms of in vivo research. In vivo studies are better suited for observing the overall effects of an oil on a living subject. While there are many reasons to believe in vivo can offer us conclusive insights about the nature of the oil being tested, there can be limitations and significant difference between the animal model and application to a human model.[3]

Clinical trials can provide a strong level of evidence. In a clinical trial, a specific therapy is tested under strictly controlled conditions to determine whether or not a treatment works without the influence of other factors not being tested. These factors may include a person's gender, their beliefs, or any other medication they may be on. Usually these trials involve individuals who will be randomly assigned to receive either the treatment being studied or standard care. Sometimes a placebo is used instead of standard care.[3]

I agree with Harris who states that many of the research papers investigating the bioactivity of essential oils and aromatherapy conclude that the results are very encouraging and that more clinical trials are required. Unfortunately, he states that, for the majority, this step is never taken.[4]

As the interest in aromatherapy continues to grow, I hope that more clinical trials will be conducted to validate many of the traditional claims made about aromatherapy.

Actions

Actions commonly cited in aromatherapy

These are the actions of essential oils that are listed in popular and commonly used aromatherapy books. Many of these claims may not have undergone intensive clinical studies. Many of these actions are based on traditional use. The Advisory Committee on Complementary Medicines (ACCM) has adopted the following definition of the term 'traditional use' intended for the purposes of regulatory affairs:

> *Traditional use refers to documentary evidence that a substance has been used over three or more generations of recorded use for a specific health related or medicinal purpose.*[5,6]

I, therefore, believe that some of these actions may be valid based on the assumption that aromatherapy meets the criteria of traditional use over three or more generations.

Actions supported by clinical studies

Based on the studies that I have reviewed and traditional evidence available, these are the actions of essential oils that can be supported by reliable clinical studies. As more studies become available, I am confident that this list will increase.

Comment

In this section, I provide my comments and observations regarding the use of the essential oil in aromatherapy. To support my comments, I may often draw upon the wisdom of other aromatherapists and researchers.

Aromatherapy Uses

Clinical aromatherapy

Where applicable, the clinical aromatherapy uses are divided into categories such as analgesic, cardiovascular system, children's remedy, detoxification, digestive system, integumentary system, lymphatic system, musculoskeletal system, nervous system, psychological, reproductive system, respiratory system, skin care and urinary system.

Energetics, psyche and subtle uses

Energetics

The energetics of the essential oils described in these monographs are drawn on the principles of TCM. In preparing this section, I am grateful to Gabriel Mojay and Peter Holmes. Having a background in TCM, I have always had an affinity with their work. They eloquently and succinctly combined important principles of TCM with aromatherapy to provide us with a holistic and integrative perspective of the therapeutic use of essential oils.

Personality

This section examines the relationship between scent and personality. It is known that individuals are often drawn towards the scent of a particular essential oil based on their personality.

In preparing this section, I am indebted to Valerie Ann Worwood for introducing aromatherapists to the concept of describing the characteristics of individual essential oils according to human personality types. The association of scent with personality types has always fascinated me.

This inspired me to qualify as a certified Myers Briggs MBTI® practitioner. In these monographs, I have assigned one of the 16 Myers-Briggs personality types to the more commonly used essential oils in aromatherapy. In assigning a personality type to the essential oil, I have based it on my experience and the responses I have had from students in my classes. A more extensive study based on much larger numbers will be needed to statistical verify the relationships between the personality types and the essential oils.

In volume II of *The Complete Guide to Aromatherapy*, we will examine the rationale behind the relationship of the essential oils and the Myers-Briggs personality types.

I will provide a very brief explanation of the Myers-Briggs personality types for those that may not be familiar with the terminology. It is based on a system to help us understand personality based on the idea that we have a preference to the ways in which we do things. Each personality type has 4 pairs of preferences. Within each pair, we tend to favour one over the other most of the time. The four pairs of opposite preferences are:

Extravert (E) and Introvert (I) – the energising preference

This preference refers to where we prefer to focus our attention and what energises us.

- Extraverts (E) focus their attention outward and get their energy from being with other people and from the things they do.
- Introverts (I) focus their attention inward and get their energy from their inner world of ideas and thoughts.

I have observed that essential oils which energise us, and are uplifting are preferred by extroverts. This includes citrus aromas, leafy aromas, spicy and rich floral aromas.

I have observed that essential oils that help us to focus inwardly, are relaxing, and help us to meditate are preferred by introverts. This includes woody aromas, light floral aromas, some leafy oils and resin oils.

Sensing (S) and Intuition (N) - the perceiving preference

This preference refers to how we prefer to take in information.

- Sensing (S) pays attention to information taken in directly from the five senses and focus on what is or what was. They focus on here-and-now reality.
- Intuition (N) perceives the world through their imagination and abstract thought. They pay attention to their sixth sense. They rely on hunches and insights and focus on what might be.

This is perhaps the most challenging preference to classify oils as all essential oils help us focus on the here-and-now moment and to engage our sense of smell. Hence, we can think of all essential oils as having a sensing quality. I like to think of this as being aware of our initial reaction to the aroma. Some essential oils awaken our intuition while others keep us focused on the present.

I have observed that essential oils with strong and stimulating aromas tend to be preferred by people with a preference to sensing and aromas which have a delicate, light and balanced aroma are preferred by those with a preference to the intuitive preference.

Thinking (T) and Feeling (F) – the decision-making preference

This preference refers to how we evaluate information and make decisions.

- Thinking (T) make decisions based on a logical and objective way.
- Feeling (F) make decisions based on what is important to them and in a personal way and on their values.

When explaining the difference between thinking and feeling I often ask – 'Where do you feel the scent – in your heart or head?'

If the energy of the aroma invigorates the mind then it will be preferred by persons with a thinking preference. If the energy awakens and warms the heart then it will be preferred by persons with feeling preference.

General fresh sweet citrus, florals, resin and woody aromas are preferred by those with a feeling preference, while herbaceous, leafy, spicy and sharp citrus are preferred by those with a thinking preference.

Judging (J) or Perceiving (P) – the lifestyle preference

These are the two lifestyle orientation preferences.

- Judging (J) tend to like closure and want to have things decided as soon as possible. They live in an organised and planned way.
- Perceiving (P) tend to be more spontaneous and flexible and keep their options open.

How does the aroma of the oil make you feel? Does it help you feel carefree and relaxed or does it instil a sense of discipline and commitment? Does it give you focus and make you feel goal oriented and focused on work?

Those with a preference to perceiving will generally be attracted to the sweet citrus, floral, sweet resin and earthy aromas while those with a judging preference will be attracted to spicy, herbaceous, resiny, woody, and sharp citrus aromas.

Subtle

This section investigates the subtle or spiritual influences of essential oils. In preparing this section, I am indebted to all the aromatherapists who have developed a unique framework that integrates the practice of aromatherapy with energy healing. I would like to acknowledge the work of the following aromatherapists – Patricia Davis, author of *Subtle Aromatherapy*, Valerie Ann Worwood, author of *The Fragrant Heavens*, Joni Keim Loughran & Ruah Bull, authors of *Aromatherapy and Subtle Energy Techniques*, and Robbi Zeck, author of *The Blossoming Heart*.

They provide us with incredible healing insights to the use of essential oils as a catalyst for personal transformation, and to promote emotional and spiritual wellbeing.

Dosage and Administration

Blending

Aromatherapy

This section provides a list of essential oils that can be blended with the essential oil for a range of conditions. The list of essential oils recommended for blending is by no means exhaustive. You only need to choose two or three essential oils from the list to support the desired therapeutic outcome. Detailed blending instructions will be provided in volume II of *The Complete Guide to Aromatherapy* in the chapter on essential oil blending.

Perfumery

This section provides advice to those of us wishing to refine our blending skills and create natural perfumes using essential oils. In preparing this section, I am indebted to the invaluable perfume blending advice provided by Steffen Arctander, author of *Perfume and Flavor Materials of Natural Origin.*

Mode of administration

The mode of administration refers to the method of application of the essential oils. The modes of administration include baths – full body bath, foot bath, sitz bath; topical application – massage, ointment, skin care; and inhalation – direct inhalation, diffuser, oil vaporiser. In some cases, I have also provided advice on the potential use of the oil by ingestion. For detailed instructions on each of the modes of administration refer to *Chapter 7 – Use.*

Safety Profile

General safety

This section lists any potential hazards of the essential oil. In preparing the section on safety, I am indebted to Robert Tisserand & Rodney Young, authors of the 2nd edition of *Essential Oil Safety*. They have prepared the most comprehensive and authoritative resource on the safe use of essential oils.

Contraindications

This section lists and discusses any contraindications where an essential oil should not be used.

Toxicity

Where applicable, this section lists and discusses toxicity concerns of the essential oil.

Regulatory guidelines

Some essential oils have GRAS status. GRAS is a list of substances 'generally recognized as safe' for use in food flavouring. It must be noted that the amounts generally recommended and used in food flavouring are much lower than a therapeutic dose required for the essential oil.

References

1. *The Plant List.* Version 1.1. Retrieved from http://www.theplantlist.org/
2. Harris B. *Editorial.* International Journal of Aromatherapy, 2006; 16(2): 55.
3. Western Sydney University. *Finding and evaluating complementary medicine evidence.* Retrieved Jan 11, 2018, from https://www.westernsydney.edu.au/nicm/health_information/evaluating_the_evidence/module_three
4. Harris R. *Phytotherapeutic uses of essential oils.* In Baser KHC, Buchbauer G. eds. *Handbook of essential oils – science, technology and applications.* 2nd edn. CRC Press, Boca Raton, 2016: 381-431.
5. *General guidelines for methodologies on research and evaluation of traditional medicine.* World Health Organization, Geneva, 2000. Retrieved from http://apps.who.int/medicinedocs/en/d/Jwhozip42e/
6. *Guidelines for levels and kinds of evidence to support indications and claims.* Therapeutic Goods Administration, Woden, 2011. Retrieved from https://www.tga.gov.au/publication/guidelines-levels-and-kinds-evidence-support-indications-and-claims

Amyris

Identification

Botanical name

Amyris balsamifera L.

Synonyms

West Indian sandalwood, West Indian rosewood, candlewood, torchwood

Family

Rutaceae

Botany and origins

Amyris balsamifera is a small tree 3-6 m which grows in northern parts of South America, in Central America and throughout the West Indies.[1]

The oil is known to remain in the timber for many years. When distilled, fence posts of amyris timber decades old yielded a small quantity of excellent quality essential oil.[2] It is not related to either *Santalum album* or *Santalum spicatum*.

Method of extraction

Amyris oil is steam distilled from the wood of *A. balsamifera*. The oil from the fresh wood is usually of an inferior quality compared to oil distilled from wood that is allowed to season for up to six months.[2]

Characteristics

Amyris oil is a pale yellow or brownish yellow viscous liquid with a subtle woody, sweet balsamic scent. It has a slightly oily-sweet, balsamic top note, reminiscent of guaiacwood. The odour varies considerably, depending on the age of the oil and the age of the wood prior to distillation.[1]

Chemical composition

Amyris oil consists primarily of sesquiterpene hydrocarbons and oxygenated sesquiterpenes.

Adulteration

Amyris oil is often fractionated. Certain fractions are sold separately, while other fractions are cut with Virginian cedarwood.[1]

Amyris oil is used to adulterate vetiver oil produced in Haiti. According to Arctander, the 'rule' is that 5% amyris oil is added to all locally produced vetiver oils before these are exported from Haiti.[1]

Pharmacopoeias and standards

The purity, composition and physico-chemical properties of amyris oil are defined in the ISO Standard 3525: 2008 Oil of Amyris.

History and Traditional Uses

Food, perfumery and flavouring

Amyris oil is used in perfumery as a fixative, but its woody scent is considered to be much more inferior to that of sandalwood oil.[1]

Therapeutics

Pharmacology and clinical studies

Antimicrobial activity

Compared with *S. album* and *S. spicatum*, amyris oil exhibited weak or no activity against a range of bacteria.[3] However, another study reported that amyris oil had good antimicrobial activity against several multi-drug-resistant microorganisms, and that it possessed antioxidant activity.[4] Another study reported that amyris oil was as effective as lemon oil and exhibited moderate activity against antimycobacteria such as *M. tuberculosis* and *M. avium*.[5]

Actions

Actions commonly cited in aromatherapy

Antiseptic, balsamic, sedative[6]

Actions supported by clinical studies

None

Comment

Review of the traditional uses and clinical data cannot confirm any clinical applications for amyris oil in aromatherapy.

Aromatherapy Uses

Clinical aromatherapy

Amyris oil lacks any of the santalols, which are considered the most pharmacologically active compounds found in *S. album* or *S. spicatum*, therefore it is incorrect to suggest that it has a similar chemical profile to other sandalwood oils and that it shares similar properties.

Energetics, psyche and subtle uses

Subtle aromatherapy

Keim Loughran & Bull suggest using amyris oil to support the development of the right brain in order to increase creativity.[7]

Dosage and Administration

Blending

Aromatherapy

Amyris is not commonly used in aromatherapy, however It could be used when an inexpensive woody base note is required. It blends well with essential oils such as Atlas or Virginian cedarwood, and could be used to intensify the rich earthy scent of vetiver or patchouli.

Perfumery

Amyris oil is often used in soap perfumes. It blends well with citronella, lavender and oakmoss oils.[1]

Mode of administration

Bath

Full body bath, foot bath

Topical

Compress, massage, ointment, skin care

Inhalation

Direct inhalation, diffuser, oil vaporiser

Safety Profile

General safety

Amyris oil is non-toxic, non-irritant and non-sensitising.[6]

Contraindications

No known contraindications.

Regulatory guidelines

While amyris oil is not listed in any of the regulatory guidelines, we can consider it to be safe for use in aromatherapy.

References

1. Arctander S. *Perfume and flavor materials of natural origins.* Allured Publishing, Carol Stream, 1994.
2. Weiss EA. *Essential oil crops.* CAB International, London, 1997.
3. Jivovetz L et al. *Comparative study on the antimicrobial activities of different sandalwood essential oils of various origins.* Flavour and Fragrance Journal, 2006; 21(3):465-468. Cited in Quintessential Aromatics Ltd database, 2013.
4. Dahiya P, Manglik A. *Evaluation of antibacterial, antifungal and antioxidant potential from Amyris balsamifera against multi drug resistant clinical isolates.* Asian Journal of Pharmaceutical and Clinical Research. 2013; 6 - Suppl 5: 57-60. Cited in Quintessential Aromatics Ltd database, 2013.
5. Alves JA et al. *Antimycobacterial activity of some commercially available plant-derived essential oils.* Chemistry of Natural Compounds, 2015; 51(2):353-355. Cited in Quintessential Aromatics Ltd database, 2013.
6. Lawless J. *The encyclopaedia of essential oils.* Element Books, Shaftesbury, 1992.
7. Keim Loughran J, Bull R. *Aromatherapy and subtle energy techniques.* Frog Limited, Berkeley, 2000.

Angelica

Identification

Botanical name

European angelica: *Angelica archangelica L.*

Himalayan angelica: *Angelica glauca* Edgew.

Synonyms

European angelica: *Angelica officinalis,* garden angelica, angel's herb, root of holy spirit[1]

Himalayan angelica: Smooth angelica[1]

Family

Apiaceae (Umbelliferae)

Botany and origins

There are over 30 different types of angelica.[2]

The two most commonly used angelica oils in aromatherapy are from the European and Himalayan angelica plants.

A. glauca is reported on the IUCN Red List of Threatened Species as an endangered species. The report states that the harvesting of the plant from its natural habitat is occurring at levels that are not sustainable. Wild population during the last 10 years has declined by 70%. Unfortunately, there are no solid conservation action programs to support this species or to stop its population decline.[3]

Angelica is a stout biennial or perennial herb which grows up to 2 m high with a large rhizome. It is cultivated in Belgium, Holland, France, Germany, Hungary and northern India.[2]

An essential oil is produced from the roots and the seeds. This monograph will focus on the root oil as it is the most frequently available and used oil.

Method of extraction

Angelica root oil is steam-distilled from the dried roots of *A. archangelica.*

Characteristics

Angelica root oil is a pale yellow to orange-brown coloured liquid. Its viscosity varies according to the root material used for distillation and the age of the essential oil. Beneath the peppery top note is a rich, somewhat herbaceous-earthy, woody base note of unique tenacity and great diffusive power. The base note is also slightly musky-animal-like with a spicy undertone.[4]

It is preferable that the oil be distilled from roots that are not more than two years old. The oil from older roots is different to that of young roots, but not inferior. The monoterpene hydrocarbons have resinified in oil from older roots and it has little or no peppery top note.[4]

Chemical composition

The chemistry of angelica root essential oil is complex. The oil contains up to 70% monoterpene hydrocarbons, small quantities of esters, alcohols, coumarins and lactones.

The major constituents of angelica root oil from Italy were α-pinene (21.3%), δ-3-carene (16.4%) and α-phellandrene (8.7%).[5]

Several reports are available on the chemical profile of *A. archangelica* oil from angelica growing in different parts of the world, showing α-pinene, limonene, *p*-cymene, δ-3-carene, α-phellandrene, β-phellandrene and bornyl acetate as the major constituents. However, an analysis of the oil extracted from *A. archangelica* roots in the Himalaya identified dillapiole and nothoapiole as the major constituents. These have never been reported before. It was suggested that great variations in the composition of the essential oil may be attributed to the existence of chemotypes, and adaptation of the species to the particular habitat.[6]

The furanocoumarins found in angelica oil are omelliferone, archangelicine, angelicine and bergaptene. These constituents are responsible for angelica root oil's phototoxicity. Coumarins have a strong affinity with the nervous system and can raise the threshold above which one registers nervous stress.[7]

The major chemical constituents in *A. glauca* essential oil from the roots are β-phellandrene, (Z)-ligustilide, methyl octane, limonene, β-pinene, thujene, (*Z*)-3-butylidene-phthalide, (*E*)-ligustilide and citronellyl acetate.[1]

The chemical composition of European angelica root oil was reported as follows:

α-pinene (24.0%), camphene (1.3%), β-pinene (1.25%), sabinene (0.76%), δ-3-carene (10.1%), α-phellandrene and myrcene (7.6%), limonene (13.2%), β-phellandrene (10%), *cis*-ocimene (1.25%), *trans*-ocimene (2.68%), *p*-cymene (9.8%), terpinolene (0.16%), copaene (1.91%), cryptone (0.5%), β-bisabolene (0.72%), humulene monoxide (0.41%), tridecanolide (0.45%), pentadecanolide (0.37%).[8]

Adulteration

Angelica root oil is a very expensive oil and has a low yield. The oil is subject to adulteration with synthetic monoterpenes.[9] In the past, angelica root oil was also adulterated with copaiba balm, gurjun balsam, lovage root oil and amyris oil.[10]

Pharmacopoeias and standards

At the time of writing, the purity, composition, physico-chemical properties and therapeutic use of angelica root oil are not defined in any pharmacopoeia monograph or standard.

History and Traditional Uses

History

The virtues of angelica have been known for centuries. Folklore testifies to its merits as a protection against contagion, for purifying the blood and for curing every conceivable malady. It was held as a sovereign remedy for poisons and all infectious maladies.[11]

Culpeper describes the properties of angelica root:

> *The stalks and roots are candied and eaten fasting, are good preservatives in time of infection, and will warm and comfort a cold stomach ... A water distilled from the root, as steeped in wine and distilled, and drank two or three spoonfuls at a time easeth all pains and torments coming of cold and wind, and taken with some of the root in powder, helpeth the pleurisy, as also all other diseases of the lungs and breast, as coughs, phthisic and shortness of breath.*[12]

Angelica was closely linked with Christian beliefs. According to one legend, angelica was revealed in a dream by an angel to cure the plague. Another explanation for the name of this plant is that it blooms on the day of Michael the Archangel, and it is used as a preservative against evil spirits and witchcraft.[11]

Traditional medicine

In India, *A. glauca* root is given to women after

delivery of a baby for vitality and strength.[1]

In Ayurveda, the roots of *A. glauca* are used in the treatment of dyspepsia, constipation, infantile atrophy, dysentery and menorrhagia.[1]

In folk medicine, the roots of *A. archangelica* are used as an antiseptic, expectorant, diuretic and antiemetic, as well as for toothaches, wounds, rheumatism, skin rashes, fever and headache.[1]

Herbal

Most old herbals refer to angelica as a purifying agent, easing rheumatism and gout, warming, comforting and sudorific, and it is particularly effective in drying out the body and expelling toxins. The powdered root is extensively used in herbal preparations to treat bronchitis, pleurisy and other diseases of the lungs. It is also recommended for menstrual regulation.[2]

The German Commission E recommends angelica root herb extract for loss of appetite, peptic discomfort, such as mild spasms of the gastrointestinal tract, feeling of fullness and flatulence.[13]

Angelica sinensis (dong quai), a species related to *A. archangelica*, is traditionally used in TCM for the treatment of dysmenorrhea.[9] A tea made from the root of *A. archangelica* has been used as a folk remedy for stomach cancer.[14]

A

Food, perfumery and flavouring

The roots of *A. glauca* are also used for seasoning curry. In the Kumaun and Garhwal regions of Uttarakhand, the roots are used in dal or curry flavouring to enhance taste.[1]

The oil is used as a fragrance ingredient in soaps, detergents, creams, lotions and perfumes.[2]

Angelica root oil is used in Benedictine, chartreuse and Cointreau type liqueurs.[4]

Therapeutics

Pharmacology and clinical studies

Antimicrobial activity

A. glauca and *A. archangelica* root essential oils have been reported to exhibit antibacterial and antifungal properties.[1,2,15]

The oil of *A. archangelica* root from Italy showed good antimicrobial activity against *Clostridium difficile, Clostridium perfringens, Enterococcus faecalis, Eubacterium limosum, Peptostreptococcus anaerobius* and *Candida albicans*. The oil had a weaker antimicrobial activity against bifidobacteria and lactobacilli, which are useful in the intestinal microflora.[5]

Anxiolytic activity

The anxiolytic effects of angelica oil were demonstrated in three anxiety models using mice.[16]

Withdrawal symptoms

A study investigated the effect of inhalation of black pepper or angelica on the nicotine habits of students, staff and faculty on a US college campus. The participants had to inhale one drop of essential oil on a tissue for two minutes whenever they craved nicotine. Both black pepper and angelica oils reduced the level of nicotine craving and allowed a longer delay before next using tobacco. Black pepper reduced the level of craving more than angelica; however, angelica allowed for further delay than black pepper. It was suggested that aromatherapy may be useful in nicotine withdrawal.[17]

Actions

Actions commonly cited in aromatherapy

Antiseptic, antispasmodic, carminative, cholagogue, depurative, diaphoretic, digestive, diuretic, emmenagogue, expectorant, nervine, stomachic, tonic[18,19]

Actions supported by clinical studies

Antimicrobial

Comment

I disagree with Lis-Balchin who states that angelica root oil has a pervasive, unpleasant aroma that does not lend itself to use as a fragrance.[9] The earthy spicy aroma of angelica root oil is divine!

Fischer-Rizzi beautifully describes angelica root when she states that the source of the angelica's strength and rejuvenation is from the earth, providing us with the physical vitality or earthy strength.[20]

However, Lis-Balchin is correct in saying that none of the traditional uses of angelica root essential oil have been documented. Most of the information available is for the whole herbal extract.[9]

Aromatherapy Uses

Clinical aromatherapy

Digestive system

The oil is an excellent tonic for the digestive system.[21]

Fischer-Rizzi states that it is an effective, bitter tasting medicine for a weak stomach or weak digestive system, as well as for dyspepsia and flatulence. For this purpose, she suggests that we take 1 to 3 drops internally, two to three times a day before a meal. However, she says not to use honey, as the bitterness of the oil has an important reflexive effect on the stomach.[20]

Lymphatic system

Angelica root oil is reputed to have excellent detoxifying and diuretic properties.[18,21] Used in a massage oil, it improves lymph drainage, and relieves rheumatism and arthritis, fluid retention and cellulite.[21]

Nervous system

Angelica root oil is well known for its tonic effect on the nervous system.[21] It is recommended for weakness and nervousness and for convalescents and elderly people.[19]

It is ideal for fatigue and stress-related disorders:

> *Angelica aids people with an upset nervous system who urgently need to rebuild body and soul. The oil helps soothe all kinds of weakness. It's like super-growth fertiliser you might feed a sickly plant. The essential oil of angelica root will help you rediscover your own inner strength and stamina.*[20]

Psychological

Fischer-Rizzi suggests placing 1 drop of angelica root oil in the palm of your hand, rubbing both hands together briskly and then holding your hands under your nose and breathing deeply. You will immediately feel enlivened and notice its strengthening effect. She suggests this is great whenever you feel faint, nauseous, weak or are suffering from anxiety.[20]

Respiratory system

It is an expectorant and may be used for chronic bronchial asthma, sinus infections, chronic respiratory problems and coughs.[21,22,23]

Skin care

Angelica root essential oil is not commonly used in skin care.

Energetics, psyche and subtle uses

Energetics

Angelica root is *warming* and *drying*. Holmes states that the oil strengthens *Yang* and is restoring. It strengthens the *Stomach* and *Spleen* and eliminates *excess damp*. It awakens the appetite, relieves abdominal distention and dispels mucous *damp*.[22]

It is beneficial in all *Yin excess* conditions such as *cold*, *damp* and phlegm congestion in the lungs, intestines and uterus.[22]

Personality

Fischer-Rizzi suggests that angelica root will assist people who are afraid or weak, or who lack perseverance and have a tough time making decisions. She perfectly describes the effect of angelica root on our psyche:

> *Don't give up! Stick with it – nothing has been lost. Don't be afraid- begin to rebuild. You are strong – nothing will knock you down.*[20]

According to Myers-Briggs personality types, the angelica root personality is likely to be an ISFP. ISFPs are easy going, likable and have an attitude of live and let live. They are often quiet, reserved and modest and do not like attention. They prefer to live in the present moment and appreciate the simple things in life. Harmonious relationships are important. They are loyal, gentle, compassionate and often put other's need before their own. They can be highly motivated when their work contributes to something they care deeply about or believe in. They enjoy helping people develop practical skills. They are flexible and adaptable. They feel restricted by excessive rules, inflexible structure and bureaucracy. They have very little desire to control or compete. They do very well in emergency situations.

Subtle

It has been suggested that the oil helps the user to be more open to angelic powers. Davis relates the physical appearance of the angelica plant to its subtle qualities:

> *The living angelica plant speaks to us eloquently … Underground it forms strong and solid roots, above ground the whole seems to aspire heavenward; the powerful stems soar to two metres in height, topped by a mass of delicate greenish-white flowers so ethereal in appearance as to seem almost insubstantial.*[24]

The oil is recommended for strengthening the mind and spirit:

> *The source of angelica's strength is the earth, since the plant itself has been strongly influenced by the elements of the soil. As an essential oil, angelica has a fiery temperament and lends us more physical vitality or earthly strength than cosmic or spiritual energy. Angelica is particularly suited to people who need solid grounding or who search for reality.*[20]

Angelica root assists in bringing us into conscious relationship with the angelic realm so we can receive its teachings and benefit from its wisdom.[21,25]

Worwood states that angelica root will encourage strength, stamina, comfort and focus, and help keep us grounded.[26]

Zeck states that angelica root can assist in strengthening our resolve and give us the strength to follow through with our convictions. It allows us to stand our ground and to assert and express our truth with confidence.[27]

Dosage and Administration

Blending

Aromatherapy

To alleviate anxiety and stress-related conditions, consider blending angelica root oil with essential oils such as bergamot, Atlas cedarwood, everlasting, lavender, lemon, lemongrass, patchouli, sandalwood or vetiver.

As a tonic to promote strength and keep us grounded, consider blending angelica root oil with essential oils such as Atlas cedarwood, ginger, patchouli, sandalwood, spikenard or vetiver.

As a digestive tonic, consider blending angelica root oil with essential oils such as black pepper, sweet fennel, ginger or sweet orange.

Fischer-Rizzi suggests using angelica root oil with lemongrass in a vaporiser to strengthen the mind and spirit.[20]

Perfumery

Arctander states that angelica root oil is highly esteemed in perfumery. However, it can be overpowering and requires much skill to blend. It blends well with patchouli, opopanax, costus, clary sage, vetiver and oakmoss absolute. It is used in heavy chypre, oriental, citrus and fougère style perfumes.[4]

Mode of administration

Bath

Full body bath, foot bath

Topical

Compress, massage, ointment

Inhalation

Direct inhalation, diffuser, oil vaporiser

Safety Profile

General safety

The oil is non-toxic and non-irritant. The furanocoumarins present in angelica root essential oil sensitises the skin to UV light. It is considered phototoxic.[13,24,28]

Tisserand & Young state that no information is available for Himalayan angelica root oil, but as it has no furanocoumarins it is not considered to be phototoxic. They also state that there are no known hazards or contraindications.[28]

Contraindications

Herbal preparations of angelica root are contraindicated in pregnancy as it is a uterine stimulant and an emmenagogue.[30]

Davis and Tisserand & Young do not state that the oil is contraindicated during pregnancy; however, Lawless states that it should not be used during pregnancy.[18,21,28]

Regulatory guidelines

Angelica root essential oil has GRAS status.

IFRA standard recommends a maximum limit of 0.8% for leave-on products. There is no restriction for wash-off products.[29]

References

1. Joshi RK. *Angelica (Angelica glauca and A. archangelica) oils.* In Preedy VR. ed. *Essential oils in food preservation, flavor and safety.* Academic Press, London, 2016: 203-208.
2. Khan I, Abourashed E. *Leung's encyclopedia of common natural ingredients used in food, drugs and cosmetics.* 3rd edn. John Wiley & Sons, New Jersey, 2010.
3. Ved D, Saha D, Ravikumar K, Haridasan K. *Angelica glauca.* The IUCN Red List of Threatened Species 2015: e.T50126564A50131275. doi: 10.2305/IUCN.UK.2015-2.RLTS.T50126564A50131275.en
4. Arctander S. *Perfume and flavor materials of natural origin.* Allured Publishing, Carol Stream, 1994.
5. Fraternale D et al. *Essential oil composition and antimicrobial activity of Angelica archangelica L. (Apiaceae) roots.* Journal of Medicinal Food, 2014; 17(9): 1043-1047. doi: 10.1089/jmf.2013.0012
6. Chauhan RS et al. *Variation in the essential oil composition of Angelica archangelica from three different altitudes in Western Himalaya, India.* Industrial Crops and Products, 2016: 94: 401-404. doi: 10.1016/j.indcrop.2016.08.044
7. Whitton S. *Herb of angels.* Aromatherapy Quarterly, 1993.
8. Lawrence BM. *Essential oils 1976-1978.* Allured Publishing, Wheaton, 1979.
9. Lis-Balchin M. *Aromatherapy science – a guide for healthcare professionals.* Pharmaceutical Press, London, 2006.
10. Schmidt E, Wanner J. *Adulteration of essential oils.* In Baser KHC, Buchbauer G. eds. *Handbook of essential oils – science, technology and applications.* 2nd edn. CRC Press, Boca Raton, 2016: 707-745.
11. Grieve M. *A modern herbal – Vol. I.* Dover Publications, New York, 1971.
12. Potterton W. ed. *Culpeper's colour herbal.* Foulsham, Great Britain, 1983.

A

13. Blumenthal M et al. *The complete German commission E monographs: therapeutic guide to herbal medicines*. American Botanical Council, Austin, 1998.
14. Duke J. *Handbook of medicinal herbs*. CRC Press, Boca Raton, 1987.
15. Dean SG, Ritchie G. *Antibacterial properties of plant essential oils*. International Journal of Food Microbiology, 1987; 5: 165-180. Cited in Quintessential Aromatics database, 2013.
16. Min L et al. *The effects of angelica essential oil in social interaction and hole-board tests*. Pharmacology, Biochemistry and Behavior, 2005; 81(4): 838-842. Cited in Quintessential Aromatics database, 2013.
17. Cordell B, Buckle J. *The effects of aromatherapy on nicotine craving on a U.S. campus: A small comparison study*. Journal of Alternative and Complementary Medicine, 2013; 19(8): 709-713. Cited in Quintessential Aromatics database, 2013.
18. Lawless J. *The encyclopaedia of essential oils*. Element Books, Shaftesbury, 1992.
19. Lavabre M. *Aromatherapy workbook*. Healing Arts Press, Rochester, 1997.
20. Fischer-Rizzi S. *Complete aromatherapy handbook*. Sterling Publishing, New York, 1990.
21. Davis P. *Aromatherapy an A-Z*. 2nd edn. C.W. Daniel Company, Saffron Walden, 1999.
22. Holmes P. *The energetics of western herbs – Vol. I*. Artemis Press, Boulder, 1989.
23. Evans WC. *Trease and Evans pharmacognosy*. 15th edn. WB Saunders, Edinburgh, 2002.
24. Davis P. *Subtle aromatherapy*. C.W. Daniel Company, Saffron Walden, 1991.
25. Keim Loughran J, Bull R. *Aromatherapy anointing oils*. Frog, Berkeley, 2001.
26. Worwood VA. *The fragrant heavens*. Transworld Publishers, London, 1999.
27. Zeck R. *The blossoming heart – aromatherapy for healing and transformation*. Aroma Tours, East Ivanhoe, 2004.
28. Tisserand R, Young R. *Essential oil safety*. 2nd edn. Churchill Livingstone, Edinburgh, 2014.
29. International Fragrance Association. *IFRA standard – angelica root oil*. 2015. Retrieved from http://www.ifraorg.org/en-us/standards-library#.WgaZjhO0P-Y
30. McGuffin M et al. *American herbal products association's botanical safety handbook*. CRC Press, Boca Raton, 1997.

Aniseed and Star Anise

Identification

Botanical name

Aniseed: *Pimpinella anisum* L.

Star Anise: *Illicium verum* JD Hook

Synonyms

Aniseed: anise, *Anisum vulgare*, *A. officinarum*

Star anise: Chinese anise, Chinese star anise

Family

Aniseed: Apiaceae (Umbelliferae)

Star anise: Illiciaceae

Botany and origins

Aniseed is an annual herb, usually less than 0.6 m high. The seeds are reddish-brown, ribbed and aromatic, with a distinctive licorice-like smell and taste. It is native to Greece and Egypt, now widely cultivated in Spain and many other countries throughout the world.[1]

Star anise is an evergreen tree usually 4-6 m high, but may grow up to 12 m. It is indigenous to South East Asia and is extensively cultivated in southern China, Vietnam, India and Japan. The part of the plant used is the dried, ripe fruit that consists of five to 13 (usually eight) seed-bearing woody follicles attached to a central axis in the shape of a star, hence the name star anise. China is the major producer of star anise.[1]

Japanese star anise should not be confused with true star anise. It is obtained from a related species, *Illicium lanceolatum*, which grows in southern China, Taiwan and Japan. It is described as a smaller, deformed version of the Chinese star anise.[1]

Method of extraction

Aniseed oil is distilled from the dried ripe fruit (seeds) of *P. anisum*. Star anise is steam-distilled from the fresh or partly dried whole or comminuted fruits of *I. verum*.

Characteristics

Aniseed oil is a clear to very pale yellow coloured oil with an intensely sweet clean odour, truly reminiscent of the crushed seeds. A very common description used is that of a 'licorice-like odour'.[2]

Chemical composition

The main chemical constituent is anethole, a phenyl propane derivative. It also contains methyl chavicol or estragole, which is a phenolic ether.

These constituents account for aniseed's excellent antispasmodic properties.[3]

Most pharmacopoeias allow the use of both aniseed and star anise essential oils indiscriminately, as the anethole content is up to 90–95% in both oils.[1]

The chemical composition of *P. anisum* oil was reported as follows:

trans-anethole (76.7-93.0%), estragole (0.5-6.1%), anisaldehyde (0.1-3.5%), linalool (0.1-1.5%), α-terpineol (0.1-1.5%), and *cis*-anethole (<0.5%).[4]

The chemical composition of *I. verum* oil was reported as follows:

trans-anethole (71.19%), feniculin (14.56%), estragole (5.04%), limonene (1.68%), linalool (0.69%), β-caryophyllene (0.63%), *trans*-α-farnesene (0.68%), anisaldehyde (0.41%), nerolidol (0.3%), cinnamyl acetate (0.25%), *cis*-ocimene (0.32%).[5]

Adulteration

Aniseed oil is often adulterated with the less expensive star anise oil or with synthetic anethole.[6]

Pharmacopoeias and standards

The purity, composition, physico-chemical properties and therapeutic use of aniseed essential oil are defined in several pharmacopoeia monographs and standards:

- ISO 3475:2002 Oil of Aniseed (*Pimpinella anisum* L.)
- German Commission E
- European Pharmacopoeia
- Draft Community Herbal Monograph on *Pimpinella anisum* L., Aetheroleum. European Medicines Agency
- WHO Monographs on Selected Medicinal Plants–Vol. 3.

History and Traditional Uses

History

Aniseed was cultivated by the ancient Egyptians as a medicine and culinary spice, and was thought to 'refresh the heart'. It was well known to the Greeks and Romans as a 'pick-me-up'. Combined with orris root, it was used by Edward IV for scenting linen and clothes.[7]

The oil was mixed with spirits of wine to create a liqueur anisette, which was recommended for bronchitis and spasmodic asthma.[8]

Arctander states that once Chinese star anise oil entered the market, it replaced aniseed fruit oil so effectively that even the pharmacopoeias acknowledged the use of the two oils indiscriminately.[2]

Traditional medicine

Aniseed has been used as aromatic carminatives, stimulants and expectorants. It is also used as an oestrogenic agent to increase milk secretion, promote menstruation, facilitate childbirth and increase libido. Chinese star anise has been used in TCM for similar purposes for more than 1,300 years.[1]

Herbal

According to the British Herbal Pharmacopoeia, the aniseed fruits have expectorant, antispasmodic, carminative and parasiticidal properties. An infusion of the dried fruits three times a day is recommended for the treatment of bronchial catarrh, persistent cough, spasmodic cough and flatulent colic.[9]

The German Commission E recommends the comminuted aniseed fruits as an infusion for the treatment of dyspeptic complaints and catarrh of the respiratory system.[10]

Aniseed oil has been extensively used for the treatment of hard, dry coughs where expectoration is difficult. It is used in lozenges, and the seeds have been used for smoking to promote expectoration.[8]

Food, perfumery and flavouring

Both aniseed and star anise are used as domestic spices.[1]

Aniseed oil is used in flavours for candy, liqueurs, cough drops, alcoholic beverages, tobacco, baked goods, spice blends, canned foods and pickles.[1,2,7] It is an important ingredient in the flavouring of licorice candy.[2]

Many countries in the Mediterranean region, such as Turkey, Greece, Spain, Italy and France, have traditional alcoholic beverages based on aniseed such as anis, arak, pastis, ouzo, sambuca and raki.

Nowadays the use of aniseed essential oil in flavouring has been mostly replaced by synthetic anethole.[2]

Therapeutics

Pharmacology and clinical studies

Many pharmacological studies involving aniseed essential oil have been published. A systemic review of these studies will not be attempted. Rather, I have chosen a selection of studies that support the traditional and clinical uses.

Anticarcinogenic activity

A study investigated the antioxidant and cytotoxic activities of *I. verum* oil in vitro. The oil displayed promising antioxidant activity and distinct antimetastatic activity against colon cancer cells. It was concluded that the cytotoxic effect of *I. verum* oil may be due to multiple mechanisms such as the induction of apoptosis and inhibition of key steps of metastasis.[11]

Anti-inflammatory activity

Anethole, the main constituent of aniseed oil, has been shown to block both inflammation and carcinogenesis. It was suggested that anethole suppressed TNF-mediated signalling, which is associated with both inflammation and carcinogenesis.[12]

Antimicrobial activity

Aniseed oil exhibits in vitro inhibitory activities against a range of bacteria and fungi known to be pathogenic to humans.[4] The oil inhibited the growth of *Aspergillus flavus, A. niger, Fusarium oxysorum* and *Penicillium* spp.[13]

An in vitro study found that the oil did not inhibit the growth of *Bacillus cereus, Escherichia coli, Pseudomonas aeruginosa* and *Staphylococcus aureus*, but did inhibit *Aspergillus aegyptiacus, Penicillium cyclopium* and *Trichoderma viride*.[13]

However, another study examining the antibacterial activity of *I. verum* oil against 18 bacteria and 12 fungal species found that the oil inhibited the majority of bacterial species, including *Bacillus anthracis, Citrobacter, Enterobacter* and *Escherichia* species, *Staphylococcus aureus* and *Pseudomonas aeruginosa*. All the fungi were completely inhibited.[14]

Antinociceptive activity

An in vivo study demonstrated that anethole has no sedative effect, but has an antinociceptive effect on mice pretreated with anethole.[15]

Antispasmodic activity

Aniseed oil exerts spasmolytic effects on smooth muscles of different organs (tracheal, jejunum and ileum) by antagonising the activity of contraction-inducing agents.[4]

Antiviral activity

Star anise oil was tested for its antiviral activity against *Herpes simplex* virus type 1 (HSV-1) in vitro. Star anise oil reduced viral activity by more than 99%.[16]

Bronchodilatory activity

Aniseed oil exerts bronchodilatory effects in vitro.[4]

Expectorant activity

Anethole has been reported to exhibit spasmolytic properties, to stimulate respiratory secretions and expectoration.[17]

The secretolytic and expectorant effects of aniseed oil may be due to the content of anethole.[4]

Oestrogenic activity

The oestrogenic activity of anethole is well documented.[1] Anethole is a methyl ether of oestrone, and seems to have potent oestrogenic activity. Research suggests that the active oestrogenic compounds are polymers of anethole, such as dianethole and photoanethole.[1,18]

Another study found that essential oils containing (*E*)-anethole as the major compound displayed oestrogenic activity, but it also stated that the oestrogenic activity of aniseed oil is not only due to the presence of anethole. Other components other than anethole may be responsible for contributing towards the oestrogenic activity.[19]

Pediculicidal activity

Aniseed oil was tested in vitro against lice and was found to be effective in the laboratory when applied in an alcoholic solution and followed by a rinse the following morning in an essential oil/vinegar/water solution.[20]

Another study compared a natural remedy which contained coconut oil, aniseed oil and ylang ylang oil with a commercial formulation containing permethrin, malathion, piperonyl butoxide and isododecane. Of 940 children, aged six to 14 years examined for head lice, 199 were infested with lice and eggs and 164 were infested only with lice. 92.3% of children were successfully treated with the natural remedy, while 92.2% of children were successfully treated with the commercial chemical treatment. There were no significant side effects associated with either formulation.[21]

Actions

Actions commonly cited in aromatherapy

Antimicrobial, antispasmodic, aphrodisiac, carminative, emmenagogue, expectorant, galactagogue, stimulant, stomachic[7,22]

Actions supported by clinical studies

Antimicrobial, antispasmodic, carminative, expectorant

Comment

Review of the traditional and clinical data supports the use of aniseed oil for the treatment of mild spasmodic gastrointestinal complaints, including bloating and flatulence, and as an expectorant in cough associated with a cold.[4]

However, the oestrogenic activity described for *trans*-anethole could not be confirmed for aniseed alcohol extracts on the basis of epidemiological data. It was stated that it is not expected that *trans*-anethole could exert oestrogenic effects when taken as a herbal infusion at recommended posology. It was also stated that the data on the oestrogenic activity of *trans*-anethole demonstrated in vitro

A

and in laboratory animals at high concentrations is not considered to be relevant to human exposure given the recommended doses and conditions of use.[23]

Aromatherapy Uses

Clinical aromatherapy

Digestive system

Aniseed is well known for its effect on the digestive system as a carminative, digestive and antispasmodic. It may be used to relieve dyspepsia, colic and flatulence.[1,7,22,24]

Respiratory system

As it is both an expectorant and antispasmodic, it is excellent for any asthmatic or respiratory condition associated with copious white phlegm, coughing, wheezing or chronic bronchial asthma.[1,7,9,10]

The expectorant action of *P. anisum* is better than caraway or sweet fennel; on the other hand, the carminative effect is much less than that of sweet fennel or caraway.[25]

Skin care

Aniseed is generally not used in skin care.

Energetics, psyche and subtle uses

A

Energetics

According to the principles of TCM, aniseed is considered *warming* and *drying*. Aniseed also has a strong affinity with the Earth Element and the ability to eliminate *damp*. *Excess damp* is often associated with digestive problems and excess phlegm. Aniseed also helps to disperse *cold* phlegm, which helps to alleviate cough associated with copious expectoration of phlegm.

Aniseed strengthens the *Qi* of the *Spleen* – the main organ in TCM responsible for transforming food and drink into *Qi* and *Blood*. It is therefore ideally suited as a tonic for those suffering from overwork, chronic illness and weak constitution.[26]

Aniseed is indicated for problems associated with disharmony of the Earth Element. We may feel ungrounded, experience obsessive thoughts, experience apprehension and worry, which leads to apathy, lethargy and poor concentration.

Aniseed is recommended in Ayurveda for controlling excess *Kapha* and for nourishing *Vata*.

Personality

The warm spicy scent of aniseed oil has an uplifting and comforting effect on the mind. It is good for introverted, melancholic or fearful people who tend to be withdrawn or frigid.[27]

Subtle

Worwood suggests that aniseed will be of assistance to those who insist they have no need for prayer and are strong and defiant. Aniseed will make the conscious mind aware that there is a conductor of the universe.[28]

Keim Loughran & Bull recommend using aniseed oil during times of mental confusion that is plagued by obsessive, negative or limiting thoughts. The oil will also assist us in changing any aspect of our life that is inhibiting our personal and spiritual growth.[29]

Dosage and Administration

Blending

Aromatherapy

For the relief of indigestion, consider blending aniseed oil with essential oils such as sweet orange, cardamom, sweet fennel seed, ginger or peppermint.

For the relief of bronchial congestion, consider blending aniseed oil with essential oils such as Atlas cedarwood, cajeput, 1,8-cineole-rich eucalypts, peppermint eucalyptus, fragonia, frankincense, ginger or pine.

Perfumery

Aniseed is typically not used in perfumery; it is mainly used in flavours.[2]

Mode of administration

Bath

Full body bath, foot bath

Topical

Massage, ointment

Inhalation

Direct inhalation, diffuser, oil vaporiser

Ingestion

Many herbalists suggest taking aniseed essential oil internally. Holmes suggests 2-4 drops in a little warm water.[26] The German Commission E suggests 0.3 g essential oil as a bronchial expectorant for upper respiratory tract congestion and dyspeptic complaints.[10]

Schnaubelt suggests that the preferred mode of use is internal and that:

> *A drop of anise oil on a teaspoon of sugar will restore equilibrium to an acutely out-of-whack autonomic nervous system.*[30]

The British Herbal Pharmacopoeia recommends a posology of 0.05-0.2 mL of aniseed oil, three times a day for the symptomatic treatment of mild, spasmodic gastrointestinal complaints, including bloating and flatulence, and as an expectorant in cough and cold.[9]

The use in children and adolescents is not recommended due to the lack of adequate data for safety assessment and because of the presence of estragole. The duration of administration should not be more than two weeks.[4]

Safety Profile

General safety

Information regarding the safe use of aniseed is conflicting. Some sources suggest that aniseed is highly toxic:

> *... very toxic and dangerous, causing a muscular numbness followed by paralysis. It can be more dangerous than pure alcohol, and should never be left where children might find it.*[31]

It is difficult to believe that aniseed is so toxic, knowing that herbalists are recommending its use internally and the only contraindications identified are the occasional allergic reactions of the skin.

Tisserand & Young state that old or oxidised aniseed or star anise oils should be avoided topically. They also explain that we should be concerned about the estragole content.[6]

Tisserand & Young state that aniseed and star anise are potentially carcinogenic. This is based on the estragole content. The oils may inhibit blood clotting and may have an effect on the reproductive hormone modulation.[6]

Oestrogenic activity of *trans*-anethole has been demonstrated in vitro and in laboratory animals, but not in humans. The EMA states that preparations containing aniseed oil might affect hormone therapy or oral contraception in women, therefore aniseed oil is also not recommended during pregnancy and lactation.[4]

Contraindications

Tisserand & Young state that aniseed should be avoided by all routes during pregnancy, breastfeeding, endometriosis, oestrogen-dependent cancers and children under five. They recommend caution when using aniseed orally if the individual is taking diabetes medication, suffers from renal insufficiency, has edematous disorders, is on anticoagulant medication, has just had major surgery, has peptic ulcers, suffers from haemophilia or has other bleeding disorders.[6]

People with known sensitivity to aniseed, to Apiaceae plants such as caraway, celery, coriander, dill and fennel, or to anethole should avoid the use of aniseed preparations. A common allergen called Bet v 1, also bound to fennel, possibly accounts for the observed cross-sensitivity found in subjects showing allergic symptoms such as rhinitis, angioedema, asthma, wheezing, urticaria, eczema, abdominal pain, vomiting and diarrhoea.[23]

Regulatory guidelines

Aniseed and star anise have GRAS status. RIFM recommended safety of use limits for aniseed and star anise at 2%.

Tisserand & Young report that IFRA recommends a maximum dermal use level for estragole of 0.01% for a leave-on or wash-off preparation for the body or face.[6]

References

1. Khan I, Abourashed E. *Leung's encyclopedia of common natural ingredients used in food, drugs and cosmetics*. 3rd edn. John Wiley & Sons, New Jersey, 2010.
2. Arctander S. *Perfume and flavor materials of natural origin*. Allured Publishing, Carol Stream, 1994.
3. Schnaubelt K. *Advanced aromatherapy*. Healing Arts Press, Rochester, 1995.
4. Committee on Herbal Medicinal Products. *Assessment report on Pimpinella anisum L.* European Medicines Agency, London, 2006. Doc ref. EMEA/HMPC/137421/2006
5. Cu JQ et al. *GC/MS analysis of star anise oil.* Journal of Essential Oil Research, 1990; 2(2): 91-92.
6. Tisserand R, Young R. *Essential oil safety*. 2nd edn. Churchill Livingstone, Edinburgh, 2014.
7. Lawless J. *The encyclopaedia of essential oils.* Element Books, Shaftesbury, 1992.
8. Grieve M. *A modern herbal — Vol. I.* Dover Publications, New York, 1971.
9. *British herbal pharmacopoeia*. British Herbal Medicine Association, Bournemouth, 1983.
10. Blumenthal M et al. *The complete German commission E monographs: therapeutic guide to herbal medicine*. American Botanical Council, Austin, 1998.
11. Asif M et al. *Anticancer attributes of Illicium verum essential oils against colon cancer.* South African Journal of Botany, 2016; 103: 156-161. Cited in Quintessential Aromatics database, 2013.
12. Chainy GBN et al. *Anethole blocks both early and late cellular responses transduced by tumor necrosis factor: Effect on NF-κB, AP-1, JNK, MAPKK and apoptosis*. Oncogene, 2000; 19(25): 2943-2950. Cited in Quintessential Aromatics database, 2013.
13. *WHO monographs on selected medicinal plants — Vol. 3*. World Health Organization, Geneva, 2007.

A

14. Sharma VD et al. *Antimicrobial activity of essential oil of Illicium verum Hook.* Indian Journal of Microbiology, 1985; 25 (3/4): 221-222. Cited in Quintessential Aromatics database, 2013.
15. Ritter AM et al. *Effects of anethole in nociception experimental models.* Evidence-Based Complementary and Alternative Medicine, 2014. doi: 10.1155/2014/345829. Cited in Quintessential Aromatics database, 2013.
16. Astani A. et al. *Screening for antiviral activities of isolated compounds from essential oils.* Evidence-Based Complementary and Alternative Medicine, 2011. doi: 10.1093/ecam/nep187. Cited in Quintessential Aromatics database, 2013.
17. Bruneton J. *Pharmacognosy.* 2nd edn. Lavoisier Publishing, Paris, 1999.
18. Balacs T. *Hormones and health.* The International Journal of Aromatherapy, 1993; 5(1): 18-20.
19. Tabanca N et al. *Estrogenic activity of isolated compounds and essential oils of Pimpinella species from Turkey, evaluated using a recombinant yeast screen.* Planta Medica, 2004; 70(4): 728-735. Cited in Quintessential Aromatics database, 2013.
20. Veal L. *The potential effectiveness of essential oil as a treatment for head lice, Pediculus humanus capitis.* Complementary Therapies in Nursing & Midwifery, 1996; 2(4): 97-101. Cited in Quintessential Aromatics database, 2013.
21. Mumcuoglu KY et al. *The in vivo pediculicidal efficacy of a natural remedy.* Israeli Medical Association Journal, 2002; 4(10): 790-793.
22. Lavabre M. *Aromatherapy workbook.* Healing Arts Press, Rochester, 1997.
23. *Pimpinella – Anise oil (Anisi aetheroleum).* Retrieved Mar 5, 2017, from https://herbalref.com/pimpinella-anise-oil-anisi-aetheroleum
24. Davis P. *Aromatherapy A-Z.* 2nd edn. C.W. Daniel Company, Saffron Walden, 1999.
25. Weiss RF. *Herbal medicine.* Beaconsfield, England, 1988.
26. Holmes P. *The energetics of Western herbs — Vol. II.* Artemis Press, Boulder, 1989.
27. Lawless J. *Aromatherapy and the mind.* Thornsons, London, 1994.
28. Worwood VA. *The fragrant heavens.* Transworld Publishers, London, 1999.
29. Keim Loughran J, Bull R. *Aromatherapy anointing oils.* Frog, Berkeley, 2001.
30. Schnaubelt K. *Medical aromatherapy.* Frog, Berkeley, 1999.
31. Ryman D. *Aromatherapy.* Judy Piatkus, Great Britain, 1991.

A

Aniseed myrtle

Identification

Botanical name

Syzygium anisatum (Vickery) Craven & Biffin

Synonyms

Backhousia anisata Vickery, aniseed tree

Family

Myrtaceae

Botany and origins

A rare tree that grows in subtropical rainforest confined to the Nambucca and Bellingen valleys of northern New South Wales.[1]

The aniseed myrtle tree has rough, corky brown bark with tapering lanceolated leaves, and grows to a height of 50 m. The flowers are creamy white and appear in late spring and summer.[1]

In the past, most of the aniseed myrtle leaf that was sold to processors and restaurants was harvested from the wild. However, market demand for a consistent year-round supply, combined with concerns over the environmental impact of accessing rainforest systems, have led to cultivated plantations fully replacing wild harvest.[2]

Method of extraction

Aniseed myrtle oil is extracted by steam distillation of the leaves of *S. anisatum.*

Characteristics

Aniseed myrtle oil is a colourless, mobile oil with a distinctive aniseed aroma.

Chemical composition

Two chemotypes have been identified, the first has a high concentration of (*E*)-anethole or *trans*-anethole, and the second is high in methyl chavicol (estragole).[3]

The chemical composition of aniseed myrtle oil was reported as follows:[3]

Constituent	Anethole chemotype	Methyl chavicol chemotype
(*E*)- anethole	71.2–93.7%	5.0–15.3%
methyl chavicol	21.1-42.8%	55.8-75.0%

Commercial applications of aniseed myrtle oil are now restricted to the species with high anethole content.[3]

Adulteration

Not reported.

Pharmacopoeias and standards

At the time of writing, the purity, composition, physico-chemical properties and therapeutic use of aniseed myrtle essential oil are not defined in any pharmacopoeia monograph or standard.

History and Traditional Uses

History

As the trees are so rare, there is little known about the traditional uses of aniseed myrtle. It has been reported that the trees were harvested during World War II, when aniseed flavouring was in short supply.[2]

Compared with lemon myrtle, aniseed myrtle is considered a 'slow mover' for Australian primary producers. The market for aniseed myrtle products is far less developed than that for lemon myrtle in all categories, such as spice, tea, value-added food products, soaps and cosmetics.[4]

Traditional medicine

Aniseed myrtle leaves have been traditionally used by the indigenous people of Australia for therapeutic applications.[3]

Food, perfumery and flavouring

It is commonly used within the bush food industry and in herbal teas where an aniseed flavour is required. Aniseed myrtle is a rich source of methyl chavicol, a material highly sought after by the flavour and fragrance industry.[1]

Therapeutics

Pharmacology and clinical studies

Antimicrobial activity

Studies have confirmed that aniseed myrtle essential oil has broad-spectrum antibacterial activity against *Escherichia coli*, methicillin-resistant *Staphylococcus aureus* (MRSA), *Staphylococcus epidermis*, *Enterobacter aerogenes*, *Proteus vulgaris*, *Salmonella typhimurium*, *Salmonella enteritidis* and *Enterococcus faecalis*.[3]

Actions

Actions commonly cited in aromatherapy

Antibacterial, antifungal, antispasmodic, carminative, insect repellent

Actions supported by clinical studies

Antimicrobial

Comment

The chemistry and pharmacology of (*E*)-anethole and estragole, the two main constituents of aniseed myrtle, are well documented. It would be reasonable to assume that the uses of aniseed myrtle in aromatherapy would be similar to those of *P. anisum* essential oil.

Aromatherapy Uses

Clinical aromatherapy

Nervous system

Schnaubelt explains that methyl chavicol stabilises an overactive sympathetic nervous system and restores a healthy balance between the sympathetic and parasympathetic nervous systems, so it has excellent antispasmodic effects.[5]

Energetics, psyche and subtle uses

Subtle

Zeck explains that aniseed myrtle helps us to assimilate life experiences and brings ideas into fruition. The oil will help to reawaken your imaginative quest and bring your vision into manifestation to enable you to move forward in life.[6]

Dosage and Administration

Blending

Aromatherapy

For the temporary relief of bronchial congestion, consider blending aniseed myrtle oil with essential oils such as Atlas cedarwood, cajeput, 1,8-cineole-rich eucalypts, peppermint eucalyptus, fragonia, frankincense, ginger or pine.

Perfumery

Aniseed myrtle is typically not used in perfumery; it is mainly used in flavours.

Mode of administration

Bath

Full body bath, foot bath

Topical

Compress, massage, ointment

Inhalation

Direct inhalation, diffuser, oil vaporiser

Safety Profile

General safety

(*E*)-anethole is prone to oxidation, which may be skin sensitising.[7]

Contraindications

Tisserand & Young state that methyl chavicol may be a reproductive hormone modulator; therefore aniseed myrtle should be contraindicated during pregnancy, breastfeeding, endometriosis, oestrogen-dependent cancers and children under 5 years of age. They also caution oral use for people taking diabetes or anticoagulant medication, who have had major surgery, suffer from peptic ulcers or suffer from haemophilia and other bleeding disorders.[7]

Regulatory guidelines

Aniseed myrtle oil is not listed in any regulatory guidelines.

References

1. Webb M. *Bush sense.* Self-published, Australia, 2000.
2. RIRDC. *Focus on anise myrtle.* Research & Development Corporation Industry Overview. 2014. Pub. No.14/110. Retrieved from http://www.agrifutures.com.au/publications/focus-on-anise-myrtle/
3. Sultanbawa Y. *Anise myrtle (Syzygium anisatum) oils.* In Preedy VR. ed. *Essential oils in food preservation, flavor and safety.* Academic Press, London, 2016: 215-219.
4. Clarke M. *Australian native food industry stocktake.* Research & Development Corporation Industry Overview. 2012. Pub No.12/066. Retrieved from http://www.agrifutures.com.au/publications/australian-native-food-industry-stocktake/
5. Schnaubelt K. *Advanced aromatherapy.* Healing Arts Press, Rochester, 1995.
6. Zeck R. *The blossoming heart – aromatherapy for healing and transformation.* Aroma Tours, East Ivanhoe, 2004.
7. Tisserand R, Young R. *Essential oil safety.* 2nd edn. Churchill Livingstone, Edinburgh, 2014.

Balsam, Peru

Identification

Botanical name

Myroxylon balsamum (L.) Harms var. *pereirae* (Royle) Harms

Synonyms

Myroxylon pereirae, Peruvian balsam, Indian balsam, black balsam.[1]

Family

Fabaceae (Leguminosae)

Botany and origins

It is a large and beautiful tree that is valued for its wood. Every part of the tree, including the leaves, abounds in a resinous juice. It also has extremely fragrant flowers. The balsam is a pathological exudate obtained from the exposed lacerated wood after strips of the bark have been removed.[2]

Guenther states that fully grown trees not less than 40-50 years old can be tapped twice a month. The yield on each extraction is approximately 4 to 6 oz of balsam. Trees over 60 years old produce up to 8 oz, whereas trees younger than 25 years yield an inferior quality balsam.[3]

The name 'Balsam of Peru' is derived from the fact that it was shipped from Peru. Peru balsam is produced almost exclusively in El Salvador.[2] The principal areas producing Peru balsam are located northeast of San Salvador, the capital of El Salvador.[3] Peru balsam remains an important export for El Salvador.[4]

The collection of the balsam does not put the tree or the forests in any danger because the tree is never cut down, and the balsam, which is a natural exudate of the tree, does not cause the tree irreparable damage.[5]

Method of extraction

Because the tree does not naturally exude a resin, the method to obtain the balsam is to remove the bark. Once the bark is removed, incisions are then made into the exposed surface of the sapwood. The surface of the sapwood is then scorched with a torch to induce flow. The surface is then wrapped in a cloth, referred to as a *trupp* (rag). After eight to 10 days, the cloth that is saturated with balsam is removed and boiled in water for about one hour. The balsam, which is heavier than water, will settle at the bottom of the container where it can be separated.[3,4]

In its crude form, the balsam solidifies into a dark-brown semi-solid mass. The balsam contains 25-30% resin and 70-75% volatile compounds. Two products that are produced from Peru balsam are a rectified essential oil and a resinoid (an alcoholic extract from the balsam).[5]

The essential oil is obtained from the balsam by distillation. A resin-free oil is produced from the crude balsam by high vacuum dry distillation.[2]

Characteristics

Peru balsam oil has a rich, sweet, balsamic, vanilla-like odour.[2] Peru balsam has also been described as possessing attractive, warm, soft characteristics, with some smoky and sensual bottom notes.[5]

Chemical composition

The chemical composition of Peru balsam was reported as follows:[5]

Constituent	Essential oil	Resinoid
benzyl alcohol	0.41%	1.11%
trans-nerolidol	5.28%	4.64%
benzoic acid	2.04%	3.22%
vanillin	0.26%	0.47%
benzyl benzoate	59.67%	49.68%
cinnamic acid	3.57%	11.69%
cis-benzyl cinnamate	1.32%	1.03%
trans-benzyl cinnamate	26.23%	23.39%

Adulteration

As Peru balsam is semi-solid at room temperature, it is often diluted and adulterated with benzyl benzoate, benzyl alcohol and other low-cost solvents.[2]

Pharmacopoeias and standards

At the time of writing, the purity, composition, physico-chemical properties and therapeutic use of Peru balsam essential oil are not defined in any standard. Peru balsam is the subject of a German Commission E Monograph.

History and Traditional Uses

History

Peru balsam was first mentioned in Europe in the writing of Nicolas Monardes in 1565. Monardes explained that the resin was produced by a tree in New Spain that the Indians called *xilo*.[4]

The resin was considered so important in religious ceremonies during the sixteenth century that Popes Pius IV and V declared that it could be used as a substitute for the consecrated sacramental oil used in baptism, ordination and extreme unction. Their edicts stated that the destruction of Peru balsam trees was sacrilegious.[4]

The resin was once listed in the US Pharmacopoeia. In 1967, a study of wound healing in a US Army hospital confirmed that Peru balsam may help reduce scar tissue formation and aid healing. However, nowadays it is primarily used for its aroma in ointments, cosmetics, perfumes and soaps.[4]

Traditional medicine

Peru balsam was once used by the Incas for embalming, and indigenous Colombians continue to use it to treat wounds and stop bleeding. It is still used locally in some regions of South America to treat asthma, catarrh, rheumatism, diarrhoea and haemorrhoids, and as an antiseptic dressing for ulcerated wounds.[4]

Herbal

Peru balsam has been extensively used in topical preparations for the treatment of wounds, indolent ulcers, scabies, haemorrhoids, pruritus, eczema and bed sores.[1]

The German Commission E recommends Peru balsam for topical preparations for infected or poorly healing wounds, burns, ulcers, frostbite, bruises and haemorrhoids.[6]

Peru balsam was also used in the past for all chronic conditions of the mucous tissues such as catarrh, gonorrhoea, mucous inflammation of the stomach and bowels, chronic diarrhoea, dysentery and leucorrhoea.[7]

Food, perfumery and flavouring

Peru balsam is used as a fixative and fragrance component in soaps, detergents, creams, lotions and perfumes, and the oil is extensively used as a flavour ingredient in many foods, alcoholic and non-alcoholic beverages, frozen dairy desserts, candy, baked goods, and gelatins and puddings.[1]

Other uses

It is used in dentistry for treating socket, (post-extraction alveolitis) and as a component in certain dental impression materials.[1]

Therapeutics

Pharmacology and clinical studies

Antimicrobial activity

Peru balsam oil was very effective in eradicating *Pseudomonas* spp. and *Staphylococcus aureus* biofilms. Peru balsam was just as effective as cassia and red thyme essential oils and had higher efficacy than certain antibiotics.[9]

Actions

Actions commonly cited in aromatherapy

Antibacterial, anti-inflammatory, antiseptic, expectorant, parasiticide, skin cell regenerator, stimulant[1,6,8]

Actions supported by clinical studies

Antibacterial, antiseptic, promotion of granulation process

Comment

Review of traditional uses and clinical data support the use of Peru balsam oil in topical preparations for the treatment of pruritus, eczema, infected and poorly healing wounds, ulcers and haemorrhoids. However, it is critical that Peru balsam essential oil is free of the sensitising constituents found in the balsam.

Aromatherapy Uses

Clinical aromatherapy

Integumentary system

Peru balsam oil is recommended for the treatment of scabies, for infected and poorly healing wounds, and for skin diseases such as pruritus and the later stages of acute eczema.[1]

The crude balsam is a common contact allergen, which may cause dermatitis. It is not commonly used in aromatherapy, but it has been suggested for dry and chapped skin, eczema, rashes, sores and wounds.[8]

B

Nervous system

Peru balsam oil is recommended for the relief of nervous tension and stress.[8]

Respiratory system

Peru balsam oil is recommended for the relief of asthma, bronchitis and coughs.[8]

Energetics, psyche and subtle uses

Personality

According to Myers-Briggs personality types, the Peru balsam personality is likely to be an ENFP. ENFPs are outgoing, lively and spontaneous. They are very enthusiastic and their joy for life can be contagious. They have a rich imagination and active mind. Their thoughts are always wandering and their mood constantly changing. They can be inspiring and charismatic leaders. They are always involved or in love with someone or something new. They know how to establish instant rapport and make people feel comfortable. They love emotional intensity and enjoy expressing their feelings. They can be charming and flirtatious. They relate with warmth to many people and can appear overly enthusiastic, positive and optimistic.

Subtle

Worwood states that the soft, sweet, warm fragrance of Peru balsam fills the spaces in our heart that have remained cold, untouchable and unreachable. It opens our heart without recrimination and when in sorrow, it comforts us and provides relief from pain.[10]

Peru balsam promotes feelings of safety and being nurtured. It is also said to promote sensuality and confidence.[11]

Dosage and Administration

Blending

Aromatherapy

Peru balsam oil can be used whenever you need a rich warm floral balsamic base. It blends well with rich floral essential oils such as rose absolute or jasmine absolute, resin essential oils such as frankincense or benzoin, and with essential oils such as clove, ginger, cinnamon bark, which have a warm intense spicy aroma.

To alleviate dry, chapped and damaged skin, consider blending Peru balsam oil with essential oils such as everlasting, cistus, lavender or sandalwood.

To alleviate the symptoms of anxiety, nervous tension and stress, consider blending Peru balsam with essential oils such as bergamot, frankincense, lavender, sweet orange, patchouli, rose absolute, sandalwood or ylang ylang.

Perfumery

Arctander describes Peru balsam as one of the best fixatives among all essential oils. He states that the tenacity in odour of this oil is outstanding. He explains that it can be incorporated in almost any type of perfume base at concentrations from less than 1% up to 5%.[2]

It blends well with delicate florals and precious wood oils. It also complements heavy sweet florals such as ylang ylang or jasmine. It imparts depth and a natural sweet spicy note to rose, and would impart a warm balsamic body to amber or oriental style perfumes.[2]

Mode of administration

Bath

Full body bath, foot bath

Topical

Compress, massage, ointment, skin care

Inhalation

Direct inhalation, diffuser, oil burner

Safety Profile

General safety

The crude balsam is well known to cause allergies and sensitisations.[1,6,8] Tisserand & Young list coniferyl benzoate, coniferyl alcohol, benzyl isoferulate and resorcinol monobenzoate as some of the sensitising compounds found in Peru balsam. However, they explain that ultra-high vacuum distillation should strip most of the coniferyl benzoate out of the resin.[12]

Contraindications

No contraindications known.

Regulatory guidelines

The European Commission's Scientific Committee on Consumer Products released an opinion on Peru balsam in 2006, stating the balsam should not be used as a fragrance ingredient; however, the distillate of Peru balsam may be used as a fragrance ingredient in cosmetics up to a maximum concentration of 0.4% in the finished product.[13]

References

1. Khan I, Abourashed E. *Leung's encyclopedia of common natural ingredients used in food, drugs and cosmetics*. 3rd edn. John Wiley & Sons., New Jersey, 2010.
2. Arctander S. *Perfume and flavor materials of natural origin*. Allured Publishing, Carol Stream, 1994.
3. Guenther E. *The essential oils – Vol. V*. Robert E. Krieger Publishing, Malabar, 1952.
4. Langenheim JH. *Plant resins – chemistry, evolution, ecology and ethnobotany*. Timber Press, Portland, 2003.
5. Frances A et al. *Peru balsam: getting to the source, El Salvador*. Perfumer & Flavorist, 2014; 39: 36-39.
6. Blumenthal M et al. *The complete German commission E monographs: therapeutic guide to herbal medicine*. American Botanical Council, Austin, 1998.
7. Lis-Balchin M. *Aromatherapy science – a guide for healthcare professionals*. Pharmaceutical Press, London, 2006.
8. Lawless J. *The encyclopaedia of essential oils*. Element Books, Shaftesbury, 1992.
9. Kavanaugh NL, Ribbeck K. *Selected antimicrobial essential oils eradicate Pseudomonas spp. and Staphylococcus aureus biofilms*. Applied and Environmental Microbiology, 2012; 78(11): 4057-4061. Cited in Quintessential Aromatics database, 2013.
10. Worwood VA. *The fragrant heavens*. Transworld Publishers, London, 1999.
11. Keim Loughran J, Bull R. *Aromatherapy and subtle energy techniques*. Frog, Berkeley, 2000.
12. Tisserand R, Young R. *Essential oil safety*. 2nd edn. Churchill Livingstone, Edinburgh, 2014.
13. *Opinion on Peru balsam*. European Commission Health & Consumer Protection Directorate-General, Brussels, 2006. Retrieved from https://ec.europa.eu/health/ph_risk/committees/04_sccp/docs/sccp_o_055.pdf

B

Basil

Identification

Botanical name

Ocimum basilicum L.

Synonyms

Sweet basil, common basil

Family

Lamiaceae (Labiatae)

Botany and origins

Basil is an annual herb, which grows to about 0.5 m in height. It is native to tropical Asia and Africa, but it is cultivated as a popular garden annual herb worldwide. It is believed to have been introduced to ancient Greece by Alexander the Great (356-323 BC).[1]

The genus *Ocimum* L. consists of 70 species and subspecies found in tropical and subtropical regions of Asia, Africa, and central and southern America, as well as the Mediterranean.[2]

The chemical composition of the oil varies significantly depending on genetic factors, geographic factors, geographical origins, nutritional status and the part of the plant used (stem, leaf or flower).[2]

The two most commonly available basil oils are:

The true sweet basil oil, also known as French, European or sweet basil. This oil has a higher percentage of linalool. This oil is generally regarded as safe to use in aromatherapy.

Exotic or Réunion basil, which is distilled in the Comoro Islands, Madagascar, Thailand and occasionally in the Seychelles. This oil has a higher percentage of methyl chavicol.[3]

According to an extensive analysis of over 200 individual basil plants, five chemotypes of basil oil have been identified:

- linalool
- methyl chavicol
- methyl eugenol
- (*E*)-methyl cinnamate
- eugenol.[4]

The (*E*)-methyl cinnamate chemotype is commonly referred to as cinnamon basil. The botanical name of holy basil, otherwise commonly known as sacred basil or tulsi basil, is *Ocimum tenuiflorum* L.[5]

Method of extraction

Basil oil is steam-distilled from the leaves and flowering tops of *Ocimum basilicum*.

Characteristics

Sweet basil oil is a pale yellow or almost colourless mobile liquid with a sweet-spicy, slightly green, fresh top note, a balsamic-woody undertone and a lasting sweetness.[6]

Exotic basil oil is a pale yellow to pale green mobile liquid with a slightly coarse-herbaceous, camphoraceous top note, and it displays an intense aniseed-like sweetness associated with the methyl chavicol content.[6]

B

Chemical composition

Estragole is also known as methyl chavicol. There are some safety concerns with the estragole content of basil, therefore in aromatherapy, it is preferable to use the linalool chemotype. The methyl chavicol chemotype is preferred in the manufacture of expensive perfumes, whereas the linalool chemotype is preferred in food flavouring and less expensive perfumes.[7]

The phenolic ethers found in basil confirm basil's antispasmodic properties, which make it ideal for the treatment of spasmodic abdominal pain and asthmatic conditions.[8]

The chemical composition of basil oil was as follows.[9]

Compound	Origin		
	Comoro Is.	France	Egypt
α-pinene	0.18%	0.11%	0.25%
camphene	0.06%	0.02%	0.07%
β-pinene	0.25%	0.07%	0.43%
myrcene	0.12%	0.13%	0.35%
limonene	2.64%	2.04%	4.73%
cis-ocimene	2.52%	0.03%	0.63%
camphor	0.37%	1.43%	0.57%
linalool	1.16%	40.72%	45.55%
methyl chavicol	85.76%	23.79%	26.56%
α-terpineol	0.84%	1.90%	1.09%
citronellol	0.65%	3.57%	1.76%
geraniol	0.03%	0.38%	0.2%
methyl cinnamate	0.05%	0.34%	0.25%
eugenol	0.74%	5.90%	5.90%

Adulteration

Arctander states that it is not uncommon for the less expensive exotic basil to be 'doctored' with the addition of linalool and sold as French basil.[6]

Pharmacopoeias and standards

The purity, composition and physico-chemical properties of basil essential oil are defined in ISO 11043:1998 Oil of Basil, methyl chavicol type (*Ocimum basilicum* L.).

History and Traditional Uses

History

The name basil originates from the Greek word, *basileus*, which means 'royal' or 'king-like' because of the royal fragrance of the herb.[1]

In India, basil is dedicated to Vishnu and is regarded as the incarnation of his wife, Lakshmi, goddess of fortune and beauty. The basil species that we are referring to in India is *Ocimum sanctum*, also called tulsi. Tulsi is called upon for life and death, for various acts of life, and above all for giving children to those who want them. According to tradition, basil protects from unfortunate destinies and evil spirits.[10]

The sixteenth century herbalist John Gerard wrote:

> *The smell of basil … taketh away sorrowfulness and maketh a man merry and glad.*[11]

Basil was recommended by Pliny against jaundice and epilepsy, and as a diuretic. It was also known as an aphrodisiac. In the Middle Ages it was prescribed for melancholy and depression.[12]

Herbal

The German Commission E recommends preparations of basil herb for feelings of fullness and flatulence, and for the stimulation of appetite and digestion.[12]

Basil has long been used in popular medicine as an anti-inflammatory and analgesic, and for the treatment of symptoms associated with diarrhoea, constipation, indigestion and cough.[2]

Food, perfumery and flavouring

Basil herb is a commonly used additive to tomato-based sauces. The herb is extensively used as a spice.

The oil is used as a flavouring ingredient in many major food products, usually at very low levels – below 0.005%.[3]

Basil oil is used as a fragrance ingredient in perfumes, soaps and personal care products.[3]

Therapeutics

Pharmacology and clinical studies

Many pharmacological studies involving basil oil have been published. A systemic review of these studies will not be attempted. Rather, I have chosen a selection of studies that support the traditional and clinical uses.

Antidepressant activity

In a study carried out on five patients aged 31 to 59 years with clinical depression, each received a 30-minute aromatherapy massage using a blend of essential oils of sweet orange, geranium and basil twice per week for four weeks. The results of the study found that there was a subjective and objective improvement in depressive states.[13]

Antifungal activity

Basil ct. methyl chavicol oil was found to have potent antifungal properties.[14,15,16]

An in vitro study examining basil oil from Egypt confirmed that the oil had significant antifungal activity. Complete inhibition of *Aspergillus flavus* growth was observed at 1000 ppm oil concentration, while marked inhibition of aflatoxin B1 production was observed at all oil concentrations tested (500, 750 and 1000 ppm).[17]

Another study examined basil oil from India against 22 species of fungi, including *Aspergillus parasiticus, A. fumigatus* and *A. niger.* The oil inhibited the growth of all fungal strains and was found to be fungistatic at low concentrations. The oil was more efficacious than commercial fungicides and fumigants.[18]

Anti-inflammatory activity

The anti-inflammatory activity of basil oil and its major component estragole was investigated in an in vivo test using mice. The smallest dose of basil oil (50 mg/kg) showed efficacy in reduction of the inflammatory process.[19]

Antimicrobial activity

Sweet basil oil and basil ct. methyl chavicol oil were tested for their antimicrobial activity against a range of gram-positive and gram-negative bacteria, yeasts and moulds using the agar well diffusion method. Both essential oils displayed antimicrobial activity against most of the microorganisms except for *Clostridium sporogenes, Flavimonas oryzihabitans* and three species of *Pseudomonas*. The study also confirmed the effectiveness of washing fresh lettuce with 0.1% (v/v) of basil ct. methyl chavicol, with survival of natural microbial flora comparable to that affected by 125ppm of chlorine.[20]

The results of an in vitro study confirmed that basil essential oil had antibacterial activity against all of the clinical strains from *Escherichia coli,* including extended-spectrum β-lactamase positive bacteria.[21]

Antispasmodic activity

An in vitro test examining the antispasmodic activity of sweet basil oil found that it had an initial spasmogenic action followed by a spasmolytic action on electrically stimulated smooth muscle of the guinea pig.[15]

Anxiolytic activity

The anxiolytic and antidepressant effects of inhaled basil oil were studied in vivo on rats performing the elevated plus-maze and forced swimming tests. The results found that the exposure to basil oil significantly improved the behaviour of the animals, indicating an anxiolytic and antidepressant activity.[22]

A study investigated the anxiolytic and sedative effect of the essential oil and hydro-alcoholic extract of basil in mice utilising an elevated plus maze and locomotor activity meter. The oil and the extract were administered intraperitoneally. The results of the study found that the anxiolytic and sedative effect of the essential oil was higher than the hydro-alcoholic extract with the same dose. The major components of the basil essential oil used were methyl chavicol (42.8%), geranial (13.0%), neral (12.2%) and β-caryophyllene (7.2%).[23]

Insecticidal activity

O. basilicum and *O. sanctum* and their major components, methyl chavicol (73%) and eugenol (44%), were tested against *Anopheles stephensi, Aedes aegypti* and *Culex quinquefasciatus* mosquito species. Both oils were found to have insecticidal activity.

O. basilicum and methyl chavicol were more effective as they gave a 100% mortality rate at lower concentrations. *Anopheles stephensi* was the most susceptible to all the tests, while *Culex quinquefasciatus* was the most resistant.[24]

The insecticidal activity of 34 essential oils was

screened against the house fly *Musca domestica* L. under laboratory conditions. Basil oil was one of eight essential oils that was found to be lethal at 13 μg/fly.[25]

Actions

Actions commonly cited in aromatherapy

Antidepressant, antiseptic, antispasmodic, carminative, cephalic, digestive, emmenagogue, expectorant, febrifuge, nervine, restorative, stomachic, sudorific[26,27]

Actions supported by clinical studies

Antifungal, antimicrobial, anxiolytic, digestive, insecticidal, nervine

Comment

Traditional uses for basil oil support claims as a carminative, and for the relief of digestive ailments such as flatulence and feelings of distension. There is also documented evidence for the antifungal and anti-inflammatory activity of the oil.

However, it appears that stronger antimicrobial and antispasmodic activities are attributed to the methyl chavicol chemotype, which should be used with care in aromatherapy.

Schnaubelt describes basil as having a balancing effect on the autonomic nervous system. He states that the European basil is less harsh than the exotic basil, and has less dramatic effects.[28]

Basil oil has always been well known in traditional medicine to restore mental and cognitive functions. It has also been considered a tonic and to have a restorative action on many body functions.

B

Aromatherapy Uses

Clinical aromatherapy

Digestive system

Basil oil is useful in digestive disorders such as vomiting, gastric spasms, nausea, dyspepsia and hiccups.[7,26]

Immune system

Basil's sudorific and febrifuge properties mean it may be used for reducing all types of fever. In Ayurvedic medicine, it is combined with black pepper for malarial fever.[26,29]

Musculoskeletal system

Basil oil is recommended for the relief of gout, muscular aches and pains, and rheumatism.[26]

Nervous system

Basil oil is reputed to clear the head, relieve intellectual fatigue, and give the mind strength and clarity. It may be used in all types of nervous disorders, especially those associated with weakness, indecision or hysteria.[8]

Basil oil is recommended for those in need of protection, due either to debilitating illness and low resistance levels, nervous exhaustion, a constitutional weakness or a change in life resulting in feelings of vulnerability.[11]

Mailhebiau states that *Ocimum basilicum* is remarkably relaxing, due to its high methyl ether content.

> *We recommend it for people with schizoid tendencies as it soothes, calms and relaxes; it is the anti-stress essence par exellence.*[10]

It is recommended as a carminative and sedative for digestive insomnia – people who 'digest' their worries during the night.[10]

Reproductive system

Basil oil is recommended for delayed menstruation, scanty periods and abdominal cramps.[8,26]

Respiratory system

Basil's antispasmodic property has a beneficial action on the respiratory system and is used for the relief of sinus congestion, asthma, bronchitis, influenza and whooping cough.[26,29]

Skin care

Basil oil has been used in low dilutions to improve the tone and appearance of the skin.[29]

Energetics, psyche and subtle uses

Energetics

Basil is a *warming* oil which tonifies *Yang* and strengthens the *Shen*. It is recommended for people who are physically or mentally exhausted, suffer from nervous depression or have become complacent and melancholic.[8]

It warms the *Lungs* and expels phlegm and relieves coughing. According to the principles of the Five Elements, basil's strong invigorating action on the mind and digestive system associates it with the Wood, Fire and Earth Elements.

Personality

Worwood describes basil personalities as the entrepreneurs of the world. They see opportunities everywhere. They have ambition and drive and are determined to achieve their goals. She explains that they can be very direct and blunt, particularly if you don't always understand them. They may seem patronising at times, but they mean no harm. They love taking on responsibility and the power of being a boss.[30]

Worwood also describes basil personalities as the protectors of ideas, imagination and free will. She also states that they are drawn to the mysterious and can be very spiritual.[30]

According to Myers-Briggs personality types, the basil personality is likely to be an ENTJ. ENTJs are dynamic, energetic, confident and competent. They naturally move into positions where they can take charge. They enjoy confrontation and they like to engage in intellectually stimulating exchanges. They like and respect people who challenge them and have little or no respect for those that don't. They have an improvement plan for everything, including their leisure. They like to set goals and provide directions. They see obstacles as challenges. They dislike inefficiency, incompetence and indecisiveness. They are competitively driven and often considered to be workaholics. They can be very honest and direct and do not hesitate to express themselves. When stressed they can have explosive outbursts or be judgemental on themselves and others.

Subtle

Worwood recommends basil to encourage positivity, assertiveness, decisiveness, clarity and strength. Basil opens our heart to those who have lost their self through constant sacrifice to others.[31]

Zeck states that the sharp spicy scent of basil will bring balance and clarity to our inner emotions and allow us to take a risk to express ourselves. She compares basil with the power of positive thinking and states that it will generate a sense of security as we express ourselves in a positive manner.[32]

Dosage and Administration

Blending

Aromatherapy

For the relief of indigestion, consider blending sweet basil oil with essential oils such as aniseed, ginger, sweet orange or peppermint.

To alleviate mental fatigue, consider blending sweet basil oil with essential oils such as black pepper, ginger, lemon, peppermint, pine or rosemary.

The German Commission E provides us with some interesting basil oil combinations:

- For wound treatment, rheumatic discomfort, colds, bruises and painful joints - a blend of basil oil, rosemary oil, cinnamon oil and peppermint oil.[12]
- For nasal catarrh, temporary shortness of breath, fatigue, cough, congestion, muscle pain, nerve pain, lumbago, sprains, flatulence and travel fatigue - a blend of basil oil, anise oil, lemon oil, sweet fennel oil, clove oil, peppermint oil, juniper berry oil, citronella oil, bergamot oil, Siberian pine oil, rosemary oil, orange peel oil, cinnamon oil, spearmint oil, wintergreen oil, nutmeg oil and wild thyme oil.[12]

  I consider this way too many oils in one blend, however, it gives you a good idea of the essential oils that blend well with basil.

Perfumery

In perfumery, sweet basil oil is often used in chypre, modern aldehydic and green perfume types. It blends well with essential oils such as bergamot, clary sage, lime and oakmoss absolute.[6]

Mode of administration

Bath

Due to the risk of skin sensitisation, I prefer not to use any of the basil oils in a bath.

Topical

Compress, massage, ointment, skin care

Inhalation

Direct inhalation, diffuser, oil vaporiser

Safety Profile

General safety

Avoid topical use of basil oil with a high content of methyl cinnamate and methyl chavicol as it will be an irritant to people with sensitive skin.[12,15] However, Tisserand & Young classify basil ct. linalool as a weak dermal sensitiser rather than a moderate one.

The Council of Europe currently recommends that the level of methyl chavicol in food products should not exceed 0.05 mg/kg.[3]

Tisserand & Young state that *O. gratissimum*, commonly known as pungent basil, typically has a high eugenol and methyl eugenol content. This means that oral dosages of the oil may inhibit blood clotting, thereby having possible drug interaction with anticoagulant medication. It may potentially be carcinogenic and be a low to moderate skin and mucous membrane irritant and sensitiser.[5]

Contraindications

Basil oil is contraindicated during pregnancy.[12,15] However, I believe that this contraindication should refer only to the estragole chemotype basil.

Tisserand & Young state that there are no known contraindications for the linalool chemotype basil. However, they state that the estragole chemotype is potentially a carcinogen based on the estragole and methyl eugenol content, and should not be taken in oral doses. They have set a dermal limit of 0.1% based on the typical content of estragole and methyleugenol.[5]

The German Commission E states that the high estragole basil oils should not be used during pregnancy or nursing, by infants or small children, or over extended periods of time.[12]

Regulatory guidelines

Sweet basil oil has GRAS status.

References

1. Li QX, Chang CL. *Basil (Ocimum basilicum L.) oils*. In Preedy VR. ed. *Essential oils in food preservation, flavor and safety*. Academic Press, London, 2016: 231-238.
2. Sakkas H, Papadopoulou C. *Antimicrobial activity of basil, oregano and thyme essential oils.* Journal of Microbiology and Biotechnology, 2001; 27(3): 429-438. doi: 10.4014/jmb.1608.08024
3. Khan I, Abourashed E. *Leung's encyclopedia of common natural ingredients used in food, drugs and cosmetics*. 3rd edn. John Wiley & Sons, New Jersey, 2010.
4. Lawrence BM. *Essential oils: From agriculture to chemistry*. The World of Aromatherapy III Conference Proceedings, NAHA, Seattle, 2000: 8-26.
5. Tisserand R, Young R. *Essential oil safety*. 2nd edn. Churchill Livingstone, Edinburgh, 2014.
6. Arctander S. *Perfume and flavour materials of natural origin*. Allured Publishing, Carol Stream, 1994.
7. Bruneton J. *Pharmacognosy*. 2nd edn. Lavoisier Publishing, Paris, 1999.
8. Holmes P. *The energetics of Western herbs — Vol. II*. Artemis Press, Boulder, 1989.
9. Lawrence BM. *Essential oils 1979-1980*. Allured Publishing, Wheaton, 1981.
10. Mailhebiau P. *Portraits in oils*. C.W. Daniel Company, Saffron Walden, 1995.
11. Tisserand R. *The art of aromatherapy*. C.W Daniel Company, Saffron Walden, 1977.
12. Blumenthal M et al. *The complete German commission E monographs: therapeutic guide to herbal medicine*. American Botanical Council, Austin, 1998.
13. Okamoto A et al. T*he effect of aromatherapy massager on mild depression: a pilot study. Letter.* Psychiatry and Clinical Neurosciences, 2005; 59:363. Cited in Quintessential Aromatics database, 2013.
14. Ndounga M, Ouamba J. *Antibacterial and antifungal activities of essential oils of Ocimum gratissimum and O. basilicum from Congo.* Fitoterapia, 1997; 68(2): 190-191. Cited in the Aromatherapy Database, by Bob Harris, Essential Oil Resource Consultants, UK, 2000.
15. Lis-Balchin M. *Aromatherapy science — a guide for healthcare professionals.* Pharmaceutical Press, London, 2006.
16. Kamble VA, Patil SD. *Spice-derived essential oils: effective antifungal and possible therapeutic agents.* Journal of Herbs, Spices & Medicinal Plants, 2008; 14(3/4): 129-143. Cited in Quintessential Aromatics database, 2013.
17. Abou El-Soud NH et al. *Chemical composition and antifungal activity of Ocimum basilicum L. essential oil.* Macedonian Journal of Medical Sciences, 2015; 3(3): 374-379. doi: 10.3889/oamjms.2015.082
18. Dube S et al. *Antifungal, physiochemical and insect repelling activity of the essential oil of Ocimum basilicum*. Canadian Journal of Botany, 1989; 67(7): 2085-2087. Cited in Quintessential Aromatics database, 2013.
19. Rodrigues LB et al. *Anti-inflammatory and antiedematogenic activity of the Ocimum basilicum essential oil and its main compound estragole: in vivo mouse models*. Chemico-Biological Interactions, 2016; 257: 14-25. doi: 10.1016/j.cbi.2016.07.026
20. Wan J et al. *The effect of essential oils of basil on the growth of Aeromonas hydrophila and Pseudomonas fluorescens*. Journal of Applied Microbiology, 1998; 84(1): 152-158. Cited in Quintessential Aromatics database, 2013.
21. Sienkiewicz M et al. *The potential use of basil and rosemary essential oils as effective antibacterial agents*. Molecules, 2013; 18(8): 9334-9351. doi: 10.3390/molecules18089334
22. Gradinariu V et al. *Comparative efficacy of Ocimum sanctum L. and Ocimum basilicum L. essential oils against amyloid beta (1-42)-induced anxiety and depression in laboratory rats.* Phytochemistry Reviews, 2014; 14(4): 567-575. Cited in Quintessential Aromatics database, 2013
23. Rabbani M et al. *Evaluation of anxiolytic and sedative effect of essential oil and hydroalcoholic extract of Ocimum basilicum L. and chemical composition of its essential oil.* Research in Pharmaceutical Sciences, 2015; 10(6): 535-543.
24. Bhatnagar M et al. *Laboratory evaluation of insecticidal properties of Ocimum basilicum Linnaeus and O. sanctum Linnaeus plant's essential oils and their major constituents against vector mosquito species.* Journal of Entomological Research, 1993; 17(1): 21-26. Cited in Quintessential Aromatics database, 2013.
25. Pavela R. *Insecticidal properties of several essential oils on the house fly (Musca domestica L.).* Phytotherapy Research, 2008; 22(2): 274-278. Cited in Quintessential Aromatics database, 2013.
26. Lawless J. *The encyclopaedia of essential oils.* Element Books, Shaftesbury, 1992.
27. Lavabre M. *Aromatherapy workbook.* Healing Arts Press, Rochester, 1997.
28. Schnaubelt K. *Advanced aromatherapy.* Healing Arts Press, Rochester, 1995.

B

29. Davis P. *Aromatherapy A-Z.* 2nd edn. C.W. Daniel Company, Saffron Walden, 1999.
30. Worwood VA. *The fragrant mind.* Transworld Publishers, London, 1995.
31. Worwood VA. *The fragrant heavens.* Transworld Publishers, London, 1999.
32. Zeck R. *The blossoming heart – aromatherapy for healing and transformation.* Aroma Tours, East Ivanhoe, 2004.

Bay laurel

Identification

Botanical name

Laurus nobilis L.

Synonyms

Bay, laurel leaf, bay sweet, true bay and Mediterranean bay

Family

Lauraceae

Botany and origins

Laurus nobilis is an evergreen tree, up to 5-10 m high, but it is usually pruned to below 3 m. The bark on mature trees is greyish, and on younger stems it is smooth and shiny, often with a reddish tint.[1]

It is believed to have originated in Asia Minor, but is now considered native to the Mediterranean region. There are several botanical species known under the name bay. These include *Pimenta racemosa*, commonly known as West Indian bay, and *Umbellularia californica*, commonly known as California bay.[1]

It is commonly planted in gardens as a hedge and in tubs to produce fresh leaves for culinary purposes.[1]

Weiss states that the wild trees have been harvested in many Mediterranean countries for centuries to produce the dried leaves; however, he states that bay laurel oil is of relatively recent origin.[1]

Method of extraction

Bay laurel oil is produced by steam distillation of the freshly picked leaves.

Characteristics

Bay laurel oil is a pale yellow to very pale olive-green or almost colourless liquid of a fresh, strong but sweet, camphoraceous and spicy medicinal odour.[2]

Chemical composition

The composition of bay laurel oil is fascinating. It contains constituents from almost all the functional groups [oxides, esters, alcohols and phenols], which explains its wide spectrum of uses.[3]

The chemical composition of *Laurus nobilis* essential oil was as follows:[4]

1,8-cineole (40%), α-terpinyl acetate (9%), sabinene (7%), α-pinene (7%), β-pinene (4%), terpinen-4-ol (4%), α-terpineol (3%), linalool (10%), *p*-cymene (1%), γ-terpinene (1%), methyl eugenol (5%).

Weiss states that the time of harvesting may have a significant influence on the chemical profile of the oil. For example, in Israel, the 1,8-cineole content was 60% in spring and only 40% in summer.[1]

Adulteration

Bay laurel oil is often adulterated with *Eucalyptus globulus*, cajeput and other synthetic monoterpenoids.[5]

Pharmacopoeias and standards

At the time of writing, the purity, composition, physico-chemical properties and therapeutic use of bay laurel essential oil are not defined in any pharmacopoeia monograph or standard.

History and Traditional Uses

History

L. nobilis was sacred to the god Apollo in classical Greece. According to legend, when Daphne, the nymph daughter of the earth goddess Gaia, was pursued by Apollo, slayer of her bridegroom, she entreated the gods for assistance, who changed her into a laurel tree. Apollo then crowned himself with a circle of laurel leaves and declared the tree sacred to his divinity.[1]

A garland of woven laurel leaves was awarded as a symbol of honour or victory in Rome. In the Middle Ages, distinguished men were crowned with a wreath of berried laurel, hence the term Poet Laureate. University graduates were known as bachelors from the Latin *baccalaureus* (*bacco* a berry and *laureus* of laurel). They were forbidden to marry as it was believed that this would distract them from their studies.[1]

Bay laurel was said to confer the gift of prophecy. A withering laurel tree in the garden predicted a disaster.[1]

Herbal

Bay laurel has long been used in herbal medicine. An infusion of the berries was supposed to suppress profuse menstruation and hasten childbirth. Infusions of the bark and leaves were frequently prescribed to alleviate kidney disorders and respiratory problems.[1]

Food, perfumery and flavouring

The dried leaves have long been used as a spice. It is considered a vital ingredient of *bouquet garni,* which is a bundle of herbs tied together and mainly used to prepare soups, stocks and stews.[1]

Bay laurel oil is used extensively in food flavouring. Arctander describes the flavour as fresh, almost orange-like, with a rich and delicately spicy undertone that is warm and soft.[2]

Bay laurel oil is an important ingredient in a famous soap traditionally manufactured in Aleppo called *sabun bi ghar*. The soap has been produced and exported from Syria for at least 500 years.[1]

Other uses

Bay laurel oil is very effective in protecting harvested fruits of kiwi and peach against the postharvest fungi *Monilinia laxa, Botrytis cinerea* and *Penicillium digitatum*. It was noted that using essential oils to help preserve food could be a good idea, as many essential oil plants are already used as spices.[6]

B

Therapeutics

Pharmacology and clinical studies

Analgesic activity

The analgesic and anti-inflammatory properties of bay laurel oil were studied in vivo using a number of animal models. It must be noted that in this study the essential oil was injected intraperitoneally at doses of 0.03 – 0.06 ml/kg. The effect was comparable with that of the reference drug morphine at 10 mg/kg i.p. The authors of the study concluded that bay laurel essential oil possesses antinociceptive activities comparable to classic analgesic drugs.[7]

Antimicrobial activity

Bay laurel oil has been reported to have excellent bactericidal and fungicidal properties.[8,9]

Antispasmodic activity

Lis-Balchin states that bay laurel oil has an initial spasmogenic effect followed by a strong spasmolytic effect on guinea pig ileum in vitro.[5]

Insecticidal activity

Bay laurel oil has been reported to have effective spatial repellent effect on *Aedes aegypti* mosquito.[10]

Wound-healing activity

Bay laurel oil has been reported to have excellent wound-healing activities. The study involved essential oils from several plants for the first aid treatment of wounds, abscesses and burns.[11]

Actions

Actions commonly cited in aromatherapy

Antifungal, antiseptic, bactericidal, carminative, diaphoretic, digestive, expectorant, tonic[12,13]

Actions supported by clinical studies

Antifungal, antiseptic, bactericidal

Comment

Bay laurel oil is not listed in any pharmacopoeia. Review of traditional uses and clinical data support the use of bay laurel oil as an effective all-round antimicrobial essential oil for the treatment of colds and flu.

Aromatherapy Uses

Clinical aromatherapy

Digestive system

Bay laurel oil has a pronounced effect on the digestive system and may be useful as an appetite stimulant. It expels wind, settles the stomach pain and has a tonic effect on the liver and kidneys.[12,13]

Integumentary system

Bay laurel oil is recommended for conditions such as ulcers, boils, acne and abscesses. Mailhebiau recommends blending bay laurel with lavender to accelerate the process of regeneration of the epidermis.[14]

Psychological

It has been described as an excellent cerebral stimulator and nerve tonic for those who doubt themselves.[13,14]

Mojay compares bay laurel to rosemary. He recommends using it for poor concentration, lack of memory and chronic nervous debility. He states that it is ideally indicated for individuals who lack self-esteem, doubt their abilities and have no confidence.[13]

Respiratory system

Bay laurel oil is a good antiseptic for the respiratory system. It is an expectorant with mucolytic properties. It is recommended for the treatment of chronic bronchitis and emphysema.[14]

Schnaubelt recommends applying three to ten drops topically over lymph nodes to support the lymphatic system whenever one has an upper respiratory tract infection. He says that one will often have an immediate sensation of relief. He recommends ingesting one drop of bay laurel as a good way to stop the onset of a sore throat. He explains that, while there is a lack of research on its benefits, there is ample anecdotal evidence to support his claims and treatment.[3] However, in light of the methyl eugenol content, I would be very reluctant to recommend ingesting even one drop of bay laurel.

Energetics, psyche and subtle uses

Energetics

Energetically, bay laurel's principal actions are to circulate and regulate *Qi* energy and to clear *cold* phlegm.[13] Mojay explains that bay laurel oil helps renew one's belief in there's own potential. He states that the fresh and spicy aroma activates the Fire Element, which is responsible for our inner vision and passion.[13]

Personality

It is particularly beneficial for individuals who lack energy and confidence. It is well suited for people who lack self-esteem and doubt their abilities and intellect.[13]

Bay laurel symbolises power, greatness and victory. Mailhebiau states that bay laurel epitomises the warrior temperament. The bay laurel personality is ideally suited to the role as a leader. They have a strength of character and confidence, but they are more likely to use their passion to prove their strength. As a result, they may be perceived as being emotionally cold and more likely to conduct their love life as if it was a battle. However, bay laurel types can encourage people to overcome their fears and inhibitions to become ambitious and act with self-assurance.[14]

According to Myers-Briggs personality types, the bay laurel personality is likely to be an ENTJ. ENTJs are dynamic, energetic, confident and competent. They naturally move into positions where they can take charge. They enjoy confrontation and they like to engage in intellectually stimulating exchanges. They like and respect people who challenge them and have little or no respect for those that don't. They have an improvement plan for everything, including their leisure. They like to set goals and provide directions. They see obstacles as challenges. They dislike inefficiency, incompetence and indecisiveness. They are competitively driven and often considered to be workaholics. They can be very honest and direct and do not hesitate to express themselves. When stressed they can have explosive outbursts or be judgemental on themselves and others.

Subtle

Worwood beautifully describes the subtle qualities of bay laurel oil as the fragrance of victors and poets who have used imagination and inspiration to attain their goals. She explains that it encourages the gift of prophecy and creativity, enabling one to go beyond the normal activities of the brain.[15]

The oil is ideal for those with psychic tendencies who depend on intuition and inspiration for their work. It promotes confidence, insight and courage.[16]

Dosage and Administration

Blending

Aromatherapy

To provide relief from the symptoms associated with a respiratory tract infection, consider blending bay laurel essential oil with other leaf oils from herbs or trees such as cypress, 1,8-cineole-rich eucalypts, niaouli, fragonia, ravintsara, tea tree, pine, fir or spruce.

Bay laurel essential oil would make an excellent anti-flu blend when blended with ravintsara, lemon, spike lavender or tea tree.

For musculoskeletal aches and pains, consider blending bay laurel with essential oils such as black pepper, ginger, kunzea, spike lavender, sweet marjoram or rosemary.

For the relief of abdominal bloating and indigestion, consider blending bay laurel oil with essential oils such as sweet orange, grapefruit, mandarin, sweet marjoram, sweet fennel or coriander seed.

To create a purifying and space-clearing blend, consider blending bay laurel oil with essential oils such as fragonia, frankincense, lemon, cold-pressed lime or myrtle.

To help alleviate physical and emotional exhaustion, consider blending bay laurel oil with essential oils such as lemon, fir, basil or rosemary. It would also create an energising and invigorating blend if blended with spice oils such as black pepper, cardamom, sweet fennel, ginger or coriander seed.

Perfumery

Arctander states that the odour of bay laurel essential oil is not very unique or distinctive. As a result, it has never attained any significance in perfumery. However, he explains that in perfumes it blends well with citrus oils, spice oils, conifer oils such as pine, cypress and juniper, and herbaceous oils such as rosemary and clary sage. It produces very interesting notes when blended with resin oils such as frankincense or labdanum. It also blends well with lavender.[2]

Mode of administration

Bath

Full body bath, foot bath

Topical

Compress, massage, ointment, skin care

Inhalation

Direct inhalation, diffuser, oil vaporiser

Safety Profile

General safety

Bay laurel oil is generally regarded as safe. Frequent use of bay laurel oil on the skin over a longer period of time (approximately 3 weeks) can result in sensitisation and irritations.[3,12]

Tisserand & Young recommend caution when using on people with hypersensitive, diseased or damaged skin and children under 2 years of age. They recommend a dermal maximum of 0.5%.[17]

Contraindications

No contraindications known.

Toxicity

Tisserand & Young state that the methyl eugenol content classifies bay laurel as potentially carcinogenic. The study often cited involves pure methyl eugenol being administered at very high doses, as high as 150 mg/kg, to rats. The administration of such high does by gavage was responsible for significant hepatotoxicity and gastric damage.[17]

This study is also cited in an EU report that prohibits methyl eugenol from being added to food because it has a potentially carcinogenic effect.[18]

Methyl eugenol is registered as an active pesticide ingredient in the USA. It is also an insect parapheromone and is used in insect traps to attract certain species of fly. It is noted that methyl eugenol is also naturally found in edible fruits such as grapefruit and bananas at a level of less than 0.1 mg/kg.[19]

The dietary exposure to methyl eugenol may arise from:

(i) ingestion of fruits and vegetables containing methyl eugenol (minor source)

(ii) ingestion of herbs and spices containing methyl eugenol (primary source)

(iii) ingestion of essential oil and herb extracts used to flavour food and beverages

(iv) ingestion of methyl eugenol added directly as a flavouring to food and beverages.[19]

The average total dietary exposure is believed to be in the range of 8-81.3 ug per day.

The IARC Monograph for methyl eugenol states that there is sufficient evidence in experimental animals for the carcinogenicity of methyl eugenol. They also state that methyl eugenol is possibly carcinogenic to humans.[19]

The no-observable-effect-level (NOEL) for methyl eugenol in rats is in the dose-range of 1-10 mg/kg body weight/day.[17] Based on an RIFM report and on the available data, I agree with Tisserand & Young, who are concerned with the relevance of high-dose carcinogenicity testing in rats.

I would suggest that methyl eugenol is not likely to present a human cancer risk at current levels of exposure resulting from the addition of essential oils containing methyl eugenol such as bay laurel.[19]

Tisserand & Young indicate that 18 mg should be the maximum adult oral dose.[17] Therefore I would be concerned about taking one drop of bay laurel, as one drop is equivalent to 50 mg.

Regulatory guidelines

Bay laurel oil has GRAS status. In the USA, it is also permitted for direct addition to food for human consumption as a synthetic flavouring substance.[19]

In the EU, Regulation (EC) 1334/2008, which became effective in January 2011, prohibits the addition of methyl eugenol to foods, and restricts the concentration of methyl eugenol in food that has been prepared with flavourings. However, if the only food ingredients with flavouring properties that have been added are fresh, dried or frozen herbs and spices, the maximum limits for methyl eugenol do not apply.[18]

References

1. Weiss EA. *Essential oil crops*. CAB International, Wallingford, 1997.
2. Arctander S. *Perfume and flavor materials of natural origin*. Allured Publishing, Carol Stream, 1994.
3. Schnaubelt K. *Advanced aromatherapy*. Healing Arts Press, Rochester, 1995.
4. Khan I, Abourashed E. *Leung's encyclopedia of common natural ingredients used in food, drugs and cosmetics*. 3rd edn. John Wiley & Sons, New Jersey, 2010.
5. Lis-Balchin M. *Aromatherapy science – a guide for healthcare professionals*. Pharmaceutical Press, London, 2006.
6. Buchbauer G, Hemetsberger S. *Use of essential oils in agriculture*. In Baser KHC, Buchbauer

G. eds. *Handbook of essential oils – science, technology and applications*. 2nd edn. CRC Press, Boca Raton, 2016: 669-706.
7. Sayyah M et al. *Analgesic and anti-inflammatory activity of the leaf essential oil of Laurus nobilis Linn*. Phytotherapy Research, 2003; 17(7): 733-736. Cited in Quintessential Aromatics database, 2013.
8. Deans SG, Ritchie G. *Antibacterial properties of plant essential oils*. International Journal of Food Microbiology, 1987; 5: 165-180. Cited in Quintessential Aromatics database, 2013.
9. Akgül A, Kivanç M. *Chemical composition and antimicrobial effect of Turkish laurel leaf oil*. Journal of Essential Oil Research, 1989; 1(6): 277-280. Cited in Quintessential Aromatics database, 2013.
10. Drapeau J et al. *Repellent studies with Aedes aegypti mosquitoes and human olfactory tests on 19 essential oils from Corsica, France*. Flavour and Fragrance Journal, 2009; 24(4): 160-169. Cited in Quintessential Aromatics database, 2013.
11. Suntar I et al. *Comparative pharmacological and phytochemical investigation on the wound-healing effects of the frequently used essential oils*. Journal of Essential Oil Research, 2013; 26(1): 41-49. Cited in Quintessential Aromatics database, 2013.
12. Lawless J. *The encyclopaedia of essential oils*. Element Books, Shaftesbury, 1992.
13. Mojay G. *Aromatherapy for healing the spirit*. Healing Arts Press, Rochester, 1999.
14. Malhebiau P. *Portraits in oils*. C.W. Daniel Company, Saffron Walden, 1995.
15. Worwood V. *The fragrant heavens*. Transworld Publishers, London, 1999.
16. Lawless J. *Aromatherapy and the mind*. Thornsons, London, 1994.
17. Tisserand R, Young R. *Essential oil safety*. 2nd edn. Churchill Livingstone, Edinburgh, 2014.
18. *Opinion of the scientific committee on food on methyleugenol (4-allyl-1,2-dimethoxybenzene)*. European Commission Health & Consumer Protection Directorate-General. Brussels, 2001. Retrieved from https://ec.europa.eu/food/sites/food/files/safety/docs/fs_food-improvement-agents_flavourings-out102.pdf
19. International Agency for Research on Cancer. *Methyleugenol*. WHO Press, Lyon, 2013. Retrieved from https://monographs.iarc/fr/ENG/Monographs/vol101/mono101-013.pdf

Bay, West Indian

B

Identification

Botanical name

Pimenta racemosa (Mill.) JW Moore

Synonyms

Bay rum tree, bay, wild cinnamon, bay-berry; also known as myrcia oil

Family

Myrtaceae

Botany and origins

The genus *Pimenta* Lindl contains 18 aromatic trees native to tropical America and the Caribbean. The genus name is derived from the Spanish word *pimienta* meaning peppercorns. The most important commercial species are *Pimenta dioica* L. Merr., which provides the pimento spice known as allspice, and *P. racemosa* (Mill) Moore, which is the source of West Indian bay oil.[1]

West Indian bay is a small to medium size forest tree that grows up to 15 m. It is native to the West Indies and is cultivated in Venezuela, Puerto Rico and the Caribbean Islands.[1]

Method of extraction

West Indian bay essential oil is steam- or water-distilled from the leaves.

Characteristics

West Indian bay oil is a pale straw to brownish-orange in colour, with a fresh-spicy, somewhat camphoraceous topnote, and a lasting sweet-balsamic undertone.[2]

Arctander states that some people find the odour of West Indian bay oil sickly sweet and nauseating, while others describe it as fresh and pleasant.[2]

Chemical composition

The main components of West Indian bay essential oil are eugenol (up to 56%), chavicol (up to 22%), and myrcene (up to 21%).[3] The chemical composition of West Indian bay oil was reported as follows:

myrcene (31.6%), limonene (1.4%), 1,8-cineole (2.0%), *trans*-ocimene (2.1%), 3-octanone (1.0%), *p*-cymene (0.5%), 3-octanol (0.5%), 1-octen-3-ol (1.3%), linalool (3.0%), terpinen-4-ol (0.3%), caryophyllene (0.9%), methyl chavicol (0.3%), neral (0.8%), α-terpineol (0.8%), geranyl acetate (0.8%), eugenol (38.6%), chavicol (11.0%).[1]

The oil content of mature leaves is generally similar to or lower than that of young leaves, but the phenol content is higher.[1]

There are three chemotypes of *P. racemosa*: a eugenol chemotype, a citral chemotype and an anise chemotype that has a high percentage of estragole and methyl eugenol. Tisserand & Young state that only the eugenol chemotype oil is produced commercially.[4]

Adulteration

West Indian bay oil is frequently adulterated with clove leaf oil and myrcene from other sources.[2,5]

Pharmacopoeias and standards

The purity, composition and physico-chemical properties of *Pimento racemosa* essential oil are defined in ISO 3045:2004 Oil of Bay [*Pimenta racemosa* (Mill) J.W. Moore].

History and Traditional Uses

Food, perfumery and flavouring

The major use of West Indian bay leaf oil is in hair lotions, especially bay rum. Bay rum was originally produced by distilling rum over the leaves, but it is now formulated by blending the essential oil with alcohol and rum.[2]

B

Therapeutics

Pharmacology and clinical studies

Antifungal activity

Growth inhibition of fungi was compared by direct contact in broth and agar medium with the fungistatic action of their vapours using the micro-atmosphere method. *P. racemosa* was very effective by direct contact, but the vapour gave very moderate- and short-term fungistatic result.[6]

Antimicrobial activity

Three chemotypes of West Indian bay oil were tested for their antimicrobial activity. The neral/geranial and the chavicol/eugenol chemotypes possessed strong antibacterial activity against *Escherichia coli, Staphylococcus aureus* and *Enterococcus faecium*. The methyl chavicol/methyl eugenol chemotype had no bacteriostatic activity. The antifungal activity of all three chemotypes was much greater than their antibacterial effect.[7]

P. racemosa oil exhibited strong effect against *Candida albicans,* and medium to strong antimicrobial activity against the gram-positive bacteria *S. aureus* and *E. faecium* and the gram-negative bacteria *E. coli, Klebsiella pneumoniae, Proteus vulgaris* and *Salmonella* sp.[8]

Actions

Actions commonly cited in aromatherapy

Analgesic, antibacterial, antifungal, antimicrobial, antiseptic, astringent, expectorant, general stimulant[8]

Actions supported by clinical studies

Antibacterial, antifungal, antimicrobial

Comment

The high percentage of phenols in the oil suggests that West Indian bay oil has good antimicrobial activity and may be useful for the treatment of colds and flu.

Aromatherapy Uses

Clinical aromatherapy

Musculoskeletal system

West Indian bay oil may be used in massage for muscular aches and pains, strains and sprains.[9]

Respiratory system

West Indian bay oil is a good antiseptic for the respiratory system, and is recommended for the treatment of colds, flu, tonsillitis and viral infections.[9]

Skin care

West Indian bay oil is recommended in hair care as a scalp stimulant, a hair rinse for dandruff and for greasy, lifeless hair. West Indian bay oil is extensively used as a fragrance ingredient in bay rum, creams, lotions, soaps, detergents and perfumes.[9]

Dosage and Administration

Blending

Aromatherapy

For the relief of muscular aches and pains, consider blending West Indian bay oil with essential oils such as cajeput, clove bud, ginger, kunzea, peppermint or rosemary.

To alleviate the symptoms of colds and flu, consider blending West Indian bay oil with essential oils such as 1,8-cineole-rich eucalypts, peppermint eucalyptus, lemon-scented eucalyptus, fragonia, ginger, lemon, peppermint, pine, tea tree or thyme.

Perfumery

West Indian bay oil is extensively used in hair lotions, after-shave lotions, and other men's fragrances. In perfumery, it blends well with essential oils such as basil, Virginian cedarwood, clove bud, ginger, patchouli, rosemary, sandalwood and ylang ylang.[2]

Mode of administration

Bath

Full body bath, foot bath

Topical

Compress, massage, ointment, skin care

Inhalation

Direct inhalation, diffuser, oil vaporiser

Safety Profile

General safety

The high eugenol content in West Indian bay oil suggests that the oil is moderately toxic and should be used with caution. Lawless also states that it may be a mucous membrane irritant, but unlike bay laurel, it does not appear to cause dermal sensitisation or irritation.[9]

Tisserand & Young caution the oral usage of essential oils high in eugenol such as West Indian bay oil. Oils high in eugenol are MAO inhibitors, inhibit platelet activity and impair liver activity.[4]

Oral dosing is cautioned in conjunction with anticoagulant drugs, major surgery, childbirth, peptic ulcers, haemophilia and other bleeding disorders.[4]

Tisserand & Young state that essential oils with a high eugenol content may be mild dermal irritants. They recommend a dermal maximum of 0.9% based on the typical eugenol content. The oil contains very little if no methyl eugenol, so there are no concerns or warnings regarding its carcinogenic potential.

Contraindications

No contraindications known.

Regulatory guidelines

West Indian bay essential oil has GRAS status.

References

1. Weiss EA. *Essential oil crops*. CAB International, Wallingford, 1997.
2. Arctander S. *Perfume and flavor materials of natural origin*. Allured Publishing, Carol Stream, 1994.
3. Khan I, Abourashed E. *Leung's encyclopedia of common natural ingredients used in food, drugs and cosmetics*. 3rd edn. John Wiley & Sons, New Jersey, 2010.
4. Tisserand R, Young R. *Essential oil safety*. 2nd edn. Churchill Livingstone, Edinburgh, 2014.
5. Schmidt E, Wanner J. *Adulteration of essential oils*. In Baser KHC, Buchbauer G. eds. *Handbook of essential oils – science, technology and applications*. 2nd edn. CRC Press, Boca Raton, 2016: 707-745.
6. Delespaul Q et al. *The antifungal activity of essential oils as determined by different screening methods*. Journal of Essential Oil Research, 2000; 12(2): 256-266. Cited in Quintessential Aromatics database, 2013.
7. Aurore GS et al. *Antibacterial and antifungal activities of the essential oils of Pimenta racemosa var. racemosa P. Miller (J.W.Moore) (Myrtaceae)*. Journal of Essential Oil Research, 1998; 10(2): 161-164. Cited in Quintessential Aromatics database, 2013.
8. Höferl M et al. *Correlation of antimicrobial activities of various essential oils and their main aromatic volatile constituents*. Journal of Essential Oil Research, 2009; 21(5): 459-463. Cited in Quintessential Aromatics database, 2013.
9. Lawless J. *The encyclopaedia of essential oils*. Element Books, Shaftesbury, 1992.

B

Benzoin

Identification

Botanical name

Sumatra benzoin: *Styrax benzoin* Dryand

Siam benzoin: *Styrax tonkinensis* Pierre

Synonyms

Gum benjamin

Family

Styracaceae

Botany and origins

Benzoin is the balsamic resin obtained from various *Styrax* species, which are small to medium trees that grow in tropical Asia.[1]

It is the pathological exudate that is formed when the tree trunk is injured. It is produced by incising the bark, which helps produce the resin that hardens on exposure to air and sunlight.[2]

The resin can be harvested when the tree is seven years old. The resin can be collected annually for 10 to 12 years, but the first three years collection provides the finest benzoin.[3]

Sumatra benzoin is a resin produced from trees that grow in the Malay Peninsula, Sumatra and Java; while Siam benzoin is produced from trees growing in Laos, Vietnam, Cambodia, China and Thailand.[1]

Siam benzoin resinoid is considered to be of a higher quality and is preferred in fine perfumery.[2]

Siam benzoin comes in different size pebble-like, often tear-shaped pieces which are hard and brittle. It is available in several grades according to the shape of the tears. 'Selected tears' or 'tears No. 1' are considered superior for perfumery purposes. Lower grades of 'tears' are usually darker and have more insoluble matter. 'Amygdaloid' forms of Siam benzoin give a very pale tincture which is less aromatic than 'selected tears'.[2]

Method of extraction

Benzoin resinoid is prepared from the crude benzoin resin by extraction with solvents such as alcohol, followed by their subsequent removal.[2] Tisserand & Young state that there is no such thing as benzoin essential oil, only a resinoid.[4]

Benzoin tincture is usually prepared from selected 'tears' of Siam benzoin. Arctander explains that the conventional strength is 20 parts by weight of Siam benzoin macerated with enough alcohol at around 90% strength by volume. He states that the benzoin gum should be almost entirely soluble in alcohol. Therefore the tincture should represent 20% solution of the alcohol-soluble resinoid.[2]

B

Characteristics

The tincture has a sweet, balsamic-vanillin-like odour. Siam benzoin has a pleasant, sweet-balsamic aroma with a distinct note of vanillin.[2] Jouhar describes the aroma of Siam benzoin as sweet, balsamic and chocolate-like, while Sumatra benzoin has a warm, sweet, powdery aroma.[5]

Chemical composition

The major constituents found in benzoin are as follows:[6]

Constituent	Siam	Sumatra
benzyl benzoate	80%	76%
benzylaldehyde	0.4%	0.9%
methyl benzoate	1.5%	0.5%
benzoic acid	12.5%	1.7%
ethyl benzoate	1.1%	0.2%
allyl benzoate	1.5%	0.9%
cinnamic acid	-	3.5%
allyl cinnamate	-	0.5%
isobutyl cinnamate	-	0.1%
cinnamyl benzoate	-	1.4%
cinnamyl cinnamate	-	0.9%

Adulteration

Siam benzoin is most sought after and is more expensive. It is often adulterated with Sumatra benzoin. It is also 'stretched' with benzyl benzoate, copaiba balsam or amyris oil.[2]

Natural benzoin resinoid is very difficult to work with as it is a very sticky solid. To render it pourable, it is usually diluted to 50% in benzyl alcohol, benzyl benzoate, dipropylene glycol and other solvents such as diethyl phthalate.[2,4] However, diethyl phthalate is not commonly used nowadays as a diluent due to toxicity concerns.[4]

Pharmacopoeias and standards

At the time of writing, the purity, composition, physico-chemical properties and therapeutic use of benzoin essential oil are not defined in any standard. Both Siam and Sumatra benzoin are officially listed in pharmacopoeias of many countries, but only Sumatra benzoin is found in the BP.[1]

History and Traditional Uses

History

Morris states that the first documented use of benzoin dates back to the sixth century AD. The Western names gum benzoin and gum benjamin come from a corruption of the Arabic word *luban jawi*, which means incense of Java. Arab traders often referred to benzoin as Eastern frankincense.[7]

The Arabs were instrumental in expanding the trade to Europe. Benzoin was considered similar to frankincense.[8]

The Malays used benzoin as holy smoke to ward off devils, and it was burned at the rice-reaping ceremony. In India, benzoin was burned before the Trimurti, the trinity of supreme divinity – Brahma, creator of the world, Shiva, destroyer of illusion, and Vishnu, regenerator of the world.[7]

Traditional medicine

Benzoin was popular as an antiseptic, parasiticide and stimulating expectorant since the time of Marco Polo.[8]

Herbal

Benzoin tincture has long been used in skin care as an antiseptic and a styptic for cuts. It is used in Friar's Balsam and in Compound Benzoin Tincture, which is commonly used as a skin protectant or topical adhesive agent. The tincture is also used in dentistry to treat inflammation of the gums and oral herpetic lesions.[1]

Compound tincture of benzoin is used as an inhalant with steam for laryngitis and bronchitis.[3]

Food, perfumery and flavouring

Sumatra benzoin is commonly used in pharmaceutical preparations, while Siam benzoin is preferred for flavours and fragrances.[1,2,8]

Siam benzoin has antioxidative and preservative properties and is used in cosmetics. Benzoin tincture is extensively used in perfumery because it makes an excellent fixative.[1,2]

Benzoic acid, now primarily a synthetic product, was initially obtained from Sumatra benzoin. Benzoic acid and its sodium salt are extensively used as a preservative in foods, drinks, fats and pharmaceutical preparations. Medicinally, benzoic acid is used as an antifungal agent.[8]

Therapeutics

Pharmacology and clinical studies

Most of the studies for benzoin pertained to benzoin tincture.

Allergen

All the studies I reviewed reported contact dermatitis from skin adhesion sprays containing benzoin tincture. One report recommended that benzoin no longer be recommended as a skin adhesive.[9]

Tincture of benzoin was patch tested on 477 patients at the Contact Dermatitis Clinic at the Skin and Cancer Foundation in Melbourne. The results showed that 45 out of 477 patients had a positive reaction to compound tincture of benzoin and 14 of the patients had a bad strong reaction.[10]

Antibacterial activity

Lis-Balchin reports that benzoin had low anti-bacterial activity against five different bacteria.[6]

Actions

Actions commonly cited in aromatherapy

Anti-inflammatory, antiseptic, astringent, carminative, deodorant, expectorant, sedative, styptic, vulnerary[11,12]

Actions supported by clinical studies

Anti-inflammatory, expectorant, vulnerary

Comment

Benzoin has been used for many years in food, perfumery and medicine with minimal sensitisation potential. However, there has been an increasing number of dermal contact allergic and sensitisation responses. RIFM recommends that only the benzoin that has had the allergens removed be used in consumer products. Lis-Balchin explains that these grades are commonly not available to aromatherapists.[6]

Lis-Balchin states that benzoin is not recommended for use on the skin, although its use as a fragrance and food additive is not banned or restricted.[6] However, Tisserand & Young state that skin sensitisation presents a low risk.[4]

Benzoin tincture has been used for superficial wound infections, and has well-established uses in both allopathic and traditional forms of medicine. It has been used as an inhalant with steam for the relief of cough, laryngitis, bronchitis and upper respiratory tract conditions. It is also used for the topical treatment of itchy skin rashes, wounds and ulcers.[13]

Aromatherapy Uses

Clinical aromatherapy

Integumentary system

It is used for cuts, dermatitis, wounds, and chapped and irritated skin conditions.[11,12] Mojay recommends benzoin for chapped skin, chilblains, frostbite and cuts.[14]

Psychological

Benzoin is recommended for nervous tension and stress-related complaints.[11]

Respiratory system

Benzoin is recommended for treating asthma, bronchitis, coughs and laryngitis.[11] Mojay recommends blending benzoin with eucalyptus, tea tree and clary sage for laryngitis, applied in a base cream to the throat.[14]

Energetics, psyche and subtle uses

Energetics

Benzoin's sweet, warm resinous base note is associated with the Earth Element. Mojay considers Benzoin one of the most important aromatic ingredients for *deficient Yang Qi* of the *Spleen*. As such, it is recommended for lethargy, cold limbs, poor appetite and abdominal distention.[14]

Mojay explains that benzoin is ideal for those who feel emotionally needy and neglected. He states that benzoin is ideal for those individuals who overthink and worry. These are feelings that are usually associated with a deficiency of the Earth Element.[14]

Personality

According to Myers-Briggs personality types, the benzoin personality is likely to be an ENFP. ENFPs are outgoing, lively and spontaneous.

They are very enthusiastic and their joy for life can be contagious. They have a rich imagination and active mind. Their thoughts are always wandering and their mood constantly changing. They can be inspiring and charismatic leaders. They are always involved or in love with someone or something new. They know how to establish instant rapport and make people feel comfortable. They love emotional intensity and enjoy expressing their feelings. They can be charming and flirtatious. They relate with warmth to many people and can appear overly enthusiastic, positive and optimistic.

Subtle

Keim Loughran & Bull state that benzoin can provide psychic protection. It steadies and focuses the mind for meditation or prayer, and allows buried thoughts and feelings to come safely to consciousness so that they can be examined and processed.[15]

Benzoin provides comfort, love and support on our spiritual path to compassionate wisdom. It helps us release painful emotions and supports us when we are impatient about our progress on our spiritual path. Benzoin helps us to be aware of our emotional wounds, past and present, and begin the process of healing and releasing them. It teaches us to have compassion for ourselves and our past, helping us to grow slowly and deeply in wisdom.[16]

Worwood states that benzoin is persuasive and direct. It allows us to open the heart and mind, allowing our soul to speak. She explains benzoin can assist in making choices with the heart by helping us to reconnect with the inner sanctum of the soul.[17]

Davis states that benzoin assists us to meditate or do anything of spiritual value while experiencing anger. She explains that benzoin relates very directly to the base chakra, on which it has a strong energising effect. She recommends using benzoin when you need to increase physical strength and energy.[18]

Mojay explains that benzoin can have a stabilising influence whenever there is physical and emotional upheaval. He recommends benzoin for those who are on a spiritual journey as it will help them to steady and focus the mind for meditation or prayer.[14]

Zeck states that benzoin brushes away resistance to change, and recommends using it when we are faced with the challenge of accepting new situations that require us to abandon a familiar position. She explains that benzoin will help us acknowledge and integrate what has changed in our life.[19]

B

Dosage and Administration

Blending

Aromatherapy

To promote wound healing, consider blending benzoin resinoid with essential oils such as cistus, everlasting, frankincense, lavender or myrrh.

To alleviate anxiety, nervous tension and stress, consider blending benzoin resinoid with essential oils such as bergamot, frankincense, geranium, lavender, sweet orange, patchouli, sandalwood, vetiver or ylang ylang.

For the relief of bronchitis, coughs and sore throats, consider blending benzoin resinoid with essential oils such as aniseed, 1,8-cineole-rich eucalypts, cajeput, Atlas cedarwood, fragonia, myrrh, pine, sandalwood or thyme.

Perfumery

Benzoin resinoid is extensively used in perfumery where its fixative effect is much appreciated. Arctander states that it can have a pronounced odour-depressing effect upon perfumes in which it is incorporated. This effect is associated with the fixative effect, which is enhanced by the rich sweetness and deep balsamic notes of the resinoid. Benzoin tincture is often added to alcohol for 'prefixation' prior to the preparation of colognes.[2]

Mode of administration

Bath

Full body bath, foot bath

Topical

Compress, massage, ointment, skin care

Inhalation

Direct inhalation, diffuser, oil vaporiser

Safety Profile

General safety

Benzoin is non-toxic, non-irritant; however, there is a low risk of the tincture being a possible sensitiser.[11]

Benzyl benzoate and benzyl alcohol are listed in the EU as allergens; however, the risk of reaction from either is considered negligible. Tisserand & Young recommend caution for dermal application for people with hypersensitive, diseased or damaged skin, and for children under 2 years of age. They state that the maximum dermal use level is 2%.[4]

Contraindications

No contraindications known.

Regulatory guidelines

Benzoin has GRAS status.

References

1. Khan I, Abourashed E. *Leung's encyclopedia of common natural ingredients used in food, drugs and cosmetics*. 3rd edn. John Wiley & Sons, New Jersey, 2010.
2. Arctander S. *Perfume and flavor materials of natural origin*. Allured Publishing, Carol Stream, 1994.
3. Grieve M. *A modern herbal – Vol. I.* Dover Publications, New York, 1971.
4. Tisserand R, Young R. *Essential oil safety*. 2nd edn. Churchill Livingstone, Edinburgh, 2014.
5. Jouhar AJ. *Poucher's perfumes, cosmetics and soaps – Vol. 1: The raw materials of perfumery*. 9th edn. Springer-Science+Business Media, Dordrecht, 1991.
6. Lis-Balchin M. *Aromatherapy science – a guide for healthcare professionals*. Pharmaceutical Press, London, 2006.
7. Morris E. *Fragrance – The story of perfume from Cleopatra to Chanel*. Products of Nature and Art, New York, 1984.
8. Langenheim JH. *Plant resins – chemistry, evolution, ecology, and ethnobotany*. Timber Press, Portland, 2003.
9. Rademaker M, Kirby JDT. *Contact dermatitis to a skin adhesive*. Contact Dermatitis, 1987; 16(5): 297-298. Cited in Quintessential Aromatics database, 2013.
10. Scardamaglia L et al. *Compound tincture of benzoin: a common contact allergen?* Australasian Journal of Dermatology, 2003; 44(3): 180-184. Cited in Quintessential Aromatics database, 2013.
11. Lawless J. *The encyclopaedia of essential oils*. Element Books, Shaftesbury, 1992.
12. Lavabre M. *Aromatherapy workbook*. Healing Arts Press, Rochester, 1997.
13. Cincu Marsalic RN, Agrawal A, Dange N, Goel A. *Tincture benzoin as an antiseptic and adhesive for preoperative surgical preparation*. Neurology India, 2007; 55(1): 88-89.
14. Mojay G. *Aromatherapy for healing the spirit*. Healing Arts Press, Rochester, 1999.
15. Keim Loughran J, Bull R. *Aromatherapy and subtle energy techniques*. Frog, Berkeley, 2000.
16. Keim Loughran J, Bull R. *Aromatherapy anointing oils*. Frog, Berkeley, 2001.
17. Worwood VA. *The fragrant heavens*. Transworld Publishers, London, 1999.
18. Davis P. *Aromatherapy A-Z*. 2nd edn. C.W. Daniel Company, Saffron Walden, 1999.
19. Zeck R. *The blossoming heart – aromatherapy for healing and transformation*. Aroma Tours, East Ivanhoe, 2004.

Bergamot

Identification

Botanical name

Citrus bergamia Risso & Poit

Synonyms

Citrus aurantium subsp. *bergamia*

Family

Rutaceae

Botany and origins

Bergamot was named for the first time by Pierre Antoine Poiteau and Joseph Antoine Risso in 1818.[1]

Both the botany and origins of bergamot are a little vague. According to Holmes, the Arabs introduced a range of citrus fruits in Malta and Sicily during the early tenth century, and he explains that the name 'bergamot' may also originate from the now defunct language of Sicilian Arabic.[2]

Imbesi & De Pasquale state that several theories regarding the origin of the name exist. They suggest that the most likely theory is that the bergamot resembles the bergamot pear, which in Turkish is referred to as *beg-armudi*, which means 'the prince's pear'. They say that bergamot is a native of India where the fruit was called *limbu* in Punjabi, *niboo* in Bengali and *neamboo* in Hindi. It is still used in these regions against scurvy, dyspepsia, and as an antiemetic, antipyretic and antiseptic.[3]

It has been suggested that bergamot is a hybrid between bitter orange and lemon, or that it is a mutation of the latter. Others suggest that it is a hybrid between bitter orange and lime (*Citrus aurantifolia*) or a cross between citron (*C. medica*) and orange, which itself is a cross between grapefruit (*C. x paradisi*) and mandarin (*C. reticulata*).[1]

Bergamot is a small evergreen tree that can grow up to 12 m tall. It is propagated by grafting, and the best results are obtained by using bitter orange, which produces sturdy long-living trees.[1]

Bergamot is cultivated almost exclusively in a narrow coastal strip in the southern part of Calabria, Italy. Nowadays it is also cultivated on the Ivory Coast, and in Guinea, Morocco and Corsica.[4]

Arctander says that only the expressed oil from the peel of the fruit is of interest. He explains that the pulp or juice is of little value as it is not edible, and the leaves and twigs may be distilled to yield a bergamot-petitgrain oil.[4]

Method of extraction

Bergamot oil is produced by cold expression from the peel of the slightly unripe bergamot fruit from *C. bergamia.*

Characteristics

Bergamot oil is a green to olive-green coloured mobile liquid with a warm fruity-sweet aroma and a fresh citrus note. This is followed by an oily-herbaceous and somewhat balsamic body and dryout. The colour of the oil fades on aging, particularly when the oil is exposed to light.[4]

Chemical composition

The chemical profile of bergamot oil according to the *Farmacopea Ufficiale Italiana* (12th edn.) was reported as follows:

limonene (30-50%), linalyl acetate (23-35%), linalool (6-15%), sabinene (0.5-2.0%), γ-terpinene (6.0-18.5%), β-pinene (5.0-10.0%), α-pinene (0.2-0.7%), geranial (<0.5%), geranyl acetate (0.1-7.0%) and caryophyllene (0.2-5.0%).[5]

The major components in Italian bergamot oil were reported as follows:

limonene (37.2%), linalyl acetate (30.1%), linalool (8.8%), γ-terpinene (6.8%), β-pinene (6.2%) and another 55 compounds.[1]

It has been reported that different rootstocks can change the chemical composition of bergamot oil. It has been suggested that lemon can be considered an alternative to bitter orange as a rootstock.[1]

The non-volatile components that are responsible for the phototoxicity of bergamot include: bergamottin (0.08-0.68%), citropten (0.01-0.35%), bergapten (0.11-0.33%), bergaptol (0-0.19%), 5-methoxy-7-geranoxycoumarin (0.04-0.15%), psoralen (0-0.0026%).[6]

Compared to other citrus essential oils, bergamot oil has a significantly lower amount of limonene (30-50%) and higher amounts of linalool and linalyl acetate.

Adulteration

Bergamot oil is adulterated by the addition of natural or synthetic compounds such as methyl N-methylanthranilate; the addition of synthetic linalool, limonene and linalyl acetate; the addition of less expensive citrus oil and their terpenes obtained from sweet orange, and the addition of the non-volatile residues of citrus oils such as grapefruit and lime.[7]

Pharmacopoeias and standards

The purity, composition, physico-chemical properties and therapeutic use of bergamot oil are defined in several pharmacopoeia monographs and standards:

- ISO 3520:1998 Oil of Bergamot [*Citrus aurantium* l. subsp. *Bergamia* (Wight et Arnott) Engler]
- *Bergamotto Essenza.* Farmacopea Ufficiale Italiana
- German Commission E
- Martindale: The Complete Drug Reference
- Assessment Report on *Citrus bergamia* Risso et Poiteau, aetheroleum. European Medicines Agency.

History and Traditional Uses

History

Bergamot was cultivated as an ornamental at the end of the seventeenth century. It is believed to have been first cultivated for the fragrance of its fruits towards 1750 near Reggio Calabria. The first documented use of bergamot essential oil in perfumery was in 1693 in *Le Parfumeur Francois,* printed in Lyon. It was used in a perfume called *Essence de Cedre ou Bergamotte.*[3]

Weiss states that bergamot essential oil was one of the main ingredients used in the original eau de cologne made by the Feminis family in the sixteenth century. Bergamot expressed oil was well established in Italy by the mid-eighteenth century.[8]

Traditional medicine

Bergamot oil was popular in the eighteenth century in Italy as a cicatrisant to treat burns or varicose veins, as an analgesic and antimicrobial, and for treating furunculosis, pediculosis and dandruff.[3]

In the second half of the eighteenth century, a few drops of the oil were added to lime tea or coffee as an antimalarial agent. It has long been used as a treatment for scabies. Internally, 2-5 drops were used as a sedative.[3]

It was commonly used in the eighteenth century to improve the smell of medicinal ointments and unguents, and to prepare tooth-powder, hair oils and cosmetic preparations. In medicine, it was used in an alcoholic solution or in preparations for massaging in cases of chronic rheumatism.[3]

B

In 1932, Spinelli provided extensive in vitro and in vivo evidence that bergamot oil could be used as an antiseptic for use in surgery. It was as effective as a 10% iodine tincture to sterilise the skin on which it was applied. Along with asepsis, there was complete absence of local irritation or symptoms attributable to absorption of the essential oil.[3]

In 1940, it was reported to effectively treat soldiers affected with scabies.[3]

Food, perfumery and flavouring

The juice obtained from the endocarp after the essential oil has been extracted is often discarded because of its bitter taste. It is, however, now being used to fortify fruit juice in place of synthetic additives.[5]

Bergamot oil is used in food, provided the bergaptens are removed. Bergamot oil is well known for its use to flavour Earl Grey tea. It is also used in frozen dairy desserts, candy, baked goods, gelatins and puddings. The highest average maximum use level in food flavouring is 0.02%.[9]

Therapeutics

Pharmacology and clinical studies

Many pharmacological studies involving bergamot essential oil have been published. A systemic review of these studies will not be attempted. Rather, I have chosen a selection of studies that support the traditional and clinical uses.

Antifungal activity

Bergamot oil exhibits in vitro inhibitory activity against clinically relevant *Candida* species. The authors concluded that the data from their clinical trial supports the potential role for the topical treatment of candida infections.[5]

Bergamot oil exhibited antifungal activity against 21 fungal species. It was particularly effective against *Aspergillus niger, Fusarium solani, F. sporotrichioides, F. oxysporum, Curvularia lunata, Verticillium dahliae,* and *Myrothecium verrucaria.*[1]

Antimicrobial activity

Several in vitro studies have identified bergamot oil as an effective antimicrobial. Turkish bergamot oil was reported to have antimicrobial activities against *Escherichia coli, Staphylococcus aureus, Bacillus cereus, Listeria monocytogenes, Kluyveromyces fragilis, Rhodotorula rubra* and *Candida albicans*. The results of bergamot essential oil inhibitory activity were reported to be similar to those obtained with synthetic antimicrobials such as nystatin, ketoconazole and clotrimazole. In another study, bergamot essential oil exhibited higher zones of inhibition than other citrus peel oils.[1]

A study found that a vaporised blend of citrus oils (orange and bergamot, 1:1 v/v) was very effective at reducing environmental bacterial contamination. The study found that the citrus vapour reduced vancomycin-resistant *Enterococcus sp.* (VRE) and methicillin-resistant *Staphylococcus aureus* (MRSA) on stainless steel surfaces by as much as 99.5%. The authors suggest that citrus vapour has the potential for application in a clinical environment as a secondary disinfectant to reduce surface contamination by VRE and MRSA.[10]

Anxiolytic activity

A study using 109 patients found that bergamot oil was effective in reducing preoperative anxiety. The authors concluded that aromatherapy may be a useful part of a holistic approach to reducing preoperative anxiety before ambulatory surgery.[11]

Another study measured the endocrinological, physiological and psychological effects of bergamot essential oil by inhalation on 41 healthy females using a randomised crossover study design. The study demonstrated that bergamot essential oil had psychological and physiological benefits in a relatively short time.[12]

Cardiovascular activity

A controlled, randomised study using 52 subjects identified the benefits of aromatherapy on blood pressure and stress responses for patients with essential hypertension. A blend of lavender, ylang ylang and bergamot was used by inhalation once daily for 4 weeks. The results of the study found that inhalation of essential oils was considered an effective nursing intervention that reduced psychological stress responses and serum cortisol levels, as well as the blood pressure of clients with essential hypertension.[13]

Bergamottine (5-geranyloxypsoralen), the non-volatile residue of the bergamot essential oil, was found to have significant antiarrhythmic activity. The results demonstrated that it possessed the characteristics of an antiarrhythmic drug with calcium-antagonist properties (class 4).[14,15]

Another study found the activity of bergamottin was comparable to that of verapamil.[16]

Neuroprotective activity

The effects of bergamot oil on excitotoxic neuronal damage were investigated in vitro. The study was performed in human neuroblastoma cells exposed to N-methyl-D-aspartate (NMDA). The results of the study found that bergamot essential oil reduced neuronal damage caused in vitro by excitotoxic stimuli, and that this neuroprotection was associated with prevention of injury-induced engagement of critical death pathways.[17]

Psychoneuroimmunological activity

A study done back in 1995 found that bergamot oil blended with lemon and orange oils was very effective as an antidepressant. The study involved 20 depressed male inpatients who were all receiving antidepressant medication. They were divided into two groups; one group was given antidepressants alone and the other group was exposed to the citrus fragrance whilst having their medication reduced weekly until their depression remitted (within 4-11 weeks). By the end of 11 weeks, 9 of the 12 patients in the citrus fragrance group had reduced their antidepressant drug intake to zero, whilst the other three had reduced their dosage by 50-75%. On the other hand, all the subjects in the antidepressant alone group still needed their usual doses of antidepressants at remission. The researchers stated that urinary cortisol and dopamine levels were significantly high in both groups before treatment, and both were reduced by the treatment. However, they said that the levels were significantly lower in the citrus fragrance group. They also found that the citrus fragrance caused high values of natural killer cell activity to return to almost normal range. The results suggest that the use of citrus fragrances such as bergamot may improve the homeostatic balance more than treatment with just antidepressants. The authors concluded that bergamot could be of psychoneuroimmunological benefit.[18]

Sedative activity

A blend of lavender and bergamot was used to determine the benefits of essential oils following transdermal absorption. Parameters such as blood pressure, pulse rate, breathing rate and skin temperature were recorded. In addition, subjects had to rate their emotional condition in terms of relaxation, vigour, calmness, attentiveness, mood and alertness in order to assess behavioural response. 40 volunteers participated in the study. Compared to the placebo, the blend of lavender and bergamot caused significant decreases of pulse and systolic and diastolic blood pressure. At an emotional level, the subjects rated themselves as feeling 'more calm' and 'more relaxed' than the subjects in the control group. It was stated that this study provided evidence for the use of bergamot and lavender in medicine for treating depression or anxiety in humans.[19]

The effects of bergamot oil on the release of amino acid neurotransmitters in rat hippocampus have been studied by both in vivo and in vitro tests. The researchers concluded that bergamot oil contains volatile fractions of unidentified monoterpene hydrocarbons that were able to stimulate glutamate release by transporter reversal and by exocytosis, depending on the dose administered.[20]

Actions

Actions commonly cited in aromatherapy

Analgesic, antidepressant, antimicrobial, antiseptic, antiviral, carminative, cicatrisant, deodorant, digestive, febrifuge, sedative, stomachic, tonic, vermifuge, vulnerary[21,22]

Actions supported by clinical studies

Antimicrobial, antiseptic, anxiolytic

Comment

Review of traditional and clinical data suggests the use of bergamot oil for improving mood and reducing symptoms of stress-induced disorders such as anxiety and depression.

Holmes states that bergamot oil promotes balance and that it can be both stimulating and sedating. This is best explained by the sweet citrus that has a balancing and relaxing effect, while the fresh, pungent citrus aroma has a stimulating, uplifting effect. He explains that bergamot is one of the few essential oils that is an autonomic nervous system regulator, managing to reduce the swing between sympathetic and parasympathetic systems.

Holmes says that the chemical profile of bergamot oil gives us a very good understanding of bergamot's balancing qualities. Not only is the oil dominated by esters, which are inherently balancing, but it also includes even more relaxing monoterpene alcohols and the more stimulating monoterpene hydrocarbons.[2]

Aromatherapy Uses

Clinical aromatherapy

Antiviral

Bergamot oil inhibits herpes simplex I virus that causes cold sores. It is particularly effective in combination with tea tree and lavender for the treatment of cold sores, chicken pox and shingles.[21]

Digestive system

Bergamot oil is particularly beneficial for nervous indigestion and loss of appetite due to emotional stress.[21]

Integumentary system

Bergamot oil's antiseptic and vulnerary actions makes it useful for treating wounds, burns, herpes and varicose ulcers. Bergamot oil is also recommended for treating eczema and psoriasis.[2]

B

Psychological

Holmes says that bergamot oil promotes emotional stability. He recommends bergamot oil for reducing irritability, moodiness, frustration, mood swings and emotional instability. Bergamot oil can also be used to alleviate negative thinking, repetitive thinking, pessimism and mild depression.[2]

Mojay compares bergamot to lavender:

> *... bergamot oil encourages the release of pent up feelings – feelings that can lead not only to depression but to insomnia, anxiety and sudden mood swings. It helps, in addition, to redirect nervous energy away from unproductive or addictive behaviour, helping us to rediscover spontaneity and optimism. Bergamot oil helps us to relax and 'let go'.*[23]

Holmes suggests that bergamot oil can promote optimism and set the stage for true emotional transformation. He states that bergamot oil is 'exceptionally harmonising'. He describes it as being able to close the gap between mind, body and emotions. Bergamot is ideal for treating stress-related conditions with symptoms that fluctuate between hyper- and hypo-functioning.[2]

Skin care

Bergamot oil is typically recommended for oily congested skin.[2,21] However, bergamot oil is phototoxic, so please exercise caution when using it in skincare.

Urinary system

Bergamot oil is recommended for the treatment of cystitis and urinary tract infections. It can be used in the very early stages of cystitis to prevent the infection spreading. This can be done by adding no more than three drops of bergamot oil to a bath and using it as a local wash.[24]

Energetics, psyche and subtle uses

Energetics

Bergamot oil is *cooling* and refreshing. The fresh, fruity, floral aroma contributes to the oil's gently relaxing, yet distinctly uplifting qualities. The energetic qualities of bergamot relate directly to its ability to harmonise *Liver Qi*. This helps to maintain the free and even flow of energy through the body.[23]

Whenever the *Liver Qi* is constrained, we feel irritable, anxious and frustrated, and experience mood swings.[2]

Holmes explains that bergamot oil regulates the *Qi* and harmonises the *Shen*. Whenever the *Liver Qi* is constrained and the *Shen* experiences disharmony, we may experience confusion, irritability, mood swings and frustration. On the other hand, when the *Heart Qi* is constrained and the *Shen* experiences disharmony, we may experience restlessness, insomnia, palpitations, irritability, anxiety and depression.[2]

Mojay describes the antidepressant properties of bergamot according to the principles of TCM:

> *Depression due to stagnant Qi-energy is therefore the result of accumulated stress or repressed anger — the key emotion of the Liver and Wood Element. Anger and frustration turned inwards oppress the Ethereal Soul (Hun) and block the free-flow of Qi, depressing mind and spirit.* [23]

Bergamot oil has a strong affinity with the Wood and Fire Elements. In Ayurveda, bergamot oil helps to calm excessive *Pitta* and balance and nourish *Vata*.

Personality

Fischer-Rizzi perfectly describes the character of bergamot:[25]

> *Thanks to bergamot's sunny and warming disposition, the oil helps people regain self-confidence, and it uplifts and refreshes the spirit. The gentle fragrance, like a bouquet of flowers, evokes joy and warms the heart.*

The personality of bergamot is young, fresh, caring and considerate. She says that bergamot types may not necessarily be young in age, but they will always be young at heart and have a joyful approach to life. They do not allow the negative things in life to drag them down. They generally are very confident and have a strong positive attitude. They often find themselves in any role in which they can display their charismatic personality, or in the caring professions that require large amounts of energy, skill and enthusiasm. The bergamot personality is very good with children as their energy levels are very compatible.[26]

When bergamot personality types become stressed, they may suffer from depression; however, they rarely allow anyone to really see just how down they can be or how sad they are feeling. Worwood says that nobody may suspect that behind the mask, a bergamot may be inwardly crying with emotional pain, only the empathy that they display towards others who are feeling distressed may give them away.[26]

According to Myers-Briggs personality types, the bergamot personality is likely to be an ENFP. ENFPs are outgoing, lively and spontaneous. They are very enthusiastic and their joy for life can be contagious. They have a rich imagination and active mind. Their thoughts are always wandering and their mood constantly changing. They can be inspiring and charismatic leaders. They are always involved or in love with someone or something new. They know how to establish instant rapport and make people feel comfortable. They love emotional intensity and enjoy expressing their feelings. They can be charming and flirtatious. They relate with warmth to many people and can appear overly enthusiastic, positive and optimistic.

Subtle

Worwood beautifully describes the subtle qualities of bergamot:

> *It brings eternal youth and happiness, even to those who have put aside their problems, ignoring them until they have become so overwhelming that the person feels that they cannot ask for help … we may cry inside, our hearts aching, but bergamot will lighten the heart, and dispel self-criticism and blame. To any soul, bergamot brings freshness and illumination, lifting us from stagnation, bringing an awareness that the light will rescue us and take us ever forward to the realms of peace and joy.*[27]

If your spirit is flat, sad or depressed, Zeck says that bergamot will help heal and cheer our soul, encouraging us to explore our deeper inner most feeling.[28]

Holmes beautifully summarises the subtle qualities of bergamot:

> *Ultimately, then, we can say that bergamot's highest gift is to assist in staying with our own experience and to be ever open, curious and in wonder of each moment of life as it arises, each now as it unfolds – without the burden of previous feelings and concepts. As a light-filled refresher of the mind and soul, bergamot simply suggests that to experience life in a balanced way, we need to start by accepting the experience of each moment for what it is, without prior expectations.*[2]

The green colour of bergamot has an affinity with the heart chakra. It is useful when the heart chakra is affected by grief.[29]

B

Dosage and Administration

Blending

Aromatherapy

Bergamot oil has a calming and relaxing influence and it can also be an uplifting and energising oil. The pleasant, refreshing citrusy and floral aroma of bergamot gives it a beautiful uplifting and yet relaxing quality. Lavabre states that bergamot oil is a blend enhancer.[22]

To alleviate fatigue, lethargy and mental exhaustion, consider blending bergamot oil with essential oils such as basil, geranium, ginger, lemon, lemongrass, cold-pressed lime, peppermint or rosemary.

To alleviate anxiety, nervous tension and stress, consider blending bergamot oil with essential oils such as coriander seed, frankincense, lavender, geranium, mandarin, neroli, sweet orange, sandalwood or ylang ylang.

To create an antiseptic blend for use in a vaporiser, consider blending bergamot oil with essential oils such as bay laurel, cajeput, lemon, 1,8-cineole-rich eucalypts, lemon-scented eucalyptus, fragonia, manuka, myrtle, pine or tea tree.

Fischer-Rizzi recommends using bergamot oil for balancing those essential oils with good psychological effect but with an odour that some people may consider unpleasant or too strong such as cypress, cistus, everlasting, frankincense or yarrow.[25]

Perfumery

Bergamot oil is used extensively in perfumery for its sweet freshness, especially in citrus-based colognes, chypres, fougères and modern fantasy style perfumes. Unlike other citrus oils, Arctander states that bergamot essential oil has a certain fixative effect when used in fairly high concentrations.[4]

Mode of administration

Bath

Full body bath, foot bath, sitz bath, douche

Topical

Massage, ointment, skin care

Inhalation

Direct inhalation, diffuser, oil vaporiser

Safety Profile

General safety

Bergamot essential oil may be photosensitising. This means that if it is applied to the skin at certain concentrations, burning can occur if the skin is exposed to ultraviolet light. Bergamot oil should not be used at more than 0.4% dilution on the skin, or the person should not go outside during the daylight for 12-18 hours after topical application. This warning applies only to leave-on products such as perfumes, oils, lotions and balms and that there is no risk from wash-off products such as soaps, shampoos and body washes.[6]

Organophosphorus and organochlorine pesticides, phosphorated plasticisers, chloroparaffins and phthalate ester contamination have been found in bergamot essential oils produced in Calabria in the crop years 1999 and 2000.[30] While this report is from 2004, it does highlight the importance of using only certified organic essential oils.

Contraindications

No contraindications known.

Regulatory guidelines

Bergamot oil has GRAS status. IFRA recommends a maximum limit of 0.4% bergamot essential oil in topical products for application to skin exposed to sun.[6]

References

1. Avila-Sosa R et al. *Bergamot (Citrus bergamia) oils.* In Preedy VR. ed. *Essential oils in food preservation, flavor and safety.* Academic Press, London, 2016: 247-252.
2. Holmes P. *Aromatica: a clinical guide to essential oil therapeutics — Vol. I.* Singing Dragon, London, 2016.
3. Imbesi A, De Pasquale A. *Citrus species and their essential oils in traditional medicine.* In Dugo G, Di Giacomo A. eds. *Citrus – the genus Citrus.* Taylor & Francis Group, London, 2002: 577-601. (Medical and Aromatic Plants – Industrial Profiles; 26)
4. Arctander S. *Perfume and flavor materials of natural origin.* Allured Publishing, Carol Stream, 1994.
5. Committee on Herbal Medicines Products. *Assessment report on Citrus bergamia Risso et Poiteau, antheroleum.* European Medicines Agency, London, 2011. Doc ref. EMA/HMPC/56155/2011
6. Tisserand R, Young R. *Essential oil safety.* 2nd edn. Churchill Livingstone, Edinburgh, 2014.
7. Bonaccorsi I, Schipilliti L, Dugo G. *Adulteration of bergamot oil.* Retrieved Mar 12, 2017 from https://www.researchgate.net/publication/258119288_Adulteration_of_Bergamot_Oil
8. Weiss EA. *Essential oil crops.* CAB International, Wallingford, 1997.
9. Khan I, Abourashed E. *Leung's encyclopedia of common natural ingredients used in food, drugs and cosmetics.* 3rd edn. John Wiley & Sons, New Jersey, 2010.
10. Laird K et al. *Reduction of surface contamination and biofilms of Enterococcus sp. and Staphylococcus aureus using a citrus-based vapour.* Journal of Hospital Infection, 2012; 80(1): 61-66. Cited in Quintessential Aromatics database, 2013.
11. Ni CH et al. *The anxiolytic effect of aromatherapy on patients awaiting ambulatory surgery: a randomized controlled trial.* Evidence-Based Complementary and Alternative Medicine, 2013. Cited in Quintessential Aromatics database, 2013.
12. Watanabe E et al. *Effects of bergamot (Citrus bergamia (Risso) Wright & Arn.) essential oil aromatherapy on mood states, parasympathetic nervous system activity, and salivary cortisol levels in 41 healthy females.* Forschende Komplementarmedizin, 2015; 22(1): 43-49. Cited in Quintessential Aromatics database, 2013.
13. Hwang JH. *The effects of the inhalation method using essential oils on blood pressure and stress responses of clients with essential hypertension.* Journal of Korean Academy of Nursing, 2006; 36(7): 1123-1134. Cited in Quintessential Aromatics database, 2013.
14. Occhiuto F et al. *Investigations to characterise the antiarrhythmic action of bergamottine, a furocoumarin isolated from bergamot oil.* Phytotherapy Research, 1997; 11(6): 450-453. Cited in Quintessential Aromatics database, 2013.
15. Occhiuto F et al. *Cardiovascular properties of the non-volatile total residue from the essential oil of Citrus bergamia.* International Journal of Pharmacology, 1996; 34(2): 128-133. Cited in Quintessential Aromatics database, 2013.
16. Occhiuto F et al. *Antianginal and antiarrhythmic effects of bergamottine, a furocoumarin isolated from bergamot oil.* Phytotherapy Research, 1996; 10(6): 491-496. Cited in Quintessential Aromatics database, 2013.
17. Corasaniti MT et al. *Cell signaling pathways in the mechanisms of neuroprotection afforded by bergamot essential oil against NMDA-induced cell death in vitro.* British Journal of Pharmacology, 2007; 151(4): 518-529. Cited in Quintessential Aromatics database, 2013.
18. Komori T et al. *Effect of citrus fragrance on immune function and depressive states.* Neuroimmunomodulation, 1995; 2(3): 170-180. Cited in Quintessential Aromatics database, 2013.
19. Hongratanaworakit T. *Aroma-therapeutic effects of massage blended essential oils on humans.* Natural Product Communications, 2011; 6(8): 1199-1204. Cited in Quintessential Aromatics database, 2013.
20. Morrone LA et al. *The essential oil of bergamot enhances the levels of amino acid neurotransmitters in the hippocampus of rats: implication of monoterpene hydrocarbons.* Pharmacological Research, 2007; 55(4): 255-262. Cited in Quintessential Aromatics database, 2013.
21. Lawless J. *The encyclopaedia of essential oils.* Element Books, Shaftesbury, 1992.
22. Lavabre M. *Aromatherapy workbook.* Healing Arts Press, Rochester, 1997.
23. Mojay G. *Aromatherapy for healing the spirit.* Healing Arts Press, Rochester, 1999.
24. Davis P. *Aromatherapy: an A-Z.* 2nd edn, C.W Daniel Company, Saffron Walden, 1999.
25. Fischer-Rizzi S. *Complete aromatherapy handbook.* Sterling Publishing, New York, 1990.
26. Worwood VA. *The fragrant mind.* Transworld Publishers, London, 1995.

27. Worwood VA. *The fragrant heavens.* Transworld Publishers, London, 1999.
28. Zeck R. *The blossoming heart – aromatherapy for healing and transformation.* Aroma Tours, East Ivanhoe, 2003.
29. Davis P. *Subtle aromatherapy.* C.W. Daniel Company, Saffron Walden, 1991.
30. Di Bella G et al. *Pesticide and plasticizer residues in bergamot essential oils from Calabria (Italy).* Chemosphere, 2004; 56(8): 777-782. Cited in Quintessential Aromatics database, 2013.

Birch, sweet

Identification

Botanical name

Betula lenta L.

Synonyms

Black birch, cherry birch, mahogany birch, southern birch[1]

Family

Betulaceae

Botany and origins

The tree grows up to about 25 m high, with dark reddish-brown bark. The tree grows wild throughout the southeastern United States up to southern Canada.[1] There are numerous species of birch; it should not be confused with the European white birch (*Betula alba*), which is used to produce birch tar oil that is used in chronic skin diseases.[2]

B

Method of extraction

Sweet birch essential oil is steam-distilled from the bark of *B. lenta* that has been macerated in warm water. During maceration, the enzyme system present hydrolyses gaultherin, which in turn releases the methyl salicylate.[2]

Characteristics

The oil of sweet birch is colourless or pale yellow, occasionally with a reddish tint. The oil has a distinct methyl salicylate odour typical of that found in wintergreen.[1]

Chemical composition

Sweet birch oil is almost entirely composed of methyl salicylate – at least 98%. It is almost identical in composition to wintergreen oil.[2]

Adulteration

Arctander states that sweet birch oil has completely lost its importance, and what the trade offers today under the label of sweet birch essential oil may very well be methyl salicylate from a chemical factory.[1]

Pharmacopoeias and standards

At the time of writing, the purity, composition, physico-chemical properties and therapeutic use of sweet birch essential oil are not defined in any pharmacopoeia monograph or standard.

It is currently official in Food Chemicals Codex monographed under methyl salicylate together with wintergreen oil.[2] This means your chances of getting authentic birch oil are very remote.

History and Traditional Uses

Traditional medicine

Native Americans used the bark in a herbal infusion for stomach ache, diarrhoea, pneumonia and pulmonary problems.[2]

Herbal

Sweet birch oil is used in antiarthritic and antineuralgic ointments and salves.[2]

Food, perfumery and flavouring

It has limited use in perfumery, but is extensively used as a flavouring agent in root beer, chewing gum and toothpaste.[1,2]

Therapeutics

Pharmacology and clinical studies

Analgesic activity

The topical application of applied rubefacients containing salicylates may be efficacious in the treatment of acute pain. However, trials of musculoskeletal and arthritic pain suggest moderate or poor efficacy. A study concluded that efficacy estimates for rubefacients are unreliable owing to a lack of good clinical trials.[3]

Actions

Actions commonly cited in aromatherapy

Analgesic, anti-inflammatory, antirheumatic, antiseptic, astringent, depurative, diuretic, rubefacient, tonic[4]

Actions supported by clinical studies

Analgesic, anti-inflammatory, antirheumatic

Comment

I understand the concerns of many aromatherapists who state that sweet birch oil should not be used in aromatherapy; however, I also agree with Lavabre who states that sweet birch oil is excellent for treating arthritic and rheumatic pain.[5]

Aromatherapy Uses

Clinical aromatherapy

Detoxification

Lavabre recommends using sweet birch oil for the treatment of accumulated toxins and fluid retention.[5]

Musculoskeletal system

Considering that methyl salicylate is extensively used in many commercial analgesic and antiarthritic ointments and balms, I believe that birch oil may be useful in aromatherapy for topical applications for the relief of short-term acute musculoskeletal pain.

Energetics, psyche and subtle uses

Subtle

Keim Loughran & Bull recommend using sweet birch oil for releasing fear and promoting courage.[7]

Dosage and Administration

Blending

Aromatherapy

For acute pain management of musculoskeletal conditions, consider blending sweet birch oil with essential oils such as black pepper, cajeput, ginger, kunzea, spike lavender, pine or peppermint.

Mode of administration

Bath

I would not recommend using sweet birch oil in a bath

Topical

Massage, ointment

Inhalation

Direct inhalation, diffuser, oil vaporiser

Safety Profile

General safety

Many aromatherapists state that sweet birch oil should not be used in aromatherapy.

Contraindications

Tisserand & Young recommend that the dermal maximum of 2.4% be applied for methyl salicylate, as long as all the contraindications listed below are observed.[6]

Methyl salicylate applied topically or orally can inhibit platelet aggregation and potentiate the action of warfarin. Therefore, sweet birch essential oil is contraindicated with anticoagulant medication, after major surgery, or for people with haemophilia and other bleeding disorders. It should not be used during pregnancy and breastfeeding. It should not be used by or given to children. It should not be given to people with salicylate sensitivity.[6]

Toxicity

Methyl salicylate is the major constituent of sweet birch oil; hence it is considered to have the same level of toxicity as wintergreen oil. There is no evidence of mutagenicity or carcinogenicity linked to methyl salicylate.[6]

Tisserand & Young cite a study that shows when volunteers applied 5 g of an ointment containing 12.5% methyl salicylate twice daily, the salicylate recovered from the urine was 15.5% on day one of application and 22% on days, two, three and four.[6]

The signs of poisoning are as follows:

> *Numerous cases of methyl salicylate poisoning have been reported in humans with a 50-60% mortality rate. Signs of poisoning include nausea, vomiting, acidosis, convulsions, tachycardia, rapid and labored breathing. There is often enlargement of the heart, congestion of the lungs, liver and kidneys and generalized lymphoid hyperplasia.*[6]

Death results from cardiovascular collapse and respiratory failure after a period of unconsciousness. Most of these fatalities reported involved high doses, but doses as small as 4 mL of methyl salicylate have been fatal in infants.[6]

The lowest lethal dose was reported in women at 355 mg/kg, in men at 101 mg/kg and in children at 228 mg/kg.[8]

Regulatory guidelines

Methyl salicylate-rich oils such as sweet birch and wintergreen have GRAS status.

References

1. Arctander S. *Perfume and flavour materials of natural origin*. Allured Publishing, Carol Stream, 1994.
2. Khan I, Abourashed E. *Leung's encyclopedia of common natural ingredients used in food, drugs and cosmetics*. 3rd edn. John Wiley & Sons, New Jersey, 2010.
3. Mason L et al. *Systemic review of efficacy of topical rubefacients containing salicylates for the treatment of acute and chronic pain*. BMJ, 2004; 328. doi: 10.1136/bmj.38040.607141.EE
4. Lawless J. *The encyclopaedia of essential oils*. Element Books, Shaftesbury, 1992.
5. Lavabre M. *Aromatherapy workbook*. Healing Arts Press, Rochester, 1997.
6. Tisserand R, Young R. *Essential oil safety*. 2nd edn. Churchill Livingstone, Edinburgh, 2014.
7. Keim Loughran J, Bull R. *Aromatherapy and subtle energy techniques*. Frog, Berkeley, 2000.
8. Alsaad A et al. *Toxicology and teratology of the active ingredients of professional therapy MuscleCare products during pregnancy and lactation: a systemic review*. BMC Complementary & Alternative Medicine, 2015; 15: 40. doi: 10.1186/s12906-015-0585-8

Black pepper

B

Identification

Botanical name

Piper nigrum L.

Synonyms

Pepper

Family

Piperaceae

Botany and origins

Piper nigrum is a native of southern India and Indonesia. It has been cultivated in the same areas for over 2,000 years. The main pepper producers are India, Indonesia and Malaysia. Pepper oil is produced only from black pepper berries.[1]

Only a very small percentage of the black pepper seeds produced is distilled to produce an essential oil.[2]

It is a perennial vine climbing to about 5 m. The inflorescence is a spike of about 20-30 sessile flowers, which develop into sessile fruits. The fruits on a spike do not mature together, and when a few fruits are ripe the spike is harvested. Ripe fruits are removed and allowed to ferment, or are soaked in running water to remove the pericarps. The seeds are dried and powdered to give us white pepper of commerce.[1]

Black peppers are more pungent and are produced from the unripe fruits on the harvested spikes. These are sun dried, usually after soaking in hot water. The pungency is due to the presence of various resins and a yellow crystalline alkaloid called piperine.[1]

Method of extraction

The essential oil of black pepper is produced by the steam distillation of the dried, crushed but not quite ripe fruits of the pepper vine, *Piper nigrum*.

Characteristics

The essential oil of black pepper is a clear to pale greenish coloured mobile liquid. It has a fresh, dry-woody, warm-spicy odour reminiscent of dried black pepper.[2]

It was believed that black pepper oil which is green was of a higher quality; however, Arctander and Weiss say this is not so.[1,2] They claim that the green colour is simply due to the presence of azulenes. If this is so, I would suggest that the green-coloured black pepper oil would be of higher quality for use in aromatherapy.

Chemical composition

Black pepper essential oil is rich in monoterpene hydrocarbons and sesquiterpene hydrocarbons. Monoterpene hydrocarbons are known for their analgesic, antiseptic and tonic properties, while sesquiterpene hydrocarbons may account for black pepper's antiviral properties.

The composition of black pepper oil can vary considerably according to origin and method of preparation. The greatest variation is within the monoterpene hydrocarbon group as follows:

limonene (0-40%), β-pinene (5-35%), α-phellandrene (1-27%), β-phellandrene (0-19%), sabinene (0-20%), δ-3-carene (trace to 15%), myrcene (trace to 10%).[1]

The chemical composition of black pepper oil from Sarawak was reported as follows:

α-pinene (5.8%), camphene (0.1%), β-pinene (10.4%), δ-3-carene (20.2%), limonene (17.1%), γ-terpinene (0.2%), *p*-cymene (0.8%), terpinolene (1.0%), δ-elemene (2.5%), α-copaene (2.3%), β-elemene (0.4%), β-caryophyllene (27.8%), α-humulene (1.4%), δ-cadinene (0.8%), caryophyllene oxide (0.6%).[1]

Adulteration

Black pepper essential oil is often adulterated with turpentine oil, α-phellandrene from less expensive sources, limonene from orange terpenes and clove leaf terpenes.[3]

Pharmacopoeias and standards

The purity, composition and physico-chemical properties of black pepper essential oil are defined in ISO 3061:2008 Oil of Black Pepper (*Piper nigrum* L.)

History and Traditional Uses

History

Pepper has been esteemed as a spice in India since time immemorial and dispersed in trade throughout the world. Pepper was so important that the search for the source of the spice and the control of the trade was a significant factor influencing world exploration and history.[1]

The word originates from the Latin *piper* which in turn comes from the Sanskrit *pippali*. Black pepper is one of the oldest known spices, being described by Theophrastus in the fourth century BC. By the Middle Ages, pepper was of great importance in Europe to season and preserve meats, and to overcome odours of rancid food. Peppercorns were very expensive and accepted as currency.[1]

Pepper arrived in Java with the early Hindu colonists, and its widespread cultivation dates from at least AD 500. Marco Polo describes pepper cultivation in Java when he visits in 1280, of Chinese sailing vessels loading up to 6,000 baskets, and of the abundance of pepper on the Malabar Coast of India. The wealth of Venice and Genoa in the thirteenth century was mostly due to the spice trade. Portugal's desire to obtain part of this lucrative business was responsible for Vasco da Gama circumnavigating Africa and arriving at Calicut on the Malabar Coast of west India on 20 May 1498. This enabled Portugal to secure a monopoly of the spice trade, which it maintained for a century.[1]

Early in the seventeenth century, the Dutch acquired pepper-producing areas in Java and Sumatra. The demise of the Dutch dominance coincided with the entry of the USA into the Far Eastern spice trade. In 1797, Captain Jonathan Carnes of Salem, Massachusetts, sailed a schooner *Rajah* into New York harbour carrying $100,000 worth of black pepper from Sumatra. For the next 50 years, ships from Salem and Boston played an important role in expanding the world pepper trade. Early in the nineteenth century, the British introduced pepper plants to Malaysia.[1]

Traditional medicine

Pepper is used in TCM and Ayurvedic medicine for its carminative, warming and eliminative properties.[4]

According to the fifth century Syriac *Book of Medicine*, black pepper was used for the treatment of diarrhoea and fever. It was also recommended to enhance the effect of other herbs. It was used with long pepper to treat gangrene, heart disease, indigestion, insect bites, diseases of the lungs and liver, and toothaches. It is mentioned in an Ayurveda materia medica from 600-300 BC. It was combined with long pepper (*Piper longum*) and Ginger (*Zingiber officinalis*) and called *trikatu*, meaning three acrids. It was used to balance psychophysical components of the body in order to prevent disease.[5]

The essential oils from various spices including black pepper were developed in the middle ages by the Arabs, who were the first to recognise their therapeutic potential. Black pepper oil was used for the preservation of food, and as an antiseptic and fragrance. It was also used as an analgesic, sedative, anti-inflammatory, spasmolytic and local anaesthetic.[5]

Herbal

Black peppercorns are used as a diaphoretic, carminative and diuretic. It stimulates the taste buds and produces a reflex increase in gastric secretion. It has allegedly been used in treatment of cancer.[4]

It is used in herbal medicine as a carminative to alleviate flatulence. It also promotes urine and stimulates the kidneys.[6]

Food, perfumery and flavouring

Both black and white pepper seeds are used extensively as domestic spices. They are widely used as flavour ingredients in many food products.[4]

The oil of black pepper is primarily used in flavour work as a modifier for other spice flavours where the pungency is not needed. Seasonings, spice sauces and dressings, meat and other canned food are often flavoured with black pepper and other spice oils.[2]

Therapeutics

Pharmacology and clinical studies

A few pharmacological studies involving black pepper essential oil have been published. A systemic review of these studies will not be

B

attempted. Rather, I have chosen a selection of studies that support the traditional and clinical uses.

Aged care

A one-month randomised, controlled study evaluated the effects of olfactory stimulation of black pepper essential oil on the risk factors associated with pneumonia in elderly patients in an aged care facility. Latency of the swallowing reflex, the number of swallowing movements, serum substance P, and blood flow to the regional cerebral reflex were measured.

The study found that black pepper improved the latency of the swallowing reflex with an increase of serum substance P. The number of swallowing movements also increased. The researchers also confirmed that inhalation of black pepper increased blood flow in the right orbitofrontal cortex, resulting in improvement of the reflexive swallowing movement. They suggested that this might be beneficial in older post-stroke patients with dysphagia, regardless of their level of consciousness or physical and mental state.[7]

Another study investigated the effects of olfactory stimuli (using black pepper and lavender oils) on postural control in older adults (78 +/- 6 years) who had no evident neurological ailments. The results of the study suggested that olfactory stimulation may improve posture stability in older adults by decreasing the velocities of postural adjustments during normal sway.[8]

Black pepper oil was investigated for its potential biological role in the prevention of Alzheimer's disease.

The results of an in vitro study indicated that black pepper exhibited strong AChE inhibitory activity and strong COX-2 inhibition. These findings suggest that black pepper oil may be beneficial in lowering the risk of Alzheimer's disease via AChE inhibition and anti-inflammatory activity via COX-2 inhibition.[9]

Antibacterial activity

The essential oil of *P. nigrum* was found to have antibacterial properties.[10]

Anti-inflammatory activity

Oral administration of black pepper oil significantly increased superoxide dismutase, glutathione, glutathione-S-transferase and glutathione reductase enzyme levels in the blood of mice, and glutathione enzymes in the liver. The study found that black pepper oil significantly reduced acute inflammation and possessed antinociceptive properties.[11]

Antivirulence activity

An in vitro study confirmed that black pepper oil has potential use as an antivirulent against persistent *Staphylococcus aureus* infections. *S. aureus* is a major human pathogen that produces diverse virulence factors such as alpha-toxin. Biofilm formation is another drug resistance mechanism of *S. aureus*. This study also confirmed that black pepper oil inhibited biofilm formation.[12]

Skin elasticity

As we get older, the elasticity of our skin is significantly reduced by elastase activity. A study examined the role of essential oils for their anti-elastase activity. The activity of two elastase enzymes – porcine pancreatic enzyme and human neutrophil elastase (HNE) – was monitored in vitro in the presence of 12 essential oils. Black pepper was one of the oils found to be an effective inhibitor of the elastase enzymes. The authors suggested that because HNE is activated by UVA radiation, essential oils may play a role in the prevention of photoaging. It was suggested that massage with essential oils can be expected to help prevent cutaneous wrinkling and aging.[13]

Spasmogenic activity

Black pepper oil was spasmogenic on isolated jejunum at concentrations exceeding 70 ug/ml.[14]

Withdrawal symptoms

A study investigated the effects of inhaling the vapour of black pepper essential oil on 48 cigarette smokers. The results reported craving for cigarettes was significantly reduced using black pepper relative to two other control conditions. The researchers also found that the symptoms of anxiety were also alleviated. The intensity of sensations in the chest was also significantly higher for black pepper. It was stated that the respiratory tract sensations are important in alleviating smoking withdrawal symptoms.[15]

Another study involving the inhalation of one drop of black pepper oil on a tissue for two minutes when a participant was craving nicotine found that the oil was effective in reducing the craving for nicotine and allowed a longer delay before next use of tobacco. The researchers stated that aromatherapy may be useful for nicotine withdrawal. No pharmacological mechanism was provided.[16]

Actions

Actions commonly cited in aromatherapy

Analgesic, antiseptic, antispasmodic, carminative, diaphoretic, diuretic, febrifuge, laxative, rubefacient, stomachic, tonic[17,18,19]

Actions supported by clinical studies

Analgesic, antioxidant, rubefacient

Comment

Black pepper essential oil is not listed in any pharmacopoeia. There is also very little data for any of its pharmacological activity. I believe that some of the properties attributed to black pepper essential oil are for the black peppercorns.

However, the chemical profile of black pepper oil suggests that the oil may be effective as an analgesic when used topically. I would like to see further studies conducted to assess the potential role of black pepper oil in aged care.

Aromatherapy Uses

Clinical aromatherapy

Circulatory system

Black pepper oil is recommended for the treatment of anaemia, and as a stimulant of the spleen, which is involved in the production of new blood cells and for the treatment of bruises.[17] It is also recommended for the treatment of chilblains.[19]

Digestive system

Black pepper's stomachic, antispasmodic and carminative properties make it an excellent choice for treating disorders of the digestive system.[17] It is recommended for atonic dyspepsia, constipation, flatulence and loss of appetite.[5]

Musculoskeletal system

Black pepper oil is recommended in a massage blend for the relief of rheumatism and arthritis, muscular aches and pains, tired and aching limbs, and muscular stiffness. It can be used before training or a performance to prevent pain and stiffness and possibly improve performance.[17]

Skin care

Black pepper essential oil is generally not used in skin care.

Energetics, psyche and subtle uses

Energetics

The *warming* qualities of black pepper indicate that it is the ideal essential oil to use to dispel any *cold* pathology. In TCM, *cold* is associated with poor digestive function, the onset of an infection with headaches, chills, fatigue, fluid congestion, and general aches and pains.[18]

According to the principles of the Five Elements, black pepper oil has a strong affinity with the Earth and Water Elements. It helps to eliminate damp, which weakens the Earth Element and eliminates excess cold, which weakens the Water Element. It tonifies the *Yang Qi* and warms the *Kidneys*. Whenever we experience *Kidney Yang deficiency*, we experience low sex drive, and suffer from lower back pain, fatigue and apathy.

Excess damp leads to *Stomach-Spleen damp-cold* condition, which is associated with chronic diarrhoea, abdominal pain and cold limbs. *Excess damp* also leads to *Lung cold-damp* condition, which is associated with cough and copious amounts of mucus and phlegm.

Black pepper will strengthen the *Zhi*, the spirit of the *Kidneys*, which is our willpower. The *Zhi* is the willpower we draw upon to survive ordeals, overcome obstacles and persevere against hardships.

Personality

The personality of black pepper is associated with that of a stern older person. Black pepper personalities are often extremely dictatorial, self-righteous and tend to take responsibility for everyone in their family circle. While black pepper is a warming oil, a black pepper personality is not easily able to express feelings of love.[20]

Worwood explains that black pepper personalities can have a total lack of empathy for other people, and can have a complete lack of lateral thinking as they are usually only interested in themselves and their families.[20]

They prefer jobs that give them power and money. They are likely to excel at being lawyers, judges, solicitors, bankers, accountants, financial advisers, or a life in the military services. They will not be happy unless they are in charge.[20]

According to Myers-Briggs personality types, the black pepper personality is likely to be an ISTJ. ISTJs are very stable, responsible and dependable. They are very private. They like to be punctual and precise, and are very orderly. They have good concentration and are difficult to distract. They find it hard to relax as they think that things that help relax are non-productive. They enjoy being in nature. They can be overly detail-oriented, are devoted hard workers, and are very thorough and accurate in everything they do. They like to have strict rules and procedures and tend to be inflexible. They are modest and unassuming and make loyal friends. They may have difficulties expressing feelings of warmth and tenderness to loved ones. They can make quick critical judgement of others.

Subtle

Black pepper oil will help us 'get a move on' at times when our lives feel 'stuck'.[21]

Black pepper is the scent of strength and fortitude. It gives us the courage to move forward and to venture into places unknown. [22] It also dissolves energy blockages caused by anger and frustration.[23]

Dosage and Administration

Blending

Aromatherapy

For muscular aches and pains, consider blending black pepper oil with essential oils such as cajeput, fragonia, kunzea, lemongrass, spike lavender, sweet marjoram, nutmeg, pine or rosemary.

For mental fatigue, consider blending black pepper oil with essential oils such as basil, clove bud, cardamom, lemon, ginger, lemongrass, cold-pressed lime, lemon myrtle or peppermint.

For physical and emotional strength and confidence, consider blending black pepper oil with essential oils such as basil, cardamom, clove bud, cinnamon bark, sweet fennel, ginger, lemon, cold-pressed lime, peppermint or rosemary oil.

Perfumery

In perfumery, black pepper provides interesting effects with eugenol, which is found in clove oil. Arctander suggests that it blends well in rose-based perfumes and when creating an oriental style fragrance.[2]

B

Mode of administration

Bath

Full body bath, foot bath

Topical

Compress, massage, ointment

Inhalation

Direct inhalation, diffuser, oil vaporiser

Safety Profile

General safety

Black pepper oil is non-irritating and non-sensitising. There are no contraindications. It has been said that excessive use can overstimulate the kidneys.[5,17] However, I could not find any clinical evidence to confirm this.

Because of the combined monoterpene hydrocarbon content (limonene, α-pinene and δ-3-carene), it is prone to oxidisation. Tisserand & Young advise us that old or oxidised black pepper oil should be avoided as it may be a skin sensitiser.[24]

Contraindications

No contraindications known.

Regulatory guidelines

Black pepper oil has GRAS status. RIFM has set the safety limit for topical use at 4%.[6]

References

1. Weiss EA. *Essential oil crops.* CAB International, Wallingford, 1997.
2. Arctander S. *Perfume and flavor materials of natural origin.* Allured Publishing, Carol Stream, 1994.
3. Schmidt E, Wanner J. *Adulteration of essential oils.* In Baser KHC, Buchbauer G. eds. *Handbook of essential oils – science, technology and applications.* 2nd edn. CRC Press, Boca Raton, 2016: 707-745.
4. Khan I, Abourashed E. *Leung's encyclopedia of common natural ingredients used in food, drugs and cosmetics.* 3rd edn. John Wiley & Sons, New Jersey, 2010.
5. Abdulazeez M et al. In Preedy VR. ed. *Essential oils in food preservation, flavor and safety.* Academic Press, London, 2016: 277-285.
6. Lis-Balchin M. *Aromatherapy science – a guide for healthcare professionals.* Pharmaceutical Press, London, 2006.
7. Ebihara T et al. *A randomised trial of olfactory stimulation using black pepper oil in older people with swallowing dysfunction.* Journal of American Geriatric Society, 2006; 54(9): 1401-1406. Cited in Quintessential Aromatics database, 2013.
8. Freeman S et al. *Olfactory stimuli and enhanced postural stability in older adults.* Gail & Posture, 2009; 29(4): 658-660. Cited in Quintessential Aromatics database, 2013.
9. Lomarat P et al. *In vitro biological activities of black pepper essential oil and its major components relevant to the prevention of Alzheimer's disease.* Thai Journal of Pharmaceutical Sciences, 2015; 39(3): 94-101. Cited in Quintessential Aromatics database, 2013.
10. Jain SR, Kar A. *The antibacterial activity of some essential oils and their combinations.* Planta Medica, 1971; 20(2): 118-123. Cited in the Aromatherapy Database, by Bob Harris, Essential Oil Resource Consultants, UK, 2000.
11. Jenna K et al. *Antioxidant, anti-inflammatory and antinociceptive properties of black pepper essential oil (Piper nigrum Linn).* Journal of Essential Oil Bearing Plants, 2014; 17(1): 1-12. Cited in Quintessential Aromatics database, 2013.
12. Lee K et al. *Anti-biolfim, antihemolysis, and anti-virulence activities of black pepper, cananga, myrrh oils and nerolidol against Staphylococcus aureus.* Applied Microbiology and

Biotechnology, 2014; 98(22): 9447-9457. Cited in Quintessential Aromatics database, 2013.
13. Mori M et al. *Inhibition of elastase activity by essential oils in vitro.* Journal of Cosmetic Dermatology, 2002; 1(4): 183-187.
14. Ramadan A et al. *Some pharmacodynamic effects and antimicrobial activity of essential oils of certain plants used in Egyptian folk medicine.* Veterinary Medicine Journal Giza, 1994; 42(1): 263-270. Cited in the Aromatherapy Database, by Bob Harris, Essential Oil Resource Consultants, UK, 2000.
15. Rose JE, Behm FM. *Inhalation of vapor from black pepper extract reduces smoking withdrawal symptoms.* Drug & Alcohol Dependence, 1994; 34(3): 225-229. Cited in Quintessential Aromatics database, 2013.
16. Cordell B, Buckle J. *The effects of aromatherapy on nicotine craving on a U.S campus: a small comparison.* Journal of Alternative and Complementary Medicine, 2013; 19(8): 709-713. Cited in Quintessential Aromatics database, 2013.
17. Davis P. *Aromatherapy A-Z.* 2nd edn. The C.W. Daniel Company, Saffron Walden, 1999.
18. Holmes P. *The energetics of Western herbs — Vol. II.* Artemis Press, Boulder, 1989.
19. Lawless J. *The encyclopaedia of essential oils.* Element Books, Shaftesbury, 1992.
20. Worwood VA. *The fragrant mind.* Transworld Publishers, London, 1995.
21. Davis P. *Subtle aromatherapy.* C.W. Daniel Company, Saffron Walden, 1991.
22. Worwood VA. *The fragrant heavens.* Transworld Publishers, London, 1999.
23. Keim Loughran J, Bull R. *Aromatherapy and subtle energy techniques.* Frog, Berkeley, 2000.
24. Tisserand R, Young R. *Essential oil safety.* 2nd edn. Churchill Livingstone, Edinburgh, 2014.

Boronia absolute

Identification

Botanical name

Boronia megastigma Ness ex Bartlett

Synonyms

Brown boronia

Family

Rutaceae

Botany and origins

Boronia is a genus of about 95 species occurring throughout Australia. Western Australia has 49 species. It is now cultivated in Tasmania. Only *Boronia megastigma* is currently harvested for its oil.[1]

Boronia is a bushy evergreen shrub, up to 2 m tall, which bears an abundance of fragrant flowers with an unusual colouring. The petals are brown on the outside, yellow on the inside.

Method of extraction

The flowers and foliage can be steam-distilled, but are usually extracted with food-grade hexane to produce a concrete, and again extracted to produce an absolute. The concrete yield is variable and averages about 1%, with an absolute yield of around 60%.[1]

Characteristics

Boronia absolute is a green viscous liquid with a fresh, fruity, spicy aroma and a rich, tenacious floral undertone.[1] Arctander describes boronia absolute as a fresh, fruity-green, sweet tea-like, slightly spicy-herbaceous odour. The main body note has a rich tenacious floral undertone of warm woody-sweet character.[2]

Chemical composition

The principle constituents of boronia absolute are ionone, eugenol, triacontane, phenols, ethyl alcohol and ethyl formate.[1]

Adulteration

Boronia absolute is subject to adulteration with ionones, eugenol, methyl eugenol and sesquiterpene fractions of ylang ylang.[2]

Pharmacopoeias and standards

At the time of writing, the purity, composition, physico-chemical properties and therapeutic use of boronia absolute are not defined in any pharmacopoeia monograph or standard.

History and Traditional Uses

Food, perfumery and flavouring

The main use for boronia absolute is in food flavourings, with a small amount used in high-class perfumes.[1,2] Tisserand & Young state that this expensive absolute is not likely to be used in significant quantities.[3]

It contains β-ionone and other ingredients which have excellent odour enhancement characteristics.[2] Boronia absolute is considered one of the most unique perfume and flavour materials because it contains ionones. It is used in high-class chypre and fougère perfumes. Because of its persistence and intensity, the absolute is valued as an addition to quality perfumes.[2]

Therapeutics

Pharmacology and clinical studies

No information available.

Actions

Actions commonly cited in aromatherapy

No information available.

Actions supported by clinical studies

None

Comment

Boronia absolute is not used in aromatherapy. It has such an interesting aroma, which makes it a very interesting aromatic raw material for someone to use in perfume creation.

Aromatherapy Uses

It has not been traditionally used in aromatherapy.

Dosage and Administration

Blending

Perfumery

Boronia absolute blends well with essential oils such as bergamot, clary sage, sandalwood and floral essential oils.[2]

Mode of administration

Topical

Massage

Inhalation

Direct inhalation, diffuser, oil vaporiser

Safety Profile

General safety

Tisserand & Young state that no known hazards or contraindications are reported. No information could be found regarding adverse skin reactions. Ionones tend to be non-reactive on the skin.[3]

Contraindications

No contraindications known.

Regulatory guidelines

It has been approved for flavouring in food use.[4]

References

1. Weiss EA. *Essential oil crops*. CAB International, Wallingford, 1997.
2. Arctander S. *Perfume and flavor materials of natural origin*. Allured Publishing, Carol Stream, 1994.
3. Tisserand R, Young R. *Essential oil safety*. 2nd edn. Churchill Livingstone, Edinburgh, 2014.
4. Khan I, Abourashed E. *Leung's encyclopedia of common natural ingredients used in food, drugs and cosmetics*. 3rd edn. John Wiley & Sons, New Jersey, 2010.

B

Buchu

Identification

Botanical name

Buchu (diosphenol ct.): *Agathosma betulina* (PJ Bergius) Pillans

Buchu (pulegone ct.): *Agathosma crenulata* (L) Pillans

Synonyms

Bookoo, buku, diosma, bucku and bucco, *Barosma betulina, Barosma crenulata*[1,2]

Family

Rutaceae

Botany and origins

Buchu is a low aromatic shrub, usually less than 2 m high with opposite or alternate leaves that are finely toothed at the margin.[3] It grows wild in South Africa. Only a small fraction of the total harvested buchu leaves are used for the distillation of essential oil.[4]

There are two types of buchu leaves – round or short buchu from *A. betulina* and long buchu from *A. crenulata*. They differ in the relative compositions of their volatile oils.[3]

Method of extraction

The essential oil of buchu is steam-distilled from the dried leaves of *A. betulina* or *A. crenulata*.

Characteristics

Buchu oil is a yellowish to brownish-yellow liquid, oily and somewhat viscous, depending on the age of the oil and the dryness of the plant material prior to distillation. The odour is very peculiar; a strong, bitter-sweet, somewhat minty-camphoraceous, root-like, penetrating odour, reminiscent of pennyroyal.[4]

Chemical composition

Tisserand & Young state that there are two chemotypes of buchu – buchu (diosphenol ct.) and buchu (pulegone ct.).[5]

The chemical composition of buchu oils was reported as follows:[2]

Constituent	A. crenulata	A. betulina
limonene	24.1%	26.8%
menthone	3.6%	10.8%
isomenthone	11.8%	26.6%
isopulegone	6.6%	0.8%
pulegone	46.7%	3.3%
cis-acetylthio-*p*-menthan-3-one	4.9%	trace
trans-acetylthio-*p*-menthan-3-one	0.4%	trace
diosphenol	0.3%	15.4%
p-diosphenol	0.2%	12.5%
cis-3-mercapto-*p*-menthan-3-one	1.2%	0.6%
trans-3-mercapto-*p*-menthan-3-one	1.5%	2.8%

Adulteration

Lis-Balchin states that buchu oil is often adulterated with solvents, and that blending with different species accounts for most of the adulteration.[2]

Burfield states that buchu oil is often adulterated with monoterpene sulphides such as *p*-menthan-8-thiol-3-one.[6]

Pharmacopoeias and standards

At the time of writing, the purity, composition, physico-chemical properties and therapeutic use of buchu oil are not defined in any pharmacopoeia monograph or standard.

History and Traditional Uses

History

The first recorded use of buchu was in 1653. The South African bushmen and other tribes had been using buchu in traditional ceremonies, as an insect repellent, as a perfume, for the healing of sores, for relief from rheumatism and as a pick-me-up tonic.[3]

Herbal

Buchu leaf herb is listed in the German Commission E, but it states that buchu leaf's use as a urinary tract anti-inflammatory and diuretic is not recommended since its effectiveness is not well documented.[3]

Herbal preparations of buchu leaf are used for the treatment of cystitis, urethritis, nephritis and catarrh of the bladder; however, the effectiveness of the claimed applications has not been documented.[7]

Buchu leaf is also listed in the British Herbal Pharmacopoeia as a urinary antiseptic for the treatment of genitourinary tract infections; however, buchu leaves are contraindicated during pregnancy.[1]

Food, perfumery and flavouring

Buchu essential oil is used for the flavouring of black currant, but *A. betulina* is preferred because of its higher diosphenols that are considered to be more desirable flavour components. The level at which it is used is very low, with the maximum highest percentage at about 0.002% (15.4 ppm).[3]

Buchu leaf oil is occasionally used in perfumery to create a chypre base and to create diffusive fresh quality in colognes. However, because of its very penetrating aroma, it is used at a very low percentage.[4]

Therapeutics

Pharmacology and clinical studies

Antibacterial activity

Lis-Balchin states that neither *A. betulina* nor *A. crenulata* essential oil demonstrated antimicrobial action against *Enterococcus hirae* and *Pseudomonas aeruginosa*, and very little activity was observed against *Escherichia coli* and *Staphylococcus aureus*. There is little use for these oils as antimicrobial agents.[2]

Antifungal activity

No antifungal activity reported.[2]

Actions

Actions commonly cited in aromatherapy

Antiseptic, carminative, diuretic, insecticide[1]

Actions supported by clinical studies

None

Comment

I agree with Lis-Balchin who says that, while buchu is extensively used in herbal medicine, the presence of pulegone in *A. crenulata* and diosphenol in *A. betulina* make buchu essential oils toxic. She states that both buchu oils are hazardous in aromatherapy massage, and suggests that their use as a fragrance is rather doubtful as they have an unpleasant aroma.[2]

Aromatherapy Uses

Buchu oil is not recommended for use in aromatherapy.[1,5]

Dosage and Administration

Blending

No blending advice has been provided for buchu oil.

Mode of administration

Bath

Buchu oil is not recommended for use in a bath.

Massage

Buchu oil is not recommended for use in massage.

Inhalation

Buchu oil is not recommended for use as an inhalation.

Safety Profile

General safety

As the essential oil from *A. crenulata* contains pulegone, it is likely to have similar toxicity to that of pennyroyal oil. It is not recommended for use in aromatherapy.

Tisserand & Young state that the maximum dermal use of *A. crenulata* is 1.4%.[5]

Contraindications

A. crenulata and *A. betulina* are contraindicated during pregnancy and breastfeeding.[5] *A. crenulata* may be an abortifacient and hepatotoxic.[5]

Regulatory guidelines

Buchu leaf essential oil has GRAS status.

References

1. Lawless J. *The encyclopaedia of essential oils.* Element Books, Shaftesbury, 1992.
2. Lis-Balchin M. *Aromatherapy science – a guide for healthcare professionals.* Pharmaceutical Press, London, 2006.
3. Khan I, Abourashed E. *Leung's encyclopedia of common natural ingredients used in food, drugs and cosmetics.* 3rd edn. John Wiley & Sons, New Jersey, 2010.
4. Arctander S. *Perfume and flavour materials of natural origin.* Allured Publishing, Carol Stream, 1994.
5. Tisserand R, Young R. *Essential oil safety.* 2nd edn. Churchill Livingstone, Edinburgh, 2014.
6. Burfield T. *The adulteration of essential oils – and the consequences to aromatherapy and natural perfume practice.* Presented to the International Federation of Aromatherapists Annual AGM, London, 2003.
7. Blumenthal M et al. *The complete German commission E monographs: therapeutic guide to herbal medicine.* American Botanical Council, Austin, 1998.

B

Buddha wood

Identification

Botanical name

Eremophila mitchellii Benth.

Synonyms

False or bastard sandalwood tree, Australian desert rosewood

Family

Myoporaceae

Botany and origins

Buddha wood occurs in the arid areas of New South Wales, Queensland and South Australia. The tree is often confused with *Santalum lanceolatum*, which is commonly referred to as Queensland sandalwood. It was named after Sir Thomas Mitchell, a nineteenth-century explorer and botanist. The origins of *Eremophila* comes from to love (*phila*) and a lonely place or desert (*eremos*).[1,2]

Buddha wood is an evergreen and often resinous shrub to small tree up to 10 m in height. It has dark, rough bark, with hairless leaves that are bright green and aromatic. The tree is considered a woody weed despite the fact that it is indigenous to Australia.[1]

Method of extraction

Buddha wood oil is either steam-distilled, or extracted with hexane followed by high vacuum distillation.[3]

Characteristics

Buddha wood essential oil has a fresh incense top

note with a woody aroma similar to sandalwood, a hint of peppery spice and a smoky leathery back note.[1] Weiss states that the oil is not a substitute or alternative for true sandalwood oil.[4] The oil has a tendency to polymerise.[3]

Chemical composition

The main constituents found in Buddha wood essential oil are three closely related sesquiterpene ketones: eremophilone (30-60%), 2-hydroxyeremophilone (6-25%) and 2-hydroxy-2-dihydroeremophilone (11-30%).[1]

Tisserand & Young state that there are many sesquiterpene compounds present in the oil that have not been fully characterised.[3]

Adulteration

Not reported.

Pharmacopoeias and standards

At the time of writing, the purity, composition, physico-chemical properties and therapeutic use of Buddha wood essential oil are not defined in any pharmacopoeia monograph or standard.

History and Traditional Uses

Traditional medicine

Australian Aborigines would use the twigs in smoking ceremonies to promote a feeling of general wellbeing.[5]

There are several reports on the biological activity and ethnopharmacology of *E. mitchellii* in literature. It is reported that the plant has been used by the Aboriginal people as a treatment for rheumatism.

Other uses

A 1951 study found that the wood oil was also found to be virtually non-toxic as a fly spray, but when combined with pyrethrins, it produced a marked increase in fly mortality in comparison to the pyrethrins alone.[6]

The interest in the commercial production of Buddha wood oil is due to its insecticidal and termiticidal properties. The oil has shown promise for remedial application as a fumigant, in chemical soil barriers, and for the treatment and preservation of timber.[6]

Therapeutics

Pharmacology and clinical studies

Antimicrobial activity

Studies have identified the oil as having antimicrobial activity against *Candida albicans* and five bacteria. No inhibition was observed against *Pseudomonas aeruginosa*.[6]

Insecticidal activity

The insecticidal activity of *E. mitchellii* oil was evaluated against two species of termites – *Nasutitermes exitiosus* and *Coptotermes acinaciformis*. The steam-distilled wood oil exhibited toxicity, repellency and antifeedant activity against both species. It was determined that eremophilone and 8-hydroxy-1(10)-dihydroeremophilone were found to be the key actives responsible for the oil's insecticidal activity.[7]

Actions

Actions commonly cited in aromatherapy

Analgesic, anti-inflammatory, fixative[1,2]

Actions supported by clinical studies

None

Comment

Buddha wood oil contains some very rare sesquiterpenes whose pharmacology has not yet been identified. Preliminary studies have shown that eremophilane sesquiterpenes inhibit P388D1 cancer cell growth in vitro.[6] It would be great to see more research into its bioactivity.

Buddha wood oil has an intriguing aroma profile that would make it a very useful oil in perfumery.

B

Aromatherapy Uses

Clinical aromatherapy

Musculoskeletal system

It has been claimed that Buddha wood oil can be used to relieve muscular aches and pains due to its anti-inflammatory properties. It is also reputed to have a somewhat analgesic effect.[1,2]

Dosage and Administration

Blending

Aromatherapy

For the relief of muscular aches and pains, consider blending Buddha wood oil with essential oils such as black pepper, cajeput, ginger, kunzea, spike lavender, pine or rosemary.

Perfumery

Buddha wood's aroma suggests that it would be excellent for its fixative qualities in blends. It adds a very unique woody aroma to anyone looking for a more masculine or woody blend.

Mode of administration

Bath

Full body bath, foot bath

Topical

Compress, massage, ointment

Inhalation

Direct inhalation, diffuser, oil vaporiser

Safety Profile

General safety

Tisserand & Young state that there are no known hazards or contraindications. There is also no information on acute toxicity for Buddha wood oil or any of its known constituents.[3]

Contraindications

No contraindications known.

Regulatory guidelines

Buddha wood oil is not defined in any regulatory guideline.

References

1. Australian Botanical Products. *Eremophila mitchellii oil*. Retrieved Apr 2, 2017, from https://www.apb.com.au/catalogue/australian-natives-A-M/eremophila-mitchelli-oil.html
2. Rose J. *Australian Buddha wood oil*. Retrieved Sep 28, 2017, from http://www.aromaticplantproject.com/articles_archive/Australian_Essential_Oils.html#17
3. Tisserand R, Young R. *Essential oil safety*. 2nd edn. Churchill Livingstone, Edinburgh, 2014.
4. Weiss EA. *Essential oil crops*. CAB International, Wallingford, 1997.
5. Richmond GS. *A review of the use of Eremophila (Myoporaceae) by Australian aborigines*. Journal of the Adelaide Botanic Gardens, 1993; 15(2): 101-107.
6. Beattie KD et al. *Chemical composition and cytotoxicity of oils and eremophilanes derived from various parts of Eremophila mitchellii Benth. (Myoporaceae)*. Phytochemistry, 2011; 72(4/5): 400-408. doi: 10.1016/j.phytochem.2010.12.011
7. Leach D. *Fighting termites – a natural chemical from an Aussie tree*. Jul 6, 2010. Retrieved Apr 2, 2017, from http://www.sciencepublic.com.au/conferences/raci/termites

C

Cabreuva

Identification

Botanical name

Myrocarpus fastigiatus Allemão

Synonyms

Cabureicica

Family

Fabaceae (Leguminosae)

Botany and origins

Cabreuva is a tropical tree which grows up to 12 m tall, with a very hard wood which is resistant to moisture and mould growth. The wood is highly regarded and is used for ornamental lumber and furniture. It is extremely hard to cut or saw.[1] Cabreuva tree is related to the trees which produce Peru balsam and copaiba balsam. It is found growing wild in Brazil, Paraguay and Argentina.[1]

Method of extraction

The essential oil is produced from the steam distillation of waste wood from the lumber mills.[1]

Characteristics

The oil is a pale yellow, somewhat viscous, possessing a sweet-woody, very delicate and slightly floral odour. It has excellent tenacity.[1]

Chemical composition

The chemical composition of cabreuva oil was reported as follows:

nerolidol (>65%), farnesol (2.5%), bisabolol and other sesquiterpene alcohols.[2]

Adulteration

Cabreuva oil is often adulterated with *oleo vermelho* essential oil which is distilled from *Myrospermum erythroxylon*.[1]

Pharmacopoeias and standards

At the time of writing, the purity, composition, physico-chemical properties and therapeutic use of cabreuva essential oil are not defined in any pharmacopoeia monograph or standard.

History and Traditional Uses

History

The wood is highly appreciated for carving and furniture making. For some time, cabreuva oil was used as a starting material for the isolation of the sesquiterpene alcohol, nerolidol – the main constituent found in the oil. This sesquiterpene is now produced synthetically.[1]

Traditional medicine

The resin from the tree was traditionally used by the natives to heal wounds, ulcers and scars.[3]

Food, perfumery and flavouring

Cabreuva essential oil is not commonly used in perfumery.[1]

Therapeutics

Pharmacology and clinical studies

No information available.

Actions

Actions commonly cited in aromatherapy

Antiseptic, balsamic, cicatrisant[3]

Actions supported by clinical studies

None

Comment

At the time of writing, there are no clinical or pharmacological studies to confirm any of the actions of cabreuva essential oil.

Aromatherapy Uses

Clinical aromatherapy

Cabreuva oil is not commonly used in aromatherapy.

Integumentary system

Cabreuva oil has been suggested for the treatment of cuts, scars and wound healing.[3]

Energetics, psyche and subtle uses

Subtle

Keim Loughran & Bull state that cabreuva oil helps to balance all the energy centres. It also helps to cleanse, seal and protect the auric field to promote healthy boundaries.[4]

Dosage and Administration

Blending

Perfumery

Arctander states that the scent of cabreuva oil is often underestimated. He explains that its tenacity and distinct 'precious wood' aroma, with a slightly green dry floral note, would make it very unique in all perfumes, but it is not commonly used in perfumery.[1]

Mode of administration

Bath

Full body bath, foot bath

Topical

Compress, massage, ointment, skin care

Inhalation

Direct inhalation, diffuser, oil vaporiser

Safety Profile

General safety

Cabreuva oil is non-toxic, non-irritating and non-sensitising.[3,5]

Contraindications

No contraindications known.

Regulatory guidelines

Cabreuva oil is not defined in any regulatory guidelines.

References

1. Arctander S. *Perfume and flavor materials of natural origin*. Allured Publishing, Carol Stream, 1994.
2. Lawrence BM. *Essential oils 1981-1987.* Allured Publishing, Wheaton, 1989.
3. Lawless J. *The encyclopaedia of essential oils.* Element Books, Shaftesbury, 1992.
4. Keim Loughran J, Bull R. *Aromatherapy and subtle energy techniques*. Frog, Berkeley, 2000.
5. Tisserand R, Young R. *Essential oil safety*. 2nd edn. Churchill Livingstone, Edinburgh, 2014.

C

Cajeput

Identification

Botanical name

Melaleuca cajuputi Powell

Synonyms

Cajuput, river tea tree, swamp tea tree, weeping tea tree, punk tea tree, *M. leucadendron* var. *cajeputi*, also known in Malaysia and Indonesia as *kayaputi* and *cajeputi*[1]

Family

Myrtaceae

Botany and origins

M. cajuputi is a medium-sized tree to 30 m, with a single trunk to 1.5 m, but several stems may grow from the original rootstock. The trees often have small crowns, especially in pure stands, with smaller branches and often slender twigs. The bark is whitish, papery, thin and flaking.[1]

The cajeput tree is occasionally referred to as 'tea-tree' or 'ti-tree' on the islands between Australia and Indonesia. The name cajeput originates from the tree's Indonesian and Malay name – *kaya* (wood) and *pitih* (white).[1]

C

Weiss explains that there are no economically viable plantations of *M. cajuputi*, and all commercial oils supplies are currently from wild trees. The branches are cut, stripped of leaves and transported to portable stills. He also explains that the trees can be harvested annually as vigorous regeneration of the leaves has been noted.[1] It has been reported that cajeput is now being cultivated in Indonesia.[2]

Williams states that *M. quinquenervia* and *M. cajuputi* can be difficult to tell apart. To make matters more challenging, both trees have the common name cajeput applied to them. However, she explains that cajeput oil originating from South East Asia generally comes from *M. cajuputi*, whereas the oil from New Caledonia is extracted from *M. quinquenervia*.[3]

Method of extraction

Cajeput essential oil is steam-distilled from the fresh leaves and twigs of *M. cajuputi*.

Characteristics

Cajeput essential oil is a colourless to pale yellow or greenish coloured liquid, with a powerful fresh, eucalyptus-like and camphoraceous odour. The oil also has a characteristic fruity-sweet body note with soft tones in the dryout. Arctander states that the green colour is not an indication that the essential oil is genuine.[4]

Chemical composition

The chemical composition of cajeput essential oil was reported as follows:

α-pinene (38.9%), β-pinene (1.5%), myrcene (0.5%), α-terpinene (0.2%), limonene (2.9%), 1,8-cineole (21.1%), γ-terpinene (1.0%), *p*-cymene (3.1%), terpinolene (0.8%), linalool (0.3%), terpinen-4-ol (1.9%) and α-terpineol (3.3%).[5]

Adulteration

Cajeput is often adulterated with cheaper eucalyptus oils, or combinations of eucalyptus oils with small quantities of terpinyl acetate, terpinyl propionate and terpineol esters.[4] Holmes states that it is commonly blended with oils from other *Melaleuca* species.[6]

Pharmacopoeias and standards

At the time of writing, the purity, composition, physico-chemical properties and therapeutic use of cajeput essential oil are not defined in any pharmacopoeia monograph or standard.

Holmes states that, because there is no internationally accepted quality standard for cajeput, the chemical composition of the oil can vary significantly; however, it is likely that this is because of all the different subspecies found in different countries and the possible blending with other *Melaleuca* species.[6]

History and Traditional Uses

History

Cajeput has been traditionally used for its antiseptic, carminative and local analgesic properties by Australian Aborigines:

> *Cajeput has been used by local aborigines on Groote Eylandt for the treatment of aches and pains. The leaves are crushed in the hand and rubbed on. Sometimes young leaves and twigs are crushed and steeped in hot water; the liquid is used to bathe the affected area and the rest is poured over the head. Crushed leaves are sniffed to cure headache.*[7]

Weiss states that cajeput oil is considered a panacea in India, Malaysia, Indonesia and other South East Asian countries. It is also widely and effectively used for the treatment of intestinal worms. It is also used as an insect repellent and insecticide.[1]

It was considered particularly valuable for colds, flu and chronic rheumatism, and was prescribed for cholera. It was first introduced to Europe in the seventeenth century. Until the Dutch gained territory in the Moluccas, it remained a very rare and expensive oil in France.[8]

Cajeput oil was first mentioned in *The Natural History of Simple Drugs* by Dr Guibourt in 1876. He described its properties as antiseptic for intestinal problems, dysentery, enteritis, urinary complaints, cystitis and infections of the urethra.[8]

Other uses

While cajeput oil is used in South East Asia as a general household remedy for colds, throat diseases, pains and headaches, it has found very little use in Europe and America, as its main constituents are similar to those found in eucalyptus oil. Arctander suggests that cajeput does not present any advantages over eucalyptus oil, except for its slightly milder-sweet aroma.[4] However, the chemistry of cajeput oil is more comparable to tea tree rather than eucalyptus.

Therapeutics

Pharmacology and clinical studies

Antibacterial activity

Clinical studies have confirmed that cajeput oil has significant antimicrobial activity against a range of bacteria.[9]

Antifungal activity

Cajeput oil was investigated for its inhibitory properties against 24 fungal species, including *Aspergillus flavus, A. fumigatus, Microsporum gypseum* and *Trichophyton mentagrophytes*. The researchers stated that cajeput oil completely inhibited several fungi, and had a pronounced effect on all the other species.[10]

Actions

Actions commonly cited in aromatherapy

Analgesic, antimicrobial, antiseptic, antispasmodic, expectorant, febrifuge, stimulant, sudorific, vermifuge[11]

Actions supported by clinical studies

Antifungal, antimicrobial, antiseptic, expectorant

Comment

Review of traditional and clinical data suggests that cajeput's antibacterial and antimicrobial properties make it beneficial for colds, coughs and catarrhal conditions. The German Commission E recommends cajeput oil for headaches, nerve pain, neuralgia, rheumatism and lumbago.[12]

The 1,8-cineole content also indicates that cajeput oil would be effective as an expectorant, and would be beneficial for catarrhal conditions, sore throats and bronchial discomforts.

Aromatherapy Uses

Clinical aromatherapy

Digestive system

Cajeput oil soothes colic and inflammation of the intestines such as enteritis, dysentery, gastric spasm and intestinal parasites.[12]

Integumentary system

Cajeput oil is used to alleviate itching due to insect bites, and to relieve eczema and psoriasis.[12]

Musculoskeletal system

Cajeput oil is used in a massage oil or an ointment for all painful conditions, especially arthritis and rheumatism. Its pain relieving properties make it useful in massage for neuralgia, gout, sciatica, lumbago, sports injuries, muscle stiffness, and general aches and pain.[6,12,13]

Psychological

Holmes recommends cajeput oil to alleviate lethargy, mental confusion, and lack of concentration and loss of motivation. He explains that renewed motivation in turn enhances the immune functioning, which is a link between the body and the psyche. It can be very useful for those recovering from chronic illness.[6]

Respiratory system

Cajeput oil is recommended for catarrhal conditions such as asthma, sinusitis, sore throats, chronic bronchitis, coughs, colds and flu. A steam inhalation with cajeput oil is recommended for cleansing the congested nasal passages. It has analgesic properties that will help to reduce the discomfort of sore throats.[11,12,13,14,15]

Skin care

Cajeput oil is recommended for the treatment of oily skin.[6,11]

Energetics, psyche and subtle uses

Energetics

Cajeput oil is described as having a hot, stimulating nature and it is recommended for *cold* and *deficient* conditions.[6]

Holmes states that cajeput oil warms the *Lungs*, expels phlegm and relieves coughing. It is used to eliminate *Lung* phlegm-*cold* and *damp*, which is associated with coughing, wheezing and mucous congestion. He also recommends cajeput to tonify the *Qi*, raise *Yang Qi* and strengthen the *Shen*. Therefore it is recommended for mental fatigue and confusion, poor focus and headaches.[6] Cajeput oil also has a strong affinity with the Metal Element.

Dosage and Administration

Blending

Aromatherapy

The German Commission E has listed 43 individual formulae for the approved use of cajeput essential oil. Some of the interesting and practical formulae for aromatherapy uses include:

- Cajeput oil, sage oil, clove oil, eucalyptus oil – for poorly healing and infected wounds and leg ulcers.
- Cajeput oil, peppermint oil, eucalyptus oil – for colds, nasal catarrhs, pain of nerves and limbs, lumbago, arthritis and first aid for toothache.
- Cajeput oil, peppermint oil, eucalyptus oil, juniper oil, wintergreen oil – for cooling, calming, pain-relieving, promoting blood circulation, sprains and strains, contusions, dislocation, calf cramps and protection from insect bites.
- Cajeput oil, eucalyptus oil, menthol, clove bud oil, peppermint oil, juniper berry oil, cinnamon oil, lemon balm oil, wintergreen oil, star anise oil – internally for shortness of breath and bronchial asthma. Externally for rheumatic discomforts, lumbago, migraine and insect bites.[12]

For the relief of pain associated with arthritis and rheumatism, consider blending cajeput oil with essential oils such as black pepper, clove bud, ginger, kunzea, peppermint, pine, rosemary or wintergreen.

For the relief of respiratory congestion associated with bronchial congestion, colds and flu, consider blending cajeput oil with essential oils such as 1,8-cineole-rich eucalypts, fragonia, kunzea, manuka, peppermint, pine, tea tree or thyme.

Perfumery

Cajeput is not typically used in perfumery.

Mode of administration

Bath

Full body bath, foot bath

Topical

Compress, massage, ointment, skin care

Inhalation

Direct inhalation, steam inhalation, diffuser, oil vaporiser

C

Safety Profile

General safety

Cajeput is non-toxic and non-sensitising. However, Davis states that it can irritate the skin, therefore it needs to be well diluted and never allowed to come into contact with mucous membranes.[15]

Contraindications

Do not apply to or near the face of infants and children.[16]

Regulatory guidelines

Cajeput essential oil has GRAS status.

References

1. Weiss EA. *Essential oil crops*. CAB International, Wallingford, 1997.
2. Brophy J, Craven L, Doran J. *Melaleucas – their botany, essential oils and uses.* Australian Centre for International Agricultural Research (ACIAR), Canberra, 2013.
3. Williams C. *Medicinal plants in Australia – Vol. 2 Gums, resins, tannins and essential oil,* Rosenburg Publishing, Dural, 2011.
4. Arctander S. *Perfume and flavour materials of natural origin*. Allured Publishing, Carol Stream, 1994.
5. Williams L. *The composition and bactericidal activity of the oil of Melaleuca alternifolia.* The International Journal of Aromatherapy, 1989; 1(3): 15.
6. Holmes P. *Aromatica: a clinical guide to essential oil therapeutics – Vol. I.* Singing Dragon, London, 2016.
7. Lassak EV, McCarthy T. *Australian medicinal plants.* Methuen Australia, North Ryde, 1983.
8. Ryman D. *Aromatherapy*. Judy Piatkus, Great Britain, 1991.
9. Lis-Balchin M. *Aromatherapy science – a guide for healthcare professionals.* Pharmaceutical Press, London, 2006.
10. Dubey NK, Kishore N, Singh SK. *Antifungal properties of the volatile fraction of Melaleuca leucadendron.* Tropical Agriculture, 1983; 60(3): 227. Cited in Quintessential Aromatics database, 2013.
11. Lawless J. *The encyclopaedia of essential oils.* Element Books, Shaftesbury, 1992.
12. Blumenthal M et al. *The complete German commission E monographs: therapeutic guide to herbal medicine.* American Botanical Council, Austin, 1998.
13. Khan I, Abourashed E. *Leung's encyclopedia of common natural ingredients used in food, drugs and cosmetics.* 3rd edn. John Wiley & Sons, New Jersey, 2010.
14. Schnaubelt K. *Medical aromatherapy*. Frog, Berkeley, 1999.

15. Davis P. *Aromatherapy A-Z*. 2nd edn. C.W. Daniel Company, Saffron Walden, 1999.

16. Tisserand R, Young R. *Essential oil safety*. 2nd edn. Churchill Livingstone, Edinburgh, 2014.

Camphor

Identification

Botanical name

Cinnamomum camphora L.

Synonyms

Hon-sho, true camphor

Family

Lauraceae

Botany and origins

Cinnamomum camphora is a tall evergreen tree with large glossy green leaves. It is native to China, Japan and Taiwan, but has now been introduced to many other countries.[1]

It flourishes in warm-temperate to semitropical regions. The highest camphor content can be found in wood and leaves of trees growing in direct light. Shaded trees or leaves usually have a lower oil and camphor content.[1]

Prior to World War I, a high proportion of the camphor traded was obtained from wild trees principally on Taiwan (then Formosa), with smaller production in Japan. It was not until the decline in the number of wild trees threatened the industry's future that plantations of camphor trees were established.[1]

When harvesting for camphor, the whole tree is cut down and reduced to chips and distilled to obtain a crude oil, which undergoes further rectification to obtain the various fractions.[1]

Method of extraction

True camphor oil is produced by steam distillation from the wood, root stumps and branches of *C. camphora*, also known as hon-sho.[2]

Along with the crude oil, a solid, partly crystalline mass of crude camphor is extracted. The essential oil is separated from the crude camphor by filter pressing. This yields the crude camphor oil that is subsequently rectified under vacuum, yielding another 50% of crude camphor.[2]

The remaining 50% of the filter-pressed crude camphor oil is now free of camphor. It contains light terpenes, cineole, safrole, terpineol and sesquiterpene alcohols.[2]

These constituents are separated into various fractions that are referred to as:

- White camphor – the light fraction containing cineole and monoterpenes.
- Brown camphor – the medium to heavy fraction which contains up to 80% safrole and some terpineol.
- Blue camphor – the heavy fraction which contains sesquiterpenes.[2]

White camphor has the lowest boiling point and does not contain any safrole. However, it contains around 30 to 50% camphor. This is the oil that has commonly been sold in aromatherapy as camphor.[2]

Without a doubt, oils from *C. camphora* have caused much confusion, and the nomenclature remains in dispute. Depending on its origin, oil from *C. camphora* has been referred to as:

- Hon-sho (true camphor) – this is the camphor chemotype, from the wood.
- Ravintsara – this is the 1,8-cineole chemotype, from the leaf from Madagascar.
- Ho leaf oil (ho-sho) – this is the linalool chemotype, from the leaf.

I describe ravintsara and ho leaf essential oils in separate monographs. The focus of this monograph will be hon-sho or true camphor, otherwise referred to as white camphor.

Schnaubelt states that the chemical differences between these oils are greater than one might expect as a result of climatic or geographic variation alone.[3]

Characteristics

White camphor oil is a clear mobile fluid with a fresh, sharp camphoraceous odour.

Chemical composition

The chemical composition of white camphor oil was reported as follows:

α-pinene (3.7%), camphene (1.64%), β-pinene (1.26%), sabinene (1.47%), phellandrene (0.17%), limonene (2.71%), 1,8-cineole (4.75%), γ-terpinene (0.24%), *p*-cymene (0.14%), terpinolene (0.3%), furfural (0.16%), camphor (51.5%), linalool (0.68%), bornyl acetate (0.02%), terpinen-4-ol (0.57%), caryophyllene (1.49%), borneol (0.02%),

C

piperitone (2.41%), geraniol (0.63%), safrole (13.4%), cinnamaldehyde (0.08%), methyl cinnamate (0.08%), eugenol (0.12%).[4]

Brown camphor contains approximately 80% safrole and yellow camphor contains 10 to 20% safrole and 15 to 23% camphor.[5]

Adulteration

White camphor oil is rarely adulterated because it is inexpensive; however, it is often fractionated and used to adulterate camphor-containing oils such as rosemary, Spanish sage and spike lavender.[6]

Pharmacopoeias and standards

At the time of writing, the purity, composition, physico-chemical properties and therapeutic use of camphor essential oil are not defined in any standard. White camphor oil is listed in the German Commission E and the British Herbal Pharmacopoeia.

History and Traditional Uses

History

Weiss provides us with a detailed history of camphor. He states that Europeans became aware of camphor via Arab traders. Sarapion, a Greek governor of the Thebaid area of the Red Sea Coast in 150 BC, described the process of refining camphor he had obtained from Arab, Ibn Amram. The Arab merchant Sinbad in the ninth century described the method for obtaining camphor from the Riha Peninsula by making incisions in trees and collecting the solid exudate.[1]

C

Camphor became commonly known in European medicine by the twelfth century. Hildegarde recommended its use under the name *ganphora* as a counterirritant in the treatment of rheumatism and inflamed joints.[1]

In China, camphor was well known and established in traditional medicine. Camphor was introduced to Japan from China in the seventeenth century.[1]

It was originally believed that camphor could only be obtained from the trunk or branches of mature trees; however, in the nineteenth century, leaves were distilled to produce camphor oil. Since 1988, the production of camphor oil from the leaf in China has been supported by the government.[1] The leaf oil is usually high in linalool and is often referred to as ho leaf oil.

Traditional medicine

White camphor has a long-standing traditional use in the treatment of respiratory tract infections. It is attributed with antiseptic, bactericidal, diuretic, expectorant, rubefacient, stimulant and vermifuge properties.[7]

White camphor oil is recommended for the treatment of acne, skin inflammations, oily skin, arthritis, muscular aches and pains, rheumatism, and respiratory conditions such as bronchitis, coughs and colds.[7]

Herbal

The German Commission E recommends white camphor oil externally for muscular rheumatism, catarrhal diseases, diseases of the respiratory system and cardiac symptoms. It is recommended internally for hypotonic circulatory regulation disorders and catarrhal diseases of the respiratory system. Camphor preparations should not be used in the facial regions of infants and small children, especially in the nasal area. A dosage of 10-20 % is recommended in semisolid preparations and 1-10% in camphor spirit.[8]

Please note that the American Association of Poisons Control Center states that camphor-containing products cannot exceed 11% camphor.[9]

Food, perfumery and flavouring

White camphor is often fractionated, producing minor components that are used in formulating synthetic perfumes. The pinene fraction is a base material for synthesis of terpineol and borneol.[2]

Other uses

Weiss states that the introduction of synthetic camphor has diminished the importance of camphor essential oil obtained from the distillation of the wood of *C. camphora*.[1]

Fractions of white camphor are used for the perfuming of detergents and low-cost household products, disinfectants and insecticides.[2]

Synthetic camphor is prepared from turpentine oil. The action of hydrogen chloride on pinene is converted into bornyl chloride, which on treatment with sodium acetate, yields isobornyl acetate. Hydrolysis of this to isoborneol and subsequent oxidation gives camphor.[10]

Therapeutics

Pharmacology and clinical studies

Antifungal activity

An in vitro study found that camphor oil has moderately effective antifungal activity against *Candida albicans*.[11] Camphor oil was found to have broad-spectrum antifungal activity against *Aspergillus flavus*.[12]

Antimicrobial activity

An in vitro study found that camphor essential

oil was more effective in inhibiting methicillin-resistant *Staphylococcus aureus* (MRSA) and methicillin-sensitive *Staphylococcus aureus* (MSSA) growth than vancomycin, which is currently the standard treatment.[13]

Antinociceptive activity

The success of camphor oil as a counterirritant and rubefacient for topical preparations is well documented. It has a mild anaesthetising effect and circumscribed sensation of heat when applied topically.

The analgesic activity of camphor is associated with its capacity of activating TRPV1, a member of the transient receptor channel superfamily, which leads to excitation and desensitisation of sensory nerves. The sensation of heat associated with the topical application of camphor is a consequence of this activation.[14]

It is stated that capsaicin shares the same action with camphor, but performs it more slowly and less completely. However, camphor's efficacy is lower.[14]

Antitussive activity

The antitussive, nasal decongestant and expectorant action of camphor has been well documented and studied. The nasal decongestant activity is associated with the stimulation of cold receptors in the nose. The inhalation of camphor vapour increases the nasal sensation of airflow by the induction of cold sensation in the nose, despite not actually affecting nasal resistance to airflow.[14]

Actions

Actions commonly cited in aromatherapy

Anti-inflammatory, antiseptic, antiviral, bactericidal, diuretic, expectorant, rubefacient, stimulant, vermifuge[7]

Actions supported by clinical studies

Antibacterial, antifungal, antinociceptive, antitussive, expectorant

Comment

Lis-Balchin states that camphor oil is not greatly acknowledged in aromatherapy, considering that camphor oil can be found in many commercial products, that are very effective respiratory and muscular balms. She concludes that there should be no problem with the use of camphor oil when it is used in very low dilutions.[15]

Pure camphor essential oil is difficult to obtain in many parts of the world. If you do intend using camphor, please ensure that it is stored in a container with a child-resistant cap and a restrictive flow device to ensure no accidental ingestion of large doses.

Aromatherapy Uses

Clinical aromatherapy

Musculoskeletal system

White camphor oil is recommended for arthritis, muscular aches and pains, rheumatism and sprains.[7]

Respiratory system

White camphor oil is recommended for the relief of respiratory tract infections such as bronchitis, coughs, colds and flu.[7]

Skin care

White camphor essential oil is recommended for use in skin care for treating acne, inflammations and oily skin problems.[7]

Dosage and Administration

Blending

Aromatherapy

For the relief of arthritis, musculoskeletal aches and pains, consider blending white camphor oil with essential oils such as black pepper, cajeput, 1,8-cineole-rich eucalypts, fir, ginger, kunzea, spike lavender, peppermint, pine, rosemary or tea tree.

For the relief of the symptoms of colds and flu with bronchial congestion, consider blending white camphor oil with essential oils such as cajeput, Atlas cedarwood, 1,8-cineole-rich eucalypts, pine, peppermint, tea tree or thyme.

Perfumery

Camphor oil is not used in perfumery.

Mode of administration

Bath

Full body bath, foot bath

Topical

Compress, massage, ointment, skin care

Inhalation

Direct inhalation, diffuser, oil vaporiser

Safety Profile

General safety

The camphor content of white camphor oil suggests that it may be convulsant and neurotoxic.[5] Lawless states that as long as white camphor essential oil does not contain safrole, it is relatively non-toxic, non-sensitising and non-irritating.[7]

Camphor preparations should not be used in the facial region of infants and small children, especially around the nasal area.[8]

The safrole content of yellow and brown camphor oil indicates that it is carcinogenic and hepatotoxic. Yellow and brown camphor oil should not be used in aromatherapy.[5,7] Brown and yellow camphor are not normally commercially available.[16]

Contraindications

Zuccarini warns us that special care must be taken during pregnancy, due to the fact that camphor crosses the placental barrier. Camphor should be avoided in children who have a history of febrile convulsions or other predisposing factors for convulsions.[14]

Toxicity

The mechanism by which camphor produces toxicity is unknown. However, absorption from the gastrointestinal tract occurs rapidly, and detectable serum concentrations will be found within minutes of ingestion. Within 5 to 15 minutes, patients may complain of mucous membrane irritation, nausea, vomiting and abdominal pain. Generalised tonic-clonic convulsions are also one of the first signs of significant toxicity and can occur soon after ingestion. Headaches, dizziness, confusion, agitation, anxiety, hallucinations, myoclonus and hyperreflexia are also experienced. Death is usually the result of respiratory failure or convulsions.[9]

C

A case has been reported where low dose dermal exposure over many years led to granulomatous hepatitis. Camphor also crosses the placenta. Fetal deaths, as well as uneventful deliveries, have been reported following camphor poisoning in the mother during the later stages of pregnancy.[9]

Most camphor products involving reports of toxicity have been camphorated oil, which is usually 20% camphor in cottonseed oil, or camphor spirits, usually 10% camphor in alcohol.[14]

A case was reported in which one teaspoon of camphorated oil, equivalent to about 1 mL of camphor, was lethal to a 16-month-old child and a 19-month child.[5]

Following a large amount of accidental ingestions by people mistaking camphorated oil for castor oil, the FDA ruled in 1983 that camphorated oil could no longer be sold over the counter (OTC). As a result of this ruling and improvements in the medical management of patients poisoned with camphor, fatal poisonings are now rare. Currently, OTC camphor-containing products cannot exceed 11% camphor. However, cases of severe toxicity and convulsions are still reported to occur even with the lower concentration products that remain on the market.[14]

The main problems associated with camphor toxicity in humans is that camphor-containing products and their perception as unhazardous medicines have been readily available.[14]

Cases of camphor poisoning and intoxication in humans are relatively frequent, mostly due to accidental ingestion. More than 100,000 cases of ingestion exposures to camphor-containing products were recorded between 1990 and 2003, causing a range of symptoms such as convulsions, lethargy, ataxia, severe nausea, vomiting and coma.[14]

Zuccarini explains that almost all the reports of poisoning from camphor-containing products are connected with improper use or accidental ingestion. He states that camphor does not represent a threat when used within indicated doses. He also recommends that camphor, in all its forms as camphorated oil, can be safely used at the recommended doses for topical application.[14]

I would reiterate that it is imperative to ensure that camphorated oil is sold in childproof closures with restrictive flow devices to ensure the risk of accidental ingestion is negligible.

Regulatory guidelines

White camphor oil has GRAS status.

The Council of Europe (1970) included camphor oil in the list of temporarily admissible flavouring substances provided no safrole is present.[17]

Brown camphor is not included in the listings of the FDA.

References

1. Weiss EA. *Essential oil crops*. CAB International, Wallingford, 1997.
2. Arctander S. *Perfume and flavor materials of natural origin*. Allured Publishing, Carol Stream, 1994.
3. Schnaubelt K. *Medical aromatherapy*. Frog, Berkeley, 1999.
4. Lawrence BM. *Essential oils 1979-1980*. Allured Publishing, Wheaton, 1981.
5. Tisserand R, Balacs T. *Essential oil safety*. Churchill Livingstone, Edinburgh, 1995.
6. Schmidt E, Wanner J. *Adulteration of essential oils*. In Baser KHC, Buchbauer G. eds. *Handbook of essential oils – science, technology and applications*. 2nd edn. CRC Press, Boca Raton, 2016: 707-745.
7. Lawless J. *The encyclopaedia of essential oils*. Element Books, Shaftesbury, 1992.

8. Blumenthal M et al. *The complete German commission E monographs: therapeutic guide to herbal medicine*. American Botanical Council, Austin, 1998.
9. Manoguerra AS et al. *Camphor poisoning: an evidence-based practice guideline for out-of-hospital management*. Clinical Toxicology; 2006; 44(4): 357-370. doi: 10.1080/15563650600671696
10. Evans WC. *Trease and Evans pharmacognosy*. 15th edn. WB Saunders, Edinburgh, 2002.
11. Devkatte AN et al. *Potential of plant oils as inhibitors of Candida albicans growth*. FEMS Yeast Research, 2005; 5(9): 867-873. Cited in Quintessential Aromatics database, 2013.
12. Mishra AK et al. *Fungistatic properties of essential oil of Cinnamomum camphora*. International Journal of Pharmacognosy, 1991; 29(4): 259-262. Cited in Quintessential Aromatics database, 2013.
13. Sharma PR et al. *Ten highly effective essential oils inhibit growth of methicillin resistant Staphylococcus aureus (MRSA) and methicillin sensitive Staphylococcus aureus (MSSA)*. International Journal of Pharmacy and Pharmaceutical Sciences, 2013; 5(1): 52-54. Cited in Quintessential Aromatics database, 2013.
14. Zuccarini P. *Camphor: risks and benefits of a widely used natural product*. Journal of Applied Science and Environmental Management, 2009; 13(2): 69-74.
15. Lis-Balchin M. *Aromatherapy science – a guide for healthcare professionals*. Pharmaceutical Press, London, 2006.
16. Tisserand R, Young R. *Essential oil safety*. 2nd edn. Churchill Livingstone, Edinburgh, 2014.
17. Opdyke DLJ. *Monographs on fragrance raw materials*. Pergamon Press, Oxford, 1979.

Caraway seed

Identification

Botanical name

Carum carvi L.

Family

Apiaceae (Umbelliferae)

Botany and origins

Caraway is a delicate biennial which grows to 60 cm high, with pale-green, finely defined leaves on hollow stems bearing white umbel-shaped flowers.[1] The plant is native to Europe and western Asia. Caraway is cultivated in The Netherlands, Denmark, Poland, Russia, Hungary, Germany, England, Spain, Tunisia, India and Pakistan.[2]

Method of extraction

The oil is steam-distilled from the dried, crushed ripe seeds.

Characteristics

Caraway seed oil is a pale yellow to brownish, mobile liquid with an intensely spicy odour reminiscent of caraway seeds.[2]

Chemical composition

Eighteen compounds, comprising more than 97% of the composition of the oil, have been identified in caraway essential oil.[3]

The chemical composition of caraway seed oil was reported as follows:

myrcene (0.4%), limonene (43.9-45.7%), dihydrocarvone (0.2-0.5%), carvone (51.9-53.9%), dihydrocarveol (0.6-1.2%), carveol (0.2-0.7%).[4]

According to the European Pharmacopeia, caraway seed oil should contain β-myrcene (0.1 to 1%), limonene (30 to 45%), carvone (50 to 65%) and a maximum of 2.5% each of *trans*-dihydrocarvone and *trans*-carveol.[5]

Adulteration

Adulteration of caraway seed oils occurs with the addition of synthetic *d*-carvone and *d*-limonene. Arctander states that adulteration can take place with caraway chaff oil, which is distilled from the waste materials from the threshing of the caraway seeds. He explains that this oil contains more terpenes and less carvone.[2]

Pharmacopoeias and standards

The purity, composition and physico-chemical properties of caraway seed oil are defined in ISO 8896: 2016 Essential Oil of Caraway.

Both essential oil and the fruit are the subjects of an assessment report for the European Medicines Agency and the German Commission E.

History and Traditional Uses

History

Caraway was one of the earliest cultivated herbs in Asia, Africa and Europe. The medicinal use of caraway seeds has been widespread in several ethnomedical systems from Northern Europe to the Mediterranean regions, Russia, Iran, India, Indonesia and North America.[4]

Caraway is acknowledged as one of the world's oldest spices, with evidence of the seeds having been found in the remains of food dating back to 3000 BC in the Mesolithic era. The ancient Egyptians buried their dead with it. The early Greeks and Romans valued it for both medicinal and culinary purposes. The name is said to come from a former province in Asia Minor called Caria.[1]

Caraway has been called by different names, mainly derived from the Latin *cuminum* and the Greek *karon*, which was adapted into Latin as *carum*. The Sanskrit term for caraway is *karavi*. The English term caraway dates back to at least 1440 and is believed to be of Arabic origin – *al-karawaya*.[3]

Caraway seeds were commonly used in the Middle Ages as an aid to digestion by adding them to bread, cakes and baked fruit.[1]

Traditional medicine

Aqueous extracts of caraway have been used in traditional medicine as an aperitif, tranquilliser, carminative, diuretic, emmenagogue, galactagogue, spasmolytic, gastric stimulant and aphrodisiac. In Ayurveda, it is used for treating stomach ailment, diarrhoea and dysentery.[3]

C

Herbal

It has traditionally been used for dyspepsia, intestinal colic, menstrual cramps, poor appetite and bronchitis.[6] It is listed in the British Herbal Pharmacopoeia for the promotion of breast milk and for flatulent colic in children.[7]

Both the essential oil and the fruit are listed in the German Commission E for the treatment of dyspeptic problems such as mild spastic conditions of the gastrointestinal tract, bloating and fullness.[8]

Food, perfumery and flavouring

The oil is also used as a fragrant component to toothpaste, mouthwash products, cosmetics and perfumes.[6,9] The seeds are still extensively used as a domestic spice, especially in bread, cakes and cheeses.[6]

Therapeutics

Pharmacology and clinical studies

Many pharmacological studies involving caraway seed oil have been published. A systemic review of these studies will not be attempted. Rather, I have chosen a selection of studies that support the traditional and clinical uses.

Anticarcinogenic activity

A study investigating the effect of caraway seed oil on colon carcinogenesis induced by 1,2-dimethylhydrazine (DMH) in rats concluded that caraway seed oil inhibited colon lesions, mediated by interference of caraway seed oil components in the activities of the main hepatic xenobiotic metabolising enzymes.[10]

Studies have indicated that carvone may have chemopreventative activity. In one study, carvone induced an increase in the activity of the detoxifying enzyme glutathione S-transferase (GST). Compounds that increase GST detoxification are considered potential inhibitors of carcinogenesis.[11]

Anticolitic activity

A study investigated the effects of caraway seed oil in an immunological model of colitis in rats induced by trinitrobenzene sulfonic acid. The oil was administered orally and intraperitoneally. The result confirmed that caraway seed oil was effective and possessed anticolitic activity irrespective of the dose and route of administration.[12]

Antimicrobial activity

Antimicrobial activity in vitro has been reported for caraway seed oil.[5] Caraway seed oil exhibited medium antimicrobial activity and carvone was recognized as one of the active components.[13]

Caraway seed oil is reported to exhibit good inhibitory antimicrobial activity against *Staphylococcus aureus, Escherichia coli, Salmonella typhi, Shigella dysenteriae* and *Vibrio cholerae*.[14]

Antioxidant activity

An in vivo study of the antioxidant activity of caraway seed oil confirmed that the oil strongly inhibited lipid peroxidation.[15]

Antispasmodic activity

A fixed combination of peppermint and caraway seed oil taken orally in capsule form was found to be effective as an antispasmodic. The combination is commercially available as an enteric-coated capsule. It was evaluated in a randomised, placebo-controlled, double-blind clinical trial. The results concluded that the oil combination had a demonstrated efficacy, with a significant reduction in symptoms of patients suffering from functional dyspepsia.[16] Another controlled crossover study confirmed that this same combination of peppermint and caraway seed oil caused smooth muscle relaxation.[17]

Antiulcerogenic activity

Caraway seed oil demonstrated antibacterial activity against gram-negative bacterium

Helicobacter pylori and its clinical isolates. *H. pylori* is recognised as the primary etiological factor associated with the development of gastric and peptic ulcer disease, along with chronic gastritis.[18]

Insecticidal activity

A study confirmed that caraway seed oil was insecticidal to house flies. It was concluded that essential oils should be considered in the use of pro-ecological preparations against insects.[19]

Actions

Actions commonly cited in aromatherapy

Antimicrobial, antiseptic, antispasmodic, astringent, carminative, digestive, diuretic, emmenagogue, expectorant, galactagogue, spasmolytic, stimulant, stomachic, tonic, vermifuge[9,20,21]

Actions supported by clinical studies

Antimicrobial, carminative, digestive, spasmolytic

Comment

Many of the uses mentioned by aromatherapists for caraway seed oil are taken directly from herbal uses. In several European pharmacopoeias, caraway fruit and the essential oil have been described as having carminative and spasmolytic properties. The European Medicines Agency assessment report recommends both the fruit and oil for the symptomatic relief of digestive disorders such as bloating and flatulence. The essential oil is recommended for topical application on the abdominal area at a 2% dilution.[5]

Aromatherapy Uses

Clinical aromatherapy

Digestive system

Caraway seed oil is principally used as a carminative and stomachic. It has a calming effect on stomach disorders and is recommended to settle the digestion and stimulate the appetite. It provides relief from diarrhoea and general bowel complaints.[6,9]

Energetics, psyche and subtle uses

Energetics

Mojay explains that caraway seed oil promotes the flow of *Qi* to the *Stomach*. He describes caraway seed oil as *hot*, sweet and invigorating. This helps to strengthen the *Yang Qi* of the *Spleen*, which helps support the *Spleen*'s energetic function of transformation and helping to eliminate *damp*. This means that caraway seed oil is indicated for abdominal distention, indigestion, nausea and flatulence.[20]

According to the principles of the Five Elements, caraway seed oil strengthens the Earth Element. Mojay recommends it to stay balanced and centred. It helps convey a feeling of confidence.[20]

According to the principles of Ayurveda, caraway would help balance excess *Kapha* dosha and stimulate *Pitta* dosha.

Subtle

Mojay explains that caraway seed oil is ideal for individuals who have been brought up in unstable emotional environments:

> *Though he or she may seek, as a sentimental ideal, the stability they were denied when young, the memories of a fluctuating childhood remain with them unconsciously, and find expression whenever emotional intimacy demands commitment. Their tendency is to shy away from such situations.*[20]

Caraway seed oil is needed whenever a restless search for quick and easy solutions threatens to undermine our steadiness and firm resolve.[20]

Dosage and Administration

Blending

Aromatherapy

Caraway seed oil is not commonly used in aromatherapy; however, the German Commission E provides approved combinations of caraway seed oil blended with aniseed oil and fennel oil for the treatment of dyspepsia. Another blend recommended for dyspepsia is caraway seed oil with peppermint oil.[8]

For the relief of indigestion and dyspepsia, consider blending caraway seed oil with essential oils such as aniseed, basil, coriander seed, sweet fennel, ginger, sweet orange, peppermint, rosemary or turmeric.

Perfumery

Arctander states that caraway oil is not commonly used in perfumery blending; however, it blends well with cassia for a soap perfume. He suggests that minute quantities of caraway seed oil may be added to jasmine bases and tabac bases.[2]

Mode of administration

Bath

Full body bath, foot bath

Topical

Compress, massage, ointment

Inhalation

Direct inhalation, diffuser, oil vaporiser

Ingestion

Caraway seed oil capsules are used in the

treatment of gastrointestinal complaints, often in conjunction with peppermint oil.[22]

The German Commission E suggests using 3-6 drops of the caraway seed oil internally for the treatment of dyspeptic problems such as mild spastic conditions of the gastrointestinal tract, flatulence, bloating and fullness.[8]

Safety Profile

General safety

Caraway seed oil is non-toxic and non-sensitising; however, it may cause dermal irritation in concentration. While the IFRA standard for carvone in leave-on products is 1.2%, Tisserand & Young state that caraway seed oil requires no restriction.[22]

Contraindications

No contraindications known; however, individuals with known sensitivities and allergies to plants from the Apiaceae family should avoid the use of caraway seed oil.[5]

Regulatory guidelines

Caraway seed oil has GRAS status.

References

1. Hemphill I. *Spice notes.* Pan MacMillan, Sydney, 2000.
2. Arctander S. *Perfume and flavor materials of natural origin.* Allured Publishing, Carol Stream, 1994.
3. Rasooli I, Allameh A. *Caraway (Carum carvi L.) essential oils.* In Preedy VR. ed. *Essential oils in food preservation, flavor and safety.* Academic Press, London, 2016: 287-293.
4. Lawrence BM. *Essential oils 1981-1987.* Allured Publishing, Wheaton, 1989.
5. Committee on Herbal Medicinal Products (HMPC). *Assessment report on Carum carvi L. fructus and Carum carvi L. aetheroleum.* European Medicines Agency, London, 2014. Doc ref. EMA/HMPC715093/2013.
6. Khan I, Abourashed E. *Leung's encyclopedia of common natural ingredients used in food, drugs and cosmetics.* 3rd edn. John Wiley & Sons, New Jersey, 2010.
7. *British herbal pharmacopoeia.* British Herbal Medicine Association, Bournemouth, 1983.
8. Blumenthal M et al. *The complete German commission E monographs: therapeutic guide to herbal medicine.* American Botanical Council, Austin, 1998.
9. Lawless J. *The encyclopaedia of essential oils.* Element Books, Shaftesbury, 1992.
10. Dadkhah A et al. *Inhibitory effects of dietary caraway essential oils on 1,2-dimethylhydrazine-induced colon carcinogenesis is mediated by liver xenobiotic metabolising enzymes.* Nutrition and Cancer, 2011; 63(1): 46-54. Cited in Quintessential Aromatics database, 2013.
11. Zheng GG et al. *Anethofuran, carvone and limonene: potential cancer chemoprotective agents from dill weed oil and caraway oil.* Planta Medica, 1992; 58(4): 338-341. Cited in Quintessential Aromatics database, 2013.
12. Keshavarz A et al. *Effects of Carum carvi L. (caraway) extract and essential oil on TNBS-induced colitis in rats.* Research in Pharmaceutical Sciences, 2013; 8(1): 1-8. Retrieved Sep 9, 2017, from https://www.ncbi.nlm.nih.gov/pmc/articles/PMC3895295/
13. Seidler-Lozykowaka K et al. *Microbiological activity of caraway (Carum carvi L.) essential oil obtained from different origins.* Acta Scientiarum. Agronomy, 2013; 35(4): 495-500.
14. Syed M et al. *Antimicrobial activity of the essential oils of the Umbelliferae family, Part V. Carum carvi, Petroselinum crispum and Dorema ammoniacum oils.* Pakistan Journal of Science & Industrial Research, 1987; 30(2): 106-109. Cited in Quintessential Aromatics database, 2013.
15. Samojlik I et al. *Antioxidant and hepatoprotective potential of essential oils of coriander (Coriandrum sativum L.) and caraway (Carum carvi L.) (Apiaceae).* Journal of Agricultural and Food Chemistry, 2010; 58(15): 8848-8853. Cited in Quintessential Aromatics database, 2013.
16. Holtmann G et al. *Effect of a fixed combination of peppermint oil and caraway oil on symptoms of quality of life in patients suffering from functional dyspepsia.* Phytomedicine, 2003; 10 (Suppl 4): 56-57. Cited in Quintessential Aromatics database, 2013.
17. Micklefield et al. *Effect of peppermint oil and caraway oil on gastroduodenal motility.* Phytotherapy Research, 2000; 14(1): 20-23. Cited in Quintessential Aromatics database, 2013.
18. Johri RK. *Cuminum cyminum and Carum carvi: an update.* Pharmacognosy Reviews, 2011; 5(9): 63-72. Retrieved Sep 9, 2017, from https://www.ncbi.nlm.nih.gov/pmc/articles/PMC3210012/
19. Gora J et al. *The possibilities of essential oils utilisation for the limitation of some insect populations or their repellency.* Programme Abstracts – 24th International Symposium on Essential Oils, 1993. Cited in Quintessential Aromatics database, 2013.
20. Mojay G. *Aromatherapy for healing the spirit.* Healing Arts Press, Rochester, 1999.
21. Lavabre M. *Aromatherapy workbook.* Healing Arts Press, Rochester, 1997.
22. Tisserand R, Young R. *Essential oil safety.* 2nd edn. Churchill Livingstone, Edinburgh, 2014.

C

Cardamom

Identification

Botanical name

Elettaria cardamomum (L.) Maton

Synonyms

Green cardamom, small cardamom

Family

Zingiberaceae

Botany and origins

Cardamom is a perennial herb with lance-shaped leaves borne on long sheathing stems, up to 4 m high. It is native to tropical Asia and is now cultivated in Sri Lanka, India, Guatemala and El Salvador.[1] Guatemala is the largest producer of cardamom in the world, followed by India.[2]

The parts used are the dried, nearly ripe fruits with seeds. The small black seeds of cardamom are embedded in a thin papery outer shell or pod. They have a pleasant aroma and a characteristic, slightly pungent taste.[2]

Numerous varieties of cardamom grow in the world and are cultivated in Madagascar, east and west Africa, Central Africa, China, Thailand and Indonesia. However, these have little or no importance as a source of essential oil.[3]

Method of extraction

Cardamom oil is produced by the steam distillation of the seeds of *E. cardamomum*. The seeds are enclosed in husks and should not be removed from the almost odourless hulls until prior to distillation.[3]

Characteristics

Cardamom oil is an almost colourless or pale yellow liquid, which darkens when exposed to sunlight. The odour of cardamom is warm-spicy, with a slightly penetrating camphoraceous-cineole-like odour. It becomes balsamic-woody with a sweet and almost floral dryout.[3]

Essential oil produced from the 'green' types of cardamom smells more of cineole than the oil produced from the bleached or pale yellow coloured cardamom seeds.[3]

Chemical composition

The chemical composition of cardamom oil was reported as follows:

α-pinene (1.5%), β-pinene (0.2%), sabinene (2.8%), myrcene (1.6%), α-phellandrene (0.2%), limonene (11.6%), 1,8-cineole (36.3%), γ-terpinolene (0.5%), linalool (3.0%), linalyl acetate (2.5%), terpinen-4-ol (0.9%), α-terpineol (2.6%), α-terpinyl acetate (31.3%), citronellol (0.3%), nerol (0.5%), geraniol (0.5%), methyl eugenol (0.2%), *trans*-nerolidol (2.7%).[4]

The composition of cardamom oil from south India is mainly α-terpinyl acetate (56.7%), 1,8-cineole (15.13%), α-terpineol (4.67%) and limonene (4.05%).[2]

The major components that impart the sweet flavour to the oil are α-terpinyl acetate, geranyl acetate, nerol and α-terpineol, while 1,8-cineole imparts the harsh medicinal aroma.[2]

Adulteration

Arctander states that adulteration of cardamom oil takes place on a big scale. 1,8-cineole from eucalyptus or camphor oil is often used to adulterate cardamom oil.[3] Adulteration is also done by the addition of α-terpinyl acetate and linalool.[5]

Pharmacopoeias and standards

The purity, composition and physico-chemical properties of cardamom essential oil are defined in ISO 4733:2004 Oil of Cardamom [*Elettaria cardamomum* (L.) Maton].

History and Traditional Uses

History

Cardamom is reputed to be one of the oldest spices known. Hemphill states that the Greek word *kardamomum* was used to describe the superior grade, and the ancient Semitic word *amomum* is a term used to describe 'very spicy'. In the first century AD it had become one of the most popular oriental spices in the Roman cuisine.[6]

Cardamom is valued as one of the most expensive spices in the world after saffron and vanilla due to its unique flavour and aroma. It was one of the most important spices traded between ancient civilisations throughout western Asia (Middle East) to ancient Egypt, Greece and Rome.[2]

According to Mojay, the name *cardamom* is thought to have originated from the Arab word *hehmama*, a derivation of the Sanskrit term for something hot and pungent. The seeds have remained an important culinary spice not only in India but all over the world.[7]

Despite having many uses as a spice and traditional medicine in India, about 60% of the world's cardamom is exported to the Middle

East where cardamom is mainly used in coffee preparation.[2]

Traditional medicine

Cardamom has been used in Ayurveda for over 3,000 years.[2] It was brought to Europe by the Greeks in the fourth century BC.[1]

Greek physicians used cardamom for the treatment of coughs, abdominal pain, spasms and sciatica. In the Greco-Arab (Unani) system of traditional medicine, cardamom is considered a powerful stimulant, carminative, stomachic and diuretic.[2]

Cardamom is a well-known remedy to treat impotence and improve low sexual response.[2]

Herbal

The German Commission E recommends cardamom seeds for the treatment of dyspepsia.[8]

Food, perfumery and flavouring

The spice is an important ingredient in genuine East Indian curry powder. Cardamom oil is also used in the canning industry for pickles, meat sauces and seasoning. Cardamom is used as a flavouring ingredient in the popular Indian tea known as chai.[1]

Saudi Arabia has the highest per capita consumption of cardamom, where the spice is used in the preparation of *gahwa*, a blend of cardamom seed powder and coffee with a ratio varying between 30:70 to 50:50 (w/w). It is also very popular in other Arab countries such as Kuwait, Oman and Qatar.[2]

C

Therapeutics

Pharmacology and clinical studies

Many pharmacological studies involving cardamom essential oil have been published. A systemic review of these studies will not be attempted. Rather I have chosen a selection of studies that support the traditional and clinical uses.

Analgesic activity

Cardamom oil was found to have significant analgesic activity, and had a suppressive action on carrageenan-induced oedema in animal studies, exerting its effect by reducing the synthesis of eicosanoid mediators of inflammation.[9]

Antiemetic activity

A randomised study was conducted with patients who experienced nausea in the postanaesthesia care unit using ginger essential oil; a blend of essential oils of ginger, spearmint, peppermint and cardamom; and isopropyl alcohol. The study confirmed that postoperative nausea was significantly reduced with inhalation of ginger oil and the blend of essential oils. It was suggested that aromatherapy could be used as an inexpensive and non-invasive treatment for postoperative nausea.[10]

A clinical trial using an inhalation of a blend of ginger, cardamom and tarragon essential oils in equal parts investigated whether the negative effects of anaesthesia could be alleviated. The results found that 75% of cases had a favourable outcome by completely blocking nausea or vomiting within 30 minutes.[11]

Antifungal activity

An in vitro test confirmed that cardamom essential oil had considerable antifungal effect against seven pathogenic moulds.[12]

Antimicrobial activity

An in vitro test confirmed that cardamom essential oil had moderate antimicrobial effect against a range of gram-positive, gram-negative and pathogenic bacteria.[13]

Other studies have confirmed that cardamom essential oil displayed strong antibacterial activity against microorganisms such as *Listeria monocytogenes, Staphylococcus aureus, Escherichia coli, Yersinia entercolitica, Pseudomonas aeruginosa, Lactobacillus plantarum, Aspergillus niger, Geotrichum candidum* and *Rhodotorula*.[2]

An in vitro study investigated the effects of cardamom essential oil and antibiotics against methicillin-resistant *S. aureus*. Antagonistic interactions were noted, particularly with 1,8-cineole. The researchers suggested that using 1,8-cineole-rich oils could diminish the antibacterial activity of amoxicillin or ciprofloxacin in infections with *S. aureus* isolate.[14]

Antispasmodic activity

Cardamom oil has been reported to have antispasmodic activity on excised mouse intestine.[1]

Gastroprotective activity

Cardamom oil significantly inhibited gastric lesions induced by ethanol and aspirin, but not those induced by pylorus ligation in rats.[15]

Hepatoprotective activity

The influence of essential oils on the activity of the hepatic carcinogen-metabolising enzymes of P-450, aryl hydrocarbon hydroxylase and GST was investigated in mice. Cardamom essential oil significantly elevated GST activity. It was suggested that cardamom oil has potential as a 'blocking agent' in chemoprotective strategies.

Cardamom oil also elevated hepatic levels of acid-soluble sulphydryl, which augmented the antioxidant defence mechanism.[16]

Insecticidal activity

At a concentration of 1000 ppm, four essential oils — coriander seed, cardamom, rosemary and sandalwood — had insecticidal activity ranging from 68% to 98% at 1 hour after treatment.[17]

Skin permeation enhancer

The effects of the cardamom oil as a penetration enhancer on percutaneous absorption was investigated using three drugs – indomethacin, piroxicam and diclofenac. The penetration index of piroxicam was extremely increased by a 1% solution of cardamom oil. The researchers confirmed that the skin permeation enhancing effects of cardamom was dependent on the kind of drug, pH value of the solvent system and the concentration of cardamom oil.[18]

Actions

Actions commonly cited in aromatherapy

Antiseptic, antispasmodic, carminative, cephalic, digestive, diuretic, expectorant, general tonic, stimulant, stomachic[7,19]

Actions supported by clinical studies

Antimicrobial, antispasmodic, digestive, hepato-protective, stomachic

Comment

Review of traditional uses and clinical data support the use of cardamom oil for the relief of indigestion and symptomatic treatment of nausea and vomiting.

Aromatherapy Uses

Clinical aromatherapy

Digestive system

Cardamom is recommended for the treatment of digestive complaints such as colic, cramps, dyspepsia and flatulence.[19,20,21]

Schnaubelt explains that cardamom oil contains the acetylcholine antagonist borneol, which is important in disrupting the pathways that trigger nausea and vomiting. He explains that it also prevents the formation of intestinal gas, reduces pain, and that it has a relaxing effect on a spasmodic colon and can help alleviate painful diarrhoea.[22]

Nervous system

Cardamom oil has been described as a cephalic and a gentle tonic of the nervous system.[7] It is also recommended for nervous exhaustion and depression.[20]

Respiratory system

Cardamom oil is recommended for catarrhal conditions of the respiratory system such as chronic bronchitis.[20]

Skin care

Cardamom is generally not used in skin care.

Energetics, psyche and subtle uses

Energetics

Cardamom oil is a *Qi* tonic. It has a *warming* quality, which makes it an excellent choice as a digestive stimulant and as a remedy for mucolytic *damp* catarrhal conditions of the respiratory and digestive system.[7]

Cardamom oil strengthens *Spleen Qi*, the main organ responsible for transforming food and drinks into *Qi* and *Blood*. Cardamom oil is recommended whenever there is a *Spleen Qi deficiency*. Typical symptoms associated with *Spleen Qi deficiency* include feelings of lethargy, poor appetite and loose stool.[7]

According to the principles of the Five Elements, cardamom is indicated for problems associated with the Earth Element. The external pathogenic factor that weakens the Earth Element is *damp*. *Excess damp* leads to lethargy, indigestion, abdominal distention and worry. Cardamom's *warming* property helps to expel *dampness*. The spirit associated with the Earth Element is the *Yi*, which is associated with our intellect and ability to think clearly.

Cardamom oil is ideal for individuals with poor concentration, overthinking and burdened by worries.[7]

Personality

The cardamom personality is strong, forthright, motivating and enthusiastic; they instill inspiration in others and tend to make good leaders.[23]

Worwood states that cardamom personality types often wear an air of detachment most of the time, and that nothing seems to worry them. She explains that they are good in leadership roles, provided that they can learn to delegate. They are often good teachers. While they are not creative, they have the stamina to carry ideas forward. As a result, they can achieve much more than a creative personality type.[23]

According to Myers-Briggs personality types, the cardamom personality is likely to be an ESTJ. ESTJs love responsibility and control. They love to be in charge. They are good at making objective decisions. They love challenges and know how to get things done. They have an opinion for everything and are rarely at a loss for words. ESTJs like to spend their free time in ways that are productive. They are good at seeing what is illogical, inconsistent and impractical. They are willing to make sacrifices in order to honour their commitments. They tend to be workaholics and drive themselves and others very hard. They like to be involved in community service organisations and volunteer activities. They enjoy spending time with their friends and family.

Subtle

Worwood recommends cardamom whenever we need clarity, motivation, focus, courage and confidence. She explains that cardamom oil gives us wisdom when we are overburdened with responsibilities. She suggests that we use it to give us strength and encouragement whenever we need to offer our friendship to a person in need. It is ideal when we are burdened by worries and responsibilities that test our endurance.[24]

Keim Loughran & Bull state that cardamom oil helps us to accept life as it is while encouraging an enthusiasm for it. They also recommend using it to help teach others with a grounded, clear, heart-centred perspective.[25]

Mojay states that cardamom oil helps to restore our 'appetite for life'.[7] Worwood states that cardamom gives us wisdom when we are overburdened with responsibilities, and when we need to tap into our generosity of spirit to allow our hearts to be open and expansive in order to be gracious in our dealings with others.[24]

C

Dosage and Administration

Blending

Aromatherapy

For mental fatigue and dispelling worrying thoughts, consider blending cardamom oil with essential oils such as bergamot, black pepper, ginger, frankincense, lemon, sweet orange or rosemary.

To alleviate nausea and vomiting, consider blending cardamom oil with essential oils such as ginger, peppermint or spearmint.

To alleviate mucous congestion of the respiratory system, consider blending cardamom oil with essential oils such as aniseed, peppermint eucalyptus, 1,8-cineole-rich eucalypts, Atlas cedarwood, sweet fennel, fragonia, frankincense, ginger, lemon, myrtle, niaouli, pine or thyme.

Perfumery

In perfumery, cardamom oil imparts a warm, sweet spicy note which complements floral bases. Cardamom oil blends well with bergamot, frankincense, ylang ylang and labdanum. Arctander states that coriander seed oil is an excellent modifier for cardamom oil in perfumery, and that this combination imparts warmth in oriental style and chypre perfumes.[3]

Mode of administration

Bath

Full body bath, foot bath

Topical

Compress, massage, ointment

Inhalation

Direct inhalation, diffuser, oil vaporiser

Safety Profile

General safety

Cardamom oil is non-toxic, non-irritant and non-sensitising.[19,26]

Contraindications

No contraindications known.

Regulatory guidelines

Cardamom essential oil has GRAS status.

References

1. Khan I, Abourashed E. *Leung's encyclopedia of common natural ingredients used in food, drugs and cosmetics*. 3rd edn. John Wiley & Sons, New Jersey, 2010.
2. Anwar F et al. *Cardamom (Elettaria cardamomum Maton) oils*. In Preedy VR. ed. *Essential oils in food preservation, flavor and safety*. Academic Press, London, 2016: 295-301.
3. Arctander S. *Perfume and flavor materials of natural origin*. Allured Publishing, Carol Stream, 1994.
4. Lawrence BM. *Essential oils 1976-1978*. Allured Publishing, Wheaton, 1979.
5. Schmidt E, Wanner J. *Adulteration of essential oils*. In Baser KHC, Buchbauer G. eds. *Handbook of essential oils – science, technology and applications*. 2nd edn. CRC Press, Boca Raton, 2016: 707-745.
6. Hemphill I. *Spice notes*. Pan Macmillan Australia, Sydney, 2000.
7. Mojay G. *Aromatherapy for healing the spirit*. Healing Arts Press, Rochester, 1999.
8. Blumenthal M. et al. *The complete German commission E monographs: therapeutic guide to herbal medicine*. American Botanical Council, Austin, 1998.
9. Al-Zuhair H, El-Sayeh B, Ammen HA, Al-

Shoora H. *Pharmacological studies of cardamom oil in animals*. Pharmacological Research, 1996; 34(1/2): 79-82. Cited in the Aromatherapy Database, by Bob Harris, Essential Oil Resource Consultants, UK, 2000.
10. Hunt R et al. *Aromatherapy as treatment for postoperative nausea: a randomized trial*. Anesthesia and Analgesia, 2013; 117(3): 597-604. Cited in Quintessential Aromatics database, 2013.
11. De Pradier E. *A trial of a mixture of three essential oils in the treatment of postoperative nausea and vomiting*. International Journal of Aromatherapy, 2006; 16(1): 15-20. Cited in Quintessential Aromatics database, 2013.
12. Badei AZM. *Antimycotic effect of cardamom essential oil against mycotoxigenic moulds in relation to its chemical composition*. Chemie, Mikrobiologie, Technologie der Lebensmittel, 1992; 14: 177-182. Cited in Quintessential Aromatics database, 2013.
13. Badei AZM et al. *Evaluation of chemical, physical and antimicrobial properties of cardamom essential oil*. Bulletin of the Faculty of Agriculture, University of Cairo, 1991; 42(1): 183-198. Cited in Quintessential Aromatics database, 2013.
14. Gradinaru AC et al. *Interactions between cardamom essential oil and conventional antibiotics against Staphylococcus aureus clinical isolates*. Farmacia, 2014; 62(2): 1214-1222. Cited in Quintessential Aromatics database, 2013.
15. Jamal A et al. *Gastroprotective effect of cardamom, Elettaria cardamomum Maton, fruits in rats*. Journal of Ethnopharmacology, 2006; 103(2): 149-153. Cited in Quintessential Aromatics database, 2013.
16. Banerjee S et al. *Influence of certain essential oils on carcinogen-metabolising enzymes and acid-soluble sulphydryls in mouse liver*. Nutrition and Cancer, 1994; 21(3): 263-269. Cited in Quintessential Aromatics database, 2013.
17. Kang S et al. *Spray adulticidal effects of plant oils against house mosquito, Culex pipiens pallens (Diptera: Culicidae)*. Journal of Pesticide Science, 2009; 34(2): 100-106. Cited in Quintessential Aromatics database, 2013.
18. Huang YB et al. *Cardamom oil as a skin permeation enhancer for indomethacin, piroxicam and diclofenac*. International Journal of Pharmaceutics, 1995; 126(1/2): 111-117. Cited in Quintessential Aromatics database, 2013.
19. Lawless J. *The encyclopaedia of essential oils*. Element Books, Shaftesbury, 1992.
20. Holmes P. *The energetics of Western herbs – Vol. I*. Artemis Press, Boulder, 1989.
21. Lavabre M. *Aromatherapy workbook*. Healing Arts Press, Rochester, 1997.
22. Schnaubelt K. *The healing intelligence of essential oils*. Healing Arts Press, Rochester, 2011.
23. Worwood VA. *The fragrant mind*. Transworld Publishers, London, 1995.
24. Worwood VA. *The fragrant heavens*. Transworld Publishers, London, 1999.
25. Keim Loughran J, Bull R. *Aromatherapy anointing oils*. Frog, Berkeley, 2001.
26. Tisserand R, Young R. *Essential oil safety*. 2nd edn. Churchill Livingstone, Edinburgh, 2014.

Carrot seed

Identification

Botanical name

Daucus carota L.

Synonyms

Oil of carrot

Family

Apiaceae (Umbelliferae)

Botany and origins

Carrot is an annual or biennial herb with erect multi-branched stems up to 1.5 m high. The common, cultivated carrot has an edible fleshy orange-red taproot.[1] The essential oil is produced in France, The Netherlands and Hungary.[2]

Method of extraction

Carrot seed oil is steam-distilled from the dried seed of the common carrot. A carrot root oil is obtained by solvent extraction of the red fleshy root of the common edible carrot root. It has a high concentration of carotenes.[2] A carrot seed absolute and CO_2 extract are also produced.[3]

Characteristics

Carrot seed oil is a yellow or amber-coloured to pale orange-brown liquid with a peculiar dry-woody, somewhat root-like, earthy odour. The top note is sweet and fresh, but the tenacious undertone and dryout is very heavy, earthy and slightly spicy.[2]

Chemical composition

The chemical composition of carrot seed essential oil cultivated in Turkey was reported as follows:

α-pinene (0.67%), camphene (0.04%), sabinene (0.1%), β-pinene (0.52%), myrcene (0.17%), limonene (0.43%), linalool (0.34%), daucene (8.74%), Z-α-farnesene (0.19%), *trans*-α-bergamotene (2.41%), *epi*-β-santalene (0.15%), (Z,Z)-α-farnesene (5.86%), germacrene D (2.34%), *ar*-curumene (0.23%), β-selinene (2.2%), α-selinene (0.89%), bicyclogermacrene (1.87%), β-bisabolene (1.9%), carotol (66.78%), daucol (0.45%).[4]

Adulteration

Carrot seed oil is often adulterated with *d*-limonene and α-pinene.[2]

Pharmacopoeias and standards

At the time of writing, the purity, composition and physico-chemical properties of carrot seed essential oil are not defined in any pharmacopoeia monograph or standard.

History and Traditional Uses

History

Carrot is better known for its edible root than its essential oil. Most of the historical references refer to the carrot root and not the essential oil from the seed.

Herbal

Carrot seeds are used in herbal medicine as a diuretic and emmenagogue, and for flatulence. In TCM, carrot seeds were used to treat chronic dysentery and as an anthelmintic.[1]

Food, perfumery and flavouring

Carrot seed oil is used as a fragrance component in soaps, detergents, creams, lotions and perfumes. Carrot root oil is used in some sunscreen preparations and as a source of β-carotene and vitamin A.[1]

Therapeutics

Pharmacology and clinical studies

Antibacterial activity

Carrot seed oil inhibits the in vitro growth of *Campylobacter jejuni* and *Helicobacter pylori*. When mice were injected with *H. pylori*, oral administration of the oil cleared the bacteria in 20-30% of cases.[5]

The oil also exhibited a high antimicrobial activity against *Staphylococcus aureus* and *Candida albicans*.[6]

Larvicidal activity

Carrot seed oil exhibited a 100% larval mortality rate at a 0.01% dose.[7] Another study also confirmed the larvicidal activity of carrot seed oil. When used at 0.1mg/mL the larvicidal mortality was greater than 90%.[8]

Actions

Actions commonly cited in aromatherapy

Carminative, cytophylactic, depurative, diuretic, emmenagogue, hepatic, stimulant[9,10]

Actions supported by clinical studies

Antibacterial, larvicidal

Comment

Carrot seed essential oil is often recommended in skin care preparations for its anti-aging properties, and is often referred to as a regenerator of the liver. Unfortunately, there is not much research on carrot seed oil and very little reference to carrot seed oil in traditional herbal literature.

The chemistry of carrot seed oil cannot be compared with that of other seed oils. The main component of carrot seed essential oil is carotol, and its level varies between 40-70%. I would like to see more clinical studies to confirm the benefits of carrot seed essential oil as a hepatoprotective essential oil, and on its use in skin care.

Aromatherapy Uses

Clinical aromatherapy

Detoxification

It is highly regarded for its hepatic, depurative and diuretic properties. Carrot seed oil is an excellent regenerator of liver cells, and should be prescribed after the acute phase of hepatitis, a violent bilious attack, drug poisoning, but not at the critical moment of the pathology. Mailhebiau recommends a blend with rosemary ct. verbenone, lemon and peppermint.[11]

Integumentary system

The excellent depurative property of carrot seed oil means that it can be used to treat eczema, psoriasis and ulcerative conditions of the skin.[11,12,13]

Carrot seed oil is excellent as a cellular regenerator for the skin. It revitalises the hypodermis and is recommended for the treatment of aged skin, dermatitis, skin irritations, skin rashes and wrinkles.[10,11,12] For this purpose, Mailhebiau recommends blending it with lavender and wheatgerm oil.[11]

Skin care

It can be used to improve the complexion of the skin and has been described as one of the strongest revitalising essential oils. It is recommended for dull, pallid, lifeless and tired skin which is tired from environmental stress.[10]

Schnaubelt states it is commonly used in skin care as it has a revitalising effect on skin suffering from lack of tone.[14]

Energetics, psyche and subtle uses

Personality

According to Myers-Briggs personality types, the carrot seed personality is likely to be an ISTP. ISTPs are quiet and they prefer to stand back and observe. They can be difficult to understand and remain a mystery to many people. They are independent and do not like to behave to the rules of society. They appear cool, dispassionate and analytical. They can be very disorganised in things where they have no interest. They dislike supervising or being supervised. They tend to ignore rules, policies and regulations when they can get in the way of results. They tend to remain calm in a crisis. They have little need for talking or socialising. They often have poor interpersonal skills and seem detached or uncaring to those who are not close to them.

Dosage and Administration

Blending

Aromatherapy

For the treatment of psoriasis and eczema, consider blending carrot seed oil with essential oils such as German chamomile, everlasting, lavender or sandalwood.

To use as a liver tonic and regenerator, consider blending carrot seed oil with essential oils such as German chamomile, everlasting, lemon or rosemary ct. verbenone.

Perfumery

Carrot seed oil is used in perfumery for its fatty-woody note. Many oriental style perfumes and modern aldehydic or fantasy type perfumes contain traces of carrot seed oil.[2]

It blends well with citrus oils, spice oils, geranium and wood oils.

Mode of administration

Bath

Full body bath, foot bath

Topical

Compress, massage, ointment, skin care

Inhalation

Direct inhalation, diffuser, oil vaporiser

Ingestion

Schnaubelt says 1 to 3 drops of carrot seed in a glass of water can be taken sporadically as a part of a program of liver regeneration.[12]

Safety Profile

General safety

Carrot seed essential oil is non-toxic, non-irritant and non-sensitising.

Contraindications

Tisserand & Young state that carrot seed essential oil may interfere with gestation, therefore it is contraindicated for pregnancy and during breastfeeding.[15]

Regulatory guidelines

Carrot seed essential oil has GRAS status.

References

1. Khan I, Abourashed E. *Leung's encyclopedia of common natural ingredients used in food, drugs and cosmetics*. 3rd edn. John Wiley & Sons, New Jersey, 2010.
2. Arctander S. *Perfume and flavor materials of natural origin*. Allured Publishing, Carol Stream, 1994.
3. Lis-Balchin M. *Aromatherapy science – a guide for healthcare professionals*. Pharmaceutical Press, London, 2006.
4. Ozcan MM et al. *Chemical composition of carrot seeds (Daucus carota L.) cultivated in Turkey: characterization of the seed oil and essential oil*. Grasas y Aceites, 2007; 58 (4): 359-365.
5. Bergonzelli GE et al. *Essential oils as components of a diet-based approach to management of Helicobacter infection*. Antimicrobial Agents and Chemotherapy, 2003; 47(10): 3240-3246. Cited in Quintessential Aromatics database, 2013
6. Imamu X et al. *Chemical composition and antimicrobial activity of essential oil from Daucus carota sativa seeds*. Chemistry of Natural Compounds, 2007; 43(4): 495-496. Cited in Quintessential Aromatics database, 2013.
7. Sharma RN et al. *Toxicity of natural essential oils to mosquitos Aedes aegypti and Culex fatigans*. Geobios, 1994; 21(3): 162-165. Cited in Quintessential Aromatics database, 2013.
8. Seo SM et al. *Larvicidal and acetylcholine esterase inhibitory activity of Apiaceae plant essential oils and their constituents against Aedes albopictus and formation development*. Journal of Agricultural and Food Chemistry, 2015; 63(45): 9977-9986.
9. Lawless J. *The encyclopaedia of essential oils*. Element Books, Shaftesbury, 1992.
10. Lavabre M. *Aromatherapy workbook*. Healing Arts Press, Rochester, 1997.
11. Malhebiau P. *Portraits in oils*. C.W. Daniel Company, Saffron Walden, 1995.

12. Schnaubelt K. *The healing intelligence of essential oils.* Healing Arts Press, Rochester, 2011.
13. Davis P. *Aromatherapy A-Z.* 2nd edn. The C.W. Daniel Company, Saffron Walden, 1999.
14. Schnaubelt K. *Medical aromatherapy.* Frog, Berkeley, 1999.
15. Tisserand R. Young R, *Essential oil safety.* 2nd edn. Churchill Livingstone, Edinburgh, 2014.

Cassia

Identification

Botanical name

Cinnamomum cassia Blume

Synonyms

Chinese or false cinnamon

Family

Lauraceae

Botany and origins

C. cassia is a large slender tree which grows in the southeastern parts of China, in Vietnam and India. The bark of this tree is referred to all over the world as cinnamon bark or cassia cinnamon; however, we should not confuse this with true cinnamon bark.[1]

Weiss explains that commercial cassia bark and oil are available from various *Cinnamomum* spp. – *C. cassia* (Chinese cassia), *C. burmannii* (Indonesian cassia), and *C. loureiroi* (Vietnamese cassia). He also advises us not to confuse the name cassia with the genus *Cassia*, Caesalpinioideae, from which *Cassia angustifolia* provides us with senna pods.[2]

Method of extraction

Cassia oil is steam-distilled from the leaves or bark of *C. cassia*; however, Arctander states that the bark is often distilled together with the leaves, stalks and twigs and waste material collected from the collection of the bark of the cassia tree.[1]

Characteristics

Arctander describes cassia oil as being very crude. It appears as a dark brown liquid with a strong, spicy, warm and woody-resinous odour, and an intensely sweet and somewhat balsamic undertone.[1]

Chemical composition

The chemical composition of cassia bark oil is reported as follows:

cinnamaldehyde (87%), cinnamyl acetate (0.08%), benzaldehyde (4.73%), linalool (0.13%), chavicol (0.33%).[3]

Adulteration

Cassia is subject to extensive adulteration as several inexpensive synthetic aroma chemicals that have a cinnamon-like aroma are readily available.[1]

Lis-Balchin states that cassia oil is grossly adulterated. Synthetic cinnamaldehyde, which is often added, has phenyl pentadienyl as a by-product at 400-500 ppm, but it can be detected at a 2% adulteration.[4]

Weiss also states that the adulteration of Chinese cassia oil is so frequent that it is doubtful if any substantial amount of pure oil was ever available commercially.[2]

Pharmacopoeias and standards

The purity, composition and physico-chemical properties of cassia essential oil are defined in ISO 3216:1997 Oil of Cassia, Chinese type.

History and Traditional Uses

History

Cassia probably originated in the Assam region of India and reached the Middle East via early Mesopotamian civilisation, whose records on clay tablets indicate considerable knowledge of spices to flavour food as early as 2000 BC. Cassia then made its way to Europe via Egypt and then Greece and Rome. Pliny describes both cassia and cinnamon in his book *Historia Naturalis*.[2]

Cassia bark was first described in China in the fourth century BC *Elegies of Ch'u*, and is again mentioned in the third century as *kui*.[2] The Arabs and Persians knew cassia bark as *darchini*, from *dar* meaning wood or bark and *chin* meaning China.[2]

Herbal

The bark is commonly used in herbal medicine. In TCM it is commonly used as a *Yang* tonic.

Cassia is extensively used as a spice. In Sri Lanka it is used for digestive complaints such as flatulence, dyspepsia, colic, diarrhoea and nausea. The British Herbal Pharmacopoeia recommends powdered cassia bark for flatulence, dyspepsia, colic and nausea.[5]

The German Commission E recommends the powdered bark and the essential oil for loss of appetite, dyspeptic complaints, bloating and flatulence.[6]

Food, perfumery and flavouring

Cassia essential oil is extensively used as a flavouring agent in food and alcoholic beverages. It is also used extensively as a spice.[2]

Therapeutics

Pharmacology and clinical studies

Antimicrobial activity

C. cassia oil was found to have the most effective antimicrobial activity against cultures of *Trichomonas vaginalis* in an in vitro study.[7]

The antibacterial activity of *C. cassia* bark oil and cinnamaldehyde was examined using five intestinal bacterial species isolated from humans. Cinnamaldehyde inhibited *Clostridium perfringens*, *Bacteroides fragilis* and *Bifidobacterium bifidum*; however, it had little or no activity towards *Bifidobacterium longum* or *Lactobacillus acidophilus*. On the other hand, tetracycline and chloramphenicol antibiotics inhibited all the bacteria. The authors concluded that cinnamaldehyde may have beneficial selective action on intestinal flora of the human gut by inhibiting the growth of pathogenic bacteria, but having no effect on the other species.[8]

Cassia oil was found to be one of the most active antibacterial oils against a range of pathogenic bacteria. It has a minimum inhibitory concentration ≤ 0.05% (vol/vol).[9]

C. verum, *C. cassia* and pure cinnamaldehyde were equally effective in inhibiting the growth of various isolates of bacteria, fungi filamentous moulds and dermatophytes.[10]

Cassia oil was more effective in eradicating *Pseudomonas* spp. and *Staphylococcus aureus* biofilms than selected important antibiotics.[11]

Actions

Actions commonly cited in aromatherapy

Antimicrobial, carminative, spasmolytic[12]

Actions supported by clinical studies

Antimicrobial

Comment

Cassia oil is not commonly mentioned in many aromatherapy books. Many aromatherapists recommend that cassia essential oil should not be used in aromatherapy. Lis-Balchin states that this is due to the toxicity of the oil and its adulteration with many sensitisers.[4]

Considering that the chance of cassia oil being adulterated is very high, I prefer that cinnamon bark oil is used instead of cassia oil.

Aromatherapy Uses

Lawless recommends that cassia oil should not be used in aromatherapy.[12]

Dosage and Administration

Blending

Aromatherapy

Cassia oil is not recommended for use in aromatherapy.

Perfumery

Arctander states that cassia oil is rarely used in perfumery.

Mode of administration

Bath

Cassia oil is not recommended for use in aromatherapy.

Massage

Cassia oil is not recommended for use in aromatherapy.

Inhalation

Cassia oil is not recommended for use in aromatherapy.

Safety Profile

General safety

There are numerous reports of allergic reactions to topical application of cassia oil. It contains 75 to 90% cinnamaldehyde. This is the cause of the cassia's potent dermal sensitiser and irritant activity. It is not recommended for use on the skin.

Tisserand & Young caution not to use cassia oil topically on hypersensitive, diseased or damaged skin, or on children under two years of age. Based on the cinnamaldehyde content, a dermal maximum of 0.05% is recommended for cassia leaf or cassia bark oil. Based on this recommendation, I would suggest not using it at all for dermal application.[13]

Contraindications

Cassia oil is contraindicated during pregnancy and breastfeeding.[4,13]

Tisserand & Young caution the oral ingestion of cassia oil for people who are on diabetes medication or anticoagulant medication, have had

C

major surgery or have peptic ulcers, haemophilia and other bleeding disorders.[13]

Regulatory guidelines

Cassia oil has GRAS status.

References

1. Arctander S. *Perfume and flavor materials of natural origin.* Allured Publishing, Carol Stream, 1994.
2. Weiss EA. *Essential oil crops.* CAB International, Wallingford, 1997.
3. Lawrence BM. *Essential oils 1976-1978.* Allured Publishing, Wheaton, 1979.
4. Lis-Balchin M. *Aromatherapy science – a guide for healthcare professionals.* Pharmaceutical Press, London, 2006.
5. *British herbal pharmacopoeia.* British Herbal Medicine Association, Bournemouth, 1983.
6. Blumenthal M et al. *The complete German commission E monographs: therapeutic guide to herbal medicine.* American Botanical Council, Austin, 1998.
7. Viollon C et al. *Antagonistic activities, in vitro, of some essential oils and natural volatile compounds in relation to the growth of Trichomonas vaginalis.* Fitoterapia, 1996: 67(3): 279-281. Cited in Quintessential Aromatics database, 2013.
8. Lee HS, Ahn YJ. *Growth-inhibiting effects of Cinnamomum cassia bark-derived materials on human intestinal bacteria.* Journal of Agricultural and Food Chemistry, 1998; 46(1): 8-12. Cited in Quintessential Aromatics database, 2013.
9. Oussalah M et al. *Inhibitory effects of selected plant essential oils on the growth of four pathogenic bacteria: E.coli 0157:H7, Salmonella typhimurium, Staphylococcus aureus and Listeria monocytogenes.* Food Control, 2007; 18(5): 414-420. Cited in Quintessential Aromatics database, 2013.
10. Ooi LSM et al. *Antimicrobial activities of cinnamon oil and cinnamaldehyde from the Chinese medicinal herb Cinnamomum cassia Blume.* American Journal of Chinese Medicine, 2006; 34(3): 511-522. Cited in Quintessential Aromatics database, 2013.
11. Kavanaugh NL, Ribbeck K. *Selected antimicrobial essential oils eradicate Pseudomonas spp. and Staphylococcus aureus biofilms.* Applied and Environmental Microbiology, 2012; 78(11): 4057-4061. Cited in Quintessential Aromatics database, 2013.
12. Lawless J. *The encyclopaedia of essential oils.* Element Books, Shaftesbury, 1992.
13. Tisserand R, Young R. *Essential oil safety.* 2nd edn. Churchill Livingstone, Edinburgh, 2014.

C

Cedarwood

Identification

Botanical name and family

There are several cedarwood oils with different physical and chemical properties. They are often referred to in literature as cedarwood oil. The most important oils are produced from distilling the wood of a number of different junipers and cypresses rather than the true cedars.[1]

From the Pinaceae family:

- Atlas cedarwood: *Cedrus atlantica* (Endl.) Manetti ex Carrière
- Himalayan cedarwood: *Cedrus deodara* (Roxb. Ex D.Don) G.Don

From the Cupressaceae family:

- Virginian cedarwood: *Juniperus virginiana* L.
- Texas cedarwood: *Juniperus mexicana* Schiede
- Chinese cedarwood: *Cupressus funebris* Endl.
- East African cedarwood: *Juniperus procera* Hochst

Synonyms

Atlas cedarwood: Moroccan cedarwood, Atlantic cedarwood

Virginian cedarwood: cedar oil, Eastern red cedarwood

Himalayan cedarwood: Deodar cedarwood

Texas cedarwood: Mexican cedar, Mexican juniper, mountain cedar, rock cedar

Chinese cedarwood: Chinese weeping cypress

Botany and origins

Atlas cedarwood

Atlas cedarwood is believed to have originated from the famous Lebanon cedars which grow wild in Lebanon and on the island of Cyprus. These trees are now protected from being felled for essential oil distillation or lumber.[2] Nowadays, it can be found in the Atlas Mountains of Morocco and northwestern Algeria.[1]

Atlas cedarwood is related to *C. deodara* and *C. libani*. *C. deodara* is known as Himalayan cedarwood, which grows at high altitude in the mountains of Himalaya. *C. libani* is known as Lebanon cedarwood and grows wild in the mountains of Lebanon and on the island of Cyprus. Any oil offered as Lebanon cedarwood oil is most likely to be oil distilled from *C. atlantica*.[2]

However, Atlas cedarwood is now on the IUCN Red List of Threatened Species as endangered in its natural habitat. The report states that declines of up to 75% in area of its natural occupancy have been estimated in recent years. Recent droughts have led to further declines in many parts of its natural habitat, and it is likely to continue if the regional climate continues to become more arid. Without proper management measures in place, these negative effects are likely to continue.[3] Atlas cedar is now cultivated in Europe.

Virginian cedarwood

J. virginiana is a slow growing evergreen tree with a narrow, dense and pyramidal crown. It grows in a fairly continuous belt running approximately from the central part of Virginia, through North Carolina and the northern edge of South Carolina, into Tennessee, central Kentucky and northern Alabama.[4]

Himalayan cedarwood

C. deodara is a tall, evergreen tree up to 50 m high. It grows extensively on the slopes of the Himalayas in northern India, Pakistan and Afghanistan, and is often the most important conifer at elevations of 1650-2400 m.[1]

Texas cedarwood

J. mexicana is a small alpine evergreen tree up to 6 m tall. It occurs in the southern United States (Texas), Mexico and parts of Central America. In the USA, like *J. virginiana*, it invades abandoned fields and overgrazed rangelands.[1]

It is small and poor looking relative of the cypress. The oil is steam-distilled from the heartwood of this tree, which is felled exclusively for the purpose of producing the essential oil. This oil is extensively used in perfumery.[2]

Chinese cedarwood

C. funebris is an evergreen tree with a wide distribution in Guizhou, Gansu and Sichuan provinces in the People's Republic of China.[1]

East African cedarwood

J. procera is a tall tree, up to 30 m or more. It is found in the drier highland forests of east Africa, particularly Kenya, at elevations of 1000-3000 m.[1]

East African cedarwood is steam-distilled from the waste wood in the sawmills of Kenya, where the wood is extensively used for the manufacture of pencils, boxes and wood carvings.[1]

Most of the east African cedarwood oil is obtained from wild trees, but there is little information published on the extent to which essential oil production may have affected the natural resource. In Kenya there is a serious depletion of the wild trees as a result of over-exploitation for timber and oil. American oil production utilises waste wood from trees felled for timber.[1]

Method of extraction

Atlas cedarwood is steam-distilled from either the wood, stumps or sawdust. Most of the distillation takes place in Morocco and the northwestern regions of Algeria.[2]

The best quality Atlas cedarwood essential oil is obtained from distilling wood chips from trees that are 20 to 30 years old. The essential oil distilled from the heartwood is considered warmer, more balsamic and aromatic.[5]

Virginian cedarwood oil is obtained by steam distillation of the wood, sawdust, shavings and other lumber wastes of *J. virginiana*.

Characteristics

Atlas cedarwood

Atlas cedarwood oil is a yellowish to orange-yellow or deep amber-coloured viscous oil that is occasionally turbid. Its odour is described as interesting to say the least – it is not exactly pleasant, with a slightly camphoraceous-cresylic top note and a sweet, tenacious woody undertone, reminiscent of cassie and mimosa.[1]

Virginian cedarwood

Virginian cedarwood oil is a pale yellow to slightly orange-yellow coloured oil that is slightly less viscous than Atlas cedarwood. The odour is at first oily and woody, with a sweet balsamic scent typical of cedarwood lumber. The odour becomes drier and more woody, less balsamic as the oil dries out.[1]

Himalayan cedarwood

Himalayan cedarwood oil is a yellowish to brownish-yellow oil, which is somewhat viscous and has a rich, sweet-woody, almost balsamic aroma reminiscent of Atlas cedarwood. It has a slightly cresylic-camphoraceous top note, which becomes delicately sweet-woody on its dryout.[2]

Holmes states that the scent of Himalayan cedarwood is similar to Atlas cedarwood, but without the pronounced sweetness and with a stronger dry-woody note.[6]

Texas cedarwood

Texas cedarwood oil is often redistilled. The oil is pale yellow to almost clear with a clean, sweet-woody aroma, which is typical of 'pencil-sharpener' odour.[2]

East African cedarwood

East African cedarwood oil has a very dry-woody, somewhat earthy aroma. It is less balsamic than Virginian cedarwood and more reminiscent of the odour of Texas cedarwood.[2]

Chemical composition

The chemical composition of *C. atlantica* essential oil was reported as follows:

Sesquiterpenes (himachalenes 14.5%, α-himachalene 10%, β-himachalene 42%, *cis*-bisabolene 1.2%); sesquiterpene alcohols (himachalol 4%, *allo*-himachalol 2.3%); ketones (α-atlantone 2.65%, γ-atlantone 5%); oxides (himachalene oxide 1%).[5]

Guenther states that *C. atlantica* trees less than 25 years old should not be felled. Older trees will yield about 3.5% of the volatile oil, while younger trees will yield less than 1%. He states that the oil distilled from the older trees and younger trees differs considerably in regard to the odour and chemical composition. Oil produced from older trees is higher in high boiling point constituents, while oil from younger trees is richer in cedrol.[4]

The chemical composition of *C. deodara* essential oil is reported as follows:

α-himachalene (20.0-30.0%), α-cedrene (12.0-16.0%), β-himachalene (8.0-13.0%), (*E*)-α-atlantone (5.0-7.0%), deodarone (4.0-6.0%), (Z)-α-atlantone (2.0-3.0%), β-cedrene (0.5-1.5%), *allo*-himachalol (0.5-1.5%), cedrol (1.0-2.0%), himachalol (1.0-2.0%).[7]

A comparative chemical composition of *Juniperus virginiana* and *Juniperus mexicana* are reported as follows:[8]

Constituents	J. virginiana	J. mexicana
α-cedrene	20.0%	21.2%
β-cedrene	6.6%	4.9%
thujopsene	18.9%	29.0%
other sesquiterpenes	13.3%	15.5%
cedrol	31.6%	25.0%
widdrol	4.8%	4.2%

The ISO standard for Texas cedarwood oil specifies a minimum cedrol content of 20% and the standard for Virginian cedarwood oil stipulates a minimum cedrol content of 14%.[1]

Adulteration

Lis-Balchin states that all commercial cedarwood oils seem to be blended together because they have similar chemical composition. As they are relatively inexpensive, there is no real problem of adulteration with synthetic components.[9] Cedarwood oils are also adulterated by the addition of cedrol from the cheaper Chinese cedarwood oil.[10]

Pharmacopoeias and standards

The purity, composition and physico-chemical properties of cedarwood essential oils are defined in the following ISO standards:

- ISO 4724:1984 Oil of Cedarwood, Virginia (*Juniperus virginiana* Linnaeus)
- ISO 4725:1986 Oil of Cedarwood, Texas (*Juniperus mexicana* Schiede)
- ISO 9843:2002 Oil of Cedarwood, Chinese type (*Cupressus funebris* Endlicher)

History and Traditional Uses

History

Atlas cedarwood was believed to be used by the ancient Egyptians for embalming purposes, cosmetics and perfumery. The Lebanon cedar was prized as a building wood.[11] The cedar trees were mentioned in the Bible, symbolising everything that was fertile and abundant. Later, Dioscorides and Galen referred to cedar's resin being used to preserve the body from putrification.[12]

According to the Song of Solomon, cedarwood was used to build Solomon's temple. Cedarwood symbolised abundance, fertility and spiritual strength. The name *Cedrus* originates from the Arabic word *kedron*, meaning 'power'.[12]

Himalayan cedarwood is a relatively recent addition to the list of cedarwoods produced commercially. Coppen states that essential oil production began in India in the late 1950s, and most of the oil produced is consumed domestically.[1]

Herbal

Decoctions of the leaves, bark, twigs and seeds of *J. virginiana* have been used to treat various illnesses including coughs, bronchitis, rheumatism, venereal warts and skin rashes.[13]

Food, perfumery and flavouring

Virginian, Texas and Atlas cedarwood oils are all used as fragrance components or fixatives in cosmetics and household products such as soaps and detergents.[13]

Other uses

Most species of cedarwood are utilised for timber purposes. *C. deodara* is considered one of the most valuable Indian timbers and is used for railway sleepers and in construction work requiring beams, posts and frames. It is also used for making pencils. The strong odour of the wood and its oily character limits its use for indoor furniture.[1]

The wood from *J. virginiana* is highly prized for

furniture making. Older trees are preferred since they contain more of the reddish heartwood, which not only gives a beautiful surface when polished, but also yields more essential oil than wood from young trees.[2] *J. virginiana* has also been used as an insect repellent.[14]

Therapeutics

Pharmacology and clinical studies

Many pharmacological and clinical studies involving cedarwood oils have been published. A systemic review of these studies will not be attempted. Rather I have chosen a selection of studies that support traditional and clinical uses.

Alopecia areata

C. atlantica oil was used in an aromatherapy massage blend for the treatment of *Alopecia areata* – a disorder in which the hair falls out in patches producing baldness. Although the results were variable, the group using the massage blend containing Atlas cedarwood showed a significant improvement of 44%.[15]

Antifungal activity

Lis-Balchin states that the antifungal activity of all the cedarwood oils was very low.[9]

Anti-inflammatory activity

An in vitro study found that *C. deodara* oil demonstrated good inhibition of 5-lipoxygenase. This indicates that it may have anti-inflammatory activity as the mechanism of inflammation begins with the oxidation of the enzyme 5-lipoxygenase.[16]

The anti-inflammatory activity of Indian *C. deodara* was investigated in an in vivo study. The oral administration of the essential oil (50 and 100 mg/kg) one hour before the induction of inflammation significantly inhibited induced rat paw oedema. It was concluded that the membrane stabilising activity of *C. deodara* essential oil has a significant role in its anti-inflammatory activity.[17]

The study also confirmed that the essential oil suppressed delayed hypersensitivity (Type IV) reactions. It was concluded that the oil produced an inhibitory effect on humoral and cell-mediated immune responses, suggesting an immunomodulatory effect in inflammatory conditions.[18]

Antimicrobial activity

Several studies suggest that the antimicrobial activity of cedarwood oils is very low due to the high percentage of inactive sesquiterpenes.[9]

Antiulcer activity

C. deodara oil showed significant gastric antisecretory and antiulcer activity in an in vivo study involving rats.[19]

Insecticidal activity

C. atlantica oil was one of six mosquito repellent substances tested against four *Anopheles* species. Of these, *A. stephensi* was found to be the most susceptible. It has been reported that cedrol, in particular, seems to have a high toxicity to cercariae *(Schistosoma mansani)*, a parasite for humans. Himalayan cedarwood oil exhibited insecticidal activity against *Callosobruchus analis* F. and *Musca domestica* L.[14]

C. deodara oil exhibited promising larvicidal activity against the larvae of *Plutella xylostella*, the diamondback moth, a common pest of cruciferous crops. It was suggested that the oil can be utilised for sustainable pest management which has both economic and ecological benefits.[20]

Molluscicidal activity

C. atlantica oil was reported to have significant molluscicidal activity. It was suggested that the oil could be effective in combating schistosomiasis.[21]

Spasmolytic activity

Lis-Balchin reported that there was a spasmolytic action on smooth muscle of the electrically stimulated guinea pig in vitro for all cedarwood oils studied – Atlas, Chinese, Texas and Virginian. She states that the sesquiterpenes were responsible for the spasmolytic action.[9]

Actions

Actions commonly cited in aromatherapy

Antibacterial, anticatarrhal, antiseborrhoeic, antiseptic, astringent, diuretic, expectorant, insecticide, sedative, tonic[1,12,22]

Atlas cedarwood is considered a lymphatic decongestant.[6,22] Virginian cedarwood is considered an emmenagogue.[11]

Actions supported by clinical studies

Anti-inflammatory, insecticidal

Comment

In aromatherapy, the two most commonly used cedarwood oils are Virginian and Atlas.

While the odour profiles of Atlas, Himalayan and Virginian cedarwood are very different, the cedarwood oils do share similar properties. Lis-Balchin states that there is not sufficient scientific evidence available to suggest that any of the cedarwood oils can alleviate many of the conditions documented in aromatherapy.[9]

Holmes states that Atlas cedarwood has a strong calming and stabilising effect on the mind and recommends it for those individuals who feel fatigued and tense at the same time.[6]

Aromatherapy Uses

Clinical aromatherapy

Lymphatic system

Atlas cedarwood oil is reputed to encourage lymphatic drainage and stimulate the breakdown of accumulated fats. It is mildly diuretic and may be used for the treatment of cellulite and oedema.[22]

Holmes recommends blending Atlas cedarwood oil with grapefruit as a lymphatic decongestant for swollen glands and lymphatic congestion.[6]

Schnaubelt states that Atlas cedarwood oil counteracts water and lipid retention and is therefore beneficial for the treatment of cellulite.[23]

Nervous system

Atlas cedarwood and Virginian cedarwood oils may be used for reducing stress, anxiety and tension.[11,22,24,25]

Holmes explains that Atlas cedarwood oil is perfect for those who suffer from stress and tension and weakness at the same time – often associated with chronic conditions that lead to exhaustion and burnout.[6]

Psychological

Holmes states that Atlas cedarwood oil helps to calm the mind and promote emotional security. He recommends it for anxiety, fearfulness and agitation. He explains that the oil also helps to reduce repetitive and excessive thinking, worry and obsessive thoughts.[6]

Fischer-Rizzi states that Atlas cedarwood oil has a strengthening and comforting effect. She states that it calms during times of fear and nervous tension. In difficult situations, the oil may provide comfort and warmth, and help stabilise energies thrown out of balance.[24]

Respiratory system

The presence of sesquiterpene ketones gives Atlas cedarwood oil its excellent mucolytic effect. The oil may be used for treating catarrhal conditions, coughs and chronic bronchitis.[11,24,25]

The presence of 7 to 10% sesquiterpene ketones gives Atlas cedarwood oil an anti-inflammatory action, which acts in the first phase of inflammation (reduction of globulins) associated with a mucolytic effect. This also gives an effective action in certain afflictions such as hay fever. The sesquiterpene alcohols (approximately 7%) take part in decongestive action on the mucosa.[5]

Virginian cedarwood oil is also recommended for treating catarrhal conditions, coughs and chronic bronchitis.[11]

Skin care

Atlas cedarwood and Virginian cedarwood oils may be used for treatment of cystitis and urinary tract infections.[11,22,24]

Urinary system

Atlas cedarwood oil and Virginian cedarwood oils are recommended in hair and skin care for improving oily skin, acne, dandruff and seborrhoea of the scalp.[11,22,24]

They are also reputed to strengthen hair growth and alleviate dandruff.[11,24]

Energetics, psyche and subtle uses

Energetics

Atlas cedarwood oil is fortifying and strengthening and it is considered a powerful tonic of the body's *Qi*. The oil is tonifying to both the *Kidneys* and *Spleen-Pancreas,* and may be used for general lethargy, nervous debility, lower backache and poor concentration. The oil is also effective in treating conditions classified as *cold damp*. It has decongesting qualities and, combined with its antiseptic properties, it is useful for genitourinary and respiratory infections.[22]

Holmes states that Atlas cedarwood oil nourishes the *Yin*, eliminates *damp* and calms the *Shen*. *Yin deficiency* and agitated *Shen* are associated with anxiety, restlessness, debility and burnout.[6]

Mojay also explains that Atlas cedarwood oil is associated with the Water Element and helps to strengthen the function of the *Kidneys*. In TCM, the energetic function of the *Kidneys* is associated with our *Zhi* or willpower. He also explains that, while ginger stimulates the willpower into action, Atlas cedarwood oil gives us the courage and strength to hold firm, even against obstinate external forces.[22]

Holmes states that Atlas cedarwood oil also has an affinity with the Earth Element. He recommends the oil for resolving *Lung* phlegm-*damp* associated with coughing and copious mucous and sputum expectoration.[6]

Personality

Worwood describes the cedarwood personality as someone gliding through life as if they had a royal charter. They may actually appear haughty and just too grand to be approached about anything mundane, but this assumption is usually incorrect as they are a tower of strength in almost all situations.[26]

> *Cedarwood personalities instill confidence and security in people less able to cope with life's*

stresses and strains and can be a great comfort in times of trouble. This ability puts them in the role of family adviser – the person you phone to ask how to deal with your tax return, or ask how you should approach a financial dispute, however you wouldn't ask them on your choice of friends, or a new outfit.[26]

Worwood warns us that cedarwood personalities are not infallible. Often they may be wrong because of their dogmatic views. The older they get, the worse they become. They do not seem to be aware that the world has changed in the last 50 years. If you have this personality for a father or grandfather, it can be quite challenging because they often hold the family to emotional and financial ransom. They can become extremely obsessive. Everything has to be in the right place and organised.[26]

According to Myers-Briggs personality types, the Atlas cedarwood personality is likely to be an INTJ. INTJs are very responsible and dependable. They are people of very few words and tend to be private. They are punctual, precise and fastidious. They have the ability to concentrate and are difficult to distract. They prefer to work alone. They are modest, unassuming and down to earth. They can be resistant to change. They can make quick critical judgements of others. They are extremely devoted in their relationships.

Subtle

Atlas cedarwood oil can give us immovable strength in times of crisis. Steadying the conscious mind, it will help us to resist the sudden events and powerful emotions that threaten to undermine our confidence and morale.[22]

Holmes states that Atlas cedarwood oil has a stabilising influence on our energy, which is very useful when one is feeling a disconnection from their surroundings or within themselves.[6]

Zeck states that Atlas cedarwood oil brings strength and commitment when we need to make changes in our lives and move forward.[27]

Keim Loughran & Bull recommend using Atlas cedarwood oil whenever we do not feel grounded, whenever we feel negativity from other people or ourselves, and during times of spiritual confusion.[28]

Dosage and Administration

Blending

Aromatherapy

For hair and scalp care and the treatment of seborrheic dermatitis with dandruff, consider blending Atlas cedarwood oil with essential oils such as bay laurel, patchouli or rosemary.

For the relief of anxiety, nervous tension and stress, consider blending Atlas cedarwood oil with essential oils such as bergamot, clary sage, Roman chamomile, lavender, frankincense, geranium, sweet orange, sandalwood, vetiver or ylang ylang.

For insomnia, consider blending Atlas cedarwood oil with essential oils such as lavender, patchouli, sandalwood or vetiver.

For mucous congestion associated with bronchitis, consider blending any of the cedarwood oils with essential oils such as aniseed, 1,8-cineole-rich eucalypts, peppermint eucalyptus, sweet fennel, ginger, sweet marjoram, myrtle or niaouli essential oil.

As a personal insect repellent, consider blending any of the cedarwood oils with essential oils such as 1,8-cineole-rich eucalypts, lemon-scented eucalyptus, citronella, spike lavender, niaouli, peppermint or tea tree.

Perfumery

Atlas cedarwood oil is commonly used in perfumery for its fixative quality and its unique odour. It blends well with labdanum and all woody-floral essential oils.[2]

Virginian cedarwood oil is used extensively in perfumery, especially in soap perfumery. It is used as a fixative and cost-reducer for oils such as vetiver, sandalwood and patchouli.[2]

Mode of administration

Bath

Full body bath, foot bath

Topical

Compress, massage, ointment, skin care

Inhalation

Direct inhalation, diffuser, oil vaporiser

Safety Profile

General safety

Atlas cedarwood and Virginian cedarwood are considered non-toxic, non-irritant and non-sensitising.

Contraindications

Price & Price, Lawless and Fischer-Rizzi say that *C. atlantica* oil should not be used during pregnancy.[11,24,29]

C. atlantica oil is also said to have neurotoxic and abortive effects.[29]

However, Tisserand & Balacs state that Atlas cedarwood oil is safe to use and it should not be contraindicated during pregnancy.[30]

Lawless states that Virginian cedarwood should not be used during pregnancy.[11] Tisserand & Balacs state that Virginian cedarwood oil is safe to use and they do not suggest that it should be contra-indicated during pregnancy.[30]

I believe that Virginian cedarwood is one of those oils whose botanical name may have been confused with savin – *Juniperus sabina* – a highly toxic oil which is contraindicated during pregnancy.

Regulatory guidelines

Atlas cedarwood has been granted GRAS status.

References

1. Coppen J. *Flavours and fragrances of plant origin*. Food and Agriculture Organization of the United Nations, Rome, 1995.
2. Arctander S. *Perfume and flavor materials of natural origin*. Allured Publishing, Carol Stream, 1994.
3. Thomas P. *Cedrus atlantica. The IUCN Red List of Threatened Species 2013:* eT42303A2979716. http://dx.doi.org/10.2305/IUCN.IK.2013-1.RLTS.T42303A2970716.en
4. Guenther E. *The essential oils – Vol. VI*. Robert E. Krieger Publishing, Malabar, 1952.
5. Collins P. *Cedarwood*. The Aromatherapist, 1996; 3(2): 30-33.
6. Holmes P. *Aromatica: a clinical guide to essential oil therapeutics – Vol. I*. Singing Dragon, London, 2016.
7. Lawrence BM. *Progress in essential oils*. Perfumer & Flavorist, 2012; 37: 42-44.
8. Lawrence BM. *Essential oils 1979-1980*. Allured Publishing, Wheaton, 1981.
9. Lis-Balchin M. *Aromatherapy science – a guide for healthcare professionals*. Pharmaceutical Press, London, 2006.
10. Schmidt E, Wanner J. *Adulteration of essential oils*. In Baser KHC, Buchbauer G. eds. *Handbook of essential oils – science, technology and applications*. 2nd edn. CRC Press, Boca Raton, 2016: 707-745.
11. Lawless J. *The encyclopaedia of essential oils*. Element Books, Shaftesbury, 1992.
12. Lavabre M. *Aromatherapy workbook*. Healing Arts Press, Rochester, 1997.
13. Khan I, Abourashed E. *Leung's encyclopedia of common natural ingredients used in food, drugs and cosmetics*. 3rd edn. John Wiley & Sons, New Jersey, 2010.
14. Cetin H et al. *Larvicidal effect of Cedrus libani seed oil on mosquito Culex pipiens*. Pharmaceutical Biology, 2009; 47(8): 665-668. doi: 10.1080/13880200902918360.
15. Hay IC, Jamieson M, Ormerod AD. *Randomized trial of aromatherapy – successful treatment of Alopecia areata*. Archives of Dermatology, 1998; 134(11): 1349-1352. Cited in the Aromatherapy Database, by Bob Harris, Essential Oil Resource Consultants, UK, 2000.
16. Baylac S, Racine P. *Inhibition of 5-lipoxygenase by essential oils and other natural fragrant extracts*. International Journal of Aromatherapy, 2003; 13(2/3): 138-142.
17. Shinde UA et al. *Membrane stabilizing activity – a possible mechanism of action for the anti-inflammatory activity of Cedrus deodara wood oil*. Fitoterapia, 1999; 70(3): 251-257. Cited in Quintessential Aromatics database, 2013.
18. Shinde UA et al. *Preliminary studies on the immunomodulating activity of Cedrus deodara wood oil*. Fitoterapia, 1999; 70(4): 333-339. Cited in Quintessential Aromatics database, 2013.
19. Kumar A et al. *Gastric antisecretory and antiulcer activities of Cedrus deodara (Roxb.) Loud. in Wistar rats*. Journal of Ethnopharmacology, 2011; 134(2): 294-297. Cited in Quintessential Aromatics database, 2013.
20. Chaudhary A et al. *Chemical composition and larvicidal activities of Himalayan cedar, Cedrus deodara essential oil and its fractions against the diamondback moth, Plutella xylostella*. Journal of Insect Science, 2011; 11: 157. doi: 10.1673/031.011.15701
21. Lahlou MS. *Composition and molluscicidal properties of essential oils of five Moroccan Pinaceae*. Pharmaceutical Biology, 2003; 41(3): 207-210. Cited in Quintessential Aromatics database, 2013.
22. Mojay G. *Aromatherapy for healing the spirit*. Healing Arts Press, Rochester, 1999.
23. Schnaubelt K. *Medical aromatherapy*. Frog, Berkeley, 1999.
24. Fischer-Rizzi S. *Complete aromatherapy handbook*. Sterling Publishing, New York, 1990.
25. Davis P. *Aromatherapy A-Z*. 2nd edn. C.W. Daniel Company, Saffron Walden, 1999.
26. Worwood VA. *The fragrant mind*. Transworld Publishing, London, 1995.
27. Zeck R. *The blossoming heart – aromatherapy for healing and transformation*. Aroma Tours, East Ivanhoe, 2004.
28. Keim Loughran J, Bull R. *Aromatherapy anointing oils*. Frog, Berkeley, 2001.
29. Price S, Price L. *Aromatherapy for health professionals*. Churchill Livingstone, Edinburgh, 1995.
30. Tisserand R, Balacs T. *Essential oil safety*. Churchill Livingstone, Edinburgh, 1995.

Celery seed

Identification

Botanical name

Apium graveolens L.

Synonyms

None

Family

Apiaceae (Umbelliferae)

Botany and origins

Celery is an erect biennial herb, which grows up to 1 m high. It is native to southern Europe. The plant is cultivated in France, India, The Netherlands, Hungary and China. Major seed-producing countries are France and India.[1]

Method of extraction

Celery seed oil is obtained by the steam distillation of the whole or crushed seeds.

Characteristics

Celery seed oil is a pale yellow to orange-yellow liquid with a sweet, spicy aroma that is long lasting and powerful. Arctander describes celery seed oil as having one of the most diffusive odours and penetrating flavours.[1]

Chemical composition

The main constituents found in celery seed oil include:

α-pinene (1.05%), β-pinene (trace), camphene (trace), sabinene (0.76%), myrcene (0.95%), limonene (72.16%), β-phellandrene (0.02%), *p*-cymene (0.74%), pentylbenzene (0.02%), linalool (1.48%), isopulegone (0.16%), carvone (0.09%), geranyl acetate (0.04%), α-ionone (0.05%), cinnamaldehyde (0.15%), thymol (0.17%), β-selinene (12.17%), α-selinene (2.05%), caryophyllene epoxide (0.55%), butyl phthalide (2.56%), eudesmol ligustilide (2.41%).[2]

Adulteration

Limonene is often used to adulterate celery seed oil.[3]

Pharmacopoeias and standards

At the time of writing, the purity, composition, physico-chemical properties and therapeutic use of celery seed essential oil are not defined in any pharmacopoeia monograph or standard. Celery is listed in the German Commission E as an unapproved herb. It is stated that the effectiveness of the claimed applications has not been documented.

History and Traditional Uses

History

The native habitat of celery is the lowland of Italy from where it spread to Northern Europe, Egypt, Algeria and into Asia. Hemphill states that the Egyptians used celery seed around 2200 BC for medicinal purposes. Celery was first cultivated as a food plant in France in 1623.[4]

In the early eighteenth century, the Italians developed a milder strain of celery, without the bitterness, for culinary use as a vegetable. This led to the cultivated variety *A. graveolens* var. *dulce*, which we are familiar with today as vegetable celery with its thick, juicy and stringless stalks.[4]

Fazal states that celery seed is one of the lesser-known and used herbs in Western herbal medicine.[5]

Traditional medicine

Celery seeds are employed as a traditional medicine in India and other countries adopting Ayurvedic traditions for healing. The seeds have been used in the treatment of liver ailments, water retention, poor digestion and various types of arthritis.[6]

Herbal

Celery is considered one of the most alkaline of foods. It has a special affinity for the stomach, kidneys and liver and helps to neutralise acids in the body.[6]

The leaves, stalks and seeds of the plant are used for arthritis, rheumatism, gout, urinary tract inflammations. Celery is also used as a diuretic, for regulating the bowels, for glandular stimulation, gall and kidney stones, as a prophylactic for nervous agitation, for loss of appetite and exhaustion.[7]

Celery leaves contain furanocoumarin, psoralen, bergapten, xanthotoxin and isopimpinellin. Dermatitis and phototoxic skin reactions from celery in some farm and grocery store workers have been reported.[7]

Celery is referred to as an aromatic bitter tonic herb that reduces blood pressure, relieves indigestion, stimulates the uterus and acts as an anti-inflammatory. The seeds are used in India as an antispasmodic to treat asthma and bronchitis and diseases of the liver and spleen.[8]

The primary use of celery seed (and even the

stalks) is to treat arthritis, gout and rheumatic complaints. It is said to 'remove irritable deposits of calcium and uric acid in the body'.[9]

Grieve attributes celery with carminative, stimulant, diuretic, tonic and nervine properties. She also states it is useful for hysteria, and promoting restfulness and sleep.[10]

Food, perfumery and flavouring

Celery seed oil is used as a fragrance component in soaps, detergents, cosmetics and perfumes. It is also extensively used as a flavouring ingredient in many foods.[8]

Therapeutics

Pharmacology and clinical studies

Many pharmacological studies involving celery seed essential oil have been published. A systemic review of these studies will not be attempted. Rather, I have chosen a selection of studies that support the traditional and clinical uses.

Antibacterial activity

Celery seed oil was strongly inhibitory against *Escherichia coli* and moderately inhibitory against *Pseudomonas aeruginosa* and *Staphylococcus aureus*.[11]

Anticarcinogenic activity

Celery seed oil significantly increased induction of GST in mouse liver. The ability to induce detoxifying enzymes correlates to anticarcinogenic activity.[12]

Antifungal activity

Celery seed oil was found to have potent antifungal activity against a range of fungal organisms.[13]

Gastroprotective activity

Oral administration of celery seed oil inhibited HCL/ethanol-induced ulcers, similar to omeprazole. The researchers stated that the antiulcerogenic activity could be related to an increase in gastric mucosal defensive factors.[14]

Hepatoprotective activity

The influence of essential oils on the activity of the hepatic carcinogen-metabolising enzymes of cytochrome P-450, aryl hydrocarbon hydroxylase (AHH) and GST was investigated in mice. Celery seed essential oil significantly elevated GST activity. It was suggested that celery seed oil has potential as a 'blocking agent' in chemoprotective strategies.[15]

Insecticidal activity

Celery seed oil has strong larvicidal, adulticidal and repellency activity against the *Aedes aegypti* larvae and mosquito.[16]

Actions

Actions commonly cited in aromatherapy

Antirheumatic, antispasmodic, aperitif, carminative, cholagogue, depurative, digestive, diuretic, emmenagogue, galactagogue, hepatic, nervine, tonic (digestive)[17]

Actions supported by clinical studies

Antifungal, antimicrobial, digestive, larvicidal

Comment

Very few references are made to celery seed essential oil in aromatherapy books. A broad range of biological activities has been attributed to celery seed. Lis-Balchin explains that all of these mentioned uses are taken directly from herbal uses and that no scientific evidence has been provided for the aromatherapeutic benefits.[18]

However, I believe that traditional uses of celery seed do support the use of celery seed essential oil for the purpose of detoxification.

Aromatherapy Uses

Clinical aromatherapy

Detoxification

Celery seed oil is highly recommended for eliminating toxins.[19]

Digestive system

Celery seed oil has traditionally been used for the treatment of dyspepsia, flatulence and indigestion.[17]

Musculoskeletal system

Celery seed oil has been recommended for the treatment of arthritis, gout and rheumatism.[17]

Reproductive system

Celery seed oil is recommended for amenorrhoea and glandular problems.[17]

Dosage and Administration

Blending

Aromatherapy

For the relief of aches and pains associated with arthritis and rheumatism, you may consider blending celery seed oil with essential oils such as cajeput, ginger, kunzea, spike lavender, pine or rosemary.

For the relief of dyspepsia and indigestion, consider blending celery seed oil with essential oils such as coriander seed, sweet fennel, ginger, sweet orange or rosemary.

For detoxification, consider using celery seed

oil with essential oils such as coriander seed, sweet fennel, grapefruit, juniper berry, lemon or rosemary.

Perfumery

Celery seed oil has very limited use in perfumery. Arctander says that it imparts a warm note in floral and oriental compositions, in lavender bouquets and in modern fantasy and aldehydic perfumes. However, he warns us that carelessly used, its diffusive and strong odour tenacity can easily ruin a perfume.[1]

Tisserand & Young state that the French oil is preferred in perfumery.[3]

Mode of administration

Bath

Full body bath, foot bath

Topical

Compress, massage, ointment

Inhalation

Direct inhalation, diffuser, oil vaporiser

Ingestion

Schnaubelt recommends taking 1 drop of celery seed oil once or twice daily, for 3 days in a row to drain toxicity from the kidneys.[19]

Safety Profile

General safety

Celery seed oil is non-toxic and non-irritant; however, it is possibly sensitising.[17] The oil is not phototoxic.[3]

Contraindications

Lawless states that it should not be used during pregnancy; however, Tisserand & Young suggest that it should not be hazardous in pregnancy.[3,17]

Regulatory guidelines

Celery seed essential oil has GRAS status.

References

1. Arctander S. *Perfume and flavor materials of natural origin.* Allured Publishing, Carol Stream, 1994.
2. Lawrence BM. *Essential oils 1988-1991.* Allured Publishing, Carol Stream, 1993.
3. Tisserand R, Young R. *Essential oil safety.* 2nd edn. Churchill Livingstone, Edinburgh, 2014.
4. Hemphill I. *Spice notes.* Pan MacMillan, Sydney, 2000.
5. Fazal SS, Singla RK. *Review of the pharmacognostical & pharmacological characterization of Apium graveolens Linn.* Indo Global Journal of Pharmaceutical Sciences, 2012; 2(1): 36-42.
6. Asif HM et al. *Monograph of Apium graveolens Linn.* Journal of Medicinal Plants Research, 2011; 5(8): 1494-1496.
7. Al-Snafi AE. *The pharmacology of Apium graveolens – a review.* International Journal for Pharmaceutical Research Scholars, 2014; 3(1): 671-677.
8. Khan I, Abourashed E. *Leung's encyclopedia of common natural ingredients used in food, drugs and cosmetics.* 3rd edn. John Wiley & Sons, New Jersey, 2010.
9. Wood M. *The earthwise herbal – Vol.1: a complete guide to old world medicinal plants.* North Atlantic Books, Berkeley, 2008.
10. Grieve M. *A modern herbal – Vol. I.* Dover Publications, New York, 1971.
11. Baananou S et al. *Antiulcerogenic and antibacterial activities of Apium graveolens essential oil and extract.* Natural Product Research, 2013; 27(12): 1075-1083. Cited in Quintessential Aromatics database, 2013.
12. Lam LK, Zheng B. *Effects of essential oils on glutathione S-transferase activity in mice.* Journal of Agricultural and Food Chemistry, 1991; 39(4): 660-662. Cited in Quintessential Aromatics database, 2013.
13. Marongiu B et al. *Isolation of the volatile fraction from Apium graveolens L. (Apiaceae) by supercritical carbon dioxide extraction and hydrodistillation: chemical composition and antifungal activity.* Natural Product Research, 2013; 27(17): 1521-1527. Cited in Quintessential Aromatics database, 2013.
14. Baananou S et al. *Antiulcerogenic activity of Apium graveolens seeds oils isolated by supercritical CO_2.* African Journal of Pharmacy and Pharmacology, 2012; 6(10): 756-762.
15. Banerjee S et al. *Influence of certain essential oils on carcinogen-metabolising enzymes and acid-soluble sulphydryls in mouse liver.* Nutrition and Cancer, 1994: 21(3): 263-269. Cited in Quintessential Aromatics database, 2013.
16. Kumar S et al. *Larvicidal, repellent and irritant potential of the seed-derived essential oil of Apium graveolens against dengue vector, Aedes aegypti* L. (Diptera: Culicidae). Frontiers in Public Health, 2014; 2: 147. doi 10.3389/fpubh.2014.00147
17. Lawless J. *The encyclopaedia of essential oils.* Element Books, Shaftesbury, 1992.
18. Lis-Balchin M. *Aromatherapy science: a guide for healthcare professionals.* Pharmaceutical Press, London, 2006.
19. Schnaubelt K. *The healing intelligence of essential oils.* Healing Arts Press, Rochester, 2011.

Chamomile, German

Identification

Botanical name

Matricaria recutita L.

Synonyms

Blue chamomile, Hungarian chamomile, *Matricaria chamomilla, Chamomilla recutita*

Family

Asteraceae (Compositae)

Botany and origins

German chamomile is a fragrant, low annual herb, up to 0.6 m tall, with delicate feather leaves and simple daisy-like white flowers on a single stem.

It is native to Europe, particularly to central and northern Europe. It is cultivated in Hungary, Yugoslavia, Bulgaria, Russia, Germany, Belgium and Spain. Hungary is one of the main producers of the oil.[1]

Frequent changes in the interpretation of the scientific name of German chamomile have led to confusion over the past two decades. The currently accepted scientific name is *M. recutita,* though *Chamomilla recutita* and, to a lesser extent, *M. chamomilla* are commonly seen in literature.[2]

C

Method of extraction

German chamomile oil is steam-distilled from the dried flower heads of *M. recutita*. The essential oil content is highest at the beginning of flowering. Drying the flowers at 40-45°C is reported to preserve the matricarin and the essential oil is reputed to be the best.[3]

Characteristics

German chamomile is a deep inky-blue, somewhat viscous oil with an intensely sweet, herbaceous odour and a fresh fruity undertone. The pure, undiluted oil has an intense odour which some find overwhelming and unpleasant.[1]

Chemical composition

The chemical composition of German chamomile oil was reported as follows:

chamazulene (2.16-35.59%), α-bisabolol (1.72-67.25%), bisabolol oxide A (0-55.08%), bisabolol oxide B (4.35-18.93%) and bisabolone oxide A (0-63.85%).[4]

German chamomile essential oil varies in composition according to the source. Four main chemotypes have been identified as follows.[4]

Type A

α-bisabolol oxide B > α-bisabolol oxide A > α-bisabolol

Type B

α-bisabolol oxide A > α-bisabolol oxide B > α-bisabolol

Type C

α-bisabolol > α-bisabolol oxide B > α-bisabolol oxide A

Type D

α-bisabolol oxide B = α-bisabolol oxide A =α-bisabolol

The content and composition of the essential oil are dependent on the development stage of the plant. For example, the quantity of α-bisabolol, α-bisabolol oxide A and B and bisabolone oxide A reached a maximum in full bloom, whereas the farnesene content decreased rapidly with the growth and development of the flower.[5]

Adulteration

The chances of adulteration are very high as it is a low yield, high price essential oil. Typical adulterants include azulenes from other plants such as yarrow, Moroccan chamomile or synthetic azulenes.[1]

Pharmacopoeias and standards

The purity, composition and physico-chemical properties of German chamomile essential oil are defined in ISO 19332: 2007 Oil of Blue Chamomile. German chamomile is also listed in several monographs:

- Assessment Report on *Matricaria recutita L., flos* and *Matricaria recutita* L., aetheroleum. European Medicines Agency
- WHO Monographs on Selected Medicinal Plants – Vol. 1

History and Traditional Uses

History

Since antiquity, chamomile flowers have been used both internally for digestive disorders and externally for skin and mucous membrane irritations. It has been difficult to ascertain which species were used historically, as many plants within the Asteraceae family were referred to by the common name of chamomile.[5]

Traditional medicine

The healing qualities of chamomile have been known by physicians for over 2,500 years.

Hippocrates gave a description of the herb in the fifth century BC. Chamomile appeared as a medicinal plant in *De Materia Medica* written by Dioscorides in the first century AD. Saladin von Asculum mentions the blue volatile chamomile oil in 1488, and in 1500, Hieronymus Brunschwig describes the distillation of the essential oil of chamomile.[6]

Herbal

Herbal infusions of German chamomile flowers are listed in the German Commission E for topical application for the inflammation of the skin, as well as for bactericidal skin diseases. Internally, the infusion is recommended for gastrointestinal spasm and inflammatory diseases of the gastrointestinal tract.[7]

Food, perfumery and flavouring

German chamomile oil is extensively used in cosmetics and body care formulations.[2]

Therapeutics

Pharmacology and clinical studies

Many pharmacological studies involving German chamomile essential oil have been published. A systemic review of these studies will not be attempted. Rather I have chosen a selection of studies that support traditional and clinical uses.

Antifungal activity

German chamomile oil was evaluated against medically important dermatophytes and opportunistic saprophytes. The results of the study indicated that *M. recutita* is a potential candidate for designing effective antifungal formulations suitable for treatment of dermatophytosis.[8]

Anti-inflammatory activity

The anti-inflammatory properties of German chamomile oil are well-documented when used topically.[9]

The accepted wisdom is that the anti-inflammatory activity of chamomile is mainly due to chamazulene. This blue compound is formed from matricarin by steam distillation. In other words, the compound found naturally in chamomile is matricarin, and this is converted into chamazulene by the action of the steam.[3]

The antiphlogistic effects of (-)-α-bisabolol found in German chamomile have been proven in experiments on adjuvant arthritis in rats.[10]

Experiments showed that (-)-α-bisabolol had a greater effect than bisabolol oxides A and B. It was suggested that standardising the content of (-)-α-bisabolol was important to the antiphlogistic effectiveness of chamomile, but that standardising the amount of oxides present was not necessary.[10]

The anti-inflammatory and antiallergenic effects of volatile and non-volatile components of German chamomile significantly inhibited swelling induced by carrageenan in rats.[11]

Antimicrobial activity

German chamomile oil exerted significant bacteriostatic and bactericidal effects against *Staphylococcus aureus, Bacillus subtilis* and *Candida albicans*. However, even at concentrations as high as 8% v/v, complete bactericidal effect was not achieved against *Pseudomonas aeruginosa* and *Escherichia coli*.[12]

The antibacterial activity of German chamomile essential oil was evaluated against *Helicobacter pylori*. It was shown that the oil inhibited the production of urease by *H. pylori*. It is known that the level of activity of urease is very important for the survival of this microorganism in the stomach.[13]

German chamomile oil has demonstrated antibacterial activity against organisms such as *Klebsiella sp., Proteus vulgaris* and *Clostridium sporogenes*.[14]

Hepatic

German chamomile oil is rich in monoterpenes and sesquiterpenes which exhibit cholagogue and choleretic activities.[15] Both the herbal extract and essential oil have a dose-dependent spasmolytic effect on the smooth muscle of the intestine and also demonstrated liver-regenerating properties.[16,17]

Sedative activity

The vapours of German chamomile oil reduced a stress-induced increase in plasma adrenocorticotropic hormone (ACTH) levels in rats. Diazepam co-administered with inhalation of German chamomile oil further reduced ACTH levels, while flumazenil, a benzodiazepine receptor antagonist, blocked the effects of German chamomile vapour on ACTH.[18]

Actions

Actions commonly cited in aromatherapy

Analgesic, antiallergenic, anti-inflammatory, anti-spasmodic, bactericidal, carminative, cholagogue, cicatrisant, emmenagogue, hepatic, sedative, stomachic, vulnerary[19]

Actions supported by clinical studies

Anti-inflammatory, bactericidal, cholagogue, cicatrisant, hepatic, sedative, vulnerary

Comment

Schnaubelt refers to German chamomile oil as one of the most reliable anti-inflammatory agents in aromatherapy. He also states that an important, often overlooked, feature is that it neutralises toxic bacterial metabolic wastes, which are often the cause of fever during acute illness.[20]

Tisserand & Young states the blue chamomile oils are produced in many parts of the world and have greatly varying composition. Typically, those oils with the higher α-bisabolol are preferred in aromatherapy.[21]

Aromatherapy Uses

Clinical aromatherapy

Children's remedy

German chamomile is considered one of the gentlest of essential oils, and is particularly beneficial for treating children. It may be used to alleviate the pain associated with teething infants.[19,22]

Detoxification

Holmes describes German chamomile oil as a liver cell regenerator and liver restorative. It would work very well in synergy with essential oils such as everlasting, rosemary and lemon to alleviate liver congestion and to promote detoxification.[23]

C

Digestive system

German chamomile oil can be used in treating colic, dyspepsia and indigestion.[19,24] The oil stimulates the liver and gall bladder and is recommended for poor appetite and slow painful digestion.[25,26]

As it is an anti-inflammatory, Holmes suggests using German chamomile for alleviating gastritis, enteritis, IBS and stomatitis.[23]

Immune system

German chamomile oil is reputed to stimulate leukocyte production. For this purpose, Valnet recommends the internal use of German chamomile.[27]

Integumentary system

German chamomile oil can be used for wounds that are slow to heal such as open leg sores, abscesses and infected ingrown nails.[24] It is important for the treatment of eczema, urticaria and dry, itchy conditions.[19,22]

Musculoskeletal system

Holmes states that German chamomile oil has a strong anti-inflammatory effect. He recommends using it for fibromyalgia, neuralgia, tendinitis, plantar fasciitis and bursitis.[23]

German Chamomile oil can be used in a massage for muscular aches and pain, and for inflamed joints associated with rheumatoid arthritis. It is beneficial in treating sprains, inflamed tendons, and swollen painful joints in bursitis.[2,19,22]

Psychological

German chamomile oil is recommended for emotional frustration, anger, irritability, agitation, sudden fits of rage, mood swings and anxiety. It calms the mind, promotes relaxation and is recommended for nervous tension and restlessness.[23]

Reproductive system

German chamomile oil is recommended for promoting and harmonising the menses, for spasmodic dysmenorrhoea and PMS.[24,26]

Respiratory system

Holmes states that German chamomile oil is a moderate antiallergenic and can be used to alleviate allergic rhinitis, sinusitis and asthma.[23]

Skin care

German chamomile oil is beneficial for sensitive skin problems. It is a local vasoconstrictor and can reduce the redness of cheeks due to enlarged capillaries.[22]

Urinary system

German chamomile oil is especially beneficial for urinary tract infections such as cystitis. Davis recommends drinking chamomile tea and having compresses and massages over the lower abdomen with the oil. The oil should also be used in a bath.[22]

Energetics, psyche and subtle uses

Energetics

According to the principles of TCM, German chamomile oil promotes the free flow of *Qi*, which is important for relaxing the nerves, relieving spasms and easing pain. This makes it beneficial for nervous tension, insomnia, indigestion and headaches.[26,28]

German chamomile oil exerts a good stabilising effect on individuals with emotional instability. Holmes suggests that it can help us deal with life's obstacles and challenges in a lateral way, not bound by habit or fear-induced rigidity. It can help us adopt a more flexible, free-flowing spontaneous response.[23]

In TCM, all these conditions are a result of constrained *Qi* with a *Shen* disharmony, or a *deficiency* of *Heart* and *Liver Yin* with *Shen* agitation.

Holmes explains that German chamomile is excellent for nourishing the *Liver Yin*. *Liver Yin deficiency* is often associated with agitation, irritability, resentment and restless insomnia. When we encounter *Heart Yin deficiency* and *Shen* agitation, we experience anxiety, restlessness, insomnia, fearfulness and palpitations.[23]

According to the principles the Five Elements, German chamomile oil helps calm excess Wood energy. According to Ayurveda, German chamomile oil helps to calm excess *Vata* and *Pitta* doshas.

Personality

The German chamomile person is a very strong, emotional person. They have emotional depth and the ability to draw out the best in other people, but keep their own feelings to themselves. They are usually down to earth and upfront. They are always good to have around in an emotional storm, or when grieving, as they provide a strong, solid shoulder to cry on if needed.[29]

Worwood suggests that blue chamomiles are well suited to a profession involving teaching or anything to do with books. She describes them as great organisers.

> *They'll organize everything if you let them – including what you have for lunch and who you should invite to your party. If their suggestions aren't taken up, the Blues can get upset, although this doesn't last too long and is soon forgotten. This is a very contented personality, and seems to take everything in its stride.*[29]

According to Myers-Briggs personality types, the German chamomile personality is likely to be an ISFJ. ISFJs are extremely dependable, loyal and committed. They are quiet and unassuming. They are down-to-earth, practical, conscientious and very diligent. They like being with family and close friends. They find it difficult to relax as they always feel they should do something productive. They often have difficulty being direct, giving orders or asking for help. They are kind, considerate and sensitive to what others are feeling. They express their feelings through thoughtful attention to others' needs. They keep their feelings to themselves to avoid displeasing or disappointing others.

Subtle

Worwood best describes the subtle qualities of German chamomile oil when she states that the scent helps us find spiritual understanding.

> *When inhaled with purpose, it can allow a deeper knowledge of the working of the universe … when confusion seems to have become prevalent in a person's spiritual life, and the laws of the Creator seem to have no meaning to the life we live on earth, then the fragrance can often help us understand.*[30]

On the other hand, Zeck states that German chamomile oil is all about letting go of the old and stale so that the fresh and new can evolve. German chamomile oil will promote your ability to let go, relax and go with the flow when circumstances or plans change.[31]

German chamomile oil also helps us to loosen the grip on old habits, ideas and beliefs that are no longer useful in our life. She says that it allows us to explore personal freedom. This, in turn, helps us to let go of self-imposed limitations. It allows us to choose new adventures and allow our consciousness to soar to new heights.[31]

Davis states that German chamomile oil can be used to counteract agitation or overactivity in any chakra. [32] I believe that it has a very strong affinity with the throat chakra.

It should be used to heal the aura wherever heat, redness or anger is present.[32]

Dosage and Administration

Blending

Aromatherapy

German chamomile oil's rich, sweet and herbaceous aroma can help us create some intriguing blends that can be very relaxing and calming to the psyche.

For an antispasmodic blend that helps ease painful spasmodic conditions associated with the nervous system, digestive system and menstrual cramping, consider blending German chamomile oil with essential oils such as Roman chamomile, clary sage, lavender or sweet marjoram.

For a liver restorative blend for liver detoxification, consider blending German chamomile oil with essential oils such as carrot seed, everlasting, lemon or rosemary.

To alleviate nervous tension, anxiety and stress, consider blending German chamomile oil with essential oils such as bergamot, clary sage, frankincense, geranium, lavender, sweet orange, patchouli or sandalwood.

For a soothing anti-inflammatory blend for the skin, consider blending German chamomile oil with essential oils such as everlasting, lavender, patchouli or sandalwood.

Perfumery

Arctander states that German chamomile oil is used in very small percentages in high-class perfumes to introduce a warm, rich undertone which lasts through all stages of evaporation.[1]

Mode of administration

Bath

Full body bath, foot bath

Topical

Compress, massage, ointment, skin care

Inhalation

Direct inhalation, diffuser, oil vaporiser

Safety profile

General safety

German chamomile oil has been reported to be non-toxic, non-irritant and non-sensitising.[19]

Contraindications

No contraindications known.

Regulatory guidelines

German chamomile essential oil has GRAS status.

References

1. Arctander S. *Perfume and flavor materials of natural origin.* Allured Publishing, Carol Stream, 1994.
2. Khan I, Abourashed E. *Leung's encyclopedia of common natural ingredients used in food, drugs and cosmetics.* 3rd edn. John Wiley & Sons, New Jersey, 2010.
3. Balacs T, Tisserand R. *German chamomile.* The International Journal of Aromatherapy, 1998; 9(1): 15-21.
4. Lawrence BM. *Essential oils 1981-1987.* Allured Publishing, Wheaton, 1989.
5. Evans WC. *Trease and Evans pharmacognosy.* 15th edn. WB Saunders, Edinburgh, 2002.
6. Franke R, Schilcher H. *Chamomile – industrial profile.* Taylor & Francis, Boca Raton, 2005.
7. Blumenthal M et al. *The complete German commission E monographs: therapeutic guide to herbal medicine.* American Botanical Council, Austin, 1998.
8. Jamalian A et al. *Chemical composition and antifungal activity of Matricaria recutita flower essential oil against medically important dermatophytes and soil-borne pathogens.* Journal of Medical Mycology, 2012; 22(4): 308-315. Cited in Quintessential Aromatics database, 2013.
9. Fleischner AM. *Plant extracts to accelerate healing and reduce inflammation.* Cosmetic Toiletries, 1985; 100: 45–58.
10. Isaac O. *Pharmacological investigations with compounds of chamomile.* Planta Medica, 1979; 35(2): 118-124. Cited in Quintessential Aromatics database, 2013.
11. Wu Y et al. *Anti-inflammatory and anti-allergic effects of German chamomile (Matricaria chamomilla L.).* Journal of Essential Oil Bearing Plants, 2011; 14(5): 549-558. Cited in Quintessential Aromatics database, 2013.
12. Aggag ME, Yousef RT. *Study of antimicrobial activity of chamomile oil.* Planta Medica, 1972; 22(2): 140-143. Cited in Quintessential Aromatics database, 2013.
13. Shikov AN et al. *Antibacterial activity of Chamomilla recutita oil extract against Helicobacter pylori.* Phytotherapy Research, 2008; 22(2): 252-253. Cited in Quintessential Aromatics database, 2013.
14. Deans SG et al. *Antibacterial properties of plant essential oils.* International Journal of Food Microbiology, 1987; 5: 165-180. Cited in the Aromatherapy Database, by Bob Harris, Essential Oil Resource Consultants, UK, 2000.
15. Rangelov A. *An experimental characterisation of cholagogic and choleretic activity of a group of essential oils.* Folia Medica, 1989; 31(1): 46-53. Cited in the Aromatherapy Database, by Bob Harris, Essential Oil Resource Consultants, UK, 2000.
16. Acterrath-Tuckermann U et al. *Pharmacological investigations with the compounds of chamomile.* Planta Medica, 1980; 39(1): 38-50. Cited in the Aromatherapy Database, by Bob Harris, Essential Oil Resource Consultants, UK, 2000.
17. Gershbein L. *Regeneration of rat liver in the presence of essential oils and their components.* Food and Cosmetic Toxicology, 1977; 15(3): 173-181. Cited in the Aromatherapy Database, by Bob Harris, Essential Oil Resource Consultants, UK, 2000.
18. Committee on Herbal Medicinal Products (HMPC), *Assessment report on Matricaria recutita L., flos and Matricaria recutita L. aetheroleum.* European Medicines Agency, London, 2014. Doc ref. EMA/HMPC/55837/2011.
19. Lawless J. *The encyclopaedia of essential oils.* Element Books, Shaftesbury, 1992.
20. Schnaubelt K. *Medical aromatherapy.* Frog, Berkeley, 1999.
21. Tisserand R. Young R. *Essential oil safety.* 2nd edn. Churchill Livingstone, Edinburgh, 2014.
22. Davis P. *Aromatherapy: an A-Z.* 2nd edn. C.W. Daniel Company, Saffron Walden, 1999.
23. Holmes P. *Aromatica: A clinical guide to essential oils therapeutics – Vol. I.* Singing Dragon, London, 2016.
24. Fischer-Rizzi S. *Complete aromatherapy handbook.* Sterling Publishing, New York, 1990.
25. Lavabre M. *Aromatherapy workbook.* Healing Arts Press, Rochester, 1997.
26. Holmes P. *The energetics of Western herbs – Vol. II.* Artemis Press, Boulder, 1989.
27. Valnet J. *The practice of aromatherapy.* C.W. Daniel Company, Saffron Walden, 1980.
28. Mojay G. *Aromatherapy for healing the spirit.* Healing Arts Press, Rochester, 1999.

C

29. Worwood VA. *The fragrant mind.* Transworld Publisher, London, 1995.
30. Worwood VA. *The fragrant spirit.* Transworld Publisher, London, 1999.
31. Zeck R. *The blossoming heart – aromatherapy for healing and transformation.* Aroma Tours, East Ivanhoe, 2004.
32. Davis P. *Subtle aromatherapy.* C.W. Daniel Company, Saffron Walden, 1991.

Chamomile, Roman

Identification

Botanical name

Chamaemelum nobile (L.) All.

Synonyms

Anthemis nobilis, garden chamomile

Family

Asteraceae (Compositae)

Botany and origins

Roman chamomile is a pleasant-smelling perennial with feathery, fern-like leaves and branched stems of a creeping habit with daisy-like flowers.[1] It is a native of western Europe and is now cultivated in England, Belgium, France and Hungary.[2]

Roman chamomile's common name is derived from the Greek word *chamaimelon* – *chamai* meaning on the ground, and *melon* an apple, referring to its distinctive smell when fresh. The botanical name of *Anthemis* is derived from the Greek word *anthos* which means a flower. The plant's specific name of *nobilis* means noble or noted – referring to its healing virtues.[1]

Method of extraction

Roman chamomile is distilled from the flowering tops of *C. nobile.*

Characteristics

Roman chamomile is a pale-yellow coloured, mobile liquid of a sweet herbaceous, somewhat fruity-warm and tea leaf-like odour that is extremely diffusive with little tenacity.[2]

Chemical composition

While Roman chamomile shares similar properties with German chamomile, its chemical profile is very different. Roman chamomile essential oil contains very little if any chamazulene or α-bisabolol – the major constituents responsible for German chamomile's anti-inflammatory and antiallergenic properties.[3]

Arctander states that Roman chamomile has the highest number of esters found in any essential oil.[2]

The chemical composition of Roman chamomile oil was reported as follows:

α-pinene (0.5-10.0%), camphene (0.0-0.5%), β-pinene (0.0-10.0%), sabinene (0.0-10.0%), myrcene (0.0-0.5%), 1,8-cineole (0.5-25%), γ-terpinene (0.0-0.5%), caryophyllene (0.0-10.0%), propyl angelate (0.5-10.0%), butyl angelate (0.5-10.0%).[4]

Adulteration

The esters that can be found in Roman chamomile oil can all be produced synthetically, therefore the oil can be adulterated with these synthetic esters.[5]

Pharmacopoeias and standards

At the time of writing, the purity, composition, physico-chemical properties and therapeutic use of Roman chamomile essential oil are not defined in any pharmacopoeia monograph or standard.

History and Traditional Uses

History

Since antiquity, chamomile flowers have been used both internally for digestive disorders and externally for skin and mucous membrane irritations.

Grieve explained that when walked upon, its strong, fragrant scent reveals its presence before it is seen. For this reason, it was used as one of the strewing herbs in the Middle Ages and is often purposely planted in green walks in gardens.[6]

Traditional medicine

Roman chamomile has long been known for its therapeutic properties. In ancient Egypt, it was used for the treatment of fever and as a sign of dedication to the Gods. Ancient Greek texts described the extensive therapeutic uses of the herb by Hippocrates and Dioscorides. The Romans used Roman chamomile to treat intestinal and rheumatic disorders.[6]

Culpeper was familiar with the pronounced effect that chamomile had on the mind and nervous system. He suggested that it comforts both the head and the brain.[6]

C

Grieve states that chamomile tea is an old-fashioned but extremely effective remedy for hysterical and nervous affections in women, and is also used as an emmenagogue.[6]

Chamomile flowers are recommended as a tonic in dropsical complaints for their diuretic and tonic properties. The flowers may be used in a poultice and for external swelling, inflammatory pain or congested neuralgia.[7]

Herbal

Roman chamomile flowers are listed and described in several pharmacopoeias. They are listed as having carminative, antiemetic, antispasmodic and sedative properties. They are used for dyspepsia, nausea and vomiting, anorexia, vomiting of pregnancy, dysmenorrhoea, and specifically for flatulent dyspepsia associated with mental stress.[8]

Food, perfumery and flavouring

Arctander states that Roman chamomile oil is rarely used in flavour work.[2] However, it is commonly used in perfumery and skin care preparations.

Therapeutics

Pharmacology and clinical studies

Many pharmacological and clinical studies involving Roman chamomile oil have been published. A systemic review of these studies will not be attempted. Rather I have chosen a selection of studies that support the traditional and clinical uses.

Anti-inflammatory activity

Roman chamomile oil has been used topically to reduce inflammation and accelerate healing times.[9]

Roman chamomile oil has been identified as having sedative and anti-inflammatory properties. It was found that the oil from the white-headed variety was significantly more sedative than the oil from the yellow-headed variety. The white-headed variety contained significantly more angelic esters, and this may have contributed to the increased sedative and anti-inflammatory properties.[9]

Antimicrobial activity

A blended oil containing Roman chamomile, ylang ylang and lavender showed potent activity against methicillin-resistant *Staphylococcus aureus*. None of the tested oil showed significant activity when tested alone, suggesting a synergistic effect of the combined oil.[8]

Roman chamomile oil was moderately active against *Candida albicans* (minimum inhibitory concentration MIC = 0.8 mg/ml). It had strong activity against strains of gram-positive (*Staphylococcus aureus, Enterococcus faecalis*) and gram-nagative (*Escherichia coli, Proteus vulgaris, Klebsiella pneumoniae*).[10]

Anxiolytic activity

In a small study, 8 patients with primary malignant brain tumours were given aromatherapy massage during their first follow-up appointment after radiotherapy. Patients were offered either a foot, hand or neck/shoulder massage with lavender or Roman chamomile oils. The results of the study demonstrated a statistical reduction of all the physical parameters measured after massage, indicating a relaxation response; however, there was no difference between the Hospital Anxiety and Depression Scales score before and after treatment, implying there was no effect on anxiety.[11]

Another study examined the effectiveness of aromatherapy on improving the quality of life of 51 patients with advanced cancer. The study compared massage with Roman chamomile oil and massage with carrier oil only. Both groups reported that the interventions reduced stress, depression, tension, pain and anxiety. However, according to the results of the Rotterdam Symptom Checklist and the State-Trait Anxiety Inventory questionnaires, there was a statistically significant improvement in the aromatherapy group.[12]

A study using a blend of lavender, Roman chamomile and neroli essential oils examined the effects of the oils on the anxiety, sleep and blood pressure of percutaneous coronary intervention (PCI) patients in an intensive care unit (ICU). 56 patients were evenly divided to either the aromatherapy or conventional nursing group. The aromatherapy participants received 10 treatments by inhalation before and 10 treatments after, the PCI. The aromatherapy group showed significantly lower anxiety and improved sleep quality compared with the conventional nursing group. The systolic and diastolic blood pressure of both groups did not show any significant difference. It was concluded that aromatherapy effectively reduced anxiety levels and increased sleep quality of PCI patients admitted to the ICU.[13]

Dementia

Roman chamomile oil was more effective than lavender oil in a study examining the effects of essential oils on the behaviour and sleep patterns of two elderly patients with Alzheimer's disease. The small study confirmed that Roman chamomile oil promoted sleep, reduced aggressive behaviour and reduced the dependence on hypnotic medication.[14]

Sedative activity

A case study was reported in which an 18-month old infant with persistent agitation on continuous sedative and narcotic infusions with midazolam experienced a 50% reduction in benzodiazepine requirement, with signs of deep sedation after the first of two topical applications of a 7.5% essential oil blend of Roman chamomile, sandalwood and galbanum oils in a jojoba oil base.[15]

Actions

Actions commonly cited in aromatherapy

Analgesic, anti-inflammatory, antiseptic, antispasmodic, bactericidal, carminative, cholagogue, digestive, emmenagogue, febrifuge, hepatic, sedative, stomachic, sudorific, vulnerary[16,17,18]

Actions supported by clinical studies

Antimicrobial, antispasmodic, anxiolytic, sedative

Comment

The therapeutic properties of German and Roman chamomile oils are often stated to be similar.[18,19,20]

I am not sure why Roman chamomile oil is compared with German chamomile oil as their chemical composition is very different. Lis-Balchin states that Roman chamomile has very little anti-inflammatory activity compared to German chamomile.[21] However, Roman chamomile oil has such an interesting ester profile, and there is evidence that it has antispasmodic, anxiolytic and relaxation properties.

I was drawn to a description of Roman chamomile by Grieve who described it as the 'Plant's Physician':

> *... that nothing contributes so much to the health of a garden as a number of chamomile herbs dispersed about it, and that if another plant is drooping and sickly, in nine cases out of ten, it will recover if you place a herb of chamomile near it.*[6]

This gives us an incredible insight into the healing qualities of Roman chamomile.

Aromatherapy Uses

Clinical aromatherapy

Children's remedy

Fischer-Rizzi refers to Roman chamomile oil as a traditional medicine for children. She recommends the oil whenever children are feeling impatient, disagreeable, tense or have nightmares.[22]

Roman chamomile is considered one of the gentlest of essential oils and is particularly beneficial for treating children. It may be used to alleviate the pain associated with teething infants.[17,19]

Digestive system

Roman chamomile oil is used in treating colic, diarrhoea, poor appetite and indigestion.[16,17,20,23]

Nervous system

The sweet scent of Roman chamomile oil is soothing, calming and antidepressant. It is particularly beneficial for alleviating anxiety and stress.[17,19] It is used to alleviate migraines and headaches, and for insomnia.[16,17]

Reproductive system

Roman chamomile oil is very helpful for treating amenorrhoea, dysmenorrhoea and PMS.[16,22]

Respiratory system

Roman chamomile oil is recommended as an emergency remedy during an asthma attack. Schnaubelt recommends rubbing the oil in the solar plexus, wrists and temples until more specific help becomes available.[24]

Skin care

Roman chamomile oil is beneficial for sensitive, red or dry skin.[19]

Energetics, psyche and subtle uses

Energetics

According to the principles of TCM, Roman chamomile promotes the free flow of *Qi*, which is important for relaxing the nerves, relieving spasms and easing pain. This makes it beneficial for nervous tension, insomnia, indigestion and headaches.[18,23]

Tisserand associates chamomile's ability to soothe restlessness, nervous irritability or impatience with its action on the *Liver* – the emotional state of anger is associated with the choleric humour and the *Liver* according to traditional herbalists and TCM.[25]

According to the principles of the Five Elements, anger is associated with the Wood Element and the *Liver*. Roman chamomile helps to calm the Wood Element and assists the *Liver* in its function to allow *Qi* to flow freely.

Personality

Worwood describes the Roman chamomile personality like someone who is full of sunshine and joy, with a harmonious disposition and emotional life. While they are serene and gentle, they sometimes appear to be in a dreamlike state. She explains that Roman chamomiles can have a strange power over ordinary mortals, on whom they have a calming, almost mesmerizing effect. People will follow them anywhere and believe implicitly in everything they say.[26]

On the other hand, she states that the inner peace that they appear to have can be misleading because they may have inner conflict, which can torment them. As a result, they are likely to have moods swings, particularly in relationships. This can cause much emotional stress. When this happens, they tend to isolate themselves from others.[26]

Fischer-Rizzi describes the type of person who might benefit from Roman chamomile oil:[22]

> *... someone who feels grumpy, discontented or impatient, chamomile is a good remedy. It is beneficial for people who feel short tempered, self-involved, overly sensitive or rarely satisfied.*

According to Myers-Briggs personality types, the Roman chamomile personality is likely to be an INFP. INFPs are gentle, calm, easygoing and affirming. Integrity and commitment to what they believe in is essential. They like time alone for their many interests. They like learning and researching new things and interests. They are highly reflective, especially in understanding the mysteries and meaning of life. They have little need to impose their values on others. They prefer to gently influence and inspire. They value authenticity and depth in their relationships.

C

Subtle

Worwood states that Roman chamomile connects us with our inner child, allowing us to come closer to the spiritual realms for comfort and uniting. She explains that it should also be used when the spirit is sad.[27]

Keim Loughran & Bull state that Roman chamomile assists us in hearing our inner voice in order to discern our individual path. They explain that it will help us to receive the teaching that has the most meaning for us and that speaks most directly to who we are.[28]

It relates to the throat chakra and can be used to help individuals to express their highest spiritual truth.[29]

Dosage and Administration

Blending

Aromatherapy

To alleviate insomnia, consider blending Roman chamomile oil with essential oils such as lavender, neroli, sweet marjoram or sandalwood.

For the relief of anxiety, nervous tension or stress, consider blending Roman chamomile oil with essential oils such as bergamot, fragonia, frankincense, geranium, lavender, sweet orange or sandalwood.

For the relief of the symptoms associated with PMS or dysmenorrhoea, consider blending Roman chamomile oil with essential oils such as clary sage, lavender, sweet marjoram, rose or ylang ylang.

For the relief of indigestion, consider blending Roman chamomile oil with essential oils such as black pepper, coriander seed, sweet fennel, sweet marjoram or sweet orange.

Perfumery

Roman chamomile oil imparts a warm, yet fresh, note with a natural depth, which is difficult to obtain by other means. It blends well with bergamot, labdanum, neroli, clary sage and oakmoss absolute.[2]

Mode of administration

Bath

Full body bath, foot bath

Topical

Compress, massage, ointment, skin care

Inhalation

Direct inhalation, diffuser, oil vaporiser

Safety Profile

General safety

Roman chamomile oil has been reported to be non-toxic, non-irritant and non-sensitising.[17]

Contraindications

No contraindications known. Not to be used if allergies to Roman chamomile and other Asteraceae plants exist. The sensitisation potency is moderate and frequency rare.[30]

Regulatory guidelines

Roman chamomile oil has GRAS status.

References

1. Le Strange R. *A history of herbal plants.* Angus and Robertson, United Kingdom, 1977.
2. Arctander S. *Perfume and flavor materials of natural origin.* Allured Publishing, Carol Stream, 1994.
3. Bruneton J. *Pharmacognosy.* 2nd edn. Lavoisier Publishing, Paris, 1999.
4. Lawrence BM. *Essential oils 1979-1980.* Allured Publishing, Wheaton, 1981.
5. Schmidt E, Wanner J. *Adulteration of essential oils.* In Baser KHC, Buchbauer G. eds. *Handbook of essential oils – science, technology*

and applications. 2nd edn. CRC Press, Boca Raton, 2016: 707-745.
6. Grieve M. *A modern herbal – Vol. I.* Dover Publications, New York, 1971.
7. Evans WC. *Trease and Evans pharmacognosy.* 15th edn. WB Saunders, Edinburgh, 2002.
8. Committee on Herbal Medicinal Products (HMPC). *Assessment report on Chamaemelum nobile (L.) All., flos.* European Medicines Agency, 2012. Doc ref. EMA/HMPC/560906/2010.
9. Melegari M et al. *Chemical characteristics and pharmacological properties of the essential oils of Anthemis nobilis.* Fitoterapia, 1989; 59 (6); 449-455. Cited in the Aromatherapy Database, by Bob Harris, Essential Oil Resource Consultants, UK, 2000.
10. Bail S et al. *Antimicrobial activities of Roman chamomile oil from France and its main compounds.* Journal of Essential Oil Research, 2009; 21(3): 283-286. Cited in Quintessential Aromatics database, 2013.
11. Hadfield N. *The role of aromatherapy massage in reducing anxiety in patients with malignant brain tumours.* International Journal of Palliative Nursing, 2001; 7(6): 279-285. Cited in Quintessential Aromatics database, 2013.
12. Wilkinson S. *Aromatherapy and massage in palliative care.* International Journal of Palliative Nursing, 1995; 1(1): 21-30. Cited in Quintessential Aromatics database, 2013.
13. Cho MY et al. *Effects of aromatherapy on the anxiety, vital signs, and sleep quality of percutaneous coronary intervention patients in intensive care units.* Evidence-Based Complementary and Alternative Medicine, 2013. doi 10.1155/2013/381381. Cited in Quintessential Aromatics database, 2013.
14. Wolfe A, Herzeberg J. *Can aromatherapy oils promote sleep in severely demented patients?* International Journal of Geriatric Psychology, 1996; 11(10): 926-927. Cited in Quintessential Aromatics database, 2013.
15. Hedayat KM. *Reduction of benzodiazepine requirements during mechanical ventilation in a child by topical application of essential oils.* Explore, 2008; 4(2): 136-138. Cited in Quintessential Aromatics database, 2013.
16. Lavabre M. *Aromatherapy workbook.* Healing Arts Press, Rochester, 1997.
17. Lawless J. *The encyclopaedia of essential oils.* Element Books, Shaftesbury, 1992.
18. Mojay G. *Aromatherapy for healing the spirit.* Healing Arts Press, Rochester, 1999.
19. Davis P. *Aromatherapy: an A-Z.* 2nd edn. C.W. Daniel Company, Saffron Walden, 1999.
20. Khan I, Abourashed E. *Leung's encyclopedia of common natural ingredients used in food, drugs and cosmetics.* 3rd edn. John Wiley & Sons, New Jersey, 2010
21. Lis-Balchin M. *Aromatherapy science – a guide for healthcare professionals.* Pharmaceutical Press, London, 2006.
22. Fischer-Rizzi S. *Complete aromatherapy handbook.* Sterling Publishing, New York, 1990.
23. Holmes P. *The energetics of Western herbs – Vol. II.* Artemis Press, Boulder, 1989.
24. Schnaubelt K. *Medical aromatherapy.* Frog, Berkeley, 1999.
25. Tisserand R. *The art of aromatherapy.* C.W. Daniel Company, Saffron Walden, 1977.
26. Worwood VA. *The fragrant mind.* Transworld Publishers, London, 1995.
27. Worwood VA. *The fragrant heavens.* Transworld Publishers, London, 1999.
28. Keim Loughran J, Bull R. *Aromatherapy anointing oils.* Frog, Berkeley, 2001.
29. Davis P. *Subtle aromatherapy.* C.W. Daniel Company, Saffron Walden, 1991.
30. Blumenthal M et al. *The complete German commission E monographs: therapeutic guide to herbal medicine.* American Botanical Council, Austin, 1998.

Champaca absolute

Identification

Botanical name

It was previously classified as *Michelia champaca*. The accepted name is now *Magnolia champaca* (L.) Baill. ex Pierre.[1]

Synonyms

Golden champa, orange champaca, champaka, champak

Family

Magnoliaceae

Botany and origins

Magnolia champaca is a medium-sized, slender tree with beautiful fragrant deep yellow to orange flowers. It is related to magnolia. The tree is native to the Philippines and Indonesia. Champaca is cultivated in India, southeastern China and Réunion.[2]

C

The champaca tree is logged for its timber. The timber is highly desirable for furniture making and cabinetry. Cropwatch reports that it is critically endangered in Nepal and that restrictions have been imposed on harvesting for export purposes by the government of Nepal.[3]

M. champaca is classified in the IUCN Red List of Threatened Species as 'Least Concern' as it is widespread in the Indo-Malaysian tropical region. The report states that there is no specific population information or data on the decline of this species. It is used for timber, but logging is not thought to be a significant threat to the species at a global level.[4]

Method of extraction

Champaca absolute is obtained by solvent extraction of the yellow flowers of *M. champaca*. An attar is also prepared using sandalwood oil. An essential oil is also extracted from the wood.[2]

Characteristics

Champaca absolute is a dark yellow or brownish-orange viscous liquid. Arctander describes the odour as very unique. It has a delicate dry floral odour reminiscent of neroli, ylang ylang, carnation and tea rose.[2]

Chemical composition

The chemical profile of champaca absolute was reported as follows:

2-phenylethanol (25-34%), methyl linoleate (10-18%), indole (2.9-12%), methyl anthranilate (2.1-9.0%), methyl benzoate (1-5%), phenylacetonitrile (1.2-4.3%), benzyl acetate (0.1-4.0%), β-ionone (0.2-3.4%), methyl palmitate (2-3%), ionone oximes (0-3.0%), (Z)-linalool oxide (0.2-2.5%), 2-phenylethyl acetate (0.4-2.0%), benzyl alcohol (0.3-2.0)%, linalool (0.2-2.0%), α-farnesene (0.6-1.6%), α-ionone (0.1-1.65), dihydro-β-ionone (0.3-1.4%), dihydro-B-ionol (0.3-1.1%), phenylaldoxime (0.5-1.0%).[5]

Adulteration

Being such an expensive essential oil, the chances of adulteration are very high. It is often cut with ylang ylang.[2]

Pharmacopoeias and standards

At the time of writing, the purity, composition, physico-chemical properties and therapeutic use of champaca absolute are not defined in any pharmacopoeia monograph or standard.

History and Traditional Uses

History

In India the flowers are infused in a vegetable oil and the perfumed oil is used as an attar in floral bouquets in the local perfume industry.[2] Champaca flowers are used in India as an offering to the gods and goddesses. In Indian folklore, it is considered to be an incarnation of Lakshmi, the goddess of wealth and prosperity.[6]

Traditional medicine

All parts of the tree have therapeutic value. The flowers are used in combination with the seeds as an antidote to scorpion and snake bites. The juice of the leaves is blended with honey and used for treating colic. An infusion of the flowers and fruit is used for reducing fever.[7]

Food, perfumery and flavouring

Champaca absolute is extensively used in perfumery.

Therapeutics

Pharmacology and clinical studies

There has been very little research into its pharmacological or clinical uses.

Actions

Actions commonly cited in aromatherapy

Antidepressant, aphrodisiac, diuretic, emmenagogue, emollient, stimulant, stomachic and tonic[6,7]

Actions supported by clinical studies

None of the actions commonly cited in aromatherapy can be supported by clinical studies.

Comment

Champaca absolute is not commonly used in aromatherapy. However, oils with a rich floral aroma often promote emotional healing and stability. They are used whenever we feel anxiety and frustration, or suffer from acute depression, irritability and emotional confusion.

Aromatherapy Uses

Clinical aromatherapy

Psychological

Irani recommends champaca for anger and manic depression, and for its grounding effect.[6]

Lind describes the exotic sensual scent of champaca absolute as warming, indulging and gratifying, enhancing self-esteem and confidence.[7]

Reproductive system

Champaca absolute is used to alleviate amenorrhoea and dysmenorhoea.[7]

C

Skin care

Champaca absolute is cooling and moisturising on the skin.[6]

Energetics, psyche and subtle uses

Energetics

Champaca absolute regulates the *Qi* of the *Heart* and harmonises the *Shen*. Whenever we experience disharmony of the *Shen,* we may experience feelings of moodiness, anxiety, irritability, restlessness and insomnia. We lack inspiration and insight and there is no 'heart and soul' to life.

According to the principles of the Five Elements, champaca absolute strengthens and balances the Fire Element.

According to the principles of Ayurveda, champaca absolute has a strong affinity with *Pitta* dosha, reduces excess *Kapha* dosha and stimulates the *Vata* dosha.

Personality

According to Myers-Briggs personality types, the champaca personality is likely to be an ESFP. ESFPs are friendly, witty, charming and talkative. They value and nurture their relationships, and give generously, without expecting anything in return. They are spontaneous and playful, and enjoy everything they do and see. People who share their sense of fun and adventure are their favourite companions. They turn everything into a fun-filled event. They enjoy good things in life – music, dance, food, drink and entertainment. They avoid being alone. They like working in a lively and stimulating atmosphere with friendly, energetic people. They can be good at dealing with the public. They like variety and frequent change of tasks or jobs. They are enthusiastic, high-spirited and have lots of energy.

Subtle

Keim Loughran & Bull state that the scent of champaca absolute energises and balances the auric field and all the energy centres. It can be used for opening the mind to the influx of divine energy and assisting in psychic development.[8]

Dosage and Administration

Blending

Aromatherapy

To create a sensual uplifting blend, consider blending champaca absolute with essential oils such as bergamot, coriander seed, jasmine absolute, sweet orange, mandarin, rose absolute, sandalwood or ylang ylang.

Perfumery

Champaca absolute blends well with other rich floral oils, sweet spice oils such as coriander seed or clove bud, sweet citrus oils such as sweet orange and mandarin, and sandalwood.[2]

Mode of administration

Bath

Full body bath, foot bath

Topical

Compress, massage, ointment, skin care

Inhalation

Direct inhalation, diffuser, oil vaporiser

Safety Profile

General safety

Champaca absolute is non-toxic and non-irritant. No adverse skin reactions are reported and the chemical constituents indicate that it should be a low risk skin sensitiser.[5]

Contraindications

No contraindications known.

Regulatory guidelines

Champaca absolute is not defined in any regulatory guideline.

C

References

1. *The plant list – Magnolia champaca (L.) Baill. ex Pierre.* Retrieved Sep 29, 2017, from http://www.theplantlist.org/tpl1.1/record/kew-117504
2. Arctander S. *Perfume and flavor materials of natural origins.* Allured Publishing, Carol Stream, 1994.
3. Burfield T. *Updated list of threatened aromatic plants used in the aroma & cosmetic industries.* V 1. 21 Mar. 2010. Retrieved from www.cropwatch.org
4. Khela, S. *Magnolia champaca.* The IUCN Red List of Threatened Species 2014: e.T191869A15267603. doi: 10.2305/IUCN.UK.2014-3.RLTS.T191869A15267603.en.
5. Tisserand R, Young R. *Essential oil safety.* 2nd edn. Churchill Livingstone, Edinburgh, 2014.
6. Irani F. *The magic of ayurveda aromatherapy.* Subtle Energies, Sydney, 2001.
7. Lind E. *Discovering an oil.* Aromatherapy Quarterly, 1997; 55: 9-11.
8. Keim Loughran J, Bull R. *Aromatherapy and subtle energy techniques.* Frog, Berkeley, 2000.

Cinnamon

Identification

Botanical name

Cinnamomum verum J. Presl.

Synonyms

Cinnamomum zeylanicum Blume

Family

Lauraceae

Botany and origins

Cinnamon is a bushy, evergreen tree up to 15 m. The bark and leaves are strongly aromatic. Three distinct essential oils (bark, leaf and root) are produced from the cinnamon tree.

The bark of young shoots is preferred. Once the bark is removed, it is dried and becomes the cinnamon quills of commerce. Commercial cinnamon bark is a dull brown, up to 5.5 mm thick, with the inner surface somewhat darker and finely striated longitudinally. The finest quality has a delicate fragrance and tastes warm, sweet and pleasant. The presence of calcium oxalate crystals indicates low-quality bark.[1]

The species name *verum* refers to the term 'true' cinnamon.[2]

Cinnamon is often confused with *Cinnamomum cassia*, which is known as cassia. Cinnamon is native to Sri Lanka, India and South East Asia. It has been introduced to the Seychelles, Zanzibar and Indonesia. Cinnamon produces the finest bark in sunny regions with an average temperature of 27-30°C.[1]

C

Method of extraction

Cinnamon bark essential oil is obtained by steam or water distillation with cohobation. Cinnamon bark contains water-soluble volatile aromatic components, which can be recovered by extracting distillation water and adding the extract to water-distilled oil. Cinnamon leaf essential oil is obtained by similar methods.[1]

Characteristics

Cinnamon bark oil is a pale yellow to dark yellow or brownish yellow liquid with an extremely powerful, diffusive, warm-spicy and tenacious odour. The dryout note is very persistent sweet, and has a powdery dryness. Arctander also states that, in the first top notes you may find a certain fruity freshness similar to the sweet candy-like freshness of a good clove bud oil.[3]

Cinnamon leaf oil is a yellow to brownish yellow oil with a warm spicy, but rather harsh odour which lacks the rich body of the bark oil. It has some resemblance to the odour of clove leaf and clove stem oil.[3]

Chemical composition

The chemical composition of cinnamon leaf and bark oil was reported as follows:

Leaf: eugenol (80-96%), eugenyl acetate (1.0%), cinnamaldehyde (3%), benzyl benzoate (3%).[4]

Bark: cinnamaldehyde (40-50%), eugenol (4-10%), benzyl benzoate (1.0%), α-pinene (0.2%), 1,8-cineole (1.65%), linalool (2.3%), caryophyllene (1.35%).[4]

The EMA assessment report for cinnamon states that cinnamon bark oil typically contains up to 4% essential oil consisting of cinnamaldehyde (60-75%), cinnamyl acetate (1-5%), eugenol (1-10%), β-caryophyllene (1-4%), linalool (1-3%) and 1,8-cineole (1-2%).[5]

Adulteration

Adulteration of cinnamon bark oil is very common. Because the main constituents of cinnamon bark oil are very common, low-cost materials, the oil can be easily cut with synthetic version components. It is also very common to simply label the oil as cinnamon oil. Such oils are typically adulterated or blended oils.[3]

Pharmacopoeias and standards

An international (ISO) standard exists for cinnamon leaf oil – ISO 3524:2003 Oil of Cinnamon Leaf, Sri Lanka Type (*Cinnamomum zeylanicum* Blume).

There is no ISO standard for cinnamon bark oil.

Cinnamon oil is defined in several pharmacopoeia monographs:

- German Commission E
- Martindale Extra Pharmacopoeia
- European Pharmacopoeia
- European Medicines Agency Assessment Report on *Cinnamomun verum* J.S. Presl, cortex and cortices Aetheroleum
- WHO Monographs on Selected Medicinal Plants — Vol. 1.

History and Traditional Uses

History

The generic name is derived from the Arabic or Persian word *mama* via the Greek word *amomum* meaning spice. The prefix *chini* refers to its believed origins.[1]

The history of cinnamon reaches back into antiquity. It is mentioned in the Bible. In Exodus, God told Moses to take myrrh, cinnamon, olive oil and bulrushes with him from Egypt. The ancient Egyptians were known to have used cinnamon in mummification. Diodorus described how, after cleaning the body with palm wine and spices and anointing it with cedar oil and other unguents, it was then rubbed down with myrrh, cinnamon and other aromatics to preserve it.[6]

Guenther describes the ancient trade routes of cinnamon:

> *Flotilla of sturdy vessels, their sails bulging in the steady monsoon winds, winged their way across the Indian Ocean's blue billows and along Arabia's barren shores towards Egypt where the precious spice could be conveyed to sharp faced dealers from Phoenicia who supplied the Greek and Roman trade. Or the spice was carried on camel back across Mesopotamia's timeless caravan trails, now buried in sand and forgotten, from the Persian Gulf to Babylon and finally to Sidon and Tyre on the Mediterranean.*[7]

The quest for cinnamon was pursued so enthusiastically that it was the principal incentive of the Portuguese in discovering the trade route to India and Sri Lanka, thus breaking the Arab control of the Oriental spice trade.[1]

When the Portuguese arrived in Ceylon in 1505, cinnamon bark was obtained from wild trees.[1]

Ceylon was occupied by the Portuguese in 1536 and then the Dutch in 1656. The Dutch started cinnamon cultivation in 1770 and exercised a strict monopoly on cinnamon trade comparable with their monopoly of nutmeg; however, the British abolished the Dutch monopoly in 1833. The removal of the very high export duty in 1943 encouraged exports, and large shipments were made to Europe.[1]

The Dutch also introduced cinnamon into their East Indian colony – Java. Indonesia is now considered one of the major producers and exporters of cinnamon products.[1]

Weiss states that where and when cinnamon oil was first produced is not clear, but it was steam-distilled in Ceylon during the Dutch occupation. He also states that cinnamon oil was listed in a European document of the sixteenth century, where a German ordinance was published controlling its price.[1]

Traditional medicine

Cinnamon has been used for several thousand years in Eastern and Western cultures in treating an extensive range of disorders.[8]

In Ayurveda, the powdered bark is recommended for treating throat and mouth infections, urinary bladder diseases, haemorrhoids, worm infestation, rhinitis, sinusitis and heart disease. It is also used for treating all types of poisons and toxins, dysentery, painful gastrointestinal disorders with indigestion, and flatulence.[2]

Herbal

The oral use of cinnamon bark (essential oil, tea infusion or tincture) is approved by the German Commission E for loss of appetite and dyspeptic complaints such as mild, spastic condition of gastrointestinal tract, bloating and flatulence.[9]

Cinnamon has been traditionally used for stomach cramps, flatulence, nausea, vomiting, diarrhoea, infant colic and common infections, and for female reproductive problems such as dysmenorrhoea, menorrhagia, lactation and pain at childbirth. It is also commonly used as an ingredient in topical preparations for pain and inflammation.[10]

The antidiabetic effects of cinnamon bark extract have been shown in streptozotocin-induced diabetic rats. Several studies have confirmed that herbal extracts of cinnamon bark not only lower blood glucose but also cholesterol levels. Several polyphenols isolated from cinnamon such as rutin, catechin, quercetin, kaempferol and isorhamnetin displayed insulin-like activity.[11]

The approved traditional uses for cinnamon bark (as a herbal tea, liquid extract [1:1], or tincture [1:5]) are for the symptomatic treatment of mild spasmodic gastrointestinal complaints, include bloating and flatulence, and for the symptomatic treatment of diarrhoea. The essential oil in liquid dosage for oral use is approved for the same use as cinnamon bark as a herb.[5]

Food, perfumery and flavouring

Cinnamon leaf is used as a fragrance component of soaps, detergents, creams, lotions and perfumes.[12]

Cinnamon bark oil has excellent masking power, and is frequently used in pharmaceuticals for masking unpleasant medicinal tastes. In combination with sweet orange oil, lime oil and cola extract, cinnamon bark oil is an important aspect of the Coca-Cola flavour profile. Arctander states that the cinnamon note is even more pronounced in the Pepsi cola flavour profile.[3]

Therapeutics

Pharmacology and clinical studies

Many pharmacological studies involving cinnamon oil have been published. A systemic review of these studies will not be attempted. Rather, I have chosen a selection of studies that support the traditional and clinical uses.

Antidiabetic activity

In a clinical study involving mice, it was found that cinnamon bark essential oil provided significant protection against alloxan-induced renal damage, and a decrease in the fasting blood glucose was achieved at the dose of 20 mg/kg.[13]

Cinnamon oil was found to significantly decrease fasting blood glucose in an animal study. In one study, a significant decrease in plasma C-peptide, serum triglyceride, total cholesterol and blood urea nitrogen levels was measured, while serum high-density lipoprotein (HDL)-cholesterol levels significantly increased after 35 days. It was concluded that cinnamon oil may be useful for the treatment of type 2 diabetes mellitus.[14]

Antimicrobial activity

To date, the antimicrobial activity of cinnamon oil has been extensively investigated. The essential oil of cinnamon oil is considered more potent than most other tested plant extracts.[11]

Cinnamon bark oil displayed antibacterial activity in vitro against *Bacillus subtilis, Escherichia coli, Staphylococcus aureus, Salmonella typhimurium* and *Pseudomonas aeruginosa*.[15]

It is also active in vitro against the following fungi – *Aspergillus* spp., *Cladosporium werneckii, Geotrichum candidum, Kloeckera apivulata, Candida lipolytica* and *Candida albicans*.[15]

C

Cinnamon oil was found to have a very high minimum fungicidal concentration (MFC) at less than 0.15% concentration against four isolates of *C. albicans*.[16]

Cinnamon oil displayed higher efficacy in inhibiting methicillin-resistant *Staphylococcus aureus* (MRSA) and methicillin-sensitive *Staphylococcus aureus* (MSSA) growth compared to vancomycin, which is the currently used standard for treatment. The authors noted that essential oils could be useful in treating hospital patients with MRSA or MSSA infection in areas where antibiotics are not readily available.[17]

Another study also found that cinnamon oil demonstrated considerable efficacy against hospital-acquired infections and antibiotic-resistant bacteria. The authors stated that essential oils could represent an inexpensive and effective antiseptic topical treatment option for antimycotic-resistant *Candida* species.[18]

Cinnamon leaf oil was found to display very high antimicrobial activity against resistant strains of bacteria. The authors reported that the oil was bactericidal against *Staphylococcus aureus* and *Escherichia coli* at concentrations ranging from 0.31% to 105 (v/v) after one hour of contact.[19]

The in vitro antibacterial activity against nine epidermal bacteria and 11 MRSA isolates found that cinnamon bark oil exhibited antimicrobial activity against all the organisms, with the minimum inhibitory concentration values (MIC) ranging from 0.15 to 2.5 μl.[20]

Cinnamon bark oil demonstrated very effective antimicrobial activity against group B streptococci (GBS) at very low concentrations. GBS are the cause of dangerous infections both of neonatal and obstetrical sepsis.[21]

Cinnamon oil displayed very high activity against *Streptococcus mutans* in vitro. The researchers suggest that the oil can be used as a viable alternative to other antibacterial agents in the control of both bacteria and yeasts responsible for oral infections.[22]

A study found that dimethylsulphoxide (DMSO), often used as a dispersing solvent, had an inhibitory effect on the antimicrobial activity of cinnamon oil. The researchers found that, when DMSO was not present, there was a 50-fold increase in the activity of cinnamon oil. In the absence of DMSO, the essential oil solubilised in the microbial lipid membrane where it could have a greater effect on cell metabolism.[23]

Cinnamon bark oil and cinnamaldehyde demonstrated the strongest antimicrobial activity against all clinical-isolated multidrug-resistant *Pseudomonas aeruginosa* strains. The same study also confirmed that cinnamaldehyde possessed a stronger antimicrobial activity than eugenol. It was also found that a combination of cinnamon bark oil and antibiotics (colistin) demonstrated a synergistic effect.[24]

Antioxidant activity

Cinnamon oil was found to exhibit superoxide-dismutase-like activity by preventing the inhibiting capacity of pyrogallol autoxidation. In a comparative study among 26 spices, cinnamon demonstrated the highest antioxidant activity, indicating that it can be applied as an antioxidant in foods.[11]

Cinnamaldehyde is known for its antityrosinase activity. Antityrosinase agents are used in cosmetics, medicine and food due to their actions in suppressing hyperpigmentation as well as the unsightly browning effects observed in mushrooms, fruits and vegetables when they are exposed to sunlight or air.[11]

Chemoprotective activity

Cinnamaldehyde found in cinnamon bark essential oil was found to inhibit the activity of nuclear factor kappa-light-chain-enhancer of activated B cells (NF-κB) and the production of tumour necrosis factor alpha (TNF-α)-induced interleukin-8 (IL-8) in A375 cells. The researchers stated that this inhibition supports the role of cinnamaldehyde as a potential anticancer agent.[11]

Another report found that *trans*-cinnamaldehyde demonstrated potential effects in restraining tumour cell growth and in enhancing tumour cell apoptosis.[11]

Insecticidal activity

Cinnamon leaf and bark oils were investigated for their mosquito control properties against *Culex quinquefasciatus, Anopheles tessellatus* and *Aedes aegypti*. Cinnamon bark oil showed good knock-down and mortality against *Culex quinquefasciatus* (LD_{50} 0.66 μg/ml) and *Anopheles tessellatus* (LD_{50} 0.33μg/ml).[25]

In another study, cinnamon bark essential oil was slightly less effective than either d-phenothrin or pyrethrum against eggs and adult females of human head louse, *Pediculus humanus capitis*, using direct contact and vapour phase toxicity bioassays.[26]

Spasmolytic activity

Cinnamon leaf and bark oils had a spasmolytic effect on electrically stimulated guinea pig ileum in vitro.[27]

Actions

Actions commonly cited in aromatherapy

Anaesthetic, antiseptic, antispasmodic, aphrodisiac, cardiac, carminative, emmenagogue, haemostatic, insecticide, stimulant, stomachic, vermifuge[28,29,30]

Actions supported by clinical studies

Antibacterial, antifungal, antimicrobial, antioxidant, carminative, insecticide

Comment

Cinnamon as a herb has been used as a medicinal agent in many healing traditions, and is described in pharmacopoeias and in traditional systems of medicine for use in the treatment of dyspeptic conditions such as mild spastic conditions of the gastrointestinal tract, fullness, flatulence, and loss of appetite. It is also used to treat abdominal pain with diarrhoea and pain associated with amenorrhoea and dysmenorrhoea.

The EMA report states that cinnamon-based products may be considered as traditional medicinal products on the basis of the long medicinal tradition in a range of specified conditions. Cinnamon has been used for centuries for dyspeptic complaints. However, it should only be considered for symptomatic treatment after serious illness is excluded.[5]

I am reluctant to use cinnamon bark or leaf oil in topical aromatherapy preparations because of the risk associated with dermal irritancy and sensitisation.

It is interesting that the preferred mode of use is ingestion. Schnaubelt states that the internal application of cinnamon bark is well tolerated and is safe and effective, provided it is used in appropriate small dosages.[31]

Aromatherapy Uses

Clinical aromatherapy

Antimicrobial

Cinnamon bark oil is regarded as one of the strongest antibacterial agents known.[32,33] It is useful for treating viral infections and contagious diseases.

Digestive system

Cinnamon bark oil is regarded as an excellent gastrointestinal stimulant. It calms spasms of the digestive tract, and relieves conditions such as dyspepsia, colitis, flatulence, diarrhoea, nausea and vomiting. It stimulates secretions of gastric juices and is recommended for loss of appetite.[28,31,32,33,34]

The strong antimicrobial properties of cinnamon bark and leaf oil are quite effective in cleansing the intestinal tract of pathogenic bacteria. The phenylpropanoid compounds such as cinnamaldehyde and eugenol act against the pathogenic bacteria and at the same time support the intestinal flora.[31]

Nervous system

Both cinnamon bark and cinnamon leaf oils are very warming; therefore, they can be used to relieve aches and chills in the early stages of colds and flu, and the feeling of debility that often remains after the initial stage of a fever. The oil is also beneficial during convalescence.[30]

Valnet recommends using cinnamon oil for general debility, and for older people during the winter months as a tonic.[32] It is recommended for people who are devitalised, emaciated and suffering from nervous depression.[34]

Energetics, psyche and subtle uses

Energetics

In TCM, cinnamon bark oil is considered to be a *hot* and stimulating remedy. It will stimulate circulation, generate warmth, support the immune system, warm and invigorate the digestion and relieves pain.[33]

According to the principles of the Five Elements, cinnamon bark oil is associated with the Fire Element; however, it can be used to manage excessive *damp* conditions associated with the Earth Element.

Personality

Worwood describes the cinnamon character as being a larger-than-life, likeable person. They are very practical, intelligent and have a strong personality. Whether male or female, they can be aggressive; however, they like to treat all people as equal. They take life very seriously and do not like being criticised.[35]

People perceive them as being in control of their life and that everything is running smoothly – even though this may not be the case. While a cinnamon personality may always put themselves first, they take their home life seriously and will defend their family members at all cost.[35]

They love competition. They believe that material wealth is important for their happiness. As a result, Worwood explains, they may often find themselves in jobs that are not really suited to their character. Although they may not be entrepreneurial, they are happy when they are self-employed in service-related businesses that are steady and always in demand.[35]

C

Worwood also explains that they do like law and order. They consider themselves fair-minded and despise lawlessness, lying or cheating. However, they can be direct and forceful and too opinionated for their own good.[35]

According to Myers-Briggs personality types, the cinnamon personality is likely to be an ESTJ. ESTJs love responsibility and control. They love to be in charge. They are good at making objective decisions. They love challenges and know how to get things done. They have an opinion for everything and are rarely at a loss for words. ESTJs like to spend their free time in ways that are productive. They are good at seeing what is illogical, inconsistent and impractical. They are willing to make sacrifices in order to honour their commitments. They tend to be workaholics and drive themselves and others very hard. They like to be involved in community service organisations and volunteer activities. They enjoy spending time with their friends and family.

Subtle

It has been described as a physical essence, which restores a taste and vigour for life to the depressed, and the fire of courage to the belly of those who may have lost it in the maze of melancholia.[34]

Worwood states that cinnamon invites love from the higher realms into our heart. She explains that the warmth of cinnamon radiates through all space and time, transforming sorrow into love.[36]

Zeck recommends using cinnamon bark oil when we are feeling emotionally withdrawn and living in a state of separation. She claims that cinnamon bark will bring warmth, energy and a sense of connection to the present moment.[37]

Dosage and Administration

Blending

Aromatherapy

The following blends are best used in a vaporiser.

To create an invigorating, uplifting blend to alleviate fatigue and lethargy, consider blending cinnamon bark oil with essential oils such ginger, sweet orange, lemon or rosemary.

To create an antimicrobial blend, consider blending cinnamon bark oil with essential oils such as bay laurel, cajeput, clove bud, kunzea, 1,8-cineole-rich eucalypts, lemon, lemon myrtle, sweet orange, rosemary, tea tree or thyme.

Perfumery

Arctander describes the addition of cinnamon bark to a perfume as follows:

> *The warmth and dry spiciness, the immediate sweetness and tremendous diffusive power induced by the addition of fractions of one percent of this oil in a perfume composition, is highly appreciated by certain perfumers.*[3]

In perfumery, cinnamon bark oil blends well with oriental-woody notes. It especially blends well with frankincense and other resins. Aftel describes spice oils such as cinnamon as a modifier for floral notes and giving definition to resins and softer notes.[38] Cinnamon bark oil blends well with other spice oils such as cardamom, clove, nutmeg and pepper to give floral oils such as rose or jasmine absolute a rich warm deep floral intensity. However, Aftel warns us to use small doses as cinnamon can easily dominate a perfume.[38]

Mode of administration

Bath

As cinnamon bark and leaf oils may be potent skin irritants and sensitisers, I do not recommend that they be used in a bath.

Topical

Cinnamon bark oil is often not recommended for topical application.[28]

Inhalation

Direct inhalation, diffuser, oil vaporiser

Ingestion

As cinnamon bark oil is a potential skin irritant and sensitiser, the preferred mode of use is ingestion.[31,33]

Schnaubelt states that the internal application of cinnamon bark is well tolerated, safe and effective, provided it is used in appropriate small dosages. He recommends one drop of oil into one tablespoon of edible vegetable oil, and then ingesting that mixture in a gelatin capsule.[31]

The German Commission E recommends oral dose of 0.05-0.2 g for cinnamon bark oil.[9]

Safety Profile

General safety

Cinnamon bark oil has been reported to be a severe dermal irritant and sensitiser.[28,30,31,39]

Tisserand & Young state that the maximum dermal use level for cinnamon bark is 0.07%. This has been calculated based on cinnamon bark oil having approximately 75.7% cinnamaldehyde, and on IFRA's recommended limit of 0.05 % for cinnamaldehyde in any dermal preparation.[39]

Cinnamon leaf oil is a mild dermal irritant, and its eugenol content suggests that it may be hepatotoxic and may inhibit blood clotting. The dilution for cinnamon leaf oil in topical preparations should not exceed 0.6% according to IFRA.[39]

Contraindications

Tisserand & Young recommend that cinnamon bark oil not be used during pregnancy and breastfeeding. They also caution its use orally for people who are on diabetes or anticoagulant medications, have had major surgery, have peptic ulcers or any bleeding disorder.[39]

Because of the high eugenol content, Tisserand & Young express caution in using cinnamon leaf oil orally, as it may interact with pethidine, monoamine oxidase inhibitors or selective serotonin reuptake inhibitors, anticoagulant medication, major surgery, peptic ulcers and other bleeding disorders.[39]

The German Commission E states that internal use of cinnamon bark oil is contraindicated during pregnancy.[9]

Toxicity

Patients with liver pathology should avoid taking cinnamon because there may be glutathione-depleting action of cinnamaldehyde. Ingestion of large amounts of cinnamon oil (equivalent to 15-20 g of bark) can lead to gastrointestinal irritation and cause sleepiness, dizziness and a rapid pulse.[5]

Regulatory guidelines

Cinnamon bark and leaf essential oils have GRAS status.

In 2011, the European Medicines Agency published final labelling monographs on cinnamon bark and cinnamon bark essential oil.

References

1. Weiss EA. *Essential oil crops*. CAB International, Wallingford, 1997.
2. Engels G, Brinckmann J. *Cinnamon.* HerbalGram – The Journal of the American Botanical Council, 2012; 95: 1-5. Retrieved Sep 11, 2017, from http://cms.herbalgram.org/herbalgram/issue95/hg95-herbpro-cinnamon.html
3. Arctander S. *Perfume and flavor materials of natural origin.* Allured Publishing, Carol Stream, 1994.
4. Lawrence BM. *Essential oils 1976-1978.* Allured Publishing, Wheaton, 1979.
5. Committee on Herbal Medicinal Products (HMPC). *Assessment report on Cinnamomum verum J.S. Presl, cortex and cortices Aetheroleum.* European Medicines Agency, London, 2011. Doc ref. EMA/HMPC/246773/2009.
6. Manniche L. *An ancient Egyptian herbal.* British Museum Press, London, 1993.
7. Guenther E. *The essential oils – Vol. IV.* Robert E Krieger Publishing, Malabar, 1950.
8. Evans WC. *Trease and Evans pharmacognosy.* 15th edn. WB Saunders, Edinburgh, 2002.
9. Blumenthal M et al. *The complete German Commission E monographs: Therapeutic guide to herbal medicine.* American Botanical Council, Austin, 1998.
10. Braun L, Cohen M. *Herbs & natural supplements: An evidence-based guide – Vol. 2.* 4th edn. Elsevier, Chatswood, 2015.
11. Rao PV, Gan SH. *Cinnamon: A multifaceted medicinal plant.* Evidence-Based Complementary and Alternative Medicine, 2014; 2014: 642942. doi: 10.1155/2014/642942.
12. Khan I, Abourashed E. *Leung's encyclopedia of common natural ingredients used in food, drugs and cosmetics.* 3rd edn. John Wiley & Sons, New Jersey, 2010.
13. Mishra A et al. *Ameliorative effect of the cinnamon oil from Cinnamomum zeylanicum upon early stage diabetic nephropathy.* Planta Medica, 2010; 76(5): 412-417. Cited in Quintessential Aromatics database, 2013.
14. Ping H et al. *Antidiabetic effects of cinnamon oil in diabetic KK-Ay mice.* Food and Chemical Toxicology, 2010; 48(8-9): 2344-2349. Cited in Quintessential Aromatics database, 2013.
15. *WHO monographs on selected medicinal plants – Vol. 1.* World Health Organization, Geneva, 1999.

16. Devkatte A et al. *Potential of plant oils as inhibitors of Candida albicans growth.* FEMS Yeast Research, 2005; 5(6): 867-873. Cited in Quintessential Aromatics database, 2013.
17. Sharma PR et al. *Ten highly effective essential oils inhibit growth of methicillin resistant Staphylococcus aureus MRSA) and methicillin sensitive Staphylococcus aureus (MSSA).* International Journal of Pharmacy and Pharmaceutical Sciences, 2013; 5(1): 52-54. Cited in Quintessential Aromatics database, 2013.
18. Warnke PH et al. *The battle against multi-resistant strains: Renaissance of antimicrobial essential oils as a promising force to fight hospital-acquired infections.* Journal of Cranio-Maxillo-Facial Surgery, 2009; 37(7): 392-397. Cited in Quintessential Aromatics database, 2013.
19. Mayaud L et al. *Comparison of bacteriostatic and bactericidal activity of 13 essential oils against strains with varying sensitivity to antibiotics.* Letters in Applied Microbiology, 2008; 47(3): 167-173. Cited in Quintessential Aromatics database, 2013.
20. Bharti P et al. *Antibacterial, antioxidant, collagenase inhibition, urease inhibition activities and chemical composition of the essential oil and extracts of Cinnamomum zeylanicum bark.* International Journal of Phytomedicine, 2013; 5(1): 36-45. Cited in Quintessential Aromatics database, 2013.
21. Sieiniewicz M et al. *Inhibitory activity of cinnamon bark oil on group B streptococci (GBS).* Journal of Essential Oil Bearing Plants, 2014; 17(5): 981-991. Cited in Quintessential Aromatics database, 2013.
22. Chaudhari LKD et al. *Antimicrobial activity of commercially available essential oils against Streptococcus mutans.* Journal of Complementary Dental Practice, 2012; 13(1): 71-74. Cited in Quintessential Aromatics database, 2013.
23. Hill P et al. *Antimicrobial action of essential oils: the effect of dimethylsulphoxide on the activity of cinnamon oil.* Letters in Applied Microbiology, 1997; 24(4): 269-275. Cited in Quintessential Aromatics database, 2013.
24. Utchariyakiat et al. *Efficacy of cinnamon bark oil and cinnamaldehyde on anti-multidrug resistant Pseudomonas aeruginosa and the synergistic effects in combination with other antimicrobial agents.* BMC Complementary and Alternative Medicine, 2016; 16: 158. doi: 10.1186/s12906-016-1134-9.
25. Ranasinghe P et al. *Medicinal properties of 'true' cinnamon (Cinnamomum zeylanicum): a systemic review.* BMC Complementary and Alternative Medicine, 2013; 13:275. doi: 10.1186/1472-6882-13-275.
26. Yang YC et al. *Ovicidal and adulticidal activities of Cinnamomum zeylanicum bark essential oil compounds and related compounds against Pediculus humanus capitis (Anoplura: Pediculicidae).* International Journal of Parasitology, 2005; 35(14): 1595-1600. Cited in Quintessential Aromatics database, 2013.
27. Lis-Balchin M. *Aromatherapy science – a guide for healthcare professionals.* Pharmaceutical Press, London, 2006.
28. Lawless J. *The encyclopaedia of essential oils.* Element Books, Shaftesbury, 1992.
29. Lavabre, M. *Aromatherapy workbook.* Healing Arts Press, Rochester, 1997.
30. Davis P. *Aromatherapy an A-Z.* C.W. Daniel Company, Saffron Walden, 1999.
31. Schnaubelt K. *Medical aromatherapy.* Frog, Berkeley, 1999.
32. Valnet J. *The practice of aromatherapy.* C.W. Daniel Company, Saffron Walden, 1980.
33. Holmes P. *The energetics of Western herbs – Vol. I.* Artemis Press, Boulder, 1989.
34. Mailhebiau P. *Portraits in oils.* C.W. Daniel Company, Saffron Walden, 1995.
35. Worwood VA. *The fragrant mind.* Transworld Publishers, London, 1995.
36. Worwood VA. *The fragrant heavens.* Transworld Publishers, London, 1999.
37. Zeck R. *The blossoming heart – aromatherapy for healing and transformation.* Aroma Tours, East Ivanhoe, 2004.
38. Aftel M. *Essence & alchemy.* Bloomsbury Publishing, London, 2001.
39. Tisserand R, Young R. *Essential oil safety.* 2nd edn. Churchill Livingstone, Edinburgh, 2014.

C

Cistus

Identification

Botanical name

Cistus ladaniferus L.

Synonyms

Rock rose, labdanum, *Cistus ladanifer*

Family

Cistaceae

Botany and origins

Cistus, also known as rock rose or labdanum, is a resinous exudate from *C. ladaniferus*, a small, wild growing shrub, up to 3 m, with lance-shaped leaves that are viscid above and densely white woolly beneath.[1,2]

The plant originates in the mountainous coastal regions of the eastern Mediterranean countries and the Middle East. Spain is the major producer of cistus gum, while France is the major producer of the absolute.[2]

Method of extraction

The gum is obtained by boiling the leaves and twigs in water. The oil is then obtained from the gum by distillation. A concrete is produced by hydrocarbon solvent extraction of the dried plant material. An absolute is then produced from the concrete.[2]

The term labdanum refers to the resinous exudation from *C. ladaniferus*.[2] Arctander explains that the term 'cistus oil' should be used to refer to the steam-distilled oil of the entire herb – leaves, stems and flowering top. This represents the aromatic characteristics of the entire plant and not those exclusively of the resinous exudation. However, the term 'cistus oil' is also used to describe the oil obtained from the distillation of the gum.[1]

Characteristics

Cistus oil from the gum is an amber-coloured or dark yellow viscous oil with a very powerful and tenacious aroma. It is sweet and warm, yet dry and reminiscent of ambergris, with a somewhat musky-like odour. The absolute has a sweet herbaceous balsamic odour.[1]

On the other hand, cistus oil from the entire herb is a pale orange coloured liquid with a peculiar, warm-herbaceous aroma. Its odour bears some similarity to that of Roman chamomile and decaying fruits. Its tenacity is much inferior to that of cistus oil from the resin. Arctander states that this oil is produced on a very limited scale, and is rare.[1]

Guenther states that cistus oil possesses a powerful balsamic, long-lasting scent which upon dilution is reminiscent of ambergris.[3]

Chemical composition

The major chemical composition of cistus oil distilled from the fresh and dried leaves and twigs of *C. ladaniferus* harvested in Spain was reported as follows:

α-pinene (3.5%), camphene (10.3%), β-pinene (0.5%), α-*p*-menthatriene (2.9%), α-terpinene (0.7%), γ-terpinene (1.6%), limonene (2.3%), *p*-cymene (4%), α-*p*-dimethylstyrene (1.6%), *allo*-aromadendrene (1.2%), α-amorphene (1.0%), 2,2,6-trimethylcyclohexanone (5.7%), *cis*-rose oxide (0.5%), pinocamphone+benzaldehyde+camphor (1.6%), linalool (0.5%), isopinocamphone (3.5%), pinocarvone (0.6%), pinocarveol (3.4%), dodecanal (1.1%), bornyl acetate (3.7%), verbenone (2.0%).[4]

Adulteration

Arctander states that there is a possibility of adulteration of crude labdanum gum with the exhausted gum from previous distillations, or with insoluble residues from the extraction of labdanum absolutes.[1]

Pharmacopoeias and standards

At the time of writing, the purity, composition, physico-chemical properties and therapeutic uses of *C. ladaniferus* essential oil are not defined in any pharmacopoeia monograph or standard.

History and Traditional Uses

History

Cistus was imported into ancient Egypt from Crete. The resin was extensively used in Egypt as a perfume and an incense. At the time of Christ, incense was made using frankincense and myrrh from Arabia, galbanum and 'onycha'. The latter has been identified as gum labdanum, which is exuded from the leaves of cistus.[5]

Guenther describes cistus as follows:

> *One of the most unforgettable scents is that of labdanum, whose sweet, warm, balsamic odor permeates sunny patches in the pine forests that cover some of the islands in the Mediterranean or stretch along the rocky coasts of the that beautiful, blue sea.*[3]

Cistus blends well with pine, sage, lavender and thyme – recreating the scent of the Mediterranean. Guenther states that the classical Greeks and Romans must have been familiar with labdanum because it is described by Dioscorides, Herodotus and Pliny.[3]

In old perfumery literature, cistus gum was obtained by combing the hair of sheep and goats that had browsed through stands of labdanum. The sticky gum would have adhered to the wool of the animals.[3]

Traditional medicine

Cistus oil has been used in Europe since the Middle Ages. Fischer-Rizzi states that the oil was used in ointments and compresses to treat infected wounds and skin ulcers.[6]

Labdanum was traditionally used as an expectorant, in catarrh of the upper respiratory tract and for diarrhoea. It is also used as an astringent, nervine, stimulant and haemostatic.[2]

Food, perfumery and flavouring

Cistus oil is also used as a fixative in many perfumes.[2]

Therapeutics

Pharmacology and clinical studies

There has been very little research into its pharmacological or clinical uses.

Antimicrobial activity

Cistus oil is reported to have antimicrobial activities against *Staphylococcus aureus, Escherichia coli* and *Candida albicans*.[2]

Cistus oil was active against gram-positive bacteria more than gram-negative bacteria. The oil exhibited strong antibacterial activity against *S. aureus* (zone of inhibition of growth was 27 mm) with the minimum inhibitory concentration (MIC) of 250 ug/ml and *Yersinia enterocolitica* (zone of inhibition of growth was 25 mm) with MIC of 62.5 ug/ml.[7]

In one study that demonstrated antibacterial activity of *C. ladaniferus* oil, it was noted that the oil was largely dominated by α-pinene, a hydrocarbon compound that exerts no or very weak activity against several bacterial strains. It turned out that the involvement of oxygenated compounds in the oil contributed to the bacteriostatic effect of the oil on bacterial growth.[8]

C

Actions

Actions commonly cited in aromatherapy

Antimicrobial, antiseptic, astringent, emmenagogue, expectorant, sedative, vulnerary[9,10]

Actions supported by clinical studies

Antimicrobial

Comment

Cistus oil is not listed in any pharmacopoeia. Review of traditional uses and clinical data cannot confirm any clinical applications for cistus oil in aromatherapy. It is also not a commonly used essential oil in aromatherapy practice; however, it has been used since antiquity to treat infected wounds and skin ulcers. Like other resins, it is likely to have wound-healing properties. It would be great to see clinical studies to confirm these properties. Cistus oil is often used in subtle aromatherapy practice.

Aromatherapy Uses

Clinical aromatherapy

Integumentary system

The oil is well known for its wound healing, and is recommended for the treatment of ulcers and wounds.[10] Mailhebiau recommends blending cistus with *Salvia officinalis* and *Lavandula officinalis* for the treatment of bedsores. He also recommends a blend of cistus, cypress and lavender for varicose ulcers.[11] The oil has been effectively used for treating chronic skin disorders such as eczema and psoriasis.[6]

Cistus is considered one of the fastest acting oils to stop bleeding from an open wound.[12]

Lymphatic system

Cistus oil is beneficial in a massage oil for increasing lymphatic drainage. For swollen lymph nodes in the neck, Fischer-Rizzi recommends a hot compress with cistus.[6]

Skin care

Having antiseptic and astringent properties, cistus is highly recommended for treating acne or oily skin.[6] It is also recommended for mature skin and wrinkles.[9]

Energetics, psyche and subtle uses

Energetics

According to the principles of the Five Elements, the sweet, warm amber scent of cistus oil has a strong affinity with the Earth Element. It instils a deep sense of calm and tranquillity.

Personality

According to Myers-Briggs personality types, the cistus personality is likely to be an INFJ. INFJs are quiet, compassionate, concerned and tender-hearted. They often have complex personalities. They have a rich imagination and are very aware of other people's emotions. They are very committed to their inspirations and ideals and inspire insight and growth in others. INFJs like balance between time alone for their many creative projects, and time with friends and family. They prefer to spend more time with mental and emotional pursuits rather than physical ones. They can be highly demanding of themselves and others. They are often perfectionists. They like to make significant contributions to the welfare of humankind. They like to think things through carefully and are good at concentrating. They are tender and gentle in their relationships. They are very good listeners and communicate clearly when they feel comfortable. They share their feelings and emotions in private and only with a small number of friends. They often feel responsibility for other people's feelings. They can be moody and melancholic. They are very sensitive to criticism and rejection and feel deeply hurt when they are not understood. They have a strong need for harmony – they can feel tense, frustrated and even become ill when they are not able to attain it.

Subtle

Fischer-Rizzi says that the warm, deep, spicy and soothing scent of cistus oil conveys a warmth that deeply affects the soul. Cistus oil is recommended for patients who feel cold, empty or numb after a traumatic event.[6]

Cistus oil is recommended as an aid to meditation. It is centring and aids in visualising spiritual experiences and bringing them to consciousness.[6,10]

Worwood beautifully describes the subtle qualities of cistus:

> *It provides a vehicle to explore the knowing, and a means by which acknowledging the existence of universal wisdom deep within. The emotions of mortals are touched by labdanum, and it can bring to the forefront of the mind access to the soul level of all living things.*[13]

Lavabre recommends cistus for the third eye and crown chakra and suggests that it be used for psychic work and meditations.[10]

Zeck explains that the scent of cistus warms, settles and quietens the physical, mental, emotional and spiritual bodies. She states that it will comfort in times of emotional stress, shock or accident or after any traumatic event.[14]

Dosage and Administration

Blending

Aromatherapy

To provide protection and comfort in times of emotional and spiritual crisis, consider blending cistus oil with essential oils such as everlasting, frankincense, lavender or myrrh.

For the management of wounds, consider blending cistus oil with essential oils such as everlasting, frankincense, lavender or patchouli.

To enhance your meditation practice, consider blending cistus oil with essential oils such as Atlas cedarwood, frankincense, pine or sandalwood.

For the treatment of mature and damaged skin, consider blending cistus oil in a base of rosehip oil with essential oils such as everlasting, frankincense, lavender, patchouli, rose absolute or sandalwood.

Perfumery

The oil is used to create amber-based and oriental-based perfumes where it will provide tenacity, warm notes and intriguing spicy-animal notes. Arctander states that it blends extremely well with citrus oils, clary sage, oakmoss absolute, juniper berry, lavender, pine needle and opopanax oils.[1]

Mode of administration

Bath

Full body bath, foot bath

Topical

Compress, massage, ointment, skin care

Inhalation

Direct inhalation, diffuser, oil vaporiser

Safety Profile

General safety

Cistus oil is non-toxic, non-irritating and non-sensitising.[9]

Contraindications

No contraindications known.[15]

Regulatory guidelines

Cistus oil has GRAS status.

References

1. Arctander S. *Perfume and flavor materials of natural origin.* Allured Publishing, Carol Stream, 1994.
2. Khan I, Abourashed E. *Leung's encyclopedia of common natural ingredients used in food, drugs and cosmetics.* 3rd edn. John Wiley & Sons, New Jersey, 2010.
3. Guenther E. *The essential oils – Vol. VI.* Robert E Krieger Publishing, Malabar, 1952.
4. Lawrence BM. *Essential oils 1988-1991.* Allured Publishing, Carol Stream, 1993.
5. Morris E. *Fragrance – the story of perfume from Cleopatra to Chanel.* Products of Nature and Art, New York, 1984.
6. Fischer-Rizzi S. *Complete aromatherapy handbook.* Sterling Publishing, New York, 1990.
7. Benayad N et al. *Antibacterial activity of essential oil and some extracts of Cistus ladaniferus from Oulmes in Morocco.* Journal of Materials and Environmental Science, 2013; 4 (6): 1066-1071.
8. Guinoiseau E et al. *Primary mode of action of Cistus ladaniferus L. essential oil active fractions on Staphylococcus aureus strain.* Advances in Microbiology, 2015; 5(13): 881-890. doi: 10.4236/aim.2015.513092.
9. Lawless J. *The encyclopaedia of essential oils.* Element Books, Shaftesbury, 1992.
10. Lavabre M. *Aromatherapy workbook.* Healing Arts Press, Rochester, 1997.
11. Mailhebiau P. *Portraits in oils.* C.W. Daniel Company, Saffron Walden, 1995.
12. Schnaubelt K. *Advanced aromatherapy.* Healing Arts Press, Rochester, 1995.

13. Worwood VA. *The fragrant heavens.* Transworld Publishers, London, 1999.
14. Zeck R. *The blossoming heart – aromatherapy for healing and transformation.* Aroma Tours, East Ivanhoe, 2004.
15. Tisserand R, Young R. *Essential oil safety.* 2nd edn. Churchill Livingstone, Edinburgh, 2014.

Citronella

Identification

Botanical name

Ceylon citronella: *Cymbopogon nardus* L.

Java citronella: *Cymbopogon winterianus* Jowitt

Synonyms

Ceylon citronella: Sri Lanka type citronella, *Andropogon nardus* L.

Family

Poaceae (Gramineae)

Botany and origins

The genus *Cymbopogon* Spreng includes 50-60 species of tropical, perennial, coarse-growing tufted grasses, many having highly aromatic foliage. The citronella oil of international trade is obtained from *C. nardus* and *C. winterianus*. They are tufted, perennial grasses with long narrow leaves, and numerous stems arising from short rhizomatous roots. *C. nardus* is more vigorous, and has a more extensive, penetrating root system than *C. winterianus*. This root system allows the species to withstand periods of drought and to grow well in a wider range of soil types.[1]

Commercial cultivation of *C. nardus* is limited to Sri Lanka, while *C. winterianus* is commercially cultivated in Indonesia, Guatemala, Honduras, Haiti, China and, more recently, India and Vietnam.[1]

The essential oil industry generally defines the oils as Ceylon and Java types, as there are characteristic differences, the most important being the geraniol content.[1]

Method of extraction

Citronella oil is obtained from the steam distillation of the leaves of *C. nardus* or *C. winterianus*.

Characteristics

C. nardus, commonly known as Ceylon citronella, is a yellow to brownish-yellow liquid with a distinctive warm-woody and yet fresh, grassy odour.[2] It has a rose nuance and is more pleasant smelling than the Java type.[3] *C. winterianus*, commonly known as Java citronella, is a colourless to pale yellow liquid with a sweet, fresh and lemony odour.[2] Java citronella has a more pronounced aldehyde note and stronger lemon-like aroma, which Lis-Balchin describes as the image of a cheap perfumery product for household soap.[3]

Chemical composition

The main constituents found in Java and Ceylon citronella oils are as follows:[1]

Constituent	Java	Ceylon
α-pinene	-	2.6%
camphene	-	8.0%
limonene	1.3%	9.7%
cis-ocimene	-	1.4%
trans-ocimene	-	1.8%
citronellal	32.7%	5.2%
camphor	-	0.5%
β-caryophyllene	2.1%	3.2%
terpinen-4-ol	trace	0.7%
citronellyl acetate	3.0%	1.9%
geranyl formate	2.5%	4.2%
1-borneol	trace	6.6%
citronellol	15.9%	8.4%
nerol	7.7%	0.9%
geraniol	23.9%	18.0%
geranyl butyrate	trace	1.5%
methyl eugenol	trace	1.7%
elemol	6.0%	1.7%
methyl isoeugenol	2.3%	7.2%

The major difference between the two species is the citronellal and geraniol content. *C. nardus* (Ceylon type) usually contains 55-65% geraniol and 7-15% citronellal, while *C. winterianus* (Java type) contains at least 35% geraniol and a minimum of 35% citronellal.[1]

Adulteration

Lis-Balchin states that adulteration of citronella oil is unlikely since citronella grass is easy to grow and it is an inexpensive essential oil. Citronella oil is often used to adulterate geranium and rose oil.[3]

Pharmacopoeias and standards

The purity, composition and physico-chemical properties of citronella essential oil are defined in

ISO 3848:2016 Oil of Citronella, Java Type.

History and Traditional Uses

History

Citronella grass has long been used by the peoples of southern India, Sri Lanka and Java; however, its early history is not recorded.[1] Lis-Balchin states that citronella oil was originally produced solely for the perfumery and fragrance industry, so there are no traditional uses of citronella oil.[3]

Traditional medicine

Poultices of the leaves were widely used in India and Sri Lanka to treat minor cuts, abrasions and swellings. Extracts of the leaves were used as a febrifuge, stomachic, diaphoretic, diuretic, emmenagogue and vermifuge.[1,4]

Food, perfumery and flavouring

Citronella oil is used extensively in detergents, household soaps and cleaners, and to a minor extent in cheap perfumes and toiletries.[2]

Other uses

Citronella oil is used as a major source for the isolation of citronellal and geraniol. The oil is extensively used as an insect repellent.[4]

Therapeutics

Pharmacology and clinical studies

Many pharmacological studies involving citronella essential oil have been published. A systemic review of these studies will not be attempted. Rather, I have chosen a selection of studies that support the traditional and clinical uses of citronella oil.

Antifungal activity

C. winterianus oil has four distinct chemotypes – Java I, Java II, Guatemala and Burma. All oils demonstrated very high antifungal activity; however, the Burma and Java II demonstrated higher growth inhibition. The authors stated that the citronella oils with higher antifungal activity had a higher citral content.[5]

C. winterianus oil managed to strongly inhibit *Trichophyton rubrum,* and therefore shows potential as a potent antifungal compound, especially for protection against dermatophytosis.[6]

Antimicrobial activity

Citronella oil has been reported to have antibacterial and antifungal activities. *C. nardus* is reputed to be as active as penicillin against certain gram-positive bacteria.[4]

C. nardus exhibited a broad antimicrobial activity against 13 different *Escherichia coli* serotypes.[7]

Autonomic nervous system activity

A study was done to identify the effect of inhalation of a range of essential oils. The physiological responses of the autonomic nervous system were evaluated by measuring R-wave intervals on an electrocardiogram, blood pressure, blood flow in the fingertip and galvanic skin conductance. The aroma of citronella oil produced an increase in the R-R interval on the electrocardiogram, and decreased blood flow and galvanic skin conductance. The authors noted that citronella oil activated both parasympathetic and sympathetic nervous system activity.[8]

Insecticidal activity

C. nardus oil was found to give almost complete protection against *Anopheles cullicifacies* (a principal malaria carrier) for up to 11 hours. The oil was considered comparable with synthetic repellents of dimethyl and dibutyl phthalate.[9]

Another study found that *C. nardus* oil provided protection for as much as 8-10 hours against the mosquitoes *Anopheles stephensi, Culex quinquefasciatus* and *Aedes aegypti,* both in the laboratory and field.[10]

A systemic review of controlled laboratory experiments using citronella oil as a mosquito repellent found that citronella-based products are less effective than DEET (N,N-diethyl-m-toluamide) products in terms of duration of protection. On the other hand, it was found that a combination of citronella oil and vanillin provided longer protection time than citronella oil on its own.[11]

At 10% and 20% concentration, *C. nardus* showed a minimum of 90% and 95% relative protection against *Anopheles arabiensis* mosquito respectively soon after application. After three hours it offered more than 70% protection; however, it was reported that the duration of protection was not as good as DEET.[12]

Actions

Actions commonly cited in aromatherapy

Antiseptic, bactericidal, deodorant, diaphoretic, febrifuge, insecticide, tonic[13,14]

Actions supported by clinical studies

Antiseptic, bactericidal, insecticide

Comment

Citronella is not commonly used in aromatherapy. It is far more common to find citronella oil used as an active ingredient in natural insect repellents.

Aromatherapy Uses

Clinical aromatherapy

Musculoskeletal system

Citronella oil is recommended in a massage oil for the relief of arthritic and rheumatic pain, muscular pain and neuralgia.[15,16]

Nervous system

Citronella oil has a fresh invigorating scent, indicating that it may be used to alleviate nervous exhaustion and fatigue.[13,15]

Respiratory system

The high aldehyde content of citronella oil suggests that the oil has excellent antimicrobial properties. It is recommended as an inhalation against colds, flu and minor infections.[13]

Skin care

Citronella oil is well known as an insect repellent. For this purpose, it may be used in a spray, diffused into the air or applied to the skin in a massage oil.[4,13,16]

It is also recommended for excessive perspiration and oily skin conditions.[13]

Dosage and Administration

Blending

Aromatherapy

As a natural insect repellent, consider blending citronella oil with essential oils such as Buddha wood, Virginian cedarwood, 1,8-cineole-rich eucalypts, lemon-scented eucalyptus, peppermint eucalyptus, kunzea, lemongrass, lemon-scented tea tree, niaouli, palmarosa, peppermint, spike lavender or tea tree.

Perfumery

Citronella oil is not commonly used in perfumery.

Mode of administration

Bath

I do not recommend using citronella oil in a bath.

Topical

Massage, ointment, skin care

Inhalation

Direct inhalation, diffuser, oil vaporiser

Safety Profile

General safety

Citronella oil has been reported to be non-toxic, non-irritant and non-sensitising. It may cause contact dermatitis in some individuals.[13] Lis-Balchin cites studies that indicated no irritation when applied to the skin at 8%.[3]

Tisserand & Young state that the maximum dermal use level based on the geraniol content is 18.2%.[17] There is some concern regarding the methyl eugenol content; however, Tisserand & Young state that the methyl eugenol content is between 0-1.7%, therefore, they consider that citronella oil does not present a risk of carcinogenicity.[17]

However, Canada's Pest Management Regulatory Agency has phased out citronella-based insect repellents because it may contain methyl eugenol. In the EU, citronella oil is not restricted in cosmetics, but it is no longer permitted as an ingredient in products making insect repellent claims.[17]

The US Environmental Protection Agency (EPA), on the other hand, has stated the oil of citronella has been used as an insect repellent without any adverse incidents. Based on the oil's low acute toxicity, its lack of mutagenicity, its GRAS status and lack of reports of adverse effects, the oil is permitted for use in natural insect repellents.[17]

Contraindications

No contraindications known.

Regulatory guidelines

Citronella oil has GRAS status.

References

1. Weiss EA. *Essential oil crops*. CAB International, Wallingford, 1997.
2. Arctander S. *Perfume and flavor materials of natural origin*. Allured Publishing, Carol Stream, 1994.
3. Lis-Balchin M. *Aromatherapy science – a guide for healthcare professionals*. Pharmaceutical Press, London, 2006.
4. Khan I, Abourashed E. *Leung's encyclopedia of common natural ingredients used in food, drugs and cosmetics*. 3rd edn. John Wiley & Sons, New Jersey, 2010.
5. Kole C et al. *Antifungal efficacy of oil and its genetic variability in citronella*. Crop Research, 1993; 6(3): 509-512. Cited in Quintessential Aromatics database, 2013.
6. de Oliveira Pereira F et al. *Growth inhibition and morphological alterations of Trichophyton rubrum induced by essential oil from Cymbopogon winterianus Jowitt ex Bor*. Brazilian Journal of Microbiology, 2011; 42(1): 233-242. Cited in Quintessential Aromatics database, 2013.
7. Duarte MCT et al. *Activity of essential oils from Brazilian medicinal plants on Escherichia coli*. Journal of Ethnopharmacology, 2007; 111(2): 197-201. Cited in Quintessential Aromatics

database, 2013.
8. Saeki Y, Shiohara M. *Physiological effects of inhaling fragrances*. International Journal of Aromatherapy, 2001; 11(3): 118-125. Cited in Quintessential Aromatics database, 2013.
9. Ansari MA, Razdan RK. *Relative efficacy of various oils in repelling mosquitoes*. Indian Journal of Malariology, 32(3): 104-111. Cited in the Aromatherapy Database, by Bob Harris, Essential Oil Resource Consultants, UK, 2000.
10. Tyagi BK et al. *Evaluation of repellent activities of Cymbopogon essential oils against mosquito vectors of malaria, filariasis and dengue fever in India*. Phytomedicine, 1998; 5(4): 324-329. Cited in Quintessential Aromatics database, 2013.
11. Kongkaew C et al. *Effectiveness of citronella preparations in preventing mosquito bites: systematic review of controlled laboratory experimental studies*. Tropical Medicine and International Health, 2011; 16(7): 802-810. Cited in Quintessential Aromatics database, 2013.
12. Solomon B et al. *Mosquito repellent actions of the essential oils of Cymbopogon citratus, Cymbopogon nardus and Eucalyptus citriodora: evaluation and formulation studies*. Journal of Essential Oil Bearing Plants, 2012; 15(5): 766-773. Cited in Quintessential Aromatics database, 2013.
13. Lawless J. *The encyclopaedia of essential oils*. Element Books, Shaftesbury, 1992.
14. Lavabre M. *Aromatherapy workbook*. Healing Arts Press, Rochester, 1997.
15. Blumenthal M et al. *The complete German commission E monographs: therapeutic guide to herbal medicine*. American Botanical Council, Austin, 1998.
16. Schnaubelt K. *Advanced aromatherapy*. Healing Arts Press, Rochester, 1995.
17. Tisserand R, Young R. *Essential oil safety*. 2nd edn. Churchill Livingstone, Edinburgh, 2014.

Clary sage

Identification

Botanical name

Salvia sclarea L.

Synonyms

Clary, muscatel sage

Family

Lamiaceae (Labiatae)

Botany and origins

Clary sage is a biennial or perennial herb, growing 30 to 120 cm high, with greyish, velvety, heart-shaped leaves and numerous pale-blue, violet-pink or white flowers.[1] It is cultivated in central Europe, Russia, England, Morocco and the USA.[2]

Method of extraction

Clary sage oil is steam-distilled from the flowering tops and foliage of *S. sclarea*.

Characteristics

Clary sage oil is a colourless to pale-yellow or pale-olive coloured liquid with a fresh, sweet, fruity, floral and herbaceous odour. Some perfumers describe it as tobacco-like, while others as balsamic or tea-like.[2]

Arctander states that the aroma of clary sage has something in common with cistus and Moroccan chamomile oil.[2]

Chemical composition

The chemical composition of French clary sage essential oil was reported as follows:

linalool (10-20%), linalyl acetate (60-70%), caryophyllene (1.5-2.5%), α-terpineol (0.5-2.5%), geraniol (trace-1.5%), neryl acetate (0.3-1.0%), sclareol (0.5-2.0%), germacrene D (3.0-5.0%).[3]

Clary sage oil is rich in esters, which are known for their antispasmodic and sedative properties.

Adulteration

Arctander explains that, because clary sage oil is relatively expensive and the main constituents found in the oil are linalool and linalyl acetate, it is frequently adulterated by the addition of these constituents that may be synthetic or of natural source. The addition of these constituents may not be detected by the physico-chemical analysis of the oil. However, it can be detected by olfactory analysis.[2]

Pharmacopoeias and standards

At the time of writing, the purity, composition, physico-chemical properties and therapeutic use of clary sage essential oil are not defined in any pharmacopoeia monograph or standard.

History and Traditional Uses

History

The English name clary is derived from the Latin word *sclarea*, a word derived from *clarus* meaning `clear'. The name clary was gradually modified to clear eye, possibly because the herb was once used for clearing mucus from the eyes.[4]

Herbal

Culpeper suggested that a compress of the mucilage made from the seeds would reduce tumours or swellings.[1] Originally grown in southern Europe, it was planted in German vineyards. It was also used as a substitute for hops in brewing beer.[3]

The flowering tops and leaves have been used to treat catarrh and as an antiseptic and emmenagogue. The herb is also used as a stomachic in digestive disorders.[5]

Food, perfumery and flavouring

Clary sage oil is used as a fragrance component in perfumes.[5] In flavouring, the coriander-like note of clary sage oil is used in liqueurs, wine essences and grape essences. It is also used as a modifier in spice compounds.[2]

Other uses

C

Clary sage is used as a source of sclareol, which is converted to sclareolide and used as flavouring in tobaccos and in the production of an ambergris substitute.[5]

Therapeutics

Pharmacology and clinical studies

Many pharmacological studies involving clary sage essential oil have been published. A systemic review of these studies will not be attempted. Rather, I have chosen a selection of studies that support the traditional and clinical uses.

Anticonvulsive activity

Clary sage oil has been reported to show anticonvulsive activity in animals.[5]

Antidepressant activity

The antidepressant effects of a range of essential oils were investigated using a forced swim test in rats. Rats were treated by intraperitoneal injection or inhalation. Clary sage oil had the strongest antistressor effect in the forced swimming test. The researchers found that the antidepressant activity of clary sage was closely associated with modulation of the DAnergic (dopamine) pathway.[6]

After inhalation of clary sage oil, 5-hydroxytryptamine (serotonin) plasma levels significantly increased and cortisol plasma levels decreased in a study on 22 menopausal women. The change rate of cortisol was greater in the depression group than the normal group. The researchers concluded that clary sage does have antidepressant-like effect.[7]

Antifungal activity

An in vitro study confirmed that clary sage oil had potent antifungal activity.[8]

Anti-inflammatory activity

Balacs reports a clinical trial by an Italian group that has been researching the anti-inflammatory and peripheral analgesic effects of clary sage oil. In rats, clary sage oil showed a significant anti-inflammatory effect and mild analgesic action after subcutaneous injection at 259 mg/kg. The anti-inflammatory response was more marked in carrageen-induced oedema than in histamine-induced inflammation. Balacs suggests that clary sage's activity is mediated via modulation of prostaglandin synthesis rather than via histamine.[9]

Antimicrobial activity

An in vitro study found that clary sage oil was more effective in inhibiting methicillin-resistant *Staphylococcus aureus* (MRSA) and methicillin-sensitive *S. aureus* (MSSA) growth than vancomycin.[10]

The results of an in vitro test confirmed that clary sage essential oil had antimicrobial activity against *S. aureus* strains isolated from patients with wound infections. It was concluded that clary sage oil may be applied to treat wounds and skin infections.[11]

Antinociceptive activity

Capsicum-induced nociceptive response was significantly reduced by the intraplantar injection of clary sage oil in a study involving mice. The researchers found that linalool was likely to be the compound responsible for the antinociceptive effect of clary sage.[12]

Anticholinergic activity

A study investigated the acetylcholinesterase (AChE) inhibition of a range of essential oils. Alzheimer's disease is characterised by the loss of activity of the neurotransmitter acetylcholine in the cerebral cortex. It was demonstrated that clary sage essential oil gave 20.8% inhibition. It was concluded that the inhibition of AChE is more effective when synaptic acetylcholine levels are low, which is the case in Alzheimer's disease.[13]

Dysmenorrhea

A randomised, placebo-controlled trial investigated the effects of aromatherapy on menstrual cramps and symptoms of dysmenorrhoea. A blend of clary sage, *Rosa centifolia* and *Lavandula officinalis* in almond oil was applied topically by massage to the abdomen. Menstrual cramps were significantly lowered in the aromatherapy group. It was suggested that aromatherapy can be offered as part of nursing care to women experiencing menstrual cramps or dysmenorrhoea.[14]

A study compared the effect of aromatherapy massage and acetaminophen on menstrual pain in Korean high school girls. The abdomen was massaged once using a blend of clary sage, marjoram, cinnamon, ginger and geranium in a base of almond oil. The level of menstrual pain was assessed using a visual analogue scale at baseline and 24 hours later. The reduction of menstrual pain was significantly higher in the aromatherapy group than in the acetaminophen group. However, the study could not verify whether the benefits were from the aromatherapy, the massage or both.[15]

A randomised, double-blind clinical trial using a blend of lavender, clary sage and marjoram, used in a 2:1:1 ratio and diluted into an unscented cream at 3%, assessed the effectiveness of the blend on menstrual cramps for outpatients with primary dysmenorrhoea. The study found that the duration of pain was significantly reduced from 2.4 to 1.8 days after the aromatherapy intervention. The study suggests that aromatherapy massage provides relief for patients with primary dysmenorrhoea.[16]

Labour

A clinical trial involving the use of essential oils during labour found clary sage oil was beneficial for its analgesic effects and relaxing effects, and its ability to accelerate labour.[17]

Sedative activity

A double-blind, randomised, controlled trial conducted on 34 women with urinary incontinence investigated the effects of inhalation of clary sage or lavender oil on the autonomic nervous system. The results suggest that lavender oil may not be appropriate in lowering stress during urodynamic examinations, whereas clary sage oil may be potentially useful in reducing stress caused by urodynamic examination in those suffering with incontinence.[18]

Clary sage oil may be effective in the prevention and treatment of stress-induced cardiovascular disease. This was based on a study in which clary sage oil intraperitoneally injected into rats subjected to immobilisation stress contributed to their recovery from endothelial dysfunction by increasing NO production and eNOS level, as well as decreasing oxidative stress.[19]

Actions

Actions commonly cited in aromatherapy

Antibacterial, anticonvulsive, antidepressant, antifungal, antispasmodic, carminative, deodorant, digestive, emmenagogue, hypotensive, nervine, sedative, tonic, uterine[20,21]

Actions supported by clinical studies

Antidepressant, antifungal, antispasmodic, neurotonic, sedative

Comment

Lis-Balchin states that clary sage is one essential oil that has an immense reputation in aromatherapy, although no real scientific proof exists for its use.[22]

On the other hand, Holmes is adamant that clary sage is one of several essential oils that have a profound effect on the neuroendocrine functions. He explains that, because clary sage oil has a balance of alcohols and esters, it can restore weak conditions and relax tense conditions. He suggests that it is much appreciated for the relief it can bring to menstrual cramps because of its uterine spasmolytic and analgesic action. He states that clary sage oil is also useful for conditions of oestrogen accumulation, which are often associated with an aggressive type of PMS syndrome, and that low-oestrogen conditions respond well to clary sage oil, especially during menopause.[23]

Holmes explains that clary sage oil is often highly recommended in childbirth because of its uterine stimulant and relaxant action.[23]

Bowles states that clary sage oil is supposed to be an emmenagogue, but this has not yet been proven in any form of clinical trial. She explains that sclareol, a compound found in clary sage, looks very similar to the steroid molecules; however, she explains that to date it remains to be tested whether sclareol has any oestrogenic effect. The solvent extract of clary sage oil contains 38-45% sclareol.[24]

The essential oil typically contains 0.1-0.4% sclareol.[25]

Tisserand & Young cite research which indicates that sclareol has no known oestrogen-like activity; however, an isomer of sclareol, 13-epi-sclareol, was found to inhibit breast and uterine cancer in vitro by possibly interacting with oestrogen receptors.[25]

C

Aromatherapy Uses

Clinical aromatherapy

Nervous system

Clary sage oil is well known for its euphoric action.[20] It is beneficial for treating anxiety, stress, nervous tension and depression.[21,26,27,28]

Clary sage oil is well known for its ability to balance. It is strengthening yet relaxing and regarded as a general tonic for mental and nervous fatigue.[20]

Holmes explains that clary sage oil is one of the most important remedies for the nervous system. It can restore a weak, debilitated nervous system. Clary sage is recommended for chronic atonic conditions with fatigue, insomnia, stress; neurasthenia with fatigue, burnout, exhaustion; and chronic adrenal fatigue.[23]

Psychological

Holmes states that clary sage oil calms the mind, promotes relaxation and has a mild euphoric effect. He recommends it for nervous and emotional tension, anxiety, emotional shock of any kind, panic and depression with anxiety or agitation. The sweet scent fosters emotional stability, while its green scent provides a calming effect.[23]

Reproductive system

Clary sage oil is one of the most important essential oils as a women's remedy. All three phases of a woman's life stand to benefit from clary sage – the menstrual cycle, childbirth and menopause.[29]

Clary sage oil is renowned for the relief it brings to menstrual cramps because of its spasmolytic and analgesic action on the womb. Clary sage oil is also a uterine stimulant and an emmenagogue that promotes menstruation when delayed, scanty or completely absent.[21,26,27,29]

Holmes states that clary sage is a very important oil for treating PMS. Like sweet fennel, it is specifically recommended for PMS and dysmenorrhoea that is due to oestrogen deficiency. Conversely, it is beneficial in conditions of oestrogen accumulation, which is often associated with a more 'aggressive type' of PMS.[23]

Holmes suggests that clary sage oil's oestrogenic action on the system results from pituitary-gonadal stimulation. It is very likely that this oil exerts a regulating action on the pituitary gland. Clary sage is recommended for managing menopause.[29]

In childbirth, clary sage oil's relaxant effect can help the mother release some tension and anxiety usually present in pre-labour and labour, right up to the transition phase. It is suggested that clary sage oil takes the edge off the physical and emotional intensity involved in the work of riding the contraction waves.[29]

Respiratory system

Clary sage oil is recommended for treating asthma as it relaxes spasms in the bronchial tube and helps reduce anxiety and emotional tension often associated with asthma sufferers.[20,21,28]

Skin care

Clary sage oil is suggested for preventing excessive sweating. It is recommended for oily skin, greasy hair and dandruff as it reduces excessive sebum production.[20,21]

Energetics, psyche and subtle uses

Energetics

According to TCM, clary sage oil is reputed to strengthen *Qi* that is depleted and it relaxes and improves circulation of *Qi*. This means that it is both a general tonic and an excellent antispasmodic.[28]

According to the principles of the Five Elements, clary sage oil is associated with the Metal Element. Mojay explains that clary sage oil has a pronounced effect on the *Lungs* and *Lung Qi*. Clary sage oil acts on the bodily soul known as the *Po*. When the *Po* is disturbed, we are unable to 'see' clearly in the here and now. We feel distracted from our spirit and intuitive insight. Clary sage oil helps us restore lucidity to our intuition allowing inspiration to flow.[28]

Holmes states that clary sage oil has an affinity with the Fire and Wood Elements. It nourishes the *Blood* and *Yin*, helps the *Yang* energy to descend and calms the *Shen*. When the *Shen* is agitated and the *Yin Qi* is deficient, we are likely to suffer from restlessness, insomnia, night sweats and headaches. He recommends blending clary sage with vetiver, geranium and patchouli for this purpose.[23]

Personality

Clary sage personalities have the ability to probe deeply into the psyche of others. They appear pensive at times. They are gentle, melancholic and thoughtful. According to Worwood, clary sage personalities will not rest until they are sure a job is done correctly, using their psyche as well as their head. She explains that they are so adaptable, can tackle almost any job and generally prefer creative occupations.[30]

Clary sage personalities are described as very warm and friendly. They enjoy people with all their idiosyncrasies. They are never judgemental and have the ability to be comforting in times of need, especially during times of grief.[30]

Clary sage brings long-lasting inner tranquillity, and, thanks to its warmth and liveliness, it helps dispel melancholy. Fischer-Rizzi compares clary sage to a colourful clown or comedian who cheers and entertains with a sort of dance. Clary sage has been particularly recognised as useful for people involved in creative work. It opens the path to the unknown, unusual, creative and intuitive.[31]

According to Myers-Briggs personality types, the clary sage personality is likely to be an INFP. INFPs are gentle, calm, easygoing and affirming. Integrity and commitment to what they believe in are essential. They like time alone for their many interests. They like learning and researching new things and interests. They are highly reflective, especially in understanding the mysteries and meaning of life. They have little need to impose their values on others. They prefer to gently influence and inspire. They value authenticity and depth in their relationships.

Subtle

Mojay suggests that clary sage oil is able to uplift one's spirit without disconnecting one from reality. The earthy quality of its herbaceous, musky sweetness reflects its ability to both steady and calm the mind, while its gentle pungency enlivens the senses and restores clarity.[28]

Holmes states that clary sage allows us to draw on our deep emotional and energetic core. In doing so, it can have a gentle effect that will help break down and remove any protective barriers we may use when relating to others.[23]

Fischer-Rizzi states that clary sage feeds the soul and helps us get through tough times. She recommends clary sage when the pressure and stress are from external factors.[31]

Keim Loughran & Bull state that clary sage strengthens the ability to dream and assists in the development of the intuitive mind, helping us access hidden truths and insights about others, ourselves and our life experiences. They explain that dreams can be a source of great teachings, offering an avenue to heal and grow, and even to resolve our problems.[32]

Davis also suggests that clary sage helps to bring us more closely in touch with the dream world. It is reputed to encourage vivid dreams, or it may be that it encourages dream recall.[33]

Zeck explains that clary sage can be used whenever we feel stagnant and unable to have a clear understanding of what is happening in our life. She explains that it helps give us clarity and understanding of our dreams, which in turn heightens our natural intuition.[34]

Worwood explains that clary sage encourages us to be satisfied with our achievements, and it assists us in realising that most of our problems exist in the imagination, and that issues which affect us will be resolved eventually.[35]

Dosage and Administration

Blending

Aromatherapy

For dysmenorrhoea and PMS, consider blending clary sage oil with essential oils such as Roman chamomile, sweet fennel, geranium, lavender, sweet marjoram, or rose absolute or otto.

For anxiety, nervous tension and stress-related conditions, consider blending clary sage oil with essential oils such as bergamot, Virginian or Atlas cedarwood, fragonia, geranium, lavender, neroli, sweet orange, patchouli, petitgrain, sandalwood or ylang ylang.

To alleviate depression, consider blending clary sage oil with essential oils such as bergamot, geranium, neroli, sweet orange, jasmine absolute, rose absolute, sandalwood or ylang ylang.

Perfumery

Arctander states that clary sage oil is commonly used in perfumery. It is used as a modifier for essential oils such as bergamot and lavender, and often blended with cistus and frankincense. It is commonly used in chypre, fougère, oriental and tabac-type fragrances. It gives classic style cologne perfumes a unique tenacity and acts as a fragrant fixative. It also blends beautifully with coriander seed, geranium, lavender, sandalwood, clove or cedarwood.[2]

Mode of administration

Bath

Full body bath, foot bath

Topical

Compress, massage, ointment, skin care

Inhalation

Direct inhalation, diffuser, oil vaporiser

Safety Profile

General safety

Clary sage oil has been reported to be non-toxic, non-irritant and non-sensitising.[21]

Contraindications

The oil is contraindicated during pregnancy.[20,21]

However, Tisserand & Young state that there are no known contraindications.[25]

Just because clary sage oil is labelled as an emmenagogue does not imply that the oil is an abortifacient in the amounts used in aromatherapy, and as such, it should present no danger in pregnancy.[36]

Lis-Balchin also states that clary sage oil is often quoted in aromatherapy literature as being oestrogenic; however, no clear scientific evidence has been forthcoming.[22]

Regulatory guidelines

Clary sage oil has GRAS status.

References

1. Le Strange R. *A history of herbal plants*. Angus and Robertson, United Kingdom, 1977.
2. Arctander S. *Perfume and flavor materials of natural origin*. Allured Publishing, Carol Stream, 1994.
3. Lawrence BM. *Essential oils 1981-1987*. Allured Publishing, Wheaton, 1989.
4. Grieve M. *A modern herbal – Vol. I*. Dover Publications, New York, 1971.
5. Khan I, Abourashed E. *Leung's encyclopedia of common natural ingredients used in food, drugs and cosmetics*. 3rd edn. John Wiley & Sons, New Jersey, 2010.
6. Seol GH et al. *Antidepressant-like effect of Salvia sclarea is explained by modulation of dopamine activities in rats*. Journal of Ethnopharmacology, 2010; 130(1): 187-190. Cited in Quintessential Aromatics database, 2013.
7. Lee KB et al. *Changes in 5-hydroxytryptamine and cortisol plasma levels in menopausal women after inhalation of clary sage oil*. Phytotherapy Research, 2014; 28(11): 1599-1605. Cited in Quintessential Aromatics database, 2013.
8. Džamić A et al. *Chemical composition and antifungal activity of Salvia sclarea (Lamiaceae) essential oil*. Archives of Biological Sciences, 2008; 60(2): 233-237. Cited in Quintessential Aromatics database, 2013.
9. Balacs T. *Research reports*. The International Journal of Aromatherapy, 1998; (8)4: 41-43.
10. Sharma PR et al. *Ten highly effective essential oils inhibit growth in methicillin resistant Staphylococcus aureus (MRSA) and methicillin sensitive Staphylococcus aureus (MSSA)*. International Journal of Pharmacy and Pharmaceutical Sciences, 2013; 5(1): 52-54. Cited in Quintessential Aromatics database, 2013.
11. Sienkiewicz M et al. *The effect of clary sage on staphylococci responsible for wound infections*. Postępy Dermatologii i Alergologii, 2015; 32(1): 21-26. doi:10.5114/pdia.2014.40957.
12. Sakurada T et al. *Intraplantar injection of bergamot essential oil into the mouse hindpaw. Effects on capsaicin-induced nociceptive behaviors*. International Review of Neurobiology, 2009; 85: 237-248. Cited in Quintessential Aromatics database, 2013.
13. Perry N et al. *European herbs with cholinergic activities: potential in dementia therapy*. International Journal of Geriatric Psychology, 1996; 11(12): 1063-1069. Cited in Quintessential Aromatics database, 2013.
14. Han SH et al. *Effect of aromatherapy on symptoms of dysmenorrhea in college students: a randomized placebo-controlled clinical trial*. Journal of Alternative and Complementary Medicine, 2006; 12(6): 535-541. Cited in Quintessential Aromatics database, 2013.
15. Hur MH et al. *Aromatherapy massage on the abdomen for alleviating menstrual pain in high school girls: a preliminary controlled clinical study*. Evidence-Based Complementary and Alternative Medicine, 2012; 2012: 187163. doi: 10.1155/2012/187163.
16. Ou MC et al. *Pain relief assessment by aromatic essential oil massage on outpatients with primary dysmenorrhea: a randomized, double-blind clinical trial*. Journal of Obstetrics and Gynaecology Research, 2012; 38(5): 817-822. Cited in Quintessential Aromatics database, 2013.
17. Burns E, Blamey C. *Soothing scents in childbirth*. The International Journal of Aromatherapy, 1994; 6(1): 24-28.
18. Seol GH et al. *Randomized controlled trial for Salvia sclarea or Lavandula angustifolia: differential effects on blood pressure in female patients with urinary incontinence undergoing urodynamic examination*. Journal of Alternative and Complementary Medicine, 2013; 19(7): 664-670. doi: 10.1089/acm.2012.0148.
19. Yang HJ et al. *Effects of Salvia sclarea on chronic immobilization stress induced endothelial dysfunction in rats*. BMC Complementary and Alternative Medicine. 2014; 14: 396. doi: 10.1186/1472-6882-14-396.
20. Davis P. *Aromatherapy an A-Z*. 2nd edn. C.W. Daniel Company, Saffron Walden, 1999.
21. Lawless J. *The encyclopaedia of essential oils*. Element Books, Shaftesbury, 1992.
22. Lis-Balchin M. *Aromatherapy science – a guide for healthcare professionals*. Pharmaceutical Press, London, 2006.
23. Holmes P. *Aromatica: a clinical guide to essential oil therapeutics – Vol. I*. Singing Dragon, London, 2016.
24. Bowles J. *The chemistry of aromatherapeutic oils*. 3rd edn. Allen & Unwin, Crows Nest, 2003.
25. Tisserand R, Young R. *Essential oil safety*. 2nd edn. Churchill Livingstone, Edinburgh, 2014.
26. Lavabre M. *Aromatherapy workbook*. Healing Arts Press, Rochester, 1997.

C

27. Schnaubelt K. *Medical aromatherapy*. Frog, Berkeley, 1999.
28. Mojay G. *Aromatherapy for healing the spirit*. Healing Arts Press, Rochester, 1999.
29. Holmes P. *Clary sage*. The International Journal of Aromatherapy, 1993; 5(1): 15-17.
30. Worwood VA. *The fragrant mind*. Transworld Publishers, London, 1995.
31. Fischer-Rizzi S. *Complete aromatherapy handbook*. Stirling Publishing, New York, 1990.
32. Keim Loughran J, Bull R. *Aromatherapy anointing oils*. Frog, Berkeley, 2001.
33. Davis P. *Subtle aromatherapy*. C.W. Daniel Company, Saffron Walden, 1991.
34. Zeck R. *The blossoming heart*. Aroma Tours, East Ivanhoe, 2004.
35. Worwood VA. *The fragrant heavens*. Transworld Publishers, London, 1999.
36. Tisserand R, Balacs T. *Essential oil safety*. Churchill Livingstone, Edinburgh, 1995.

Clove bud

Identification

Botanical name

Syzygium aromaticum (L) Merr & LM Perry

Synonyms

Eugenia aromatica, E. caryophyllata, E. carophyllus

Family

Myrtaceae

Botany and origins

The clove is an evergreen tree, up to 15 m high, with glossy green leaves, fragrant red flowers and purple fruits. The buds appear with a rosy-pink corolla at the tip, and as the corolla fades, the calyx slowly turns deep red. The calyxes are beaten from the tree and, when dried, provide the clove buds of commerce.[1]

It is a long-lived tree and is reported to remain productive for 150 years. The modern English name of clove is from the French *clou* meaning nail, derived from the Latin *clavus*. Clove is indigenous to the Moluccas, now part of Indonesia. The first recorded use was in the Chinese Han period 220-206 BC, where it was used to sweeten the breath.[1]

Method of extraction

Clove bud oil is water-distilled from the dried flower buds of *Syzygium aromaticum.*

The clove buds are comminuted prior to distillation. If the cloves are steam-distilled, hydrolysis takes place, and most of the natural acetyl eugenol is converted to eugenol. Compared to steam distillation, the level of hydrolysis that occurs during water distillation is minimal.[2]

The eugenol content of water distillation is typically 85-89%, while the eugenol content of steam-distilled clove bud oil is typically 91-95%.[1]

Characteristics

Clove bud oil is a clear to yellow mobile liquid, becoming brown with a strong, sweet and spicy odour.[2]

Clove leaf oil is a dark brown mobile liquid with a harsh, woody, phenolic, slightly sweet aroma. The leaf oil is often rectified and is usually a pale yellow colour with a sweeter, less harsh, dry woody odour closer to that of eugenol.[1]

Chemical composition

The composition of the bud, stem and leaf oils can be differentiated as follows:[3]

Constituent	clove leaf	clove stem	clove bud
eugenol	85-90%	87-92%	80-85%
eugenyl acetate	0-10%	3-5%	8-12%
isoeugenol	-	trace	-
sesquiterpene hydrocarbons	10-15%	6-8%	6-12%

Adulteration

Adulterants of clove bud oil are usually clove stem or leaf oil, or clove terpenes remaining after eugenol extraction.[1]

Lis-Balchin states that the price of synthetic eugenol and isoeugenol is higher than that of clove leaf or clove stem oil, therefore it is unlikely to be used to adulterate clove bud oil.[4]

Pharmacopoeias and standards

The purity, composition and physico-chemical properties of clove leaf and bud essential oils are defined in several pharmacopoeia monographs and standards:

- ISO 3141:1997 Oil of Clove Leaves [*Syzygium aromaticum* (L) Merr. Et Perry, syn. *Eugenia caryophyllus* (Sprengel) Bullock et S. Harrison]
- ISO 3142:1997 Oil of Clove Buds [*Syzygium aromaticum* (L) Merr. Et Perry, syn. *Eugenia caryophyllus* (Sprengel) Bullock et S. Harrison].

C

History and Traditional Uses

History

Cloves became known in Europe following a publication by Marco Polo in AD 1298. Venice was the leading European source of cloves and other spices in the thirteenth century. Cloves were traded in Europe via the Arabs, who for centuries had a monopoly of the sea-borne spice trade until it was broken by the Portuguese in the sixteenth century. The Portuguese had a monopoly in the trade of cloves for over a century.[1]

The Dutch subsequently broke the Portuguese monopoly, instituting their own, which they maintained with the utmost ruthlessness. In order to prevent other countries from obtaining cloves, the Dutch issued a proclamation in 1621, which ensured that all clove trees be destroyed except on Amboina and adjacent islands. This destruction of wild and cultivated trees resulted in a great loss of genetic diversity.[1]

Cloves were introduced to Zanzibar in the nineteenth century. Zanzibar, now part of Tanzania, has become the world's largest exporter of cloves.[1]

Traditional medicine

During the Renaissance, pomanders were made with cloves to keep epidemics and the plague at bay. Cloves are used in traditional medicine as a carminative, antiemetic and counterirritant. Clove tea is used to relieve nausea, and the oil is well known for its ability to alleviate toothache. In TCM, clove oil is used for diarrhoea, hernia and bad breath.[5]

Herbal

Clove buds are recommended in the German Commission E as a mouthwash for the treatment of inflammatory changes of the oral and pharyngeal mucosa and for topical analgesia in dentistry.[6]

Clove bud oil (or eugenol) is used for the symptomatic relief of toothache. The oil can be applied directly without pressure onto the carious tooth with a small piece of cotton.[5]

Food, perfumery and flavouring

The main use of cloves, both whole and ground, is as a domestic culinary spice and for the production of sauces and pickles.[1] Clove bud oil is extensively used as a fragrance component in soaps, detergents, creams, lotions and perfumes. Clove leaf oil is primarily used in soaps and low-cost perfumes.[5] Many spice blends, including curry, contain powdered cloves. Many herbal and bitter liqueurs contain clove macerates.[7]

Other uses

Indonesia is one of the largest consumers of clove buds. The comminuted clove buds are used to the extent of up to 8% in Indonesian *kretek* cigarettes.[1,2]

Therapeutics

Pharmacology and clinical studies

Many pharmacological studies involving clove essential oil have been published. A systemic review of these studies will not be attempted. Rather, I have chosen a selection of studies that support the traditional and clinical uses.

Acaricidal activity

Human scabies is considered a debilitating skin condition caused by *Sarcoptes scabiei*. Scabies is often treated with topical creams such as permethrin and oral ivermectin. Recent reports of acaricide tolerance in scabies in northern Australia prompted efforts to better understand the resistance mechanisms and identify potential new acaricides. In this study, three essential oils were tested for their acaricidal properties. Results showed that clove oil and eugenol were highly toxic against scabies mites. Eugenol demonstrated levels of toxicity comparable to benzyl benzoate, the positive control acaricide, killing mites within an hour of contact.[8]

Analgesic activity

Clove oil has long been used as a local analgesic for the relief of toothache.[6,7] Eugenol, like other phenols, acts to depress sensory receptors involved in pain perception. The mechanism of action involves a pronounced inhibition of prostaglandin biosynthesis resulting from blockages of both the cyclooxygenase and lipoxygenase pathways.[9,10]

Anticarcinogenic activity

Many in vitro studies have confirmed that clove bud extract and eugenol have chemoprotective and anticarcinogenic activity.[11]

Clove oil and eugenol displayed a 40-80% inhibition of melanin production in B16 melanoma cells in an in vitro study at 100-200 mcg/mL. However, at higher concentrations, the essential oil displayed cytotoxicity. It was concluded that further studies were required to establish safe therapeutic dosages.[11]

Antidepressant activity

A study investigated the safety and antidepressant activity of clove oil. The results confirmed the safety of clove oil, and suggested that its antidepressant activity might be attributed to the improvement in the hippocampal pERK1/2-

pCREB-BDNF pathways in rats exposed to chronic unpredictable mild stress.[12]

Antifungal activity

A study reported broad-spectrum antifungal activity of clove oil against *Candida albicans*.[13]

Clove oil was found to present significant antifungal activity. An in vivo study confirmed that the topical application of clove oil to guinea pigs (twice a day for 20 days) completely cured dermatophyte infection in 60% of cases.[14]

Antimicrobial activity

The EMA report states that the majority of publications on the pharmacological effects of clove spice, clove essential oil and eugenol deal with the antimicrobial effects.[7]

Eugenol inhibits the growth of 30 *Helicobacter pylori* strains tested, at a concentration of 2 µml / ml after nine and 12 hours of incubation. A lower pH-value increased the activity. The bacteria did not develop any resistance even after 10 passages grown at subinhibitory concentrations. The authors concluded that eugenol may prevent the growth *of H. pylori*.[7]

Clove oil was superior to rosemary oil when tested against several gram-positive and gram-negative bacteria, as well as against two fungi. When clove oil and rosemary oil were blended, a synergistic effect was observed against *C. albicans* and antagonism for *Aspergillus niger*.[15]

Another study confirmed that the vapour of clove oil was effective against the growth of gram-negative and gram-positive bacteria. The researchers concluded that essential oils in a vapour phase could be used as a preservative method to prevent microorganism proliferation.[16]

Many studies comparing a range of essential oils have identified clove oil as exhibiting the strongest activity against a range of bacteria.[17,18]

Antiviral activity

In vitro studies have confirmed that clove bud essential oil had inhibitory activity on hepatitis C virus protease. Another study confirmed significant activity against herpes simplex virus type I.[11]

Pediculicidal activity

A study reported that the pediculicidal activity of clove bud and clove leaf oil and eugenol was almost identical and comparable to that of pyrethrum and δ-phenothrin.[19]

Spasmolytic activity

A saturated aqueous solution of clove oil had a significant spasmolytic effect on electrically stimulated guinea pig ileum in vitro.[4]

Actions

Actions commonly cited in aromatherapy

Analgesic, anthelmintic, antiseptic, antispasmodic, antiviral, carminative, expectorant, larvicidal, stimulant, stomachic, vermifuge[20]

Actions supported by clinical studies

Acaricidal, analgesic, antifungal, antibacterial, antiseptic, antispasmodic, antiviral, carminative, pediculicidal, stomachic

Comment

Review of traditional uses and clinical data support the use of clove bud oil for the temporary relief of toothache due to dental cavity, and symptomatic treatment of minor inflammations in the mouth or throat.

Clove oil is not commonly used in aromatherapy as it is considered a local irritant, and allergic reactions may also be possible. However, when applied correctly, clove oil can be considered clinically safe.

Aromatherapy Uses

Clinical aromatherapy

Antiseptic

Clove bud oil has excellent antiseptic properties because of the high proportion of eugenol. It may be used for the prevention of colds and flu.[20,21,22] A 1% emulsion of clove bud oil has antiseptic strength three to four times greater than phenol.[22]

Digestive system

Clove bud oil is a carminative and antispasmodic, helping stimulate digestion, restoring appetite and relieving flatulence.[20,22]

Musculoskeletal system

Clove bud oil can be used in a massage oil, liniment or balm to help relieve arthritis, rheumatism and sprains.[20]

Nervous system

Clove bud oil is a physical and mental tonic, and should be used in conjunction with peppermint to ward off drowsiness.[21,23]

Skin care

While clove bud oil may be used as an insect repellent, it is generally not used in skin care as it is a potential dermal irritant and sensitiser.

Toothache

The dental value of cloves is well known.[20,21,23,24]

Clove bud oil has a minor anaesthetic effect.

The use of clove bud oil for the relief of toothache is only a temporary measure. Dental attention should be sought as soon as possible. Repeat administration after 20 minutes then every 2 hours thereafter if necessary. A small piece of cotton wool or tip of cotton bud should be soaked in undiluted oil or in a diluted solution. The cotton bud or cotton wool should be accurately directed to the decayed part of the tooth, avoiding contact with the gums.[7]

Energetics, psyche and subtle uses

Energetics

According to TCM, clove oil is *warming* and it tonifies *Qi*. It may be used to generate warmth and to eliminate any condition associated with *cold*.

Personality

The rich spicy aroma of clove oil suggests that the clove personality is dynamic, self-assured and full of energy.

According to Myers-Briggs personality types, the clove personality is likely to be an ESTJ. ESTJs love responsibility and control. They love to be in charge. They are good at making objective decisions. They love challenges and know how to get things done. They have an opinion for everything and are rarely at a loss for words. ESTJs like to spend their free time in ways that are productive. They are good at seeing what is illogical, inconsistent and impractical. They are willing to make sacrifices in order to honour their commitments. They tend to be workaholics and drive themselves and others very hard. They like to be involved in community service organisations and volunteer activities. They enjoy spending time with their friends and family.

Subtle

Worwood states that clove bud oil prepares us for action. It helps us move forward and make things happen. It awakens our senses and provides us with the confidence we need to handle tough times and not be afraid. The scent of clove discourages inhibiting thoughts.[25]

Zeck states that clove bud oil helps us to loosen our attachment to material things and to our ideas about how life is or should be lived. It will help us to remove any obstacles and to declutter our life and liberate us from false attachments.

Dosage and Administration

Blending

Aromatherapy

Clove bud oil is considered a blend modifier, so please use it sparingly in aromatherapy. Considering it has the potential to be a dermal irritant and sensitiser, please use sparingly in topical applications. When blended with other spice oils and rich floral oils, it creates a sensual warm aromatherapy blend.

For the relief of indigestion and abdominal distension, consider blending clove bud oil with essential oils such as caraway, coriander seed, sweet fennel, ginger, spearmint or peppermint.

To create a rich, spicy floral blend, consider blending clove bud oil with essential oils such as cardamom, cinnamon bark, nutmeg, black pepper, carnation absolute, rose absolute or ylang ylang.

For the relief of musculoskeletal aches and pains, consider blending clove bud oil with essential oils such as black pepper, cajeput, peppermint eucalyptus, ginger, kunzea, spike lavender, nutmeg, pine or rosemary.

For an effective antimicrobial blend for a vaporiser, consider blending clove bud oil with essential oils such as bay laurel, fragonia, lavender, lemongrass, lemon, manuka, oregano, tea tree or thyme.

Perfumery

Clove bud oil blends well with certain deep-sweet florals such as carnation absolute, rose absolute, jasmine absolute and ylang ylang to create a unique richness and body to the blend. Arctander also explains that clove bud oil is often an important ingredient in oriental style perfumes.[2]

Clove leaf oil is often used in 'low-cost' spicy style perfumes and in scenting soaps.[2]

Mode of administration

Bath

As clove bud oil is a potential irritant, I would not recommend using it in a bath; however, it may be used in a wash off product.

Topical

Massage, ointment

Inhalation

Direct inhalation, diffuser, oil vaporiser

Safety Profile

General safety

Clove bud oil has been reported to be a potential skin irritant and sensitising agent.[20] IFRA and Tisserand & Young recommend a maximum dermal limit of 0.5%.[26]

Contraindications

No contraindications known.

Toxicity

At high doses (0.5 mL/kg), clove oil is toxic, especially in young children, in whom it causes CNS depression, hepatic necrosis, convulsions or major haemostatic abnormalities.[10]

A near-fatal ingestion of clove oil was reported involving a two-year-old boy who had drunk between 5 –10 ml of clove oil.[27]

Regulatory guidelines

Cloves and their derivatives have been granted GRAS status.[5]

References

1. Weiss EA. *Essential oil crops*. CAB International, Wallingford, 1997.
2. Arctander S. *Perfume and flavor materials of natural origin*. Allured Publishing, Carol Stream, 1994.
3. Lawrence BM. *Essential oils 1976-1978*. Allured Publishing, Wheaton, 1979.
4. Lis-Balchin M. *Aromatherapy science – a guide for healthcare professionals*. Pharmaceutical Press, London, 2006.
5. Khan I, Abourashed E. *Leung's encyclopedia of common natural ingredients used in food, drugs and cosmetics*. 3rd edn. John Wiley & Sons, New Jersey, 2010.
6. Blumenthal M et al. *The complete German commission E monographs: therapeutic guide to herbal medicine*. American Botanical Council, Austin, 1998.
7. Committee on Herbal Medicinal Products (HMPC). *Assessment report on Syzygium aromaticum (L.) Merill et L.M. Perry, flos and Syzygium aromaticum (L.) Perry, floris aethroleum*. European Medicines Agency, 2011. Doc ref. EMA/HMPC/534946/2010.
8. Pasay C et al. *Acaricidal activity of eugenol based compounds against scabies mites*. PLoS ONE, 2010; 5(8): 1-9. Cited in Quintessential Aromatics database, 2013.
9. Tyler V. *Herbs of choice: the therapeutic use of phytomedicinals*. Pharmaceutical Products Press, Binghamton, 1994.
10. Bruneton J. *Pharmacognosy*. 2nd edn. Lavoisier Publishing, Paris, 1999.
11. Braun L, Cohen M. *Herbs & natural supplements: an evidence-based guide – Vol. 2*. 4th edn. Elsevier, Chatswood, 2015.
12. Liu BB et al. *Essential oil of Syzygium aromaticum reverses the deficits of stress-induced behaviors and hippocampal p-ERK/p-CREB/brain-derived neurotrophic factor expression*. Planta Medica, 2015; 81(3): 185-192. Cited in Quintessential Aromatics database, 2013.
13. Khan MSA, Ahmad I. *In vitro influence of certain oils on germ tube formation, cell surface hydrophobicity, and production of proteinase and hemolysin in Candida albicans*. Journal of Natural Pharmaceuticals, 2012; 3(2): 110-117. Cited in Quintessential Aromatics database, 2013.
14. Ramadan ANA et al. *Some pharmacodynamics effects and antimicrobial activity of essential oils of certain plants used in Egyptian folk medicine*. Veterinary Medicine Journal, Giza, 1994; 42(1): 263-270. Cited in Quintessential Aromatics database, 2013.
15. Fu Y et al. *Antimicrobial activity of clove and rosemary essential oils alone and in combination*. Phytotherapy Research, 2007; 21(10): 989-994.
16. Goñi P et al. *Antimicrobial activity in the vapour phase of a combination of cinnamon and clove essential oils*. Food Chemistry, 2009; 116(4): 982-989. Cited in Quintessential Aromatics database, 2013.
17. Singh BS, Singh G. *Antibacterial activity of the essential oils of three medicinal plants*. Indian Drugs, 1978; 15(11): 227-229. Cited in Quintessential Aromatics database, 2013.
18. Din M et al. *Biological activity – based assessment of essential oil emulsions*. Journal of Food Processing and Preservation, 2015; 39(6): 1452-1456. Cited in Quintessential Aromatics database, 2013.
19. Yang YC et al. *Ovicidal and adulticidal effects of Eugenia caryophyllata bud and leaf oil compounds on Pediculus capitis*. Journal of Agricultural and Food Chemistry, 2003; 51(17): 4884-4888. Cited in Quintessential Aromatics database, 2013.
20. Lawless J. *The encyclopaedia of essential oils*. Element Books, Shaftesbury, 1992.
21. Lavabre M. *Aromatherapy workbook*. Healing Arts Press, Rochester, 1997.
22. Valnet J. *The practice of aromatherapy*. C.W. Daniel Company, Saffron Walden, 1980.
23. Malhebiau P. *Portraits in oils*. C.W. Daniel Company, Saffron Walden, 1995.
24. Davis P. *Aromatherapy: an A-Z*. 2nd edn. C.W. Daniel Company, Saffron Walden, 1999.
25. Worwood VA. *The fragrant heavens*. Transworld Publishers, London, 1999.
26. Tisserand R, Young R. *Essential oil safety*. 2nd edn. Churchill Livingstone, Edinburgh, 2014.
27. Hartnoll G et al. *Near fatal ingestion of oil of cloves*. Archives of Diseases in Childhood, 1993; 69(3): 392-393.

Coriander seed

Identification

Botanical name

Coriandrum sativum L.

Synonyms

The herb is often referred to as cilantro and Chinese parsley.

Family

Apiaceae (Umbelliferae)

Botany and origins

Coriander is a strong-smelling herb, up to 0.8 m high, with bright green delicate leaves and a profusion of small, umbrella-shaped, pale-pink to whitish flowers, which produce the seeds.[1]

Coriander leaves are also referred to as cilantro. They have an intense, fresh green aroma. Upon drying, the seeds are small and almost spherical, 5 mm in diameter.[1]

Coriander is native to Europe and western Asia. It is now cultivated throughout the world. Most of the essential oil is produced in Russia, Poland, Hungary, The Netherlands, France and England.[2]

C

Method of extraction

An essential oil is obtained by steam distillation of the crushed seeds. An essential oil is also obtained by steam distillation of the leaves. Arctander explains that extraction of coriander seed oil from the seeds is difficult. The seed only contains 0.7% essential oil. It also contains 25% fixed oil (fatty oil). As the seed is very bulky, 1 tonne of crushed seeds in a 4,500 litre still will only yield 7 kg of coriander essential oil. Furthermore, coriander essential oil is slightly soluble in water.[2]

Characteristics

Coriander seed oil is a colourless to pale yellow liquid with a pleasant, sweet, somewhat woody-spicy aroma. The oil has a delightful floral-balsamic undertone with a peppery-woody top note.[2]

Chemical composition

The chemical composition of coriander seed oil was reported as follows:

α-pinene (9.3-11.0%), camphene (1.4-1.6%), β-pinene (0.8-0.9%), sabinene (0.7-0.8%), myrcene (1.9-2.0%), limonene (3.4-3.5%), γ-terpinene (11.4-12.1%), *p*-cymene (6.9-7.1%), linalool (56.9-58.4%), camphor (0.9-1.1%), α-terpineol (0.9-1.3%), geraniol (1.7-2.2%), geranyl acetate (0.8-1.1%).[3]

An essential oil is also produced from the fresh leaves. It contains a high proportion of decyl aldehyde, which imparts an intense green aroma.[2]

Adulteration

As the main constituents of coriander seed are readily available in synthetic form, the oil is frequently prone to adulteration. Arctander states that certain distillers even make it a rule to 'cut' their coriander oil with 20% synthetic linalool prior to resale.[2]

Coriander seed oil is also adulterated with 1,8-cineole from eucalyptus or camphor oil, α-terpinyl acetate and linalool.[4]

Pharmacopoeias and standards

The purity, composition and physico-chemical properties of coriander seed essential oil are defined in ISO 3516:1997 Oil of Coriander Fruits (*Coriandrum sativum* L.).

History and Traditional Uses

History

Coriander is considered one of the most ancient of herbs. It is mentioned in the Bible, and its seeds have been found in the tombs of the pharaohs. It was a popular herb with the Greeks, Hebrews and Romans of antiquity.[1]

The name *coriandrum*, used by Pliny, is derived from Latin *koros*, meaning 'bed bug'. This is because the aroma of the fresh leaf resembled that of a bug.[5]

Traditional medicine

All parts of the coriander plant are highly valued for the treatment of different disorders in the traditional folk medicine systems of different cultures.

In Ayurvedic medicine, coriander seeds have been employed in the treatment of arthritis and other inflammatory diseases. In the northern areas of Pakistan, the whole plant of coriander is used as a traditional medicine to treat flatulence, dysentery, diarrhoea, cough, stomach complaints, jaundice and vomiting. In Turkey, an infusion of the seeds is used as a digestive and carminative agent to enhance appetite.[6]

The fruits are used as an aromatic carminative, stomachic and antispasmodic – usually in the form of an infusion. In TCM, coriander seeds are used as a stomachic, and for the treatment of measles, dysentery and haemorrhoids.[7]

In Saudi Arabia, Jordan and Morocco, infusion of

coriander seeds is used as an antidiabetic agent.[6]

Herbal

The German Commission E recommends coriander seed for dyspeptic complaints and loss of appetite.[8]

Food, perfumery and flavouring

The whole dried seeds are ground and commonly used as a condiment or spice in the Mediterranean region, and it is a major ingredient of curry powder in Indian food. The seeds are also used to flavour many foods such as fish and meat, bakery and confectionary products.[6]

The fresh leaves are commonly known as cilantro or Chinese parsley, and are extensively used in Indian, Thai and Vietnamese cuisines.[6]

Coriander seed oil is used as a fragrance component in soaps, cosmetics and perfumes. It is also used in flavouring tobacco. The seeds and oil are extensively used as flavour ingredients in all types of food products, including alcoholic and non-alcoholic beverages.[7]

Therapeutics

Pharmacology and clinical studies

Many pharmacological studies involving coriander seed essential oil have been published. A systemic review of these studies will not be attempted. Rather, I have chosen a selection of studies that support the traditional and clinical uses.

Analgesic activity

Coriander seed oil was found to exhibit an analgesic effect (37.5 mg/kg) similar in efficacy to the aspirin control (50 mg/kg).[9]

It has been reported that linalool, the major constituent of coriander seed oil, plays a major role in its analgesic activity, while other studies found the contribution of glutamatergic system in antinociception elicited by linalool in mice.[6]

Anticarcinogenic activity

Coriander seed oil has been shown to have anticarcinogenic activity. The in vitro antitumour and immunomodulating activities of coriander seed extracts on breast cancer cell lines suggest its potential application and use in cancer prevention and inhibition of metastasis.[6]

Antifungal activity

Coriander seed oil has potent antifungal activity against a range of different *Candida* species.[10,11]

Antimicrobial activity

Coriander seed oil has been reported to inhibit a broad spectrum of microorganisms, and has proven efficacy as an antibacterial agent.[6]

A study examined the antimicrobial and antibiofilm activity of coriander seed oil and its major constituent linalool, as well as their effect in the quorum sensing (QS) system and their potential as antioxidants. The results confirmed that both compounds had anti-campylobacter activity, inhibited in vitro biofilm formation and promoted biofilm dispersion even at sub-MIC concentrations, and interfered with the QS system through the inhibition of violacein production.[12]

A study found that a blend of coriander seed and cumin seed essential oils showed a synergistic interaction both in antimicrobial and antioxidant activity. The authors also confirmed that the coriander and cumin combination did not show any cytotoxic effect both in brine shrimp lethality, as well as human normal colon cell line assays. The results suggest that coriander – cumin combination might be an effective natural antimicrobial and antioxidant agent in pharmaceuticals and food industries.[13]

A range of essential oils were evaluated for their antimicrobial activity against 11 different bacterial and 3 fungal strains belonging to species reported to be involved in food poisoning and food decay. Coriander seed oil displayed the best antibacterial activity, while thyme and spearmint oils were more effective to inhibit the fungal species.[14]

Antioxidant activity

It was confirmed that coriander seed oil and linalool were shown to have radical scavenging properties and lipid peroxidation inhibition ability, which could make them potential alternatives to synthetic antioxidants.[14]

Digestive activity

It has been stated that the digestive stimulant action may be mediated through the stimulation of the liver to secrete more bile enriched in bile acids, and the stimulation of enzyme activities that support digestion, both pancreatic and intestinal in origin.[6]

Hepatoprotective activity

The influence of essential oils on the activity of the hepatic carcinogen-metabolising enzymes of cytochrome P-450, aryl hydrocarbon hydroxylase (AHH) and glutathione S-transferase (GST) was investigated in mice. Coriander seed essential oil significantly elevated GST activity. It was suggested that coriander seed oil has potential as a 'blocking agent' in chemoprotective strategies.[15]

Hypotensive activity

Coriander seed oil displayed angiotensin

converting enzyme (ACE) inhibition with an IC50 value of 34.8 μg/mL and possessed strong DPPH radical scavenging activity. The research suggests that the oil could potentially be used for the management of hypertension as an ACE inhibitor.[14]

Insecticidal activity

At concentrations of 1000 ppm, four essential oils – coriander seed, cardamom, rosemary and sandalwood – had insecticidal activity ranging from 68% to 98% at 1 hour after treatment against house mosquito, *Culex pipiens pallens*.[16]

Larvicidal activity

Coriander seed oil is reported to have strong larvicidal activity against the mosquito, *Ochlerotatus caspius*.[17]

Sedative activity

The extracts and essential oil of coriander seed possess sedative-hypnotic activity. However, the aqueous extract of coriander seeds has a much stronger effect than its hydroalcoholic extract or essential oil. The results of this study support the use of coriander seeds as a sedative.[18]

Actions

Actions commonly cited in aromatherapy

Analgesic, antispasmodic, aperitif, bactericidal, carminative, depurative, digestive, revitalising, stimulant, stomachic[19,20,21]

Actions supported by clinical studies

Analgesic, antifungal, antimicrobial, bactericidal, digestive, hepatoprotective

Comment

Coriander seed oil has a long history of use as a traditional medicine. Numerous traditional uses for coriander seed essential oil support claims as a carminative and for the relief of digestive ailments such as flatulence and feelings of distension.

Many in vitro and in vivo studies suggest that the extract and essential oil of coriander seeds possess numerous biological properties. It would be exciting to see further investigations for its medicinal use as an antidiabetic, hypoglycaemic and chemoprotective agent.

Aromatherapy Uses

Clinical aromatherapy

Digestive system

Coriander seed oil alleviates dyspepsia, flatulence and nausea. It stimulates the appetite and is recommended for the treatment of anorexia nervosa.[20,21]

Musculoskeletal system

Coriander seed oil is recommended for the treatment of arthritis, gout, muscular aches and pains, and rheumatism.[20,21]

Nervous system

Coriander seed oil has a neurotonic effect and is recommended for general debility, mental fatigue and nervous exhaustion.[19,21]

Energetics, psyche and subtle uses

Energetics

Mojay describes coriander seed oil as *warm* and *dry* in nature. He explains that it shares the same digestive and carminative properties found in all other essential oils from the Apiaceae family. It helps to circulate *Qi* to the *Stomach*. As a result, it is beneficial for the relief of indigestion, abdominal distention and flatulence.[19]

Mojay also explains that coriander seed oil can be used to circulate the *Qi* and disperse *cold*. *Cold* causes painful obstruction, which is often associated with osteoarthritis, neuralgia and rheumatic pain.[19]

It also strengthens the function of the *Spleen* and *Stomach*, which is associated with the Earth Element. It helps to resolve *damp* and alleviate abdominal distension. It also invigorates the Intellect *(Yi)*, the spirit associated with the Earth Element, and is recommended for general debility, mental fatigue and nervous exhaustion.[19]

Coriander seed also has an affinity with the Fire Element. The combination of a warm, woody and peppery aroma indicates that the oil can both calm and uplift the *Shen*. Whenever the *Shen* is weak, we may experience nervous depression, which is often accompanied by worry and anxious overthinking.[19]

Personality

Worwood describes the coriander personality as a sincere, imaginative, optimistic, warm and inviting person. They enjoy expressing themselves and are very expressive. She states that they are usually very creative. They are passionate in whatever they do. Worwood states that if there were an animal equivalent to the coriander personality it would be the chameleon. She explains that they can adopt different appearances and behaviours at a moment's notice.[22]

Mojay states that coriander seed oil is ideally suited to creative people who find it difficult to cope with predictability and routine.[19]

C

According to Myers-Briggs personality types, the coriander seed personality is likely to be an ESFP. ESFPs are friendly, witty, charming and talkative. They value and nurture their relationships, give generously, without expecting anything in return. They are spontaneous, playful and enjoy everything they do and see. People who share their sense of fun and adventure are their favourite companions. They turn everything into a fun-filled event. They enjoy good things in life – music, dance, food, drink and entertainment. They avoid being alone. They like working in a lively and stimulating atmosphere with friendly, energetic people. They can be good at dealing with the public. They like variety and frequent change of tasks or jobs. They are enthusiastic, high-spirited and have lots of energy.

Subtle

Coriander seed oil should be used to encourage creativity, and to promote imagination, motivation, optimism, sincerity, expressiveness and enthusiasm. Worwood states that the scent of coriander seed is fresh and helps us seek new horizons. She recommends it for seekers who wish to experience all things before they feel sure of themselves and of the future journey to their soul.[23]

Keim Loughran & Bull say that, in times of ill health, our beliefs about the nature of the illness, the reason for it, how long it will last and the likely outcome have a great influence. They explain that coriander seed essential oil increases our confidence about the timing of healing. When we are more open to the possibility of a more rapid recovery, our focused intention and belief in ourselves can make a real difference.[24]

Dosage and Administration

Blending

Aromatherapy

The pleasant, sweet, woody-spicy scent of coriander seed oil blends well with most essential oils. Coriander seed oil is a blend enhancer. A blend enhancer has a pleasant scent and will give a lift and add personality to modify your blend without overpowering it.

For example, it could be used to add warmth and depth to any floral blend using rose absolute, jasmine absolute or ylang ylang. It helps to soften strong spicy aromas of ginger, clove bud, cinnamon bark or nutmeg. It gives a gentle, pleasant warmth to citrus oils such as bergamot, mandarin and sweet orange. The spicy floral aroma complements the rich, earthy and woody scented oils such as patchouli, sandalwood and vetiver.

For digestive support and the relief of indigestion, consider blending coriander seed oil with essential oils such as black pepper, sweet fennel, ginger, mandarin, sweet orange or spearmint.

To encourage creativity and promote motivation and optimism, consider blending coriander seed oil with essential oils such as bergamot, ginger, frankincense, neroli, sweet orange or rosemary.

Perfumery

Arctander states that the warm, sweet note of coriander seed oil blends well with clary sage and bergamot to create cologne style perfumes. It also blends well with essential oils such as cypress, ginger, neroli, petitgrain and sandalwood. It blends well with jasmine absolute, frankincense and cinnamon to create interesting oriental style perfumes.[2]

Mode of administration

Bath

Full body bath, foot bath

Topical

Compress, massage, ointment, skin care

Inhalation

Direct inhalation, diffuser, oil vaporiser

C

Safety Profile

General safety

Coriander seed oil is non-toxic, non-irritant and non-sensitising.[21]

Contraindications

No contraindications known.[25]

Regulatory guidelines

Coriander seed oil has GRAS status.

References

1. Hemphill I. *Spice notes.* Pan MacMillan, Sydney, 2000.
2. Arctander S. *Perfume and flavor materials of natural origin.* Allured Publishing, Carol Stream, 1994.
3. Lawrence BM. *Essential oils 1988-1991.* Allured Publishing, Carol Stream, 1993.
4. Schmidt E, Wanner J. *Adulteration of essential oils.* In Baser KHC, Buchbauer G. eds. *Handbook of essential oils – science, technology and applications.* 2nd edn. CRC Press, Boca Raton, 2016: 707-745.

5. Grieve M. *A modern herbal – Vol. I.* Dover Publications, New York, 1971.
6. Laribi B et al. *Coriander (Coriandrum sativum L.) and its bioactive constituents.* Fitoterapia, 2015; 103: 9-26.
7. Khan I, Abourashed E. *Leung's encyclopedia of common natural ingredients used in food, drugs and cosmetics.* 3rd edn. John Wiley & Sons, New Jersey, 2010.
8. Blumenthal M et al. *The complete German commission E monographs: therapeutic guide to herbal medicine.* American Botanical Council, Austin, 1998.
9. Afifi NA et al. *Some pharmacological activities of essential oils of certain Umbelliferous fruits.* Veterinary Medicine Journal, Giza. 1994; 42(3): 85-92. Cited in Quintessential Aromatics database, 2013.
10. Begnami AF et al. *Antimicrobial potential of Coriandrum sativum L. against different Candida species in vitro.* Food Chemistry, 2010; 118(1): 74-77. Cited in Quintessential Aromatics database, 2013.
11. Furletti VF et al. *Action of Coriandrum sativum L. essential oil upon oral Candida albicans biofilm formation.* Evidence-Based Complementary and Alternative Medicine, 2011; 2011: 985832. Cited in Quintessential Aromatics database, 2013. doi: 10.1155/2011/985832.
12. Duarte A et al. *Antioxidant properties of coriander essential oil and linalool and their potential to control Campylobacter spp.* Food Control, 2016; 61: 115-122. Cited in Quintessential Aromatics database, 2013.
13. Bag A, Chattopadhyay RR. *Evaluation of synergistic antibacterial and antioxidant efficacy of essential oils of spices and herbs in combination.* PLoS One, 2015; (10)7: e0131321. Cited in Quintessential Aromatics database, 2013. doi: 10.1371/journal.pone.0131321.
14. Zeb A. *Coriander (Coriandrum sativum) oils.* In Preedy VR. ed. *Essential oils in food preservation, flavor and safety.* Academic Press, London, 2016: 359-364.
15. Banerjee S et al. *Influence of certain essential oils on carcinogen-metabolising enzymes and acid-soluble sulphydryls in mouse liver.* Nutrition and Cancer, 1994; 21(3): 263-269. Cited in Quintessential Aromatics database, 2013.
16. Kang SH et al. *Spray adulticidal effects of plant oils against house mosquito, Culex pipiens pallens (Diptera: Culicidae).* Journal of Pesticide Science, 2009; 34(2): 100-106. Cited in Quintessential Aromatics database, 2013.
17. Knio KM et al. *Larvicidal activity of essential oils extracted from commonly used herbs in Lebanon against the seaside mosquito, Ochlerotatus caspius.* Bioresource Technology, 2008; 99(4): 763-768. Cited in Quintessential Aromatics database, 2013.
18. Emamghoreishi M, Heidari-Hamedani G. *Sedative-hypnotic activity of extracts and essential oil of coriander seeds.* Iran Journal of Medical Science, 2006; 31(1): 22-27.
19. Mojay G. *Aromatherapy for healing the spirit.* Healing Arts Press, Rochester, 1999.
20. Lavabre M. *Aromatherapy workbook.* Healing Arts Press, Rochester, 1997.
21. Lawless J. *The encyclopaedia of essential oils.* Element Books, Shaftesbury, 1992.
22. Worwood VA. *The fragrant mind.* Transworld Publishers, London, 1995.
23. Worwood VA. *The fragrant heavens.* Transworld Publishers, London, 1999.
24. Keim Loughran JK, Bull R. *Aromatherapy and subtle energy techniques.* Frog, Berkeley, 2000.
25. Tisserand R, Young R. *Essential oil safety.* 2nd edn. Churchill Livingstone, Edinburgh, 2014.

C

Cypress

Identification

Botanical name

Cupressus sempervirens L.

Synonyms

Italian cypress, Mediterranean cypress

Family

Cupressaceae

Botany and origins

The tree originates in the eastern Mediterranean countries and can be found along the coast of southern France, Italy, Corsica, Sardinia, Sicily, north Africa, Spain, Portugal and the Balkan countries. Most of the oil is distilled in southern France.[1]

It is an extremely old species of tree dating back to the Pliocene era (5.3 to 1.8 million years ago). It is an exceptionally long-lived tree; some cypress trees are believed to be 2,000 years old.[2]

Method of extraction

Cypress oil is steam-distilled from the leaves (needles) and twigs of *C. sempervirens* which are obtained by pruning the trees in autumn.

Guenther states that wooden branches should

be removed from the distillation material. The age of the branches influences the properties and composition of the oil. Young branches yield an oil with a lower specific gravity and higher optical rotation than old branches.[3]

Characteristics

Cypress is a pale yellow to almost colourless, mobile liquid with a sweet balsamic, yet refreshing odour, reminiscent of pine needles and juniper berry oil, with a unique dryout of a delicate and tenacious sweetness often compared with amber and labdanum.[1]

Chemical composition

The chemical composition of cypress oil was reported as follows:

α-pinene (20.4%), camphene (3.6%), sabinene (2.8%), β-pinene (2.9%), δ-3-carene (21.5%), myrcene and α-terpinene (1.1%), terpinolene (6.3%), linalool (0.07%), bornyl acetate (0.3%), cedrol (5.35%), δ-cadinene (1.7%).[4]

Adulteration

Arctander states that other varieties of cypress are often distilled with 'true' cypress, as the branches and other woody material are not always screened prior to distillation.[1]

Cypress is often adulterated with other evergreen essential oils. Essential oils from different cypress species are often blended together with juniper berry oil or pine needle oil, together with synthetic pinenes and camphene.[5]

Pharmacopoeias and standards

At the time of writing, the purity, composition, physico-chemical properties and therapeutic use of cypress essential oil are not defined in any pharmacopoeia monograph or standard.

History and Traditional Uses

History

Cypress was well known to the ancient Egyptians. It was burnt with juniper and pine for purifying the air in temples.[5]

It has been known in Mediterranean countries since antiquity. The Greeks and Romans planted it on temple and burial grounds. Nowadays the tree is still associated with parks and cemeteries. Guenther beautifully describes cypress:

> *It is a tree of serene beauty, blending well into the Mediterranean landscape; its dark foliage contrasts the lucid sky and etches delicate silhouettes against the blue sea.*[3]

Herbal

Ancient Greeks mashed the cones and steeped them in wine to treat dysentery, coughing up of blood and coughs.[5]

Hippocrates recommended cypress for severe cases of haemorrhoids with bleeding. Dioscorides and Galen recommended macerating the leaves in wine with a little myrrh for a fortnight. This was recommended for bladder infections and internal bleeding.[6]

Mojay states that cypress also had an equally ancient reputation for alleviating menstrual disorders.[7]

Culpeper recommended cypress for its 'drying and binding' qualities. He recommended it for conditions such as diarrhoea, dysentery and varicose veins.[8]

Traditional medicine

Guenther states that cypress oil has been used to alleviate the temporary distressing effects of whooping cough in children. For this purpose, he explains a 25% alcoholic solution of the oil should be applied four times daily on the bed linen and pillow cases. He states that the number, length and intensity of cough convulsions are significantly diminished.[3]

Valnet attributes many properties to cypress oil. He describes it as an astringent vasoconstrictor, antispasmodic, antisudorific, antirheumatic, diuretic and general restorative. He recommended it for treating haemorrhoids, ovarian disorders, menopause, whooping cough, enuresis, influenza, loss of voice, rheumatism and excessive sweating of the feet. He provides us with recipe for haemorrhoids; however, it needs to be noted that the recipe involves a herbal extract of cypress – not the essential oil.[9]

Food, perfumery and flavouring

Cypress oil is not used in food flavouring. It is used in perfumes as a modifier for pine, citrus colognes, fougères, chypre and modern aldehydic perfumes.[1]

Therapeutics

Pharmacology and clinical studies

Antimicrobial activity

Cypress oil demonstrated moderate antimicrobial activity against *Escherichia coli*, *Shigella dysenteriae*, *Bacillus subtilis* and *Staphylococcus albus*.[10]

Nootropic activity

A study examining the effect of the aroma of essential oils to mental and physical work found that cypress oil produced a favourable impression after physical work compared to that before work.[11]

Actions

Actions commonly cited in aromatherapy

Antiseptic, antispasmodic, astringent, deodorant, diuretic, haemostatic, hepatic, styptic, sudorific, venous decongestant, tonic[7,8,9,12]

Actions supported by clinical studies

Antiseptic

Comment

Lis-Balchin states that there is virtually no bioactivity data available for cypress oil.[5] I go further to say that cypress oil is not even mentioned in any modern herbal. Most of the information we know of cypress oil comes from ancient herbals. Perhaps Tisserand best summarises cypress when he states:

> *Cypress would seem to be one of the most useful oils, if only we knew more about its properties.*[8]

Aromatherapy Uses

Clinical aromatherapy

Circulatory system

Cypress oil is renowned as an excellent venous decongestant and is used for the treatment of varicose veins, oedema and haemorrhoids.[9,12,13,14,15]

Holmes describes the therapeutic properties of cypress:

> *Cypress is the only essential oil which is a true venous blood decongestant as well as an astringent … it gives a lift to the side of the circulation liable to congestive stasis, relieving resultant menstrual imbalances with heavy periods and intermenstrual bleeding. Part of cypress' blood activating action is a restorative effect on the veins themselves, useful with ailments ranging from haemorrhoids to phlebitis.*[16]

Psychological

Fischer-Rizzi recommends using cypress oil when one experiences uncontrollable crying spells. She describes the scent of cypress as soothing and suggests that cypress oil strengthens an overburdened nervous system and helps to restore calm.[14]

Reproductive system

Cypress oil is known as a menstrual regulator. It may be used to relieve painful periods. It is recommended for dysmenorrhoea, menorrhagia and menopausal problems.[12,15] It is recommended for severe hot flashes during menopause.[14]

Respiratory system

Cypress oil is reputed to be effective as a cough remedy for the management of acute and chronic bronchitis and whooping cough.[9,12,13,15]

Tisserand describes cypress oil as a powerful antispasmodic. He also recommends it for asthma, whooping cough and all spasmodic coughs.[8]

Skin care

Cypress oil is used in skin care preparations for its antiseptic and astringent properties. It is used for acne as well as oily and over-hydrated skins. It is recommended for excessive perspiration.[12,13,15] It is also recommended in a foot bath for excessive sweating of the feet.[9,14,15]

Energetics, psyche and subtle uses

Energetics

According to the principles of TCM, the main action of cypress is to regulate the flow of *Blood*. This, according to Mojay, makes it an important oil for the treatment of dysmenorrhoea and menorrhagia. Mojay also explains that cypress has a restorative and toning effect on the veins. Cypress also promotes the circulation of *Qi*. Like lavender it has a wide-ranging antispasmodic effect, which is beneficial for treating spasmodic colitis, PMS and asthma.[7]

According to the principles of the Five Elements, cypress is associated with the Metal and Water Elements. Mojay explains that cypress reinforces the bodily soul, the *Po*, the vital spirit of the *Lungs*.[7]

Personality

> *The cypress tree, standing dark and silent, is like a finger pointing to heaven! It does not indulge in needless movements, like other trees that stretch out limbs, allowing them to sway in the wind.*[14]

This description by Fischer-Rizzi gives you a clear indication of the cypress personality. Cypress represents the strength within, wisdom, and is seen as a symbol of eternity.

Worwood explains that a cypress person tends to be forceful, outspoken and firm in their views, and is seen as a strong person who is able to resolve most problems. She also states that cypress is a symbol of eternity that directs itself to the heavens, answering to no one but the great spirit. The cypress character may be the head teacher you fear or the grandparents who always make you aware of your boundaries, but always instilling discipline and respect.[17]

Mailhebiau describes the cypress personality:

> *The splendour of the cypress, a fine slender tree rising like a flame towards the starry, endless sky, represents the sacred flame of life, the unchangeable, eternal essence, and powerful evokes the spiritual archetype of cypress, a tall, fine-looking old man with the wisdom granted by a thousand years of intense, disciplined life*

... Thus cypress is associated with the idea of immortality of the soul.[2]

He suggests that anyone who has lost touch with a sense of harmony and serenity will benefit from a blend of cypress, Atlas cedarwood, rosemary and sandalwood.[2]

According to Myers-Briggs personality types, the cypress personality is likely to be an INTJ. INTJs are very responsible and dependable. They are people of very few words and tend to be private. They are punctual, precise and fastidious. They have the ability to concentrate and are difficult to distract. They are modest, unassuming and down to earth. They can be resistant to change. They can make quick critical judgements of others. They are extremely devoted in their relationships.

Subtle

Cypress oil is helpful at times of transition such as career changes and moving home, and is always helpful with painful transitions such as bereavement or ending of close relationships.[18]

Keim Loughran & Bull state that life is filled with changes and transitions. It is not the end result that is important but the journey. Cypress will assist with any and all of these life transitions.[19] Cypress helps us to have the courage to surrender our will to a higher purpose – to change, heal, transform and go through the many deaths that accompany the birth of wisdom.[19]

Worwood states that cypress has the ability to connect strongly to the human frequencies and thought-forms:

With great direction, cypress helps connection with the wisdom of the universe. It empathizes with suffering, the energies that emanate from a life in sorrow. It offers strength and energetic protection to those who need protecting, and those who are feeling vulnerable and insecure, and have lost their purpose.[20]

Mojay states that cypress has one of the most distinct and profound psychological actions to help us cope and accept even difficult change – of both an inner and outer nature. He also suggests that cypress helps to dissolve remorse, instils optimism and comforts those in bereavement.[7]

Zeck suggests that cypress brings structure, strength and a sense of protection during times of transition and change:

Major life transitions will often involve a bottoming out emotionally and spiritually, bring a sense of disenchantment and disillusionment. The past and the future seem to be dynamically opposed to the present moment.[21]

During such times, you will be required to navigate a way through a major life transition and identify the resources required for change. Cypress supports and holds the space for the soul to remain in balance. This gives us the opportunity to explore our visions, our symbols and dreams and for us to move forward.[21]

Dosage and Administration

Blending

Aromatherapy

For the treatment of oily and congested skin types, consider blending cypress oil with essential oils such as geranium, lavender, lemon, juniper berry or tea tree.

To make a deodorising blend, consider blending cypress oil with essential oils such as fragonia, geranium, palmarosa, lavender, tea tree or ylang ylang.

For the relief of poor venous circulation, consider blending cypress oil with calendula-infused oil and essential oils such as everlasting, lemon or geranium.

For the relief of bronchial congestion, consider blending cypress oil with essential oils such as cajeput, 1,8-cineole-rich eucalypts, peppermint eucalyptus, fragonia, pine or tea tree.

To make an uplifting and revitalising blend, consider blending cypress oil with essential oils such as bergamot, grapefruit, lemon, lemon-scented eucalyptus, fir, myrtle, pine, rosemary or spruce.

To guide us through a major life transition, consider blending cypress oil with essential oils such as Atlas cedarwood, fragonia, cistus, everlasting, frankincense, lavender, neroli or sandalwood.

Perfumery

Cypress oil is used in perfumery as a modifier in pine needle fragrances, in citrus colognes, fougères and chypre style perfumes and in modern aldehydic perfumes.[1]

By removing the terpenes, a concentrated cypress oil can be made in which the ambergris and labdanum-like odour of the higher boiling fractions becomes predominant.[3]

Mode of administration

Bath

Full body bath, foot bath

Topical

Compress, massage, ointment, skin care

Inhalation

Direct inhalation, diffuser, oil vaporiser

Safety Profile

General safety

Cypress oil has been reported to be non-toxic, non-irritant and non-sensitising.[12] Tisserand & Young advise that old or oxidised cypress oil should be avoided. Skin sensitisation may occur if oxidised.[22]

Contraindications

No contraindications known.

Regulatory guidelines

RIFM recommends maximum safety limit of 4%.[5]

References

1. Arctander S. *Perfume and flavor materials of natural origin.* Allured Publishing, Carol Stream, 1994.
2. Mailhebiau P. *Portraits in oils.* The C.W. Daniel Company, Saffron Walden, 1995.
3. Guenther E. *The essential oil – Vol. VI.* Robert Krieger Publishing, Malabar, 1952.
4. Lawrence BM. *Essential oils 1976-1978.* Allured Publishing, Wheaton, 1979.
5. Lis-Balchin M. *Aromatherapy science – a guide for healthcare professionals.* Pharmaceutical Press, London, 2006.
6. Ryman D. *Aromatherapy.* Judy Piatkus, Great Britain, 1991.
7. Mojay G. *Aromatherapy for healing the spirit.* Healing Arts Press, Rochester, 1999.
8. Tisserand R. *The art of aromatherapy.* C.W. Daniel Company, Saffron Walden, 1977.
9. Valnet J. *The practice of aromatherapy.* C.W. Daniel Company, Saffron Walden, 1980.
10. Siddiqi RR et al. *Antimicrobial activity of essential oils from Schinus terebinthifolius, Cupressus sempervirens, Citrus limon, Ferula asafoetida. Part 1.* Pakistan Journal of Science & Industrial Research, 1995; 38(9/10): 358-361. Cited in Quintessential Aromatics database, 2013.
11. Sugawara Y et al. *Alteration of perceived fragrance of essential oils in relation to type of work: a simple screening test for efficacy of aroma.* Chemical Senses, 1999; 24(4): 415-421. Cited in Quintessential Aromatics database, 2013.
12. Lawless J. *The encyclopaedia of essential oils.* Element Books, Shaftesbury, 1992.
13. Schnaubelt K. *Medical aromatherapy.* Frog, Berkeley, 1999.
14. Fischer-Rizzi S. *Complete aromatherapy handbook.* Sterling Publishing, New York, 1990.
15. Davis P. *Aromatherapy: an A-Z.* 2nd edn. C.W. Daniel Company, Saffron Walden, 1999.
16. Holmes P. *The energetics of Western herbs – Vol. I.* Artemis Press, Boulder, 1989.
17. Worwood VA. *The fragrant mind.* Transworld Publishers, London, 1995.
18. Davis P. *Subtle aromatherapy.* C.W. Daniel Company, Saffron Walden, 1991.
19. Keim Loughran J, Bull R. *Aromatherapy and subtle energy techniques.* Frog, Berkeley, 2000.
20. Worwood VA. *The fragrant heavens.* Transworld Publishers, London, 1999.
21. Zeck R. *The blossoming heart – aromatherapy for healing and transformation.* Aroma Tours, East Ivanhoe, 2004.
22. Tisserand R, Young R. *Essential oil safety.* 2nd edn. Churchill Livingstone, Edinburgh, 2014.

C

Cypress, blue

Identification

Botanical name

Callitris intratropica R.T. Baker & H.B. Sm.

Synonyms

Northern cypress pine, Australian blue cypress

Family

Cupressaceae

Botany and origins

The genus name, *Callitris* is from the Greek words *calli,* meaning beautiful and *treis,* meaning three, in reference to the triangular shape of the scale-like leaves that are arranged in whorls of three.[1]

Cypress pine is a native to Australia and grows in the Northern Territory, northern Western Australia, Cape York and northeastern Queensland. The tree usually grows in open forest, but is also found in heath forest, vine thickets, monsoon forest and on rainforest edges.[1]

C. intratropica is a medium to large sized tree up to 45 m in height with a highly fragrant wood.[2]

Method of extraction

Blue cypress oil is distilled from chipped bark and wood of *C. intratropica.* Blue cypress oil is extracted from plantation grown trees, not from wild harvesting.[1]

Characteristics

Blue cypress oil has a deep cobalt blue colour with a rich, resinous, woody and smoky aroma.[2]

Chemical composition

The chemical composition of blue cypress essential oil was reported as follows:

β-eudesmol (14.4%), dihydrocolumellarin (14.0%), guaiol (13.7%), δ-eudesmol (9.1%), α-eudesmol (7.6%), guaiazulene (6.2%), chamazulene (5.6%), columellarin (2.9%), callitrin (2.4%), cadelene (2.3%), β-selinene (2.2%), α-selinene (1.5%), callitrisin (1.4%), elemol (1.3%).[3]

Resinous compounds in the bark react during distillation with other aromatic compounds to create guaiazulene. It is a sesquiterpene known as azulenes, which are said to possess anti-inflammatory and antiallergenic properties.[1]

Adulteration

Not reported.

Pharmacopoeias and standards

At the time of writing, the purity, composition, physico-chemical properties and therapeutic use of blue cypress essential oil are not defined in any pharmacopoeia monograph or standard.

History and Traditional Uses

History

Williams states that a gum sourced from *C. intratropica* was used by Australian Aboriginals as a glue for making durable tools such as wooden prongs to fish spears or the hardwood head to the shaft of a bamboo spear. However, the gum had toxic properties. Ingestion was said to cause swelling of the stomach and inhaling the fumes when the gum was heated was believed to be harmful.[4]

The first recorded use of *C. intratropica* by European settlers was in 1905, by Mr Joe Cooper, who milled the timber for building purposes. At the same time, RT Barker and HG Smith wrote a paper entitled, *A Research on the Pines of Australia*, in which the characteristics and properties of *C. intratropica* were investigated and defined.[1]

The first essential oil production began in the mid-1990s.[1]

Other uses

The resin of cypress pine and other native *Callitris* species is known as Australian sandarac resin. In the past, sandarac was used as a coating for 'gastro-resistant' capsules, so that the capsules would not dissolve in the stomach.[1]

Therapeutics

Pharmacology and clinical studies

Antibacterial activity

An in vitro study confirmed that blue cypress oil was effective against a range of gram-positive and gram-negative bacteria.[5]

Anti-inflammatory activity

An in vitro study found that blue cypress oil suppressed LPS-induced PGE2 production, which suggests that the oil can be used to inhibit overactivation of macrophages followed by stimulation of inflammatory mediators.[6]

Antioxidant activity

An in vitro study confirmed that blue cypress oil had high antioxidant activity. It was stated that essential oils with antioxidant activity are of special interest in diseases of an inflammatory nature.[7]

Actions

Actions commonly cited in aromatherapy

Antibacterial, anti-inflammatory, antimicrobial, wound healing[1,2]

Actions supported by clinical studies

Anti-inflammatory, antimicrobial

Comment

This is a unique Australian essential oil that has exciting therapeutic potential. I hope that more clinical and pharmacological research will be conducted to study its bioactivity. It contains a diverse range of constituents such as monoterpene hydrocarbons, sesquiterpene hydrocarbons, sesquiterpene alcohols, sesquiterpene lactones and monoterpene alcohols.

Blue cypress oil contains a small percentage of sesquiterpene lactones, callitrisin and dihydrocallitrisin. Essential oils with lactones are often used in the treatment of chronic catarrh and bronchial congestion.[8]

Aromatherapy Uses

Clinical aromatherapy

Antiviral

Blue cypress oil is reported to have antiviral properties and has been beneficial against common warts caused by papilloma virus, shingles and cold sores.[1]

Integumentary system

Blue cypress oil has been used as a wound-healing

agent with anti-inflammatory and antibacterial properties. Webb states that it appears to be useful for skin conditions characterised by erythema (redness and skin irritation).[2]

It also has analgesic properties and has been used for pain relief and wound healing in burns.[3,4]

Musculoskeletal system

Blue cypress oil's analgesic properties have been used for pain relief for joint pain associated with arthritis.[3,4]

Psychological

Webb states that blue cypress oil is beneficial for grounding people who are flighty, nervous or emotionally distraught. The oil has a calming and reassuring effect.[2]

Dosage and Administration

Blending

Aromatherapy

For the relief of pain and inflammation associated with the musculoskeletal system, consider blending blue cypress oil with essential oils such as cajeput, kunzea, ginger, lavender or rosemary.

For the relief of sensitive and inflamed skin, consider blending blue cypress oil with essential oils such as German chamomile, everlasting, lavender, neroli or sandalwood.

Perfumery

Blue cypress oil is not commonly used in perfumery.

Mode of administration

Bath

Full body bath, foot bath

Topical

Compress, massage, ointment, skin care

Inhalation

Direct inhalation, diffuser, oil vaporiser

Safety Profile

General safety

Blue cypress oil was mildly irritating when applied to rabbits at 100%, but not irritating at 50%.[8]

No skin irritation or allergic sensitisation reactions have been reported with people using blue cypress oil. It is recommended to use diluted on the skin.[1]

Contraindications

Tisserand & Young state that the β-eudesmol found in blue cypress oil is an anti-angiogenic. There may be a link between anti-angiogenic activity and reproductive toxicity, therefore they have decided to contraindicate blue cypress oil during pregnancy and lactation.[9]

Regulatory guidelines

Blue cypress oil is not defined in any regulatory guideline.

References

1. Australian Botanical Products. *Blue cypress monograph.* Retrieved Sep 28, 2017 from http://www.abp.com.au/files/Blue_Cypress_monograph_2011_ABP_1_.pdf
2. Webb M. *Australian essential oil profile – blue cypress.* Aromatherapy Today, 2001; 19: 37-39.
3. Doimo L. *Azulenes, costols and gamma-lactones from cypress-pines (Callitris columellaris, C. glaucophylla and C. intraropica) distilled oils and methanol extracts.* Journal of Essential Oil Research, 2001; 13(1): 25-29. doi: 10.1080/10412905.2001.9699594.
4. Williams C. *Medicinal plants in Australia – Vol. 2 Gums, resins, tannins and essential oil.* Rosenburg Publishing, Dural, 2011.
5. Wanner J et al. *Chemical composition and antibacterial activity of blue cypress essential oil, Callitris intratropica R.T. Baker.* 41st International Symposium on Essential Oils, Wrocław, 2010. doi: 10.13140/2.1.3539.2320.
6. Destryana AR et al. *Antioxidant and anti-inflammatory activities of Ocotea, copaiba and blue cypress essential oils in vitro and in vivo.* Journal of the American Oil Chemists' Society, 2014; 91(9): 1531-1542. Cited in Quintessential Aromatics database, 2013.
7. Zhao Q, Bowles EJ, Zhang H-Y. *Antioxidant activities of eleven Australian essential oils.* Natural Product Communications, 2008; 3(5): 837-842. Cited in Quintessential Aromatics database, 2013.
8. Bowles EJ. *The chemistry of aromatherapeutic oils.* 3rd edn. Allen & Unwin, Crows Nest, 2003.
9. Tisserand R, Young R. *Essential oil safety.* 2nd edn. Churchill Livingstone, Edinburgh, 2014.

Dill seed

Identification

Botanical name

Anethum graveolens L.

Synonyms

European dill

Family

Apiaceae (Umbelliferae)

Botany and origins

Dill is an annual or biennial herb with a smooth, erect stem, growing up to 1 m high. It is a native to the Mediterranean region, but is now cultivated worldwide. Dill seed oil is mainly produced in Europe.[1]

Indian dill (*Anethum sowa*) is a smooth perennial herb, up to 1 m high. It is native to tropical Asia and is cultivated in India and Japan.[2]

Method of extraction

Dill seed oil is steam-distilled from the crushed, dried seeds of *Anethum graveolens*. Indian dill seed oil is obtained by the steam distillation of the crushed seed.[2]

Characteristics

Dill seed oil is a pale yellow to colourless oil with a fresh, warm-spicy aroma. Arctander describes the odour as light and fresh, warm-spicy and reminiscent of caraway and spearmint.[2] Arctander states that the odour of Indian dill seed is distinctly different from that of the European dill seed oil. He explains that Indian dill seed is more like parsley seed.[2]

Chemical composition

The chemical composition of European dill seed oil was reported as follows:

α-pinene (trace), camphene (trace), β-pinene (trace), myrcene (0.3%), α-phellandrene (0.4-1.1%), limonene (39.5-39.6%), β-phellandrene (1.2-1.3%), *cis*-ocimene (trace-0.1%), *p*-cymene (trace-0.1%), terpinolene (trace), carvone (54.6-54.8%), myristicin (trace-0.4%).[3]

The carvone content of European dill seed oil is usually higher than that of Indian dill seed oil. Indian dill seed oil also contains high levels of apiole, a compound known to be toxic.[4]

The chemical composition of Indian dill seed oil was reported as follows:

apiole (20.7-52.5%), limonene (5.9-45%), carvone (17.4-23.1%), (*E*)-dihydrocarvone (4.2-16.6%), α-phellandrene (trace – 6.5%), (*Z*)-dihydrocarvone (0.8-5.2%).[5]

Adulteration

Dill seed essential oil is often adulterated with phellandrene, distilled limonene from orange terpenes, synthetic carvone and dihydrocarvone.[6]

Pharmacopoeias and standards

At the time of writing, the purity, composition, physico-chemical properties and therapeutic use of dill seed oil are not defined in any pharmacopoeia monograph or standard.

History and Traditional Uses

History

Dill is native to the Mediterranean region and southern Russia. According to Hemphill, it was first cultivated in 3000 BC by the ancient Babylonians and Assyrians.[7]

The ancient Romans regarded dill as a symbol of vitality. Culpeper was aware of dill's excellent carminative action:

> *… it stays the hiccough, being boiled in wine, and but smelled unto being tied in a cloth. The seed is more use than the leaves, and more effectual to digest raw and vicious humours, and is used in medicines that serve to expel wind, and the pains proceeding therefrom …*[8]

The name is derived from the old Norse word *dilla*, which means to soothe or lull.[9]

Traditional medicine

Dill is a medicinal herb that has been used for more than 2,000 years. The seeds are carminative, stomachic, digestive and tranquillising, and have been traditionally used for treating stomach ailments, colic, hiccups, bad breath and flatulence. A poultice of dill seeds can be used to treat bruises, blocked milk ducts and overloaded breasts in women who are breastfeeding. Dill herb is used in Ayurvedic medicine for its digestive properties and for rheumatic conditions.[9]

Herbal

Dill seeds are used as a carminative and a flavour. Dill seeds are also used in gripe water for infants.[8,10,11] The German Commission E recommends dill seeds for the treatment of dyspepsia.[12]

Food, perfumery and flavouring

Dill seed is extensively used as a culinary spice. The seeds are extensively found in breads, condiments and relishes, and meats.[1,7,10]

Therapeutics

Pharmacology and clinical studies

Many pharmacological studies involving dill seed oil have been published. A systemic review of these studies will not be attempted. Rather, I have chosen a selection of studies that support the traditional and clinical uses.

Antifungal activity

Dill seed oil possessed strong antifungal activity against *Aspergillus niger* and *Candida albicans*.[13]

A study investigated the antifungal mechanism of dill seed essential oil against *C. albicans* and *Aspergillus flavus*. The researchers investigated the effect of the essential oil on the plasma membrane and mitochondria. The essential oil caused morphological changes in the cells of the fungi and a reduction in the quantity. The researchers concluded that the antifungal activity of dill seed oil results from its ability to disrupt the permeability barrier of the plasma membrane, and from the mitochondrial dysfunction-induced reactive oxygen species accumulation in the fungi.[14,15]

Antimicrobial activity

Dill seed oil possessed good antibacterial activity against a range of microorganisms.[16]

Antioxidant activity

Dill seed oil and its main constituents demonstrated potent NO-scavenging effect and inhibited the expression of inducible NO synthase.[17]

Antispasmodic activity

Dill seed oil was reported to have spasmolytic effects on the smooth muscles of the gastrointestinal tract.[1]

Chemopreventative activity

Fractions of dill seed oil were found to act as inducers of glutathione S-transferase (GST), one of the main detoxifying enzymes in the liver. Anethofuran and carvone also acted as inducers in the small intestinal mucosa, whereas in the colon, GST activity was significantly increased by carvone and limonene.[18]

Hypoglycaemic activity

A study demonstrated that subcutaneously injected dill seed oil into alloxan-induced diabetic rats had a significant hypoglycaemic activity within one hour.[19]

Hypolipidaemic activity

A study involving daily oral administration of dill seed oil for two weeks significantly reduced total cholesterol, triglyceride and low-density lipoprotein cholesterol. The oil also increased high-density lipoprotein cholesterol. It was concluded that dill seed oil has significant lipid-lowering effects and is a promising cardioprotective.[20]

Actions

Actions commonly cited in aromatherapy

Antispasmodic, bactericidal, carminative, digestive, emmenagogue, galactagogue, hypotensive, stimulant, stomachic[1,10]

Actions supported by clinical studies

Antifungal, carminative, digestive, hepatoprotective

Comment

Dill seed has a long history of use in traditional medicine. Traditional uses for dill seed oil support claims as a carminative and for the relief of digestive ailments such as flatulence and feelings of distension.

Further studies should be done to understand the potential chemoprotective and hypoglycaemic role of dill seed essential oil.

Aromatherapy Uses

Clinical aromatherapy

Digestive system

Dill seed oil is used as an aromatic carminative for the relief of colic, dyspepsia, flatulence and indigestion.[1,8]

Reproductive system

Dill seed oil is recommended for dysmenorrhoea and for promoting lactation.[1,8]

Energetics, psyche and subtle uses

Energetics

Dill seed oil is *warming* and *drying*. It shares the same digestive and carminative properties found in all other essential oils from the Apiaceae family. It helps to circulate *Qi* to the *Stomach*. As a result, it is beneficial for the relief of indigestion, abdominal distention and flatulence. Dill seed oil can also be used to circulate the *Qi* and disperse *cold*. *Cold* causes painful obstruction, which is often associated with osteoarthritis, neuralgia and rheumatic pain.

Miller & Miller describe the energetics of dill as cooling to neutral. According to the principles of Ayurveda, dill seed oil helps to reduce *Pitta* and *Kapha* dosha.[21]

D

Subtle

Worwood states that the sweet scent of dill seed oil helps us to remember the wonders of this world. She explains that the joy of creation is encapsulated in dill, and that it reminds us that the body is fragile and indebted to the earth. Dill seed oil gives us the clarity and vision we need to complete the tasks we undertake on our journey of life.[22]

Dill seed oil encourages tenderness, transformation and harmony, and clears the way to complete the tasks we undertake on our journey. Dill seed oil is said to clear a room of negative emotional energies such as anger, fear or jealously.[23]

Dosage and Administration

Blending

Aromatherapy

To alleviate dyspepsia and indigestion, consider blending dill seed oil with essential oils such as aniseed, basil, sweet fennel, coriander seed, sweet marjoram, sweet orange, peppermint or spearmint.

To clear negative emotional energies, consider blending dill seed oil with essential oils such as frankincense, fragonia, lavender, lemon or sandalwood.

Perfumery

Dill seed oil is not commonly used in perfumery.

Mode of administration

Bath

Full body bath, foot bath

Topical

Compress, massage, ointment

Inhalation

Direct inhalation, diffuser, oil vaporiser

Ingestion

Schnaubelt recommends one drop of dill seed essential oil for casual ingestion in a glass of water. He recommends it for childhood colic and indigestion.[24]

Safety Profile

General safety

European dill seed oil is non-toxic, non-irritant and non-sensitising.[8] Essential oils high in limonene such as dill seed oil are prone to oxidise easily. Therefore, to prevent oxidation, the oil should be stored in a dark, airtight container in a refrigerator.[25]

Contraindications

No contraindications are known for European dill seed oil. Indian dill seed oil contains apiole, and as such, it may be considered a hepatotoxin and an abortifacient. Indian dill seed oil is contraindicated during pregnancy and breastfeeding. European dill seed oil does not contain apiole.[25]

Regulatory guidelines

Dill seed oil has GRAS status.

References

1. Khan I, Abourashed E. *Leung's encyclopedia of common natural ingredients used in food, drugs and cosmetics*. 3rd edn. John Wiley & Sons, New Jersey, 2010.
2. Arctander S. *Perfume and flavor materials of natural origin*. Allured Publishing, Carol Stream, 1994.
3. Lawrence BM. *Essential oils 1981-1987*. Allured Publishing, Wheaton, 1989.
4. Denys J et al. *Characterization of essential oil of dill (Anethum graveolens L.)*. Journal of Essential Oil Research, 1995; 7(1): 11-20. doi: 10.1080/10412905.1995.9698456.
5. Lawrence BM. *Essential oils 1988-1991*. Allured Publishing, Wheaton, 1993.
6. Schmidt E, Wanner J. *Adulteration of essential oils*. In Baser KHC, Buchbauer G. eds. *Handbook of essential oils – science, technology and applications*. 2nd edn. CRC Press, Boca Raton, 2016: 707-745.
7. Hemphill I. *Spice notes*. Pan MacMillan, Sydney, 2000.
8. Grieve M. *A modern herbal – Vol. I*. Dover Publications, New York, 1971.
9. Najaran ZT et al. *Dill (Anethum graveolens L.) oils*. In Preedy VR. ed. *Essential oils in food preservation, flavor and safety*. Academic Press, London, 2016: 405-412.
10. Lawless J. *The encyclopaedia of essential oils*. Element Books, Shaftesbury, 1992.
11. Evans WC. *Trease and Evans pharmacognosy*. 15th edn. WB Saunders, Edinburgh, 2002.
12. Blumenthal M et al. *The complete German commission E monographs: therapeutic guide to herbal medicine*. American Botanical Council, Austin, 1998.
13. Jirovetz L et al. *Composition, quality control, and antimicrobial activity of the essential oil of long-time stored dill (Anethum graveolens L.) seeds from Bulgaria*. Journal of Agricultural and Food Chemistry, 2003; 51(13): 3854-3857. Cited in Quintessential Aromatics database, 2013.
14. Chen Y et al. *Antifungal mechanism of essential oil from Anethum graveolens seeds against Candida albicans*. Journal of Medical Microbiology, 2013; 62(8): 1175-1183. Cited in Quintessential Aromatics database, 2013.

D

15. Tian J et al. *The mechanism of antifungal action of essential oil from dill (Anethum graveolens L.) on Aspergillus flavus*. PLoS ONE, 2012; 7(1): e30147. Cited in Quintessential Aromatics database, 2013.
16. Syed M et al. *Antimicrobial activity of the essential oils of Umbelliferae. Part 2*. Pakistan Journal of Science & Industrial Research, 1986; 29(3): 189-192. Cited in Quintessential Aromatics database, 2013.
17. Kazemi M. *Phenolic profile, antioxidant capacity and anti-inflammatory activity of Anethum graveolens L. essential oil*. Natural Product Research, 2015; 29(6): 551-553. Cited in Quintessential Aromatics database, 2013.
18. Zheng GG et al. *Anethofuran, carvone and limonene: potential cancer chemopreventive agents from dill weed oil and caraway oil*. Planta Medica, 1992; 58(4): 338-341. Cited in Quintessential Aromatics database, 2013.
19. Essway GS et al. *The hypoglycaemic effect of volatile oil of some Egyptian plants*. Veterinary Medicine Journal, Giza, 1995; 43(2): 167-172. Cited in Quintessential Aromatics database, 2013.
20. Hajhashemi V, Abbasi N. *Hypolipidemic activity of Anethum graveolens in rats*. Phytotherapy Research, 2008; 22(3): 372-375. Cited in Quintessential Aromatics database, 2013.
21. Miller L, Miller B. *Ayurveda and aromatherapy*. Lotus Press, Twin Lakes, 1995.
22. Worwood VA. *The fragrant heavens*. Transworld Publishers, London, 1999.
23. Keim Loughran J, Bull R. *Aromatherapy and subtle energy techniques*. Frog, Berkeley, 2000.
24. Schnaubelt K. *The healing intelligence of essential oils*. Healing Arts Press, Rochester, 2011.
25. Tisserand R, Young R. *Essential oil safety*. 2nd edn. Churchill Livingstone, Edinburgh, 2014.

Elemi

Identification

Botanical name

Canarium luzonicum (Blume) A. Gray

Synonyms

Elemi gum, elemi resin, elemi oleoresin

Family

Burseraceae

Botany and origins

Elemi is a tropical tree that grows up to 30 m tall and yields a resinous exudate, which is used to produce the essential oil. Elemi is native to the Philippines and the Moluccas, where it is also cultivated.[1]

Method of extraction

The resin is extracted with a solvent to form the resinoid. Elemi oil is obtained by the steam distillation of the resin.[2]

Characteristics

Elemi oil is a colourless or pale yellow, mobile liquid with a fresh, lemon-like, peppery odour that dries out into a balsamic, slightly green-woody and sweet-spicy, pleasant note.[2]

Arctander states that elemi oil is not very stable. The oil has a high content of unstable monoterpenes that tend to form peroxides, which can present the risk of explosion when exposed to modest heating.[2]

Elemi oil also tends to resinify and polymerise readily, and the odour can accordingly become quite disagreeable.[2]

Chemical composition

The chemical composition of elemi oil was reported as follows:

α-pinene (5.4%), β-pinene (1.0%), sabinene (1.3%), limonene (26.9%), β-phellandrene (1.6%), *p*-cymene (7.7%), myrcene (1.0%), α-phellandrene (4.3%), elemol (10.65).[3]

Adulteration

Elemi oil is often adulterated with the addition of α-phellandrene and limonene.[4]

Elemi oil is frequently used as an adulterant and is often used for constructing artificial oils. Elemi oil has been found as an adulterant in lemon oil, black pepper oil, dill weed oil, angelica seed oil and numerous other oils.[1]

Pharmacopoeias and standards

At the time of writing, the purity, composition, physico-chemical properties and therapeutic uses of elemi essential oil are not defined in any pharmacopoeia monograph or standard.

History and Traditional Uses

History

Elemi resin was used by the Egyptians for embalming.[5]

Traditional medicine

Elemi has been used as a stomach stimulant and as an expectorant.[6] Local people in the Philippines have used elemi resin externally as a rubefacient and for the treatment of rheumatism. It is also used in plasters that are heated and applied to the chest to stop severe coughing.[7]

Food, perfumery and flavouring

The resinoid and oil are primarily used as fixatives and fragrance components in soaps, detergents, cosmetics and perfumes. Elemi oil is occasionally used as a flavouring ingredient in food products, alcohol and soft drinks.[1]

Guenther states that the oil was used as a suitable starting material for the isolation of α-phellandrene, which was then used for compounding other artificial essential oils. The gum was also employed for a long time in pharmaceutical plasters and ointments and to impart toughness to varnishes.[8]

Therapeutics

Pharmacology and clinical studies

At the time of writing, no pharmacological or clinical studies for elemi oil could be found.

Actions

Actions commonly cited in aromatherapy

Antiseptic, balsamic, cicatrisant, expectorant, stimulant, stomachic, tonic[9,10]

Actions supported by clinical studies

None

Comment

Lavabre says that the medicinal properties and indications of elemi oil are similar to those of frankincense and myrrh.[10]

C. luzonicum is classified in the IUCN Red List of Threatened Species as 'Vulnerable A1cd'. This means that there has been a reduction of at least 80% of the species over the last 10 years or three generations, whichever is longer, based on a decline in the area of occupancy, extent of occurrence or quality of habitat and the actual levels of exploitation.[11]

In light of its status as a vulnerable species, I would prefer not to use elemi oil in aromatherapy or perfumery.

Aromatherapy Uses

Clinical aromatherapy

Nervous system

Davis describes elemi oil as a tonic and stimulant. She states that it is helpful for anyone who is stressed, especially when the stress has led to exhaustion.[5]

Respiratory system

Catarrhal conditions respond well to elemi oil. It eases congestion of the lungs and controls excess mucus.[5,9]

Skin care

Elemi oil is recommended in skin care for aged skin, infected cuts and wounds, inflammations and wrinkles. It is drying and cooling to the skin. It may also be beneficial for the treatment of chronic skin conditions such as ulcers, fungal growths and infected wounds.[5,9]

Energetics, psyche and subtle uses

Subtle

Worwood states that elemi oil can be used in emotional healing to encourage soothing, calm, stillness, contentment, compassion and peace. Elemi wraps us in a cloak of sympathy when our spirit is most in need of comfort. Elemi is soothing yet strong; supporting our humanity; and offering strength and upliftment when we need to reconnect all parts of our being – our body, mind and spirit.[12]

Elemi also grounds us after deep meditation and balances the spiritual and worldly life.[13]

Davis describes elemi as a harmonising oil that brings mind, body and spirit into alignment with each other. She states that it is a wonderful oil to vaporise during meditation because it induces a deep calm without any drowsiness.[5]

Dosage and Administration

Blending

Aromatherapy

To alleviate catarrhal conditions, consider blending elemi oil with essential oils such as aniseed, cajeput, 1,8-cineole-rich eucalypts, frankincense, ginger and spike lavender.

To assist in meditation, consider blending elemi oil with essential oils such as frankincense, lemon, patchouli or sandalwood.

To alleviate stress associated with fatigue and exhaustion, consider blending elemi oil with essential oils such as basil, bergamot, geranium, ginger, lemon, cold-pressed lime or rosemary.

To promote emotional and spiritual healing, consider blending elemi oil with essential oils such as Peru balsam, benzoin or cistus.

Perfumery

Elemi oil is used as a freshener and top note ingredient in many perfumes to create fougère, chypre or cologne style perfumes. It can be used in a heavy-sweet floral base and is very interesting in oriental style perfumes. It blends well with cinnamon bark, frankincense, cistus, rosemary, lavender and sage oil.[2]

Mode of administration

Bath

Full body bath, foot bath

Topical

Compress, massage, ointment, skin care

Inhalation

Direct inhalation, diffuser, oil vaporiser

Safety Profile

General safety

Elemi oil is non-toxic, non-irritant and non-sensitising.[9]

Contraindications

No contraindications known.

Regulatory guidelines

Elemi oil has GRAS status.

References

1. Khan I, Abourashed E. *Leung's encyclopedia of common natural ingredients used in food, drugs and cosmetics*. 3rd edn. John Wiley & Sons, New Jersey, 2010.
2. Arctander S. *Perfume and flavor materials of natural origin*. Allured Publishing, Carol Stream, 1994.
3. Lawrence BM. *Essential oils 1981-1987*. Allured Publishing, Wheaton, 1989.
4. Burfield T. *The adulteration of essential oils – and the consequences to aromatherapy and natural perfume practice*. Presented to the International Federation of Aromatherapists Annual AGM, London, 2003.
5. Davis P. *Aromatherapy: an A-Z*. 2nd edn. C.W. Daniel Company, Saffron Walden, 1999.
6. Opdyke DLJ. *Monographs on fragrance raw materials*. Pergamon Press, Oxford, 1979.
7. Langenheim JH. *Plant resins – chemistry, evolution, ecology, ethnobotany*. Timber Press, Portland, 2003.
8. Guenther E. *The essential oils – Vol. IV*. Robert E Krieger, Malabar, 1950.
9. Lawless J. *The encyclopaedia of essential oils*. Element Books, Shaftesbury, 1992.
10. Lavabre M. *Aromatherapy workbook*. Healing Arts Press, Rochester, 1997.
11. World Conservation Monitoring Centre. *Canarium luzonicum*. The IUCN Red List of Threatened Species 1998: e.T33352A9779122. doi: 10.2305/IUCN.UK.1998.RLTS.T33352A9779122.en.
12. Worwood VA. *The fragrant heavens*. Transworld Publishers, London, 1999.
13. Keim Loughran J, Bull R. *Aromatherapy and subtle energy techniques*. Frog, Berkeley, 2000.

E

Eucalypts: 1,8-cineole-rich

This monograph examines the 1,8-cineole-rich eucalyptus oils.

Identification

Botanical name

Boland states that, of the 600 species of eucalyptus, fewer than 20 have ever been commercially exploited.[1] The species most commonly used for their high 1,8-cineole content are:

- *Eucalyptus globulus* Labill: blue gum, Tasmanian blue gum
- *Eucalyptus polybractea* R.T. Baker: blue mallee eucalyptus
- *Eucalyptus radiata* Sieber ex DC: narrow-leaved peppermint, black peppermint
- *Eucalyptus smithii* R.T. Baker: gully gum, gully ash, white top, white ironbark, Smith's gum.[1]

Family

Myrtaceae

Botany and origins

Almost all eucalyptus plants are indigenous to Australia, where they make up about 75% of all Australian tree flora.[2]

The large eucalyptus plantations in other countries have been established mainly from Australian seeds. They are now so extensive that eucalypts form a significant proportion of the forested area in countries such as Ethiopia and South Africa.[2]

Today the major eucalyptus producing countries are China, Spain, Portugal, South Africa and Chile. China is presently the world's largest producer of eucalyptus oil.[2]

The ability of some species of eucalypts to grow quickly and coppice readily has made them valuable where wood fuel is of great domestic importance. Eucalypts are known to produce the hardest, heaviest and most durable wood, known as ironbark.[2]

The genus *Eucalyptus* was named by French botanist C L L'Héritier de Brutelle, from the Greek word *eu* (well) and *kalipto* (covered), referring to the cup-like structure which is thrown off as the flower expands.[2]

The 1,8-cineole-rich eucalypts include:[1]

Species	Cineole (%)	Oil yield (%) on fresh wt basis
E. globulus	65-85%	0.7-2.4%
E. polybractea	60-93%	0.7-5.0%
E. radiata	65-75%	2.5-3.5%
E. dives (cineole variant)	60-75%	3.0-6.0%
E. smithii	70-80%	1.0-2.2%
E. vridis	70-80%	1.0-1.5%
E. eneorifolia	40-90%	approx 2.0%
E. camaldulensis	10-90%	0.3-2.8%
E. dumosa	33-70%	1.0-2.0%
E. leucoxylon	65-75%	0.8-2.5%
E. oleosa	54-52%	1.0-2.1%
E. sideroxylon	60-75%	0.5-2.5%
E. tereticornis	45%	0.9-1.0%

In this monograph, we will profile those eucalyptus species that are of commercial significance.

Eucalyptus globulus

Eucalyptus globulus is described as a majestic forest tree growing up to 70 m, with a large open crown. This species has the distinction of being the most studied of all the eucalypts. *E. globulus* hybridises moderately easily and hybrids have been reported in many countries.[2]

E. globulus is found mainly in Tasmania and southern Victoria. The species is also extensively grown in plantations in Spain, Yunnan Province of China and Chile.[1,2]

Eucalyptus polybractea

Eucalyptus polybractea is an evergreen multi-stemmed shrub, up to 8 m high. It is common to the semi-arid interior of New South Wales and Bendigo in Victoria. It flowers from March to June and sometimes again in September. The blossoms occur in clusters in leaf forks.[1,2] Australia is the only country which utilises *E. polybractea* for oil production.[2]

E. polybractea is the primary source of the cineole-rich eucalyptus oils. It is the major species under cultivation for commercial production of eucalyptus oil. It is reported to have double the oil yield and much higher cineole content than *E. globulus*. The species is ideally suited to mechanical harvesting as it coppices freely after repeated cuttings.[1,2]

Weiss states that the profitable life of an *E. polybractea* plantation could be over 100 years. Natural stands in Australia have been harvested continuously for over 70 years with no deterioration.[2]

Eucalyptus radiata

Eucalyptus radiata is considered one of the most important sources of eucalyptus oils. *E. radiata* naturally occurs in the southern NSW coastal regions. It is also cultivated in South Africa.[2]

Weiss explains that *E. radiata* oil is often incorrectly named Australiana oil or Australiana type oil.[2] It varies from a small tree with a bushy crown to a large tree of good form. There are two subspecies: *E. radiata* subsp. *radiata* and *E. radiata* subsp. *robertsonii*.[2]

Eucalyptus smithii

Eucalyptus smithii is found primarily on lower hillslopes, besides streams and at the edges of swamps, where the soil never dries completely. The species prefers good loamy soils or sandy loams with clay subsoil, and occurs in tall open forest formation with a number of other eucalypt species.[2]

E. smithii is named after HG Smith, Australia's foremost pioneer of essential oil and natural product chemistry. This tree has become more popular than *E. globulus* among planters and distillers because it is faster growing and its leaves yield more oil on steam distillation.[3]

Weiss states that the species is not cultivated in Australia, but the oil is obtained from plantations established in Swaziland, South Africa and on a smaller scale in Argentina and Uruguay. In Australia, the foliage is obtained from wild trees which are harvested annually and allowed to coppice.[2]

Method of extraction

Eucalyptus oil is steam-distilled from the fresh or partially dried leaves of the eucalypt species.

Crude *E. globulus* oil is normally rectified as it often has an unpleasant aroma due to the presence of lower aliphatic aldehydes.[2]

E

Characteristics

Eucalyptus globulus oil is a light to greenish yellow mobile liquid with an unpleasant odour, which may cause coughing and irritation when inhaled. The rectified oil has a clear, refreshing, slightly camphoraceous aroma typical of eucalyptus oil.[2]

Eucalyptus polybractea oil is yellow-brown, becoming almost colourless to pale yellow upon rectification. The rectified oil has a pronounced sweet camphoraceous aroma.[2]

Eucalyptus radiata oil is a colourless to pale yellow oil with a fresh, very powerful, peppery-camphoraceous aroma.[2]

Eucalyptus smithii oil is a colourless or very pale yellow, mobile liquid with a fresh cineole-like odour.[3]

Chemical composition

The active therapeutic and principal constituent of the eucalyptus medicinal oils is 1,8-cineole. The quality of the oil is specified by the minimum standards which are defined in the British Pharmacopoeia (BP). It requires a eucalyptus oil to contain not less than 70% 1,8-cineole and to be free of α- and β-phellandrene.[2]

Although many eucalyptus species contain 1,8-cineole in their oils, only a limited number combine a composition high in 1,8-cineole with consistently high total yields and are suitable for commercial exploitation. Rectification and blending of eucalyptus oils has, therefore, become common practice.[2]

Rectification is done by redistillation in a vacuum in which the low boiling point fractions of the oil are removed and the high boiling residues remain.[2]

Lassak & McCarthy cite work conducted by Penfold & Grant, who noticed that the high boiling residues of eucalyptus oil extracted from the rectified essential oil exhibited a greater germicidal power than the rectified oil.[4]

Many eucalyptus oils sold as BP grade are blended and redistilled.

Eucalyptus globulus

Some 100 constituents have been identified in *E. globulus* essential oil with 1,8-cineole to 60-70%. Other constituents include 15 monoterpene compounds (20-25%), 15 monoterpene alcohols (3-5%), 5 terpenoid alcohols (1-2%), 5 monoterpene esters (1-2%), 10 sesquiterpenes (3-5%), 10 sesquiterpene alcohols (1-2%) and 5 benzenoid compounds (0.5%).[2]

The main constituents according to Boland, Brophy & House are 1,8-cineole (61-69%), α-pinene (6-11%), limonene (2.0-3.0%) and *p*-cymene (0.4-10%). The oxygenated compounds include pinocarvone (0.3-1%), terpinen-4-ol (0.2-0.6%), *trans*-pinocarveol (0.5-1%) and α-terpineol (0.5-0.7%). A small amount of isovaleraldehyde (0.1-0.2%) is also present. The major sesquiterpenes detected include globulol (5.0-7.0%), viridiflorol (0.6%), spathulenol (0.3%) and α-, β- and γ-eudesmols (0.1-1.0% each). The major sesquiterpene hydrocarbons are aromadendrene (2.0%) and alloaromadendrene (0.2%).[1]

Eucalyptus polybractea

The essential oil obtained from *E. polybractea* is dominated by 1,8-cineole. The 1,8-cineole content is up to 92%. Other constituents found in the oil include monoterpene hydrocarbons α-pinene (1%), limonene (1%), *p*-cymene (2%), β-pinene (0.2%) and sabinene (0.2%). There are numerous oxygenated monoterpenes but they do not contribute much to the overall oil. They include terpinen-4-ol (0.5%), α-terpineol (0.4%) and carvone (0.2%).[2] No sesquiterpenes are detected in this oil.[2]

Eucalyptus radiata

Boland, Brophy & House say that there are possibly six chemotypes of *E. radiata*.[1]

The first is rich in monoterpenoid compounds. The major constituents are 1,8-cineole (57-71%) and α-pinene (15-21%). Other constituents include limonene (5%), *p*-cymene (0.3-1%), *trans*-pinocarveol (0.4%), α-terpineol (3%) and α-terpinyl acetate (0.1-4%). The major sesquiterpenes are globulol (0.7%), viridiflorol (0.2-0.6%), spathulenol (0.5-0.8%), nerolidol (0.3%), three eudesmols (0.1-0.2%), bicyclogermacrene (0.2%) and alloaromadendrene (0.2%). Overall Boland, Brophy & House say that 61 compounds were detected in this chemotype. Of these, 22 are sesquiterpenes accounting for less than 5% of the oil.[1]

The second chemotype has a more even distribution of monoterpenes, the major members being related to piperitone. The principal constituents are α-phellandrene (18%), 1,8-cineole (13%), *p*-cymene (14%), the menth-2-en-1-ols (8-11%), piperitone (13%), the piperitols (2-4%) and terpinen-4-ol (5%). The major sesquiterpenes are alcohol globulols (0.2%), viridiflorol (0.1%), spathulenol (0.4%) and α- and β- eudesmols (0.4-0.5%). In this chemotype, 32 compounds are present in amounts greater than 0.01%. Of these eight are sesquiterpenes accounting for less than 2% of the oil.[1]

Eucalyptus smithii

1,8-cineole (75-84%) is the major component in the essential oil of *E. smithii*. The oil also has monoterpene hydrocarbons: α-pinene (4-6%), limonene (0.2-0.6%) and *p*-cymene (0.4-2%). α-terpineol (1.5-2.5%) is the major oxygenated monoterpene.[1]

Aromadendrene (0.2-0.7%) is the only sesquiterpene hydrocarbon of any consequence, while globulol (0.6-2.4%) and α-, β- and γ-eudesmols (0.3-1.9%) are the major alcohols. 50 compounds were detected in the oil in amounts greater that 0.01%. Of these 35 are sesquiterpenes.[1]

Adulteration

Eucalyptus oils are generally not adulterated. However, it is more common for the 1,8-cineole-rich eucalyptus oils to be rectified or blended to meet BP grade.

Pharmacopoeias and standards

The purity, composition and physical-chemical properties of the 1,8-cineole-rich eucalyptus oils are defined in ISO 3065: 2011 Oil of Eucalyptus Australian Type, containing a volume fraction of 80% to 85% of 1,8-cineole.

The 1,8-cineole-rich eucalyptus oils are the subjects of many international pharmacopoeias such as:

- European Pharmacopoeia
- Committee on Herbal Medicinal Products (HMPC). *Assessment Report on Eucalyptus globulus Labill., Eucalyptus polybractea R.T. Baker and/or Eucalyptus smithii R.T. Baker, aetheroleum.*
- ESCOP 2003 Monographs
- *WHO Monographs on Selected Medicinal Plants. Volume 2.* World Health Organization, 2004.

History and Traditional Uses

History

It was Baron Ferdinand von Mueller, the first government botanist of Victoria appointed in 1853, who convinced his friend Joseph Bosisto, a Melbourne pharmacist, of the virtues of eucalyptus oils and the potential for developing an indigenous industry.[1]

In 1854, Bosisto built his first distillation plant on the banks of Dandenong Creek near Dandenong on the outskirts of Melbourne. He distilled eucalyptus oil from what was then known as *Eucalyptus amygdalina*, now known as *E. radiata*.[1]

By the 1880s the eucalyptus oil industry had firmly established itself. Bosisto received financial backing from Melbourne businessmen Alfred Felton and Frederick Grimwade, and together they formed the Eucalyptus Mallee Company. Today this company still produces eucalyptus oil which is marketed under the name Bosisto's Brand Eucalyptus Oil.[1]

Eucalyptus oil was in huge demand during World War I, as it was used to help control a meningitis outbreak and for the influenza of 1919. However, by 1930 overseas eucalyptus plantations impacted dramatically on Australian produced oil.[1]

The eucalyptus oil industry in Australia reached its peak in 1947, when total production reached almost 1,000 tonnes, of which 70% was exported. Since then the industry has declined. In 1989, the world eucalyptus oil market was about 2,000 to 3,000 tonnes per annum, of which about 5 to 10% was produced in Australia.[1]

Traditional medicine

In Australia, Aboriginal people often made eucalyptus leaves into a type of steam bath.[5]

Throughout the world, eucalyptus oil has been popularly used for treating respiratory disorders as well as colds and influenza.[5]

In folk medicine, vaporised eucalyptus oil was a common inhalation therapy for serious childhood disorders such as croup and diphtheria. The inhalation of eucalyptus oils helped to reduce the swelling of mucous membranes and loosen mucus. The resultant easing of respiratory tract congestion explained why eucalyptus oil became popular in cough and cold medicines.[5]

Grieve states that it was von Mueller who introduced eucalyptus to Europe. He was the first to suggest that the scent of the leaves resembled that of cajeput oil and that it may be useful as a disinfectant. Seeds were sent to France in 1857 and then planted in Algiers. The seeds were planted in a marshy district of Algiers that was infested with malaria. Within five years the eucalyptus trees proved to be successful. The roots of the eucalyptus trees had a powerful drying action on the soil, eliminating the risk of malaria. As a result, eucalyptus trees were cultivated in many temperate areas around Europe that had a high risk of malaria.[6]

In traditional herbal medicine, eucalyptus oil is often used internally for treating asthma, fever, flu, whooping cough, loss of appetite, dyspeptic complaints, inflammatory and infectious diseases of the kidney and bladder, diabetes and rheumatic complaints. It is often used externally for wounds, acne, poor healing ulcers, stomatitis, bleeding gums, rheumatism, neuralgia and gonorrhoea.[7]

Herbal

The German Commission E recommends eucalyptus oil internally and externally for catarrh of the respiratory system, and externally for rheumatic complaints.[8]

The WHO monograph recommends eucalyptus oil for the symptomatic treatment of catarrh and coughs, and topically as a rubefacient for the treatment of rheumatic complaints.[9]

The ESCOP monograph lists the following therapeutic indications for eucalyptus oil: internally as an adjuvant treatment of chronic obstructive respiratory complaints including bronchitis and bronchial asthma, for the symptomatic relief of colds and catarrh of the upper respiratory tract, and externally for the symptomatic treatment of colds and rheumatic complaints.[10]

Food, perfumery and flavouring

The 1,8-cineole-rich eucalyptus oils are commonly used in medicine for inhalations, soaps, gargles and lozenges.[4]

Other uses

The 1,8-cineole-rich eucalyptus oils are often used in industrial detergents, disinfectants, soaps, throat gargles and lozenges. They are also effective in insecticides and are used to a minor extent in paints and varnishes.[2]

E

Therapeutics

Pharmacology and clinical studies

Many pharmacological studies involving eucalyptus essential oils have been published. A systemic review of these studies will not be attempted. Rather, I have chosen a selection of studies that support the traditional and clinical uses.

Analgesic activity

A randomised, double-blind, placebo-controlled, crossover study examined the efficacy of a blend of eucalyptus oil and peppermint oil for the relief of headaches in 32 patients. Five different preparations were used:

- 10 g peppermint oil and 5 g eucalyptus oil
- 10 g peppermint oil and traces of eucalyptus oil
- traces of peppermint oil and 5 g of eucalyptus oil
- traces of both peppermint and eucalyptus oil
- a placebo.

The preparations and the placebo were applied topically to the forehead and temples, and the neurophysiological and psychological parameters were measured. All the participants experienced improved cognitive performance and muscle relaxation with the peppermint and eucalyptus oil preparations used, but they had no effect on the sensitivity to the headache.[18]

The analgesic properties of eucalyptus oil have been attributed to the monoterpene components. It has been suggested that because the monoterpenoid profile differs among eucalyptus species, this accounts for variations in therapeutic effect.[19]

Antifungal activity

Many studies have confirmed the antifungal activity of eucalyptus oils. At a concentration of 0.05% (V/V), eucalyptus oil could completely inhibit the activity of two different strains of *Candida albicans*. The antifungal activity of eucalyptus oil was also observed against five *Fusarium* fungal species.[8]

Anti-inflammatory activity

Eucalyptus oil was found to inhibit prostaglandin synthesis in vitro at a concentration of 37 μmol/L. The anti-inflammatory activity of *E. radiata* has been demonstrated in patients with dry weeping dermatitis. It was suggested that it was probably due to inhibition of inflammatory markers such as TNF-α, COX enzymes, 5-lipoxygenase and other leukotrienes.[19]

In another study, it was demonstrated that 1,8-cineole supported lung function four times better than controls in a double-blind clinical trial of 32 patients with severe steroid-dependent bronchial asthma. Patients were randomly assigned 200 mg 1,8-cineole three times a day for three weeks or a placebo. 12 of the 16 patients receiving 1,8-cineole remained stable despite reduced steroid doses.[19]

Antimicrobial activity

Eucalyptus oil and 1,8-cineole have been reputed to have antiseptic and expectorant properties and strong antibacterial activity against several strains of *Streptococcus*.[11,12,13]

An in vitro study examining the antimicrobial activity of *E. globulus* oil confirmed that the oil had good antimicrobial activity against gram-negative *Escherichia coli* and gram-positive bacteria *Staphylococcus aureus*. The rate of inhibition was greater on gram-positive bacterium.[14]

The essential oils of eight eucalyptus species growing in Tunisia were evaluated for their antimicrobial activities by disc diffusion and microbroth dilution methods against seven bacterium isolates – *Haemophilus influenzae, Klebsiella pneumoniae, Pseudomonas aeruginosa, Staphylococcus aureus, Streptococcus agalactiae, Streptococcus pneumoniae* and *Streptococcus pyogenes*. *Eucalyptus odorata* showed the strongest antimicrobial activity against all the microorganisms tested. The chemistry of *E. odorata* was characterised by the highest mean percentage of cryptone (20.9±1.3%), cuminal (6.6±0.6%), phellandral (6.6±0.4%), verbenone (0.9±0.2%), *p*-cymen-8-ol (2.9±0.6%), spathulenol (3.2±0.9%), carvacrol (1.7±0.3%), *p*-cymene (16.7±5.2%), terpinen-4-ol (3.0±0.8%), caryophyllene oxide (1.7±0.2%), viridiflorol (4.5±1.6%) and by the lowest level of 1,8-cineole (4.5±1.6%).[15]

This study supports a statement made by Williams that 1,8-cineole-rich eucalyptus oils have very poor antimicrobial activity. Williams cites two clinical trials, one which reported eucalyptus as having a high antimicrobial activity and one which indicated that eucalyptus oil has little to no antimicrobial activity. Williams conducted his own research, which revealed little to no antimicrobial activity against *Candida albicans, Staphylococcus aureus* and *E. coli*. He also tested 1,8-cineole and it also failed to show any zone of inhibition against a range of microorganisms.[16]

Williams concluded that the selection of eucalyptus oils for use in household disinfectants is because of price rather than efficacy of their disinfectant properties.[16] Lassak & McCarthy claim that the only reason that eucalyptus gained a reputation as an antiseptic is because of the clean, crisp smell. They suggest that the clearing effect of 1,8-cineole vapour on the nasal passage results in easier and deeper breathing. Good deep breathing and fresh air have always been associated with good health.[4]

Another clinical trial also suggests that 1,8-cineole is not responsible for the antimicrobial activity of eucalyptus oil. The activity is due to the presence of minor constituents such as the alcohols-borneol, *trans*-pinocarveol, nerol and citronellol. It was suggested that the presence of these alcohols increased antimicrobial activity provided that no unfavorable components were present such as myrtenol, geraniol and cedrol.[17]

The EMA assessment report for eucalyptus oil states that several studies concerning the antimicrobial activity of eucalyptus show that the oil has broad activity against several microbial strains, while other studies reveal no or only slight activity.[7]

Antitussive activity

A study compared the antitussive activity of eucalyptus oil with that of codeine in an in vivo study using guinea pigs. Inhalation of eucalyptus oil was found to have a significant antitussive effect relative to codeine.[19]

The antitussive activity of 1,8-cineole has also been demonstrated in humans in a single-blind crossover study. It is believed that 1,8-cineole interacts with the M-8 (TRPM8) receptor potential channel, the cooling-sensitive thermoreceptor primarily affected by menthol, which produces a cooling sensation.[19]

Another possible antitussive mechanism may be due to the effect on pulmonary C-fibres, which contain TRPM8 receptors.[19]

Antiviral activity

In vitro study has found that eucalyptus oil has potent antiviral activity against *Herpes simplex* virus type I. The antiviral activity of *E. globulus* essential oil was investigated on strains of adenovirus and mumps virus isolated from patients. In a concentration of 0.25μl/ml (0.025%), the essential oil displayed mild antiviral activity against mumps virus, but not against adenovirus.[7]

Decongestant activity

Several studies have examined the effects of eucalyptus oil as a nasal decongestant. One study found that inhalation of eucalyptus oil over a period of five minutes had no effect on nasal resistance to airflow; however, the oil did have a stimulating effect on nasal cold receptors, which gave the majority of participants in the trial the sensation of an increased airflow.[9]

A single-blind study examined the efficacy of vaporised eucalyptus oil in reducing nasal congestion in 234 patients with acute respiratory tract infections. It was reported that the essential oil was significantly more effective in reducing nasal congestion only during the first hour following treatment. In other clinical studies of patients with acute common colds, no significant differences in nasal decongestant activity were reported between the essential oil (1.3%) in petrolatum and a petrolatum placebo.[9]

Miticidal activity

When compared with detergent concentrate alone, a 30-minute pre-wash soak with eucalyptus oil/detergent formula reduced the number of live mites that could be recovered by 97%. This eliminated the need for washing in hot water and maintained low allergen levels in bedding for a longer period than those laundered alone because mites were adversely affected by the low concentration of eucalyptus oil vapour.[19]

Actions

Actions commonly cited in aromatherapy

Analgesic, antibacterial, anti-inflammatory, antineuralgic, antirheumatic, antiseptic, antispasmodic, antiviral, astringent, balsamic, cicatrisant, decongestant, deodorant, diuretic, expectorant, febrifuge, hypoglycaemic, rubefacient, vermifuge, vulnerary[20,21,22]

Actions supported by clinical studies

Analgesic, antifungal, antimicrobial, antitussive, decongestant, expectorant

Comment

There is no doubt that eucalyptus oil is a very effective and important oil for the symptomatic treatment of obstructive respiratory conditions such as bronchitis, asthma, the common cold and other conditions associated with catarrh of the upper respiratory tract.

Although it is often recommended internally and externally in Europe for these conditions, in Australia the oil is generally used externally in vaporisers, chest rubs and nasal inhalants.[19]

Many studies suggest that the crude or unrectified eucalyptus oil which is rich in minor monoterpene alcohols is pharmacologically more active.

The clean, refreshing scent of eucalyptus oil also energises and awakens our mind and psyche.

Aromatherapy Uses

Clinical Aromatherapy

Antiviral

Davis recommends using *E. radiata* to alleviate the acute pain of shingles. She recommends blending it with bergamot for the treatment of cold sores and genital herpes.[24]

E

Musculoskeletal system

Eucalyptus oil has been used to relieve insect bites and muscular aches and pains. It is indicated for rheumatic pain of a cold nature, and may be used to relieve muscular aches and pains and neuralgia.[20,22,23,24]

Nervous system

Eucalyptus oil is recommended for the treatment of headaches, neuralgia and debility.[20,23]

Psychological

The aroma of eucalyptus oil helps to dispel melancholy, revives the spirits and restores vitality and a positive outlook. Eucalyptus oil helps to disperse the negative feelings associated with such situations, and gives us, inwardly, 'room to breathe'.[22]

Mojay explains that eucalyptus oil is suited for people who feel emotionally 'hemmed in' or restricted by their surroundings – whether at home, at work or in society. They sense the possibility of achieving greater freedom and a wider life experience, but dare not seek to create this due to excessive caution, habit, fear or responsibility.[22]

Holmes states that eucalyptus oil can help us whenever we are faced with situations marked by confusion, ambiguity or negativity. The scent of eucalyptus revitalises our psyche to make us more confident to tackle any obstacle or challenge we are faced with.[23]

Respiratory system

Eucalyptus is best known as a decongestant inhalation for colds and catarrh.[24] Schnaubelt recommends using *E. radiata* oil as an inhalation and for topical use for rhinitis, flu, otitis, sinusitis and bronchitis.[25] Valnet states that spraying of a 2% emulsion containing eucalyptus oil kills off 70% of local airborne staphylococci.[26]

Balacs suggests that, during a respiratory tract infection such as a common cold, the nasal and lower respiratory passage become constricted which in turn makes breathing difficult. Research indicates that aromatic inhalations containing eucalyptus oil can significantly improve respiratory function. It has been suggested that the mechanisms of action of such respiratory congestion may be reflex, and related to nerve stimulation by the essential oils.[27]

Balacs explains that the reputation of eucalyptus oil as a decongestant relies on its ability to stimulate cold receptors in the nose. During an infection with a common cold virus, the nasal and lower respiratory passages restrict the passage of air into the lungs because of vasoconstriction. Along with menthol and camphor, eucalyptus oil and cineole have the effect of reducing surface tension between water and air in the lungs, a property which would presumably enhance the effects of the lungs' own surfactant.[27]

Skin care

Eucalyptus oil is effective as an insect repellent and is used to treat burns, blisters, cuts and wounds.[20,24]

Energetics, psyche and subtle uses

Energetics

According to TCM, eucalyptus is an exceptional remedy for clearing *Lung-phlegm* and *wind-heat*. This makes it beneficial for the onset of flu or fever, sore throat, the common cold, sinusitis and chronic bronchitis.[22,23]

Mojay classifies it as a tonic of the *Lung Qi* and recommends using it to enhance the breathing function, promoting the uptake of oxygen by the red blood cells.[22]

Holmes states that eucalyptus strengthens *Yang*, tonifies the *Lung* and *Heart Qi* and strengthens the *Shen*. Whenever we have *Yang deficiency* with *Shen weakness*, we may feel mental fogginess and fatigue, poor focus, confusion and forgetfulness.[24]

According to the principles of the Five Elements in TCM, eucalyptus oil has a strong affinity with the Metal Element. The *Lungs* are the *Yin* organ associated with the Metal Element. Eucalyptus oil not only supports the physical function of the *Lungs*, it also supports the psychological and spiritual aspects of the Metal Element, referred to as the *Po*, also known as the animal soul.

When the Metal Element is out of balance, our *Po* spirit is affected and we may experience a vague feeling that 'something isn't right', but have no clear sense why. We may experience physical pain that takes over our entire life and seems to have no identifiable cause, or we hold on to unexpressed emotional issues.

Eucalyptus helps improve our breathing and assists our ability to let go. It nurtures the *Po*, providing us with spiritual protection whenever we feel fragile and vulnerable.

Personality

Worwood describes the eucalyptus personality as a well-balanced, calm and rational person. She states that they can often appear to be very cool, logical and laid back. They are also good, solid characters who may appear to be shy. She describes them as being secretive because they don't think anyone would be interested in their private matters.[28]

They tend to be drawn to the sciences and are often found in the medical professions, but they are also likely to be accountants, bankers and solicitors. They prefer to be in professions that do not require much creative thought but have strict guidelines that they must adhere to.[28]

According to Myers-Briggs personality types, the eucalyptus personality is likely to be an ISTJ. ISTJs are very stable, responsible and dependable. They are very private; they like to be punctual and precise; and they are very orderly. They have good concentration and are difficult to distract. They find it hard to relax as they think that things that help relax are non-productive. They prefer simplicity to status. They enjoy being in nature. They are good at remembering facts and figures, can be overly detail-oriented and are devoted, hard workers. They are very thorough and accurate in everything they do. They prefer to work with machines, facts and numbers rather than with people. They like to have strict rules and procedures. They have a tendency to be inflexible. They are often resistant to change. They can make quick critical judgement of others.

Subtle

Eucalyptus may be used at a subtle level to cleanse any place where there has been conflict or where negative energies are felt.[28] Eucalyptus oil is also described as a fragrance of renewal and is recommended for those seeking new horizons.[29]

Keim Loughran and Bull explain that eucalyptus oil helps us become aware of the emotions associated with burnout and stress. They state that eucalyptus oil helps to remove the emotional energy blockages and allows us to take a deep breath and get a new perspective on the situation.[30]

Zeck recommends using eucalyptus whenever we feel overwhelmed with our life. It allows us to discover ways to respond to situations rather than overreacting when our ability to respond is diminished.[31]

Dosage and Administration

Blending

Aromatherapy

The 1,8-cineole-rich eucalyptus oils blend very well with all other leaf, spicy and citrus oils.

For the relief of muscular aches and pains and rheumatic conditions, consider blending eucalyptus oil with essential oils such as black pepper, cajeput, clove bud, fragonia, kunzea, ginger, spike lavender, rosemary or thyme.

For the relief of colds and influenza, consider blending eucalyptus oil with essential oils such as bay laurel, cajeput, *Eucalyptus dives*, *Eucalyptus citriodora*, fragonia, ginger, lemon, manuka, peppermint, pine, ravintsara, rosemary, oregano, tea tree or thyme.

For the relief of bronchial congestion, consider blending eucalyptus oil with essential oils such as aniseed, *Eucalyptus dives*, Atlas cedarwood, oregano, pine, rosemary ct. camphor or thyme.

As an insect repellent against mosquitos, consider blending eucalyptus oil with essential oils such as cajeput, *Eucalyptus citriodora*, citronella, Virginian cedarwood, lemongrass, niaouli or peppermint.

To promote mental clarity and alertness, consider blending eucalyptus oil with essential oils such as basil, lemon, lemon myrtle, lime, peppermint or rosemary.

Perfumery

The 1,8-cineole-rich eucalyptus oils are not commonly used in perfumery. They tend to be used for scenting household cleaning products and in low-cost industrial perfumes for masking certain odours.

Arctander states that it is comparatively stable in soaps and has a powerful radiation or 'lifting' effect upon other ingredients in soap perfumes.[3]

Mode of administration

Bath

Full body bath, foot bath

Topical

Compress, massage, ointment, skin care

Inhalation

Direct inhalation, steam inhalation, diffuser, oil vaporiser

Safety Profile

General safety

Eucalyptus oil has been reported to be non-toxic, non-irritant and non-sensitising.[20,22,23]

Contraindications

The WHO monograph for eucalyptus oil states that preparations of eucalyptus oil should not be administered internally to children or patients with inflammation of the gastrointestinal tract, gall bladder disease or impaired liver function. It should also not be taken internally during pregnancy.[9]

Eucalyptus oil preparations should not be applied to the face, especially the nose of infants or young children.[9]

E

Toxicity

There is some confusion and controversy regarding its safety.

The leaves of some eucalyptus are a source of food for the koalas. A koala is known to eat 10 g of 1,8-cineole a day with no adverse effects. It appears that the oil is conjugated with glucuronic acid present in the koala's blood and is excreted in a water-soluble form in urine.[4]

Unfortunately, humans are not able to metabolise 1,8-cineole in the same way as koalas. Lassak & McCarthy cite an incident where, for about the past five years, a man had been in the habit of swallowing five to 10 drops of eucalyptus oil to keep colds at bay and to make him feel good. He began to feel discomfort and pain in the region of the liver. After entering hospital for a check-up, he was informed that he suffered from cirrhosis of the liver, and that, unless he stopped drinking immediately, his condition would continue to deteriorate. This man had never drunk alcohol, and the apparent cause of his condition was the ingested eucalyptus that he had assumed would improve his health.[4]

Eucalyptus oil is scheduled as a poison in Australia. While it is freely available, it must be sold with a child-resistant closure. Balacs suggests that the evidence that eucalyptus oil is dangerous is very thin indeed:

> *There have been cases of oral poisoning, but these are most notable for the fact that remarkably large doses have been survived, usually with no permanent ill-effect. It should be noted that this author* [Balacs] *is very concerned to highlight potential toxicity wherever it exists: it does seem however, that eucalyptus and cineole are two of the least toxic materials one comes across in essential oils.*[27]

Balacs cites recorded fatalities resulting from the ingestion of eucalyptus. Some of the reports date back to 1893, and the amount of eucalyptus oil ingested ranged between 15 mL to 90 mL. As the records are old, it was not clearly recorded whether it was pure eucalyptus oil that was ingested or a blend of eucalyptus and other substances.[27]

An Australian study over an 11-year period from 1981 to 1992 recorded that 109 children were admitted to a Melbourne hospital for eucalyptus poisoning. According to the report, 31 had some degree of CNS depression, 3 were unconscious having ingested between 5 and 10 mL and 1 child who ingested about 75 mL was unconscious. Vomiting occurred in 37%, ataxia in 15% and pulmonary dysfunction in 11%.[27]

The treatment for 21% of the cases was ipecac, 57% received a nasogastric activated charcoal and 12% required no treatment. It also needs to be noted that not one child died from eucalyptus poisoning. Balacs cites a report from Queensland where 33 out of 41 children admitted to hospital with suspected eucalyptus poisoning were entirely without symptoms, despite the fact that in some cases they had consumed as much as 30 mL of oil.[27]

On the other hand, some clinical trials have suggested that 1,8-cineole has a similar neurotoxic profile to that of camphor in tests.[12,27] The clinical trial studied the effects of 1,8-cineole on cortical sodium and potassium. It was found that 1,8-cineole altered brain sodium and potassium in a similar way to camphor and was consistent with increased susceptibility to convulsions.[27]

Regulatory guidelines

Eucalyptus oil and 1,8-cineole have GRAS status.

References

1. Boland DJ, Brophy JJ, House APN. *Eucalyptus leaf oils: use, chemistry, distillation and marketing*. Inkata Press, Melbourne, 1991.
2. Weiss EA. *Essential oil crops*. CAB International, Wallingford, 1997.
3. Arctander S. *Perfume and flavor materials of natural origin.* Allured Publishing, Carol

Stream, 1994.
4. Lassak EV, McCarthy T. *Australian medicinal plants*. Methuen Australia, North Ryde, 1983.
5. Williams C. *Medicinal plants in Australia. Vol. 2: Gums, resins, tannin and essential oils*. Rosenburg Publishing, Kenthurst, 2011.
6. Grieve M. *A modern herbal – Vol. I*. Dover Publications, New York, 1971.
7. Committee on Herbal Medicinal Products (HMPC). *Assessment report on Eucalyptus globulus Labill., Eucalyptus polybractea R.T. Baker and/or Eucalyptus smithii R.T. Baker, aetheroleum*. European Medicines Agency, London, 2013. doi: EMA/HMPC/307782/2012.
8. Blumenthal M et al. *The complete German commission E monographs: therapeutic guide to herbal medicine*. The American Botanical Council, Austin, 1998.
9. *WHO monographs on selected medicinal plants – Vol 2., Aetheroleum Eucalypti*. World Health Organization. Geneva, 2004.
10. European Scientific Cooperative on Phytotherapy (ESCOP). *Eucalyptus oil – Eucalyptus aetheroleum*. In *ESCOP monographs*. 2nd edn, European Scientific Cooperative on Phytotherapy/Thieme, Stuttgart, 2003.
11. Khan I, Abourashed E. *Leung's encyclopedia of common natural ingredients used in food, drugs and cosmetics*. 3rd edn, John Wiley & Sons, New Jersey, 2010.
12. Bruneton J. *Pharmacognosy*. 2nd edn, Lavoisier Publishing, Paris, 1999.
13. Benouda A et al. *The antiseptic properties of essential oils in vitro, tested against pathogenic germs found in hospitals*. Fitoterapia, 1988; 59(2): 115-119. Cited in the Aromatherapy Database, by Bob Harris, Essential Oil Resource Consultants, UK, 2000.
14. Bachir RG, Benali M. *Antibacterial activity of the essential oils from the leaves of Eucalyptus globulus against Escherichia coli and Staphylococcus aureus*. Asian Pacific Journal of Tropical Biomedicine, 2012; 2(9): 739-742. doi: 10.1016/S2221-1691(12)60220-2.
15. Elaissi A et al. *Chemical composition of 8 eucalyptus species essential oils and the evaluation of their antibacterial, antifungal and antiviral activities*. BMC Complementary and Alternative Medicine, 2012; 12: 81. doi: 10.1186/1472-6882-12-81.
16. Williams L. *Australian eucalyptus oils*. Simply Essential, 1994; 12: 21-25.
17. Zakarya D et al. *Chemical composition – antimicrobial activity relationships of Eucalyptus essential oils*. Plantes Medicinales et Phytotherapie, 1993; 26(4): 319-331. Cited in the Aromatherapy Database, by Bob Harris, Essential Oil Resource Consultants, UK, 2000.
18. Göbel H et al. *Effect of peppermint and eucalyptus oil preparations on neurophysiological and experimental algesimetric headache parameters*. Cephalagia, 1994; 14(3): 228-234. doi:10.1046/j.1468-2982.1994.014003228.
19. Braun L, Cohen M. *Herbs & natural supplements: an evidence-based guide*. 4th edn, Elsevier, Chatswood, 2015.
20. Lawless J. *The encyclopaedia of essential oils*. Element Books, Shaftesbury, 1992.
21. Lavabre M. *Aromatherapy workbook*. Healing Arts Press, Rochester, 1997.
22. Mojay G. *Aromatherapy for healing the spirit*. Healing Arts Press, Rochester, 1997.
23. Holmes P. *Aromatica – a clinical guide to essential oil therapeutics – Vol. 1: Principles and profiles*. Singing Dragon, London, 2016.
24. Davis P. *Aromatherapy: an A-Z*. 2nd edn, C.W. Daniel Company, Saffron Walden, 1999.
25. Schnaubelt K. *Medical aromatherapy*. Frog Ltd, Berkeley, 1999.
26. Valnet J. *The practice of aromatherapy*. C.W. Daniel Company, Saffron Walden, 1980.
27. Balacs T. *Cineole-rich eucalyptus*. The International Journal of Aromatherapy, 1997; 8(2): 15-21.
28. Worwood VA. *The fragrant spirit*. Transworld Publishers, London, 1999.
29. Davis P. *Subtle aromatherapy*. C.W. Daniel Company, Saffron Walden, 1991.
30. Keim Loughran J, Bull R. *Aromatherapy anointing oils*. Frog, Berkeley, 2001.
31. Zeck R. *The blossoming heart – aromatherapy for healing and transformation*. Aroma Tours, East Ivanhoe, 2004.

Eucalyptus, broadleaf peppermint

Identification

Botanical name

Eucalyptus dives Schauer

Synonyms

Broadleaf peppermint, blue peppermint, peppermint gum, peppermint eucalyptus

Family

Myrtaceae

Botany and origins

E. dives occurs in a wide range of habitats from

foothills of the main ranges in southern NSW.[1]

It is usually a small to medium tree which grows up to 12-15 m.[1] The foliage is harvested annually from wild trees in Australia which are felled and allowed to coppice.[2]

There are three types of broadleaf peppermint eucalyptus:

- 1,8-cineole chemotype (*E. dives* var. C)
- piperitone chemotype (*E. dives* var. Type)
- phellandrene chemotype (*E. dives* var. 'A') which yields an oil with approximately 60% α-phellandrene and 2 to 8% piperitone.[1]

Method of extraction

Peppermint eucalyptus oil is steam-distilled from the freshly cut leaves and twiglets.

Characteristics

The *E. dives* type 'A' essential oil is a colourless to pale yellow mobile oil with a fresh spicy-minty and slightly camphoraceous odour.[3]

Chemical composition

The chemical composition of the piperitone chemotype *Eucalyptus dives* essential oil was reported as follows:

α-pinene (1.1%), α-phellandrene (19.52%), 1,8-cineole (0.45%), *p*-cymene (3.36%), terpinolene (2.02%), terpinen-4-ol (4.0%), piperitone (52.27%), *trans*-piperitol (0.27%), globulol/viridiflorol (6.03%).[1]

Adulteration

It is highly unlikely that *E. dives* essential oil is subject to adulteration.

Pharmacopoeias and standards

At the time of writing, the purity, composition, physico-chemical properties and therapeutic uses of peppermint eucalyptus essential oil are not defined in any pharmacopoeia monograph or standard.

History and Traditional Uses

History

The leaves of the piperitone chemotype have been used as a flavouring in Australia since colonial times, especially in combination with brewed black billy tea.[4]

Traditional medicine

The Aborigines smoked people with burning leaves for the relief of fever.[5]

Food, perfumery and flavouring

Piperitone-rich oils are used as a source of *l*-piperitone, which is chemically transformed to menthol. Menthol has a fresh, clean odour of peppermint and is used in gargles, toothpaste, liniments and food flavouring.[5]

Therapeutics

Pharmacology and clinical studies

Antibacterial activity

Peppermint eucalyptus oil had moderate antibacterial activity against *Staphylococcus aureus*.[6]

Antifungal activity

Peppermint eucalyptus oil has been found to have antifungal activity against *Candida albicans*.[7]

Actions

Actions commonly cited in aromatherapy

Analgesic, anti-neuralgic, antiseptic, decongestant, expectorant, insecticide, mucolytic, rubefacient [8,9,10]

Actions supported by clinical studies

Antiseptic, decongestant, mucolytic

Comment

Clinical studies have confirmed that peppermint eucalyptus oil has antimicrobial activity; however, very few studies have been conducted to confirm any of the other pharmacological actions often attributed to the essential oil.

Ketones are reported to be effective at reducing mucosal secretions caused by respiratory tract infections.[11] Piperitone is a relatively harmless ketone, which makes it highly effective as a mucolytic agent for bronchitis.[9]

Aromatherapy Uses

Clinical aromatherapy

Musculoskeletal system

Peppermint eucalyptus oil is recommended for the treatment of arthritis, muscular aches and pains, rheumatism, sports injuries and sprains.[10]

Nervous system

Peppermint eucalyptus oil is recommended for the treatment of headaches, neuralgia and debility.[10]

Respiratory system

E. dives ct. piperitone oil has excellent mucolytic properties. When it is blended with a 1,8-cineole-rich eucalyptus oil, it becomes a very effective expectorant. This is a great blend for providing relief to congestion associated with upper respiratory tract infections.[10]

E

Skin care

Schnaubelt recommends using *E. dives* ct. piperitone oil in skin care to calm hyperactive sebaceous glands.[9]

Dosage and Administration

Blending

Aromatherapy

For the relief of the symptoms of colds and flu associated with bronchial congestion, consider blending peppermint eucalyptus oil with essential oils such as cajeput, 1,8-cineole-rich eucalypts, lemon-scented eucalyptus, fragonia, ginger, lemon, lemon myrtle, niaouli, pine, rosalina or tea tree.

Perfumery

Peppermint eucalyptus essential oil is not commonly used in perfumery.

Mode of administration

Bath

Full body bath, foot bath

Topical

Compress, massage, ointment, skin care

Inhalation

Direct inhalation, diffuser, oil vaporiser

Safety Profile

General safety

It is non-toxic, non-irritant and non-sensitising.[9,10,12]

Contraindications

No contraindications known.

Regulatory guidelines

Eucalyptus dives essential oil is not defined in any regulatory guideline.

References

1. Boland DJ, Brophy JJ, House APN. *Eucalyptus leaf oils: use, chemistry, distillation and marketing*. Inkata Press, Canberra, 1991.
2. Weiss EA. *Essential oil crops*. CAB International, Wallingford, 1997.
3. Arctander S. *Perfume and flavor materials of natural origin*. Allured Publishing, Carol Stream, 1994.
4. Cribb AB, Cribb JW. *Useful wild plants in Australia*. Collins, Sydney, 1981.
5. Lassak EV, McCarthy T. *Australian medicinal plants*. Methuen Australia, North Ryde, 1983.
6. Dias C et al. *Antibacterial activity evaluation of 15 Eucalyptus species essential oils against clinically relevant pathogenic bacteria*. American Journal of Microbiology, 2014; 5(2): 41-48. doi: 10.3844/ajmsp.2014.41.48.
7. Beylier MF, Givaudan SA. *Bacteriostatic activity of some Australian oils*. Perfumer & Flavorist. 1979; 4(1): 23-25. Cited in Quintessential Aromatics database, 2013.
8. Webb M. *Bush sense*. Self-published, Australia, 2000.
9. Schnaubelt K. *Advanced aromatherapy*. Healing Arts Press, Rochester, 1995.
10. Lawless J. *The encyclopaedia of essential oils*. Element Books, Shaftesbury, 1992.
11. Bowles J. *The chemistry of aromatherapeutic oils*. 3rd edn. Allen & Unwin, Crows Nest, 2003.
12. Tisserand R, Young R. *Essential oil safety*. 2nd edn. Churchill Livingstone, Edinburgh, 2014.

E

Eucalyptus, ironbark

Identification

Botanical name

Eucalyptus staigeriana F.v. Muell. ex F.M. Bailey

Synonyms

Lemon-scented ironbark, Australian lemon balm

Family

Myrtaceae

Botany and origins

E. staigeriana is a medium-sized ironbark with a narrow and diffuse crown, except in open-grown specimens where the crown may be as wide as its height. It grows well in the hot sub-humid regions of north Queensland.[1]

Arctander states that this is one of the few eucalyptus oils produced exclusively outside Australia, although it is originally from Australia. He states that it is cultivated in Brazil, South Africa, the Seychelles and Guatamala.[2]

Method of extraction

Ironbark eucalyptus oil is steam-distilled from the leaves and terminal branchlets.

Characteristics

The oil of *E. staigeriana* is a pale yellow to dark yellow, somewhat oily liquid with a sweet and fresh, fruity-lemony aroma.[2]

Chemical composition

The chemical composition of *E. staigeriana* essential oil was reported as follows:

geraniol (9-18%), methyl geranate (11-18%), geranyl acetate (4-14%), limonene (1-14%), β-phellandrene (12-34%) and neral (8-12%).[3]

Over 30 of the compounds identified in amounts greater than 0.01% are monoterpenes.[3]

Adulteration

Arctander states that it is highly unlikely that ironbark eucalyptus oil is adulterated.[2]

Pharmacopoeias and standards

At the time of writing the purity, composition, physico-chemical properties and therapeutic uses of ironbark eucalyptus oil are not defined in any pharmacopoeia monograph or standard.

History and Traditional Uses

Food, perfumery and flavouring

Ironbark eucalyptus oil is used in perfumery, toiletry preparations and some flavouring.[1,2]

Other uses

Ironbark eucalyptus oil is used for scenting household cleaning products.[2]

Therapeutics

Pharmacology and clinical studies

Antimicrobial activity

An in vitro study confirmed that ironbark eucalyptus oil has strong antimicrobial activity.[4]

Antioxidant activity

An in vitro study confirmed that ironbark eucalyptus oil had very high antioxidant activity. It has been suggested that the antioxidant effect of essential oils is of special interest in diseases with an inflammatory response.[5]

Actions

Actions commonly cited in aromatherapy

Anti-inflammatory, antimicrobial, antiseptic, digestive stimulant, uplifting[6]

Actions supported by clinical studies

Antimicrobial

Comment

I am surprised that ironbark is not popular in aromatherapy as it has such a delightful lemon aroma. It has a very balanced and diverse range of chemical constituents. The aldehyde content is naturally quenched by limonene. It has a range of monoterpene hydrocarbons, monoterpene alcohols and esters that would give the oil excellent antiseptic properties, with the lower risk of dermal irritancy compared with other aldehyde rich essential oils.

Aromatherapy Uses

Clinical aromatherapy

It has a very uplifting and relaxing quality. Rhind states that the oil has anti-inflammatory, pain-relieving, and antifungal action.[7]

Dosage and Administration

Blending

Aromatherapy

Ironbark eucalyptus oil has a pleasant, light, sweet, refreshing citrus note that allows it to blend very easily with other citrus oils such as sweet orange, grapefruit, lemon, lime or mandarin.

To alleviate anxiety, stress and nervous tension, consider blending ironbark eucalyptus oil with essential oils such as Atlas cedarwood, Virginian cedarwood, fragonia, geranium, lavender, neroli, sweet orange, petitgrain or sandalwood.

For the prevention of colds and flu, consider blending ironbark eucalyptus oil with essential oils such cajeput, bay laurel, 1,8-cineole-rich eucalypts, lemon myrtle, fragonia, kunzea, lemon, manuka, kanuka or tea tree.

Perfumery

Arctander states that it has a very pleasant fresh, fruity and lemony aroma, which makes it interesting in soap perfumes and detergent fragrances.[2]

Mode of administration

Bath

Because of the high aldehyde content, I would not recommend ironbark eucalyptus oil for use in a bath.

Topical

Massage, ointment

Inhalation

Direct inhalation, diffuser, oil vaporiser

E

Safety Profile

General safety

There is no clinical data on skin sensitisation; however, due to the citral content, Tisserand & Young recommend a dermal maximum of 3.4% to avoid skin sensitisation.[8]

To avoid skin sensitisation, IFRA recommends a maximum dermal use level for citral of 0.6% for leave-on topical body care products. Because of the high (+)-limonene content, Tisserand & Young recommend that the oil is stored in dark airtight containers in a refrigerator to prevent oxidation.[8]

Contraindications

No contraindications known.

Regulatory guidelines

Ironbark eucalyptus oil is not defined in any regulatory guideline.

References

1. Boland DJ, Brophy JJ. House APN. *Eucalyptus leaf oils: use, chemistry, distillation and marketing*. Inkata Press, Canberra, 1991.
2. Arctander S. *Perfume and flavor materials of natural origin*. Allured Publishing, Carol Stream, 1994.
3. Weiss EA. *Essential oil crops*. CAB International, Wallingford, 1997.
4. Gilles M et al. *Chemical composition and antimicrobial properties of essential oils of three Australian Eucalyptus species*. Food Chemistry, 2010; 119(2): 731-737. Cited in Quintessential Aromatics database, 2013.
5. Zhao Q, Bowles EJ, Zhang HY. *Antioxidant activities of eleven Australian essential oils*. Natural Product Communications, 2008; 3(5): 837-842. Cited in Quintessential Aromatics database, 2013.
6. Webb M. *Bush sense*. Self-published, Australia, 2000.
7. Rhind JP. *Aromatherapeutic blending*. Singing Dragon, London, 2016.
8. Tisserand R, Young R. *Essential oil safety*. 2nd edn. Churchill Livingstone, Edinburgh, 2014.

Eucalyptus, lemon-scented

E

Identification

Botanical name

Corymbia citriodora Hook

Synonyms

Eucalyptus citriodora, lemon-scented gum, lemon-scented spotted gum, citron-scented gum tree

Family

Myrtaceae

Botany and origins

Like all other species of eucalyptus, lemon-scented eucalyptus originates from Australia. Its native habitat is the coastal regions of Queensland.[1] Nowadays it is cultivated in Brazil, China, India, Kenya and South Africa.[2]

Lemon-scented eucalyptus is a medium to tall tree up to 50 m in height with a single stem. The bark is smooth throughout, deciduous, bluish grey to apple-pink, sometimes red, and often blotched with all three colours.[1]

Younger leaves have a higher percentage of essential oil than mature leaves.[1]

C. citriodora is very similar *to Corymbia maculata* (Syn. *Eucalyptus maculata*), differing only in having slightly narrower crown leaves. Also, *C. maculata* foliage is not lemon-scented.[3]

Method of extraction

Lemon-scented eucalyptus oil is steam-distilled from the freshly cut leaves and twiglets.

Characteristics

Lemon-scented eucalyptus oil is a colourless to pale yellow, mobile liquid that has a strong and very fresh, rosy-citronella-like odour and a sweet, balsamic-floral dryout note.[2]

Chemical composition

The chemical composition of lemon-scented eucalyptus essential oil was reported as follows:

α-pinene (0.14%), citronellal (80.10%), linalool (0.66%), isopulegol (3.41%), iso-isopulegol (8.51%), β-caryophyllene (0.39%), citronellol (4.18%).[1]

Adulteration

It is highly unlikely that lemon-scented eucalyptus oil is subject to adulteration.

Pharmacopoeias and standards

At the time of writing the purity, composition, physico-chemical properties and therapeutic uses of lemon-scented eucalyptus essential oil are not defined in any pharmacopoeia monograph or standard.

History and Traditional Uses

History

The leaf of the tree has been utilised as an antiseptic, carminative and digestive agent.[4]

Traditional medicine

The gum exudate (kino) was used by early settlers and Aborigines as an astringent for the treatment of diarrhoea. The kino contains the antibiotic substance citriodorol.[5]

Food, perfumery and flavouring

Lemon-scented eucalyptus is one of the only eucalypt species which is used for the perfumery industry. While the oil has limited use directly as a perfume, it is rich in citronellal, which is used to produce other aromatic compounds used extensively in inexpensive perfumes, soaps and disinfectants.[2]

Other uses

Williams states that the reputation of lemon-scented eucalyptus oil as a mosquito repellent has provided the impetus for producing and marketing the oil on an international scale. In China, a locally produced mosquito repellent called Quwenling is so effective that it has largely replaced the synthetic repellent dimethyl phthalate on the market. It is made from the waste distillate after the extraction of lemon-scented eucalyptus oil. However, as with many natural insect repellents, it does have some limitations. While the initial repellency is as effective as DEET, the duration of protection is less.[4]

Therapeutics

Pharmacology and clinical studies

Eucalyptus citriodora is now classified as *Corymbia citriodora*. However, many research papers still use the name *Eucalyptus citriodora*.

Antifungal activity

Lemon-scented eucalyptus oil has been found to have antifungal activity against *Candida albicans*.[6]

E. citriodora essential oil is rich in citronellal, an aldehyde, which has excellent antifungal activity against various dermatophytes.[7]

Anti-inflammatory activity

An in vivo study confirmed that a number of aldehydes in lemon-scented eucalyptus oil had antioxidant activity that may have contributed to the anti-inflammatory effects observed when orally administered to rats. It was suggested that the oil inhibits prostaglandin biosynthesis in the same way as salicylate drugs and non-steroid anti-inflammatory drugs.[8]

Schnaubelt states that the anti-inflammatory effect is most pronounced if the oil is administered in low concentrations.[9]

Antimicrobial activity

An in vitro study confirmed that a combination of clove and *E. citriodora* essential oils possessed a synergistic activity against *S. aureus, Pseudomonas aeruginosa, Escherichia coli, C. albicans, Trichophyton mentagrophytes, Microsporum gypseum* and *Cryptococcus neoformans*. It was stated that the combination of the two essential oils exhibited significant synergistic and enhanced activity against the microorganisms, and that they should be considered for use against a wide range of skin disease-causing microorganisms.[10]

Antioxidant activity

An in vitro study confirmed that lemon-scented eucalyptus oil had very high antioxidant activity. It has been suggested that the antioxidant effect of essential oils is of special interest in disease with an inflammatory response.[11]

Insecticidal activity

A study comparing the insect repellent activity of plant extracts found that pyrethrum extract had the highest repellent activity followed by *E. citriodora* oil, *Ocimum basilicum* oil and neem oil respectively. The study confirmed that lemon-scented eucalyptus oil was not effective at the concentration of 0.0001% and 0.001%, but was effective at a concentration of 0.015%. It was found to be most effective at 1% and above, providing 97.37% protection.[12]

Another report stated that lemon-scented eucalyptus oil is very effective as an insect repellent only for a short duration of time as it only acts on mosquitos in the vapour phase. It was suggested if a volatile compound is combined with a non-volatile substance, it may be possible to block insect attack both in the air and the surface skin. The study examined the potential for improved repellent activity by combining neem oil with lemon-scented eucalyptus oil. An ideal repellent should provide initial mosquito anti-landing effect by providing an air barrier of volatile molecules and a secondary skin surface barrier. If the mosquitos penetrate the air barrier of volatile molecules, they can be then further deterred if they meet a compound on the skin that is relatively non-volatile and possesses antifeedant effect on the skin. Neem oil is classified as an antifeedant and is non-volatile. The research confirmed that this combination provided complete protection and displayed mosquito paralysis for a period of one hour.[13]

Upper respiratory tract infections

A randomised, double-blind, controlled trial investigated the clinical effects of a blend of five essential oils – *E. citriodora, Eucalyptus globulus, Mentha piperita, Origanum syriacum* and *Rosmarinus officinalis* in patients with upper respiratory tract infections. The main outcome measure was patient assessment of the change in severity of the most debilitating symptoms such as sore throat, hoarseness and cough. 60 patients participated in the trial. It was concluded that the spray application of the five essential oils provided significant and immediate improvement in the symptoms of upper respiratory tract infection; however, the effect was not significant after three days of treatment. After three days there was no difference in symptom severity between the two groups. This suggests that the essential oils possessed a local rather than a systemic effect on the upper respiratory tract.[14]

Actions

Actions commonly cited in aromatherapy

Antiseptic, antiviral, bactericidal, deodorant, expectorant, fungicidal, insecticide[15,16]

Actions supported by clinical studies

Antiseptic, antiviral, bactericidal, fungicidal, insecticide

Comment

Williams states that the oil gained its fame for having the highest level of citronellal in any plant. Essential oils rich in aldehydes are traditionally considered to be calming and sedative.[4] Aldehyde-rich oils are also considered very effective for the treatment of fungal infections.[17]

Lassak & McCarthy state that its low 1,8-cineole content limits its usefulness as a decongestant. The oil has gained a lot of attention for its effectiveness as an insect repellent.[5]

Aromatherapy Uses

Clinical aromatherapy

Musculoskeletal system

Lemon-scented eucalyptus oil is an effective anti-inflammatory for arthritis and helps to relieve muscular tension. Schnaubelt suggests that it works best when blended with everlasting oil.[8]

Nervous system

Schnaubelt states that lemon-scented eucalyptus oil's sedative qualities make it useful for the treatment of sleeplessness.[8]

Respiratory system

Lemon-scented eucalyptus oil is recommended for the temporary relief of asthma, laryngitis, colds, fever and other infectious diseases.[15,16]

Skin care

Lemon-scented eucalyptus oil is recommended for treating athletes foot and other fungal infections. It is highly recommended as an insect repellent.[15]

Energetics, psyche and subtle uses

Personality

Worwood describes the lemon-scented eucalyptus personality as being fresh, alive and loving freedom – constantly expressing new ideas and full of vitality and laughter. They have a vitality and exuberance which they bring to everything they do. They are usually very well-liked by others because they dislike disharmony, and will always be there to support you in times of emotional crisis. They are described as a tower of strength, always listening attentively and never being critical or judgemental.[18]

Dosage and Administration

Blending

Aromatherapy

To create a natural insect repellent, consider blending lemon-scented eucalyptus oil with essential oils such as basil, Atlas or Virginian cedarwood, citronella, 1,8-cineole-rich eucalypts, lemongrass, palmarosa or vetiver.

For the relief of muscular aches and pains, consider blending lemon-scented eucalyptus oil with essential oils such as black pepper, ginger, kunzea, spike lavender, peppermint, pine or rosemary.

To alleviate sleeplessness, consider blending lemon-scented eucalyptus oil with essential oils such as bergamot, lavender, neroli, sweet orange or sandalwood.

To create an uplifting and energising blend, consider blending lemon-scented eucalyptus oil with essential oils such as basil, black pepper, ginger, lemongrass, lemon myrtle, lime, pine or rosemary.

For the relief of colds and flu, consider blending

lemon-scented eucalyptus oil with 1,8-cineole-rich eucalypts or peppermint eucalyptus.

Perfumery

Lemon-scented eucalyptus oil is not commonly used in perfumery. It has an intense citrus aroma, so it should be used sparingly in any blend. I would recommend blending it with citrus oils such as lemon or sweet orange.

Mode of administration

Bath

Because of the high aldehyde content, lemon-scented eucalyptus essential oil is not recommended for use in a bath.

Topical

Massage, ointment

Inhalation

Direct inhalation, diffuser, oil vaporiser

Safety Profile

General safety

Lemon-scented eucalyptus oil is non-toxic, non-irritant and non-sensitising. However, essential oils rich in aldehydes such as citral and citronellal may cause sensitisation reactions if used undiluted.

E

Contraindications

No contraindications known.

Regulatory guidelines

Lemon-scented eucalyptus oil is not defined in any regulatory guideline.

References

1. Boland DJ, Brophy JJ, House APN. *Eucalyptus leaf oils: use, chemistry, distillation and marketing*. Inkata Press, Canberra, 1991.
2. Arctander S, *Perfume and flavor materials of natural origin.* Allured Publishing, Carol Stream, 1994.
3. Centre for Plant Biodiversity Research. *Corymbia citriodora.* Retrieved July 6, 2017, from http: www.anbg/gov.au/cpbr/cd-keys/euclid3/euclidsample/html/Corymbia_citriodora.htm
4. Williams C. *Medicinal plants in Australia – Vol. 2. Gums, resins, tannins and essential oil.* Rosenburg Publishing, Dural, 2011.
5. Lassak EV, McCarthy T. *Australian medicinal plants.* Methuen Australia, North Ryde, 1983.
6. Beylier MF, Givaudan SA. *Bacteriostatic activity of some Australian oils.* Perfumer & Flavorist, 1979; 4(1): 23-25. Cited in Quintessential Aromatics database, 2013.
7. Tabassum N, Vidyasagar GM. *Antifungal investigation of plant essential oils: A review.* International Journal of Pharmacy and Pharmaceutical Sciences. 2013; 5(2):19-28.
8. Gbenou JD et al. *Phytochemical composition of Cymbopogon citratus and Eucalyptus citriodora essential oils and their anti-inflammatory and analgesic properties on Wistar rats.* Molecular Biology Reports, 2013; 40(2): 1127-1134. doi: 10.1007/s11033-012-2155-1.
9. Schnaubelt K. *Medical aromatherapy.* Frog, Berkeley, 1999.
10. Kirui JK et al. *Combined antibacterial and antifungal activities of Eucalyptus citriodora and Syzygium aromaticum essential oils.* African Journal of Pharmacology and Therapeutics, 2014; 3(1): 29-37.
11. Zhao Q, Bowles EJ, Zhang HY. *Antioxidant activities of eleven Australian essential oils.* Natural Product Communications, 2008; 3(5): 837-842. Cited in Quintessential Aromatics database, 2013.
12. Kiplang'at KP, Mwangi RW. *Repellent activities of Ocimum basilicum, Azadirachta indica and Eucalyptus citriodora extracts on rabbit skin against Aedes aegypti.* Journal of Entomology and Zoology Studies, 2013; 1(5): 84-91.
13. Kiplang'at KP, Mwangi RW. *Synergistic repellent activity of plant essential oils against Aedes aegypti on rabbit skin.* International Journal of Mosquito Research, 2014; 1(4): 55-59.
14. Ben-Arye E et al. *Treatment of upper respiratory tract infections in primary care: a randomized study using aromatic herbs.* Evidence-Based Complementary and Alternative Medicine, 2011; 2011: 690346. doi: 10.1155/2011/690346.
15. Lawless J, *The encyclopedia of essential oils.* Element Books, Shaftesbury, 1992.
16. Lavabre M. *Aromatherapy workbook.* Healing Arts Press, Rochester, 1997.
17. Bowles EJ. *The chemistry of aromatherapeutic oils.* 3rd edn. Allen & Unwin, Crows Nest, 2003.
18. Worwood VA. *The fragrant mind.* Transworld Publishing, London, 1995.

Everlasting

Identification

Botanical name

Helichrysum angustifolium (L.) DC

Synonyms

H. italicum (Roth) G. Don, helichrysum, immortelle

Family

Asteraceae (Compositae)

Botany and origins

The genus *Helichrysum* (Miller) belongs to the Asteraceae family. It is a very large genus with approximately 600 species widespread all over the world. Approximately 25 species are native to the Mediterranean region. It is a small aromatic shrub, up to 40-50 cm high with yellow flowers, growing on dry cliffs and sandy soil. Only the essential oil extracted from the plants belonging to the *H. angustifolium* species is used in aromatherapy.[1]

The name helichrysum comes from the Greek word *helios* (sun) and *chrysos* (gold) because of the way the plant blooms, giving the impression of little golden suns.[2]

Method of extraction

Everlasting oil is steam-distilled from the flowering tops of *H. angustifolium*. The flowering tops are cut by hand. About 1 tonne of flowering tops produces 900 g to 1.5 kg of essential oil. It is therefore not surprising that it demands such a high price.[1]

Characteristics

Everlasting oil is a pale-yellow, oily liquid with a powerful and diffusive aroma, which is considered quite unique. It is described as a sweet-fruity and tea-like aroma with an outstanding tenacity.[3]

Holmes describes it has a base note with a very high intensity and excellent persistence.[4]

Chemical composition

Everlasting oil contains numerous monoterpenes and some unusual sesquiterpenes not found in other essential oils.[1]

Schnaubelt suggests that the diketones found in the oil may contribute to everlasting's amazing wound-healing properties. However, some samples of everlasting seem to have very few or no diketones. Schnaubelt speculates that this may be a consequence of harvesting the flowers too early.[5]

The chemical profile of *Helichrysum italicum* subsp. *italicum* was reported as follows:

neryl acetate (34.5-39.9%), γ-curcumene (5.1-12.9%), (+)-limonene (5.1-7.3%), neryl propionate (4.8-6.7%), *ar*-curcumene (2.3-4.6%), italidione I (3.5-4.5%), nerol (2.6-3.4%), italicene (2.4-3.4%), α-pinene (1.5-2.9%), linalool (1.5-2.8%), italidione II (0.6-2.6%), eudesm-5-en-11-ol (0-2.3%), italidione II isomer (0.6-2.0%), 4,6-dimethyloctan-3,5-dione (1.0-1.1%), 4-methylhexan-3-one (0-1.1%), isoitalicene (0.7-1.0%), 1,8-cineole (0-1.0%).[6]

Holmes states that everlasting sourced from the Balkan region has a higher sesquiterpenes content, making it possibly more effective as an anti-inflammatory, whereas the Corsican oil has a higher neryl acetate content, making it a better analgesic.[4]

Adulteration

Because of the limited availability, the risk of adulteration is high. Often the more expensive Corsican everlasting oil is mixed with the less expensive oil from the Balkans.[4] Sometimes more than one species are harvested and processed together.[6]

Pharmacopoeias and standards

At the time of writing, the purity, composition, physico-chemical properties and therapeutic use of everlasting essential oil are not defined in any pharmacopoeia monograph or standard.

E

History and Traditional Uses

History

Schnaubelt states that large quantities of everlasting oil were distilled in the former Yugoslavia. It was primarily used to fragrance pipe tobaccos. It was only in the early 1990s that aromatherapy discovered the oil. Unfortunately, its popularity grew right around the time of the Balkan war. Supply from the Balkans dried up during the war and the only remaining production was coming from Corsica. This caused the price of the oil to increase dramatically.[5]

In the last 10 years, production of everlasting from the hillsides of Croatia, Bosnia and Herzegovina has returned to the market, but the price remains high.[5]

Herbal

In herbal medicine, everlasting is used as an expectorant, antitussive, choleretic, diuretic, anti-inflammatory and antiallergenic agent. It has been used for bronchitis, asthma, whooping cough, psoriasis, burns, rheumatism, headache, migraines, allergies and liver ailments. It is usually taken in the form of a decoction or infusion.[7]

Food, perfumery and flavouring

The absolute and essential oil are sometimes used in perfumery. Everlasting extracts are used as a flavouring component in many food and beverage products.[7]

Therapeutics

Pharmacology and clinical studies

Anti-inflammatory

Everlasting oil is known to contain ketones that contribute to the anti-inflammatory process. Arzanol was identified as the major anti-inflammatory component. Studies have identified arzanol as a potent dual-inhibitor of pro-inflammatory mediators and inflammatory enzymes, providing a mechanistic rationale for the well-known anti-inflammatory activity of *H. italicum*.[1]

Antimicrobial activity

Of all the properties attributed to everlasting, the antimicrobial properties have received the most attention. *H. italicum* and *H. stoechas* showed significant activity towards *Staphylococcus aureus* and *S. epidermidis*, but were variable in activity towards gram-negative species. *H. italicum* was active against *Klebsiella pneumoniae* and *Pseudomonas aeruginosa*.[8]

One very interesting study demonstrated that *H. italicum* oil significantly reduces the multidrug resistance (MDR) of several gram-negative strains of bacteria. Many bacteria have developed effective mechanisms of resistance such as efflux pumps overexpression. Efflux pumps play an important role in bacteria resistance to antibiotics and contribute to the spread of multidrug resistant pathogen (MDR phenotype). The researchers concluded that by blocking this mechanism with efflux pump inhibitors (EPIs), it is possible to restore the effectiveness of antibiotics.[1]

Wound-healing activity

Voinchet & Giraud-Robert investigated the therapeutic effects and potential clinical applications of *H. italicum* oil combined with rosehip oil after cosmetic and reconstructive surgery. They observed that the blend had excellent anti-inflammatory and wound-healing properties, as well as reducing pain, oedema and bruising. They also highlighted that neryl acetate, a main component of the oil, contributed to pain relief. They attributed the observed effects to the occurence of italidiones. This class of molecules is also reputed to have anti-haematomal properties.[1]

Everlasting is often referred to as the 'super arnica of aromatherapy'. That is why it is referred to as a phlebotonic and is indicated for couperose skin (red veins), haematoma, thrombosis and the prevention of bruises.[9]

Actions

Actions commonly cited in aromatherapy

Anti-inflammatory, antimicrobial, antiseptic, cholagogue, cicatrisant, expectorant, hepatic, mucolytic, phlebotonic [1,2,5,9,10,11,12]

Actions supported by clinical studies

Anti-inflammatory, antimicrobial, antiseptic, cicatrisant, hepatic

Comment

Schnaubelt states that everlasting's effects have been so convincing that it has never met with any kind of criticism, despite the absence of pharmacological scientific data.[5]

Everlasting oil is a relatively new oil to the practice of aromatherapy. The essential oil's action in treating both chronic and acute skin disorders, with its combined skin-regenerating and anti-inflammatory action, means that it has secured itself a place as one of the most precious and important essential oils in aromatherapy.

Everlasting oil has also found a very important role for aromatherapists in the management of deep-seated psychological and emotional problems; however, there is a lack of studies examining the effect of everlasting on our emotional wellbeing. It would be good to have studies investigating its effect on our psyche.

Aromatherapy Uses

Clinical aromatherapy

Circulatory system

Among its chemical constituents are a group of ketone-like compounds called beta-diones. It is this group of constituents that contribute to the oil's anticoagulant properties, making it applicable in the treatment of any severe bruising that results in haematoma.[6,9,10]

Detoxification

Everlasting oil acts as a stimulant for the liver and gall bladder. Fischer-Rizzi states that the oil should be taken orally in small doses, one drop twice daily. She recommends warm compresses of everlasting and rosemary (used in a 1-to-1 ratio). She also recommends using everlasting to help drain the lymph glands and says that the oil will enhance the effects of a lymphatic draining massage.[12]

Schnaubelt states that everlasting regulates cholesterol and stimulates liver cells. He suggests the preferred mode of use for detoxification is internally in low dosages combined with lemon and rosemary ct. verbenone.[13]

First aid

Everlasting oil is highly recommended as a first aid remedy for injuries, strains, sprains and tissue trauma.[4,5,11] Schnaubelt recommends applying the oil undiluted.[5]

Musculoskeletal system

Everlasting oil can be used to alleviate pain and inflammation associated with rheumatoid arthritis.[4,10]

Psychological

Worwood recommends using everlasting to counteract stress and tension during an emotional crisis, to alleviate mental and emotional exhaustion, to alleviate loneliness and insecurity and to release emotional blockages.[13]

Holmes recommends everlasting for anxiety, suppressed anger, frustration, resentment, agitation, emotional instability, moodiness, sorrow and a negative outlook. He states that the oil promotes emotional stability and calm. He also describes everlasting as emotionally calming, softening and stabilising. It helps one cope with deep frustration and long bottled-up resentment.[4]

Respiratory system

Everlasting has been found to have strong mucolytic and expectorant properties, which makes it beneficial for treating sinus infections, bronchitis and coughs.[10]

Wound healing

Everlasting oil has exceptional healing properties on the skin – speeding cellular growth and assisting in wound healing. Price & Price attribute everlasting's remarkable healing and rejuvenating properties to the oil's cicatrisant, antimicrobial and anti-inflammatory properties.[9]

Schnaubelt states that it will disinfect the wound, but unlike other essential oils with antiseptic properties, it will not be painful. It also prevents swelling and inflammation. He explains that the oil is so mild that it can be applied neat for the immediate treatment of injuries, especially bleeding wounds.

> *Dropping this oil into a bleeding wound sanitizes the wound, speeds its closure and effectively stops the pain. Using it undiluted on wounds avoids bringing other, less suited substances, such as fatty base oils, into the wound.*[5]

However, he also explains that it can be very effective in a 1% dilution in a base oil.

It is recommended for the treatment of acne, chronic dermatitis, psoriasis, burns and dermal inflammation.[4,5,9,12] The oil is also recommended for scar reduction.[5,11]

Energetics, psyche and subtle uses

Energetics

Mojay compares the energetic qualities of everlasting, with Roman chamomile and yarrow. He states that it regulates the flow of *Qi* and clears *heat*, therefore it would be beneficial for conditions associated with the *Liver* and encourage the flow of bile.[7]

According to the principles of the Five Elements, Holmes states that everlasting has an affinity with Wood and Fire.[4] Holmes explains that everlasting oil activates *Qi* and *Blood*, settles the *Heart* and calms our *Shen*.[4] Whenever our *Shen* is agitated we are likely to suffer from anxiety, depression, headaches and insomnia.

Personality

Worwood beautifully describes the everlasting character as:

> *Ever young at heart and youthful in appearance, immortelles will have the air of eternal youth about them, even in the last stages of their journey on this earth.*[14]

She continues to describe the personality of everlasting:

> *The immortelle profile is one of quietness, introversion and youth, with a quiet knowing that comes from being sure of the spirituality of all things, and the understanding that there are greater things in heaven and earth than we can see.*[14]

Worwood suggests that the immortelle person is spiritually highly evolved, and may often appear fairy-like and have a high level of consciousness and mental agility.[14]

Friendships are very precious to an immortelle personality. They are always encouraging and helpful. They can always see other people's points of view even if they don't agree with them, and will accept other people's ways of doing things. They always try to understand other ways of thinking and doing things.[14]

Worwood states that they can appear guarded, as if protecting themselves emotionally, but this can be an inaccurate judgement because they simply do not feel the need to externalise and express their emotions to everyone.[14]

According to Myers-Briggs personality types, the everlasting personality is likely to be an INFP. INFPs are gentle, calm, easygoing and affirming. Integrity and commitment to what they believe in are essential. They like time alone for their many interests. They like learning and researching new things and interests. They are highly reflective, especially in understanding the mysteries and meaning of life. They have little need to impose their values on others. They prefer to gently influence and inspire. They value authenticity and depth in their relationships.

Subtle

Fischer-Rizzi states that everlasting increases dream activity and may help guide one towards an important stage of awareness. She states dreams become easier to remember and dreams with important messages occur more frequently.[12]

Zeck beautifully describes everlasting's subtle effects:

> *When you are knotted-up inside and unable to stop thinking, the earthy, warming aroma of everlasting unravels the tension that develops from thoughts going round and round.*[14]

Everlasting will help to ground you if you are one of the walking wounded, immobilised by your thinking and your feelings.[15]

When describing the subtle qualities of everlasting, the term 'walking wounded' is repeated by many aromatherapists. Worwood explains that the fragrance of everlasting opens hearts to the unseen energies that affect our lives here on earth. She states:

> *It has a special purpose for "the walking wounded" – those who cannot reminisce for fear of the painful emotions that may be brought to the fore. It is also for those who feel their physical self has lost touch with their soul.*[16]

Worwood states that everlasting allows us to understand that to 'truly love' also involves the acceptance of the pain of love – willingly and without compromise.[16]

Holmes explains that everlasting has a profoundly purifying and transformative effect on the emotional body and the heart as an energetic and spiritual organ.

> *It can therefore potentially heal the core emotional trauma from which distressed feelings and negative emotions arose in the first place. As such, it is also a prime remedy for the closed and deeply wounded heart, whether from loss, betrayal or any other cause.*[4]

Keim Loughran & Bull explain that everlasting dissolves emotional blockages and helps to balance the upper chakras. It resonates with the heart chakra by promoting compassion for self and others. They also say that it integrates compassion and spirituality and activates and supports the intuitive mind.[17]

It also helps to integrate the heart with the spirit, so that the information you perceive can be shared in gentle and loving service to others. The oil also grounds us in divine love and guidance, fostering understanding and compassionate insight.[17]

Everlasting oil also has a strong affinity with the third eye chakra.

Dosage and Administration

Blending

Aromatherapy

For the relief of anxiety, nervous tension and stress, consider blending everlasting oil with essential oils such as German and Roman chamomile, clary sage, frankincense, lavender, neroli, patchouli, sandalwood, sweet orange, sweet marjoram or vetiver.

For healing emotional wounds or trauma, consider blending everlasting oil with essential oils such as rock rose, lavender, neroli, rose otto or sandalwood.

Fischer-Rizzi recommends blending everlasting with cistus and lavender for treating skin allergies, eczema, rashes and psoriasis. She states that when everlasting is combined with rosemary it makes an excellent liver stimulant.[12]

As a liver tonic, consider blending everlasting oil with essential oils such as carrot seed, lemon or rosemary.

For the treatment of thrombosis, Holmes recommends blending everlasting with lemon oil.[4]

For the relief of muscle and joint pain, consider blending everlasting oil with cajeput, ginger, spike lavender, kunzea or peppermint.

Perfumery

Arctander says that, in perfumery, everlasting oil blends well with boronia absolute, Roman chamomile, cistus, lavender, oakmoss absolute and clary sage. The oil is an excellent modifier for certain types of fruity flavours where rich and deep-sweet notes are required. He also states that it blends well with citrus oils such as lemon, lime and petitgrain.[3]

Mode of administration

Bath

Full body bath, foot bath

Topical

Compress, massage, ointment, skin care

E

Inhalation

Direct inhalation, diffuser, oil burner

Ingestion

As a liver stimulant, Fischer-Rizzi and Schnaubelt suggest that everlasting be taken orally in small doses.[2,12] Fischer-Rizzi recommends taking 1 drop twice daily.[12]

Safety Profile

General safety

Everlasting oil is considered non-toxic, non-irritant and non-sensitising.[4,5,6]

Contraindications

No contraindications known.

Regulatory guidelines

Everlasting essential oil has GRAS status.

References

1. Guinoiseau E et al. *Biological properties and resistance reversal effect of Helichrysum italicum (Roth) G. Don.* In Méndez-Vilas A. ed. *Microbial pathogens and strategies for combating them: science, technology and education.* Formatex Research Center, 2013: 1073-1080.
2. Mailhebiau P. *Portraits in oils.* C.W. Daniel Company, Saffron Walden, 1995.
3. Arctander S. *Perfume and flavor materials of natural origin.* Allured Publishing, Carol Stream, 1994.
4. Holmes P. *Aromatica: a clinical guide to essential oil therapeutics – Vol. I.* Singing Dragon, London, 2016.
5. Schnaubelt K. *The healing intelligence of essential oils.* Healing Arts Press, Rochester, 2011.
6. Tisserand R, Young R. *Essential oil safety.* 2nd edn. Churchill Livingstone, Edinburgh, 2014.
7. Khan I, Abourashed E. *Leung's encyclopedia of common natural ingredients used in food, drugs and cosmetics.* 3rd edn. John Wiley & Sons, New Jersey, 2010.
8. Tsoukatou M et al. *Chemical composition of the essential oils and headspace samples of two Helichrysum species occurring in Spain.* Journal of Essential Oil Research, 1999; 11(4): 511-516.
9. Price S, Price L. *Aromatherapy for health professionals.* 4th edn. Churchill Livingstone, Edinburgh, 2012.
10. Lawless J. *The encyclopaedia of essential oils.* Element Books, Shaftesbury, 1992.
11. Mojay G. *Aromatherapy for healing the spirit.* Healing Arts Press, Rochester, 1999.
12. Fischer-Rizzi S. *Complete aromatherapy handbook.* Sterling Publishing, New York, 1990.
13. Schnaubelt K. *Medical aromatherapy.* Frog, Berkeley, 1999.
14. Worwood VA. *The fragrant mind.* Transworld Publishers, London, 1995.
15. Zeck R. *The blossoming heart – aromatherapy for healing and transformation.* Aroma Tours, East Ivanhoe, 2003.
16. Worwood VA. *The fragrant heavens.* Transworld Publishers, London, 1999.
17. Keim Loughran J, Bull R. *Aromatherapy and subtle energy techniques.* Frog, Berkeley, 2000.

F

Fennel, sweet

Identification

Botanical name

Foeniculum vulgare Mill.

Synonyms

Foeniculum officinale, Roman fennel

Family

Apiaceae (Umbelliferae)

Botany and origins

Fennel is a biennial or perennial herb that grows up to 2 m in height, with fine, feathery leaves and umbels of golden-yellow flowers. It is indigenous to Mediterranean countries such as Italy, Greece and France.[1]

There are two subspecies of fennel:[2]

- *F. vulgare* var. *amara*, known as bitter fennel
- *F. vulgare* var. *dulce*, known as sweet fennel.

Method of extraction

Fennel oil is produced from the distillation of the crushed seeds of *F. vulgare*.

Characteristics

Sweet fennel oil is a colourless to pale yellow liquid with a very sweet, but slightly earthy or peppery-spicy odour and a clean, sweet aromatic dryout. Arctander states that there is a hint of a fruity-fresh top note in fresh oils.[1]

Bitter fennel oil is a pale yellow to almost colourless liquid of a somewhat sharp and warm-camphoraceous aroma. It is initially earthy, becoming sweet, anisic and spicy.[1]

Chemical composition

The chemical composition of sweet fennel oil from Turkey was reported as follows:

α-pinene (trace-0.5%), sabinene (0.1-0.2%), myrcene (0.1%), fenchone (1.3-1.8%), (Z)-anethole (0.1%), *trans*-anethole (82.2-86.8%), methyl chavicol (4.0-4.9%), limonene (2.2-4.9%), carvone (0.8-1.3%), 1,8-cineole (0.2-4.9%), *p*-anisaldehyde (1.1-2.4%).[3]

The concentration of *trans*-anethole in sweet fennel oil varies from 50 to 90%, depending on the varieties, sources and the ripeness of the seeds.[2]

The oil of bitter fennel is reported to contain not less than 60% anethole and 15% fenchone, and not more than 6% estragole.[4]

Adulteration

Sweet fennel oil should be produced only from the fruits; however, more often the entire aerial part is used. Adulteration is also done by the addition of synthetic anethole or anethole from other sources like star anise. It is adulterated by blending it with star anise and limonene. Bitter fennel oil is often adulterated by blending with sweet fennel oil produced from the whole aerial part of the plant, or blending with star anise and fennel terpenes.[5]

F

Pharmacopoeias and standards

The purity, composition and physico-chemical properties of sweet and bitter fennel essential oil are defined in:

- ISO 17412: 2007 Oil of Bitter Fennel
- European Medicines Agency Assessment Report on *Foeniculum vulgare* Miller
- German Commission E.

History and Traditional Uses

History

The name of fennel comes from Latin *foenum*, meaning hay, and the Romans called it *foeniculum*.[6]

Fennel was well known to the ancient Egyptians, Greeks and Romans. It was cultivated for its aromatic fruits and succulent edible shoots. Pliny had high regard for its medicinal properties.[6]

The Greeks were the first to recognise its value as a slimming aid. The ancient Greek name of the herb, *marathron*, from *maraino* (to grow thin) probably refers to this property. It was said to convey longevity, and to give strength and courage. The ancient Greeks ate the seeds for this reason, and to help control their weight while training for the Olympics.[6]

The seeds were carried by Roman soldiers on long marches to chew when they did not have time to stop and cook a meal, and by devout Christians to satisfy the cravings of hunger on fasting days.[7]

During the Middle Ages, the use of fennel was entwined with witchcraft and superstition. It was used with St John's wort as protection against evil forces. It was hung inside houses and churches or above doors to protect those inside against the devil.[8]

Seventeenth-century herbalist William Coles affirms the properties of fennel:

> *... both the seeds, leaves and root of our garden fennel are much used in drinks and broths for those that are grown fat, to abate their unwieldiness and cause them to grow more gaunt and lank.*[6]

Culpeper was aware of fennel's qualities:

> *... fennel is good for breaking of wind ... to provoke urine ... to break and ease the pain of the stone ... stay the hiccough ... allay the heat and loathing of the stomach, and the gripings thereof ... open obstructions of the liver, gall and spleen ... and to ease the painful and windy swellings of the spleen ... as also in gout and cramps.*[8]

Traditional medicine

In TCM, fennel is used to treat any lower abdominal pain caused by *cold* and *damp* conditions that are often associated with symptoms such as abdominal pain, indigestion, decreased appetite and vomiting.[9]

Herbal

Bone & Mills state indications that can be supported by clinical trials for the use of fennel fruit include dyspeptic conditions of the upper gastrointestinal tract.[9]

The German Commission E recommends fennel seeds (as a herbal infusion, tincture, syrup and honey) and the essential oil for the treatment of dyspeptic complaints, bloating, flatulence and catarrhal conditions of the upper respiratory tract.[10]

The WHO monograph for fennel seed reports that it is used in traditional medicine for blepharitis, bronchitis, constipation, conjunctivitis, diabetes, dyspnoea, fever, gastritis, headache, pain, poor appetite, and respiratory and urinary tract infections.[11]

Food, perfumery and flavouring

The dried, aromatic seeds are widely used in culinary preparations for flavouring bread and pastry, in candies, alcoholic liqueurs, as well as in oral and medicinal preparations.[2]

Therapeutics

Pharmacology and clinical studies

Many pharmacological studies involving sweet fennel essential oil have been published. A systemic review of these studies will not be attempted. Rather, I have chosen a selection of studies that support the traditional and clinical uses.

Analgesic activity

There was no significant difference between the analgesic activity of sweet fennel oil and aspirin in a study involving mice. 0.25 and 0.5 mL/kg of fennel oil was administered intraperitoneally for the purposes of this study.[12]

Antidiabetic activity

Ingestion of fennel seed oil (30 mg/kg body weight) confirmed a hypoglycaemic effect and antioxidant activity in diabetic induced rats.[13]

Another study examined the effects of transdermal nanoemulsions of encapsulated fennel seed oil on diabetic induced rats. The results showed that the oil reduced plasma glucose levels and this was sustained for seven days after a single topical application of a dose of 120 mg/kg of fennel seed essential oil.[14]

Antifungal activity

An in vitro study found that fennel seed oil killed pathogens of *Trichophyton rubrum, Trichophyton mentagrophytes* and *Scytalidium dimidiatum* in 5 seconds, whilst at the minimum fungicidal concentrations it required 50 to 80 minutes. Tests also found that the oil was effective against other nail-infective fungi in a range of 0.5 to 1 ul/mL concentrations. The authors reported that the essential oil did not produce any irritation or adverse reactions at 5% concentrations on human skin when used for 3 weeks.[15]

Another in vitro study confirmed that fennel seed oil had antifungal activity against *T. rubrum, Trichophyton tonsurans, Microsporum gypseum* and *T. mentagrophytes*. Further studies revealed that the oil damaged the plasma membrane and intracellular organelles, and that it could also inhibit the mitochondrial enzyme activities of the organisms. It was also noted that the antifungal activity was better than commonly used antifungal agents such as fluconazole and amphotericin B.[16]

Antimicrobial activity

Lis-Balchin states that fennel oil has low antibacterial activity.[17] However, I have found many studies confirming the antibacterial activity of fennel oil. In one study, fennel oil inhibited the growth of *Escherichia coli* (MIC - 0.5% V/V), *Staphylococcus aureus* (MIC - 0.25%), *Salmonella typhimurium* (MIC - 1.0%) and *Candida albicans* (MIC - 0.5%).[4]

An in vitro study confirmed that fennel seed oil had antimicrobial activity against methicillin-sensitive *S. aureus* (MSSA) and resistant strains (MRSA). The researchers noted that the results were comparable with vancomycin (30 ug).[18] Other in vitro studies have found that fennel oil exhibited moderate antimicrobial activities.[19]

Antioxidant activity

An in vitro study confirmed strong antioxidant activity of fennel seed oil in comparison with butylated hydroxyanisole (BHA) and butylated hydroxytoluene (BHT).[20]

Antispasmodic activity

Fennel seed oil has been reported to have spasmolytic effects on smooth muscles of experimental animals.[2]

Fennel seed oil was found to be antispasmodic towards smooth muscle of isolated rat ileum and urinary bladder. It inhibits contractions induced by acetylcholine in a calcium-free medium. It was concluded that fennel oil inhibited calcium release from intracellular stores or blocked binding proteins.[21]

A study confirmed the bronchodilatory effects of fennel seed oil in animal studies. The researchers found that the relaxant effect of fennel essential oil was because it had an inhibitory effect on a potassium channel opening.[22]

Fennel seed oil significantly and dose-dependently reduced the intensity of oxytocin-induced contractions and prostaglandin E2-induced contractions of the isolated rat uterus.[23]

Antitumor activity

Anethole was reported to be an in vitro potential inhibitor of tumour necrosis factor (TNF)-induced cellular responses such as activation of nuclear factor kappa B (NF-kB) and other transcription factors, and also to block TNF-induced activation of the apoptotic pathway. Another study using mice cited in the EMA report states that the anticarcinogenic and cytotoxic effect of anethole was comparable with cyclophosphamide (a standard cytotoxic drug).[4]

Autonomic nervous system activity

A study found that sweet fennel oil decreased the parasympathetic nervous system, and reduced fatigue and mental stress caused by a one-hour arithmetic assignment.[24]

Choleretic activity

Fennel seed oil and anethole were found to have

F

a cholagogue and choleretic effect on rats and guinea pigs.[25,26]

Dysmenorrhoea

Seventy women, 15 to 24 years old who suffered from primary dysmenorrhoea, were involved in a clinical study to compare the effects of sweet fennel essential oil versus mefenamic acid. Fennel seed oil was administered orally. Both fennel and the drug relieved menstrual pain; however, mefenamic acid was more potent than fennel in the second and third menstrual days. Also, it must be noted that five cases withdrew from the study due to the odour of fennel, and one case reported a mild increase in the amount of her menstrual flow. The researchers suggested that fennel seed oil can be used as a safe and effective herbal drug for primary dysmenorrhoea, even though it has a lower potency than mefenamic acid in the doses used for this study.[27]

A double-blind, randomised study was conducted using 60 young women diagnosed with primary dysmenorrhoea to compare the effects of 1% and 2 % fennel seed oil with a placebo for the relief of dysmenorrhoea symptoms. The essential oil was administered orally as soon as the pain commenced, and subsequent doses taken when needed, but not in intervals less than 4 hours. Results indicated that the group taking fennel oil had a higher decrease in the level of pain severity than the placebo group. The average total bleeding in the fennel essential oil group was significantly higher, compared to the placebo group. It was suggested that the decrease in pain intensity was attributed to the oestrogenic-like activity of anethole, the main chemical component of fennel essential oil.[28]

F

Expectorant activity

Anethole and fenchone have been found to stimulate secretions of the upper respiratory tract.[2]

Bone & Mills cite a study where fennel seed oil administered by inhalation exerted a mild antitussive or cough suppressant effect on cough generated by mechanical stimulation in guinea pigs.[9]

Hepatoprotective activity

The hepatoprotective activity of fennel seed oil was confirmed in a study involving rats.[29]

Infantile colic

A randomised, double-blind, placebo-controlled trial using an emulsion of 0.1% fennel seed oil in water with a 0.4% polysorbate emulsifying agent examined the effect of the oil in treating infantile colic. The results concluded that the 0.1% fennel seed oil emulsion was superior to the placebo in decreasing the infantile colic. No side effects were reported.[30]

Larvicidal activity

Fennel seed oil exerted significant larvicidal activity against two mosquito species after 24-hour exposure.[31]

Sweet fennel seed oil exhibited larvicidal activity against the larvae of *Culex quinquefasciatus*. The oil gave 90% mortality rate within 40 minutes.[32]

Oestrogenic activity

Research suggests that polymers of anethole are active oestrogenic compounds.[2,4,33]

The EMA report for fennel seed cites several studies, which demonstrate that fennel does have oestrogenic activity. In one study, 38 women affected by idiopathic hirsutism were treated, in a double-blind, placebo-controlled study, for 12 weeks, twice a day, with a cream containing 2%, 1% and 0% of fennel fruit extract obtained with ethanol. In both treatment groups, a significant reduction of facial hair growth was observed.[4]

In another study, *trans*-anethole administered orally to immature female mice at 80 mg/kg body weight for three days significantly increased uterine weight. The results confirm that *trans*-anethole has oestrogenic activity.[4]

Bone & Mills explain that the structural resemblance of anethole to catecholamines may help explain the galactagogue activity of fennel. They explain that anethole may influence milk secretion by competing with dopamine at appropriate receptor sites, thereby reducing the inhibition of prolactin secretion by dopamine. Dianethole and photoanethole (polymers of anethole) resemble the oestrogenic compounds stilbene and diethylstilbestrol, and have demonstrated oestrogenic activity.[9]

Actions

Actions commonly cited in aromatherapy

Analgesic, anti-inflammatory, antiseptic, antispasmodic, aperitive, carminative, cholagogic, depurative, digestive stimulant, diuretic, emmenagogue, expectorant, galactagogue, splenic, stomachic[34,35,36]

Actions supported by clinical studies

Antispasmodic, carminative, digestive stimulant, expectorant, hepatoprotective, stomachic

Comment

The EMA report concluded that the traditional uses of fennel for 'dyspeptic complaints such as mild, spasmodic gastro-intestinal ailment, bloating and flatulence' and 'catarrh of the upper respiratory tract' are supported not only by expert opinion and clinical experience, but also by available data.[4]

The EMA report states that investigations available on the role of fennel in reducing pain in primary dysmenorrhoea in humans are very preliminary. It explains that the likelihood of the postulated effect is considerably increased by several studies that show fennel seed oil to exert a relaxing effect on pre-contracted smooth muscles from tracheal, ileal and uterine tissues by antagonising contraction-inducing agents.[4]

Aromatherapy Uses

Clinical aromatherapy

Digestive system

Sweet fennel oil is traditionally used as a stomachic and a carminative in treating flatulence and other digestive problems.[2,7] The oil is recommended in the German Commission E Monographs for peptic discomforts, spastic disorders of the gastrointestinal tract, feelings of fullness and flatulence.[10]

Lymphatic system

Sweet fennel oil is a diuretic and lymphatic decongestant, assisting the body to eliminate toxins. It is often used for treating fluid retention, cellulite and obesity, both as an essential oil and herbal tea.[7,34]

Reproductive system

Sweet fennel oil is recommended for regulating the menstrual cycle, particularly where periods are scanty and painful.[2,7] It may be used during menopause to reduce symptoms caused by fluctuating hormonal levels.[2]

Respiratory system

Like aniseed, sweet fennel oil is an antispasmodic and expectorant, and is recommended for catarrh of the upper respiratory tract.[2,34]

Skin care

Sweet fennel oil is recommended in skin care preparation for the treatment of dull, oily and mature skin types.[34]

Urinary system

Sweet fennel oil is a diuretic and traditionally used as a urinary tract antiseptic. It may be used for the treatment of urinary tract infections.[7]

Energetics, psyche and subtle uses

Energetics

Sweet fennel is classified as a *warming* and *drying* remedy that helps to eliminate excess *damp* and *cold*, which are associated with conditions of the digestive system, respiratory system and reproductive system. Such conditions may include dyspepsia and indigestion. Sweet fennel oil expels phlegm and is recommended for bronchial asthma and wheezing.[36,37]

Fennel seed oil is closely related to the Earth Element and the *Yi* (intellect). According to the principles of TCM, the *Yi* gives us the capacity for sustained intention, purpose, clarity of thought and integrity.

According to the principles of Ayurveda, fennel oil helps reduce excess *Kapha*.

Personality

Worwood describes the fennel personality as someone who is constantly active and always on the move:

> *They don't walk – they hurry along – leaping up the stairs rather than waiting for a lift ... they belong to swimming clubs and probably play squash at the weekend. They excel at any type of competition – at work as well as at play.*[38]

Fennel personalities tend to be very intelligent people who are quick-witted and creative, and in need of a lot of mental stimulation. Worwood also explains that fennel seed personalities are very assertive and determined. They are emotionally very active, constantly changing their emotions. One minute they are crying, the next minute they are laughing.[38]

Mojay states that fennel is suited to the type of individual who tends to overthink and overanalyse:

> *While they may easily generate concepts and ideas, they rarely communicate them or put them into practice. They may find it difficult to articulate and express themselves, feelings, too, tend to churn within. The more such emotions are locked inside, the more they intensify, building up tension that affects the bowels. The unacceptable, unexpressed thoughts and emotions that are pushed below consciousness accumulate in the intestines as nervous spasm and gas.*[36]

According to Myers-Briggs personality types, the sweet fennel personality is likely to be an ESTP. ESTPs are confident, gregarious and exciting. They like being with people who share their interests and sense of fun. Adventure is pleasurable for them. They are charming and have an infectious manner. They can be assertive. They have lots of energy and are constantly on the go. They can have an intense personality and seek recognition and success. They are often not interested in dealing with interpersonal or emotional issues.

F

Subtle

Davis refers to the traditional uses of fennel as a form of protection against witches and evil. She recommends using fennel if you feel threatened at any time by psychic attack. To do this, Davis suggests rubbing a drop or two on your hands and smoothing them over your aura at a little distance from the surface of the body.[39]

Keim Loughran & Bull state that learning to speak compassionately, appropriately and truthfully is a primary precept and moral teaching on the spiritual path. They explain that words have great power to harm or benefit others, and fennel will aid the development of direct, authentic and skillful communication. Fennel helps us to discover what we want to say and then accurately express it to others in a positive way. Fennel also protects us from being harmed by someone else's negative words, as well as thoughts and deeds.[40]

Zeck recommends sweet fennel oil to assist us in completing tasks that are not complete or require further attention. She explains that it is beneficial if we are feeling unfulfilled and we need to examine what may be holding us back from moving forward.[41]

Worwood suggests that sweet fennel oil helps bring the light of solution into the shadows of difficulty, and its extraordinary power boosts our spirituality and recharges our physical and mental bodies. She explains that this subtle strength clears and purifies the auric field of people and the environment beyond, giving protection from outside influences.[42]

F

Dosage and Administration

Blending

Aromatherapy

For the relief of indigestion, consider blending sweet fennel oil with essential oils such as black pepper, coriander seed, ginger, sweet marjoram, sweet orange, peppermint or spearmint.

For the relief of spasms and pain associated with dysmenorrhoea, consider blending sweet fennel oil with essential oils such as clary sage, geranium, ginger, lavender, sweet marjoram or rose.

To create a detoxifying blend, consider blending sweet fennel oil with essential oils such as coriander seed, juniper berry, grapefruit, lemon or rosemary.

For the relief of cough and mucous congestion associated with a cold, consider blending sweet fennel oil with essential oils such as cajeput, Atlas cedarwood, peppermint eucalyptus, 1,8-cineole-rich eucalypts, fragonia, ginger, myrtle, niaouli or thyme.

Perfumery

Sweet fennel oil is sometimes used for chypre and fougère style perfumes; however, it is more commonly used in flavour work for liqueurs, candy and cough lozenges.[1]

Mode of administration

Bath

Full body bath, foot bath

Topical

Compress, massage, ointment

Inhalation

Direct inhalation, diffuser, oil vaporiser

Ingestion

For digestive complaints, the German Commission E recommends 10 to 20 g of fennel honey syrup which is made with 0.5 g fennel oil/kg.[10]

However, oral use of fennel oil in children is not recommended.[5,10] Also, ingestion of fennel oil for a prolonged period is not recommended unless otherwise advised by a physician or pharmacist.[10]

Safety Profile

General safety

Sweet and bitter fennel seed oils are often contraindicated for use by people suffering from epilepsy or during pregnancy.[7,34]

I have a suspicion that some aromatherapists may be concerned about the fenchone content which is a ketone. As we know, some ketones are reputed to be neurotoxic. There is no pharmacological evidence to suggest that fenchone or *trans*-anethole are neurotoxic in the doses used in aromatherapy.[43] Bitter fennel oil may cause sensitisation in some individuals.[10,34,43]

An epileptic seizure was reported in a 38-year-old woman, a known epileptic patient who was under treatment and had well-controlled epilepsy. It was reported that she developed a generalised tonic-clonic seizure and remained unconscious for 45 minutes following the ingestion of a number of cakes containing an unknown quantity of fennel essential oil. The authors concluded that fennel essential oil can induce seizures and should be avoided by patients with epilepsy.[44]

Contraindications

Tisserand & Young state that bitter and sweet fennel seed oils are contraindicated during pregnancy, breastfeeding, endometriosis, oestrogen-dependent cancers, and for children under five years of age.[45]

The German Commission E states that bitter fennel seed oil should not be used during pregnancy or for infants and toddlers.[10]

The German Commission E also advised that, unless otherwise advised by a physician or pharmacist, one should not consume fennel oil internally for an extended period (several weeks).[10] It also advises that fennel oil is not recommended orally for young children. The EMA report states that the oral use of fennel oil in children and adolescents under 18 years of age is contraindicated.[4]

Tisserand & Young caution against oral administration of sweet or bitter fennel seed oils in the following circumstances – people taking anticoagulant drugs such as aspirin, heparin and warfarin, haemophilia, peptic ulcer, internal bleeding, severe hepatic or renal impairment, hypertensive or diabetic retinopathy – as it is likely to inhibit blood coagulation.[45]

Regulatory guidelines

Bitter fennel seed is not included in the listing of the FDA or FEMA. Sweet fennel seed oil has GRAS status and is approved by the FDA for food use.[46]

References

1. Arctander S. *Perfume and flavor materials of natural origin.* Allured Publishing, Carol Stream, 1994.
2. Khan I, Abourashed E. *Leung's encyclopedia of common natural ingredients used in food, drugs and cosmetics.* 3rd edn. John Wiley & Sons, New Jersey, 2010.
3. Lawrence BM. *Progress in essential oils – sweet fennel oil and extract.* Perfumer & Flavorist, Feb 25, 2016.
4. Committee on Herbal Medicinal Products (HMPC), *Assessment report on Foeniculum vulgare Miller.* European Medicines Agency, London, 2008. Doc. ref: EMEA/HMPC/137426/2006.
5. Schmidt E, Wanner J. *Adulteration of essential oils.* In Baser KHC, Buchbauer G. eds. *Handbook of essential oils – science, technology and applications.* 2nd edn. CRC Press, Boca Raton, 2016: 707-745.
6. Grieve M. *A modern herbal – Vol. 1.* Dover Publications, New York, 1971.
7. Davis P. *Aromatherapy: an A-Z.* 2nd edn. C.W. Daniel Company, Saffron Walden, 1999.
8. Le Strange R. *A history of herbal plants.* Angus and Robertson, United Kingdom, 1977.
9. Bone K, Mills S. *Principles and practice of phytotherapy.* 2nd edn. Churchill Livingstone, Edinburgh, 2013.
10. Blumenthal M et al. *The complete German commission E monographs: therapeutic guide to herbal medicine.* American Botanical Council, Austin, 1998.
11. *WHO monographs on selected medicinal plants – Vol. 3.* World Health Organization, Geneva, 2007.
12. Ozbek H et al. *Evaluation of median lethal dose and analgesic activity of Foeniculum vulgare Miller essential oil.* International Journal of Pharmacology. 2006; 2(2): 181-183. Cited in Quintessential Aromatics database, 2013.
13. El-Soud NA et al. *Antidiabetic activities of Foeniculum vulgare Mill.* Macedonian Journal of Medical Sciences, 2011; 4(2): 139-146. Cited in Quintessential Aromatics database, 2013.
14. Mostafa DM et al. *Transdermal nanoemulsions of Foeniculum vulgare Mill. essential oil: preparation, characterization and evaluation of antidiabetic potential.* Journal of Drug Delivery Science and Technology, 2015; 29: 99-106. Cited in Quintessential Aromatics database, 2013.
15. Patra M et al. *Utilization of essential oil as natural antifungal against nail-infective fungi.* Flavour and Fragrance Journal, 2002; 17(2): 91-94. Cited in Quintessential Aromatics database, 2013.
16. Zeng H et al. *In vitro antifungal activity and mechanism of essential oil from fennel (Foeniculum vulgare L.) on dermatophyte species.* Journal of Medical Microbiology, 2015; 64(1): 93-103. Cited in Quintessential Aromatics database, 2013.
17. Lis-Balchin M. *Aromatherapy science – a guide for healthcare professionals.* Pharmaceutical Press, London, 2006.
18. Mahboubi A et al. *Antimicrobial activity of rosemary, fennel and galbanum essential oils against clinical isolates of Staphylococcus aureus.* Biharean Biologist, 2011; 5(1): 4-7. Cited in Quintessential Aromatics database, 2013.
19. Shahat AA et al. *Chemical composition, antimicrobial and antioxidant activities of essential oils from organically cultivated fennel cultivars.* Molecules, 2011; 16(2): 1366-1377. Cited in Quintessential Aromatics database, 2013.
20. Singh G et al. *Chemical constituents, antifungal and antioxidant potential of Foeniculum vulgare volatile oil and its acetone extract.* Food Control, 2006; 17(9): 745-752. Cited in Quintessential Aromatics database, 2013.
21. Saleh MM et al. *Volatile oil of Egyptian sweet fennel (Foeniculum vulgare var. dulce, Alef.) and its effects on isolated smooth muscles.* Pharmaceutical & Pharmacological Letters, 1996; 6(1): 5-7. Cited in the Aromatherapy Database, by Bob Harris, Essential Oil Resource Consultants, UK, 2000.
22. Boskabady MH et al. *Possible mechanism(s) for relaxant effects of Foeniculum vulgare on guinea pig tracheal chains.* Pharmazie, 2004; 59(7):

F

561-564. Cited in Quintessential Aromatics database, 2013.
23. Ostad SN et al. *The effect of fennel essential oil on uterine contraction as a model for dysmenorrhoea pharmacology and toxicology study*. Journal of Ethnopharmacology, 2001; 76(3): 299-304. Cited in Quintessential Aromatics database, 2013.
24. Nagai H et al. *Effects of odor on humans (II): Reducing effects of mental stress and fatigue*. Chemical Senses, 1991; 16(2): 198. Cited in Quintessential Aromatics database, 2013.
25. Rangelov A. *An experimental characterisation of cholagogic and cholesteric activity of a group of essential oils*. Folia Medica, 1989; 31(1): 46-53. Cited in the Aromatherapy Database, by Bob Harris, Essential Oil Resource Consultants, 2000.
26. Rangelov A et al. *Experimental study of the cholagogic and choleretic action of some of the basic ingredients of essential oils on laboratory animals*. Folia Medica, 1988; 30(4): 30-38. Cited in the Aromatherapy Database, by Bob Harris, Essential Oil Resource Consultants, 2000.
27. Namavar JB et al. *Comparison of fennel and mefenamic acid for the treatment of primary dysmenorrhea*. International Journal of Gynaecology and Obstetrics, 2003; 80(2): 153-157. Cited in Quintessential Aromatics database, 2013.
28. Khorshidi N et al. *Clinical effects of fennel essential oil on primary dysmenorrhoea*. Iranian Journal of Pharmaceutical Research, 2003; 2(2): 89-93. Cited in Quintessential Aromatics database, 2013.
29. Őzebek H et al. *Hepatoprotective effect of Foeniculum vulgare essential oil*. Fitoterapia, 2003; 74(3): 317-319. Cited in Quintessential Aromatics database, 2013.
30. Alexandrovich I et al. *The effect of fennel (Foeniculum vulgare) seed oil emulsion in infantile colic: a randomised placebo-controlled study*. Alternative Therapies, 2003; 9(4): 58-61. Cited in Quintessential Aromatics database, 2013.
31. Pitasawat B et al. *Aromatic plant-derived essential oil: an alternative larvicide for mosquito control*. Fitoterapia, 2007; 78(3): 205-210. Cited in Quintessential Aromatics database, 2013.
32. Rana IS, Rana AS. *Efficacy of essential oils of aromatic plants as larvicide for the management of filarial vector Culex quinquefasciatus with special reference to Foeniculum vulgare*. Asian Pacific Journal of Tropical Disease, 2012; 2(3): 184-189. Cited in Quintessential Aromatics database, 2013.
33. Balacs T. *Hormones and health*. The International Journal of Aromatherapy, 1993; 5(1): 18.
34. Lawless J. *The encyclopaedia of essential oils*. Element Books, Shaftesbury, 1992.
35. Lavabre M. *Aromatherapy workbook*. Healing Arts Press, Rochester, 1997.
36. Mojay G. *Aromatherapy for healing the spirit*. Healing Arts Press, Rochester, 1999.
37. Holmes P. *The energetics of Western herbs – Vol. I*. Artemis Press, Boulder, 1986.
38. Worwood VA. *The fragrant mind*. Transworld Publishers, London, 1995.
39. Davis P. *Subtle aromatherapy*. C.W. Daniel Company, Saffron Walden, 1991.
40. Keim Loughran J, Bull R. *Aromatherapy anointing oils*. Frog, Berkeley, 2001.
41. Zeck R. *The blossoming heart – aromatherapy for healing and transformation*. Aroma Tours, East Ivanhoe, 2004.
42. Worwood VA. *The fragrant heavens*. Transworld Publishers, London, 1999.
43. Tisserand R, Balacs T. *Essential oil safety*. Churchill Livingstone, Edinburgh, 1995.
44. Skalli S, Bencheikh RS. *Epileptic seizure induced by fennel essential oil*. Epileptic Disorders, 2011; 13(3): 345-347. Cited in Quintessential Aromatics database, 2013.
45. Tisserand R, Young R. *Essential oil safety*. 2nd edn. Churchill Livingstone, Edinburgh, 2014.
46. Opdyke DLJ. *Monographs on fragrance raw materials*. Pergamon Press, Oxford, 1979.

F

Fir needle

Identification

Botanical name

There are many oils distilled from the twigs and needles of various species of the conifer family, which are commonly called fir needle oil. It is very important to know the specific botanical name. The most common fir needle oils used in aromatherapy are:

Canadian fir needle: *Abies balsamea* (L.) Mill.

Silver fir needle: *Abies alba* Mill.

Siberian fir needle: *Abies sibirica* Ledeb.

Japanese fir needle: *Abies sachalinensis* (F. Schmidt) Mast.

Synonyms

Canadian fir needle: balsam fir, fir balsam

Silver fir needle: white fir, silver spruce, white

spruce

Siberian fir needle: Russian fir, Siberian silver fir

Japanese fir needle: Japanese pine needle, Sakhalin fir

Family

Pinaceae

Botany and origins

Abies alba is a relatively small tree which grows in Austria, eastern France, Germany, Poland, Russia and Canada. The tree is planted in many European countries for lumber, wood pulp and Christmas trees.[1]

Lawrence states that over the centuries the *Abies alba* species has been reduced because of overexploitation, deforestation and afforestation with faster growing species. Recently, forest management practices across Europe have arrested this decline.[2]

Siberian fir needle oil is considered one of the most popular fir needle oils in Europe and the USA. Japanese fir needle oil is also called pine needle oil.[1]

Method of extraction

Fir needle oils are produced from the steam distillation from the leaves and twigs of various *Abies* species.

Characteristics

A. alba needle oil is a colourless to pale yellow liquid with a rich balsamic-sweet and pleasant coniferous fragrance.[1]

A. sibirica needle oil is a colourless to very pale or olive yellow oily liquid with a refreshing balsamic, slightly fatty or oily aroma, a powerful pine-forest scent and a peculiar fruity-balsamic undertone.[1]

Guenther states that *A. alba* essential oil is the most delightful and has the most pleasant aroma of all the pine, spruce and fir oils. He describes *A. alba* oil as having the characteristic scent reminiscent of sunny pine forests.[3]

Chemical composition

The chemical composition of *A. alba* essential oil was reported as follows:

santene (2.3%), tricyclene (1.6%), α-pinene (26.4%), camphene (14.8%), β-pinene (3.6%), myrcene (1.1%), δ-3-carene (6.2%), limonene (26.3%), β-phellandrene (1.5%), terpinolene (0.3-0.7%), bornyl acetate (5.4%).[2]

Adulteration

A. alba needle oil is occasionally adulterated with Siberian fir needle oil, turpentine oil or with fractions of pinene.[1]

Pharmacopoeias and standards

The purity, composition and physico-chemical properties of Siberian fir essential oil are defined in ISO 10869:2010 Oil of Fir Needle, Siberian.

History and Traditional Uses

History

Fir pine trees exude a resin called fir balsam. This was used by Native Americans for medicinal and religious purposes.[3]

Traditional medicine

Guenther states that the oil has been traditionally used in inhalations for the treatment of colds and in preparations for the treatment of rheumatism.[3]

Herbal

The German Commission E recommends fir essential oil (*A. alba* Miller) for catarrhal illness of the upper and lower respiratory tract. It is also recommended externally for rheumatic and neuralgic pains.[4]

Food, perfumery and flavouring

A. alba oil is used in perfumes for bath preparations, air fresheners, disinfectants, colognes, soap perfumes and detergents.[1]

Therapeutics

Pharmacology and clinical studies

Antimicrobial activity

The antimicrobial properties of *A. alba* oil have been investigated, and it has been found to have moderate activity to very little activity.[5]

A study confirmed that *Abies balsamea* oil was inactive against *Escherichia coli* but active against *Staphylococcus aureus*.[6]

Antitumour activity

Balsam fir needle oil was found to be active against several solid tumour cells. All the individual components of the oil were tested and all were inactive except for α-humelene. Balsam fir oil and α -humulene were evaluated on cellular glutathione content and on the production of reactive oxygen species.[7]

Insecticidal activity

Silver fir needle oil was highly repellent to mosquitos. Fruit flies were killed by essential oils of Douglas fir and silver fir.[8]

Stress reduction activity

Siberian fir needle oil reduced arousal levels on

individuals who had been working on a task using a visual display terminal. It was suggested that the oil may be useful for preventing visual display terminal-related mental health disturbances.[9]

Actions

Actions commonly cited in aromatherapy

Analgesic, antiseptic, deodorant, expectorant, rubefacient, stimulant, tonic [10,11]

Actions supported by clinical studies

Analgesic, antiseptic, expectorant, insecticidal

Comment

Fir needle essential oils have a pleasant fresh conifer and green note that may be beneficial for improving mood and reducing the symptoms of stress-induced disorders such as anxiety and depression.

There is a lack of clinical data for many of the therapeutic uses of fir needle oil in aromatherapy; however, Holmes describes Siberian fir as a nerve restorative and a pituitary-adrenal restorative.[12]

Schnaubelt explains that the chemical profile of many of the conifer needle essential oils may help us understand why they may have such properties. He explains that they have a balance of stimulating monoterpene and calming esters. He suggests that they contain hormone-mimicking, polycyclic terpenoid compounds and states that they are endocrine tonics, re-establishing hormonal balance in the pituitary, thyroid, adrenals and ovaries.[13]

F

Aromatherapy Uses

Clinical aromatherapy

Musculoskeletal system

Fir needle oil is recommended for the relief of muscular aches and pains due to rheumatism or arthritic conditions.[4,10,11]

Nervous system

Fir needle oil is recommended for alleviating anxiety and stress.[10]

Holmes suggests that Siberian fir needle oil is a pituitary-adrenal restorative, and recommends the oil for adrenal fatigue, exhaustion and low stamina. He also describes Siberian fir oil as a nervous system restorative, and recommends using the oil for mental and physical fatigue, neurasthenia, debility and depression.[12]

Psychological

Holmes states that Siberian fir needle oil promotes motivation and self-confidence. The oil is recommended when we experience loss of motivation with apathy, and when we experience low self-esteem and self-confidence. Siberian fir oil is ideal for the person who is chronically discouraged and lacks the will, motivation or stamina to preserve in the face of life's challenges.[12]

Respiratory system

Fir needle oil is recommended for catarrhal illness of the upper and lower respiratory tract.[10,11]

Fir needle oil has a strong affinity for strengthening the respiratory system. It is considered to have a restorative, decongestant and relaxant effect on the lungs and bronchi.[12]

It is best used in chronic respiratory conditions typified by weak lungs, phlegm congestion and bronchial spasm. Holmes suggests that the exceptionally high levels of bornyl acetate are responsible for the oil's exceptional antispasmodic effect on the respiratory system.[12]

However, the German Commission E states that fir needle oil is contraindicated for bronchial asthma and whooping cough, as bronchospasms can be increased.[4]

Energetics, psyche and subtle uses

Energetics

Siberian fir needle oil tonifies and regulates the *Qi*, strengthens the *Shen*, warms the *Lungs* and dispels *wind-cold*.[12]

Whenever we have *Qi deficiency* with weak *Shen*, we may experience physical and mental fatigue and we have low vitality and stamina. Whenever *wind-cold* invade the body, we may experience, aches and pains, sore throat, sinus congestion and fatigue.[12]

According to the principles of the Five Elements, it has a strong affinity with the Metal and Water Elements.[12]

Subtle

Holmes states that the aroma of Siberian fir needle oil bestows strength and vitality to the soul.[12]

Fir needle oil is said to encourage protection, clarity of mind and spirit. It allows us to achieve strength and inner unity.[14] It is considered elevating and grounding and is recommended for the third eye and crown chakras.[10]

Keim Loughran & Bull state that fir needle oil teaches us to release energy blocks caused by unbalanced emotions. They recommend using it whenever we experience strong emotions that make us feel ungrounded, or when we are afraid of what we are feeling.[15]

Dosage and Administration

Blending

Aromatherapy

For relief of bronchitis with cough, consider blending fir needle oils with essential oils such as aniseed, cajeput, cypress, peppermint eucalyptus, 1,8-cineole-rich eucalypts, niaouli, pine, ravintsara or spruce.

For the relief of muscular aches and pains, consider blending fir needle oils with essential oils such as cajeput, ginger, kunzea, spike lavender, peppermint or rosemary.

As a nervous system restorative, consider blending fir needle oils with essential oils such as bergamot, coriander seed, fragonia, lavender, lemon, cold-pressed lime or rosemary.

Perfumery

Siberian fir oil blends well with other pine or fir needle oils, oakmoss absolute, citrus oils, rosemary oil, juniper berry, patchouli, and lavender essential oils.[1]

Arctander states that *A. alba* oil is used in perfumes for bath preparations, air fresheners, disinfectants, fougère style colognes, soap perfumes and detergents. He explains that it blends well with galbanum, cistus, lavender, oakmoss absolute and rosemary essential oils.[1]

Mode of administration

Bath

Full body bath, foot bath

Topical

Compress, massage, ointment

Inhalation

Direct inhalation, diffuser, oil vaporiser

Safety Profile

General safety

Fir needle oil has been reported to be non-toxic, non-irritant and non-sensitising.[11]

It is prone to oxidation because of its high monoterpene hydrocarbon content. Skin sensitisation may occur if the oil is oxidised.[16]

Contraindications

The German Commission E states that fir needle oil is contraindicated for bronchial asthma and whooping cough, as it increases bronchial spasms.[4]

Regulatory guidelines

Siberian fir needle oil has GRAS status.

References

1. Arctander S. *Perfume and flavor materials of natural origin.* Allured Publishing, Carol Stream, 1994.
2. Lawrence BM. *Progress in essential oils: Silver fir or Abies alba oil.* Perfumer & Flavorist, 2017; 42(3): 50-57.
3. Guenther E. *The essential oils – Vol. VI.* Robert E Krieger Publishing, Malabar, 1952.
4. Blumenthal M et al. *The complete German commission E monographs: therapeutic guide to herbal medicine.* The American Botanical Council, Austin, 1998.
5. Bağci E, Diğrak M. *Antimicrobial activity of essential oils of some Abies (fir) species from Turkey.* Flavour and Fragrance Journal, 1996; 11(4): 251-256.
6. Pichette A et al. *Composition and antibacterial activity of Abies balsamea essential oil.* Phytotherapy Research, 2006; 20(5): 371-373. Cited in Quintessential Aromatics database, 2003.
7. Legault J et al. *Antitumor activity of balsam fir oil: production of reactive oxygen species induced by α-humulene as possible mechanism of action.* Planta Medica, 2003; 69(5): 402-407. Cited in Quintessential Aromatics database, 2013.
8. Gora J et al. *The possibilities of essential oils utilisation for the limitation of some insect populations or their repellency.* Programme Abstracts – 24th International Symposium on Essential Oils, 1993. Cited in Quintessential Aromatics database, 2013.
9. Matsubara E et al. *The essential oil of Abies sibirica (Pinaceae) reduces arousal levels after visual display terminal work.* Flavour and Fragrance Journal, 2011; 26(3): 204-210. Cited in Quintessential Aromatics database, 2013.
10. Lavabre M. *Aromatherapy workbook.* Healing Arts Press, Rochester, 1997.
11. Lawless J. *The encyclopaedia of essential oils.* Element Books, Shaftesbury, 1992.
12. Holmes P. *Aromatica: a clinical guide to essential oil therapeutics – Vol. I.* Singing Dragon, London, 2016.
13. Schnaubelt K. *Advanced aromatherapy.* Healing Arts Press, Rochester, 1995.
14. Worwood VA. *The fragrant heavens.* Transworld Publishing, London, 1999.
15. Keim Loughran J, Bull R. *Aromatherapy anointing oils.* Frog, Berkeley, 2001.
16. Tisserand R, Young R. *Essential oil safety.* 2nd edn. Churchill Livingstone, Edinburgh, 2014.

F

Fragonia

Identification

Botanical name

Agonis fragrans JR Wheeler & NG Marchant

Synonyms

Coarse tea tree

Family

Myrtaceae

Botany and origins

Agonis fragrans is a relatively new oil from Australia. It was first introduced to aromatherapists in 2006. It occurs naturally in the southwestern region of Western Australia. It is a small shrub growing up to 2.5 m. It is also referred to as 'coarse tea-tree' by the cut-flower industry.[1]

There is more than one chemotype; however, the Agriculture Department of Western Australia and John Day (grower and distiller) have determined the best chemotype for use. This specific chemotype is now used in aromatherapy and has been trademarked as fragonia essential oil.[1]

In 2001, The Paperbark Co. established a plantation of *A. fragrans* that is now producing, promoting and selling increasing quantities of the oil.[2] John and Peta Day explain that they chose the name fragonia with great care, and think it reflects not only the botanical name, *Agonis fragrans*, but also its beautiful characteristics and the gentle fragrance of the foliage and oil.[3]

Method of extraction

Fragonia oil is produced by steam distillation from *A. fragrans.*

Characteristics

Fragonia oil has a soft, clean, refreshing and delicate camphoraceous aroma, with a hint of a citrus note and a sweet balsamic undertone.[4]

Chemical composition

The chemical composition of fragonia essential oil was reported as follows:

α-pinene (21-27%), β-pinene (1.5-1.7%), myrcene (1.4-2.2%), limonene (2.4-2.5%), α-terpinene (1.3-3.3%), *p*-cymene (2.2-2.9%), 1,8-cineole (29-32.5%), linalool (11.7-12.4%), terpinen-4-ol (3.7-4.3%), α-terpineol (5.4-7.6%), myrtenol (3.1-4.5%), geraniol (0.5-1.2%).[1]

Adulteration

It is unlikely that fragonia oil is subject to adulteration.

Pharmacopoeias and standards

At the time of writing, the purity, composition, physico-chemical properties and therapeutic use of fragonia essential oil are not defined in any pharmacopoeia monograph or standard.

History and Traditional Uses

History

A. fragrans essential oil is a relatively new oil to the aromatherapy scene. The species itself was only described in 2001 and there is no scientific data on its chemistry and uses prior to this.

Therapeutics

Pharmacology and clinical studies

Anti-inflammatory activity

In vitro studies conducted by the School of Paediatrics and Child Health at the University of Western Australia found that fragonia oil inhibited secretion of cytokine interferon (IFN) γ production by mononuclear cells. INFγ and other pro-inflammatory cytokines are involved in the pathogenesis of inflammation, autoimmune disease and atopic dermatitis. This suggests that fragonia oil may be involved in inflammatory response to tissue injury or infection. The authors, however, recommended more studies to test this.[2]

Antimicrobial activity

The antimicrobial activity of fragonia oil was just as effective as tea tree according to research at the University of Western Australia.[2]

The MIC for fragonia are similar to other well-known antimicrobial oils such as tea tree (*Melaleuca alternifolia*), lemongrass (*Cymbopogon citratus*) and oregano (*Origanum vulgare*).[1]

Actions

Actions commonly cited in aromatherapy

Analgesic, anti-inflammatory, antimicrobial, antiseptic, decongestant, expectorant, immune stimulant[1,5,6]

Actions supported by clinical studies

While further studies are required, I am confident that the clinical studies will support the actions commonly cited in aromatherapy.

Comment

Pénoël states that when we look closely at the

chemical profile of fragonia, there are three main constituent molecular groups:

- monoterpenes – α-pinene, β-pinene, myrcene, limonene, *p*-cymene and α-terpinene
- oxides – 1,8-cineole
- monoterpenols – linalool, terpinen-4-ol, α-terpineol and myrtenol.[5]

These three main molecular groups are present in *A. fragrans* in an almost perfect proportional balance of one third each. Pénöel suggests that this makes fragonia a truly unique essential oil because of the perfectly balanced ratio of monoterpene hydrocarbons, oxides and monoterpene alcohols. He refers to fragonia as the 'golden triangle' – the symbol of balance and harmony.[5]

This is rare as many essential oils usually have one dominant group of compounds. The balanced chemical composition contributes to the oil's most pleasant aroma and diverse healing properties.

Aromatherapy Uses

Clinical aromatherapy

Analgesic

Testimonial and case studies have demonstrated the benefits of fragonia oil to relieve pain associated with arthritis and relief of muscular and joint pain within a short time of topical application. Guba states that the *p*-cymene may contribute to this effect.[1]

However, Pénöel states that there are other essential oils that have a higher percentage of *p*-cymene but do not have the same analgesic effect as fragonia. Therefore, it is likely that the analgesic action of fragonia is due to the synergistic actions of many constituents.[5]

Anti-inflammatory

An in vitro study found that fragonia oil inhibited secretion of the interferon involved in the inflammatory response to tissue injury or infection, which suggests that the oil has anti-inflammatory properties.[1,6]

Expectorant

The 1,8-cineole content makes fragonia oil an excellent expectorant, and the oil is indicated for respiratory conditions with infection and congestion.[1]

Pénöel has reported great success in treating the respiratory system with fragonia oil. It has been suggested that the monoterpenols provide antimicrobial action upon most common bacteria, while the 1,8-cineole aids the breakup of mucous secretions.[5]

Immune stimulant

Anecdotal experiences with clients reported by Pénöel suggest that fragonia oil has immune-enhancing properties. Pénöel recommends using it topically to areas of lymph nodes (neck, groin and armpits) or to larger areas of the body, such as the abdomen and back, in a 'perfusion' treatment.[1,4]

Infections

Fragonia oil is considered to be an excellent remedy for topical infections such as acne or impetigo, fungal infections such as tinea, and viral infections such as cold sores.[1]

Psychological

Once you smell fragonia you will understand what Pénöel means when he explains that the oil has a deeply calming influence on our psyche:

> *The calm feeling that you obtain is different from the effect of taking a synthetic medication ... Its power comes from its capacity to create inner peace and establish harmony from within. We live in a crazy world of constant acceleration and the disease of 'more, more, more ...' cuts us off from true meaning of life.*[5]

Fragonia induces a profound feeling of calmness and tranquillity and a genuine feeling of serenity. Pénöel also explains that fragonia oil induces a far better quality of sleep. He refers to his personal experience using fragonia:

> *Sometimes we have to go to bed very late because of too much work to finish; the use of fragonia does improve the depth and the relaxing effect of the sleep, so that in the morning there is no feeling of being tired because of too little sleep.*[5]

Guba explains that fragonia oil has a gentle, calming effect on the mind:

> *The experience of 'making peace' seems particularly reserved for those actually dealing with constrained, blocked emotions and in this case, Fragonia does appear to act as a gentle 'helper' in loosening these emotional issues for inspection and release.*[1]

Energetics, psyche and subtle uses

Energetics

The energetic qualities of fragonia oil are *cooling*. It is primarily indicated for conditions of a *hot* and inflammatory nature.

Personality

According to Myers-Briggs personality types, the fragonia personality is likely to be an INFP. INFPs are gentle, calm, easygoing and affirming. Integrity and commitment to what they believe in are essential. They like time alone for their many interests. They like learning and researching new

F

things and interests. They are highly reflective, especially in understanding the mysteries and meaning of life. They have little need to impose their values on others. They prefer to gently influence and inspire. They value authenticity and depth in their relationships.

Subtle

Zeck best describes the subtle qualities of fragonia oil when she states that fragonia is like a candle carrying the light of dignity, nurturing the spirit, and helping you to come to terms and resolve any past traumas and unresolved family issues. Fragonia gently helps remove scars from past emotional pain. She explains that it helps you build resilience and that it carries a unique energy pattern, bringing the gift of the power of love. Fragonia calls you to that place in your higher consciousness where you are connected to something far greater than yourself. It helps you become more resilient, allowing you to celebrate life despite any illness, disease or emotional discomfort.[7]

Fragonia oil allows us to see with new eyes, experience profound insight, change our perspective and attitude, or receive a vision. Fragonia helps us master the third eye chakra. It helps us to keep our mind focused on related issues, including the awareness of the benefits to be gained from transcending the purely physical world and opening ourselves up to intuitive sight and wisdom: the ability to learn from experience and emotional intelligence.[7]

F

Dosage and Administration

Blending

Aromatherapy

Fragonia oil's clean, fresh, delicate, camphoraceous aroma means that it can easily complement most other essential oils. Fragonia oil blends well with very strong scented oils as well as delicate, light floral oils.

For the relief of muscular aches and pains, consider blending fragonia oil with essential oils such as black pepper, cajeput, peppermint eucalyptus, ginger, kunzea, lavender, manuka, pine or rosemary.

For the relief of symptoms associated with colds and flu, consider blending fragonia oil with essential oils such as cajeput, 1,8-cineole-rich eucalypts, spike lavender, manuka, peppermint, tea tree or thyme ct. linalool.

For the relief of anxiety, nervous tension and stress, consider blending fragonia oil with essential oils such as bergamot, clary sage, geranium, lavender, neroli or sandalwood.

Perfumery

Fragonia is not commonly used in perfumery.

Mode of administration

Bath

Full body bath, foot bath

Topical

Compress, massage, ointment, skin care

Inhalation

Direct inhalation, diffuser, oil vaporiser

Safety Profile

General safety

The overall composition of fragonia oil means that it is a safe and non-toxic essential oil. It is safe for use on children, the elderly and during pregnancy. It should be well tolerated on the skin and may even be used undiluted.[1]

Contraindications

No contraindications known.

Regulatory guidelines

Fragonia oil is not defined in any regulatory guideline.

References

1. Guba R. *A new Australian native – fragonia essential oil.* Essential News, Vol. 20, 2008.
2. Robinson C. *A new essential oil, Agonis fragrans: chemotype selection and evaluation.* Rural Industries Research and Development Corporation, RIRDC Publication No 06/090, Kingston, 2006.
3. Day J, Day P. *Fragonia – the oil for the new millennium.* Aromatherapy Today, 2006; 36: 8-11.
4. *Fragonia – an overview,* The Paperbark Co, 2008.
5. Pénoël D. *Fragonia – the latest promising aromatic gift from Australia.* Aromatherapy Today, 2006; 36: 12-18.
6. Wallwork K. *Fragonia essential oil.* Aromatherapy Today, 2006; 36: 4-7.
7. Zeck R. *The blossoming heart – aromatherapy for healing and transformation.* Aroma Tours, East Ivanhoe, 2004.

Frankincense

Identification

Botanical name

Boswellia spp.

Synonyms

Olibanum

Family

Burseraceae

Botany and origins

Frankincense, also known as olibanum, is a natural oleo-gum-resin formed from the physiological exudate from the bark of various *Boswellia* species. For many years there has been so much confusion and little clarity about the various types of frankincense.

The most commonly used species are:

- *Boswellia sacra:* from Oman, Yemen and southern Saudi Arabia
- *Boswellia carterii* Birdwood: from Somalia
- *Boswellia frereana* Birdwood: from Somalia
- *Boswellia papyrifera:* from western Ethiopia
- *Boswellia serrata:* from western India.[1]

The trees originate from the mountainous areas of western India, southern Arabia and northeastern Africa. The trees are not cultivated, and the collection of the resin is made where the trees are most abundant. Nowadays the major frankincense producing countries are Somalia, Yemen, India and Ethiopia.[2,3]

Tisserand & Young suggests that *B. carterii* and *B. sacra* are the same plant; however, this has been disputed by some.[3]

DeCarlo states that there are two types of *Boswellia* that grow in Somalia – *Boswellia sacra* (syn *B. carterii*) and *Boswellia frereana*.[4]

It appears that *B. frereana* originated in Somalia, with small amounts coming from Oman. *B. papyrifera* is found in Eritrea, Yemen, India, Ethiopia, Kenya and Somalia. Tisserand & Young state that the frankincense oils with higher α-pinene levels (50-80%) probably indicate *B. frereana*, while lower concentrations (10-50%) indicate *B. sacra*. They state that there may also be a α-thujene chemotype for *B. sacra*.[3]

It is reported that the best frankincense occurs on trees growing in the narrow strip of Oman's desert plateau that borders the mountains of the former South Yemen, where the trees have ideal soil conditions and tropical sun, accompanied by heavy dew from the monsoons.[4]

The Arabic name for *B. sacra* includes numerous variants of *mogar*, whereas the Somali name is *mohar* and the most common name is *mohar madow*. In Somali, *B. frereana* is called *yagar*.[5]

Most of the resin is produced from *B. papyrifera.* However, there is very little oil in the resin of this species, so it is not commonly used for producing frankincense essential oil.[3]

The oleo-gum-resin is tapped from an incision made on the trunk of the tree. A milky-white liquid appears, which then solidifies into amber or orange-brown crystals of resin. The gum resin is then graded according to flavour, colour, shape and size. The age, appearance, moisture level and odour characteristics determine the quality of the oil.[6]

The method for harvesting frankincense has not changed much in the past several thousand years. Incisions are made in the bark of the trunk or branches, where the secretory tissues occur; the resin exudes and is collected when it hardens sufficiently.[5]

Cropwatch lists several *Boswellia* species that are listed in the IUCN Red List of Threatened Species 2008. *B. sacra* is the only frankincense species on the list which is of commercial importance.[7]

F

Method of extraction

Frankincense essential oil is produced from the steam distillation of the resin of various *Boswellia* species. A resinoid absolute of frankincense is also produced for the perfume industry by solvent extraction.[3]

Characteristics

The essential oil of *B. carterii* is colourless to yellowish-green or amber-green, with a diffusive, fresh-terpene-like, almost green-lemon-like aroma. It has a slight peppery note with a rich, sweet-woody, balsamic undertone.[2]

Lis-Balchin says that the scent of frankincense oil can be tenacious; however, this depends on the distillation procedure. It can also have a cistus-like, amber-type, balsamic dryout note.[8]

Chemical composition

The chemistry of frankincense oil is very complex. It has more than 20 monoterpenes and 28 sesquiterpenes.

The chemical composition of *Boswellia serrata* oil from India was reported as follows:

α-thujene (71.74%), α-pinene (5.22%), thuja-2,4(10)-diene (0.4%), sabinene (5.2%), β-pinene (0.37%), myrcene (0.91%), α-phellandrene (2.24%), δ-3-carene (3.86%), α-terpinene (0.38%), limonene (1.64%), β -phellandrene (0.49%), *cis*-β-ocimene (0.6%), *p*-cymene (1.66%), *trans*-β-ocimene (0.27%), γ-terpinene (0.79%), terpinolene (0.26%), α-thujone (0.13%), terpinene-4-ol (0.67%), methyl chavicol (1.37%), β-bourbonene (0.32%), germacrene D (0.17%), valencene (0.13%), kessane (0.12%).[9]

The chemical composition of *Boswellia carterii* oil from Somalia was reported as follows:

α-thujene (trace – 10%), α-pinene (30-60%), sabinene (trace – 8%), β-pinene (trace – 14%), β- myrcene (trace – 10%), limonene (2-15%), viridiflorol (trace - 10%).[10]

Adulteration

Frankincense oil is subject to frequent adulteration. The residue from the distillation of frankincense oil is subject to hydrocarbon solvent extraction to yield an 'olibanum resin'. This resin has no commercial value as it is odourless; however, it is frequently used as a cutting ingredient in frankincense essential oil. It improves the fixative value of the oil but it impairs the odour of the oil.[2]

Pharmacopoeias and standards

At the time of writing, the purity, composition, physico-chemical properties and therapeutic use of frankincense essential oil are not defined in any pharmacopoeia monograph or standard.

Frankincense gum appears in the WHO Monograph as Gummi *Boswellii/Boswellia serrata* and the European Pharmacopoeia Monograph – #2310 Indian frankincense as *Olibanum indicum*.

History and Traditional Uses

History

The name olibanum is thought to be derived from Latin, *olium libanum*, meaning oil from Lebanon. The name frankincense is derived from the old French word *franc*, meaning free, pure or abundant, and Latin *incensum*, meaning to smoke.[11]

Frankincense played a very important role in the religious and domestic lives of ancient Egyptian, Persian, Hebrew, Greek and Roman civilisations. It has always been considered an important ingredient in cosmetics, as an aromatic incense and in religious rituals of these ancient civilisations.

Frankincense is believed to be part of the oldest global supply chain. The Nabataeans, an Arab tribe, monopolised the trade nearly 2,000 years ago and maintained their lucrative competitive advantage for more than five centuries.[4]

The Egyptians obtained frankincense from the land of Punt, believed to have been a region in Somalia. The famous *kyphi*, a renowned scent used by ancient Egypt, was made with frankincense. *Kyphi* was used as an incense and also added to beverages.[12]

In ancient Egypt, a dead king had to be perfumed with incense in order to be accepted by the gods. Incense was considered the scent of the gods and it was believed that acquiring the scent of incense, the king would affirm his basic identity with the gods.[13]

Kohl, a black powder used by Egyptian women to paint their eyelids, is made from charred frankincense.[14]

According to Pliny the Elder, in ancient times, frankincense could only be harvested by specially appointed families. The resin was considered to be divine and gatherers were restricted from impure acts during harvesting of the resin.[5]

By the Roman times, transport costs and the high demand for incense far exceeded the supply of frankincense and myrrh. Frankincense and myrrh were considered such precious commodities that their value was similar to that of gold.[15]

More than 3,000 tonnes of frankincense was imported by the Romans each year. By this stage the original sacred use of frankincense to honour the gods had been transmuted into extravagant, luxurious use for mortals. Nero was said to have burned so much frankincense at the funeral of his wife that it exhausted Arabia's supply for an entire year.[15]

Frankincense is regularly mentioned in the Bible:

> *Thy two breasts are like two young roes that are twins, which feed among the lilies.*
>
> *Until the day break, and the shadows flee away, I will get me to the mountain of myrrh, and to the hill of frankincense.*[16]
>
> Song of Solomon 4:5-4:6 (King James Version)

The most famous reference to frankincense is in the Bible when it was given as a gift to the infant Jesus:

> *And when they came into the house, they saw the young child with Mary his mother, and fell down, and worshipped him: and when they opened their treasures, they presented unto him gifts; gold and frankincense and myrrh.*[16]
>
> Matthew 2:11 (King James Version)

Stoddart states that the burning of incense became very popular with the ancient Hebrews. The rituals associated with burning incense became increasingly complex, reaching their peak in the

F

temple of Herod, two decades before the birth of Christ. Incense was always burned when a burnt offering was prepared, most likely to also soften the harsh odour emanating from the slaughtered animals and burning flesh.[17]

Early Christians scorned the use of incense. Stoddart cites Lactantius who said that odours are not required by God and should not be offered to him. He explains there is little doubt that the revulsion that early Christians had to incense resulted from the heavy usage by the Jews; however, Christians soon began to use incense as a fumigant only for sanitary protection such as a burial or if a church building smelt particularly unwholesome.[17]

It is still used in many parts of the Arab world. For example, the Muslim inhabitants of the United Arab Emirates say that a dirty smelly body is vulnerable to evil; the scented person is surrounded by angels. They believe that the most useful scent for attracting angels and dispelling evil spirits is frankincense. For this reason, children, houses and mosques are censed weekly with frankincense.[18]

Traditional medicine

Holmes says that frankincense resin was a very valuable remedy in traditional Greek, Ayurveda and Chinese medicine. He says that Persian physician Ibn Sina (Avicenna) used frankincense for ulcers, tumours, fevers, dysentery and vomiting. In Ayurveda, frankincense is primarily used as a drying, astringent remedy for damp and *Kapha* conditions of the digestive, respiratory and urogenital organs.[19]

Indian frankincense, commonly referred to as *dhoop*, is considered one of the most valued herbs in Ayurveda. It was mainly used to treat arthritis, but also beneficial for diarrhoea, dysentery, ringworm, boils, fevers, skin and blood diseases, cardiovascular diseases, mouth sores, bronchitis, asthma, cough, vaginal discharges, hair loss, jaundice, haemorrhoids, irregular menses and stimulation of the liver.[6]

Herbal

Modern pharmacology suggests that the gum-resin extracts of *Boswellia serrata* have excellent antiarthritic, anti-inflammatory, analgesic and hepatoprotective properties.[20]

Food, perfumery and flavouring

Frankincense oil is used in fine perfumery in citrus-based perfumes, incense-like perfumes, oriental, floral and masculine perfumes.[2]

Therapeutics

Pharmacology and clinical studies

Many pharmacological studies involving frankincense oil have been published. A systemic review of these studies will not be attempted. Rather, I have chosen a selection of studies that support the traditional and clinical uses.

Anti-inflammatory activity

B. serrata is used in Ayurveda for treating inflammatory diseases. A number of researchers have investigated the anti-inflammatory and antiarthritic effects of the boswellic acids found in the gum. It is believed that the mechanism of action may occur via the inhibition of 5-lipoxygenase and leucite elastase. Both these enzymes play key roles in inflammatory and hypersensitivity-based diseases.[21]

Antimicrobial activity

Lis-Balchin says that frankincense's antibacterial effects are strong; however, it has poor antifungal effects.[8]

Several studies have confirmed that frankincense has pronounced activity against a range of bacteria.[22,23]

Antitumour activity

Almost all the research on frankincense and cancer is related to boswellic acid that can be found in the resin – not the essential oil. Frankincense extract contains about 50% boswellic acid, and there has been extensive research on the antitumoral activity of boswellic acid.[21,24]

Many researchers have identified boswellic acid found in the frankincense resin extract as having very strong anti-inflammatory and antitumor activity. Researchers found that more than 50% of myeloid leukaemia cells underwent apoptosis for 24 hours after treatment with 20 μg/mL boswellic acid isolated from *Boswellia carterii* resin.[25]

Another researcher examined the effects of acetyl-11-keto-β-boswellic acid (AKBA) on pancreatic cancer. The results of the study demonstrate that AKBA can suppress the growth and metastasis of human pancreatic tumours in an orthotopic nude mouse model that correlates with modulation of multiple targets.[26]

I believe that frankincense oil may not be as effective as we have made it out to be as it does not contain any boswellic acid. The herbal extract of frankincense gum would be more effective for this purpose as it contains the boswellic acids.

Boswellic acid is only found in the resin with no traces of it found in the essential oil. As Tisserand points out:

> *... boswellic acid is much too heavy a molecule to be volatile so it would be impossible to find it in the essential oil. Boswellic acid has a molecular weight in the range of 450-500. However volatile molecules all have molecular weight below 300.*[24]

It is irresponsible for anyone to claim that frankincense essential oil has antitumour activity as it does not contain any boswellic acid.

Bronchial asthma

Lis-Balchin cites a double-blind, placebo-controlled study in which bronchial asthma was reduced in 70% of 40 patients treated with the gum resin at 300 mg three times daily for six weeks.[8]

Immunostimulant

Frankincense oil exhibited a strong immunostimulant activity (90% lymphocyte transformation) when assessed by a lymphocyte proliferation assay.[27]

Actions

Actions commonly cited in aromatherapy

Analgesic, antidepressant, antiseptic, astringent, carminative, cicatrisant, cytophylactic, expectorant, sedative, vulnerary[11,28,29,30,31]

Actions supported by clinical studies

Antidepressant, antiseptic, expectorant, sedative

F

Comment

I agree with Lis-Balchin who states that, because there is so much variation in the chemical composition of frankincense depending on the source of the resin, it is very difficult to make generalisations about its bioactivity.[8]

Most of the pharmacological and clinical studies involving frankincense involve boswellic acid. Many of the therapeutic actions attributed to frankincense are due to the boswellic acid. As the essential oil does not contain any boswellic acid, we cannot confirm with confidence many of the aromatherapeutic properties that are often assigned to the essential oil.

Frankincense oil has always had a very special spiritual connection with humankind. The resin has been incorporated into the rituals and belief systems of many religions. The essential oil is often recommended to quieten the mind and assist in meditation, prayer and spiritual practices.

Aromatherapy Uses

Clinical aromatherapy

Immune system

Price & Price regard frankincense oil as being a very effective immunostimulant essential oil.[28]

Mojay states that frankincense strengthens the immune system and is especially useful in cases when the immune system is weakened because of stress and depression.[29]

Musculoskeletal system

Frankincense oil is recommended topically for the relief of joint pain and muscular aches and pains.[28]

Palliative care

Price & Price state that frankincense oil can be very helpful for palliative care. When we are confronted with our mortality, we may turn inwards and question our innermost thoughts, beliefs and values in an attempt to make sense of what is happening. Essential oils such as frankincense can provide spiritual support, bringing comfort and peace in the form of deep relaxation. This allows patients to focus on their spirituality.[28]

Psychological

Price & Price state that frankincense oil is well known for its effects on the human psyche and it is recognised as being beneficial for nervous depression.[28] Mojay states that frankincense's most important sphere of action is the nervous system. He explains that it is able to relax and yet revitalise, making it excellent for treating both nervous tension and nervous exhaustion. He refers to frankincense as an important essential oil for alleviating depression.[29]

Frankincense oil has been recommended for nervous tension, stress-related conditions, restlessness, grief, anxiety, mental confusion, nervous depression and sensory overstimulation.[19]

Holmes believes that the scent of frankincense primarily stimulates two cerebral centres:

- the raphe nucleus to release serotonin and GABA for the calming effect
- the hippocampus and amygdala to release various neurotransmitters for mental stimulant effect.[19]

He suggests that the sesquiterpenes in frankincense contribute to the oil's calming action, while the monoterpenes may be the basis for the oil's mental stimulant action.[19]

Respiratory system

Frankincense oil has traditionally been used to treat respiratory conditions such as asthma, bronchitis and catarrhal conditions.[29]

Frankincense oil has anticatarrhal and expectorant properties that make it beneficial for treating bronchitis and asthma, especially associated with nervous tension.[30]

Davis has found frankincense essential oil helpful for people with asthma because it slows and deepens breathing.[31]

Skin care

Frankincense oil is well known in skin care for its wound-healing properties. It is also recommended for treating dry and mature skin, scars and wrinkles.[11,30]

Frankincense oil has been recommended for the treatment of non-suppurating sores, wounds, chronic ulcers, swollen gums, bleeding, boils, carbuncles and abscesses.[19]

Energetics, psyche and subtle uses

Energetics

Holmes states that frankincense oil has unique energetic qualities because of the oil's complex aroma, which he describes as spicy, sweet, woody and green.[19]

He explains that the spicy component of the aroma causes energy to rise and disperse, whereas the sweet, woody and green aromas have the effect of causing energy to go down and stabilise.[19]

The sweet, woody and green note exerts a more calming, grounding and balancing effect that reduces excessive energy. This accounts for frankincense's use for nervous tension, anxiety and mental confusion. On the other hand, the spicy aspect of frankincense is generally uplifting and tonifying. This is why the oil is often recommended to alleviate fatigue, grief, depression and poor mental focus.[19]

Mojay states that frankincense is able to smooth the flow of stagnant *Qi* whenever there is stress that leads to irritability, restlessness and insomnia.[29]

In terms of the Five Elements, frankincense is often associated with the Earth Element. Frankincense oil has a strong harmonising effect on the Intellect *(Yi)*.[29] When our *Yi* is out of balance, we may experience obsessive thoughts and repetitive thought patterns, we tend to worry excessively and our thinking is confused, and we find it difficult to make logical connections between ideas or to order thoughts in logical patterns.

Frankincense also helps to harmonise the Metal Element. It has anticatarrhal and expectorant properties that alleviate respiratory congestions associated with weak *Lung Qi* and it strengthens our *defensive Qi*.

In Ayurveda, frankincense oil is perfect for balancing *Vata* dosha and calming excessive *Pitta*.

Personality

Worwood describes frankincense personalities as displaying an air of mystery and secretiveness. They are often considered eccentric and prefer to use their own initiative to get something done. There is a sense of maturity, confidence and efficiency about a frankincense personality. They seem to have an understanding of the nature of the universe.[33]

While they are not necessarily religious people, they love all things spiritual and have a profound love of god in their heart. They are usually good communicators – clear and eloquent; however, they may be perceived as blunt.[33]

When they are negative, the frankincense personality can be destructive and bitter. They can be sceptical, cynical and are often inclined to be guilt-ridden, insecure and uncertain. They are liable to suffer from anxiety and stress and be short-tempered and agitated. However, as they are such an enlightened person, they are able to realise what is going on and make a concerted effort to change direction into positivity.[33]

They are typically very steady, upright citizens and will be attracted to jobs that command respect and honour. In their business dealings they have the ability to sense accurately whether a deal will turn out well or if it will be a waste of time. Worwood states that they make very good counsellors as their advice is very down to earth and practical.[33]

According to Myers-Briggs personality types, the frankincense personality is likely to be an INTJ. INTJs are very responsible and dependable. They are people of very few words and tend to be private. They are punctual, precise and fastidious. They have the ability to concentrate and are difficult to distract. They are modest, unassuming and down to earth. They can be resistant to change. They can make quick critical judgements of others. They are extremely devoted in their relationships.

Subtle

Frankincense has always had a very special spiritual connection with humankind:

> *The first perfume was incense, its earliest uses bound up in religious rites … With their complex aromatic layering, these substances are a vehicle for spiritual exaltation … The burning of aromatics opens the door between the mundane and the supernatural, an elevation of consciousness that has been incorporated into the rituals and belief systems of many religions. Indeed, incense has permeated spiritual practice as thoroughly as spiritual practice has permeated human life.*[17]

Frankincense is often recommended to quieten the mind and assist in meditation, prayer and spiritual practices. For example, Zeck states:

> *Frankincense cleanses the aura, is finely attuned to the subtle energies and paves the way to the higher self.*[34]

Worwood describes the subtle qualities of frankincense as elevating, spiritual and meditative. She explains that it holds some of the wisdom of the universe, that which is manifested in the spiritual self. She also recommends using frankincense to help ground us and reconnect us with our body in cases of spiritual shock or loss.[35]

Keim Loughran & Bull state that frankincense deepens our breath, calms and focuses our mind and opens our consciousness to make clear, direct contact with the divine. It creates a mindful, meditative state in which we can experience and integrate divine wisdom. Frankincense enhances a meditative state so that we can better receive and integrate healing energy.[36]

Davis explains that frankincense will help us cut ties with the past, especially where these may block personal growth.[37]

Mojay compares frankincense to sandalwood:

> *... like sandalwood, it is an ideal aid to meditation, contemplation, and prayer, ceasing mental chatter and stilling the mind. Facilitating a state of single pointed concentration, it allows the spirit to soar.*[29]

Mojay states that frankincense contains the power to focus our spiritual consciousness:

> *We have allowed ourselves to become oppressed by the mundane or tied to the past – indeed, restricted or weighed-down by any form of over-attachment – frankincense can help us break free. This it will achieve through encouraging tranquillity, insight and spiritual self-discipline, allowing the ego-self and trans-personal self to work in unison.*[29]

I have always felt that frankincense oil can be used for the lower chakras – base chakra and solar plexus; however, at the same time it helps balance all the upper chakras. Holmes' explanation sheds some light on paradox:

> *By promoting both an upward and downward movement of energy, here is an oil that creates connection between the lower and upper body parts, thereby generating a dynamic balance between them. Energetically we can say that frankincense connects the lowest chakra with the middle and upper chakras.*[19]

He also explains that frankincense helps integrate the personality by creating connections between the different aspects of our individual self.[19]

This explains why frankincense induces the state of contemplation that religions around the world have engaged in their ceremonies for thousands of years. Frankincense can lead to a state that can be the doorway to transcendent liberation from the physical body.[19]

F

Dosage and Administration

Blending

Aromatherapy

For inflammation and joint pain, consider blending frankincense oil with essential oils such as black pepper, clove bud, everlasting, ginger, spike lavender, sweet marjoram or rosemary.

To help calm and slow down breathing, consider blending frankincense oil with essential oils such as fragonia, neroli or sandalwood.

To help alleviate catarrhal conditions, associated with bronchitis or asthma, consider blending frankincense oil with essential oils such as Atlas cedarwood, cajeput, fragonia, spike lavender, myrtle, pine or spruce.

To promote wound healing, consider blending frankincense oil with essential oils such as German chamomile, everlasting, lavender, myrrh, patchouli or sandalwood.

To promote mental clarity, focus and cognitive enhancement, consider blending frankincense oil with essential oils such as bergamot, coriander seed, fragonia, lemon, cold-pressed lime, pine, spruce or rosemary.

To assist in meditation and mindfulness practice, consider blending frankincense oil with essential oils such as Roman chamomile, lemon, myrtle, myrrh, neroli, patchouli, pine and sandalwood.

Perfumery

Aftel describes frankincense as having a soft, incense-like odour. In perfumes, it is used as an important fixative in spicy, exotic and flowery perfumes. It also blends well with citrus oils. It does have a very diffusive lighter base note. It can blend with milder notes without dominating them.[38]

Arctander says the olibanum oil modifies the sweetness of sweet orange and bergamot oil to give citrus colognes a delightful effect. He states that frankincense also blends well with rather difficult 'fresh' perfume notes such as verbena. It is an important ingredient in many oriental style perfumes, floral perfumes and citrus colognes.[2]

Mode of administration

Bath

Full body bath, foot bath

Topical

Massage, ointment, skin care

Inhalation

Direct inhalation, diffuser, oil vaporiser

Safety Profile

General safety

Frankincense oil is considered non-toxic, non-irritant and non-sensitising.[11]

Contraindications

No contraindications known.

Regulatory guidelines

Frankincense oil has been approved for food use.[6]

References

1. Lawrence BM. *Essential oils 1992-1994.* Allured Publishing, Carol Stream, 1995.
2. Arctander S. *Perfume and flavor materials of natural origin.* Allured Publishing, Carol Stream, 1994.
3. Tisserand R, Young R. *Essential oil safety.* 2nd edn. Churchill Livingstone, Edinburgh, 2014.
4. DeCarlo A, Ali S. *Sustainable sourcing of phytochemicals as a development tool: the case of Somaliland's frankincense industry.* Institute for Environmental Diplomacy & Security, The University of Vermont, March 2014. Retrieved from http://www.uvm.edu/ieds/sites/default/files/Somaliland_3_27_14.PDF
5. Langenheim JH. *Plant resins – chemistry, evolution, ecology, and ethnobotany.* Timber Press, Portland, 2003.
6. Khan I, Abourashed E. *Leung's encyclopedia of common natural ingredients used in food, drugs and cosmetics.* 3rd edn. John Wiley & Sons. New Jersey, 2010.
7. Burfield T. *Frankincense – a brief catch-up.* Retrieved Aug 13, 2016, from www.cropwatch.org
8. Lis-Balchin M. *Aromatherapy science – a guide for healthcare professionals.* Pharmaceutical Press, London, 2006.
9. Southern Cross University. *Perfect Potion Boswellia serrata oils – certificate of analysis.* 2016.
10. Southern Cross University. *Perfect Potion Boswellia carterii oils – certificate of analysis.* 2016.
11. Lawless J. *The encyclopaedia of essential oils.* Element Books, Shaftesbury, 1992.
12. Manniche L. *An ancient Egyptian herbal.* British Museum Press, London, 1993.
13. Classen C. *World of sense – exploring the senses in history across cultures.* Routledge, London, 1993.
14. Grieve M. *A modern herbal – Vol. I.* Dover Publications, New York, 1971.
15. Lyttelton C. *The scent trail – a journey of the senses.* Bantam Press, London, 2007.
16. https://www.kingjamesbibleonline.org
17. Stoddart DM. *The scented ape – the biology and culture of human odour.* Cambridge University Press, Cambridge, 1990.
18. Classen C, Howes D, Synnott A. *Aroma – the cultural history of smell.* Routledge, London, 1994.
19. Holmes P. *Frankincense oil.* The International Journal of Aromatherapy, 1998/1999; 9(4): 156-161.
20. Siddiqui MZ. *Boswellia serrata, a potential anti-inflammatory agent: an overview.* Retrieved Aug 13, 2016, from http://www.ncbi.nlm.nih.gov/pmc/articles/PMC3309643
21. *Frankincense – a cropwatch bibliography.* Cropwatch, 2010; 1(11). Retrieved Aug 13, 2016, from www.cropwatch.org
22. Wahab A et al. *The essential oil of olibanum.* Planta Medica, 1987; 53(4): 382-384.
23. Al-Saidi S et al. *Composition and antibacterial activity of the essential oils of four commercial grades of Omani Luban, the oleo-gum resin of Boswellia sacra FLUECK.* Chemistry and Biodiversity, 2012; 9(3): 615-624.
24. Tisserand R. *Frankincense oil and cancer in perspective.* Retrieved Mar 3, 2016 from http://tisserandinstitute.org/frankincense-oil-and-cancer-in-perspective/
25. Xia L et al. *Boswellic acid acetate induces apoptosis through caspase-mediated pathways in myeloid leukemia cells.* Molecular Cancer Therapeutics, 2005; 4(3): 381-388.
26. Park B et al. *Boswellic acid supresses growth and metastasis of human pancreatic tumors in an orthotopic nude mouse model through modulation of multiple targets.* PLoS ONE, 2011; (6)10: e26943. doi: 10.1371/journal.pone.0026943
27. Mikhaeil BR et al. *Chemistry and immunomodulatory activity of frankincense oil.* Zeitschrift fur Naturforschung Teil C, 2003; 58(3/4): 230-238.
28. Price S, Price L. *Aromatherapy for health professionals.* 4th edn. Churchill Livingstone, Edinburgh, 2012.
29. Mojay G. *Aromatherapy for healing the spirit.* Healing Arts Press, Rochester, 1999.
30. Lavabre M. *Aromatherapy workbook.* Healing Arts Press, Rochester, 1997.
31. Davis P. *Aromatherapy: an A-Z.* 2nd edn. C.W. Daniel Company, Saffron Walden, 1999.
32. Schnaubelt K. *Medical aromatherapy.* Frog, Berkeley, 1999.
33. Worwood VA. *The fragrant mind.* Transworld Publishers, London, 1995.
34. Zeck R. *The blossoming heart – aromatherapy for healing and transformation.* Aroma Tours, East Ivanhoe, 2004.
35. Worwood VA. *The fragrant heavens.* Transworld Publishers, London, 1999.
36. Keim Loughran J, Bull R. *Aromatherapy and subtle energy techniques.* Frog, Berkeley, 2000.

37. Davis P. *Subtle aromatherapy*. C.W Daniel Company, Saffron Walden, 1991.

38. Aftel M. *Fragrant – the secret life of scent*. Riverhead Books, New York, 2014.

Galangal

Identification

Botanical name

The two most important species are:

- lesser galangal (*Alpinia officinarum* Hance)
- greater galangal (*Alpinia galanga* Willd).

Both plants are members of the ginger family and their rhizomes resemble ginger.[1]

Synonyms

Galanga oil, false ginger oil

Family

Zingiberaceae

Botany and origins

G

The genus *Alpinia* is a large genus of the *Zingiberaceae* family, consisting of almost 250 species. Plants from this genus have been utilised as traditional medicines, food and spices in many countries such as China, Japan and India.[2]

The name galangal comes from the Arabic *khalanjan*, which originates from a Chinese word for ginger, *liang-jiang*. Two different species are in common use – smaller (or lesser) galangal (*A. officinarum* Hance), a perennial herb native to southern China; and greater galangal (*A. galanga*), a stemless perennial herb of southeastern Asia, native to Java.[1,3]

Galangal is a tropical plant with long, green, blade-like leaves and ginger-like rhizomes. Greater galangal is the one used most in South East Asian cooking, growing to 2 m tall, with greenish-white, orchid-shaped flowers with dark-red veined tips. The knobbly, underground rhizomes have a thin, orange-brown skin with lighter and darker 'tiger-stripe' rings, while the inside is creamy, pale yellow flesh. The aroma of the greater galangal rhizome is reminiscent of ginger with a sharp, sinus-penetrating aroma and a biting hot clean taste.[3]

Lesser galangal is smaller. It grows to around 1 m high; the rhizomes are orange-red to rusty brown with similar stripes. The flesh is pale brown inside. Hemphill states that this variety has medicinal applications and is seldom used in cooking.[3]

However, most of the technical and pharmacological studies that I surveyed from India, Sri Lanka and China indicate that *A. galanga* is the most commonly used plant for medicinal purposes.

A. galanga is cultivated in many tropical areas of Asia. It is cultivated in India, Thailand, Indonesia, China and Malaysia. The herb is propagated by rhizomes and grows best in shaded areas away from direct sunlight. It requires well-drained soils to grow in and is usually propagated by dividing and replanting the rhizomes during spring. The four- to six-year-old plants are harvested for their rhizomes at the end of the growing season. The rhizomes are unearthed in early autumn and late summer in China, where the plant is extensively cultivated. Harvested rhizomes are carefully washed and cut into segments and then dried for storage and processing into herbal medicine.[4]

Method of extraction

The essential oil is steam-distilled from the roots of *A. officinarum* or *A. galanga*.

Characteristics

A. officinarum oil is a yellowish to olive-brown, occasionally pale-olive or pale-yellow, liquid possessing a fresh, spicy-camphoraceous and spicy-woody odour reminiscent of bay laurel, cardamom and ginger oils. The essential oil from the dried rhizomes has a richer spicy-woody aroma.[5]

Chemical composition

The main constituents found in the essential oil of *A. galanga* rhizome collected from Yunnan, China was reported as follows:

α-pinene (10.89%), camphene (4.14%), β-pinene (14.36%), 1,8-cineole (22.63%), fenchol (1.72%), borneol (8.41%), α-terpineol (8.59%), geraniol (2.13%).[6]

It is interesting to note the differences between *A. galanga* rhizome oils from other regions. For example, the oil from Indonesia had higher α- and β-pinenes (18.6%) and 1,8-cineole (47.3%), while the Malaysian oil is characterised by sesquiterpenoids with β-farnesene (18.2%) and β-bisabolene (16.2%). On the other hand, *A. galanga* from southern India contained 1,8-cineole (33.0 -30.2%), camphor (5.0-14%), α-terpineol (2.3-9.35%), α-fenchyl acetate (1.1-12.7%) and

(*E*)-methyl cinnamate (2.6-5.3%) as the main components, whereas *A. galanga* from northeast India had 1,8-cineole as the major component at 76.5%.[6]

These results suggest the existence of chemotypes of this species, and further studies on plant cultivation and essential oil standardisation are needed.

Ly et al. state that the essential oil in the rhizome of *A. galanga* (greater galangal) has been investigated by many researchers, while the oil in the rhizome of *A. officinarum* (lesser galangal) has only been studied by Lawrence et al.[1]

Ly et al. compared the *A. officinarum* oil from the fresh rhizome with that from the dried rhizome. The main components in the fresh rhizome were 1,8-cineole (50%), exo-2-hydroxy-1,8-cineole acetate (11.2%), β-caryophyllene (6.4%), α-pinene (1.7%), β-pinene (2.6%), β-bisabolene (2.6%), chavicol (2.0%), limonene (2.0%), terpin-4-ol (1.6%), chavicol acetate (1.2%) and methyl eugenol (1.0%).[1]

On drying the rhizomes, the monoterpene fraction (including hydrocarbon and oxygenated compounds) decreased in content, while the sesquiterpene and aromatic compound fractions increased.[1]

The main components of the oil from dried rhizomes were β -bisabolene (9.6%), 1,8-cineole (8.2%), chavicol acetate (5.9%), chavicol (5.3%), eugenol acetate (3.7%), α-farnesene (3.3%), methyl eugenol (3.3%), β-caryophyllene (2.9%), α-bisabolol (2.6%), spathulenol (2.5%), farnesyl acetate (2.4%) and 4-hydroxycinnamyl acetate (2.3%).[1]

It is interesting that the ratio of hydrocarbons to oxygenated constituents (0.72) for the dried sample is almost double that for the fresh rhizome (0.33), in spite of the disappearance of monoterpene hydrocarbons from the dried rhizome. Ly et al. suggest that this could be an aid in evaluating whether fresh or dried rhizome was used to produce the oil.[1]

The composition of *A. officinarum* oil was compared with *A. galanga* oil. It was noted that a similar pattern occurred in which the 1,8-cineole in the oil from fresh rhizomes was much higher than in the oil from the dried rhizome. Many of the other compounds were similar. However, it was noted that 1′-acetoxychavicol acetate was not found in *A. officinarum* oil. This may, therefore, be an effective way to distinguish lesser galangal from greater galangal oil.[1]

Adulteration

No information could be found on the adulteration of galangal oil. However, it is important to know whether the fresh or dried rhizomes have been used to extract the essential oil. There is a significant difference in the ratio of the main chemical constituents found in essential oil from the dried and fresh rhizomes. There is also a significant variance in the chemistry of galangal oil according to the country of origin, and other factors such as time of harvest and climatic and seasonal variations.

Pharmacopoeias and standards

At the time of writing, the purity, composition, physico-chemical properties and therapeutic uses of galangal essential oil are not defined in any pharmacopoeia monograph or standard.

A. galanga rhizome is the subject of many Ayurveda and Chinese pharmacopoeias and monographs.[7]

History and Traditional Uses

History

Galangal is a pungent and aromatic rhizome, which is used as a flavouring agent as well as traditional medicine in South East Asia. Galangal root was known to ancient Indians for its medicinal and culinary purposes. It has been used as a spice for over a thousand years, especially in curries.[8,9]

The roots have been used in Europe as a spice for over a thousand years, having been introduced by Arab or Greek physicians. However, it is now rarely used except in China, India and Russia. It is used in Russia for flavouring vinegar and the liqueur *nastoika*. It is a favourite spice and medicine in Lithuania and Estonia.[9]

Traditional medicine

In Ayurveda, galangal has been used to improve appetite, taste and voice. It is useful for the management of *Vata* diseases. In Unani system, rhizomes have been used as a stomachic, aphrodisiac, tonic, diuretic, expectorant and carminative. It is useful for headache, rheumatic pain, sore throat, stuttering, pain in the chest, diabetes, burning of the liver and diseases of the kidneys.[4]

In China and Thailand, it is used as a folk medicine for stomach health. Galangal has been used in traditional medicine for its carminative, emmenagogue, aphrodisiac, antipyretic, anti-inflammatory and antispasmodic activities.[10]

Herbal

The rhizome is currently listed in the British Herbal Pharmacopoeia for the treatment of dyspepsia, flatulence, colic, nausea and vomiting.[11]

Food, perfumery and flavouring

It has been reported that greater galangal rhizomes are used in the preparation of meat dishes and curries in its natural form, or for flavouring foods as a dried herb, whereas lesser galangal is used mainly as a medicine.[1] However, Chauhan et al. state that greater galangal rhizomes are commonly used in traditional Indian medicine.[12]

Therapeutics

Pharmacology and clinical studies

Many pharmacological studies involving galangal essential oil have been published. A systemic review of these studies will not be attempted. Rather, I have chosen a selection of studies that support the traditional and clinical uses.

Analgesic activity

The anti-inflammatory and analgesic effects of *A. galanga* oil have been extensively studied. Topical preparations containing alcoholic extract of the rhizome have shown significant analgesic effect in formalin test. A randomised, double-blind, placebo-controlled study was conducted in 261 patients with osteoarthritis of the knee and moderate to severe pain. The highly concentrated extract was found to have, statistically a significant effect in reducing the symptoms of osteoarthritis.[4]

G

Antifungal activity

The ethanolic extracts of galangal rhizomes posed fungicidal activity against a wide range of human pathogenic fungi.[13]

Antimicrobial activity

The antimicrobial activity of essential oils from fresh and dried rhizomes of *A. galanga* was investigated. The essential oils from dried *A. galanga* rhizomes were more effective against the tested microorganisms.[14]

Antitumour activity

A. galanga oil was found to cause antitumour activity. Active compounds from *A. galanga* such as 1′-acetoxychavicol acetate and 1′-acetoxyeugenol acetate were isolated as antitumour principles against sarcoma 180 ascites in mice.[4]

1′-acetoxychavicol acetate has been reported to act as an antitumour agent as well as an inhibitor of chemically induced carcinogenesis.[4]

Antiviral activity

It was reported that a methanolic extract of *A. galanga* showed potent inhibitory activity against human immunodeficiency virus type-1 (HIV-1) and human cytomegalovirus (HCMV).[4]

Gastroprotective activity

The antisecretory and cytoprotective actions of *A. galanga* are responsible for its antiulcer activity. An ethanolic extract of *A. galanga* significantly reduced gastric secretion. It was suggested that these properties may be responsible for the antiulcer activity of *A. galanga*.[4]

Actions

Actions commonly cited in aromatherapy

Antiseptic, bactericidal, carminative, diaphoretic, stimulant, stomachic[8]

Actions supported by clinical studies

Analgesic, antifungal, anti-inflammatory, antimicrobial, carminative, gastroprotective

Comment

A. galanga rhizome is not the subject of any European Pharmacopeia; however, it is extensively referenced in Indian and Chinese pharmacopoeias. Galangal oil is not commonly used in aromatherapy; however, review of traditional uses and clinical data support the use of galangal essential oil for the treatment of gastrointestinal complaints and the relief of musculoskeletal conditions such as arthritis.

Aromatherapy Uses

Clinical aromatherapy

Digestive system

Galangal oil is especially beneficial for digestive complaints such as flatulence, dyspepsia and nausea.[8]

Energetics, psyche and subtle uses

Energetics

The properties of galangal are *warming*. It helps dispel *cold* conditions associated with the digestive system and the respiratory system.

Galangal oil also stimulates the *Yang Qi* of the *Kidneys*, making it beneficial for relieving lower back pain associated with muscular fatigue and fatigue.

According to TCM and the Five Elements, galangal helps strengthen the *Zhi*. The *Zhi* is responsible for our willpower and determination. Whenever our *Zhi* is weak, we tend to lack the personal drive and optimism to take action, even though we may have clear plans and intentions. We may procrastinate and doubt ourselves and wait for others to spur us on. We may feel disconnected from our physical body and we may shy away from vigorous and sustained activity.

Subtle

Keim Loughran & Bull state that galangal oil will help our personal willpower to become healthy, clear and balanced. It is said to develop personal integrity.[15]

Dosage and Administration

Blending

Aromatherapy

For the relief of indigestion, consider blending galangal oil with essential oils such as caraway seed, coriander seed, sweet fennel, ginger, sweet orange, peppermint or rosemary.

To alleviate musculoskeletal aches and pains, consider blending galangal oil with essential oils such as bay laurel, black pepper, cajeput, clove bud, lemon-scented eucalyptus, ginger, kunzea, spike lavender, pine or rosemary.

For the relief of physical and emotional exhaustion, consider blending galangal oil with essential oils such as basil, bay laurel, cardamom, clove bud, sweet fennel, lemon, lemongrass, lemon myrtle, lime, peppermint, pine or rosemary.

Perfumery

Galangal oil is rarely used in perfumery. It could be used to introduce interesting notes in oriental bases, woody perfumes and spicy perfumes. It blends well with citrus oils, spice oils, herbaceous oils, fresh pine needle oils, rich earthy scented oils such as patchouli and vetiver, and warm resins such as benzoin, myrrh and opopanax.[5]

Mode of administration

Bath

Full body bath, foot bath

Topical

Compress, massage, ointment

Inhalation

Direct inhalation, diffuser, oil vaporiser

Safety Profile

General safety

Galangal essential oil is non-toxic, non-irritant and non-sensitising.[8]

Contraindications

No contraindications known.[16]

Regulatory guidelines

Galangal essential oil has GRAS status.

References

1. Ly TN, Yamauchi R, Kato K. *Volatile components of the essential oils in galangal (Alpinia officinarum Hance) from Vietnam.* Food Science Technology Research, 2001; 7(4): 303-306.
2. Zhang W et al. *The genus Alpinia: a review of its phytochemistry and pharmacology.* World Journal of Traditional Chinese Medicine, 2016; 2(1): 26-41.
3. Hemphill I. *Spice notes.* Pan Macmillan Australia, Sydney, 2000.
4. Chudiwal AK, Jain DP, Somani RS. *Alpinia galanga Willd – an overview on phyto-pharmacological properties.* Indian Journal of Natural Products and Resources, 2010; 1(2): 143-149.
5. Arctander S. *Perfume and flavor materials of natural origin.* Allured Publishing, Carol Stream, 1994.
6. Wu Y et al. *Composition of the essential oil from Alpinia galanga rhizomes and its bioactivity on Lasioderma serricorne.* Bulletin of Insectology, 2014; 67(2): 247-254.
7. Arambewela L, Wijesinghe A. *Sri Lankan medicinal plant monographs and analysis – Vol. 10: Alpinia galanga.* National Science Foundation, Colombo, 2006.
8. Lawless J. *The encyclopaedia of essential oils.* Element Books, Shaftesbury, 1992.
9. Grieve M. *A modern herbal – Vol. I.* Dover Publications, New York, 1971.
10. Kaushik D et al. *Current pharmacological and phytochemical studies of the plant Alpinia galanga.* Journal of Chinese Integrative Medicine, 2011; 9(10): 1061-1065.
11. *British herbal pharmacopoeia.* British Herbal Medicine Association, Bournemouth, 1983.
12. Chauhan SK et al. *Development of pharmacognostic profile of Alpinia galanga, Willd. (Zingiberaceae).* International Journal of Pharmacological Research, 2015: 5(3): 57-61.
13. Subramanian P, Nishan M. *Biological activities of greater galangal, Alpinia galanga – a review.* Journal of Botanical Sciences, 2015: S1: 15-19.
14. Raviraja Shetty G, Monisha S. *Pharmacology of an endangered medicinal plant Alpinia galanga – a review.* Research Journal of Pharmaceutical, Biological and Chemical Science, 2015; (61): 499-511.
15. Keim Loughran J, Bull R. *Aromatherapy and subtle energy techniques.* Frog, Berkeley, 2000.
16. Tisserand R, Young R. *Essential oil safety.* 2nd edn. Churchill Livingstone, Edinburgh, 2014.

Galbanum

Identification

Botanical name

Ferula galbaniflua Boiss & Buhse

Synonyms

Ferula gummosa, galbanum resin, galbanum oleoresin

Family

Apiaceae (Umbelliferae)

Botany and origins

Several species of *Ferula* are used as a source of galbanum. *F. galbaniflua* is a large perennial with a smooth stem, shiny ovate leaves and small flowers. It contains resin ducts that exude an oleoresin. The dried resinous exudate is collected by making incisions at the base of the stem.[1]

There are two types of galbanum resin: a soft or 'Levant' galbanum resin which is a viscous liquid, and hard galbanum (Persian galbanum) which is solid. The former contains more volatile oil and is used for the production of the essential oil.[2]

Galbanum is native to the Middle East and western Asia. It is cultivated in Iran, Turkey and Afghanistan. Normally the resin is distilled either in Europe or the USA.[3]

G

Method of extraction

The oil is obtained by steam distillation of the root exudation of *F. galbaniflua*.

Characteristics

Galbanum is a clear to pale yellow or green, or olive-brown, mobile liquid, which possesses a powerful green, leaf-like odour with a woody, pine-needle-like and balsamic undertone. Arctander describes the scent of galbanum as that of green peppers or a tossed green salad.[2]

Chemical composition

The chemical composition of galbanum oil was reported as follows:

tricyclene (2.3%), α-pinene (9.6%), camphene (0.2%), β-pinene (53.7%), sabinene (1.4%), myrcene (2.9%), δ-3-carene (13.1%), limonene (1.8%), (*Z*)-β-ocimene (2.3%), (*E*)-β-ocimene (1.3%), terpinolene (0.5%), (*E*,*Z*)-1,3,5-undecatriene (0.5%), (*E*,*E*)-1,3,5-undecatriene (0.2%).[4]

It was noted that galbanum oil contained an additional 98 components making up 10.2% of the total essential oil; however, none of these were identified.[4]

Adulteration

Adulteration of galbanum oil is common. It is often diluted with pinene, galbanol and camphene; however, Arctander states that these can be easily detected by an experienced perfumer during an olfactory examination of the oil.[2]

Pharmacopoeias and standards

The purity, composition and physico-chemical properties of galbanum essential oil are defined in the ISO 14716:1998 Oil of Galbanum.

History and Traditional Uses

History

It was used by ancient civilisations as incense, and in Egypt for cosmetics and in the embalming process.[1,5]

It is mentioned in the Bible as an ingredient for a sacred incense:

> *And the Lord said unto Moses, take unto thee sweet spices, stactes and onycha, and galbanum; these sweet spices with pure frankincense: of each shall there be a like weight: and thou shalt make it a perfume, a confection after the art of the apothecary, tempered together, pure and holy: and thou shalt beat some of it very small, and put of it before the testimony in the tabernacle of the congregation, where I will meet with thee: it shall be unto you most holy. And as for the perfume which thou shalt make, ye shall not make to yourselves according to the composition thereof: it shall be unto thee holy for the Lord.*[6]
>
> Exodus 30:34-30:37 (King James Version)

Herbal

It is often used in a similar way to asafoetida – for the treatment of wounds, inflammations and skin disorders, and for respiratory, digestive and nervous system ailments.[3]

Food, perfumery and flavouring

It is used extensively as a green component, especially in floral, herbaceous and conifer perfumes. It is used as a flavour component in many food products.[3,7]

Therapeutics

Pharmacology and clinical studies

There has been very little research into the pharmacological or clinical uses of galbanum essential oil.

Antimicrobial activity

When compared with rosemary and fennel oils, galbanum exhibited the best antimicrobial activity against MRSA and MSSA.[8]

Actions

Actions commonly cited in aromatherapy

Anti-inflammatory, antimicrobial, antiseptic, aphrodisiac, balsamic, carminative, cicatrisant, emmenagogue, expectorant, hypotensive, restorative, tonic[1,3,5]

Actions supported by clinical studies

None of the actions commonly cited in aromatherapy can be supported by clinical studies.

Comment

Galbanum is an ancient aromatic resin that has traditional uses in incense and for wound healing; however, a review of traditional uses and clinical data could not confirm any clinical applications for galbanum oil in aromatherapy.

Galbanum oil has a pleasant fresh green note that may be beneficial for improving mood and reducing the symptoms of stress-induced disorders such as anxiety and depression.

Aromatherapy Uses

Clinical aromatherapy

Integumentary system

Although galbanum oil is not commonly used in aromatherapy, it has been recommended in skin care for the treatment of abscesses, acne, boils, cuts and inflammations that are slow to heal.[1,5]

Nervous system

Galbanum oil may be useful for reducing stress-related conditions and nervous disorders.[1] It can be used to induce feelings of calm, stability, direction, concentration and focus.[9]

Respiratory system

It is beneficial for alleviating asthma, bronchitis, catarrh and chronic coughs.[1]

Energetics, psyche and subtle uses

Subtle

Worwood refers to galbanum as a sacrificial fragrance that allows for the shedding of old ideas and outmoded behaviour and attitudes.[10]

Keim Loughran & Bull explain that it will help shed light on life's purpose and the inner self. It communicates to the deeper layers of self, allowing a gradual unfolding of truth for those who have been blinded by success and ambition, allowing a sense of balance with the physical and spiritual self.[9]

Dosage and Administration

Blending

Aromatherapy

For the relief of stress, anxiety, depression and nervous tension, consider blending galbanum oil with essential oils such as bergamot, fragonia, geranium, fir needle, frankincense, lavender, sweet orange, neroli, pine or rosemary.

For the relief of bronchitis and catarrhal conditions, consider blending galbanum oil with essential oils such as Atlas cedarwood, cajeput, 1,8-cineole-rich eucalypts, peppermint eucalyptus, sweet fennel, ginger, frankincense, pine or rosemary.

To promote wound healing, consider blending galbanum oil with essential oils such as German chamomile, everlasting, lavender, frankincense, myrrh or patchouli.

Perfumery

Galbanum is an essential ingredient in perfumery for creating chypre, fougère, pine, forest or mossy type perfumes. It is always used in very modest concentrations.[2]

Arctander states that it can introduce a very interesting note to a floral composition, especially when a leafy character is essential to create a truly natural feeling. It blends very well with lavender, clary sage and violet leaf.[2]

Mode of administration

Bath

Full body bath, foot bath

Topical

Compress, massage, ointment, skin care

Inhalation

Direct inhalation, diffuser, oil vaporiser

Safety Profile

General safety

Galbanum oil is non-toxic, non-irritant and non-sensitising.[1]

Contraindications

No contraindications known.[1]

Regulatory guidelines

Galbanum oil has FEMA approval for use as food flavouring.[11]

References

1. Lawless J. *The encyclopaedia of essential oils.* Element Books, Shaftesbury, 1992.
2. Arctander S. *Perfume and flavor materials of natural origin.* Allured Publishing, Carol Stream, 1994.
3. Khan I, Abourashed E. *Leung's encyclopedia of common natural ingredients used in food, drugs and cosmetics.* 3rd edn. John Wiley & Sons, New Jersey, 2010.
4. Lawrence BM. *Progress in essential oils – galbanum.* Perfumer & Flavorist, 2007; 32: 49-51.
5. Davis P. *Aromatherapy: an A-Z.* 2nd edn. C.W. Daniel Company, Saffron Walden, 1999.
6. *King James Bible online.* Retrieved from https://www.kingjamesbibleonline.org
7. Langenheim JH. *Plant resins – chemistry, evolution, ecology and ethnobotany.* Timber Press, Portland, 2003.
8. Mahboubi A et al. *Antimicrobial activity or rosemary, fennel and galbanum essential oils against clinical isolates of Staphylococcus aureus.* Biharean Biologist, 2011; 5(1); 4-7. Cited in Quintessential Aromatics database, 2013.
9. Keim Loughran J, Bull R. *Aromatherapy and subtle energy techniques.* Frog, Berkeley, 2000.
10. Worwood VA. *The fragrant heavens.* Transworld Publishing, London, 1999.
11. Burdock GA. *Fenaroli's handbook of flavor Ingredients.* 6th edn. CRC Press, Boca Raton, 2009.

Geranium

G

Identification

Botanical name

Pelargonium spp.

Synonyms

Rose geranium, pelargonium. However, James states that the term geranium should not be used to label the essential oil produced from the *Pelargonium* species.[1]

Family

Geraniaceae

Botany and origins

It appears that we have confused the *Geranium* and *Pelargonium* species. Lis-Balchin explains:

> *The genera Geranium and Pelargonium are invariably confused by the general public and also plant sales personnel, health food shop workers and alternative medicine practitioners, especially aromatherapists.*[2]

Lis-Balchin goes on to explain that geranium oil is extracted from the leaves of some *Pelargonium* species and cultivars, but its paramedical effects are often equated with those of the genus *Geranium* such as *Geranium robertianum* and *G. maculatum.* The latter are native to Europe and were used as herbal medicines for hundreds of years. They were described by Gerard (1633), Culpeper (1652) and Grieve (1937).[2]

This confusion existed before Linnaeus introduced his binomial system of classification in 1753. Both genera were then placed under the genus *Geranium* and although they were correctly reclassified in 1820 under two separate genera, acceptance by the general public as well as nursery retailers was and still is minimal.[2]

The *Pelargonium* species are native to South Africa and were introduced to European botanical gardens as early as 1600, where they were used as ornamental plants. They have medicinal properties that were only known to the Hottentots, Zulus and the local Boers in South Africa.[2]

Miller states that the genus *Pelargonium* includes about 270 distinct species, and the majority of these are found in southern Africa. She states that the genus is almost unequal in the plant kingdom for the enormous diversity created to adapt to these different habitats.[3]

The genera *Geranium* and *Pelargonium* are classified in the family Geraniaceae and like the three other genera included in Geraniaceae, they also have a similar elongated fruit with five mericarps, each containing a single seed.[3]

The cultivars grown to produce geranium oil have been developed from species such as *Pelargonium capitatum, P. graveolens* and *P. radens.*[3,5]

However, Demarne states that these are not natural species. We now know that the true *P. radens* and *P. graveolens* are mint-scented species, while *P. capitatum* species is very poor in essential oil and has a very faint rose scent. All these natural species are said to have originated from southern Africa.[5]

Demarne states that the cultivars of geranium should be named *'Pelargonium* hybrids of *P. capitatum* x *P. radens'* or *'Pelargonium* hybrids of *P. capitatum x P. graveolens'.*

The oil composition, in particular, depends on the *P. capitatum* parent, which transmits the ability to synthesise geraniol and citronellol rather than isomenthone.[5]

He also states that most of the world's geranium oil is now produced mainly in China, Egypt, Réunion and India. China is now the biggest producer of geranium oil. Egypt is the second biggest producer.[5]

Lis-Balchin explains that the botanical name, *P. graveolens*, is another misnomer. While she states this is true for some geranium oil originating out of Africa, it is doubtful, as this species has a more distinctive peppermint aroma. She states the main source of geranium oil is a cultivar known as *Pelargonium* cv. 'Rose', which gives rise to the commercial 'geranium oil – Bourbon', and what we often refer to as Rose geranium originated from hybridisation in England, probably in the eighteenth century. This cultivar was then exported to the south of France and Réunion and more recently to China. The 'Rose' cultivar is likely to be a hybrid between *P. capitatum* x *P. radens*.[2]

Other *Pelargonium* species grown in gardens for their fragrant leaves include *P. citriodorum* (citron-scented), *P. fragrans* (nutmeg-scented) and *P. tomentosum* (peppermint-scented).[6]

A number of geranium oils are available and they are usually distinguished by a country of origin prefix: Reunion, Chinese, Egyptian or Moroccan.[6]

Bourbon geranium, which is produced on Réunion is considered the most important and the most desirable of all the geranium oils.[6]

According to Tisserand & Young, the name 'rose geranium' was reserved for geranium from Réunion, which was from the cultivar commonly referred to as Bourbon geranium. However, this geranium from Réunion is now only produced in very small quantities and is no longer sold on the open market.[4]

It is interesting that Lis-Balchin states that the term 'rose geranium' implies either a particular cultivar or sometimes the fact that rose petals were distributed on top of geranium leaves during the distillation.[7]

However, Lis-Balchin then contradicts herself when she states a further misconception: the name 'rose geranium' has been interpreted by some aromatherapists as meaning that geranium was distilled over rose. She explains that this would be rather difficult as geranium leaves would smother the rose petals.[8]

An oil from Bulgaria known as zdravetz oil is distilled from *Geranium macrorrhium*. Zdravetz oil is a pale olive green or pale yellowish-green, somewhat viscous liquid, which at room temperature is normally 30% liquid and 70% crystals. The crystals begin to dissolve at 32°C. The main constituents of zdravetz oil are sesquiterpenes (up to 90%), of which about half are germacrone.[6]

Method of extraction

Geranium oil is steam-distilled from the leaves and branches of various *Pelargonium* species.

Characteristics

The aroma of geranium will vary according to the geographic origin. Bourbon geranium is a greenish-olive oil with a pronounced green, leafy-rosy scent. The odour of freshly distilled Bourbon geranium has a peculiar, rather obnoxious top note which is partly due to dimethyl sulphide. It is produced during the rapid decaying of the plant material immediately prior to the distillation. The unpleasant top note will disappear after proper aeration or aging of the oil.[9]

Moroccan geranium is usually darker to medium yellow colour, and the Egyptian geranium is yellow to yellow-greenish colour. Both have a sweet, rosy, herbaceous odour somewhat similar to Réunion geranium.[6]

The Chinese geranium is dark green, often with a brownish or brownish-yellow tinge, and the odour is harsher than Bourbon geranium and is often more lemony and rosy, with a sweet-herbaceous note.[6]

Pelargonium plants grown at higher elevation in subtropical climates frequently produce an essential oil that is lighter than oil from the same cultivar at lower altitudes. Weiss also noted that harvesting the plants when they are in full bloom tended to produce an oil with a lower geraniol and citronellol content than cutting it prior to blooming.[6]

Chemical composition

There can be quite some difference in the chemical composition of geranium essential oil from different places of origins:[6]

Constituent	Bourbon	Chinese	Egyptian
linalool	12.90%	3.96%	9.47%
citronellol	21.28%	40.23%	27.40%
nerol	1.24%	0.67%	0.88%
geraniol	17.45%	6.45%	18.00%
citronellyl formate	8.37%	11.35%	6.74%
geranyl formate	7.55%	1.92%	4.75%
geranyl butyrate	1.34%	0.98%	1.48%
geranyl tiglate	1.04%	1.32%	1.06%
isomenthone	7.20%	5.70%	5.39%
guaia-6,9-diene	3.90%	4.40%	0.27%

Demarne states that the citronellol is usually higher in Chinese oil (38-40%) and Egyptian oil (31-33%) than in Bourbon oil (19-21%). On the other hand, geraniol and linalool are higher in Bourbon oil (geraniol 16-19% and linalool 7-10%) than Egyptian oil (geraniol 12-15% and linalool 5-6 %) and Chinese oil (geraniol 7-10% and linalool 2-3%).[5]

The ratio of linalool+geraniol/citronellol varies from 0.3 (Chinese oil) to 0.6 (Egyptian oil) and 1.4 (Bourbon oil). The amount of geranyl formate and citronellyl formate is proportional to their corresponding alcohols in the oils, and isomenthone is slightly higher in Bourbon oil (8-9%) than the other oils.[5]

Adulteration

Weiss states that geranium oils from all origins are frequently adulterated. The finer the original quality the more common the occurrence.[6]

Lis-Balchin states that geranium oil can easily be adulterated. Because it mainly contains citronellol and geraniol and their esters, it can easily be concocted from cheaper essential oils and synthetic aromatic ingredients, and be adjusted to the recommended ISO standards. The odour of such oils tend to be more appreciated by perfumers than the real essential oil.[2]

G

Pharmacopoeias and standards

The purity, composition and physico-chemical properties of geranium oil are defined in ISO 4731:2012 Essential Oil of Geranium (*Pelargonium* x ssp.).

History and Traditional Uses

History

Pelargoniums first reached Europe some 350 years ago:

> *In Europe, it became fashionable for rich people to build glass houses to accommodate plants from warmer climates that would not have survived frosts. The lifting of tax on glass in 1851 had an impact on this activity. Pelargoniums became popular subjects for hybridizing, because cross-pollination was not difficult, and they have the advantage of growing all the year around, so there is no dormancy to interrupt the work. The length of the flowering period was also a bonus and inspired gardeners to use the results of the breeding work as long lasting summer bedding.*[1]

By the time of Queen Victoria, pelargoniums, or 'geraniums' as they were popularly known, were very fashionable plants. The misnomer of 'geranium' originated because the seed of the pelargonium is very similar to the seed of the geranium. The botanists at the time decided that the pelargoniums were, in fact, closely related to European geraniums, and named them accordingly.[1]

However, as science progressed, this was found not to be true, and it was later on that the term 'pelargonium' was applied to these plants; however by then it was too late – the word 'geranium' was well and truly part of the English language for what we now know as a 'zonal pelargonium'.[1]

The interest in growing rose-scented leaf geranium dates from the mid-nineteenth century. At this time, real rose from *Rosa damascena* was very rare and expensive. This situation forced French perfumers to look for new essential oils with a rose scent such as geranium. The geranium plant requires lots of sunshine and well-drained soils rich in organic matter. It does not like frosts and temperatures below 2 °C as they are harmful to the growth and even the survival of the plant. Geranium was also a labour-intensive crop, hence by 1850 the cultivation and production of rose geranium moved from southern France to the French colonies of Northern Africa and the Indian Ocean.[5]

The first geranium plants grown for the French perfume industry were planted in Algeria in 1847, and in the 1880s extensive plantations were established on Réunion. Geranium oil is also produced in other parts of the world such as Kenya, Tanzania, India, China and Egypt.[6]

Herbal

The confusion existing over the therapeutic activity of geranium oil originates from transcribing Culpeper's and other herbal texts that only refer to *Geranium robertianium*, which has a completely different chemical composition to the geranium oil of today.[2]

The first reference to the true geranium is in Dioscorides' *De Materia Medica*, as *geranion* from the Greek *geranos*, a crane, because of the shape of the long-beaked fruit. The plant and its fragrant leaves were used by the Romans.[6]

Valnet recommends using geranium internally for various forms of debility (deficiency of adrenal cortex), diarrhoea, sterility, diabetes, urinary stones, gastric ulcers and jaundice.[10]

Lis-Balchin states that the medicinal properties of geranium oil (from *Pelargonium*) are, therefore, not only largely unsubstantiated, but based solely on the properties attributed to the mainly water-soluble extracts of the geranium species known as herb robert.[2]

Lawless states:

> *The British plant herb Robert (Geranium*

robertianum) and the American cranesbill (G. maculatum) are the most widely used types in herbal medicine today. Having been used since antiquity, they have many properties in common with the rose geranium, being used for conditions such as dysentery, haemorrhoids, inflammations, metrorrhagia and menorrhagia. The root and herb cranesbill is specifically indicated in the British Herbal Pharmacopoeia for diarrhea and peptic ulcer.[11]

Unfortunately, geranium oil from the *Pelargonium* species does not have any of the properties commonly associated with *G. robertianum*.

Tisserand describes geranium as:

> *A mild diuretic, and used internally for stones of the urinary passages. It is also of value in jaundice, and its bitter taste indicates an effect on the small intestine. We can see this in its pronounced action on diarrhea/enteritis; it may be effective against gall stones.*[12]

Once again, these are all properties of herb robert, which have nothing at all to do with the essential oil that we refer to as geranium that is extracted from the *Pelargonium* species.

It is interesting that many other aromatherapy authors seem to be aware of the difference between herb robert and *Pelargonium* species; however, they still attribute medicinal properties of herb robert to geranium essential oil. For example, Lavabre states:

> *Old herbals mention geranium of Herb Robert (Geranium robertianum), which grows wild in the temperate zones of the globe. This plant is totally different from the pelargonium used for the extraction of essential oils.*[13]

Lavabre also attributes the properties of herb robert such as haemostatic, cicatrisant, antidiabetic, diuretic and stimulant of the adrenal cortex to geranium oil.[13]

Rhind quotes Lawless, who states that geranium can be used for the treatment of oedema, poor circulation, cellulitis, sore throats, premenstrual syndrome and menopause, and to stimulate the adrenocortical glands.[14]

Continually repeating what previous aromatherapists have said about geranium only perpetuates the myths and misinformation. Lis-Balchin states that it simply shows a lack of understanding of the origins of geranium oil:

> *The worst misnomer shows the total misconception of the genus as in many aromatherapy books and journals, Geranium maculatum, Geranium robertianum and other Geranium species are implicated either directly or indirectly. This arose due to the unfortunate original mistake made by aromatherapy book authors, who read up the medicinal properties of true 'geranium' from the many Herbals and thought that those were attributable to the Pelargonium species.*[2]

Food, perfumery and flavouring

Geranium oil is extensively used in perfumery and as a fragrance component in all types of cosmetic products such as soaps, creams, lotions and perfumes.[9,15]

Therapeutics

Pharmacology and clinical studies

Many pharmacological studies involving geranium essential oil have been published. A systemic review of these studies will not be attempted. Rather, I have chosen a selection of studies that support the traditional and clinical uses.

Analgesic activity

A double-blind crossover clinical study found that geranium oil was associated with a significant reduction in pain. I am concerned with this study because geranium oil was used at 100%, 50% and 10% solutions. The authors noted that the pain reduction was dose dependent. It is not surprising that the study also reported 20 minor adverse reactions among seven patients for five treatments. All the adverse reactions were considered not serious and were all resolved in an hour.[16]

Antimicrobial activity

Geranium oil has been reported to exhibit antifungal and antibacterial activities in vitro.[15,17]

Lis-Balchin states that the antimicrobial activity of geranium is variable according to the chemical composition of the oil. She cites an antifungal study which tested 16 samples of geranium oil. *Aspergillus niger* was inhibited by 0 to 94%, *A. ochraceus* was inhibited by 12 to 95% and *Fusarium culmorum* was inhibited by 40 to 86%.[7]

Geranium oil was found to be a very effective antifungal when tested against *Candida albicans*. Unfortunately, the botanical origins of the oil were not stated.[18]

Anti-neuro-inflammatory activity

Another study found that geranium oil has an anti-neuro-inflammatory effect on microglial cells. Microglial cells are important immune cells in the brain, and their activation is involved in neurodegenerative diseases such as Alzheimer's disease. The study demonstrated that geranium oil inhibited nitric oxide (NO) production, as well as the expression of the pro-inflammatory enzymes cyclooxygenase-2 (COX-2) and induced nitric oxide synthase in primary cultures of activated microglial cells. When the major constituents of the oil at their natural concentration were tested, none of them could inhibit NO production. The result also suggests a possible synergistic interaction between the major constituents.[19]

Anxiolytic activity

Clinical studies have confirmed that inhalation of geranium essential oil is very effective in reducing anxiety.[20]

Female reproductive system

Often studies involve geranium oil blended with other essential oils and used in massage. Typically, in such studies it difficult to ascertain if the effects were from geranium oil or from the massage. One such study involved investigating the effects of aromatherapy massage on alleviating menopausal symptoms. While the study found that aromatherapy massage may be an effective treatment of menopausal symptoms such as hot flushes, depression and pain in climacteric women, it was unfortunate that it could not be identified if the benefits were from the essential oils or from the massage. Also, the study used a blend of essential oils of lavender, rose geranium, rose and jasmine in an evening primrose oil base, so it was not possible to identify if geranium oil was of any benefit or not.[21]

Another study involving massage with a blend of essential oils containing geranium oil found that aromatherapy massage was very effective in reducing menstrual pain. The study concluded that the reduction in menstrual pain was significantly higher in the aromatherapy group than the acetaminophen group; however, it could not be verified whether the positive effects were from the essential oils, the massage or both.[22]

G

Lymphoedema

A study using a blend of essential oils containing geranium oil found that, while the massage was effective in reducing symptom associated with lymphoedema, the group using the essential oil blend did not appear to experience any improvement compared to the group just using massage.[23]

Psychophysiological activity

Electroencephalograms can be used to measure brainwave responses to aromas. This technique is referred to as contingent negative variation (CNV). This can be used to determine whether an odour is stimulating, sedating or neutral. A study was able to differentiate brainwave patterns stimulated by odours from those caused by sight and sound. They were found to be independent of the level of consciousness, psychological state or degree of arousal of the subjects being tested. The study also found that factors such as age, sex or culture did not influence the results. One study found that geranium had a stimulating effect.[24]

However, other studies using CNV found that geranium had a sedative effect.[25]

Spasmolytic activity

Lis-Balchin has extensively researched the spasmolytic activity of geranium oil. She tested 32 different *Pelargonium* species, hybrids and cultivars grown in the UK. All the oils were found to be spasmolytic. The mechanism of action was also discussed. It was suggested that their effect might involve an action on calcium flux into the smooth muscles. Apart from citronellol and geraniol, it was not known which other components were responsible for the spasmolytic activity.[26]

In another study, 16 commercial geranium oil samples from Réunion, China, Egypt and Morocco were examined for their antimicrobial activity and for their spasmolytic and antioxidant properties. While the antimicrobial activity varied, all samples were spasmolytic. The components geraniol, citronellol, linalool, isomenthone, guaia-6,9-diene and citronellyl formate were all identified as spasmolytic.[16]

Actions

Actions commonly cited in aromatherapy

Antidepressant, anti-inflammatory, antiseptic, astringent, cicatrisant, deodorant, diuretic, haemostatic, stimulant (adrenal cortex), styptic, tonic, vermifuge, vulnerary[11,27,28,29]

Actions supported by clinical studies

Analgesic, antidepressant, antimicrobial, anxiolytic

Comment

Lis-Balchin states that the numerous aromatherapy uses for geranium oil, both in massage or inhalation, have not been correctly validated. However, she does explain that there is every reason to accept the scientific evidence that massage in itself can relax, and that inhalation of a pleasant aroma and its action through the limbic system can also have a relaxing effect.[7]

Many stress-related conditions such as dermatitis, asthma, intestinal problems and headaches may be indirectly alleviated by the use of geranium oil. Based on traditional aromatherapy use and clinical studies, I believe geranium essential oil would be effective in aromatherapy treatments to alleviate stress and anxiety.

Aromatherapy Uses

Clinical aromatherapy

Detoxification

I believe that this property attributed to geranium oil is incorrect as this is associated with herb robert. Many aromatherapists have successfully used geranium oil many times in detoxification treatments. I have also used geranium oil in detoxification blends. Typically, I would blend geranium oil with essential oils such as juniper berry, rosemary, sweet fennel, lemon or grapefruit. All these essential oils have excellent hepatic and diuretic properties. It is likely that the benefits may have come from these other essential oils.

Therefore, the following statement that I made in the second edition of *The complete guide to Aromatherapy* is likely to be incorrect:

> *Geranium oil is a diuretic and has a stimulating effect on the lymphatic system. It is beneficial for treating cellulite, fluid retention and oedema of the ankles.*[30]

Holmes describes geranium as a liver decongestant and detoxicant. He recommends it for liver congestion, metabolic toxicosis and high blood cholesterol, and suggests that it can also be used as a lymphatic and venous decongestant for lymphatic stasis with swollen glands, varicose veins, haemorrhoids with pruritus, and phlebitis.[28] All these properties relate to herb robert and not geranium essential oil.

Integumentary system

Holmes states that it has excellent skin-regenerating and anti-inflammatory actions. As such it can be used for both acute and chronic skin conditions.[28]

Geranium oil is reputed to have excellent astringent properties, which make it useful for treating wounds and bruises.[11,13,27]

It is recommended for its anti-inflammatory properties for conditions such as eczema and psoriasis, and is used for treating acne.[11,13] Mojay suggests that it is an anti-inflammatory essential oil to be compared with lavender and German chamomile. He recommends geranium oil for psoriasis and eczema. He also states that it can be used for skin infections such as acne, impetigo and athlete's foot.[29]

I could not find any clinical evidence or pharmacological studies to confirm the anti-inflammatory properties of geranium oil.

Psychological

The most effective use of geranium oil in aromatherapy is the influence that it has on our psyche. Mojay states that geranium conveys a feeling of calm strength and security. He suggests that geranium is beneficial for both chronic and acute anxiety, particularly where it is associated with nervous exhaustion due to stress and overwork.[29]

Holmes best sums up geranium's influence on our psychological wellbeing – emotional balance, stability and calm. He states that geranium is a key oil for bracing emotional instability, and that it can be helpful for moodiness and mood swings. It is also recommended for emotional despondency associated with low self-esteem, insecurity, mood swings, chronic anxiety, irritability and feeling emotionally withdrawn.[28]

Reproductive system

I believe that this property often attributed to geranium oil is incorrect as it is often associated with herb robert:

> *It has often been said that geranium oil may be a stimulant of the adrenal cortex, whose hormones are essentially regulating and balancing. This is why geranium oil is recommended for conditions where fluctuating hormones are a problem. In particular, geranium oil may be used to relieve premenstrual tension and menopause.*[30]

I believe that the aroma of geranium may help to alleviate emotional stress that may accompany fluctuating hormones and menstrual problems; therefore it may still be beneficial in a blend for menstrual problems. Once again geranium is often blended with essential oils such as sweet fennel, rose or clary sage, which may have a more direct influence on the hormones.

Skin care

It is popular in skin care, not only for its delightful aroma, but for its action in balancing the production of sebum. This makes it valuable for skin that is either dry, oily or combination skin.[11,12,13]

Rhind recommends geranium oil for inflammations of the skin, pain, soft tissue damage and bruising.[31]

Energetics, psyche and subtle uses

Energetics

Mojay states that, according to the principles of TCM, geranium oil is unique. It is considered *cool* and *moist*. It clears *heat* – therefore it is able to calm the *mind*, relax the nerves and reduce feelings of anxiety. It also has the ability to strengthen *Qi*.[29]

He states that it can help to convey a feeling of calm strength and security, and recommends using it for both chronic and acute anxiety, especially when one is feeling nervous exhaustion due to stress and overwork.[29]

While it perfectly complements lavender in any blend for stress, Mojay describes the difference between lavender and geranium as follows:

> *While lavender oil is suited to the individual in whom emotions overwhelm the mind, geranium oil is for those whose rationality and personal drive deny the place of feeling and impression. The oil therefore helps to reconnect us to our feeling-life – to our emotional sensitivity, relaxed spontaneity, and healthy thirst for pleasure and enjoyment. With this comes a greater capacity for intimate communication – one in which being able to receive and experience is as important as the power to give and express.*[29]

According to the principles of the Five Elements, geranium oil has a strong affinity with the Wood Element. According to Ayurveda, geranium would help to balance the *Vata* and cool the *Pitta*.

Personality

Worwood refers to geranium as a mothering personality – a person who is always ready to take care of someone or something. Geranium personalities are able to create a sense of security and stability wherever they go. They are friendly and comforting, warm and generous, although not in any way extroverted or over-talkative. They are often very popular personalities simply because they have this amazing ability to make people feel worthy and wanted.[32]

G

However, she warns that geranium personalities are often taken advantage of because of their generosity. They never consciously look for thanks or appreciation but get it naturally. They have the ability to wash away your tension and stress just by being there for you. They also tend to take on too much, not leaving enough space for themselves.[32]

Mojay states that geranium is the ideal remedy for the workaholic perfectionist and for the person who has forgotten imagination, intuition and sensory experience.[29]

According to Myers-Briggs personality types, the geranium personality is likely to be an ENFJ. ENFJs are caring and concerned. They have charming and enthusiastic personalities and get on well with everyone. They are excellent communicators and natural leaders, and are good at motivating others. They respect a variety of opinions and are good at creating team spirit. They like to be reassured of their value by receiving praise, respect and affirmations. They often have many 'shoulds' and 'should nots'.

Subtle

Keim Loughran & Bull state that geranium oil is ideal for the individual who does not have enough time, their life is so frantic and busy, they are unable to find moments of stillness and relaxation and are often overwhelmed by too much to do. This also impairs the ability to nurture creativity, relationships and connection with body, mind and spirit.[33]

Geranium is a profoundly feminine oil that helps us create and identify what truly nurtures and sustains us. It helps us to relax and calm our body, mind and spirit, so that we can connect with ourselves, other people and the environment around us. It enables us to balance stillness and movement, and spontaneity and structure. Geranium creates a quiet balanced place where life emerges naturally, creatively and joyfully.[33]

Worwood beautifully describes the subtle healing qualities of geranium:

> *When the spirit is hidden, like a frightened child, within, geranium offers its warm hand of comfort, opening our hearts and memories and healing the pain.*[34]

Worwood also states that geranium resonates with Mother Earth. It signifies the archetypal energy of goddess culture and encompasses the energy of the feminine, reproduction, birth and rebirth.[34]

Zeck states that the refreshing scent of geranium minimises extreme feelings and emotions, helping us to feel more balance and harmony. She recommends using geranium when we are feeling out of sync with the rhythm of nature. She states that geranium will help us connect with the rhythm of life, especially when we are disconnected from our own rhythms.[35]

Dosage and Administration

Blending

Aromatherapy

Geranium's distinctive complex aroma is both rosy floral and green and herbaceous. This rich complex aroma is what makes geranium such a perfect oil for balancing our psychological wellbeing.

Lavabre refers to geranium as a blend equaliser. It helps to fill the gap and helps your blend flow harmoniously.[13]

To alleviate anxiety, nervous tension and stress, consider blending geranium oil with essential oils such as bergamot, German chamomile, Roman chamomile, fragonia, lavender, lemon, mandarin, neroli, sweet orange, patchouli, rose otto or absolute, sandalwood, vetiver or ylang ylang.

For a mentally uplifting and invigorating blend, consider blending geranium oil with essential oils such as basil, black pepper, cardamom, clove bud, ginger, grapefruit, lemon, cold-pressed lime, peppermint, pine, rosemary, spruce or peppermint.

To alleviate depression, consider blending geranium oil with essential oils such as bergamot, coriander seed, jasmine absolute, lavender, lemon, sweet orange, mandarin, neroli, rose otto, sandalwood or ylang ylang.

For congested and oily skin, consider blending geranium oil with essential oils such as cypress, grapefruit, lavender, lemon or juniper berry.

Perfumery

Geranium oil is extensively used in perfumery. Its floral sweetness, delightful freshness and delicate warm-rosy tonalities blend so well with other floral components used in perfumery.[9]

Mode of administration

Bath

Full body bath, foot bath

Topical

Compress, massage, ointment, skin care

Inhalation

Direct inhalation, diffuser, oil vaporiser

Safety Profile

General safety

Geranium oil has been reported to be non-toxic, non-irritant and non-sensitising. However, cases of dermatitis in hypersensitive individuals caused by geranium oil have been documented.[11]

Contraindications

No contraindications known.

Regulatory guidelines

Geranium essential oil has GRAS status.

References

1. James J. *Cultivation and sales of Pelargonium plants for ornamental use in the UK and worldwide.* In Lis-Balchin M. ed. *Geranium and Pelargonium.* Taylor & Francis Group, London, 2002: 80-91. (Medical and Aromatic Plants – Industrial Profiles; 27).
2. Lis-Balchin M. *History of nomenclature, usage and cultivation of Geranium and Pelargonium species.* In Lis-Balchin M. ed. *Geranium and Pelargonium.* Taylor & Francis Group, London, 2002: 5-10. (Medical and Aromatic Plants – Industrial Profiles; 27).
3. Miller DM. *The taxonomy of Pelargonium species and cultivars, their origins and growth in the wild.* In Lis-Balchin M. ed. *Geranium and Pelargonium.* Taylor & Francis Group, London, 2002: 49-79. (Medical and Aromatic Plants – Industrial Profiles; 27).
4. Tisserand R, Young R. *Essential oil safety.* 2nd edn. Churchill Livingstone, Edinburgh, 2014.
5. Demarne FE. *'Rose-scented geranium' a Pelargonium grown for the perfume industry.* In Lis-Balchin M. ed. *Geranium and Pelargonium.* Taylor & Francis Group, London, 2002: 193-211. (Medical and Aromatic Plants – Industrial Profiles; 27).
6. Weiss EA. *Essential oil crops.* CAB International, Wallingford, 1997.
7. Lis-Balchin M. *Aromatherapy science – a guide for health professionals.* Pharmaceutical Press, London, 2006.
8. Lis-Balchin M. *Geranium oil and its use in aromatherapy.* In Lis-Balchin M. ed. *Geranium and Pelargonium.* Taylor & Francis Group, London, 2002: 234-246. (Medical and Aromatic Plants – Industrial Profiles; 27).
9. Arctander S. *Perfume and flavor materials of natural origin.* Allured Publishing, Carol Stream, 1994.
10. Valnet J. *The practice of aromatherapy.* C.W Daniel Company, Saffron Walden, 1980.
11. Lawless J. *The encyclopaedia of essential oils.* Element Books, Shaftesbury, 1992.
12. Tisserand R. *The art of aromatherapy.* C.W. Daniel Company, Saffron Walden, 1977.
13. Lavabre M. *Aromatherapy workbook.* Healing Arts Press, Rochester, 1997.
14. Rhind JP. *Essential oils – a handbook for aromatherapy practice.* 2nd edn. Singing Dragon, London, 2012.
15. Khan I, Abourashed E. *Leung's encyclopedia of common natural ingredients used in food, drugs and cosmetics.* 3rd edn. John Wiley & Sons, New Jersey, 2010.
16. Greenway FL et al. *Temporary relief of postherpetic neuralgia pain with topical geranium oil.* American Journal of Medicine, 2002; 115(7): 586-587. Cited in Quintessential Aromatics database, 2013.
17. Lis-Balchin M. *Bioactivity of geranium oils from different commercial sources.* Journal of Essential Oil Research, 1996; 8(3): 281-290.
18. Devkatte AN et al. *Potential of plant oils as inhibitors of Candida albicans growth.* FEMS Yeast Research, 2005; 5(9): 867-873. Cited in Quintessential Aromatics database, 2013.
19. Elmann A et al. *Anti-neuro-inflammatory effects of geranium oil in microgial cells.* Journal of Functional Foods, 2010; 2(1): 17-22. Cited in Quintessential Aromatics database, 2013.
20. Morris N et al. *Anxiety reduction by aromatherapy: anxiolytic effects of inhalation of geranium and rosemary.* International Journal of Aromatherapy, 1995; 7(2): 33-39. Cited in from Quintessential Aromatics database, 2013.

G

21. Hur MH et al. *Aromatherapy massage affects menopausal symptoms in Korean climacteric women: a pilot-controlled clinical trial.* Evidence-Based Complementary and Alternative Medicine, 2008; 5(3): 325-328. Cited in Quintessential Aromatics database, 2013.
22. Hur MH et al. *Aromatherapy massage on the abdomen for alleviating menstrual pain in high school girls: a preliminary controlled clinical study.* Evidence-Based Complementary and Alternative Medicine, 2012. Cited in Quintessential Aromatics database, 2013. doi: 10.1155/2012/187163.
23. Barclay J et al. *Reducing the symptoms of lymphoedema: is there a role for aromatherapy?* European Journal of Oncology Nursing, 2006; 10(2): 140-149. Cited in Quintessential Aromatics database, 2013.
24. Manley CH. *Psychophysiological effect of odor.* Critical Reviews in Food Science and Nutrition, 1993; 33(1): 57-62. Cited in Quintessential Aromatics database, 2013.
25. Torii S. et al. *Contingent negative variation and the psychological effects of odor.* In Van Toller S, Dodds GH eds. *Perfumery: The psychology and biology of fragrance.* Chapman & Hall, New York, 1988: 107-120.
26. Lis-Balchin M et al. *The spasmolytic activity of the essential oils of scented Pelargoniums (Geraniaceae).* Phytotherapy Research, 1997; 11(8): 583-584. Cited in Quintessential Aromatics database, 2013.
27. Davis P. *Aromatherapy: an A-Z.* 2nd edn. C.W. Daniel Company, Saffron Walden, 1999.
28. Holmes P. *Aromatica: a clinical guide to essential oil therapeutics – Vol. I.* Singing Dragon, London, 2016.
29. Mojay G. *Aromatherapy for healing the spirit.* Healing Arts Press, Rochester, 1999.
30. Battaglia S. *The complete guide to aromatherapy.* The International Centre of Holistic Aromatherapy. 2nd edn. Brisbane, 2003.
31. Rhind JP. *Aromatherapeutic blending.* Singing Dragon, London, 2016.
32. Worwood VA. *The fragrant mind.* Transworld Publishers, London, 1995.
33. Keim Loughran J, Bull R. *Aromatherapy anointing oils.* Frog, Berkeley, 2001.
34. Worwood VA. *The fragrant heavens.* Transworld Publishers, London, 1999.
35. Zeck R. *The blossoming heart – aromatherapy for healing and transformation.* Aroma Tours, East Ivanhoe, 2004.

G

Ginger

Identification

Botanical name

Zingiber officinale Roscoe

Synonyms

Another member of the same family, *Languas officinarum,* is known as ginger root or Chinese ginger.[1]

Family

Zingiberaceae

Botany and origins

Ginger is a tropical perennial herb growing 0.6 to 1.2 m high, with reed-like stems, lanceolate leaves and purple flowers. The stem grows directly from the thick tuberous rhizome, from which both the spice and essential oil are produced.[1]

Originally from India, ginger is now cultivated in India, China, most of South East Asia, many Pacific Ocean islands, Australia and the tropical regions of Africa.[1]

Method of extraction

Ginger oil is produced by steam distillation, occasionally by water and steam distillation, of the dried, unpeeled, ground rhizomes of *Z. officinale.*

An oleoresin is produced by solvent extraction of the dried and unpeeled rhizome of *Z. officinale,* since peeled ginger loses most of its essential oil content.[2]

Supercritical fluid extraction dissolves the aromatic and pungent principles from the powdered rhizomes in liquid carbon dioxide under pressure. Weiss states that this technique produces an extract that is considered near to the true ginger flavour and pungency.[1]

Characteristics

Ginger oil is a pale-yellow to light-amber-coloured mobile liquid. Its odour is warm, but fresh-woody, spicy with a slight fresh top note. The sweet and heavy undertone is tenacious, sweet and rich, almost balsamic-floral.[3]

Ginger oleoresin is a dark brown or very dark-amber-coloured, viscous liquid, with a warm-spicy, sweet aroma.[3]

Much of the scent of ginger is due to the essential oil. However, its sharp, pungent taste is from the gingerols and shogaol found in the CO_2 extract, whereas the steam-distilled essential oil is warm, gentle and soft without the sharp components.[4]

Chemical composition

Some 100 constituents have been identified in distilled ginger oil. The main components are sesquiterpene hydrocarbons (50-66%), oxygenated sesquiterpenes (up to 17%), and the rest is made up of monoterpene hydrocarbons and oxygenated monoterpenes.[1]

The chemical composition of a range of distilled ginger oils was reported as follows:[1]

Constituent	Australia	Sri Lanka	India
α-pinene	trace	0.2-3.3%	0.4%
camphene	trace	0.9-14.1%	1.1%
geranial	3-20%	1.0-7.7%	1.4%
nerol	1-10%	2.5-10.1%	0.2%
1,8-cineole	-	2.1-12.23%	-
ar-curcumene	6-10%	5.7-17.7%	17.7%
zingiberene	20-28%	0.3-1.2%	35.6%
(*Z*)-β-farnesene	-	0.5-1.2%	-
β-sesquiphellandrene	7-11.0%	trace-0.3%	-
β-bisabolene	5-9%	20.1-60.4%	0.2%
β-eudesmol	-	1.0-5.4%	-

Australian ginger oil typically has a higher citral (geranial) content than most other ginger oils. This gives the oil a distinctly fresh, lemon-like aroma. This is probably due to more careful drying of the rhizomes.[1]

It has been reported that the citrus-like aroma of ginger oil (which is due to citral) is characteristic of oil distilled from fresh or quickly dried ginger, whereas commercial oils distilled from sun-dried ginger lack the lemony note.[5]

Ginger oil distilled from dry material is characterised by a higher proportion of sesquiterpene hydrocarbons. The major sesquiterpene hydrocarbons are zingiberene, *ar*-curcumene, β-bisabolene, (-)-β-sesquiphellandrene and (*E*,*E*)-α-farnesene.[5]

Both zingiberene and (-)-β-sesquiphellandrene can be oxidised to *ar*-curcumene in essential oil stored under unfavourable conditions. It is believed that high levels of *ar*-curcumene may, therefore, be an indicator of degraded oil, but could also possibly reflect distillation conditions.[5]

Ginger oleoresin and CO_2 ginger extract contain mainly the pungent principles gingerols and shogaols, as well as zingerone. Shogaols and zingerone are dehydration and degradation products of gingerols.[6]

It was reported that CO_2 extraction provides us with the most effective method of extracting the principal components responsible for the pungent characteristics of ginger, gingerols, as heat decomposition does not occur.[1,7]

It was found that oleoresin of ginger extracted with solvents such as ethanol or acetone lacks the strong aroma due to the loss of volatile components during the evaporation process of the solvents. On the other hand, ginger extract obtained by high-pressure CO_2 contains both the aromatic and pungent components that best resemble the flavour profile of the starting material. It was found that the 6-gingerol content could be controlled by manipulating CO_2 extraction conditions.[7]

The compounds responsible for the biological activity of ginger extracts are gingerols, shogaols, 6-paradol, 6-gingerdiol, gingerenone A, zingerone, diarylheptanoids, hexahydrocurcumin and its derivatives (curcuminoids).[2,6]

The main chemical constituents in a certified organic CO_2 ginger extract from Indonesia were as follows:

neral (1.5%), geranial (2.6%), *ar*-curcumene (19.9%), α-zingiberene (19.6), α-farnesene (4.5%), β-bisabolene (10.1%), sesquiphellandrene (16.1%), zingerone (0.03%), total gingerols (20.4%), total shogaols (4.3%).[8]

Adulteration

Adulteration of ginger oil is not common.[9]

Pharmacopoeias and standards

The purity, composition and physico-chemical properties of ginger essential oil are defined in ISO 16928:2014 Essential Oil of Ginger. Ginger root and its oil are also listed in several monographs:

- German Commission E
- Overview of Comments Received on Community Herbal Monograph on *Zingiber officinale* Roscoe, Rhizome. European Medicines Agency
- WHO Monographs on Selected Medicinal Plants – Vol. 1.

History and Traditional Uses

History

The Latin term *zingiber* derives from the ancient Tamil root, *ingiver*, meaning ginger rhizome. The term *ingiver* spread to ancient Greece and Rome through the Arab traders, and from there to Western Europe. In second century AD Rome, ginger was one of the very few commodities on which a duty was levied at Alexandria, the port of entry. In the Middle Ages, ginger was considered a privileged good. During the thirteenth and fourteenth centuries, next to pepper, ginger was the most common and most precious of spices.[1]

Ginger is a vital ingredient in Chinese, Japanese and Indian cuisines, as well as in the cuisines of many other Asian countries.[10]

Traditional medicine

Ginger has been valued as a spice and medicinal plant since ancient times in India and in China. In India, it was referred to as *mahaoushadha* and *vishwabheshaja*, literally meaning the great medicine and the universal cure respectively. Ginger was mentioned in the ancient Ayurvedic texts of *Charaka Samhitha* and *Susrutha Samhitha*. [10]

In TCM, ginger is divided into three preparation types: *sheng-jiang* – the fresh raw rhizome; *gan-jiang* – the dried raw rhizome; and *pao-jiang* – the dried, quick-fried rhizome. All three are considered warming remedies with particular affinity to the digestive system and lungs. The fresh rhizome is considered the most dispersing of the three. It is used to disperse the external pathogens, *cold* and *wind cold*, which are often characterised by colds and flu, headaches, general aches and pain, nasal congestion and a runny nose. In comparison, the dried rhizome is used for *cold* conditions associated with poor appetite and weak digestion, cold limbs, vomiting and diarrhoea. The dried rhizomes are also better suited to individuals who have atony (lack of muscle tone), congestion or debility. The fried rhizome is considered a stronger remedy and is also applied topically to stop bleeding.[11]

G

Herbal

Ginger is used universally in traditional medicine, as well as in modern medicine for the treatment of nausea and vomiting associated with pregnancy, and for the prevention of travel and seasickness. Many countries have approved ginger as a nonprescription drug for the prevention of motion sickness. It is also recognised as an anti-inflammatory drug beneficial for the treatment of rheumatoid arthritis and osteoarthritis.[10]

The German Commission E recommends using the rhizome powder for gastrointestinal distress and to prevent motion sickness (2 g/day). It is described as having antiemetic, positive inotropic and stimulant effects on intestinal peristalsis, salivary and gastric secretions.[12]

The WHO monograph for ginger root reports that it is used in traditional medicine for the treatment of dyspepsia, flatulence, colic, vomiting, diarrhoea, spasms and other stomach complaints. It is also used for the treatment of colds and flu, to stimulate the appetite, and as an anti-inflammatory agent for the treatment of migraines and rheumatic and muscular disorders.[13]

Ginger has been shown to reduce pain associated with periods in women at doses of 1 g daily. The 2-month placebo-controlled trial found that ginger was as effective as ibuprofen and mefenamic acid.[14]

The results of a systemic review and meta-analysis of randomised clinical trials provided evidence for the effectiveness of ginger in treating primary dysmenorrhoea. The research clearly demonstrates that 750-2000 mg/day of dried powdered ginger during the first 3-4 days of the menstrual cycle provided very promising potential treatment for pain and discomfort associated with primary dysmenorrhoea.[15]

Food, perfumery and flavouring

Ginger oleoresin is preferred for flavouring foods and beverages. It is used as a flavouring agent in baking goods, spice blends, meat sauces, candy, throat lozenges and carbonated soft drinks.[3]

Therapeutics

Pharmacology and clinical studies

Many pharmacological studies involving ginger essential oil and ginger CO_2 extract have been published. A systemic review of these studies will not be attempted. Rather, I have chosen a selection of studies that support the traditional and clinical uses.

Antiemetic activity

Clinical trials have identified that ginger has antiemetic properties. Most of the trials revealed an activity superior to that of a placebo for motion sickness, postoperative nausea or morning sickness (at the usual of 1 g per day). The antiemetic action may be a consequence of the direct stimulating effect on the gastrointestinal tract.[16]

A single-blind, controlled, randomised crossover study assessed the efficacy of inhaling ginger oil for the management of nausea, vomiting and health-related quality of life in breast cancer patients undergoing chemotherapy. The evidence from this study found that inhaling ginger essential oil was not effective for alleviating nausea. However, the study confirmed that there was a significant improvement in the health-related quality of life.[17]

However, another double-blind trial involving 744 cancer patients found that oral supplementation of dried ginger powder at a daily dose of 0.5–1.0 g significantly reduced the severity of acute chemotherapy-induced nausea in adult cancer patients.[18]

6-gingerol and 6-shogaol are implicated in ginger's anti-nausea properties, as they are found to suppress gastric contraction and increase both gastrointestinal motility and spontaneous peristaltic activity. Davis explains that this then reduces the gastrointestinal feedback to the central chemoreceptors, thus reducing the feeling of nausea.[2]

Postoperative nausea is a common complication of anaesthesia and surgery. Antiemetic medication may reduce postoperative nausea but does not reliably prevent it. A randomised trial examined the benefits of aromatherapy in reducing postoperative nausea. Inhalation of ginger oil was found to be effective as a treatment for postoperative nausea.[19]

Anti-inflammatory activity

The oral consumption of dried, powdered ginger taken for between 3 months and 2.5 years by patients with rheumatoid arthritis and osteoarthritis was able to provide relief of pain and swelling. The researchers suggested that the effects of ginger could be related to the inhibition of prostaglandin and leukotriene biosynthesis.[2]

6-gingerol and four gingerdione derivatives were identified as the main active compounds that are able to inhibit the biosynthesis of thromboxane and prostaglandin. The results of an in vitro assessment of two different supercritical fluid extracted ginger oils at Southern Cross University found that both essential oils had significant anti-inflammatory activity. All of the known compounds – 6-gingerol, 8-gingerol, 10-gingerol and [6]-shogaol – in ginger oil displayed potent anti-inflammatory activity. 10-gingerol, for example, had over twice the inhibitory activity of aspirin at 100 μM concentration.[2]

When administered orally, ginger oil exhibited anti-inflammatory activity in rats with induced severe chronic adjuvant arthritis.[9]

Oral administration of ginger oil for one month significantly increased superoxide dismutase, glutathione and glutathione reductase enzyme levels in the blood of mice and glutathione-S-transferase, glutathione peroxidase and superoxide dismutase enzymes in the liver. Ginger oil produced significant reduction in acute inflammation produced by carrageenan and dextran, and formalin induced chronic inflammation.[20]

Antimicrobial activity

Lis-Balchin cites studies that confirm the antibacterial activity of ginger is very low. However, she states that the sesquiterpenes from ginger rhizomes have in vitro activity against rhinovirus IB.[9]

The antimicrobial activities of the essential oil and oleoresins of ginger were examined using various food-borne pathogenic fungal and bacterial species. The essential oil and the oleoresin both had good to moderate inhibitory activity; however, the essential oil was found to be better than the oleoresin.[21]

Cardiovascular system

A considerable number of pharmacological studies involving the digestive, central nervous and cardiovascular systems have been reported for gingerol and shogaol. It has been identified that these constituents have potent inhibitory action against prostaglandin synthetase, which corresponds with anti-inflammatory and anti-platelet aggregation.[22]

Digestive activity

The pungent principles (6-gingerol and 10-gingerol) present in an extract of ginger were found to increase bile secretion and were responsible for the cholagogic effect of ginger. These pungent principles were also reported to enhance gastrointestinal motility. A number of sesquiterpenes (β-bisabolene, *ar*-curcumene and α-zingiberene), 6-gingerol and 6-shogaol have been identified as having antiulcer effects in rats.[23]

Hepatic activity

Clinical trials have shown that the oleoresin is a cholesterol-lowering agent. Gingerol has been found to be a cholagogue and hepatoprotective agent.[16,22]

Actions

Actions commonly cited in aromatherapy

Analgesic, carminative, expectorant, febrifuge, rubefacient, stimulant, stomachic, sudorific and tonic[24,25]

Actions supported by clinical studies

I believe that the ginger CO_2 extract is likely to have all the above actions commonly cited in aromatherapy. It is unlikely that the distilled ginger oil has many of the actions commonly cited in aromatherapy.

Comment

As a medicinal herb, ginger may be prepared by either decocting the fresh root or by preparing an alcoholic tincture or fluid extract with it. A tincture is considered the most complete preparation as it contains the essential oil constituents as well as the pungent alcohols, shogaol and gingerol found in the oleoresin.[26]

While it may be tempting to suggest that the essential oil and herbal extract have similar properties, Holmes points out that, because the distilled essential oil contains no pungent components, the essential oil cannot have diaphoretic properties. He states that it is a waste of time using ginger essential oil as a diaphoretic at the onset of a cold.[26]

The oleoresin and CO_2 extract may be of interest to aromatherapists as they contain more of the pungent and warming components found in the herb. Gingerol and shogaol may have a local irritant effect on mucous membranes, and it is possible that vascular stimulation that follows from taking ginger comes either from direct action on metarterioles or by reflex from sensory receptors at other sites.[27]

Aromatherapy Uses

Clinical aromatherapy

Cardiovascular system

Mojay describes ginger oil as a circulatory stimulant and tonic of the heart. He recommends it for poor circulation, cold hands and feet, cardiac fatigue and angina pectoris.[27]

Digestive system

Ginger oil is indicated for indigestion, flatulence, nausea and chronic gastritis.[24] Mojay states that it should be blended with Roman chamomile and sweet orange to relieve travel and morning sickness.[28]

Schnaubelt states that ginger oil is a choleretic and it helps stimulate the production of bile from the liver.[29]

Immune system

Holmes describes ginger as an antiviral and immunostimulant agent, and suggests using the oil or a tincture of ginger to treat the onset of colds and flu. He states that it has been shown to stimulate both T-lymphocytes and cell-mediated immunity. However, he explains that it is less useful once the infection has set in and becomes bacterial.[24]

Musculoskeletal system

Ginger oil may be used in a compress or massage for rheumatism, arthritis and muscular pain of a cold, contracting type.[25,28]

Psychological

Holmes recommends using ginger whenever we have poor motivation, low willpower, feel discouraged, suffer from burnout or confusion, or feel emotionally empty and cold. He states that it will promote motivation, courage and self-confidence. He also states that it will promote alertness and stimulate the mind, and recommends using ginger oil for lethargy, mental apathy and poor concentration.[24]

Zeck recommends using ginger when our body has become depleted of physical and emotional energy. When there has been a loss of energy on a physical and emotional level, this may lead to feelings of melancholy and grief for oneself. Ginger will help build your strength and energy to succeed.[30]

Respiratory system

Ginger oil is recommended for catarrhal conditions, coughs, sinusitis and sore throats.[24]

Schnaubelt explains that ginger oil suppresses coughs and has an expectorant action on the bronchi and lungs.[29]

Energetics, psyche and subtle uses

Energetics

The properties of ginger are described as *warming*. Not only is this *warming* quality beneficial for stimulating arterial circulation, but it also helps dispel *cold* conditions associated with the digestive system, respiratory system and reproductive system.[24,28]

It has a *warming* and stimulating effect on the *Lungs* and is ideally suited to treat chronic bronchitis. Ginger's ability to tonify the *Yang Qi* of the *Kidneys* makes it beneficial for relieving lower back pain associated with muscular fatigue.[28]

Holmes states that low sex drive, frigidity, fatigue, cold skin and extremities, and apathy are also associated with *Kidney Yang Qi deficiency*.[24]

Ginger oil helps to dispel *Lung phlegm-cold* and *damp* conditions, which are associated with cough and copious expectoration of phlegm.[24]

According to TCM and the Five Elements, ginger will help strengthen the *Zhi*. The *Zhi* is responsible for our willpower and determination. Whenever our *Zhi* is weak, we may have clear plans and intentions, but lack the personal drive and optimism to take action. We may procrastinate and doubt ourselves and wait for others to spur us on. We may feel disconnected from our physical body and we may shy away from vigorous and sustained activity.[28]

According to the principles of Ayurveda, ginger has a strong stimulating effect on the *Pitta* dosha, and as such it is commonly advised to avoid ginger if you have strong *Pitta* dosha. Ginger is ideally suited to reduce excess *Kapha*.

Personality profile

A ginger personality is a strong silent type. The character of ginger is warming, strengthening and encouraging.[31]

G

Worwood states that this personality can be very strong, masculine and forceful; however, they are always respectful of other people's personal space and they will never be possessive. Ginger personalities make good listeners; however, they are not good conversationalists. She states that a ginger personality will expect you to do your own thing, just as they expect you to leave them alone to do theirs.[31]

Mojay states that ginger is ideal for those who have clear plans and good intentions, but who lack the personal drive and optimism to manifest initiative and take real or immediate action.[28]

According to Myers-Briggs personality types, the ginger personality is likely to be an ISTJ. ISTJs are very stable, responsible and dependable. They are very private. They like to be punctual and precise, and are very orderly. They have good concentration and are difficult to distract. They find it hard to relax as they think that things that help relax are non-productive. They enjoy being in nature. They can be overly detail-oriented, are devoted hard workers, and are very thorough and accurate in everything they do. They like to have strict rules and procedures and tend to be inflexible. They are modest and unassuming and will make loyal friends. They may have difficulties expressing feelings of warmth and tenderness to loved ones. They can make quick critical judgement of others.

Subtle

The scent of ginger will increase determination and clarity. It is recommended for conditions associated with loss of motivation, will or inner strength, especially when these present as apathy, listlessness, indecision, confusion and disconnection.[26]

Keim Loughran & Bull state that ginger strengthens us on all levels so that we have the courage and confidence to identify what we want and then to create it. It invites abundance, helping us to tap into the richness of the universe. It helps us believe that we deserve to experience abundant life.[32]

Holmes states that ginger will infuse warmth and passion into the soul and the feeling life. He recommends ginger whenever we become apathetic, unmotivated and discouraged to the point of indifference, emotional coldness and downright depression. Ginger will help those individuals who have become emotionally withdrawn to become more fully present and passionate about the things they truly and deeply care for.[24]

Worwood describes ginger as a fragrance of valour and courage. It will give strength and courage to those who are faint-hearted and weak.[33]

Ginger has a very strong affinity with the solar plexus chakra. This is the chakra that helps to strengthen our self-confidence and willpower.

Dosage and administration

Blending

Aromatherapy

For the relief of colds and flu associated with bronchial congestion, consider blending ginger oil with essential oils such cajeput, 1,8-cineole-rich eucalyptus oils, lemon-scented eucalyptus, peppermint eucalyptus, fragonia, kunzea, lemon myrtle, manuka, myrtle, peppermint, pine or tea tree.

For the relief of muscular aches and pains, consider blending ginger CO_2 extract with essential oils such as black pepper, cajeput, kunzea, fragonia, peppermint, pine or rosemary.

For the relief of nausea and travel sickness, consider blending ginger oil or ginger CO_2 extract with essential oils such as cardamom or peppermint.

To alleviate hiccups, consider blending ginger CO_2 extract with essential oils such as cardamom, sweet fennel or peppermint.

Perfumery

Ginger oil adds a warm, sensual note to any floral oil. It blends well with ylang ylang, rose absolute or jasmine absolute to create a rich oriental floral style perfume. Warm spice oils such as ginger blend well with the vibrant citrus oils such as lemon, grapefruit, mandarin or sweet orange. Ginger oil blends well with amyris, Virginian or Atlas cedarwood, cardamom, coriander seed and sandalwood to create a spicy woody masculine style perfume.

In flavour composition, the CO_2 ginger extract blends very well with sweet orange and lime essential oils.[4]

Mode of administration

Bath

Distilled ginger essential oil can be used in full body bath, foot bath; however, avoid using CO_2 ginger extract in a bath as it may cause dermal irritation.

Topical

Compress, massage, ointment

Inhalation

Distilled ginger essential oil – direct inhalation, diffuser, oil vaporiser

The pungent components in CO_2 ginger extract can be irritating to the sinuses, so I do not recommend using it in a diffuser.

Safety Profile

General safety

There are no known hazards or contraindications associated with ginger oil. Ginger oil is non-toxic and non-irritant. When tested at 4% on 25 volunteers, it had neither irritating nor sensitising effect.[34]

Contraindications

No contraindications known.

Regulatory guidelines

Ginger essential oil has GRAS status.

References

1. Weiss EA. *Essential oil crops*. CAB International, Wallingford, 1997.
2. Davis C, Herse J. *New value-added opportunities for natural therapeutic products in the Australian ginger industry*. Horticulture Australia, 2003.
3. Arctander S. *Perfume and flavor materials of natural origin*. Allured Publishing, Carol Stream, 1994.
4. Schnaubelt K. *The healing intelligence of essential oils*. Healing Arts Press, Rochester, 2011.
5. Wohlmuth H. *Phytochemistry and pharmacology of plants from the ginger family, Zingiberaceae*. Southern Cross University, Lismore, 2008.
6. Vernin G, Parkanyi C. *Chemistry of ginger*. In Ravindran PN, Nirmal Babu K. ed. *Ginger – The genus Zingiber*. CRC Press, Boca Raton, 2005: 87-180.
7. Yonei Y et al. *Extraction of ginger flavor with liquid or supercritical carbon dioxide*. The Journal of Supercritical Fluids, 1995; 8: 156-161.
8. Southern Cross University. *Perfect Potion ginger CO_2 extract – certificate of analysis*. 2017.
9. Lis-Balchin M. *Aromatherapy science – a guide for healthcare professionals*. Pharmaceutical Press, London, 2006.
10. Ravindran PN, Nirmal Babu K. *Introduction*. In Ravindran PN, Nirmal Babu K. ed. *Ginger – The genus Zingiber*. CRC Press, Boca Raton, 2005: 1-14.
11. Bone K, Mills S. *Principles and practice of phytotherapy*. 2nd edn. Churchill Livingstone, Edinburgh, 2013.
12. Blumenthal M et al. *The complete German commission E monographs: therapeutic guide to herbal medicine*. American Botanical Council, Austin, 1998.
13. *WHO monographs on selected medicinal plants – Vol. 1*. World Health Organization, Geneva, 1999.
14. *Ginger*. Retrieved Sep 18, 2017, from https://examine.com/supplements/ginger/
15. Daily JW et al. *Efficacy of ginger for alleviating the symptoms of primary dysmenorrhea: a systemic review and meta-analysis of randomized clinical trials*. Pain Medicine, 2015; 16(12): 2243-2255. doi: 10.1111/pme.12853.
16. Bruneton J. *Pharmacognosy*. 2nd edn. Lavoisier Publishing, Paris, 1999.
17. Lua PL et al. *Effects of inhaled ginger aromatherapy on chemotherapy-induced nausea and vomiting and health-related quality of life in women with breast cancer*. Complementary Therapies in Medicine, 2015; 23(3): 396-404.
18. Ryan JL et al. *Ginger (Zingiber officinale) reduces acute chemotherapy –induced nausea: a URCC CCOP study of 576 patients*. Support Care in Cancer, 2012; 7(12): 1479–1489.
19. Hunt R et al. *Aromatherapy as treatment for postoperative nausea: a randomized trial*. Anesthesia and Analgesia, 2013: 117(3): 597-604. Cited in Quintessential Aromatics database, 2013.
20. Jeena K et al. *Antioxidant, anti-inflammatory and antinociceptive activities of essential oil from ginger*. Indian Journal of Physiology and Pharmacology, 2013: 57(1): 51-62. Cited in Quintessential Aromatics database, 2013.
21. Singh G et al. *Chemistry, antioxidant and antimicrobial investigations on essential oil and oleoresins of Zingiber officinale*. Food and Chemical Toxicology, 2008; 46(10): 3295-3302. Cited in Quintessential Aromatic database, 2013.
22. Evans WC. *Trease and Evans pharmacognosy*. 15th edn. WB Saunders, Edinburgh, 2002.
23. Yamahara J et al. *The anti-ulcer effect in rats of ginger constituents*. Journal of Ethnopharmacology, 1988; 23(2/3): 299-304.
24. Holmes P. *Aromatica: a clinical guide to essential oil therapeutics – Vol. I*. Singing Dragon, London, 2016.
25. Lawless J. *The encyclopaedia of essential oils*. Element Books, Shaftesbury, 1992.
26. Holmes P. *Ginger oil*. The International Journal of Aromatherapy, 1996; 7(4): 16.
27. Mills S. *The essential book of herbal medicine*. Arkana Penguin Books, England, 1991.
28. Mojay G. *Aromatherapy for healing the spirit*. Healing Arts Press, Rochester, 1999.
29. Schnaubelt K. *Advanced aromatherapy*. Healing Arts Press, Rochester, 1995.
30. Zeck R. *The blossoming heart – aromatherapy for healing and transformation*. Aroma Tours, East Ivanhoe, 2004.
31. Worwood VA. *The fragrant mind*. Transworld Publishers, London, 1995.
32. Keim Loughran J, Bull R. *Aromatherapy and subtle energy techniques*. Frog, Berkeley, 2000.

G

33. Worwood VA. *The fragrant heavens.* Transworld Publishers, London, 1999.

34. Tisserand R, Young R. *Essential oil safety.* 2nd edn. Churchill Livingstone, Edinburgh, 2014.

Grapefruit

Identification

Botanical name

Citrus paradisi Macf.

Synonyms

Citrus racemosa, Citrus decumana var. *racemosa, Citrus maxima* var. *racemosa,* shaddock fruit[1]

Family

Rutaceae

Botany and origins

Citrus paradisi is a hybrid between *C. maxima* (pomelo) and *C. sinensis* (sweet orange). Grapefruit is the only citrus species native to the New World, and probably originated in the West Indies from a natural cross between introduced parents sometime in the seventeenth century.[1]

The oil is produced in the USA, the West Indies, Brazil, Israel and Nigeria.[2]

Grapefruit is a large, vigorous tree that grows up to 30 m, with a single trunk, many branches, and a round to blunt conical shape if left unpruned. The fruit is large, up to 15 cm diameter, generally spherical but often compressed laterally, light yellow to orange. The shape and colour of the fruit are dependent on the cultivar.[1]

The difference between the essential oil from the white- and red-fleshed cultivars is that the former generally has a higher aldehyde content and lower evaporative residue than the latter, which also contains a small percentage of linalool.[1]

Method of extraction

Grapefruit oil is expressed from the peels of the grapefruit.

Characteristics

The oil is a mobile, yellowish to greenish yellow or pale orange-yellow oil with a fresh-citrus and sweet odour.[2] The characteristic grapefruit aroma and flavour is reported to be due to nootkatone.[3]

Chemical composition

The chemical composition of grapefruit essential oil was reported as follows:

α-pinene (0.38%), β-pinene (0.02%), sabinene (0.42%), myrcene (1.37%), *d*-limonene (84.0%), citronellal (0.1%), decanol (0.4%), linalool (0.1%), nootkatone (0.1%).[1]

While the major constituent of grapefruit oil is limonene, it is nootkatone that gives grapefruit its characteristic taste. Over 100 compounds have been detected, with monoterpenes accounting for about 95%; including *d*-limonene up to 95%.[1]

The percentage of non-volatiles in grapefruit oil is high compared with sweet orange or mandarin oil. Weiss also states that substantial variation exists in the peel oil from cultivars grown in the same region, and from cultivars grown in different regions.[1]

Like most other citrus oils, grapefruit oil is not very stable and deteriorates easily upon exposure to moisture, air and daylight.[2]

Adulteration

Grapefruit oil is rarely adulterated; however, there are different qualities of the oil, and it is important to get freshly produced and carefully stored oil. Cold-pressed grapefruit oil can be adulterated by the addition of lower quality steam-distilled grapefruit, grapefruit terpenes and sweet orange and its terpenes.[1,2]

The presence of δ-3-carene in grapefruit oil is an indication that it has been diluted with sweet orange oil products.[4]

Pharmacopoeias and standards

The purity, composition and physico-chemical properties of grapefruit are defined by ISO 3053:2004 Oil of Grapefruit (*Citrus* x *paradisi* Macfad.), obtained by Expression.

History and Traditional Uses

History

Arctander states that grapefruit did not exist 400 years ago, and it was still a rarity around the beginning of the twentieth century.[2]

Food, perfumery and flavouring

Grapefruit oil is extensively used as a flavour in soft drinks and as a fragrance component in soaps, detergents and personal care products.[3]

Therapeutics

Pharmacology and clinical studies

Antimicrobial activity

An in vitro study demonstrated that grapefruit essential oil had antifungal activity against a wide range of moulds commonly associated with food spoilage such as *Aspergillus niger, Aspergillus flavus, Penicillium chrysogenum* and *Penicillium verrucosum*.[5]

Studies indicate that grapefruit oil has considerable antimicrobial activity when tested against *Candida albicans, A. niger* and the generally difficult to inhibit *Pseudomonas aeruginosa*.[1]

Grapefruit oil was tested on methicillin-resistant *Staphylococcus aureus* (MRSA) and methicillin-sensitive *S. aureus* (MSSA) from hospital patients using the disk diffusion method. Grapefruit oil showed higher effectiveness in inhibiting MRSA and MSSA growth than vancomycin, which is the currently used standard antibiotic for treatment. The authors concluded that essential oils such as grapefruit could be beneficial towards treating hospital patients with MRSA and MSSA infections in areas where antibiotics are not readily available.[6]

Stress reduction activity

Olfactory stimulation from the scent of various essential oils has an effect on the sympathetic nervous system dysfunctions associated with lifestyle diseases such as hypertension was investigated. The researchers found that grapefruit oil caused increases in adrenaline and noradrenaline levels, but that the changes were not statistically significant.[7]

G

Actions

Actions commonly cited in aromatherapy

Antidepressant, antiseptic, depurative, disinfectant, diuretic, hepatoprotective, stimulant[8,9]

Actions supported by clinical studies

Antimicrobial, antiseptic, hepatoprotective

Comment

Review of the clinical research for grapefruit oil suggests that it has considerable antimicrobial activity. The actions of grapefruit oil have been described as being similar to that of lemon oil. The *d*-limonene content of grapefruit indicates that grapefruit oil has hepatoprotective properties similar to lemon oil.

Aromatherapy Uses

Clinical aromatherapy

Lymphatic system

Grapefruit oil is a lymphatic stimulant and is indicated for cellulite, obesity and water retention.[10,11,12]

Psychological

Grapefruit oil has an uplifting and reviving effect, which makes it valuable for treating stress, depression and nervous exhaustion. It is recommended for people who are depressed and lethargic, particularly in winter.[12]

Skin care

Grapefruit oil is beneficial for treating oily skin and acne, and has a tonic effect on the skin and scalp.[12]

Energetics, psyche and subtle uses

Energetics

Grapefruit oil is *cooling*, cleansing and decongesting. It is beneficial for both an overheated *Liver* and sluggish lymphatic system. Symptoms associated with an overheated *Liver* include abdominal distension, constipation, nausea and a feeling of general irritability.[10]

Mojay states that grapefruit oil, like all citrus oils, has the ability to smooth the flow of stagnant *Qi* which is associated with the Wood Element. This helps to alleviate feelings of frustration, irritability, stress and tension.[10]

According to the principles of the Five Elements, grapefruit oil also helps to reduce excess *damp* associated with the Earth Element. *Damp* conditions are often associated with chronic indigestion, abdominal bloating, lethargy, heaviness of the body and water retention.

According to the principles of Ayurveda, grapefruit oil would strengthen *Vata* and *Pitta* and help to reduce *Kapha*. [13]

Personality

The grapefruit personality is described as a warm, happy person who is bursting with energy, loves life and people. They can be great motivators and have so much 'get up and go' without being overbearing. Worwood also describes grapefruit personalities as clear thinkers. They make wonderful healers because of their infectious enthusiastic personality, because they are naturally attuned to their spiritual selves.[14]

Under pressure, they tend to resort to 'comfort eating' as a means of dealing with difficult situations. Mojay explains that such people often have high expectations of everything, however, whenever reality fails to meet their goals and desires, they tend to react with anger, blame and self-criticism. Grapefruit oil helps to clear psychological heat that results from deep-seated frustration and self-blame.[10]

According to Myers-Briggs personality types, the grapefruit personality is likely to be an ENTP. ENTPs are energetic, enthusiastic and confident. Many are nonconformists. They are innovative and have excellent analytical ability, and are resourceful in solving problems. They like variety and change. Because they have so many interests, they feel that life is too short. They feel relaxed when they do new things. They enjoy travelling to exotic places. They can be inspirational and rise to leadership positions because of their quick mind. They work best when interacting with many people. They are optimistic, charming and quick-witted. They value their freedom and independence. They seek growth, excitement and continuous improvement in their relationships. They enjoy debating and they like to have the last say. They may deny emotional pain and keep busy to avoid dealing with their feelings. They can be arrogant, argumentative and insensitive.

Subtle

Worwood states that grapefruit oil awakens the human spirit from a slumber – it is energising and enlivening. She explains that it can reconnect the mind, body and soul.[15]

Zeck recommends using grapefruit oil whenever you are feeling drained, strung out or depressed. She explains that the light fruity aroma of grapefruit lifts the spirits and radiates optimism. Grapefruit helps us focus our thoughts on the positive aspects of our life.[16]

Keim Loughran & Bull state that the scent of grapefruit oil dissolves emotional energy blocks associated with feelings of frustration and self-blame. It also promotes confidence and increases mental clarity and intuition.[17]

Dosage and Administration

Blending

Aromatherapy

For the relief of stress, anxiety and nervous tension, consider blending grapefruit essential oil with bergamot, geranium, lavender, lemon, neroli, sweet orange or sandalwood.

To alleviate fatigue and feelings of apathy, consider blending grapefruit oil with basil, black pepper, cardamom, coriander seed, ginger, lemon, lime, sweet orange or rosemary.

To create a detoxification blend, consider blending grapefruit oil with essential oils such as juniper berry, everlasting, sweet fennel, lemon, sweet orange or rosemary.

Perfumery

Grapefruit oil is typically not used in perfumery; however, it would add a fresh, uplifting top note to any perfume.

Mode of administration

Bath

Full body bath, foot bath

Topical

Compress, massage, ointment, skin care

Inhalation

Direct inhalation, diffuser, oil vaporiser

Safety Profile

General safety

Grapefruit oil is reported to be non-toxic, non-irritating and non-sensitising.[3,8] Old and oxidised grapefruit oil should be avoided.[18]

Contraindications

IFRA recommends that for application to the skin exposed to the sun, expressed grapefruit oil be limited to a maximum of 4% in products for the skin.[18]

Regulatory guidelines

Grapefruit essential oil has GRAS status.

G

References

1. Weiss EA. *Essential oil crops*. CAB International, Wallingford, 1997.
2. Arctander S. *Perfume and flavor materials of natural origin*. Allured Publishing, Carol Stream, 1994.
3. Khan I, Abourashed E. *Leung's encyclopedia of common natural ingredients used in food, drugs and cosmetics*. 3rd edn. John Wiley & Sons, New Jersey, 2010.
4. McHale D. *Adulteration of citrus oil*. In Dugo G, Di Giacomo A. eds. *Citrus – the genus Citrus*. Taylor & Francis Group, London, 2002: 496-517.
5. Viuda-Martos M et al. *Antifungal activity of lemon (Citrus lemon L.), mandarin (Citrus reticulate L.), grapefruit and orange (Citrus sinensis L.) essential oils*. Food Control, 2008; 19(12): 1130-1138. Cited in Quintessential Aromatics database, 2013.
6. Sharma PR et al. *Ten highly effective essential oils inhibit growth of methicillin resistant*

Staphylococcus aureus (MRSA) and methicillin sensitive Staphylococcus aureus (MSSA). International Journal of Pharmacy and Pharmaceutical Sciences, 2013; 5(1): 52-54. Cited in Quintessential Aromatics database, 2013.
7. Haze S et al. *Effects of fragrance inhalation on sympathetic activity in normal adults.* Japanese Journal of Pharmacology, 2002; 90(3): 247-253. Cited in Quintessential Aromatics database, 2013.
8. Lawless J. *Aromatherapy and the mind.* Thornsons, London, 1994.
9. Rhind JP. *Aromatherapeutic blending.* Singing Dragon, London, 2016.
10. Mojay G. *Aromatherapy for healing the spirit.* Healing Arts Press, Rochester, 1999.
11. Lavabre M. *Aromatherapy workbook.* Healing Arts Press, Rochester, 1997.
12. Davis P. *Aromatherapy: an A-Z.* 2nd edn. The C.W. Daniel Company, Saffron Walden, 1999.
13. Miller L, Miller B. *Ayurveda and aromatherapy.* Lotus Press, Twin Lakes, 1995.
14. Worwood VA. *The fragrant mind.* Transworld Publishers, London, 1995.
15. Worwood VA. *The fragrant heavens.* Transworld Publishers, London, 1999.
16. Zeck R. *The blossoming heart – aromatherapy for healing and transformation.* Aroma Tours, East Ivanhoe, 2004.
17. Keim Loughran J, Bull R. *Aromatherapy and subtle energy techniques.* Frog, Berkeley, 2000.
18. Tisserand R, Young R. *Essential oil safety.* 2nd edn. Churchill Livingstone, Edinburgh, 2014.

Guaiacwood

G

Identification

Botanical name

Bulnesia sarmientoi Lorentz ex. Griseb.

Synonyms

Champaca wood, oil of guaiac

Family

Zygophyllaceae

Botany and origins

Guaiacwood is a small, wild tropical tree which grows up to 4 m tall, and is native to South America, growing in Brazil, Paraguay and Argentina.[1]

B. sarmientoi is listed by CITES in Appendix II as species that are not necessarily now threatened with extinction, but may become so unless trade is closely controlled.[2,3]

Method of extraction

Guaiacwood oil is steam-distilled and occasionally water-distilled from the wood and sawdust from the Palo Santo tree.[1]

Characteristics

Guaiacwood oil is a soft or semi-solid mass, yellowish to greenish yellow or pale amber in colour. It is often described as having a delicate, sweet, 'tea rose' odour. The oil may also have a 'smoked ham' aroma, which is not desirable.[1]

Chemical composition

The chemical composition of guaiacwood oil was as follows:

guaiol (42-72%), bulnesol, δ-bulnesene, β-bulnesene, α-guaiene, β-patchoulene and guaioxide. The main constituent of guaiacwood oil is a sesquiterpene called guaiol.[4]

Adulteration

Guaiacwood oil is occasionally adulterated with copaiba balsam. It has often been used as an adulterant for rose absolute, amyris oil, sandalwood oil, costus oil and oakmoss resin.[1]

Pharmacopoeias and standards

At the time of writing, the purity, composition, physico-chemical properties and therapeutic use of guaiacwood essential oil are not defined in any pharmacopoeia monograph or standard.

History and Traditional Uses

History

The wood is very hard and extensively used for ornamental carving.[1]

Herbal

Guaiacwood essential oil should not be confused with the guaiac wood mentioned in the German Commission E and British Herbal Pharmacopoeia. These pharmacopoeias refer to *Guaiacum officinale*, from which a gum and resin is used for the treatment of rheumatic complaints.[5,6]

The oil is used as a starting material for the synthesis of guaiazulene, which has anti-inflammatory properties.[4]

Food, perfumery and flavouring

The oil is a low-cost fixative and modifier, and an

excellent blender in woody-floral perfumes, soap compounds and high-class perfumes. It is also used for the isolation of guaiol from which guaiyl acetate can be manufactured. This is used for the creation of tea rose perfumes.[1]

Therapeutics

Pharmacology and clinical studies

At the time of writing, no pharmacological or clinical studies for guaiacwood oil could be found.

Anti-inflammatory activity

Guaiazulene, obtained from guaiacwood by dehydration of guaiol, has been demonstrated to have anti-inflammatory activity in animal studies.[5]

Actions

Actions commonly cited in aromatherapy

Anti-inflammatory, antioxidant, antirheumatic, antiseptic, diaphoretic, diuretic[7]

Actions supported by clinical studies

None of the actions commonly cited in aromatherapy can be supported by clinical studies.

Comment

There is no information regarding the therapeutic properties of guaiacwood essential oil. There has been some confusion with the therapeutic actions of the herbal extracts of *Guaiacum officinale* and *Guaiacum sanctum*, which are listed in both the German Commission E and British Herbal Pharmacopoeia.

Guaiazulene, obtained by dehydration of guaiol, is used in commercial topical preparations for its anti-inflammatory properties; however, guaiazulene is not naturally found in the oil.[4]

Aromatherapy Uses

Clinical aromatherapy

Lawless states that guaiacwood oil may be used for the treatment of arthritis and gout.[7] However, I believe that this may be incorrect and refer to *G. officinale*.

Energetic, psyche and subtle uses

Subtle

Guaiacwood oil is used to balance and heal all the energy centres so that a person can follow their spiritual path with clarity and integrity. The oil assists in finding one's life work and purpose.[8]

Dosage and Administration

Blending

Aromatherapy

While guaiacwood essential oil may have little aromatherapeutic benefits, it imparts a delicate woody floral to any aromatherapy blend where a pleasant long-lasting fixative is required.

Perfumery

It blends especially well with rose otto and rose absolute; essential oils such as amyris, geranium, neroli, palmarosa and sandalwood; and spice oils such as nutmeg and ginger.[1]

The success to using guaiacwood in perfumery, according to perfumers Jan and Ramanauskas, is to use a very small amount. They state that when a perfume blend is overdosed with guaiacwood it imparts a distinct smokiness of bacon, but when employed with skill it adds a very interesting, slightly smoky black tea note. They recommend using it in warm floral style perfumes, and suggest that it goes well in oriental, leathery and woody style perfumes. They explain that in masculine notes you can use it at higher levels, and that it blends well with amber dry woody notes. It also brings depth and body to lemon fragrances.[9]

Mode of administration

Topical

Massage, ointment

Inhalation

Direct inhalation, diffuser, oil vaporiser

Safety Profile

General safety

Guaiacwood oil is non-toxic, non-irritant and non-sensitising.[2,7] There is no recommended IFRA restriction for the use of guaiacwood oil.

Contraindications

No contraindications known.

Regulatory guidelines

Guaiacwood oil has GRAS status.

G

References

1. Arctander S. *Perfume and flavor materials of natural origin.* Allured Publishing, Carol Stream, 1994.
2. Tisserand R, Young R. *Essential oil safety.* 2nd edn. Churchill Livingstone, Edinburgh, 2014.

3. Burfield T. *Updated list of threatened aromatic plants used in the aroma & cosmetics industries.* V1.21 March 2010.
4. Khan I, Abourashed E. *Leung's encyclopedia of common natural ingredients used in food, drugs and cosmetics.* 3rd edn. John Wiley & Sons, New Jersey, 2010.
5. Blumenthal M et al. *The complete German commission E monographs: therapeutic guide to herbal medicine.* American Botanical Council, Austin, 1998.
6. *British herbal pharmacopoeia.* British Herbal Medicine Association, Bournemouth, 1983.
7. Lawless J. *The encyclopaedia of essential oils.* Element Books, Shaftesbury, 1992.
8. Keim Loughran J, Bull R. *Aromatherapy and subtle energy techniques.* Frog, Berkeley, 2000.
9. Gleason J. *Comparing notes: complexity, performance and natural effects.* Perfumer & Flavorist, 2009; 34: 47.

Ho Leaf (Linalool ct.)

H

Identification

Botanical name

Cinnamomum camphora (L.) J. Presl.

Synonyms

Ho-sho (fragrant camphor tree), shiu, shiu-sho

Family

Lauraceae

Botany and origins

C. camphora is a tall evergreen, growing up to 30 m. It is widely cultivated in Taiwan, Japan and China. Guenther states that there are three distinct chemotypes of *C. camphora*. They are as follows:

- Hon-sho – camphor chemotype
- Ho-sho – linalool chemotype
- Yu-sho – cineole chemotype.[1]

He explains that the three chemotypes are morphologically identical and can only be identified by the oil yield.[1]

Ho leaf oil used in aromatherapy is the linalool chemotype.

Burfield & Sheppard-Hanger state that ho wood oil is often a blend of essential oils produced from the steam distillation of the wood of *Cinnamomum* species such as *C. camphora* L. var. *linaloolifera* and *C. camphora* Sieb. var. *glavescens* Hayata. The more sweet-camphoraceous leaf and branch oils of these species often have a linalool content as low as 15%; however, the oil is often fractionated and rectified to produce an oil with a high *l*-linalool and negligible camphor content.[2]

Burfield & Sheppard-Hanger state that the Chinese authorities have introduced a ban on tree felling of certain species of *Cinnamomum* because of climatic concerns. This has caused the price of ho oils to increase. They also state that there are potential problems of exhaustion of the *Cinnamomum* species as there is no policy of tree replanting.[2]

Method of extraction

Ho leaf oil is steam-distilled from the leaf of *C. camphora*.

Characteristics

Ho leaf oil is a clear oil with a clean, sweet, floral-woody and delicate odour. Arctander states that there is little or no change in the odour during evaporation on a perfume blotter. High-grade ho leaf oil should contain no camphor-like notes, and it should have a clean linalool scent – no other essential oil comes close to the scent of pure linalool.[3]

Chemical composition

The chemical composition of ho leaf oil from camphor tree cultivated in southern Brasil was reported as follows:

linalool (93.14%), camphor (0.46%), *l*-borneol (0.2%), γ-elemene (0.27%), β-caryophyllene (0.64%), α-humulene (0.22%), germacrene D (0.3%), (*E*)-nerolidol (0.11%).[4]

Tisserand & Young state that ho leaf ct. linalool oil may contain methyl eugenol, which is potentially carcinogenic. However, it is very high in linalool and nerolidol, which are anticarcinogenic compounds. Consequently, they state that there is no need to set any dose limit.[5]

Adulteration

Synthetic linalool and linalyl acetate are frequently used to adulterate ho leaf ct. linalool oil.[6]

Pharmacopoeias and standards

At the time of writing, the purity, composition, physico-chemical properties and therapeutic use of ho leaf ct. linalool essential oil are not defined in any pharmacopoeia monograph or standard.

History and Traditional Uses

History

Kerr states that the linalool chemotype was not considered of any importance as there was no use for it until the 1920s.[7]

Food, perfumery and flavouring

Ho leaf oil is used in perfumery, and for the isolation of linalool and the production of linalyl esters.[6]

Therapeutics

Pharmacology and clinical studies

Antibacterial activity

In vitro studies have confirmed the antibacterial activity of ho leaf oil against a range of bacterial species.[6]

Antifungal activity

Ho leaf oil exhibited fungicidal activity against *Aspergillus niger*, *Aspergillus ochraceus* and *Fusarium culmorum*.[6]

Miticidal activity

Eighty-two essential oils were tested for their miticidal activity on mites such as *Dermatophagoides pteronyssinus*, *Dermatophagoides farinae* and *Tyrophagus putrescentiae*. Ho leaf oil was found to have a very powerful miticidal activity.[8]

Sedative activity

Lis-Balchin states that evidence exists that linalool has sedative properties and is a relaxant.[6] Considering that ho leaf ct. linalool has a high linalool content, we can assume that the oil may be used as a sedative.

Actions

Actions commonly cited in aromatherapy

Antibacterial, antifungal, antimicrobial, antiviral, tonic[2]

Actions supported by clinical studies

Antimicrobial, insecticidal, relaxant

Comment

Many aromatherapy books do not mention ho leaf oil; however, Lis-Balchin and Kerr state that ho leaf oil would make a great substitute for rosewood oil due to the similarity in chemical composition, especially since the production of rosewood oil is leading to the destruction of rainforests in the Amazon.[6,7]

Aromatherapy Uses

Clinical aromatherapy

Psychological

Ho leaf oil has an uplifting and enlivening effect, which is helpful to balance the emotions. It is recommended when one is feeling weary and overburdened with problems. It has an overall calming effect without inducing any drowsiness.[7]

Skin care

Kerr suggests using ho leaf oil as a tissue regenerator, making it beneficial for treating aged skin. He also states that it is ideal for people with dry, sensitive and inflamed skin.[7]

Dosage and Administration

Blending

Aromatherapy

For the relief of anxiety, nervous tension and stress-related conditions, consider blending ho leaf oil with essential oils such as bergamot, geranium, lavender, sweet orange, neroli, patchouli, rose otto, sandalwood or ylang ylang.

For the relief of dry and sensitive skin, consider blending ho leaf oil with essential oils such as everlasting, lavender, neroli, patchouli, rose otto or sandalwood.

Perfumery

Arctander states that ho leaf oil is used in perfumery as a modifier, blender, sweetener or floraliser.[3]

Mode of administration

Bath

Full body bath, foot bath

Topical

Compress, massage, ointment, skin care

Inhalation

Direct inhalation, diffuser, oil vaporiser

Safety Profile

General safety

There are no contraindications for ho leaf oil. Some texts may have confused camphor oil with ho leaf oil, which comes from the same species.

Ho leaf oil applied topically at full strength under occlusion was moderately irritating to rabbits. When tested at 10% in petrolatum, it produced no irritation after a 48-hour closed patch test on human subjects.[9]

Contraindications

No contraindications known.[5]

Regulatory guidelines

No FEMA number has been assigned to ho leaf oil; however, the Council of Europe includes ho leaf oil in the list as a food additive.[9]

References

1. Guenther E. *The essential oils – Vol. IV.* Robert E Krieger Publishing, Malabar, 1950.
2. Burfield T, Sheppard-Hanger S. *Substituting for rosewood oil ... a look at other high linalool containing oils.* Aromatherapy Today, 2003; 26: 30-37.
3. Arctander S. *Perfume and flavor materials of natural origin.* Allured Publishing, Carol Stream, 1994.
4. Frizzo CD et al. *Essential oils of camphor tree (Cinnamomum camphora Nees & Eberm) cultivated in southern Brazil.* Brazilian Archives of Biology and Technology, 2000; 43(3): 313-316. doi: 10.1590/S1516-89132000000300011.
5. Tisserand R, Young R. *Essential oil safety.* 2nd edn. Churchill Livingstone, Edinburgh, 2014.
6. Lis-Balchin M. *Aromatherapy science – a guide for healthcare professionals.* Pharmaceutical Press, London, 2006.
7. Kerr J. *Ho leaf/Rosewood.* Aromatherapy Today, 1998; 7: 6-9.
8. Watanabe F et al. *Killing activities of the volatiles emitted from essential oils for Dermatophagoides pteronyssinus, Dermatophagoides farinae and Tyrophagus putrescentiae.* Shoyakugaku Zasshi, 1989; 43(2): 163-168. Cited in Quintessential Aromatics database, 2013.
9. Opdyke DLJ. *Monographs on fragrance raw materials.* Pergamon Press, Oxford, 1979.

Hyssop

H

Identification

Botanical name

Hyssop ct. linalool: *Hyssopus officinalis* var. *decumbens*

Hyssop ct. pinocamphone: *Hyssopus officinalis*

Synonyms

Creeping hyssop

Family

Lamiaceae (Labiatae)

Botany and origins

Hyssop is a perennial aromatic small sub-shrub, which grows up to 0.5 m high, with slender herbaceous stems arising from a woody base, bearing whorls of small purplish-blue flowers.

It is native to southern Europe and has been cultivated as a culinary herb and medicinal herb for hundreds of years. The major producing countries include France, Hungary and The Netherlands

Method of extraction

Hyssop oil is steam-distilled from the leaves and flowering tops of *H. officinalis* or *H. officinalis* var. *decumbens*.

Characteristics

Hyssop oil is a pale yellow or faintly greenish yellow to almost colourless oil, with a powerful, sharp, sweet-camphoraceous odour and a warm, spicy undertone.[1]

Chemical composition

It is important to distinguish between the oil of *H. officinalis* and *H. officinalis* var. *decumbens*. The latter is free of the potentially toxic ketones, whereas the oil of *H. officinalis* contains a high percentage of pinocamphone.[2]

The chemical composition of *H. officinalis* essential oil produced from plants collected in the Piedmont region (Italy) was reported as follows:

α-pinene (0.6%), β-pinene (11.1%), sabinene (1.5%), myrcene (2.1%), limonene (12.2%), pinocamphone (1.7%), isopinocamphone (43.3%), β-bourbonene (1.4%), caryophyllene oxide (0.5%).[3]

The main chemical components found in *H. officinalis* var. *decumbens* oil from the high Provence Alps in France was reported as follows:

linalool (49.6%), 1,8-cineole (13.3%), limonene (5.4%), β-caryophyllene (2.8%), β-pinene (3.0%) and α-pinene (2.4%).[4]

Isopinocamphone and pinocamphone were present in very low amounts.[4]

The composition of *H. officinalis* oil from the north of Iran has a very interesting and unusual chemical profile:

1,8-cineole (0.31%), linalool (0.56%), *cis*-sabinol (1.75%), camphor (6.76%), terpinen-4-ol (0.28%), myrtenal (0.43%), bornyl acetate (1.42%), myrtenyl acetate (74%), α-cubebene (0.53%), β-bourbonene

(1.46%), β-caryophyllene (2.1%), α-caryophyllene (0.64%), germacrene (3.36%), cubenol (0.33%), δ-cadinene (0.47%), spathulenol (2.14%), caryophyllene oxide (2.13%), elemol (0.46%).[5]

The exceptionally high myrtenyl acetate content could not be explained. It was suggested that the composition of *H. officinalis* oil may vary considerably within a single species from one season to another, and due to climatic factors and agrotechnical factors such as fertilisation, water supply and the stage of plant development at the time of harvesting.[5]

Adulteration

Hyssop oil is occasionally adulterated with cedar leaf oil, camphor oil or camphor oil fractions, lavandin oil, myrtle oil or sage oil.[1]

Pharmacopoeias and standards

The purity, composition and physico-chemical properties of hyssop oil are defined in ISO 9841:2013 – Essential oil of hyssop (*Hyssopus officinalis* L. ssp. *officinalis*).

History and Traditional Uses

History

The name comes from the Greek word, *hyssopus*, itself derived from the Hebrew word *ezob*, meaning good-scented herb. Both the flowers and leaves have been highly valued since antiquity for their therapeutic properties, and it was one of the bitter herbs mentioned in the Old Testament. Hippocrates prescribed it for pleurisy and bronchitis.[6]

It was commonly used in the Middle Ages for its therapeutic properties. Culpeper recommended:

> *It is good to wash inflammations, and takes away the blue and black marks that come by strokes, bruises or falls ... it is an excellent medicine for the quinsy, or swelling in the throat, to wash and gargle it ... The hot vapours of the decoction taken by a funnel in the ears, eases the inflammation and singing noise of them ... It is good for falling sickness (epilepsy), expectorates tough phlegm, and is effectual in all cold griefs, or diseases of the chest and lung.*[7]

Herbal

Hyssop herb is used for sore throats, coughs, colds, digestive disorders, intestinal ailments and menstrual complaints. It is a diaphoretic and may be used externally for treating skin irritations, burns, bruises and frostbite.[8]

Hyssop herb is currently listed in the British Herbal Pharmacopoeia as a specific for bronchitis and the common cold.[9] The German Commission E states that hyssop herb is used for the gentle stimulation of circulation, for intestinal catarrhs, for diseases of the respiratory system, digestive disorders, intestinal ailments, menstrual complaints, heart problems and eye pain.[10]

Food, perfumery and flavouring

Hyssop oil is used in perfumery, and in flavour work as a replacement for the herb in pickles, meat sauces and seasonings. It also gives an interesting bouquet to alcoholic beverages, particularly the 'chartreuse' style liqueurs.[1]

Therapeutics

Pharmacology and clinical studies

Antimicrobial activity

The essential oils of *H. officinalis* var. *decumbens* and *H. officinalis* were tested for their antimicrobial activity. At concentrations of 1% or higher, both essential oils possessed antibacterial activity; however, *H. officinalis* var. *decumbens* was more effective.[11]

Another in vitro study confirmed that *H. officinalis* var. *decumbens* essential oil exhibited stronger antimicrobial activity than *H. officinalis*. Both oils strongly inhibited the *Candida* species, with an MIC range of 0.15-1.25 v/v.[12]

Antiviral activity

H. officinalis oil exhibited high antiviral activity against acyclovir-sensitive herpes simplex virus (HSV) type 1 strain KOS and acyclovir-resistant clinical isolates.[13]

An in vitro study confirmed that *H. officinalis* oil exhibited antiviral activity against herpes simplex virus type 2 (HSV-2). A dose-dependent viricidal activity was demonstrated. The results of the study indicated that *H. officinalis* oil affects HSV-2 before adsorption by interacting with the viral envelope.[14]

Epileptogenic activity

An in vitro study using slices of rat cerebral cortex examined the effects of varying concentrations of reputedly epileptogenic essential oils and their major ketones component. The results clearly indicated an inhibitory action on oxygen consumption and cellular respiration of the cerebral cortex in the presence of essential oils and their ketone components. The inhibition was present even at small doses and increased with time and dose. *H. officinalis* oil was the most inhibitory oil. It was assumed that the respiratory inhibition is the initial part of a process, leading to metabolic and electrolyte imbalance that in turn creates tissue hypoxia and increases the risk of epileptiform seizures.[15]

Spasmolytic activity

H. officinalis var. *decumbens* oil has a spasmolytic effect on the electrically stimulated smooth muscle of the isolated guinea pig ileum.[16]

Actions

Actions commonly cited in aromatherapy

Antibacterial, antiseptic, antispasmodic, cicatrisant, digestive, emmenagogue, expectorant, febrifuge, hypertensive, nervine, sudorific, vulnerary[17,18,19]

Actions supported by clinical studies

Antibacterial, antifungal, antispasmodic, antiviral

Comment

Schnaubelt states that it is important in aromatherapy to use *H. officinalis* var. *decumbens*, as it is free of the potentially toxic ketones.[2] He explains that in the past, distillers in Provence would produce *H. officinalis* var. *decumbens* essential oil from wildcrafted plants. However, recently *H. officinalis* var. *montana intermedia* has been cultivated. This variety also has a minimal ketone content, making it very safe for aromatherapy uses. It is considered to be a very powerful, non-toxic, antiviral essential oil which can be used on children and adults. Schnaubelt states that it can be dabbed undiluted directly onto herpes lesions or fever blisters in the mouth. He also explains that the oil alleviates nervous depression, anxiety and asthma-related symptoms.[20]

H

Aromatherapy Uses

Clinical aromatherapy

Circulatory system

Hyssop oil has a regulatory effect on the circulation and helps raise low blood pressure.[18,21] It is recommended in a cold compress for the treatment of bruises.[17,21]

Digestive system

Hyssop oil is a tonic to the digestive system. It acts as an appetite stimulant and mild laxative, relieves stomach cramps and expels wind.[8,19]

Immune system

Hyssop oil is recommended for colds and flu.[17,20] *H. officinalis* var. *decumbens* oil is reputed to have potent antiviral effects and is suitable for treating herpes.[22]

Nervous system

Hyssop oil has an invigorating effect on the mind, and is recommended for poor concentration, mental fatigue and nervous debility.[19,23]

Lawless states that hyssop oil can alleviate anxiety, nervous tension and stress-related conditions.[17] Schnaubelt states that it is useful for nervous depression.[20]

Reproductive system

Hyssop oil relieves menstrual problems associated with water retention during periods, and is effective for treating amenorrhoea and leucorrhoea.[8,17,23]

Respiratory system

Hyssop oil has a special affinity with the respiratory system. It liquefies mucus and relieves bronchial spasms. It is effective for treating colds, sore throats, influenza, bronchitis and asthma.[2,18,20,21,23]

Skin care

Hyssop oil is recommended for the treatment of bruises, cuts, dermatitis, eczema, inflammation and wounds.[17]

Energetics, psyche and subtle uses

Energetics

Hyssop is described as *hot* and stimulating and is a tonic of *Yang Qi* and *defensive Qi*. It strengthens and warm the *Lungs*, and is recommended for chronic bronchitis, poor vitality, breathlessness and immune deficiency.[19,23]

Hyssop oil strengthens and balances the Metal Element and invigorates the *Po*.[19]

The *Po* teaches us life's lessons through grief and loss. This can be a difficult path that some people cannot follow – those people who cannot let go of their hurts cannot grow, become wiser and learn from their difficulties.

Subtle

Fischer-Rizzi states that the scent of hyssop oil rejuvenates our spirits without letting us lose touch with reality. She explains that a muddled mind becomes more organised and concentration improves.[24]

Hyssop is reputed to be a cleansing herb and is recommended to cleanse any area in which you are planning to meditate or use for healing purposes.[25]

Keim Loughran & Bull recommend using hyssop oil to clear negative energy and to provide protection from other people's negative moods and emotions. It also eases feelings of grief.[26]

Worwood describes hyssop as a holy herb that uplifts the spirit to the realms of divine wisdom. She suggests that it purifies and cleanses, awakens closed hearts and minds, and promotes tolerance and understanding. It also promotes unconditional love and acceptance and the comprehension needed for the ultimate oneness with the universe.[27]

Mojay states that hyssop has traditionally been considered the herb of protection. It has been used to defend one from negative influences and 'evil spirits'. It would benefit the person who is easily affected by others' moods and emotions, and who quickly attracts and absorbs any tension in the environment.[19]

Dosage and Administration

Blending

Aromatherapy

For the relief of colds and flu associated with bronchial congestion, consider blending *H. officinalis* var. *decumbens* oil with essential oils such as aniseed, cajeput, 1,8-cineole-rich eucalypts, ginger, pine, ravintsara, tea tree or thyme.

To alleviate nervous exhaustion, consider blending *H. officinalis* var. *decumbens* oil with essential oils such as basil, geranium, lemon or rosemary.

To dispel bruises, consider blending *H. officinalis* var. *decumbens* oil with essential oils such as black pepper, ginger, lavender, lemon or rosemary.

For the treatment of cold sores, consider blending *H. officinalis* var. *decumbens* oil with bergamot or tea tree oil.

Perfumery

Hyssop oil is used in perfumery to provide a rich body, warm-spicy-herbaceous note with personality. It is often used in citrus colognes, fougère, amber and light-aldehydic style perfumes. Hyssop oil blends well with lemon, lavender, rosemary, myrtle, bay laurel, sage and clary sage essential oils.[1]

Mode of administration

Bath

Full body bath, foot bath, sitz bath

Topical

Compress, massage, ointment, skin care

Inhalation

Direct inhalation, steam inhalation, diffuser, oil vaporiser

Safety Profile

General safety

H. officinalis var. *decumbens* contains very little of the hazardous ketones and is considered relatively safe to use.[2,17,28]

Contraindications

Hyssop oil should not be used during pregnancy or on individuals with epilepsy.[17,19,21]

There are no known hazards or contraindications for *H. officinalis* var. *decumbens* oil.[29]

Toxicity

The German Commission E cites three cases of poisoning resulting in clonic or clonic-tonic spasms. In adults, the dose involved was 10 and 30 drops, and in a six-year-old child the dosage was two to three drops over several days. These cases would relate to the pinocamphone-rich hyssop oils.[10]

Tisserand & Young state that the pineocamphone-rich hyssop oil is a neurotoxin and should not be used at all during pregnancy and breastfeeding, or for children under 2 years of age. They also state that it should not be taken orally. They recommend that the maximum percentage for dermal application be limited to 0.3%.[29]

Regulatory guidelines

Hyssop oil has GRAS status.

References

1. Arctander S. *Perfume and flavor materials of natural origin*. Allured Publishing, Carol Stream, 1994.
2. Schnaubelt K. *Medical aromatherapy*. Frog, Berkeley, 1999.
3. Lawrence BM. *Progress in essential oils – hyssop oil*. Perfumer & Flavorist, 2008; 33:52-53.
4. Fathiazad F, Hamedeyazdan S. *A review on Hyssopus officinalis L.: composition and biological activities*. African Journal of Pharmacy and Pharmacology. 2011; 5(17): 1959-1966. doi: 10.5897/AJPP11.527.
5. Fathiazad F et al. *Phytochemical analysis and antioxidant activity of Hyssopus officinalis L. from Iran*. Advanced Pharmaceutical Bulletin, 2011; 1(2): 63-67. doi: 10.5681/apb.2011.009.
6. Le Strange R. *A history of herbal plants*. Angus and Robertson, United Kingdom, 1977.
7. Grieve M. *A modern herbal – Vol. I*. Dover Publications, New York, 1971.
8. Khan I, Abourashed E. *Leung's encyclopedia of common natural ingredients used in food, drugs and cosmetics*. 3rd edn. John Wiley & Sons, New Jersey, 2010.
9. *British herbal pharmacopoeia*. British Herbal Medicine Association, Bournemouth, 1983.
10. Blumenthal M et al. *The complete German commission E monographs: therapeutic guide to herbal medicine*. American Botanical Council, Austin, 1998.
11. Renzini G et al. *Antibacterial and cytotoxic activity of Hyssopus officinalis L. oils*. Journal of

Essential Oil Research, 1999; 11(5): 646-654. Cited in Quintessential Aromatics database, 2013.
12. Mazzanti G et al. *Antimicrobial properties of the linalol-rich essential oil of Hyssopus officinalis L. var. decumbens*. Flavour and Fragrance Journal, 1998; 13(5): 289-294. Cited in Quintessential Aromatics database, 2013.
13. Schnitzler P et al. *Susceptibility of drug-resistant clinical Herpes simplex virus type 1 strains to essential oils of ginger, thyme, hyssop and sandalwood*. Antimicrobial Agents and Chemotherapy, 2007; 51(5): 1859-1862. Cited in Quintessential Aromatics database, 2013.
14. Koch C et al. *Inhibitory effect of essential oils against herpes simplex virus type 2*. Phytomedicine, 2008; 15(1/2): 71-78. Cited in Quintessential Aromatics database, 2013.
15. Steinmetz MD et al. *The activity of essential oils of sage, thuja, hyssop and certain components on respiration of cerebral cortex slices in vitro*. Plantes Medicinales et Phytotherapie, 1985; 19(1): 35-47. Cited in Quintessential Aromatics database, 2013.
16. Mazzanti G, Lu M, Salvatore G. *Spasmolytic action of the essential oil from Hyssopus officinalis L. var. decumbens and its major components*. Phytotherapy Research, 1998; 12(S1): S92-S94. Cited in Quintessential Aromatics database, 2013.
17. Lawless J. *The encyclopaedia of essential oils*. Element Books, Shaftesbury, 1992.
18. Lavabre M. *Aromatherapy workbook*. Healing Arts Press, Rochester, 1997.
19. Mojay G. *Aromatherapy for healing the spirit*. Healing Arts Press, Rochester, 1999.
20. Schnaubelt K. *The healing intelligence of essential oils*. Healing Arts Press, Rochester, 2011.
21. Davis P. *Aromatherapy: an A-Z*. 2nd edn. C.W. Daniel Company, Saffron Walden, 1999.
22. Schnaubelt K. *Advanced aromatherapy*. Healing Arts Press, Rochester, 1995.
23. Holmes P. *The energetics of Western herbs – Vol. I*. Artemis Press, Boulder, 1989.
24. Fischer-Rizzi S. *Complete aromatherapy handbook*. Sterling Publishing, New York. 1990.
25. Davis P. *Subtle aromatherapy*. C.W. Daniel Company, Saffron Walden, 1991.
26. Keim Loughran J, Bull R. *Aromatherapy and subtle energy techniques*. Frog, Berkeley, 2000.
27. Worwood VA. *The fragrant heavens*. Transworld Publishers, London, 1999.
28. Tisserand R, Balacs T. *Essential oil safety*. Churchill Livingstone, Edinburgh, 1995.
29. Tisserand R, Young R. *Essential oil safety*. 2nd edn. Churchill Livingstone, Edinburgh, 2014.

Jasmine absolute

Identification

Botanical name

Jasminum grandiflorum L.

Synonyms

Jasminum officinale, Jasminum officinale L. var. *grandiflorum*

Family

Oleaceae

Botany and origins

The *Jasminum* species are evergreen deciduous shrubs or shrubby climbers with white, pink or yellow very fragrant flowers. Jasmine is native to the Indian and South East Asian region.[1]

There are more than 200 species of jasmine cultivated in the subtropics worldwide. The three most important commercially cultivated species used for essential oil production are:

- *J. auriculatum*
- *J. grandiflorum*
- *J. sambac*.[1]

J. auriculatum is native to southern India and has adapted to regions with high temperatures and above average rainfall.[1]

J. grandiflorum is native to northern Iran, Afghanistan and Kashmir, and has been introduced and is commercially cultivated in many countries, principally around the Mediterranean. It has adapted to a milder climate.[1]

Grasse, a town in the south of France, became the principal supplier of jasmine absolute; however, due to the high costs of production, most jasmine cultivation is now in countries such as Algeria, Morocco, Egypt and India.[1] The major jasmine absolute producing countries are Egypt and India. Egypt produces approximately 70-80% of the world's jasmine absolute.[2]

J. sambac is native to southern India and has a long history of cultivation in India. It is commonly referred to as *mogra*.[1]

Method of extraction

Jasmine absolute is produced by alcohol extraction of jasmine concrete, which is prepared by extraction with hydrocarbon solvents or by enfleurage. The enfleurage process has been beautifully described In Patrick Suskind's novel, *Perfume*:

> *Jasmine season began at the end of July, the perfume of this flower was both so exquisite and so fragile that not only did the blossoms have to be picked before sunrise, but they also demanded the most gentle and special handling. Warmth diminished their scent; suddenly to plunge them into hot macerating oil would have completely destroyed it. The souls of these noblest of blossoms could not be simply ripped from them, they had to be methodically coaxed away. In a special impregnated room, the flowers were strewn on glass plates smeared with cool oil or wrapped in oil soaked clothes, there they would die slowly in their sleep. It took three or four days for them to wither and exhale their scent into the adhering oil. Then they were carefully plucked off and new blossoms spread out.*
>
> *This procedure was repeated a good, ten, twenty times, and it was September before the pomade had drunk its fill and the fragrant oil could be pressed from the clothes. The yield was considerably less than with maceration.*
>
> *But in purity, it was unequalled, the jasmine oil radiated the sticky sweet, erotic scent of the blossoms with lifelike fidelity.*[3]

This well-known method of extraction which has been employed for over 200 years is today becoming increasingly impractical and uneconomical due to the high costs of labour.[4]

Today, most jasmine absolute is commonly obtained by solvent extraction, via the concrete from the flowers of *J. grandiflorum* cultivated in Egypt, Italy, Morocco and India, and of *J. sambac* from China and India.[1]

The flowers open in the early morning and there is a rapid and significant loss of essential oil once the buds have opened. For example, one of the constituents, indole, dropped by 0.6-0.8 mg/100 g of flowers in the first hours after the buds open.[1]

Flowers are usually picked by hand as a suitable method for mechanical harvesting has not been commercially developed. Flowers must be processed without delay. Approximately 1,000 kg of jasmine flowers will yield 2.5-3.5 kg of concrete, and half this amount as an absolute.[1]

Weiss states that a large cheap workforce is essential to harvest jasmine flowers. This is one of the reasons that Egypt has become a significant supplier of jasmine.[1]

Characteristics

Jasmine absolute is a dark orange (on aging reddish-brown), somewhat viscous liquid, and it possesses an intensely floral, warm, rich and highly diffusive odour with a peculiar waxy-herbaceous, oily-fruity and tea-like undertone.[4]

Arctander describes the scent of jasmine absolute from the traditional enfleurage method as being only faintly reminiscent of jasmine absolute from concrete or of the jasmine flower itself. It resembles the odour of orange flower absolute – warm, sweet, heavy, tenacious, fatty-floral, slightly herbaceous and deep-fruity, but less indolic sharp than the odour of jasmine flower itself.[4]

Chemical composition

The chemical composition of jasmine absolute was reported as follows:

benzyl acetate (22.09%), linalool (6.44%), benzyl alcohol (0.92%), farnesene (1.86%), indole (2.5%), benzyl benzoate + phytol (24.55%), *cis*-jasmone (2.6%), methyl anthranilate (2.04%), methyl jasmonate (2.99%), phytol acetate (10.25%), eugenol (1.66%), isophytol+jasmone lactone (9.77%).[1]

While the main volatile component of jasmine is benzyl acetate, minor constituents such as indole and *cis*-jasmone significantly contribute to the typical jasmine fragrance.

There is a significant difference between the main volatiles emitted by living and picked flowers. For instance, indole and benzyl acetate, which occur in relatively high concentration in the headspaces of living jasmine flowers, decrease significantly in the headspace of picked flowers. The linalool content also rises from 3% to 30% of the total volatiles.[1]

Jasmine absolute produced from a pomade varies in odour from jasmine absolute produced from concrete. Generally, the indole note is more pronounced in the pomade-absolute than in the absolute from concrete.[4]

Adulteration

Because of jasmine absolute's high price and very low yield during extraction, adulteration is very common. It is commonly adulterated with synthetic components such as indole, cinnamic aldehyde, *cis*-jasmone, farnesene, benzyl benzoate, benzyl acetate and fractions of ylang ylang.[4,5]

Pharmacopoeias and standards

At the time of writing, the purity, composition, physico-chemical properties and therapeutic use of jasmine absolute are not defined in any pharmacopoeia monograph or standard.

History and Traditional Uses

History

Jasmine's fragrant flowers have been used since antiquity for personal adornment and in religious ceremonies.[1]

The word jasmine is derived from the Arabic word meaning *Yasmin* or 'gift from God'. In India, *jasmine sambac* is commonly known as 'Queen of the Night', because the scent is stronger during the hours of darkness. The jasmine flower has been symbolically used throughout the centuries.

In the Philippines, *J. sambac* is traditionally called *sampaguita* meaning 'I promise you', and its flower is a symbol of fidelity, purity and eternal love.[2]

In China, the jasmine flower symbolises the sweetness of women, while in India it symbolises divine hope. In the fifteenth century jasmine was cultivated for its fragrant flowers in the gardens of the emperors of China, Afghanistan, Iran and Nepal. It was not until around 1600 when jasmine was brought to Spain by the Moors and first made its appearance in Europe.[1]

J. sambac, also known as Tuscan jasmine, was introduced into India by the Duke of Tuscany about 1691. Jasmine reached China along the Silk Road and the use of its flowers to flavour tea, *mo-li-hau-cha*, originated there. Such teas now use *J. paniculatum* flowers.[1]

J

Traditional medicine

As a medicinal plant, jasmine has traditionally been considered an aphrodisiac and relaxant.[5]

Jasmine species were mentioned in ancient Indian Ayurvedic literature. The oil was traditionally used in treatment of various conditions such as arthritis, hepatitis, conjunctivitis, gastritis and diarrhea.[2]

In China, the flowers of *J. officinale* var. *grandiflorum* are mainly used to treat hepatitis, pain due to liver cirrhosis, and abdominal pain due to dysentery, while the flowers of *J. sambac* are used to treat conjunctivitis, skin ulcers and tumours, as well as abdominal pain due to dysentery.[6]

Herbal

Jasmine has long been used for its effect on the reproductive system. It can be used as an aphrodisiac and to assist in childbirth.[1,5]

Food, perfumery and flavouring

Jasmine is extensively used in perfumes, body care preparations, soaps, air fresheners and skin care products.[2]

Dried jasmine flowers from *J. sambac* are used as an ingredient of Chinese jasmine tea.[5]

Therapeutics

Pharmacology and clinical studies

Many pharmacological studies involving jasmine absolute have been published. A systemic review of these studies will not be attempted. Rather, I have chosen a selection of studies that support the traditional and clinical uses.

Antimicrobial activity

A limited number of studies have investigated jasmine absolute's antimicrobial activity. An in vitro study confirmed that *J. sambac* oil showed good antifungal activity against *Aspergillus flavus, Trichophyton mentagrophytes, T. tonsurans, T. verrucosum, Epidermatophyton floccosum* and *Microsporum nanum*.[2]

The antimicrobial activity of jasmine absolute is often associated with the linalool content.[2]

Antispasmodic activity

An in vitro study utilising guinea pig ileum demonstrated that jasmine absolute had a spasmolytic activity. It was suggested that the spasmolytic activity was mediated through cAMP.[6]

Childbirth

A six-month trial was conducted involving 500 women at a maternity hospital using essential oils such as chamomile, clary sage, eucalyptus, jasmine, frankincense, lavender, lemon, mandarin, peppermint and rose. The oils were administered by inhalation, bath and massage. A high level of overall satisfaction by mothers and midwives was noted on the use of essential oils during labour.[7]

Nootropic activity

The effect on the pentobarbital sleep time by olfactory stimulation using various odorants was investigated in mice. The study found that jasmine shortened the sleep time. The researchers concluded that olfactory stimulation associated with odour inhalation influences pentobarbital sleep time.[8]

A study clearly identified excitatory effects for jasmine and sedative effects for lavender in a human vigilance test.[9]

During the vigilance test taken by 24 subjects, lavender significantly increased reaction time, whereas jasmine significantly decreased reaction time compared to the control group in which no essential oil was inhaled. The results confirmed that lavender had a sedative effect while jasmine had an excitatory effect on behaviour.[10]

Jasmine oil shortened the pentobarbital-induced sleeping time of mice to 77% of the control group.

The researchers identified *cis*- and *trans*-phytol as the components responsible for this effect.[11]

A study investigating the effect of aromatherapy massage with jasmine oil on humans found that jasmine oil caused significant increases in breathing rate, blood oxygen saturation and systolic and diastolic blood pressure, which indicated an increase of autonomic arousal. At an emotional level, subjects in the jasmine group rated themselves as more alert and less relaxed than subjects in the control group. This provides evidence for the use of jasmine for the relief of depression and uplifting mood in humans.[12]

A single-blind clinical trial found that ten-pin bowling in the presence of the odour of jasmine improved scores by 26.7%. The authors stated that the possible mechanisms of action include mood regulation, enhanced alertness and concentration, anxiolysis, increased self-confidence and improved hand-eye coordination.[13]

Another study was designed to determine if certain odours could increase humans' ratings and tolerance of pain. The results indicated that peppermint and jasmine odour significantly decreased ratings of pain over time and increased overall pain tolerance. The participants reported reduced mental, physical and temporal workload requirements, decreased effort and frustration, and increased performance and vigor.[14]

Actions

Actions commonly cited in aromatherapy

Antidepressant, antiseptic, antispasmodic, aphrodisiac, parturient, sedative, uterine[15,16,17,18]

Actions supported by clinical studies

Antidepressant, antispasmodic, aphrodisiac

Comment

Fischer-Rizzi gives us the best description of jasmine absolute when she states that no other essential oil is capable of changing our mood so intensely, and that it offers little choice other than optimism. She explains that the fragrance penetrates the deepest layers of our soul, opening the doors to our emotions.[17]

Aromatherapy Uses

Clinical aromatherapy

Psychological

The therapeutic value of jasmine absolute is inseparable from the exquisite, comforting sweetness of its aroma, and the effect it has on the mind and emotions. Jasmine is considered one of the most effective essential oils for nervous anxiety, restlessness and depression.[19]

The fragrance of jasmine diminishes fear; it is helpful in enhancing self-confidence and defeating pessimism.

Mojay explains that jasmine is ideal whenever fear and vulnerability, or anxiety and depression, cut us off from our ability to share physical pleasure and affection. Jasmine can reawaken our passion and reunite it with love, providing us with support and reassure us.[19]

Holmes describes jasmine as a depression fighter equal to melissa, basil and ylang ylang. Jasmine acts best on depression of the *Yang deficiency*. This includes symptoms such as apathy, chilliness, fatigue, weakness and restlessness.[20]

Jasmine absolute has been described as a powerful antidepressant of a stimulating nature. It is recommended when depression has given rise to lethargy.[21]

Reproductive system

Jasmine absolute is one of the most useful oils to use during childbirth. If it is used as a massage oil on the abdomen and lower back in the early stages of labour, it will relieve the pain and strengthen the contractions. It helps with the expulsion of the placenta after delivery and aids postnatal recovery.[15,21] It can be used to relieve spasms of the uterus, and delayed and painful menstruation.[15,17]

Skin care

Jasmine absolute is particularly useful in skin care and is used to treat dry and irritated skin.[15,20]

Energetics, psyche and subtle uses

Energetics

Jasmine absolute regulates the *Qi* of the *Heart* and harmonises the *Shen*. Whenever we experience disharmony of the *Shen* we may experience feelings of moodiness, anxiety, irritability, restlessness and insomnia. We lack inspiration and insight and there is no 'heart and soul' to life.

According to the principles of the Five Elements, jasmine strengthens and balances the Fire Element.

According to the principles of Ayurveda, jasmine has a strong affinity with *Pitta* dosha, it reduces excess *Kapha* dosha and stimulates the *Vata* dosha.

Personality

Worwood describes the jasmine personality as the passionate seductress, gentle and charismatic, bewitching all those who come into her presence.[22]

While Worwood is describing the female jasmine personality, she states that the male jasmine man is equally charming, charismatic and at ease with his femininity. Jasmine is a no-holds-barred personality. Jasmine personalities are joyful, happy people, comfortable with themselves. They can be unnerving if you are not used to them, particularly at work.[22]

According to Myers-Briggs personality types, the jasmine personality is likely to be an ESFP. ESFPs are friendly, witty, charming and talkative. They value and nurture their relationships, give generously, without expecting anything in return. They are spontaneous, playful and enjoy everything they do and see. People who share their sense of fun and adventure are their favourite companions. They turn everything into a fun-filled event. They enjoy good things in life – music, dance, food, drink and entertainment. They avoid being alone. They like working in a lively and stimulating atmosphere with friendly, energetic people. They can be good at dealing with the public. They like variety and frequent change of tasks or jobs. They are enthusiastic, high-spirited and have lots of energy.

Subtle

Lavabre best summarises the subtle qualities of jasmine when he says that it releases inhibition, liberates imagination, develops exhilarating playfulness and has the power to transcend physical love fully releasing both male and female sexual energy.[16]

Mojay recommends jasmine for depression which results from unconscious restraint and repression – an approach to life based on values discordant with the individual soul and its true desires.[19]

Zeck recommends using jasmine when you are faced with seemingly unresolved emotional challenges and feeling fearful. She states that the exotic beauty of jasmine will dissolve those fears and provide divine inspiration.[23]

Worwood states that jasmine softly embraces the spirit and the heart. This promotes a greater understanding of the conscious mind. She explains that jasmine's purpose is to provide us with our personal haven – this allows us to find a greater resonation with our higher self. She explains that our aspirations may not always be what is required to follow a spiritual journey. Often our dreams and wishes for others may deflect them from our spiritual journey. Jasmine helps us to understand and accept this.[24]

According to Keim Loughran & Bull, jasmine promotes love and sensuality. It also connects our spirituality and sexuality, and promotes creativity and artistic development.[25]

J

Dosage and Administration

Blending

Aromatherapy

To alleviate depression, consider blending jasmine absolute with essential oils such as bergamot, black pepper, coriander seed, geranium, ginger, grapefruit, lavender, sweet orange, rose absolute, sandalwood or ylang ylang.

For the relief of anxiety, stress and nervous tension, consider blending jasmine absolute with essential oils such as bergamot, coriander seed, geranium, lavender, neroli, sweet orange, patchouli, sandalwood or ylang ylang.

For the relief of PMS and dysmenorrhoea, consider blending jasmine absolute with essential oils such as Roman chamomile, clary sage, sweet fennel, geranium, lavender, sweet marjoram or ylang ylang.

Perfumery

Arctander states that whenever a floral note is required eight times out of ten the perfumer will use a jasmine base. Jasmine is often blended with rose to create the heart and soul of any floral based perfume. He gives us some practical advice when he explains that the practising student perfumer is often surprised when they learn how little jasmine absolute has to be used to create a floral note.[4]

Mode of administration

Bath

Full body bath, foot bath

Topical

Compress, massage, ointment, skin care

Inhalation

Direct inhalation, diffuser, oil vaporiser

Safety Profile

General safety

Jasmine absolute is non-irritating, non-sensitising and non-toxic. However, Khan & Abourashed have cited coniferyl acetate and coniferyl benzoate as allergenic components of the jasmine absolute.[6]

IFRA recommends a dermal limit of 0.7% for jasmine absolute.[26]

Contraindications

No contraindications known.

Regulatory guidelines

Jasmine absolute has GRAS status.

References

1. Weiss EA. *Essential oil crops.* CAB International, Wallingford, 1997.
2. Ahmed N et al. *Jasmine (Jasminum sambac L. Oleaceae).* In Preedy VR. ed. *Essential oils in food preservation, flavor and safety.* Academic Press, London, 2016: 487-494.
3. Suskind P. *Perfume: The story of a murderer.* Penguin Books, London, 1986.
4. Arctander S. *Perfume and flavour materials of natural origin.* Allured Publishing, Carol Stream, 1994.
5. Lis-Balchin M. *Aromatherapy science – a guide for healthcare professionals.* Pharmaceutical Press, London, 2006.
6. Khan I, Abourashed E. *Leung's encyclopedia of common natural ingredients used in food, drugs and cosmetics.* 3rd edn. John Wiley & Sons. New Jersey, 2010.
7. Burns E, Blamey C. *Using aromatherapy in childbirth.* Nursing Times, 1994; 90(9): 54-60. Cited in Quintessential Aromatics database, 2013.
8. Tsuchiya T et al. *Effects of olfactory stimulation on sleep time induced by pentobarbital administration in mice.* Brain Research Bulletin, 1991; 26(3): 397-401. Cited in Quintessential Aromatics database, 2013.
9. Ilmberger I et al. *Effects of essential oils on human attentional processes.* Programme Abstracts – 24th International Symposium on Essential Oils, 1993. Cited in Quintessential Aromatics database, 2013.
10. Karamat E et al. *Excitatory and sedative effects of essential oils on human reaction time performance.* Chemical Senses, 1992; 17(6): 876. Cited in Quintessential Aromatics database, 2013.
11. Kikuchi A et al. *Stimulant-like ingredients in absolute jasmine.* Chemical Senses, 1989; 14(2): 304. Cited in Quintessential Aromatics database, 2013.
12. Hongratanaworakit T. *Stimulating effect of aromatherapy massage with jasmine oil.* Natural Product Communications, 2010; 5(1): 157-162. Cited in Quintessential Aromatics database, 2013.
13. Hirsch A et al. *The effects of the aroma of jasmine on bowling score.* International Journal of Essential Oil Therapeutics, 2007; 1(2): 79-82. Cited in Quintessential Aromatics database, 2013.
14. Raudenbush B et al. *Effect of odorant administration on pain and psychophysiological measures in humans.* North American Journal of Psychology, 2004; 6(3): 361-370. Cited in Quintessential Aromatics database, 2013.
15. Lawless J. *The encyclopaedia of essential oils.* Element Books, Shaftesbury, 1992.
16. Lavabre M. *Aromatherapy workbook.* Healing Arts Press, Rochester, 1997.
17. Fischer-Rizzi S. *Complete aromatherapy handbook.* Sterling Publishing, New York, 1990.
18. Holmes P. *Jasmine.* The International Journal of Aromatherapy, 1998; 8(4): 8-12.
19. Mojay G. *Aromatherapy for healing the spirit.* Healing Arts Press, Rochester, 1999.
20. Holmes P. *The energetics of Western herbs – Vol. I.* Artemis Press, Boulder, 1989.
21. Davis P. *Aromatherapy: an A-Z.* 2nd edn. C.W. Daniel Company, Saffron Walden, 1999.
22. Worwood VA. *The fragrant mind.* Transworld Publishers, London, 1995.
23. Zeck R. *The blossoming heart – aromatherapy for healing and transformation.* Aroma Tours, East Ivanhoe, 2004.
24. Worwood VA. *The fragrant heavens.* Transworld Publishers, London, 1999.
25. Keim Loughran J, Bull R. *Aromatherapy and subtle energy techniques.* Frog, Berkeley, 2000.
26. Tisserand R, Young R. *Essential oil safety.* 2nd edn. Churchill Livingstone, Edinburgh, 2014.

Juniper berry

Identification

Botanical name

Juniperus communis L.

Synonyms

Common juniper

Family

Cupressaceae

Botany and origins

The shrub, *Juniperus communis,* grows wild throughout central Europe. It is a small tree reaching the height of 12 m, with blue-green needle-like leaves, greenish-yellow flowers and small round berries. The berries take about three years to mature.[1]

The best juniper berries are collected in Northern Italy, Austria, Czech Republic, Hungary, Croatia, Serbia and France.[1]

Schnaubelt states that the Corsican variety of mountain juniper referred to as *Juniperus communis* var. *montana* is naturally high in limonene and almost free of sabinene, the terpene hydrocarbon that is responsible for causing kidney irritation.[2]

Method of extraction

The best juniper berry oil is steam-distilled from the crushed, dried or partly dried ripe berries. Arctander states that most commercial juniper berry oil is derived from the fermented fruits as a by-product of the central European juniper-brandy manufacturing process.[1]

Characteristics

Juniper berry oil is a clear or very pale yellow mobile oil, having a fresh, yet warm, rich-balsamic, woody-sweet and pine-needle-like odour. The oil derived from fermented fruits is usually a more turpentine-like, pinene-like odour, with no sweet balsamic notes.[1]

Chemical composition

The chemical composition of juniper berry oil was reported as follows:

α-pinene (33.7%), camphene (0.5%), β-pinene (1.1%), sabinene (27.6%), myrcene (5.5%), α-phellandrene (1.3%), α-terpinene (1.9%), γ-terpinene (3.0%), 1,4-cineole (4%), β-phellandrene (1.3%), *p*-cymene (5.5%), terpinen-4-ol (4.0%), bornyl acetate (0.4%), caryophyllene (0.6%), and trace amounts of limonene, camphor, linalool, linalyl acetate, borneol and nerol.[3]

J

The EMA assessment report states that the composition of juniper berry essential oil depends on the source. The composition range of juniper berry essential oil according to the 2008 European pharmacopoeia is as follows:

α-pinene (24.1-55.4%), β-pinene (2.1-6.0%), β-myrcene (7.3-22.0%), sabinene (1.4-28.8%), limonene (2.3-10.9%), terpinene-4-ol (0.7-17.0%), α-terpineol (up to 1.7%), α-thujene (0.6-1.9%), caryophyllene (1.3-2.3%).[4]

Adulteration

Arctander states that juniper berry oil is very frequently adulterated. He explains that one could say that commercial juniper berry oil is rarely the true distillate from the berries. The most frequent additive is the inferior oil from the fermented berries. Other adulterants include pinene, camphene, turpentine oil fractions, juniper wood and twig oils.[1]

The EMA assessment report states that juniper berry oil should be prepared from ripe berries only. The essential oil should not be prepared with any needles or wood from the trees.[4]

Juniper berry oil is also adulterated with *Juniperus oxycedrus*.[5]

Pharmacopoeias and standards

The purity, composition, physico-chemical properties and therapeutic uses of juniper berry essential oil are defined in several pharmacopoeia monographs and standards:

- ISO 8897:2010 Oil of Juniper Berry (*Juniperus communis* L.)
- European Pharmacopoeia
- British Pharmacopoeia
- Martindale Extra Pharmacopoeia.

History and Traditional Uses

History

In ancient Rome, Pliny the Elder used juniper berry for relieving aches and pains of rheumatism. Roman physicians prescribed preparations of berries for stomach and chest pains, flatulence, coughs and colds, tumors and uterine disorders.[6]

Juniper branches were also burned in temples as purifying herbs. In medieval Europe, juniper wood was burned to banish evil spirits and to ward off the plague. In England, branches of juniper were often strewn on floors to sweeten the smell of the rooms and to cleanse the air of infection and disease. It was also believed that juniper would provide protection against witches.[6]

Native Americans also believed that juniper possessed purifying and protecting powers. For example, the Cheyenne burned juniper in ceremonies to ease the fear of thunder, while the Navajo burned juniper to produce 'good luck smoke' for hunters.[6]

Medieval herbalists recommended juniper as an antidote against poisons and as a cure for a wide range of conditions from flatulence to feeble-mindedness.[6]

Culpepper was well aware of juniper's diuretic and detoxifying properties:

> *It is a remedy for dropsy, brings down the terms, helps fits of the mother, expels wind and strengthens the stomach. It provokes the urine and is good for gout and sciatica, and strengthens the limbs.*[7]

Mojay states that the English name *juniper* is derived from the Latin *juniores* meaning young berries.[8]

Traditional medicine

In Western traditional medicine, juniper berries were used to relieve indigestion and flatulence and to stimulate the appetite. Juniper berries were also recommended to relieve the aches of rheumatism, dropsy, bronchitis and some types of cancer.[6]

Davis states that juniper was traditionally used in France as a tonic, especially for convalescence.[9]

Herbal

The berries and extract are used as ingredients in diuretic and laxative preparations. The berries are used as a carminative and diuretic, to treat flatulence, colic, intestinal worms and gastrointestinal infections.[10]

The German Commission E recommends a daily dosage of 2-10 g of the dried berries for dyspepsia; however, warns that prolonged use may cause kidney damage and that it is contraindicated during pregnancy.[11]

Juniper berries are recommended for acute and chronic cystitis and topical application for rheumatic pain in the joints or muscles.[12,13]

Food, perfumery and flavouring

The oil is used as a fragrance component in soaps, detergents, creams, lotions and perfumes.[10]

Other uses

Juniper berries are used for making gin.[1,10]

Therapeutics

Pharmacology and clinical studies

Many pharmacological studies involving juniper berry oil have been published. A systemic review of these studies will not be attempted. Rather, I have chosen a selection of studies that support the traditional and clinical uses.

Antiglycation activity

A study investigating the antiglycation properties of essential oil from the berries and branchlets of juniper berries found that the oil had promising inhibitory activity in haemoglobin and glycation assays. It was suggested that juniper oil has antiglycation properties and could be used for the prevention and treatment of diabetic complications.[14]

Anti-inflammatory activity

An in vitro study found that *J. communis* oil demonstrated good inhibition of 5-lipoxygenase. This indicates that it may have anti-inflammatory activity, as the mechanism of inflammation begins with the oxidation of the enzyme 5-lipoxygenase.[15]

Antimicrobial activity

Juniper oil exhibited bactericidal activity against gram-positive and gram-negative bacterial species, with MIC values between 8 and 70% (v/v). The oil also had strong fungicidal activity against yeast, yeast-like fungi and dermatophytes.[16]

High concentrations of juniper oil inhibited the growth of microorganisms. The results indicated that juniper oil was comparable with the antibiotic gentamycin. The same study also found that *Escherichia coli* was the only bacteria tested that was completely resistant to juniper essential oil. However, it was also recommended that further studies be done to confirm the safety of using high concentrations for humans.[17]

Anticholinergic activity

Inhalation of juniper oil significantly decreased the acetylcholinesterase activity and exhibited antioxidant potential in rat studies. It was suggested that juniper oil may be beneficial to manage oxidative stress associated with Alzheimer's disease by decreasing the activity of acetylcholinesterase and antioxidative mechanism.[18]

Antispasmodic activity

Juniper oil has an antispasmodic effect on isolated guinea pig ileum.[12]

Diuretic activity

Juniper berries and juniper oil stimulate the glomerular filtration rate of the kidney; however, they are known to irritate the renal epithelium and could cause hematuria.[19]

It is believed that the toxicity depends on the hydrocarbon content of the essential oil. Juniper berry oil contains high levels of α- and β-pinenes, which are known irritants to the urinary tract. Higher levels of pinenes would result from co-distillation of the needles, branches and unripe berries with ripe berries. It has been concluded that oil distilled from the ripe berries can be safely used in diuretic therapy.[20]

Elastase activity

The activity of two elastase enzymes, porcine pancreatic enzyme and human neutrophil elastase, were examined in vitro in the presence of 12 essential oils. Juniper oil demonstrated very high anti-elastase activity. The authors state that as we get older the elasticity of the skin is decreased because of these enzymes. It was concluded that massage using essential oils such as juniper oil may help prevent skin aging.[21]

Actions

Actions commonly cited in aromatherapy

Anticatarrhal, antirheumatic, antiseptic, antispasmodic, astringent, carminative, cicatrisant, decongestant, depurative, expectorant, lymphatic decongestant, nervine, rubefacient, sedative, stomachic, sudorific, tonic (nervous system), vulnerary[8,9,22,23]

Actions supported by clinical studies

Antirheumatic, antiseptic, carminative, diuretic

Comment

The EMA assessment report states that juniper berry oil should be limited to the stimulation of diuresis and dyspepsia. The former is sustained by tradition and by experimental evidence, the latter only by tradition.[4]

Holmes suggests that juniper oil is one of the few essential oils that have a good fluid decongestant effect – meaning that it has excellent diuretic property.[24] However, the use of juniper berry as a diuretic is no longer recommended by some authors. The EMA assessment report for juniper berry oil states that there is a lack of systematically obtained clinical safety and toxicity data for juniper. Many references give contradictory information based on interpretation by authors and not on clinical evidence. Schilcher & Heil are not convinced of the renal toxicity of *Juniperus* oil, because quite a lot of sources may have just copied the doubtful renal side effects.[4]

Lis-Balchin states that true juniper berry oil is rare, as the fermented berries, which produce an inferior oil, are more economical and abundant. Therefore, when using juniper berry oil, please be wary of commercially produced oil where the source of the berries cannot be verified.[12]

J

Aromatherapy Uses

Clinical aromatherapy

Detoxification

Juniper berry oil is well known for its diuretic and lymphatic decongestant properties. It is recommended for clearing toxins and resolving toxaemia, and to reduce levels of uric acid in the body, thus being beneficial for cellulite and rheumatic conditions.[9,22,23,24]

Digestive system

Juniper berry oil is recommended for chronic indigestion associated with bloating and abdominal pain.[24]

Integumentary system

Juniper berry oil is recommended for skin conditions that result as an accumulation of toxins in the body such as weeping type eczema, acne and psoriasis.[9,22,23]

Muscular system

Juniper berry oil is recommended as a neuromuscular stimulant and analgesic, and can be used for chronic painful rheumatic and arthritic conditions, for fibromyalgia, neuralgia and lower back pain.[24]

Psychological

Juniper berry oil is recommended for nervous and intellectual fatigue.[23] Holmes recommends juniper berry oil to dispel lethargy, apathy, gloominess, negative thoughts, mental disorientation, confusion and loss of instinctive self-confidence. He states we should think of juniper as a mental detoxifier as much as a physiological one. He recommends it for individuals with low perseverance and willpower, who become easily discouraged and apathetic.[24]

Skin care

Juniper berry oil is recommended for oily skin types.[9,24] It is ideal for tired devitalised skin and for congested skin.[8,24]

Urinary system

Juniper berry oil is recommended for treating cystitis, pyelitis and urinary stones. However, if there is blood or pus in the urine or a fever, do not delay in getting medical assistance.[9]

Energetics, psyche and subtle uses

Energetics

The energetic qualities of juniper berry oil are warming and stimulate *Yang* energy.[8,24] The oil is considered a powerful tonic of the body.[8] Its warming and invigorating effect benefits tiredness, poor circulation, cold hands and feet, and lower backache.[8]

Juniper berry oil is ideal for conditions associated with *cold* and *damp*. *Cold* and *damp* conditions are typically characterised by poor circulation, genitourinary tract infections, digestive problems such as diarrhoea and poor appetite, and accumulation of toxins.[8,24]

According to the principles of the Five Elements, juniper berry oil is associated with the Water Element.[8,24] Mojay states that juniper berry oil helps to strengthen our *Zhi*. The *Zhi* represents our willpower, ambition and self-actualisation. Our *Zhi* helps us break through psychological stagnation and strengthen our will power.[8]

When the Water Element is out of balance, our *Zhi* spirit is affected. Typical signs and symptoms may include a feeling of absolute despair, the inability to face fears which interferes with expression of true self, an inability to move on or take on life, and a complete disintegration of the nervous system.

Personality

The juniper personality is described as having a profound spiritual ease; they have no concern for human authority, preferring to be directed by their intuition or religious beliefs. Worwood describes juniper as the personality of spring. They are not afraid to enjoy themselves, therefore they often appear immature because they take delight in new experiences and knowledge.[25]

Juniper personalities are best suited to professions that allow them freedom of thought and speech. They prefer work where they can be left on their own. They can have difficulty choosing a romantic partner because they need someone who understands why they need to withdraw into themselves for inner reflection without feeling excluded.[25]

According to Myers-Briggs personality types, the juniper berry personality is likely to be an INTP. INTPs are quiet, reserved and highly independent. They like to be precise. They have a natural curiosity to understand the universe and to examine its universal truths and principles. They may be good at developing complex systems and conceptual models, but prefer to leave the implementation to others. They have high standards of intellectual and professional competence. They can have difficulty explaining their deep thoughts so that others can understand. They dislike supervising others or resolving conflict. They appear to be concerned with their thoughts, interests and work and can neglect their relationships. They prefer calm, conflict-free atmosphere. They can appear to be formal and distant with strangers and acquaintances, but are generally open-minded and accepting of people once they know them.

Subtle

The fresh clean scent of juniper is associated with purification.[9,22,23] It is no wonder that it has been used since ancient times for spiritual purification. It may be used for driving out negative influences.[8]

Mojay suggests that juniper helps us to break through psychological stagnation and helps us to consolidate willpower. He suggests that it is suited to someone who is feeling burdened and deeply absorbed in their own thoughts – thoughts which revolve around worries, pressures and unpleasant memories.[8]

Holmes states that juniper berry oil has a good stabilising and centring effect, and recommends using it when we feel mental spaciness, lack of embodiment and our energy is dispersed. It will help to promote strength, empowerment and instinctive self-confidence. He also states that juniper berry refreshes the mind and helps to resolve negative and confused thoughts and mental fogginess. He explains that we should think of juniper berry oil as a mental detoxifier as much as a physiological one.[24]

Zeck recommends using juniper oil whenever you need to purify the room and dispel unwanted or negative thoughts and cleanse your body. She states that juniper helps to reduce negativity associated with bad habits, beliefs and behaviours that are robbing you of your joy of life.[26]

Keim Loughran & Bull state that juniper clears the body, mind and spirit of the damaging perceptions that interfere with our confidence and sense of self-worth. It releases old thoughts, strengthens our intuition and deepens trust in our inner voice. Juniper teaches that a clear mind prepares us to listen to our spirit and integrate what we have heard. Juniper is one of the primary oils for protecting us from the negativity of others. Through this energetic detoxification, we are free to grow in spiritual wisdom.[27]

Worwood states that juniper will allow us to complete tasks and learn lessons. It clears obstructions on our pathway to the divine spirit. She explains that juniper's fragrance is cleansing and purifying when inhaled, and subtle changes occur at a physical, mental and spiritual level. It encourages inner vision, strength, vitality, sincerity, enlightenment and humility.[28]

Dosage and Administration

Blending

Aromatherapy

For the relief of pain associated with musculoskeletal and rheumatic conditions, consider blending juniper berry oil with essential oils such as black pepper, cajeput, fir, ginger, kunzea, spike lavender, pine or rosemary.

For the relief of dyspepsia, consider blending juniper berry oil with essential oils such as aniseed, black pepper, cardamom, sweet fennel, ginger, sweet orange or rosemary.

To treat oedema, consider blending juniper berry oil with essential oils such as sweet fennel, grapefruit or lemon.

To create a detoxifying blend, consider blending juniper berry oil with essential oils such as carrot seed, sweet fennel, grapefruit, lemon, sweet orange or rosemary.

Perfumery

Juniper berry oil is used in perfumery for its fresh-balsamic aroma as a modifier for pine needle oils. It is also used with citrus oils in room spray perfumes, fougères, chypres and spice perfumes.[1]

Mode of administration

Bath

Full body bath, foot bath

Topical

Compress, massage, ointment, skin care

Inhalation

Direct inhalation, diffuser, oil vaporiser

Safety Profile

General safety

Juniper berry oil has been reported to be non-toxic, non-irritant and non-sensitising. Juniper berry oil is contraindicated during pregnancy or for those with kidney disease.[9,22] It must be remembered that this refers to the internal use of herbal extracts of juniper berries.[13,19]

I agree with Tisserand & Balacs who state that there is a good chance that juniper oil may have been confused with savin, whose botanical name is *Juniperus sabina*.[29]

Juniper berry is very high in α-pinene. As a result, it is prone to oxidation. Skin sensitisation may occur if the oil is oxidised. Tisserand & Young state that there is no reason to consider unoxidised juniper berry oil as being hazardous.[30]

J

Contraindications

No contraindications known.

Regulatory guidelines

Juniper berry essential oil has GRAS status.

References

1. Arctander S. *Perfume and flavor materials of natural origin.* Allured Publishing, Carol Stream, 1994.
2. Schnaubelt K. *The healing intelligence of essential oils.* Healing Arts Press, Rochester, 2011.
3. Lawrence BM. *Essential oils 1981-1987.* Allured Publishing, Wheaton, 1989.
4. Committee on Herbal Medicinal Products (HMPC). *Assessment report on Juniperus communis L., aetheroleum.* European Medicines Agency, London, 2011. Doc ref. EMA/HMPC/12401/2010.
5. Schmidt E, Wanner J. *Adulteration of essential oils.* In Baser KHC, Buchbauer G. eds. *Handbook of essential oils – science, technology and applications.* 2nd edn. CRC Press, Boca Raton, 2016: 707-745.
6. Foster S, Johnson RL. *Desk reference to nature's medicine.* National Geographic Society, Washington DC, 2006.
7. Grieve M. *A modern herbal – Vol. II.* Dover Publications, New York, 1971.
8. 8. Mojay G. *Aromatherapy for healing the spirit.* Healing Arts Press, Rochester, 1999.
9. Davis P. *Aromatherapy: an A-Z.* 2nd edn. C.W. Daniel Company, Saffron Walden, 1999.
10. Khan I, Abourashed E. *Leung's encyclopedia of common natural ingredients used in food, drugs and cosmetics.* 3rd edn. John Wiley & Sons, New Jersey, 2010.
11. Blumenthal M et al. *The complete German commission E monographs: therapeutic guide to herbal medicine.* American Botanical Council, Austin, 1998.
12. Lis-Balchin M. *Aromatherapy science – a guide for healthcare professionals.* Pharmaceutical Press, London, 2006.
13. British Herbal Medicine Association's Scientific Committee. *British herbal pharmacopoeia 1983.* British Herbal Medicine Association, West York, 1983.
14. Asgary S et al. *Inhibition of protein glycation by essential oils of branchlets and fruits of Juniperus communis subsp. hemisphaerica.* Research in Pharmaceutical Sciences, 2014; 9(3): 179-185. Cited in Quintessential Aromatics database, 2013.
15. Baylac S, Racine P. *Inhibition of 5-lipoxygenase by essential oils and other natural extracts.* International Journal of Aromatherapy, 2003; 13(2/3): 138-142. Cited in Quintessential Aromatics database, 2013.
16. Pepeljnjak S et al. *Antimicrobial activity of juniper berry essential oil (Juniperus communis L., Cupressaceae).* Acta Pharmaceutica, 2005; 55(4): 417-422. Cited in Quintessential Aromatics database, 2013.
17. Singh RS et al. *Antimicrobial activity of essential oils of Juniperus communis against bactericidal and fungal species.* International Journal of Essential Oil Therapeutics, 2010; 4(3/4): 92-94. Cited in Quintessential Aromatics database, 2013.
18. Cioanca O et al. *Anti-acetylcholinesterase and antioxidant activities of inhaled juniper oil on amyloid beta (1-42)-Induced oxidative stress in the rat hippocampus.* Neurochemical Research, 2015; 40(5): 952-960. Cited in Quintessential Aromatics database, 2013.
19. Bruneton J. *Pharmacognosy.* 2nd edn. Lavoisier Publishing, Paris, 1999.
20. Mediherb Monitor. No.7, December 1993.
21. Mori M et al. *Inhibition of elastase activity by essential oils in vitro.* Journal of Cosmetic Dermatology, 2002; 1(4): 183-187. Cited in Quintessential Aromatics database, 2013.
22. Lawless J. *The encyclopaedia of essential oils.* Element Books, Shaftesbury, 1992.
23. Lavabre M. *Aromatherapy workbook.* Healing Arts Press, Rochester, 1997.

24. Holmes P. *Aromatica: a clinical guide to essential oil therapeutics – Vol. I.* Singing Dragon, London, 2016.
25. Worwood VA. *The fragrant mind.* Transworld Publishers, London, 1995.
26. Zeck R. *The blossoming heart – aromatherapy for healing and transformation.* Aroma Tours, East Ivanhoe, 2004.
27. Keim Loughran J, Bull R. *Aromatherapy anointing oils.* Frog, Berkeley, 2001.
28. Worwood VA. *The fragrant heavens.* Transworld Publishers, London, 1999.
29. Tisserand R. Balacs T. *Essential oil safety.* Churchill Livingstone, Edinburgh, 1995.
30. Tisserand R. Young R. *Essential oil safety.* 2nd edn. Churchill Livingstone, Edinburgh, 2014.

Kanuka

Identification

Botanical name

Kunzea ericoides (A. Rich.) Joy Thomps

Synonyms

White tea tree, *Leptospermum ericoides*

Family

Myrtaceae

Botany and origins

A small bushy tree with pointed leaves on full branches, kanuka is indigenous to New Zealand. All material is hand harvested from sustainable and naturally regenerating stands of kanuka on the East Cape of New Zealand. It is often confused with manuka.

Method of extraction

Kanuka oil is steam-distilled from the freshly cut plant material.

Characteristics

Kanuka oil has a sweet, herbaceous aroma, similar to that of manuka.

Chemical composition

The chemical composition of kanuka oil remains consistent throughout New Zealand; however, two chemotypes have been identified. The most common chemotype is low in *p*-cymene, while the less common chemotype has higher levels of (>5%) *p*-cymene.[1]

A chemical composition of kanuka oil from the North Island was reported as follows:

α-pinene (61.6%), *p*-cymene (2-5%), other monoterpenes (<3%), sesquiterpenes (<2%), 1,8-cineole (6.0%), viridiflorol (3.2%), α -terpineol (1.1%).[2]

Adulteration

Lis-Balchin states that the admixing of different trees and shrubs would give the oil variable chemical composition, which may compromise the therapeutic efficacy of the oil.[3]

Pharmacopoeias and standards

At the time of writing, the purity, composition, physico-chemical properties and therapeutic use of kanuka essential oil are not defined in any pharmacopoeia monograph or standard.

History and Traditional Uses

History

Maori folklore attributes the kanuka as the 'male' tree and manuka the 'female.'[2] Maoris have traditionally used manuka and kanuka for their medicinal properties. Infusions of the leaves were drunk as a tea for many internal complaints.[4]

Traditional medicine

Traditional medical applications of kanuka and manuka include internal or external sedatives, reducing fever and cough suppressants. A decoction of the seed capsules can also be used to treat inflammation. A decoction of the leaves can also be used to alleviate dysentery, diarrhoea and colic pain. A poultice from the pounded capsules of the plants was used to dry open wounds or runny sores and to treat scalds and burns.[5]

Therapeutics

Pharmacology and clinical studies

Antimicrobial activity

An in vitro study confirmed that kanuka and manuka significantly inhibited a range of fungi and bacteria. The fungicidal properties of the oil were confirmed with a minimum inhibitory concentration ranging from 0.78% to 3.13%. The oils also displayed excellent bactericidal activity with 100% inhibition of the examined bacteria. In terms of inhibiting effects on fungal growth, kanuka oil was superior to manuka oil.[5]

Mucositis

A study examined the effects of an essential oil mouthwash on radiation, induced mucositis of the oropharyngeal area during treatment for head and neck cancers. 19 patients participated in the randomised, placebo-controlled study, involving the use of a gargle containing two drops of a 1:1 mix of manuka and kanuka in water, which reported delayed onset of mucositis and reduced pain and oral symptoms relative to the placebo (gargling with water). The study confirmed that manuka and kanuka oil used in a gargle can provide relief on the development of radiation-induced mucositis.[6]

Actions

Actions commonly cited in aromatherapy

Antibacterial, antifungal, anti-inflammatory

Actions supported by clinical studies

Antibacterial, antifungal

Comment

I am not sure why kanuka is often referenced in literature alongside manuka, considering that it has a totally different chemical profile to manuka. The chemistry of manuka oil is complex with monoterpenes, sesquiterpenes and triketones, whereas the kanuka oil is predominantly composed of the monoterpene hydrocarbon – α-pinene.

K

Aromatherapy Uses

Clinical aromatherapy

Musculoskeletal system

Kanuka oil is useful for muscular pain relief and to relieve swelling. It may be used for sprains, strains and sports injuries. *p*-cymene in kanuka oil is responsible for the oil's analgesic properties.[2]

Respiratory system

Kanuka oil is beneficial for all types of respiratory tract infections and can be used to relieve coughs, colds and flu.

Skin care

Kanuka oil may be used in skin care preparations for anti-acne preparations and preparations for prevention of body and foot odour.

Energetics, psyche and subtle uses

Energetics

I would recommend kanuka oil for dispersing *wind cold* conditions. *Wind cold* is characterised as the onset of respiratory tract infections, with aches and pains, chills and a dislike for cold. Kanuka oil also tonifies the *Qi* and strengthens the *Shen*. Whenever we have *Qi* deficiency and our *Shen* is weak, we experience fatigue, lethargy, poor focus and depression.

Subtle

Keim Loughran & Bull state that kanuka oil balances all the energy centres and increases feelings of joy.[7]

Dosage and Administration

Blending

Aromatherapy

For the relief of musculoskeletal aches and pains, consider bending kanuka oil with essential oils such as black pepper, cajeput, ginger, kunzea, spike lavender, pine or rosemary.

For the relief of the symptoms of colds and flu, consider blending kanuka oil with essential oils such as 1,8-cineole-rich eucalypts, fragonia, peppermint eucalyptus, lemon-scented eucalyptus, lemon, lemon myrtle, manuka, pine, tea tree or thyme.

Perfumery

Kanuka oil is not commonly used in perfumery.

Mode of administration

Bath

Full body bath, foot bath

Topical

Compress, massage, ointment, skin care

Inhalation

Direct inhalation, diffuser, oil vaporiser

Safety Profile

General safety

Kanuka is non-toxic and non-irritant; however, it may be a mild sensitiser. Tisserand & Young state that kanuka oil has high α-pinene content and is, therefore, prone to oxidation. It should be stored in dark, airtight containers in a refrigerator.[8]

Contraindications

No contraindications known.

Regulatory guidelines

Kanuka oil is not defined in any regulatory guideline.

References

1. *Essential oil production from manuka and*

kanuka. Crop & Food Research Broadsheet, No. 116, 2000.
2. Maddocks-Jennings W et al. *A fresh look at manuka and kanuka essential oils from New Zealand*. The International Journal of Aromatherapy, 2005; 15(3): 141-146.
3. Lis-Balchin M. *Aromatherapy science – a guide for healthcare professionals*. Pharmaceutical Press, London, 2006.
4. Anthony C. *Aromatherapy in New Zealand: indigenous use of essential oils from native plants, manuka and kanuka essential oils*. Proceedings of the Australasian Aromatherapy Conference, Sydney, 1996.
5. Chen CC et al. *Investigations of kanuka and manuka essential oils for in vitro treatment of disease and cellular inflammation caused by infectious microorganisms*. Journal of Microbiology, Immunology and Infection, 2016; 49(1): 104-111. Cited in Quintessential Aromatics database, 2013.
6. Maddocks-Jennings W et al. *Evaluating the effects of the essential oils Leptospermum scoparium (manuka) and Kunzea ericoides (kanuka) on radiotherapy induced mucositis: a randomized, placebo controlled feasibility study*. European Journal of Oncology Nursing, 2009; 13(2): 87-93. Cited in Quintessential Aromatics database, 2013.
7. Keim Loughran J, Bull R. *Aromatherapy and subtle energy techniques*. Frog, Berkeley, 2000.
8. Tisserand R, Young R. *Essential oil safety*. 2nd edn. Churchill Livingstone, Edinburgh, 2014.

Kunzea

Identification

Botanical name

Kunzea ambigua (Sm.) Druce

Synonyms

Australian kunzea, tick bush, Tasmanian spring flower

Family

Myrtaceae

Botany and origins

Kunzea is a tall, erect woodland tree, which grows up to 5 m, although it is typically smaller. It has small white flowers and is found in the northeast region of Tasmania and the southeast mainland of Australia. Kunzea is a wild harvested plant from natural stands of kunzea maintained in plantation-like settings.[1] It is closely related to the bottlebrushes and *Leptospermum* species. There are about 40 species occurring in all states of Australia. One species occurs in New Zealand.[2]

Method of extraction

Kunzea oil is steam-distilled from the aerial parts of *Kunzea ambigua*.

Characteristics

Kunzea oil is a clear, mobile liquid with a pleasant, fresh and slightly spicy aroma.[3] It is also described as having a fresh, invigorating scent reminiscent of the Australian bush.[4]

Chemical composition

A total of 64 compounds have been identified in kunzea essential oil. Kunzea oil contained 70% monoterpenes including α-pinene (48.3%), 1,8-cineole (14.5%) and α-terpineol (1.9%). Kunzea oil from other *K. ambigua* plants had significantly different content – α-pinene (0.6-62.5%), 1,8-cineole (0-14%), spathulenol (0.5-12.2%), globulol (0.5-22.6%) and viridiflorol (0.3-3.8%).[5]

Therefore, we can expect some variability in the pharmacological activity of the essential oil.

Adulteration

It is unlikely to be adulterated; however, there appears to be a significant variation in the percentage of the major chemical components. More studies are needed to establish the ideal chemical profile of kunzea essential oil to ensure the desired therapeutic efficacy.

Pharmacopoeias and standards

At the time of writing, the purity, composition, physico-chemical properties and therapeutic use of kunzea essential oil are not defined in any pharmacopoeia monograph or standard.

History and Traditional Uses

History

Webb explains that early pioneers noted that native animals that slept under this species were often infected by ticks and other mites from the bush – hence the common name of 'tick bush'; however, he suggests that the native animals were, in fact, seeking relief from infestations by brushing up against, sleeping or lying under this species.[3]

K

Therapeutics

Pharmacology and clinical studies

Antifungal activity

A study confirmed the effectiveness of kunzea oil for the treatment of onychomycosis, a fungal infection of the nails caused by dermatophytes, yeasts and moulds. The study compared the efficacy of kunzea with the commercial preparation amorolfine. It was established that kunzea oil displayed similar efficacy to that of the commercial product.[6]

Anti-inflammatory activity

Topical applications of kunzea oil were found to provide anti-inflammatory effect on the skin to manage psoriasis.[7]

Antimicrobial activity

Kunzea oil appears to possess potentially useful in vitro antimicrobial activity; however, more work is required to establish the optimum antimicrobial potential of kunzea.[8]

Insecticidal activity

Kunzea oil was evaluated and compared with citronella oil for its insecticidal property. It was found to have comparable insecticidal properties to citronella. However, the authors concluded that essential oils are significantly less repellent than DEET and should not be used in regions prone to mosquito-borne disease.[9]

An in vitro study tested the insecticidal properties of kunzea by exposing head lice with a 5% or 100% solution of the essential oil. Head lice exposed to both the 5% and 100% solution resulted in 100% mortality within 120 minutes. The researchers concluded that kunzea oil shows great potential as an effective alternative to current active ingredients contained within commercial pediculicide formulations.[10]

Actions

Actions commonly cited in aromatherapy

Analgesic, antiarthritic, antifungal, anti-inflammatory, antimicrobial, antiseptic, insecticidal, relaxant[1,3,4]

Actions supported by clinical studies

Antifungal, antimicrobial, insecticidal

Comment

Anecdotal evidence suggests that kunzea oil has excellent analgesic properties. It would be great to see clinical trials to investigate the efficacy of kunzea's analgesic properties. Aromatherapists have speculated that the anti-inflammatory and analgesic properties may be due to some very interesting sesquiterpene compounds found in kunzea essential oil.

Aromatherapy Uses

Clinical aromatherapy

Analgesic

Kunzea oil has also been found to be beneficial to ease the pain from insect bites, minor burns, recurring shingles and headaches. It is also highly recommended for the treatment of arthritis, muscular pain and soft tissue injuries. Webb suggests a dab of the neat essential oil on insect bites for immediate pain relief.[4]

Integumentary system

Webb cites anecdotal feedback from users of kunzea oil who state it has been helpful for the treatment of eczema, dermatitis, rashes and leg infections.[3]

Nervous system

Kunzea oil is recommended for the temporary relief of nervous tension, stress and mild anxiety.[3]

Energetics, psyche and subtle uses

Energetics

The energetic qualities of kunzea oil are *cooling*. It is indicated for conditions of a *hot* and inflammatory nature.

Subtle

Zeck states that kunzea oil helps to alleviate deep emotional pain as a result of suppression. Kunzea oil assists in the release of physical and emotional pain, and in transforming the immediate shock of accidents.[11]

Dosage and Administration

Blending

Aromatherapy

For the relief of anxiety, stress and nervous tension, consider blending kunzea oil with essential oils such as bergamot, geranium, fragonia, lavender, lemon, lime, grapefruit, neroli, sweet orange or sandalwood.

For the relief of muscular aches and pains, consider blending kunzea oil with essential oils such as black pepper, cajeput, clove bud, ginger, spike lavender, lemongrass, pine, rosemary or peppermint.

To alleviate sensitive and inflamed skin, consider blending kunzea oil with essential oils such as

K

German chamomile, everlasting, lavender, neroli or sandalwood.

Perfumery

Kunzea oil is not commonly used in perfumery.

Mode of administration

Bath

Full body bath, foot bath

Topical

Compress, massage, ointment, skin care

Inhalation

Direct inhalation, diffuser, oil vaporiser

Safety Profile

General safety

Kunzea oil is non-toxic and a non-irritant; however, it may be a mild sensitiser. People with sensitive skin should do a patch test first.[1]

Contraindications

No contraindications known.

Regulatory guidelines

Kunzea oil is not defined in any regulatory guideline.

References

1. Guba R. *Kunzea essential oil.* Essential News, Vol. 19, 2006.
2. Australian Native Plants Society. *Kunzea ambigua*. Retrieved Sep 29, 2017, from http://anpsa.org.au/k-amb.html#
3. Webb M. *Bush sense.* Self-published, Australia, 2000.
4. Webb M. *Australian essential oil profile – kunzea.* Aromatherapy Today, 2002; 21:34-37.
5. Thomas J et al. *An examination of the essential oils of Tasmania Kunzea ambigua, other Kunzea spp. and commercial kunzea oil.* Journal of Essential Oil Research, 2010; 22(5): 381-385. doi: 10.1080/10412905.2010.9700351.
6. *RIRDC completed projects in 2008-2009 and research in progress as at June 2009 – essential oils and plant extracts*. Rural Industries Research and Development Corporation, Barton, 2009. RIRDC Publication No. 09/098.
7. Thomas J et al. *An evaluation of the clinical efficacy of kunzea oil formulations in the therapeutic management of psoriasis in adults.* Proceedings of the APSA Annual Conference, Hobart, 2009.
8. Thomas J. *Kunzea oil: investigation of composition, bioactivity and therapeutic potential*. University of Tasmania, 2012.
9. Thomas J et al. *Evaluation of repellent properties of volatile extracts from Australian native plant Kunzea ambigua against Aedes aegypti (Diptera: Culcidae).* Journal of Medical Entomology, 2009; 46(6): 1387-1391. doi: 10.16031033.046.0619.
10. Williams CR et al. *Can kunzea oil (Kunzea ambigua) control head lice (Pediculus humanus capitis)?* Parasitology Open, 2016; 2(3): 1-5. doi: 10.1017/pao.2015.2.
11. Zeck R. *The blossoming heart – aromatherapy for healing and transformation*. Aroma Tours, East Ivanhoe, 2004.

L

Lavender

Identification

Botanical name

Lavandula angustifolia Mill.

Synonyms

True lavender, common lavender, *Lavandula officinalis* Chaix, *Lavandula vera* DC

Family

Lamiaceae (Labiatae)

Botany and origins

Lavender is an aromatic evergreen sub-shrub with linear or lance-shaped leaves. It grows up to 0.9 m high and is a native of the Mediterranean region.

The *Lavandula* genus has approximately 30 species that grow around the world. The four main species of lavender are:[1]

- *Lavandula angustifolia* – true lavender
- *Lavandula latifolia* – spike lavender
- *Lavandula* x *intermedia* – lavandin
- *Lavandula stoechas* – maritime lavender.

Most lavender grown for essential oil production comes from *L. angustifolia* P. Miller, *L. officinalis* Chaix or *L. vera* de Candolle, which is referred to as true lavender.[1]

Approximately half of the true lavender produced now comes from cultivated clones such as 'Maillette'. This gives a 40 to 50% higher yield than population lavender (grown from seed).

Harris states that population lavender has a superior fragrance and commands a higher price than cloned lavender and lavender from other countries. Lavandulol and its ester lavandulyl acetate are said to contribute to the aroma of this oil.[1]

Clonal crops are made via cuttings. Healthy plants are cut down near ground level and cultivated in a nursery before planting in spring. Price & Price explain the population plants produce a lavender oil which is much richer in chemical constituents; however, the cloned plants produce an oil of a much more consistent quality from year to year.[2]

The main producers of true lavender are Bulgaria and France. Smaller producers include Australia, Argentina, England, Hungary, Japan, Morocco, Italy, Algeria, India and Russia.[3]

Arctander states lavender grown and distilled at a higher altitude (from 600 to 1500 m) has a reputation of being the best quality lavender. This is because distilleries located at higher altitudes distil the oil at 92-93°C instead of 100°C. This produces an oil with a higher ester content. Even at this small decrease of temperature, hydrolysis of the natural linalyl esters takes place at a much slower rate. A rapid distillation at a slightly reduced pressure will also produce an oil with a higher linalyl ester content.[3]

L

Grieve discusses in great detail the ideal method of cultivating lavender and the best time to harvest the plant. She recommends the blooms be fully developed, as this will produce an essential oil with a high ester content. She suggests very cold weather prevents the esters from developing, and the most refined lavender oil is distilled from the flowers that have been stripped from the stalk. This, however, leads to a very expensive lavender oil.[4]

Lavandin is a hybrid of true lavender and spike lavender. The lavandin plant is larger and much more robust than true lavender. It is ideally suited to large-scale cultivation and harvesting methods. It is very popular with the fragrance industry as it yields twice the amount of oil as true lavender, and it is commonly used in soaps, detergents and cosmetics.[1]

Most commonly available and produced lavender oils are from the clonal varieties such as the lavender 'Maillette' or lavender 'Matheronne' oil.[5]

The main clones of lavandin in France are:

- abrial
- super
- sumian
- grosso.[5]

Lavender has been grown in Australia since 1921 when CK Denny established a lavender plantation in northern Tasmania from French seed stock. Over the years, Bridestowe Lavender Farm has undertaken considerable cultivar selection of *Lavandula angustifolia* to produce a consistently high-quality lavender oil of international repute. Bridestowe estate produces 1-1.5 tonnes of oil annually, much of which is exported.[6]

Method of extraction

All lavender oils are steam-distilled from the freshly cut flowering tops and stalks of the lavender plant.

Characteristics

True lavender oil is a colourless or pale-yellow liquid with a sweet, floral, herbaceous, refreshing aroma and a pleasant balsamic-woody undertone.[3]

Lavandin oil is a pale yellow to almost colourless liquid with a strong herbaceous, very fresh camphoraceous top note and a woody-herbaceous middle note.[3]

Lavender 'Maillette' oil has a fresh, floral, herbaceous and sweet aroma. It may be the most familiar lavender scent when we inhale the different lavenders. It will never surprise you with any unusual notes as it is from a clonal variety designed to give us a consistently rich lavender aroma, batch after batch.

Tasmanian lavender oil has a unique aroma profile compared to the French lavenders. There is nothing like it. It has a light, fresh, green top note with a herbaceous, floral body note and a pleasant woody base note.

Chemical composition

The composition of lavender oil varies significantly from species to species and from one country to another.

The major components of lavender oil are linalyl acetate, linalool, *cis*-ocimene and lavandulyl acetate. Those of spike lavender are linalool, 1,8-cineole and camphor, and of lavandin are linalool, linalyl acetate, camphor, 1,8-cineole and borneol.[7]

There are more than 100 constituents in lavender oil, more than 80 in lavandin and approximately 60 in spike lavender. Lavender oil is the most variable in qualitative composition.[7]

The major constituents of lavender, lavandin and spike lavender was reported as follows:[7]

Constituent	Lavender oil	Lavandin oil	Spike lavender oil
linalyl acetate	12-54%	19-26%	0-1.5%
linalool	10-50%	20-23%	26-44%
cis- and/or *trans*-ocimene	1.0-17%	1.0-3.0%	0-0.3%

Constituent (continued)	Lavender oil	Lavandin oil	Spike lavender oil
lavandulol	0.1-14%	0.5-0.8%	0.2-1.5%
1,8-cineole	2.1-3.0%	10%	25-36%
camphor	0-0.2%	12%	5.3-14.3%
α- and β-pinene	0.02-0.3%	0.6-0.9%	1.6-3.6%
borneol	1.0-4.0%	2.9-3.7%	0.8-4.9%
caryophyllene and/or its oxide	3.0-8.0%	2.7-6.0%	0.1-0.3%
myrcene	0.4-1.3%	1.2-1.5%	0.2-0.4%
farnesene	Trace	1.1%	0.2-0.3%
germacrene D	0.2-0.9%	1.0-1.2%	-
camphene	0.1-0.2%	0.3-0.6%	0.2-1.8%
limonene	0.2-0.4%	0.9-1.5%	1.0-2.2%

The ISO standards for French lavender, lavandin abrialis and lavandin grosso are as follows:[8]

Constituent	L. angustifolia	Lavandin abrialis	Lavandin grosso
	ISO 3515	ISO 3054	ISO 8902
octan-3-one	Tr-2.0%	-	-
d-limonene	0-0.5%	-	-
trans-β-ocimene	2.0-6.0%	-	-
cis-β-ocimene	4-10%	1.5-3.5%	-
1,8-cineole	0-1.5%	6-11%	4.0-7.0%
linalool	25-38%	28-38%	25-35%
camphor	0.0-0.5%	7-11%	6-8%
lavandulol	>0.3%	0.5-1.5%	0.3-0.5%
lavandulyl acetate	2.0%	1.0-2.0%	1.5-3.0%
terpinen-4-ol	2.0-6.0%	0.0-1.0%	2.0-4.0%
α-terpineol	0-1.0%	0-1.0%	-
borneol	-	1.5-3.5%	1.5-3.0%
linalyl acetate	25-45%	Tr-1.6%	1.5-3.0%

Schnaubelt states the following are typical markers for authentic population lavender:[9]

- The sum of linalool and linalyl acetate is never more than 80% in authentic fine lavender.
- The sum of *cis*- and *trans*- ocimenes should be at least 9%.
- Lavandulyl acetate is a compound that is specifically telling because it cannot be purchased inexpensively on the market, but is made by nature in lavender essential oil. Its concentration should be at least 4.5% in fine lavender.
- The concentration of camphor should be below 0.5%.

Comparative chemical composition of various *L. angustifolia* essential oils was reported as follows:[10]

Constituent	Lavender 'Maillette'	Population lavender	Bulgarian lavender	Tasmanian lavender
octan-3-one	-	-	0.24%	3.10%
3-octanonal	-	-	-	0.68%
d-limonene	0.11%	0.50%	1.33%	0.28%
trans-β-ocimene	1.12%	5.12%	0.39%	0.82%
cis-β-ocimene	-	3.67%	0.29%	4.10%
1,8-cineole	-	0.92%	3.61%	0.05%
trans-linalool oxide	-	0.25%	-	0.45%
terpinolene	-	-	-	0.36%
linalool	35.70%	29.19%	40.01%	36.66%
camphor	0.48%	0.41%	3.10%	0.17%
lavandulol	-	1.04%	0.75%	0.67%
terpinen-4-ol	0.07%	2.48%	0.12%	2.06%
α-terpineol	0.44%	0.96%	0.15%	0.56%
linalyl acetate	43.39%	35.62%	39.44%	34.00%
lavandulyl acetate	-	3.75%	0.09%	1.89%
β-caryophyllene	-	4.78%	-	2.38%
α-santalene	-	-	-	1.03%
(*E*)- β-farnesene	-	1.95%	-	0.50%

Adulteration

Lavender is one of the most commonly adulterated essential oils. Adulteration of true lavender is achieved by:

- addition of lavandin oil
- substitution by lavandin oil
- addition of synthetic linalool and linalyl acetate
- addition of linalool and linalyl acetate from other natural sources.[1]

Schnaubelt states that French export data indicates that approximately 250 tonnes of so-called fine lavender oil is exported annually. However, the statistics of the lavender association growers indicates that only 20 tonnes are distilled.[9]

Figure that out!

Unfortunately, Schnaubelt states that we cannot even trust the gas chromatograms to confirm the purity, as lavender oil is often artfully reconstructed by mixing the main components of linalool and linalyl acetate with less expensive lavandin oils to be then sold off as expensive lavender oil.[9]

Authentic and genuine lavender oils should carry certification from the official regulatory authorities called AOC, *Appellation d'Origine Controllée*. This authenticates the origin of the lavender plants in the same way that cheeses, wines and other agricultural products are regulated.[5]

Prior to World War I, lavender oil was produced almost exclusively from wild plants growing in the French and Italian Alps. Today most of the large cultivations of lavender in the Provence region are different lavandin hybrids – *grosso, super, sumian* and *abrialis*.[9]

In the 1930s, farmers found that they could cross fine *L. angustifolia* with the sturdier *L. latifolia* to produce hybrids which produced substantially more oil. Schnaubelt points out that this oil is not too bad if it is organic, but it does reflect the human intention for higher yields and a more robust fragrance.[9]

Pharmacopoeias and standards

The purity, composition and physico-chemical properties of true lavender are defined in several standards and monographs. The following pharmacopoeias and composition standards are available:

- ISO 3515:2002 Oil of Lavender (*Lavandula angustifolia* Mill.)
- ISO 8902:2009 Oil of Lavandin Grosso (*Lavandula angustifolia* Mill. X *Lavandula latifolia* Medik.), French Type
- ISO 3054:2017 Oil of Lavandin Abrial (*Lavandula angustifolia* Mill. X *Lavandula latifolia* Medik.), French Type
- European Pharmacopoeia
- German Commission E
- WHO Monographs on Selected Medicinal Plants – Vol. 3
- Assessment report on *Lavandula angustifolia Miller, aetheroleum* and *Lavandula angustifolia* Miller, flos. European Medicines Agency.

L

History and Traditional Uses

History

Lavandula comes from *lavare*, meaning 'to wash' in Latin. Lavender essential oil has been widely used as a toilet water and is one of the most common ingredients in potpourri and sachets.[4]

Castle & Lis-Balchin state that it is impossible to identify whether many of the ancient texts were referring to *L. vera* or *L. spica*. Lavender was first mentioned for its healing qualities by Dioscorides (40-90 AD). He attributed lavender with laxative and invigorating properties and advised using it as a tea. Galen also included lavender oil as an antidote for poisons and bites, while Pliny suggested that it was best for making perfumes. Pliny also advocated lavender for bereavement as well as promoting menstruation.[11]

Hildegard of Bingen (1098-1179) was the first person in the Middle Ages to clearly distinguish between *L. vera* and *L. spica*. She described lavender as hot and dry, having very little moisture and recommended it as a treatment for lice. She also recommended decoction of lavender for pulmonary congestion, and to promote rest and sleep she suggested a bath steeped in lavender.[11]

Culpeper recommended a decoction of lavender flowers to help prevent falling sickness (epilepsy), and giddiness or turning of the brain. He also explained that it strengthened the stomach and freed the liver and spleen from obstructions.[11]

Traditional medicine

Grieve describes lavender as a restorative tonic against fainting, palpitations of a nervous nature, giddiness, spasms and colic. She recommends a few drops of lavender oil in a hot foot bath to relieve fatigue, and outwardly applied, she recommends it for the relief of toothache, neuralgia, sprains and rheumatism. She also recommended anointing lavender to the temples and forehead for headaches.[4]

Lavender's antiseptic properties were well known by the French Academy of Medicine, where it was used in the swabbing of wounds, and the treatment of sores, varicose ulcers, burns and scalds. It was René-Maurice Gattefossé who observed the healing effects of lavender oil when he burned his hand in a laboratory accident. Lavender is still regularly associated with and used for the treatment of burns and for healing the skin.[4]

Lavender is reportedly used as an antispasmodic, carminative, stimulant, diuretic, sedative, tonic and stomachic. It is used for conditions such as spasms, colic, giddiness, nervous headache, migraine, toothache, sprains, neuralgia, rheumatism, acne, pimples, sores, nausea and vomiting.[12]

Herbal

The German Commission E recommends lavender flowers internally for mood disturbances such as restlessness or insomnia, functional abdominal complaints and for balneotherapy to treat functional circulatory disorders.[13]

Braun & Cohen cite studies in which methanolic and aqueous extracts of *Lavandula officinalis* demonstrated potent sedative and hypnotic activities in vivo. It was stated that this provided an explanation for its therapeutic use in the treatment of anxiety and insomnia.[14]

Food, perfumery and flavouring

Lavender oil is extensively used as a fragrance component in cosmetics, soaps, detergents and perfumes.[12]

Therapeutics

Pharmacology and clinical studies

Many pharmacological studies involving lavender oil have been published. A systemic review of these studies will not be attempted. Rather I have chosen a selection of studies with emphasis on those studies that support the traditional uses. Many of the pharmacological studies involving lavender oils have focused on the linalool and linalyl acetate components.

Analgesic activity

A randomised controlled study using 66 subjects examined the effects of inhalation of lavender oil or linalyl acetate on pain relief and lower urinary tract symptoms (LUTS), following the removal of indwelling urinary catheters from patients after colorectal cancer. Patients inhaled 1% lavender, 1% linalyl acetate or a control for 20 minutes. The blood pressure, heart rate, LUTS and visual analogue scales of pain magnitude and quality of life regarding urinary symptoms were measured before and after inhalation. There was a significant difference in pain magnitude and urinary residual sense of indwelling catheters observed among the three groups, with the inhalation of linalyl acetate being significantly more effective than inhalation of lavender or control.[15]

In a triple-blind, randomised, placebo-controlled trial, 60 pregnant women admitted to a general hospital for cesarean section were divided randomly into two groups. After the cesarean, the lavender group inhaled 3 drops of 10% lavender oil and the placebo group inhaled 3 drops of placebo after the start of the postoperative pain, 4, 8 and 12 hours later, for 5 minutes. Patient's pain was measured by the visual analogue scale (VAS) score before and after each intervention. Patients in the lavender group had less postoperative pain than the placebo group. The decreased heart rate and the patient's level of satisfaction with analgesia were significantly higher in the lavender group (P=0.001). In the placebo group, the use of diclofenac for complete analgesia was also significantly higher than the lavender group (P=0.008).[16]

After using the drug and comparing it with before, there was more decrease in the VAS score in the lavender group than the placebo group; these values were significant four, eight and 12 hours after the first intervention. In the lavender group the level of satisfaction with the drug was 90%, while in the placebo group, a 50% satisfaction was reported. In the lavender group, 43.3% used diclofenac for completing analgesia, whereas 76.7% of the placebo group used diclofenac suppositories.[16]

A randomised controlled trial was conducted with 80 patients in the cardiac surgery intensive care unit who had a chest tube for at least 24 hours after coronary artery bypass grafting. Patients were randomised to receive cold application, inhalation with lavender, cold application with lavender, or none of the interventions. Patients in all the treatment groups had significantly lower pain intensity and anxiety compared with the control group, 5, 10 and 15 minutes after the chest tube removal procedure.

It was concluded that aromatherapy with lavender together with the cold application was an effective treatment for reducing pain and anxiety associated with post-coronary artery bypass grafting chest tube removal.[17]

Another randomised clinical trial conducted on 56 participants examined the effect of lavender oil on the early hours of postpartum period on maternal pains, fatigue and mood. 29 were in the aromatherapy group who received lavender and 27 in the control group. The findings showed that inhalation of lavender in the early hours of postpartum can reduce the mother's pain and fatigue and improve their mood. It was also noted that the study had some limitations, such as the sample size being small, the study being done for only a short period (24 hours after delivery) and the effect of the intervention not being assessed for the subsequent days or weeks.[18]

Anti-inflammatory activity

At 0.1%, lavender oil was found to suppress TNF-α-induced neutrophil adherence.[14] One clinical trial examined the anti-inflammatory properties of lavender oil on experimentally induced bronchial asthma in mice. An increase in airway resistance was inhibited in the group using lavender compared to the control group. The lavender group also has less mucin hyperplasia than the control group; furthermore, the lavender group showed lower interleukin and cytokine levels in the lung tissues. The authors concluded that lavender may be useful as an alternative medicine for bronchial asthma.[19]

Antimicrobial activity

Lis-Balchin states lavender oil's antimicrobial activity is moderate in contrast to the considerable antimicrobial status credited to lavender by aromatherapists. She explains that this is not surprising considering there is so much chemical variability in the different lavender oils.[20]

In vitro, lavender oil reversed bacterial resistance to piperacillin in multidrug-resistant *Escherichia coli*. The authors suggest this was via alterations of outer membrane permeability and bacterial quorum sensing inhibition.[21]

Other studies have confirmed that when lavender was blended with other essential oils, the antimicrobial activity was enhanced. The authors concluded that *L. angustifolia* in combination with *Citrus sinensis* (sweet orange) demonstrated the best antimicrobial effects.[22]

Studies have confirmed that lavender oil has variable antifungal activity. An in vitro study compared the antifungal activity of lavender oil and clotrimazole (a conventional chemical drug used to treat vaginal candidiasis) on isolated *Candida albicans* from vaginal candidiasis. The study found that after 48 hours there was no difference in the lavender group and clotrimazole.[23]

Antispasmodic activity

Linalool, one of lavender oils major components, demonstrated antispasmodic activity when tested on an in vitro preparation of guinea-pig ileum smooth muscle.[20]

Anxiolytic activity

Lavender's anxiolytic effects have been well documented. A clinical trial using aromatherapy massage with lavender and geranium found aromatherapy effective for reducing anxiety and decreasing heart and respiratory rates among patients who had been hospitalised with personality disorders.[24]

An anxiolytic effect was observed when lavender and sweet orange essential oils were administered via a vaporiser to mice without affecting locomotor activity. It was suggested that the effect was not mediated through the GABA-A/benzodiazepine complex.[14]

L

Oral preparations of lavender oil were also effective as adjuvant therapy for moderate to severe depression and for generalised anxiety disorder. The authors of the clinical trial found that Silexan (a new oral lavender oil capsule preparation that has been standardised for 20-45% linalool and 25-46% linalyl acetate) was just as effective as lorazepam for adults with generalised anxiety disorder, and has no potential for drug abuse.[25] It was noted that no sedation was reported; however, after six weeks there was significant reduction in depression (57.4% of sample), sleep disorders (51.1%), restlessness (61.7%) and anxiety (44.7%).[26]

The oral ingestion of lavender (80 mg as Silexan) results in an increase in serum linalool, with a half-life of four hours following acute administration and nine hours following repeated daily oral ingestion.[27]

Oral lavender preparations (80 mg/day) showed a significant beneficial influence on the quality and duration of sleep, and improved general mental and physical health without causing any undesirable side effects in 221 patients suffering from anxiety disorders.[28]

One study investigated the molecular mechanism of action of lavender oil's anxiolytic activity. The researchers found that lavender oil bears some similarities with the established anxiolytic pregabalin. Lavender oil inhibits voltage dependent calcium channels in synaptosomes, primary hippocampal neurons and stably overexpressing cell lines in the same range as pregabalin. The researchers concluded that they have provided a pharmacological and molecular rationale for the clinical use of oral application of lavender oil in patients suffering from anxiety.[29]

To examine the effect of Silexan (a soft gel capsule with 80 mg of standardised lavender oil) on serotonin-1A receptor binding, 17 healthy men undertook two positron emission tomography measurements following the daily intake of 160 mg Silexan or placebo for a minimum of 8 weeks in a randomised, double-blind, crossover designed study.[30]

The positron emission tomography found that serotonin-1A receptor binding potential was shown to be significantly reduced following the intake of Silexan compared with a placebo. It was proposed that the anxiolytic effects of Silexan involves the serotonin-1A receptor.[30]

The anxiolytic and antidepressant activity attributed to lavender may be due to an antagonism on the NMDA-receptor and inhibition of serotonin transporter (SERT). Lavender essential oil exerted affinity for the glutamate NMDA-receptor in a dose-dependent manner. In addition, lavender and linalool were able to bind the SERT, whereas it did not show affinity for GABA-A/benzodiazepine receptor.[31]

Cardiovascular activity

Mixed clinical results exist for lavender's traditionally reported role as a hypotensive. One publication reported that the aroma of lavender decreased respiration, heart rate and blood pressure. Another confirmed the reduction in breathing rate and subjective calmness, while both heart rate and diastolic blood pressure increased. It is likely that these differences are reflective of a hedonic effect (whether the scent is 'liked' or 'not liked' by the person).[27]

Dementia

The role of lavender oil for the management of Alzheimer's disease (AD) has been extensively researched. One such study used a range of psychometric tools to measure the cognitive function and concentration of AD patients exposed to a blend of lemon and rosemary in the morning, and lavender and orange in the evening. Sweet orange activates the parasympathetic nervous system, while rosemary and lemon are known to relieve depression and improve concentration. The study concluded that aromatherapy can improve cognitive function in AD patients.[32]

Another study found that dermally applied lavender oil did not improve symptoms in patients with dementia[33], while another study found that 60% of patients with severe dementia had reduced agitated behaviour with vaporised lavender.[34]

Lavender combined with sweet marjoram, patchouli and vetiver essential oils in a cream base and applied by massage 5 times per day for 4 weeks to 56 residents with moderate to severe dementia in an aged care facility demonstrated a significant but small improvement in mini-mental tests, increased alertness and less resistance, compared to the use of a massage cream without essential oils.[35]

On the other hand, another study examined whether the scent of lavender oil alone was enough to decrease the frequency of agitated behaviour in patients with dementia. There is significant evidence that people with dementia have impaired olfactory ability. The results of this study found that the use of aromatherapy by inhalation did not decrease agitation in patients with severe dementia. It has suggested that the cutaneous application of the essential oil may be necessary to achieve the effects reported in previous controlled studies.[36]

This was confirmed by another single-blind, randomised, controlled trial examining the role of aromatherapy (3% lavender oil spray) with and without hand massage on 67 people with dementia who had a history of disruptive behaviour. The study found that, despite a downward trend in behaviours displayed, none of the aromatherapy interventions significantly reduced the disruptive behaviour.[37]

Neurodegenerative Alzheimer's disease is associated with profound deficits in synaptic transmission and synaptic plasticity. In one study, the effect of aqueous extracts of lavender on the induction of long-term potentiation (LTP) in the hippocampus was evaluated. Lavender effectively restored LTP in the Alzheimer's group. It was concluded that the positive effect of the lavender extract on the plasticity of synaptic transmission supports its behavioural effects on the improvement of impaired spatial memory in mice with Alzheimer's disease.[38]

A study in which lavender oil was diffused twice daily in an adult day care centre confirmed that the oil reduced the frequency of agitation in elderly patients with dementia in the 70-85 age group; however, it did not show any statistical difference in the frequency of other behaviours such as restlessness, wandering, anger and anxiety.[39]

Headaches

A placebo-controlled clinical study suggests that the inhalation of lavender oil may be an effective and safe treatment in the acute management of migraine headaches.[40]

Menstrual pain and PMS

A study found that lavender oil used in a massage oil significantly reduced pain associated with menstruation to a greater degree than the placebo. There was a 38% reduction in pain with lavender oil massage compared to only 9.8% reduction in pain with the placebo group.[41]

A study examined the effects of aromatherapy massage with lavender on the severity of dysmenorrhoea in 80 nursing and midwife students in Iran. A significant decrease in visual analogue scale after the lavender massage was reported in comparison to the placebo massage. There was a significant statistical difference on the effect of the lavender massage than that of the massage without lavender oil.[42]

The results of a randomised crossover study involving 17 women in their 20s confirmed that short-term inhalation of lavender oil could be used to alleviate premenstrual emotional symptoms and could, at least in part, contribute to the improvement of parasympathetic nervous system activity.[43]

Sedative activity

The sedative activity of lavender oil and its main constituents, linalool and linalyl acetate, has a dose-dependent effect in mice and has been shown to reverse caffeine-induced hyperactivity. Another study confirmed that lavender oil had a modulating effect on adrenocorticotrophic hormone, catecholamine and gonadotrophic levels in mice.[14]

In human trials, inhalation of lavender oil has induced states of relaxation and sedation, altered EEG responses, enhanced sleep and improved alertness on waking. Lavender has also significantly decreased heart rate and increased high frequency spectral components to produce calm and vigorous mood states in healthy volunteers.[14]

Many animal and human studies confirm that lavender oil has anxiolytic, mood-stabilising, sedative and neuroprotective activities.[44]

Sleep-enhancing activity

Lavender oil is best known for its sleep-enhancing

properties and results from many clinical trials suggest this.[45]

A systematic search to examine the evidence on lavender oil to improve sleep was conducted, and the major databases including AMED, BNI, Cochrane CENTRAL, EMBASE, MEDLINE, PsycINFO and PubMed were systematically reviewed up to April 2012. Eight eligible studies were found of which 4 were randomised controlled studies. Most of the studies had small samples and methodological limitations. It was suggested that early results appear promising, but that they should be viewed with caution. It was suggested that more rigorous trials are needed to investigate the true effect of lavender oil inhalation on sleep.[45]

While lavender oil has long been used for the treatment of insomnia and there have been quite a few published studies on aromatherapy and insomnia, Buckle warns us not to use too much lavender in a diffuser as it could exacerbate a person's insomnia. She also suggests that, in some elderly people, the scent of lavender could be disliked due to negative associations.[46]

A study examined the effects of 12 weeks of aromatherapy on self-reported sleep and heart rate variability (HRV) in midlife women with insomnia. 67 women aged 45-55 were recruited for the study. The aromatherapy group received lavender inhalation for 20 minutes each time, twice a week for 12 weeks. The control group received health education for sleep hygiene with no intervention. The study demonstrated that lavender inhalation had a persistent short-term effect on HRV with an increase in parasympathetic modulation. The participants receiving the aromatherapy also experienced a significant improvement in sleep quality after the intervention. It was also noted that the lavender group did not confer any long-term benefit on HRV.[47]

Another study investigated the effects of lavender oil on sleep and assessed the responses to gender difference. 31 young healthy sleepers (16 men and 15 women, aged 18 to 30 years) completed three consecutive overnight sessions in a sleep laboratory: one adaptation, one stimulus and one control night. Subjects received an intermittent presentation of lavender or a control (distilled water) stimulus between 23:10 and 23:40 h. Lavender increased the percentage of deep or slow wave sleep in men and women. All subjects reported a higher vigour the morning after lavender exposure, supporting the restorative slow-wave sleep. Lavender also increased stage 2 (light) sleep, and decreased rapid eye movement (REM) sleep and the amount of time to reach wake after first falling asleep (wake after sleep onset latency) in women, with the opposite effects in men. It was concluded that lavender serves as a mild sedative and has practical application for promoting sleep in young men and women.[48]

A randomised controlled trial using 79 college students with self-reported sleep issues compared the effectiveness of lavender and sleep hygiene on sleep quality. Both the lavender and the sleep hygiene group demonstrated better sleep quality after two weeks. The lavender group also reported feeling refreshed upon waking. The sleep quality did not differ between the two groups.[49]

Wound-healing activity

In wound-healing models, lavender oil accelerates re-epithelialisation and wound closure via enhanced epidermal growth factor secretion.[50]

A study demonstrated that topical application of lavender oil promoted collagen synthesis and differentiation of fibroblasts, accompanied by uptake regulation of transforming growth factor-β (TGF-β). The results of the study suggest that lavender has the potential to promote wound healing in the early phase by acceleration of formation of granulation tissue, tissue remodelling by collagen replacement and wound contraction through up-regulation of TGF-β.[51]

Guba used a blend of essential oils including 4% lavender oil on 18 patients with skin ulcers or wounds. In most cases where the formulation was applied daily, healing took 5 days to 12 weeks. There were no adverse reactions reported.[52]

Other activities

An in vitro study provided some evidence that lavender oil and linalool had an antiproliferative effect on human prostate cancer. The antitumour activity was associated with cell proliferation inhibition and apoptosis induction in xenograft tumours.[53]

One study confirmed that lavender oil had cardioprotective effect through inhibiting oxidative stress and the inflammatory pathway in the rat model with infarct-like myocardial injury. It was suggested that lavender oil may be helpful in prevention or attenuation of heart injury in patients with high risk of myocardial infarction or ischemic heart disease.[54]

Actions

Actions commonly cited in aromatherapy

Analgesic, anticonvulsive, antidepressant, anti-inflammatory, antirheumatic, antiseptic, antispasmodic, antiviral, bactericide, carminative, cholagogue, cicatrisant, cordial, cytophylactic, decongestant, deodorant, emmenagogue, fungicide, hypotensive, nervine, restorative, sedative, sudorific, vulnerary[20,55,56,57]

Actions supported by clinical studies

Analgesic, anticonvulsive, antidepressant, anti-inflammatory, antirheumatic, antiseptic, antispasmodic, bactericide, carminative, cholagogue, cicatrisant, cytophylactic, emmenagogue, fungicide, hypotensive, nervine, restorative, sedative, sudorific, vulnerary

Comment

A number of controlled trials and observational studies confirm that inhalation of lavender oil has a relaxing effect and is able to reduce anxiety and improve mood, concentration and sleep.

Schnaubelt explains that the complex chemistry of an essential oil can help explain the multitude of properties attributed to the oil. Linalool, the main component of lavender, simultaneously inhibits HMG CoA reductase, reduces spasms, is anticonvulsant and modifies autonomic nervous system activity to name a few. These effects of linalool are then layered with at least an equal number of physiological effects of linalyl acetate, another main component. In addition to the web of physiological activities present in linalool and linalyl acetate alone, there are the effects of various monoterpene hydrocarbons. Myrcene, for example, acts as a free radical scavenger and induces liver detoxification enzymes.[9]

L. angustifolia oil contains mainly alcohols and esters. These components contribute to lavender's relaxing properties. Price & Price say it is also recommended for respiratory ailments such as asthma, spasmodic coughing, influenza, and bronchitis.[2] I suggest that lavandin or spike lavender with a higher 1,8-cineole and camphor content would be more suitable for respiratory ailments.

L. latifolia oil contains fewer esters and has a slightly lower alcohol content. It contains up to 30% of the oxide 1,8-cineole and about 15% of the ketone camphor. This makes it a very effective expectorant, especially useful for chest and throat infections. Topically it is excellent for headaches, neuralgia, and muscular aches and pains.[2]

Holmes suggests that lavandin oil is less bioactive than lavender oil; however, he states that it is especially useful for treating mental-emotional conditions when used in diffusers and massage. He also states that it may be appropriate in cases where a milder treatment is required – especially for children and the elderly.[57]

Buckle compared the properties of true lavender and lavandin. She did this because at the time (1993), and unfortunately still to this day, lavandin had been considered as having little therapeutic value. She made a 2% solution of *L. angustifolia* and *L. x intermedia*, which were simply labelled lavender A and lavender B. The therapists and patients were blind to which lavender they were testing. Interestingly, lavandin was twice as effective as true lavender in eliciting a positive relaxation response. Unfortunately, no reason for this was given.[46]

Aromatherapy Uses

Clinical aromatherapy

Cardiovascular system

Lavender oil is often recommended for lowering blood pressure and palpitations.[57]

Integumentary system

Lavender oil is commonly associated with burns and healing of the skin. It has antiseptic, analgesic and cytophylactic properties that will ease the pain of a burn, prevent infection and promote rapid healing.

Lavender oil is beneficial for conditions involving inflammation such as acne, dermatitis, eczema, psoriasis, boils and wounds.[55,56,58,59]

Musculoskeletal system

Lavender oil is very beneficial for the relief of muscular aches and pain, arthritis, rheumatism and lumbago.[55,57,58] I would recommend the 1,8-cineole and camphor-rich lavender oils such as spike lavender and lavandin.

Nervous system

Lavender oil has a harmonising effect on the nervous system. Holmes explains this in terms of lavender's ability to deal with stress. Stress that becomes counterproductive on the physiological level involves either the sympathetic or parasympathetic nervous system. Sympathetic hyperfunctioning is triggered by physical stress, whereas parasympathetic hyperfunctioning is triggered more by emotional stress. Both types of stress reactions will produce symptoms such as spasms, cramps, pains, nervous tension, irritability and mental distraction.[59]

Holmes states that lavender oil can inhibit both sympathetic or parasympathetic nervous system functions, therefore lavender can assist our responses to unproductive stress of any kind. Likewise, lavender will tend not to interfere with productive stress – a normal part of life.[59]

Lavender oil can exert a sedative or a stimulant action, depending on one's actual needs. It will act as a sedative in conditions of mental and emotional agitation and unrest, calming the mind, comforting feelings and alleviating fears, while it is uplifting and revives the spirits for someone feeling emotionally depleted and depressed.[59]

Lavender oil is regarded as the first choice in the treatment of insomnia, especially when the insomnia is due to mental stress and anxiety.[57,58] It is recommended for the treatment of migraines and headaches.[55,56]

Psychological

Fischer-Rizzi states that the scent of lavender oil instantly melts away any nagging thoughts and stresses that make you feel anxious and tense. She perfectly describes lavender's effect on our psyche:

> *The fragrance of lavender is like fresh, tangy mountain air that's happy and free. Its fragrance imparts a feeling of inner freedom that allows one to let go of compulsions and anger. Lavender helps one undo negative self-talk; thinking becomes clearer, and balanced decisions may be made. The essential oil helps reduce mental ramblings that keep people from falling asleep.*[60]

Holmes describes the unique ability of lavender to calm, balance and uplift:

> *Lavender is generally indicated for all types of distressed and stuck emotions. Individuals who get repeatedly stuck in unproductive emotional postures, who are unable to put the brakes on their volatile tempers, will stand to benefit the most from this potentially transformative oil. The net result of lavender's ability to generate emotional renewal is a refreshed, equanimous state where everything is poise and composure.*[57]

Holmes states that lavender promotes emotional stability and renewal, and recommends it for emotional confusion, irritability, anger, moodiness, mood swings and depression.[57] Typically oils rich in monoterpene alcohols and esters have relaxing and uplifting qualities, therefore I would recommend using any of the *L. angustifolia* oils.

Reproductive system

Lavender oil is valuable for relieving PMS and menstrual pain. Davis recommends gently massaging a massage oil with lavender into the lower abdomen or using it in a hot compress.[58]

A clinical trial identified lavender as the most popular essential oil during childbirth and it was found to reduce maternal anxiety, to relieve pain and to lighten the mood.[61]

Holmes refers to lavender oil as a uterine relaxant and recommends it for spasmodic dysmenorrhoea and menstrual cramping.[57]

Typically oils rich in esters have antispasmodic properties; therefore, I would recommend lavender oils rich in linalyl acetate such as lavender 'Maillette' oil or the population lavender oils.

Respiratory system

Lavender oil is recommended for the treatment of colds and flu, bronchitis, throat infections and catarrhal conditions.[55,56,60]

Mailhebiau states that lavender oil is particularly beneficial for asthma of a nervous origin or a result of uncontrolled anxiety. He explains that it will relax the person and enable them to breathe more easily.[62]

Typically oils rich in 1,8-cineole and camphor have expectorant and mucolytic properties; therefore, I would recommend a 1,8-cineole-rich lavender such as spike lavender or some of the lavandins.

Skin care

The antiseptic, anti-inflammatory and cicatrisant properties of lavender oil make it beneficial in many skin care preparations. It can be used for all skin types. It can be used as an insect repellent and may also be used to treat insect bites – preventing the itching and scratching.[56,58]

Energetics, psyche and subtle uses

Energetics

According to the principles of TCM, lavender oil is *cooling*. Holmes states that lavender nourishes the *Yin*, activates the *Qi*, clears *heat* and calms the *Shen*. The *Shen* can be thought of as our spirit. When the *Shen* is agitated we have mental restlessness, anxiety, worry, depression and palpitations. When our *Yin* is *deficient* we suffer from fatigue, insomnia, hot spells, night sweats and headaches.[57]

Lavender also calms excessive Wood and Fire and has strong affinity with the Water Element. The Water Element nourishes the *Yin* and has a calming quality that we find in lavender oil.[57]

Mojay states that the psychological uses of lavender come from its ability to calm and stabilise the *Qi* of the *Heart*. According to TCM, the *Heart* is responsible for maintaining our overall mental-emotional equilibrium.[63]

Personality

Worwood describes lavender as the 'mother' or 'grandmother' of essential oils. She states that the lavender personality is eclectic and formidable, yet gentle and kind. She is able to care for a multitude of physical and psychological problems and, like a mother, can accomplish several jobs at the same time.[64]

Worwood states that lavender is the perfect balance between masculine and feminine traits within us all. She explains that the lavender personality seems to have an incredible amount of energy to call upon:

Embracing lavender is direct, pure of thought, brave and humble. It makes men gentle and women strong. Even in times of hardship a lavender personality bravely continues overcoming obstacles that are placed in their way, having the ability to give generously of themselves – caring for others, often with gentleness and sacrifice.[64]

They will also often find themselves being attracted to volunteer jobs helping the homeless or the disadvantaged. They are gentle personalities who will always be attracted to roles that involve being kind-hearted, humane and benevolent.[64]

Mailhebiau compares lavender to Mother Teresa:

Tireless, always even-tempered, with unfailing gentleness and devotion, Lavandula cares for and calms, listens to and remedies a thousand ills. She takes care of children, adults and elderly, animals, plants, the earth and sky. She looks after everyone with equal love and if there is anyone in the world whom she neglects, it is herself.[62]

According to Myers-Briggs personality types, the lavender personality is likely to be an ESFJ. ESFJs are warm-hearted, outgoing and friendly. They are highly sociable and become restless when separated from others. They thrive on being needed and appreciated. They are more attuned to the needs of others than their own. ESFJs enjoy busy lives. They like to be involved in community service organisations and volunteer activities. They enjoy spending time with their friends and family. They are service oriented and want to provide practical help to others. They tend to be talkative and are comfortable chatting with just about anyone. They value harmony and try not to offend or disappoint anyone.

Subtle

Worwood states that lavender embodies the protective love of Mother Earth, and says that it is energetically very active in the auric field closest to the body. She also explains the profound impact lavender can have on our psyche:

When deep sadness covers the spirit like a suffocating blanket, lavender gently lifts the weight. When inner tears fall, lavender wipes them away. When depression clouds the psyche, lavender blows it asunder. And for those with worries that trouble the spirit, lavender lifts the veil of despair.[65]

Davis recommends lavender for achieving deeper states of meditation. Lavender oil's harmonising qualities make it perfect for balancing the heart chakra and help to bring the higher and lower chakras into harmony with each other.[66]

Keim Loughran & Bull recommend lavender oil for integrating our spirituality into everyday life. Lavender can also be used to increase awareness and sensitivity to healing energy work.[67]

Zeck states that lavender oil warms the heart and calms the emotions by promoting awareness to nurture ourselves while travelling the river of life:

Where there has been self-neglect and lack of self-care wearing away the health and energy of your body, lavender brings nourishment and heartening reassurance.[68]

Dosage and Administration

Blending

Aromatherapy

Fischer-Rizzi states that little can go wrong when lavender is mixed with other essential oils. Lavender oil is compatible with most other oils. However, she explains that it does not blend harmoniously with rosemary.[60]

I suggest that lavender would blend well with rosemary. A blend of lavender, rosemary, neroli and petitgrain would create a delightful, refreshing eau de cologne perfume. Is it possible that Fischer-Rizzi means to say the two should never be blended as lavender is relaxing and rosemary is stimulating. However, I am afraid that this is also not true. A blend of lavender and rosemary would be ideal for muscular aches and pains or for someone feeling physically exhausted and emotionally drained. On the other hand, I agree that rosemary and lavender oils should not be blended if you were making a blend to alleviate insomnia.

Fischer-Rizzi also suggests that lavender has no sensual qualities, and we should beware of mixing it with sensual oils like ylang ylang or jasmine.[60] However, lavender works so well with strong florals. Lavender has a feminine quality that enhances and balances the intense sensual feminine energy of rich floral oils such as jasmine or ylang ylang.

For the relief of stress, anxiety and nervous tension, consider blending lavender oil with essential oils such as bergamot, Atlas cedarwood, clary sage, coriander seed, Roman chamomile, fragonia, geranium, neroli, sweet orange, patchouli, petitgrain, rose, sandalwood, vetiver or ylang ylang.

To alleviate insomnia, consider blending lavender oil with essential oils such as Atlas cedarwood, Roman chamomile, fragonia, sweet marjoram, neroli, sandalwood or vetiver.

To alleviate depression, consider blending lavender oil with essential oils such as bergamot, clary sage, geranium, jasmine absolute, neroli, patchouli, rose absolute or otto, sandalwood or ylang ylang.

L

For the relief of dysmenorrhoea, consider blending lavender oil with essential oils such as Roman chamomile, clary sage, geranium, sweet marjoram or rose.

For the relief of muscular aches and pains, consider blending lavender oil with essential oils such as black pepper, cajeput, clove, peppermint eucalyptus, fragonia, ginger, kunzea, sweet marjoram, nutmeg, pine, rosemary or thyme.

To alleviate headaches, consider blending lavender essential oil with cornmint or peppermint.

To promote wound healing, consider blending lavender oil with essential oils such as German chamomile, everlasting, frankincense, myrrh, patchouli or sandalwood.

For the relief of dermatitis and eczema, consider blending lavender oil with essential oils such as German chamomile, everlasting, neroli, patchouli or sandalwood.

Perfumery

Lavender oil is extensively used in fougères, chypres, amber and floral style perfumes. Arctander states that lavender oil blends well with bergamot, clary sage, citrus oils, oakmoss absolute, patchouli, rosemary and pine needle oils. He explains that it is unequalled as a popular, fresh-sweet, herbal-floral fragrance in colognes and perfumes.[3]

L

Mode of administration

Bath

Full body bath, foot bath, sitz bath

Topical

Compress, massage, ointment, skin care

Inhalation

Direct inhalation, diffuser, oil vaporiser

Safety Profile

General safety

Lavender oil is considered non-toxic, non-irritant and non-sensitising.[55]

Contraindications

No contraindications known.

Toxicity

Three case reports have been published of gynaecomastia developed in prepubertal boys aged four, seven and 10 following regular topical use of skin care products containing lavender and tea tree oils.[69]

In all three boys, gynaecomastia was resolved shortly after the use of products containing these oils discontinued. The authors concluded that repeated topical exposure to lavender and tea tree oils probably caused prepubertal gynaecomastia, a rare condition characterised by the growth of breast tissue in males, as a consequence of early exposure to sex hormones.[69]

It must be noted that the authors did state that other components in these products may also possess endocrine disrupting activity that can contribute to the gynaecomastia, but these components were not tested. They only chose to evaluate the component that was found in all the products used by the patients (lavender oil), and a chemically similar component that was found in some of the products (tea tree oil).[69]

They performed in vitro studies with lavender oil and tea tree oil and suggest that they possess weak oestrogenic and anti-androgenic activities that may have contributed to an imbalance in oestrogen and androgen pathway signalling. They also explain that prepubertal gynaecomastia is extremely rare.[69]

Interestingly, no other in vivo clinical trial on lavender and tea tree has ever found any oestrogenic effects. Kemper clearly states that in vitro testing alone is not adequate grounds for indicting traditionally used products to create public fear.[70]

It also needs to be noted that no oestrogenic compounds have ever been found in either lavender or tea tree; however, it is well known that there is a growing number of endocrine disrupters in our environment that have been shown to accumulate in adipose tissue.[70]

Kalyan also concludes that no oestrogenic compounds have yet to be found in either lavender or tea tree and states that it is, therefore, very important that we carefully interpret these findings. Kaylan also states that the report of Henley et al. indicates a very weak hormone-modulating effect, and it would be bewildering if such a low hormonal activity alone could instigate gynaecomastia.[71]

Dean reminds us that the oils were in wash-off products. The product in question was a wash-off product containing less than 1% essential oil. If you correlate this with the in vitro study performed by Henley et al., then a child weighing 20 kg would need to use approximately 40 bottles of shampoo for each application. The claim of a causative link between the use of lavender or tea tree oil products and prepubertal gynaecomastia appears to be misleading and unwarranted.[72]

Tisserand is also concerned by comments made by Begoun who opposes any fragrance, natural or synthetic, being used in a cosmetic.[73] She labels lavender as being photosensitising and cytotoxic – meaning that topical application causes skin cell death. She also states that it enhances oxidation and as a result causes skin irritancy.[74]

Tisserand explains that, over a period of years, lavender oil constituents can oxidise to hydroperoxides. These oxidation products are often slightly more skin-allergenic than the original compounds. This is why the IFRA recommends that skin care preparations with essential oils high in linalool should include an antioxidant; however, Tisserand points out that, even without an antioxidant, the shelf life of a lavender-containing product should be good for at least 12 months.[73]

Tisserand & Young point out that, considering the high usage of lavender oil on the skin in aromatherapy, the reported incidence of skin reactions is very low. They cite many studies that confirm this:

- In a 48-hour occlusive patch test on 50 Italian volunteers, undiluted lavender oil produced no adverse reactions. Similarly tested at 1% on 273 eczema patients, it produced no reactions.
- Tested at 10% on 25 volunteers, it was neither irritating nor sensitising.
- In a study of 200 dermatitis patients, none were sensitive to 2% lavender oil on patch testing.[75]

In Japan, lavender is regarded as a high-risk skin sensitiser. However, subsequent reports have suggested that this dramatic increase in sensitisation to lavender is attributed to the introduction of dried lavender flowers into the home.[75]

There are many studies that confirm that lavender oil is anti-allergenic. Tisserand & Young cite a study that shows that lavender inhibited the release of the inflammatory mediators TNF and histamine.[75]

A Japanese study found that lavender oil inhibited the generation of singlet oxygen, which causes the most damage in response to UVA / UVB radiation. This suggests that regular use of lavender oil in skin preparations could suppress the aging effects of sunlight on the skin. Another study found that lavender oil has excellent antioxidant activity, suggesting that it could inhibit degenerative such change as skin cancer, sun damage and the effects of aging.[75]

Regulatory guidelines

Lavender essential oil has GRAS status.

Reference

1. Harris R. *Lavenders of Provence.* The World of Aromatherapy III Conference Proceedings, NAHA, Seattle, 1999; 75-81.
2. Price S, Price L. *Aromatherapy for health professionals.* 4th edn. Churchill Livingstone, Edinburgh, 2012.
3. Arctander S. *Perfume and flavor materials of natural origin.* Allured Publishing, Carol Stream, 1994.
4. Grieve M. *A modern herbal l – Vol. II.* Dover Publications, New York, 1971.
5. Société Coopérative Agricole des Plantes à Parfum de Provence (SCA3P). *Huile essentielle de lavande: Catalogue des huiles essentielles de Provence.* Retrieved Oct 10, 2017, from http://www.sca3p.com/en/essential-oils-provence/catalalogue-en/lavender-lavandula-angustifolia-perfumery-cosmetics-aromatherapy
6. Southwell I. *Australian standards for oil of Australian lavandin cultivars.* Rural Industries Research and Development Corporation, Barton, 2012. RIRDC Publication No11/133.
7. Harborne JB, Williams CA. *Phytochemistry of the genus Lavandula.* In Lis-Balchin M. ed. *Lavender – the genus Lavandula.* Taylor & Francis Group, London, 2002: 86-99.
8. Lis-Balchin M. *Lavender essential oil.* In Lis-Balchin M. ed. *Lavender – the genus Lavandula.* Taylor & Francis Group, London, 2002: 117-123.
9. Schnaubelt K. *The healing intelligence of essential oils.* Healing Arts Press, Rochester, 2011.
10. Southern Cross University. *Perfect Potion lavender oils – certificate of analysis.* Perfect Potion, Brisbane, 2016.
11. Castle J, Lis-Balchin M. *History of usage of Lavandula species.* In Lis-Balchin M. ed. *Lavender – the genus Lavandula.* Taylor & Francis Group, London, 2002: 35-50.
12. Khan I, Abourashed E. *Leung's encyclopedia of common natural ingredients used in food, drugs and cosmetics.* 3rd edn. John Wiley & Sons, New Jersey, 2010.
13. Blumenthal M et al. *The complete German commission E monographs: therapeutic guide to herbal medicine.* American Botanical Council, Austin, 1998.
14. Braun L, Cohen M. *Herbs & natural supplements: an evidence-based guide – Vol. 2.* Elsevier, Chatswood, 2015.
15. Yu SH, Seol GH. *Lavandula angustifolia Mill. oil and its active constituent linalyl acetate alleviate pain and urinary residual sense after colorectal cancer surgery: a randomised controlled trial.* Evidence-Based Complementary and Alternative Medicine, 2017; 2017: 3954181. doi: 10.1155/2017/3954181.

L

16. Olapour A et al. *The effect of inhalation of aromatherapy blend containing lavender essential oil on caesarean postoperative pain.* Anesthesiology and Pain Medicine, 2013; 3(1): 203-207. doi: 10.5812/aapm.9570.
17. Hasanzadeh F et al. *The effect of cold application and lavender oil inhalation in cardiac surgery patients undergoing chest tube removal.* EXCLI Journal, 2016; 15: 64-74. doi: 10.17179/excli2015-748.
18. Vaziri F et al. *Effect of lavender oil aroma in the early hours of postpartum period on maternal pains, fatigue and mood: a randomized clinical trial.* International Journal of Preventive Medicine, 2017; 8: 29. doi: 10.4103/ijpvm.IJPVM_137_16.
19. Ueno-lio T et al. *Lavender essential oil inhalation suppresses allergic airway inflammation and mucous cell hyperplasia in a murine model of asthma.* Life Sciences, 2014; 108(2): 109-115.
20. Lis-Balchin M. *Aromatherapy science – a guide for healthcare professionals.* Pharmaceutical Press, London, 2006.
21. Yap PS et al. *Membrane disruption and anti-quorum sensing effects of synergistic interaction between Lavandula angustifolia (lavender oil) in combination with antibiotic against plasmid-conferred multi-drug-resistant Escherichia coli.* Journal of Applied Microbiology, 2014; 116(5): 1119-1128.
22. de Rapper S et al. *The in vitro antimicrobial activity of Lavandula angustifolia essential oil in combination with other aroma-therapeutic oils.* Evidence-Based Complementary and Alternative Medicine, 2013; 2013: 852049. doi: 10.1155/2013/852049.
23. Behmanesh F et al. *Antifungal effect of lavender essential oil (Lavandula angustifolia) and Clotrimazole on Candida albicans: an in vitro study.* Scientifica, 2015; 2015: 261397. doi: 10.1155/2015/261397.
24. Domingos T da S, Braga EM. *Massage with aromatherapy: effectiveness on anxiety of users with personality disorders in psychiatric hospitalisation.* Revista da Escola de Enfermagem da USP, 2015; 49(3): 450-456.
25. Woelk H, Schläfke S. *A multi-center, double-blind, randomised study of the lavender oil preparation Silexan in comparison to Lorazepam for generalized anxiety disorder.* Phytomedicine, 2010; 17(2): 94-99.
26. Uehleke B et al. *Phase II trial on the effects of Silexan in patients with neurasthenia, post-traumatic stress disorder or somatization disorder.* Phytomedicine, 2012; 19(8-9): 665-71. doi: 10.1016/j.phymed.2012.02.020.
27. *Lavender.* Retrieved Apr 3, 2016 from http://examine.com/supplements/lavender/
28. Kasper S et al. *Silexan, an orally administered Lavandula oil preparation, is effective in the treatment of 'subsyndromal' anxiety disorder: a randomized, double-blind, placebo controlled trial.* International Clinical Psychopharmacology, 2010; 25(5): 277-287.
29. Schuwald AM et al. *Lavender oil-potent anxiolytic properties via modulating voltage dependent calcium channels.* PLoS ONE, 2013; 8(4): e59998. doi: 10.1371/journal.pone.0059998.
30. Baldinger P et al. *Effects of silexan on the serotonin-1A receptor and microstructure of the human brain: a randomized, placebo-controlled, double-blind, cross-over study with molecular and structural neuroimaging.* International Journal of Neuropsycholopharmacology, 2015; 18(4): pyu063. doi: 10.1093/ijnp/pyu063.
31. López V et al. *Exploring pharmacological mechanisms of lavender (Lavandula angustifolia) essential oil on central nervous system targets.* Frontiers in Pharmacology, 2017; 8: 280. doi: 10.3389/fphar.2017.00280.
32. Jimbo D et al. *Effect of aromatherapy on patients with Alzheimer's disease.* Psychogeriatrics, 2009; 9: 173-179.
33. O'Connor DW et al. *A randomized, controlled cross-over trial of dermally-applied lavender (Lavandula angustifolia) oil as a treatment of agitated behaviour in dementia.* BMC Complementary and Alternative Medicine, 2013; 13: 315.
34. Holmes C et al. *Lavender oil as a treatment for agitated behaviour in severe dementia: a placebo controlled study.* International Journal of Geriatric Psychiatry, 2002; 17(4): 305-308.
35. Bowles EJ et al. *Effects of essential oils and touch on resistance to nursing care procedures and other dementia-related behaviours in a residential care facility.* International Journal of Aromatherapy, 2002; 12(1): 22-29.
36. Snow AL et al. *A controlled trial of aromatherapy for agitation in nursing home patients with dementia.* The Journal of Alternative and Complementary Medicine, 2004; 10(3): 431-437. doi: 10.1089/1075553041323696.
37. Fu CY et al. *A randomised controlled trial of the use of aromatherapy and hand massage to reduce disruptive behaviour in people with dementia.* BMC Complementary Alternative Medicine, 2013; 13: 165. doi: 10.1186/1472-6882-13-165.
38. Soheili M et al. *Lavandula angustifolia extract improves deteriorated synaptic plasticity in an animal model of Alzheimer's disease.* Iranian Journal of Basic Medical Sciences, 2015; 18(11): 1147-1152. PMCID: PMC4764119.
39. Moorman Li R. *Evaluating the effects of diffused lavender in an adult day care center for patients with dementia in an effort to decrease behavioural issues: a pilot study.* Journal of Drug Assessment, 2017; 6(1): 1-5. doi: 10.1080/21556660.2016.1278545.
40. Sasannejad P et al. *Lavender essential oil in the treatment of migraine headache: a placebo-controlled clinical trial.* European Neurology, 2012; 67(5): 288-291.

L

41. Apay SE et al. *Effect of aromatherapy massage on dysmenorrhea in Turkish students.* Pain Management Nursing, 2012; 13(4): 236-240. doi: 10.1016/j.pmn.2010.04.002.
42. Bakhtshirin F et al. *The effect of aromatherapy massage with lavender oil on severity of primary dysmenorrhea in Arsanjan students.* Iranian Journal of Nursing and Midwifery Research, 2015; 20(1): 156-160. PMC4325408.
43. Matsumoto T et al. *Does lavender aromatherapy alleviated premenstrual emotional symptoms?: a randomized crossover trial.* BioPsychoSocial Medicine, 2013; 7: 12. doi: 10.1186/1751-0759-7-12.
44. Koulivand PH et al. *Lavender and the nervous system.* Evidence-Based Complementary and Alternative Medicine, 2013; 2013: 681304. doi: 10.1155/2013/681304.
45. Fismer KL, Pilkington K. *Lavender and sleep: a systematic review of the evidence.* European Journal of Integrative Medicine, 2012; 4(4): e436-e447. doi: 10.1016/j.eujim.2012.08.001.
46. Buckle J. *Clinical aromatherapy – essential oils in practice.* 2nd edn. Churchill Livingstone, Edinburgh, 2003.
47. LW Chien et al. *The effect of lavender aromatherapy on autonomic nervous system in midlife women with insomnia.* Evidence-Based Complementary and Alternative Medicine, 2012; 2012: 740813. doi: 10.1155/2012/740813.
48. Goel N et al. *An olfactory stimulus modifies nighttime sleep in young men and women.* Chronobiology International, 2005; 22(5): 889-904. doi: 10.1080/07420520500263276.
49. Lillehei AS et al. *Effect of inhaled lavender and sleep hygiene on self-reported sleep issues: a randomized controlled trial.* Journal of Alterative and Complementary Medicine, 2015; 21(7): 430-438. doi: 10.1089/acm.2014.0327.
50. Koca Kutlu A et al. *A comparison study of growth factor expression following treatment with transcutaneous electrical nerve stimulation, saline solution, povidone-iodine and lavender oil in wounds healing.* Evidence-Based Complementary Alternative Medicine, 2013; 2013: 361932. doi: 10.1155/2013/361832.
51. Mori HM et al. *Wound healing potential of lavender oil by acceleration of granulation and wound contraction through induction of TGF-β in a rat model.* BMC Complementary and Alternative Medicine, 2016; 16: 144. doi: 10.1186/s12906-016-1128-7.
52. Guba R. *Wound healing: a pilot study using an essential oil-based cream to heal dermal wounds and ulcers.* The International Journal of Aromatherapy, 1998/1999; 9(2): 67-74.
53. Zhao Y et al. *In vitro and in vivo efficacy studies of Lavender angustifolia essential oil and its active constituents on the proliferation of human prostate cancer.* Integrative Cancer Therapies, 2017; 16(2): 215-226. doi: 10.1177/1534735416645408.
54. Sadeghzadeh J et al. *Lavandula reduces heart injury via attenuating tumor necrosis factor-alpha and oxidative stress in a rat model if infarct-like myocardial injury.* Cell Journal, 2017; 19(1): 84-93. doi: 10.22074/cellj.2016.4148.
55. Lawless J. *The encyclopaedia of essential oils.* Element Books, Shaftesbury, 1992.
56. Lavabre M. *Aromatherapy workbook.* Healing Arts Press, Rochester, 1997.
57. Holmes P. *Aromatica: a clinical guide to essential oil therapeutics – Vol. I.* Singing Dragon, London, 2016.
58. Davis P. *Aromatherapy: an A-Z.* 2nd edn. C.W. Daniel Company, Saffron Walden, 1999.
59. Holmes P. *Lavender.* The International Journal of Aromatherapy, 1992; 4(2): 20-22.
60. Fischer-Rizzi S. *Complete aromatherapy handbook.* Sterling Publishing, New York, 1990.
61. Burn E, Blamey C. *Soothing scents in childbirth.* The International Journal of Aromatherapy, 1994; 6(1): 24-28.
62. Mailhebiau P. *Portraits in oils.* C.W. Daniel Company, Saffron Walden, 1995.
63. Mojay G. *Aromatherapy for healing the spirit.* Healing Arts Press, Rochester, 1999.
64. Worwood VA. *The fragrant mind.* Transworld Publishers, London, 1995.
65. Worwood VA. *The fragrant heavens.* Transworld Publishers, London, 1999.
66. Davis P. *Subtle aromatherapy.* C.W. Daniel Company, Saffron Walden, 1991.
67. Keim Loughran J, Bull R. *Aromatherapy and subtle energy techniques.* Frog, Berkeley, 2000.
68. Zeck R. *The blossoming heart – aromatherapy for healing and transformation.* Aroma Tours, East Ivanhoe, 2004.
69. Henley DV et al. *Prepubertal gynecomastia linked to lavender and tea tree oils.* New England Journal of Medicine, 2007; 356(5): 479-485.
70. Kemper K et al. *To the editor: Prepubertal gynecomastia linked to lavender and tea tree oils.* The New England Journal of Medicine, 2007; 356: 2541-2544.
71. Kalyan S. *To the editor: Prepubertal gynecomastia linked to lavender and tea tree oils.* The New England Journal of Medicine, 2007; 356: 2541-2544.
72. Dean CJ. *To the editor: Prepubertal gynecomastia linked to lavender and tea tree oils.* The New England Journal of Medicine, 2007; 356: 2541-2544.
73. Tisserand R. *Lavender oil – skin savior or skin irritant?* Retrieved Apr 1, 2016 from http://roberttisserand.com/2011/08/lavender-oil-skin-savior-or-skin-irritant/
74. *Lavender extract and oil.* Retrieved Oct 9, 2017 from http://www.paulaschoice.com/ingredient-dictionary/plant-extracts/lavender-extract-and-oil.html
75. Tisserand R, Young R. *Essential oil safety.* 2nd edn. Churchill Livingstone, Edinburgh, 2014.

Lavender, spike

Identification

Botanical name

Lavandula latifolia Medic.

Synonyms

Lavandula spica DC, aspic

Family

Lamiaceae (Labiatae)

Botany and origins

Spike lavender is an aromatic evergreen sub-shrub with linear or lance-shaped leaves. It grows up to 1 m high and is native to the Mediterranean region. It is easy to distinguish from other lavender species as it has long spatula-shaped leaves and long flowering spikes with greyish blue flowers.[1] Price & Price state that spike lavender is a much larger plant than true lavender.[2] Spike lavender grows wild around the Mediterranean countries, particularly Spain, France and Italy. Spain is the major producer of the oil.[3]

Method of extraction

Spike lavender oil is steam-distilled from the flowering tops of *L. latifolia.* Most spike lavender is distilled from wild plants.[1]

L

Characteristics

Spike lavender oil is a pale yellow to almost clear-coloured mobile liquid, with a fresh camphoraceous and herbaceous odour and a somewhat dry-woody undertone.[3]

Chemical composition

The main difference between spike lavender and true lavender is the high camphor and 1,8-cineole content of spike lavender. The chemical composition of spike lavender from Spain was reported as follows:

α-pinene (1.7%), camphene (0.5%), β-pinene (1.5%), myrcene (1.4%), 1,8-cineole (23.5%), *p*-cymene (0.6%), camphor (20.0%), linalool (32.4%), terpinen-4-ol (1.5%), borneol (4.6%), geraniol (1.8%).[4]

The composition of true lavender (*L. angustifolia*) and spike lavender essential oils extracted from plants grown in the southeast of Spain were compared. Linalool (37-54%), linalyl acetate (21-36%) and (*E*)-β-caryophyllene (1-3%) were the most abundant constituents for true lavender, while the most abundant constituents for spike lavender were linalool (35-51%), 1,8-cineole (26-32%), camphor (10-18%), α-pinene (1-2%), α-terpineol (1-2%) and α-bisabolene (1-2%).[5]

Adulteration

Lis-Balchin states that synthetic camphor is often added to lavandin oil, or synthetic linalool and linalyl acetate and sold off as spike lavender. Spike lavender is also cut with Spanish sage oil, rosemary oil, lavandin oil, eucalyptus oil or their fractions.[6]

Pharmacopoeias and standards

The purity, composition and physico-chemical properties of spike lavender essential oil are defined in ISO 4719: 2012 Essential Oil of Spike Lavender (*Lavandula latifolia* Medikus), Spanish type.

History and Traditional Uses

History

Commonly called aspic, it is considered the 'male lavender' in contrast to *L. angustifolia*, which is referred to as the 'female lavender'. The term 'aspic' comes from the Greek term meaning 'Egyptian cobra', and it earned this name as it was historically used against the venom of the asp.[7]

Spike lavender oil was considered too camphoraceous and never worth more than 1/5 the value of true lavender. However, many herbalists from the Middle Ages considered spike lavender as the medicinal lavender. For example, Culpeper described the oil of spike lavender as being so fierce and piercing in its qualities that it must be used cautiously. He stated that just a few drops are sufficient, and that the oil is not safe when the body is full of illnesses (blood and tumours) because it is too heating.[8]

Culpeper recommended spike lavender for a variety of ailments such as pains of the head and brain, falling sickness, dropsy, cramps and convulsions.[7]

Hildegard of Bingen states that spike lavender is hot and dry; however, she explains that its heat is healthy. She explains that whoever cooks this lavender in wine or, if he has no wine, honey and water and frequently drinks it when it is warm, will lessen the pain in his liver and lungs, and the stuffiness in his chest.[9]

Traditional medicine

Spike lavender oil was an ingredient in the famous *oleum spicae*, which was used for the treatment of old sprains and stiff joints.[7]

Food, perfumery and flavouring

Spike lavender oil has limited use in perfumery; however, it is often used to scented soap.[3]

Therapeutics

Pharmacology and clinical studies

Antibacterial activity

In vitro study found that spike lavender oil displayed antibacterial effect against 19 out of 25 different bacterial species and 12 out of 20 *Listeria monocytogenes*.[6]

Antifungal activity

An in vitro study confirmed that spike lavender oil had excellent antifungal activity against *Aspergillus niger* and moderate activity against *Fusarium culmorum*.[6]

Spasmolytic activity

Spike lavender oil has been reported as having spasmolytic effects on the smooth muscles when tested on electrically stimulated smooth muscle guinea pig ileum in vitro.[6]

Actions

Actions commonly cited in aromatherapy

Analgesic, antidepressant, antiseptic, cholagogue, cicatrisant, decongestant, emmenagogue, insecticide, rubefacient, vulnerary[10,11]

Actions supported by clinical studies

Antibacterial, antifungal, antiseptic, rubefacient

Comment

The properties and uses of spike lavender oil in aromatherapy are usually referenced as being similar to true lavender. This is confusing, considering that the chemistry and odour profile of spike lavender is significantly different to true lavender.

However, many of the pharmacological activities of *L. angustifolia* oil have been attributed to linalool, and considering that spike lavender oil does have a similar percentage of linalool, it is likely that spike lavender does share some similar activities with true lavender oil.

The high percentage of 1,8-cineole and camphor contribute to spike lavender's mucolytic and expectorant activity, making it a very useful oil for respiratory tract infections and congestion. The camphor content also suggests that spike lavender oil may also have good analgesic qualities. Without the ester, linalyl acetate, it is unlikely that spike lavender would have the same balancing and relaxing quality of true lavender.

Aromatherapy Uses

Clinical aromatherapy

Analgesic

Mailhebiau suggests blending spike lavender oil with peppermint oil for treating headaches, and blending it with sage oil for treating late or painful periods. He also states that, blended with rosemary oil, spike lavender becomes an excellent anti-inflammatory and efficient painkiller in cases of rheumatism.[12]

Integumentary system

Franchomme and Pénoël state that spike lavender oil is very well tolerated by the skin and is indicated for severe burns.[2] Spike lavender oil may be used as an insect repellent.[11]

Respiratory system

Spike lavender oil is valued for its expectorant and mucolytic properties.[11,12,13] Spike lavender is especially useful in chest and throat infections for children and adults.[2]

Energetics, psyche and subtle uses

Energetics

Spike lavender oil is stimulating and *warming*.[14] According to the principles of TCM, spike lavender is likely to tonify the *Qi* and strengthen the *Shen*. It also warms the *Lungs* and expels *cold* and *damp* conditions, which are associated with chronic cough and phlegm. It helps to dispel *wind cold*, which is often associated with sinus congestion, aches and pain and general fatigue.

Personality

Mailhebiau compares the spike lavender personality with that of Jean-Jacques Rousseau.[12] This comparison is easy to appreciate when one reads the following statement made by Rousseau:

> *I used to rise with the sun and was happy; I used to go for walks and was happy … I walked in the woods and over the hillsides, wandered through the valleys, read and was idle; I worked in the garden, picked fruit, helped with the cleaning, and happiness followed me everywhere.*[12]

Mailhebiau explains that Rousseau was an anti-establishmentarian who loved to challenge the false values of his time. He compares the physical characteristics of the spike lavender person to an old student from May 1968, who has come down from his barricades to go and climb hills – long-haired and bearded, who away from pollution, carries on a self-sufficient lifestyle as a likeable fringe-person and questions – not without reason – social values and the advanced technologies, which he does not shirk from using if the need arises.[12]

Subtle

Mailhebiau suggests that spike lavender oil is a good essence for bringing people back to a more natural lifestyle. He explains that spike lavender is a good counterweight to insane rationalism, which is only bearable in the eyes of those for whom the earth is simply an object of fleeting profits.[12]

Dosage and Administration

Blending

Aromatherapy

As a natural insect repellent, consider blending spike lavender oil with essential oils such as Atlas cedarwood, citronella, lemon-scented eucalyptus, 1,8-cineole-rich eucalypts, niaouli, peppermint, lemon-scented tea tree or tea tree.

For the relief of muscular aches and pains, arthritic and rheumatic pain, consider blending spike lavender oil with essential oils such as black pepper, cajeput, peppermint eucalyptus, fragonia, ginger, kunzea, peppermint or rosemary.

For the relief of bronchitis and chest and throat infections, consider blending spike lavender oil with essential oils such as aniseed, Atlas cedarwood, cajeput, sweet fennel, 1,8-cineole-rich eucalypts, peppermint eucalyptus, fragonia, lemon, niaouli, pine, ravintsara, rosemary or thyme.

For the relief of headaches and neuralgia, consider blending spike lavender oil with essential oils such as cajeput, kunzea, lavender, sweet marjoram or peppermint.

To alleviate general fatigue, poor circulation and debility, consider blending spike lavender oil with essential oils such as black pepper, coriander seed, ginger, lemon, peppermint or rosemary.

As a general antiseptic for healing topical skin infections and bedsores, consider blending spike lavender oil with essential oils such as everlasting, *Lavandula angustifolia*, sage or tea tree.

Perfumery

Arctander states that spike lavender oil has a freshness that makes it applicable in many styles of perfume such as lavender style, fougère style, pine and woody style perfumes, oriental styles or cologne style perfumes. He explains that spike lavender blends well with other essential oils that have a high 1,8-cineole or camphor content. This includes oils such as rosemary, sage, eucalyptus, lavandin or lavender. It also blends well with petitgrain, spice oils, pine needle oils, cedarwood or patchouli oil.[3]

Mode of administration

Bath

Full body bath, foot bath, sitz bath

Topical

Compress, massage, ointment, skin care

Inhalation

Direct inhalation, diffuser, oil vaporiser

Safety Profile

General safety

Spike lavender oil is non-toxic, non-irritating and non-sensitising.[10]

Contraindications

Lawless and Tisserand & Young state that there are no contraindications known.[10,15]

However, Holmes states that spike lavender oil is contraindicated in fevers, epilepsy and during pregnancy.[14]

Toxicity

It may be mildly neurotoxic based on the camphor content.[15] The camphor content varies between 10% and 20% and the 1,8-cineole content varies between 25% and 35%. Tisserand & Young state that, since linalool is an anticonvulsant, it may mitigate the neurotoxicity of the camphor in spike lavender oil.[15]

Regulatory guidelines

Spike lavender oil has been granted GRAS status.

References

1. Harris R. *Lavenders of Provence*. The World of Aromatherapy III Conference Proceedings. NAHA, Seattle, 1999; 75-81.
2. Price S, Price L. *Aromatherapy for health professionals*. 4th edn. Churchill Livingstone, Edinburgh, 2012.
3. Arctander S. *Perfume and flavor materials of natural origin*. Allured Publishing, Carol Stream, 1994.
4. Lawrence BM. *Essential oils 1981-1987*. Allured Publishing, Wheaton, 1989.
5. Carrasco A et al. *Lavandula angustifolia and Lavandula latifolia essential oils from Spain: aromatic profiles and bioactivities*. Planta Medica, 2016; 82(1/2): 163-170. doi: 10.1055/s-0035-1558095
6. Lis-Balchin M. *Aromatherapy science – a guide for healthcare professionals*. Pharmaceutical Press, London, 2006.
7. Grieve M. *A modern herbal – Vol. II*. Dover

Publications, New York, 1971.
8. Castle J, Lis-Balchin M. *History of usage of Lavandula species.* In Lis-Balchin M. ed. *Lavender – the genus Lavandula.* Taylor & Francis Group, London, 2002: 35-50. (Medical and Aromatic Plants – Industrial Profiles; 29).
9. Hildegard von Bingen. *Hildegard von Bingen's physica.* Trans. Throo P. Healing Arts Press, Rochester, 1998.
10. Lawless J. *The encyclopaedia of essential oils.* Element Books, Shaftesbury, 1992.
11. Lavabre M. *Aromatherapy workbook.* Healing Arts Press, Rochester, 1997.
12. Mailhebiau P. *Portraits in oils.* C.W. Daniel Company. Saffron Walden, 1995.
13. Davis P. *Aromatherapy: an A-Z.* 2nd edn. C.W. Daniel Company, Saffron Walden, 1999.
14. Holmes P. *Aromatica: a clinical guide to essential oil therapeutics – Vol. I.* Singing Dragon, London, 2016.
15. Tisserand R, Young R. *Essential oil safety.* 2nd edn. Churchill Livingstone, Edinburgh, 2014.

Lemon

Identification

Botanical name

Citrus x *limon* (L.) Osbeck

Synonyms

Expressed lemon oil

Family

Rutaceae

Botany and origins

Lemon species are divided into two groups with either smooth or rough-skinned fruit. Some taxonomists regard the two as distinct species: the smooth as *C. limon* and the rough (citronelle) as *C. jambhiri* Hodg. Others consider the rough lemon as a lime x citron hybrid.[1]

The lemon tree is believed to be a native of southeastern China. It is believed to have arrived in Europe via Persia and the Middle East with the returning Crusaders in the twelfth century.[1] However, Holmes states that the lemon tree was brought by the Moors to Sicily and Spain during the tenth-century medieval al-Andalus era.[2]

Columbus brought lemon and orange seeds on his second voyage to the West Indies in 1493. Little did he know he would be founding the world's largest lemon industry by the twentieth century.[3]

The lemon tree fruits all year round, the fruits appearing with a deep green colour and ripening to a bright yellow. Lemon oil is mostly cultivated in California and Florida and in Southern Europe.[4]

Nowadays the principal production areas of lemon oil are Italy, Spain, Israel, Argentina and the USA.[1]

Method of extraction

Lemon oil is obtained from the peel of lemons by cold expression. Weiss states that the rough lemon fruit has virtually no commercial use except as a seed source. Lemon peel will yield approximately 2.2% essential oil; however, cold pressing normally returns only 66-75% of the oil.[1]

Steam distilling produces a higher yield; however, the distilled oil has different characteristics and is considered inferior.[1]

Characteristics

Lemon oil is a yellow to greenish yellow or pale yellow mobile liquid of a very light, fresh and sweet odour, truly reminiscent of the ripe peel.

There should be no turpentine-like, harsh terpene notes. The odour of lemon oil is not very lasting. However, good lemon oil should retain its fresh lemon aroma practically unchanged on a blotter until there is no odour left at all.[4]

Chemical composition

Expressed lemon oil is comprised mostly (up to 70%) of limonene, a monoterpene hydrocarbon. The chemical composition of lemon was reported as follows:

α-pinene (1.8-3.6%), camphene (0-0.1%), β-pinene (6.1-15.0%), sabinene (1.5-4.6%), myrcene (1.0-2.1%), α-terpinene (0-0.5%), linalool (0-0.9%), β-bisabolene (0.56%), limonene (62.1-74.5%), *trans*-α-bergamotene (0.37%), nerol (0.04%), neral (0.76%).[5]

Adulteration

Expressed lemon oil is frequently adulterated with distilled lemon oil, lemon terpenes, *d*-limonene (natural isolate or synthetic from pinene), synthetic dipentene, or synthetic or isolated citral.[4]

Pharmacopoeias and standards

The purity, composition and physico-chemical properties of lemon essential oil are defined in ISO 855: 2003 Oil of Lemon. Lemon oil is also listed in the European Pharmacopoeia.

L

History and Traditional Uses

History

Lemon juice was considered to be a remedy for scurvy. English ships were required by law to carry sufficient lemon or lime juice for every seaman to have once daily after being at sea for 10 days or more.[6]

The juice was used as a diaphoretic and diuretic. Lemon juice is highly recommended in acute rheumatism and sometimes given to counteract narcotic poisons. The juice is a good astringent and is said to be the best cure for severe, obstinate hiccups and is helpful in jaundice and palpitation of the heart.[6]

Food, perfumery and flavouring

Lemon oil is extensively used in pharmaceuticals as a flavouring agent and as a fragrance ingredient in soaps, detergents and perfumes.[7]

Therapeutics

Pharmacology and clinical studies

Many pharmacological studies involving lemon essential oil have been published. A systemic review of these studies will not be attempted. Rather, I have chosen a selection of studies that support the traditional and clinical uses.

L

Air purifier

In a study, lemon oil vaporised in the air was effective in killing 40% of airborne microbes after 20 minutes and 90% after three hours.[8]

Alzheimer's disease

A clinical trial in Japan examined the effects of aromatherapy on patients with Alzheimer's disease. Researchers investigated the effects of essential oils in 28 elderly people, 17 of whom had Alzheimer's. Rosemary and lemon essential oils were used in the morning and lavender and orange in the evening. All patients showed significant improvement in personal orientation related to cognitive function based on the assessment tools typically used for assessing the stages of dementia.[9]

Anticarcinogenic activity

A review article on the role of *d*-limonene confirms that it has well-established chemoprotective activity against many types of cancer. Evidence from a phase I clinical trial shows a partial response in a patient with breast cancer, and stable disease for more than six months in three patients with colorectal cancer. The author states that *d*-limonene induces phase I and phase II carcinogen metabolising enzymes (cytochrome P450), which metabolise carcinogens to less toxic forms and prevent the interaction of chemical carcinogens with DNA.[10]

Schnaubelt explains that limonene inhibits phase I liver detoxification enzymes, while simultaneously inducing phase II enzymes. This means that the production of potentially toxic or even carcinogenic compounds which can sometimes occur in the phase I process are slowed and the accelerated phase II process removes them instantly.[11]

He explains that limonene selectively inhibits the reproduction of tumour cells via the inhibition of HMG CoA reductase.[11]

Antidepressant activity

Studies suggest that the aroma of citrus essential oils can restore stress-induced immunosuppression. It is well known that the dysregulation of the neuroendocrine and immune function is associated with psychosomatic or psychiatric disorders. In one study, researchers created a citrus fragrance using lemon, orange and bergamot essential oils and *cis*-4-hexanol (an aroma chemical with a green grassy smell). 20 depressed male inpatients receiving antidepressant medications were divided into two groups. One group was given antidepressants alone and the other group was exposed to the citrus blend continuously, while having their medication reduced weekly until their depression remitted (within 4 to 11 weeks). The Hamilton Rating Scale for Depression and the Self-Rating Depression Scale were used to evaluate psychiatric states. Both scores were improved in both groups. By the end of 11 weeks, 9 of the 12 patients in the citrus blend group had reduced their antidepressant drug intake to zero, while the other three had reduced their dosage by 50-75%. On the other hand, all subjects in the antidepressant group still needed their usual dose of antidepressants at remission. Urinary cortisol and dopamine levels were significantly lower after the treatment in the citrus blend group. The citrus blend group also had a significantly higher NK cell activity compared to the antidepressant group.[12]

The researchers suggested that the use of citrus fragrances in the treatment of depression could be of psychoneuroimmunological benefit, although caution was recommended with the interpretation of this study due to the small size.[12]

Antifungal activity

Lemon oil has exhibited high antifungal activity in vitro against *Candida albicans*.[13]

An in vitro study demonstrated that lemon oil had antifungal activity against a wide range of moulds commonly associated with food spoilage such as *Aspergillus niger, Aspergillus flavus, Penicillium chrysogenum* and *Penicillium verrucosum*.[14]

Antimicrobial activity

Lemon oil has exhibited antimicrobial properties.[15]

Anxiolytic activity

The anxiolytic action of lemon, lavender and rose oil was examined using an elevated plus-maze task, a forced swimming test and an open field task in mice. Lemon oil had the strongest antistress effect in all three behavioural tasks. The pharmacological mechanisms were investigated and it was found that lemon oil significantly accelerated the metabolic turnover of dopamine in the hippocampus and of 5-HT (serotonin) in the prefrontal cortex and striatum. The researchers stated that the results suggest that lemon oil possesses anxiolytic, antidepressant-like effects via suppression of dopamine activity related to enhanced 5-HTnergic neurons.[16]

Gallstone dissolution

In vitro, *d*-limonene dissolved gallstones within two hours. In patients post gallstone surgery, an infusion of 20 mL *d*-limonene every other day dissolved gallstones overlooked by surgery. In some patients, gallstone dissolution occurred after only three infusions.[10]

Gastroprotective activity

A study investigated the gastroprotective mechanism of action from lemon oil, *d*-limonene and β-pinene. The minimum inhibitory concentration (MIC) against *Helicobacter pylori* was determined in vitro. Both lemon oil and *d*-limonene demonstrated very effective gastroprotective effect. It was suggested that the gastroprotective mechanism is involved with prostaglandin E2.[18]

In a double-blind, placebo-controlled study, 13 participants suffering from mild/moderate to severe heartburn were randomised to *d*-limonene or placebo. The limonene group received 1,000 mg of *d*-limonene once a day in a capsule, while the placebo group received an identical capsule containing soyabean oil. By day 14, 86% of participants taking the *d*-limonene achieved complete relief of symptoms, compared to 29% of the participants in the placebo group.[10]

d-limonene has been shown to be effective in relieving occasional heartburn and gastroesophageal reflux disorder. In vitro studies suggest that it may neutralise the effect of gastric acid by coating the stomach wall and protecting the mucosal lining from gastric acid exposure.[10]

Neuroprotective activity

The in vitro effect of lemon oil on heat shock-induced apoptosis of both human and rat astrocytes was investigated. The results demonstrated that the astrocytes pretreated with lemon oil inhibited heat shock-induced apoptosis. Heat shock-induced DNA fragmentation (a characteristic of apoptosis) was inhibited by the lemon pretreatment, as were the condensation of nuclear chromatin, the activation of caspase-3 and the cleavage of poly-ADP-ribose polymerase (PARP). It was suggested that lemon oil may modulate apoptosis through inhibition of PARP cleavage by preventing caspase-3 activation. It was also suggested that lemon oil may have neuroprotective effects on the brain.[19]

Nootropic activity

A clinical trial tested the effect of odours on cognitive functions. Lemon oil was found to activate anticipation and attention processes. It was noted that the effect increased with increasing odour concentration. The researchers also noted that if a subject preferred a particular odour, the effect of the odour was stronger.[17]

Actions

Actions commonly cited in aromatherapy

Antidepressant, antifungal, antimicrobial, antirheumatic, antiseptic, antispasmodic, astringent, bactericidal, carminative, depurative, diaphoretic, digestive, diuretic, febrifuge, haemostatic, hypotensive, immunostimulant, rubefacient, tonic[2,20,21,22,23,24]

Actions supported by clinical studies

Antifungal, antiseptic, bactericidal, chemoprotective, hepatic

Comment

Evidence supports that many of the therapeutic properties attributed to lemon oil are due to the high *d*-limonene content, which has a strong chemoprotective and hepatoprotective activity.[10,11] This is why lemon oil has often been referred to as a detoxifier or depurative. Review of traditional uses and clinical evidence also supports the role of lemon oil in gastroprotective activity and as an effective antimicrobial agent. Many studies confirm that citrus aromas are uplifting and can be helpful to alleviate stress, anxiety and depression.

There has been some confusion regarding the properties of lemon juice, assuming that these properties also apply to the essential oil. For example, the antiscorbutic property often attributed to the oil is only a property of the lemon juice.

L

Aromatherapy Uses

Clinical aromatherapy

Circulatory system

Lemon oil is an excellent tonic for the circulatory system, reducing blood viscosity and helping to break up plaque deposits in the arteries, reducing cholesterol.[22,23,24,25]

It is an excellent remedy for tonifying the blood vessels and it may be used on varicose veins, broken capillaries, haemorrhoids and nosebleeds.[2,23,24]

Fischer-Rizzi recommends mixing lemon oil in a 1:1 ratio with cypress oil in a skin lotion or compress for treating varicose veins.[25]

Detoxification

Lemon oil can be used as a mild detoxifier and is very useful for the treatment of toxaemia or for cellulite.[21]

Schnaubelt states that lemon oil can be blended with other essential oils to support liver regeneration and detoxification. This is why he recommends that we eat citrus fruits or use essential oils that are rich in limonene, such as orange or lemon.[11]

Holmes refers to lemon oil as a liver restorative and decongestant. He recommends using it for liver and biliary congestion, metabolic and microbial toxicosis, headaches, and rheumatic and arthritic conditions.[2]

L

Immune system

Lemon oil is often referred to as having immune-stimulating properties. It is suggested that it stimulates the production of white blood cells to fight off infectious organisms.[23]

Psychological

Fischer-Rizzi states that lemon oil clears the mind and aids in the decision-making process without overstimulating the mind. In fact, it can be very calming for those who are emotionally overwrought. She describes lemon as a 'rational oil', and recommends it to calm stormy emotional outbursts or help avoid them altogether.[25]

Holmes recommends lemon oil for mental fogginess and mental fatigue with poor concentration. It is beneficial for those who wake up in the morning feeling low energy. He also recommends lemon oil for eliminating negative thinking, pessimism and depression. He best sums up lemon's influence on our psyche:

> *Lemon oil can also go a long way to dig us out of the rut of routine, habit-bound, unimaginative patterns of thinking. By creating light and clarity in the psyche, it can help shrink gloomy, negative, depressive thoughts – which can be considered a mental kind of congestive damp.*[2]

Respiratory system

Lemon oil's strong antiviral action makes it beneficial to alleviate colds and flu, especially when there is yellow or green catarrh.[20,21,22,23,24]

Skin care

Lemon oil acts as an astringent counteracting overproduction of sebum, and is especially useful for teenage problem skin. It tones aging skin and has antibacterial properties that are beneficial for the treatment of acne and boils.[21,23] It is recommended for treating warts and verrucae. For this purpose, it is best to apply the undiluted oil.[23]

Energetics, psyche and subtle uses

Energetics

Lemon oil is *cooling* and *drying* and it is recommended to clear *heat*, *dampness* and phlegm. For this reason, it is considered an excellent detoxifying essential oil.[24]

Holmes states that lemon oil strengthens and calms the *Shen* and eliminates *damp* conditions. Whenever the *Shen* is weak, we feel mental fatigue, lack focus, and may experience headaches. Whenever the *Shen* is feeling agitated, we suffer from anxiety, restless and insomnia.

Damp conditions are often associated with chronic indigestion, abdominal bloating, lethargy, heaviness of the body and water retention.[2]

Mojay explains that lemon oil acts mainly on the Earth Element as it is a pancreatic stimulant and mental decongestant.[24]

According to the Five Elements, lemon oil tonifies the Wood Element and helps to reduce *excess damp* associated with the Earth Element. According to the principles of Ayurveda, lemon oil would strengthen *Vata* and *Pitta* and help to reduce *Kapha*.

Personality

Worwood states that lemon personalities sparkle and are full of life, with a very positive approach in the form of an unshakeable confidence in everything that they do. Lemon is like a breath of fresh air, positively wonderful to have around, not too bothered by the struggles and strains of living and able to take everything quite calmly.[26]

Worwood states that, while a lemon personality may appear sweet, they can become very critical and not understand why others cannot do something as good as them. She says that they are inclined to become workaholics and will do better owning their own business where it is easier for them to set the pace.[26]

According to Myers-Briggs personality types, the lemon personality is likely to be an ENTP. ENTPs are energetic, enthusiast and confident. Many are nonconformists. They are innovative and have excellent analytical ability and are resourceful in solving problems. They like variety and change. Because they have so many interests, they feel that life is too short. They feel relaxed when they do new things. They enjoy travelling to exotic places. They can be inspirational and rise to leadership positions because of their quick mind. They work best when interacting with many people. They are optimistic, charming and quick-witted. They value their freedom and independence. They seek growth, excitement, and continuous improvement in their relationship. They enjoy debating and they like to have the last say. They may deny emotional pain and keep busy to avoid dealing with their feelings. They can be arrogant, argumentative and insensitive.

Subtle

Fischer-Rizzi describes lemon as an essential oil with high vibrations. She explains that essential oils with high vibrations lift one's spirits, especially when one may be feeling mental fatigue.[25] Worwood states that lemon oil is spiritually cleansing. It enables the entire psyche to react to the positive in mortal, as well as divine, love.[27]

Mojay compares lemon oil to rose oil. He states that lemon oil can encourage greater trust and security. It can help to open the heart by alleviating fears of emotional involvement and of losing oneself in another person.[24]

Zeck refers to lemon oil as a delightful aromatic 'spa for the brain':

> *If you are feeling confused and out of your depth, lemon's bracing and enlivening effect upon your senses will sharpen your progress, clear your head and pave the way for rational thinking.*
>
> *Confusion can bring irrational emotional outbursts and such behaviours are usually not welcomed or tolerated by others. Lemon helps to cut through confusion and is a delightfully aromatic spa for the brain.*[28]

She also explains that lemon oil will enhance rational, logical thinking and any intellectual pursuits.[28]

Keim Loughran & Bull state that lemon is a joyous and energising essential oil that helps to open and strengthen our intuition. It encourages us to be fully present, focused and clear for intuitive impressions, helping us stay grounded in the heart and the objective of the mind.[29]

Dosage and Administration

Blending

Aromatherapy

Lemon adds a refreshing top note to all aromatherapy blends. It can often be used liberally in a blend without having a strong impact on the overall aroma of the blend. The fresh, invigorating scent of lemon oil softens and complements the spicy, warm scent of oils such as ginger, black pepper, clove bud and cinnamon bark. Such blends would be quite energising and warming and may be used to alleviate fatigue.

To create a detoxification blend that can be used in a bath or massage oil, consider blending lemon oil with essential oils such as juniper berry, carrot seed, sweet fennel, sweet orange, everlasting or rosemary.

As a liver tonic, consider blending lemon oil with essential oils such as carrot seed, everlasting or rosemary ct. verbenone.

To promote mental clarity, and alleviate fatigue and tiredness, consider blending lemon oil with essential oils such as basil, black pepper, geranium, ginger, lemongrass, peppermint or spearmint.

To create a blend that is antiseptic and antimicrobial, consider blending lemon oil with essential oils such as 1,8-cineole-rich eucalypts, fragonia, lavender, manuka, niaouli, tea tree or thyme.

Perfumery

Lemon oil is extensively used in perfumes for its refreshing, sweet fruity note. Arctander says it is the most important ingredient in old-fashioned citrus-type colognes, and is used as a top note ingredient in many perfumes.[4]

Mode of administration

Bath

Full body bath, foot bath

Topical

Massage, ointment, skin care

Inhalation

Direct inhalation, diffuser, oil vaporiser

Ingestion

Schnaubelt recommends ingesting lemon essential oil to support the detoxification process. He recommends 1 drop of essential oil in a glass of water.[11]

Safety Profile

General safety

Lemon oil is non-toxic, non-irritant. Sensitisation can occur in some people, and it should not be used on the skin prior to exposure to the sun as it is phototoxic.[21,23,24,25,30]

Lemon oil is sensitising if it is oxidised. IFRA recommends that essential oils rich in limonene should only be used when the level of peroxides are kept to the lowest practical level. This can be achieved by adding antioxidants.[30]

IFRA standards recommend expressed lemon oil be limited to a maximum of 2% in products applied to the skin. This does not apply to soaps or wash-off products.[30]

Schnaubelt recommends only using lemon oil obtained exclusively from certified organically grown fruits that are pesticide-free, because most industrially cultivated citrus plantations are invariably sprayed with heavy doses of chemicals.[11]

Contraindications

If it is applied to the skin at over the maximum use level recommended by IFRA, the skin should not be exposed to sunlight or sunbed rays for 12 hours.[30]

Regulatory guidelines

Lemon essential oil has GRAS status.

L

References

1. Weiss EA. *Essential oil crops*. CAB International, Wallingford, 1997.
2. Holmes P. *Aromatica: a clinical guide to essential oil therapeutics – Vol. I.* Singing Dragon, London, 2016.
3. Guenther E. *The essential oils – Vol. III.* Robert E. Krieger Publishing Company, Malabar, 1949.
4. Arctander S. *Perfume and flavor materials of natural origin.* Allured Publishing, Carol Stream, 1994.
5. Lawrence BM. *Essential oils 1981-1987.* Allured Publishing, Wheaton, 1989.
6. Grieve M. *A modern herbal – Vol. II.* Dover Publications, New York, 1971.
7. Khan I, Abourashed E. *Leung's encyclopedia of common natural ingredients used in food, drugs and cosmetics.* 3rd edn. John Wiley & Sons, New Jersey, 2010.
8. Bardeau F. *Use of essential aromatic oils to purify and deodorise the air.* Chirugien-Dentiste de France (Paris), 1976; 46(319): 53. Cited in Quintessential Aromatics database, 2013.
9. Jimbo D, et al. *Effect of aromatherapy on patients with Alzheimer's disease.* Psychogeriatrics, 2009; 9(4): 173-179.
10. Sun J. *D-limonene: safety and clinical applications.* Alternative Medicine Review, 2007; 12(3): 259-264.
11. Schnaubelt K. *The healing intelligence of essential oils.* Healing Arts Press, Rochester, 2011.
12. Komori T et al. *Effects of citrus fragrance on immune function and depressive states.* Neuro-immunomodulation, 1995; 2(3): 174-180.
13. Szweda P et al. *Essential oils, silver nanoparticles and propolis as alternative agents against fluconazole resistant Candida albicans, Candida glabrata and Candida krusei clinical isolates.* Indian Journal of Microbiology, 2015; 55(2): 175-183. Cited in Quintessential Aromatics database, 2013.
14. Viuda-Martos M et al. *Antifungal activity of lemon (Citrus lemon L.) mandarin (Citrus reticulate L.), grapefruit and orange (Citrus sinensis L.) essential oils.* Food Control, 2008; 19(12): 1130-1138. Cited in Quintessential Aromatics database, 2013.
15. Frassinetti S et al. *Antibacterial and antioxidant activity of essential oils from Citrus spp.* Journal of Essential Oil Research, 2011; 23(1): 27-31. Cited in Quintessential Aromatics database, 2013.
16. Komiya M, Takeuchi T, Harada E. *Lemon oil vapor causes an anti-stress effect via modulating the 5-HT and DA activities in mice.* Behavioural Brain Research, 2006; 172(2): 240-249. Cited in Quintessential Aromatics database, 2013.
17. Kikuchi A et al. *Effect of odours on cardiac response patterns in a reaction time task.* Chemical Senses, 1991; 16(2): 183. Cited in Quintessential Aromatics database, 2013.
18. Rozza AL et al. *Gastroprotective mechanisms of Citrus lemon (Rutaceae) essential oil and its majority compounds limonene and β-pinene: involvement of heat-shock protein-70, vasoactive intestinal peptide, glutathione, sulfhydryl compounds, nitric oxide and prostaglandin E2.* Chemico-Biological Interactions, 2011; 189 (1/2): 82-89. Cited in Quintessential Aromatics database, 2013.
19. Koo HN et al. *Inhibitory effect of apoptosis in human astrocytes CCF-STTG1 cells by lemon oil.* Pharmacological Research, 2002; 45(6): 469-473. Cited in Quintessential Aromatics database, 2013.
20. Lavabre M. *Aromatherapy workbook.* Healing Arts Press, Rochester, 1997.
21. Lawless J. *The encyclopaedia of essential oils.* Element Books, Shaftesbury, 1992.
22. Valnet J. *The practice of aromatherapy.* C.W. Daniel Company, Saffron Walden, 1980.
23. Davis P. *Aromatherapy: an A-Z.* 2nd edn. C.W. Daniel Company, Saffron Walden, 1999.

24. Mojay G. *Aromatherapy for healing the spirit.* Healing Arts Press, Rochester, 1999.
25. Fischer-Rizzi S. *Complete aromatherapy handbook.* Sterling Publishing, New York, 1990.
26. Worwood VA. *The fragrant mind.* Transworld Publishers, London, 1995.
27. Worwood VA. *The fragrant spirit.* Transworld Publishers, London, 1999.
28. Zeck R. *The blossoming heart – aromatherapy for healing and transformation.* Aroma Tours, East Ivanhoe, 2004.
29. Keim Loughran J, Bull R. *Aromatherapy anointing oils.* Frog, Berkeley, 2001.
30. Tisserand R, Young R. *Essential oil safety.* 2nd edn. Churchill Livingstone, Edinburgh, 2014.

Lemongrass

Identification

Botanical name

West Indian lemongrass: *Cymbopogon citratus* DC

East Indian lemongrass: *Cymbopogon flexuosus* Nees ex Steud.

Synonyms

C. citratus: Guatemala lemongrass

C. flexuosus: Cochin lemongrass, native lemongrass

Family

Poaceae (Gramineae)

Botany and origins

Lemongrass oil is produced from two distinctly different species of *Cymbopogon*. *C. citratus* and *C. flexuosus* are tufted perennial grasses with numerous stiff stems arising from a short rhizomatous rootstock.[1]

C. flexuosus is a native of India and *C. citratus* is possibly a native of Sri Lanka. *C. citratus* is widely cultivated all over the world and has been named West Indian lemongrass. India is the major producer of East Indian lemongrass. The major producers of West Indian lemongrass are Guatemala, Madagascar, the Comoro Islands, Brazil, Malaysia and Vietnam.[2]

Weiss states that only young and rapidly expanding leaves synthesise and accumulate essential oils. The leaf blades have a higher oil content than the leaf sheaths, and the oil content increases from the leaf base to the tip.[1]

Arctander explains that, in many tropical regions, the production of lemongrass oil is a by-product of cattle raising. Where cattle feed is scarce, the exhaust grass from distillation can offer a good nutritive when added to molasses residues. He also explains that lemongrass exhausts the soil of nutrients, and that when it is used as feed for cattle, the cows become the perfect recycling machine returning the nutrients back to the soil.[2]

The name *cymbopogon* is derived from the Greek words *kymbe* meaning boat and *pogon* meaning beard, referring to the flower spike arrangement.[3]

Method of extraction

Lemongrass oil is steam-distilled from fresh or partly dried leaves of *C. citratus* or *C. flexuosus*.[2]

Characteristics

Lemongrass oil is a yellow or amber coloured, somewhat viscous liquid with a very strong, fresh grassy, herbaceous and citrus odour. *C. citratus* usually has an earthy undertone reminiscent of citronella oil, while *C. flexuosus* smells sweeter, distinctly more lemony, fresh and light.[2]

Chemical composition

The chemical composition of lemongrass oil was reported as follows:[1]

Constituent	C. flexuosus	C. citratus
myrcene	0.46%	8.2-19.2%
limonene	2.42%	trace
linalool	1.34%	0.8-1.1%
citronellal	0.37%	0.1%
geranyl acetate	1.95%	1.0%
nerol	0.39%	0.3-0.4%
geraniol	3.80%	0.5-0.6%
neral	30.06%	25-28%
geranial	51.19%	45.2-55.9%
citronellol	0.44%	0.1%

C. citratus oil usually has a slightly lower citral (neral + geranial) content and a significantly higher amount of myrcene.

Adulteration

As lemongrass is an inexpensive oil, it is unlikely to be adulterated with synthetics. However, it can be substituted by *Litsea cubeba* of a similar composition.[4]

Pharmacopoeias and standards

The purity, composition and physico-chemical

properties of lemongrass essential oil are defined in ISO 3217:1974 Oil of Lemongrass (*Cymbopogon citratus*).

History and Traditional Uses

History

Lemongrass was originally used as a food flavouring in Asia. The fresh leaves are crushed in water and used as a hair wash and toilet water in India.[1]

Traditional medicine

Lemongrass herb is used in Ayurveda for infectious diseases and fever, and as a sedative and insecticide.[4]

Lemongrass herb is also used in TCM to treat colds, headache, stomach ache, abdominal pain and rheumatic pain.[5]

Herbal

A decoction of lemongrass leaf is taken orally for the relief of sore throat. The tea is also used as an emetic, anti-inflammatory, diuretic and sedative. In South East Asia, the tea is taken orally as an emmenagogue.[3] The dried leaves are commonly used as a 'lemon' flavour in herbal teas.[5]

The German Commission E lists lemongrass oil for disorders and discomforts of the gastrointestinal tract, muscle pain, neuralgia, colds and various nervous disturbances, and for conditions of exhaustion.[6]

L

Food, perfumery and flavouring

It is often used as a masking fragrance in deodorants, waxes, polishes, detergents and insecticides.[1]

Lemongrass oil is used as a fragrance component in soaps and detergents.[5] However, Arctander states that lemongrass is not used in perfumes.[2]

Other uses

The leaves can also be used as a source of cellulose and paper production.

A majority of lemongrass oil is used for citral production, which is then used for perfumery and flavour use or in the synthesis of vitamin A.[1] Citral from lemongrass oil is used in the production of ionones and methyl ionones as well.[2]

Therapeutics

Pharmacology and clinical studies

Many pharmacological studies involving lemongrass essential oil have been published. A systemic review of these studies will not be attempted. Rather, I have chosen a selection of studies that support the traditional and clinical uses.

Antifungal activity

Lemongrass oil has been reported to exhibit excellent antifungal properties.[3,7,8]

Undiluted lemongrass oil was more effective than commercial fungicides such as benzoic acid, nystatin and tineafax against pathogenic fungi. It was stated that the antifungal activity was associated with the high citral content.[9]

Another in vitro study confirmed that lemongrass oil exhibited the most effective killing activity and possessed the strongest inhibitory effect on *Candida* biofilm formation. The oil was also found to inhibit germ tube formation, which might affect adherence.[10]

Lemongrass oil exhibited significant antifungal activity against *Candida albicans, Candida tropicalis* and *Aspergillus niger*. It has been suggested that the strong inhibitory effect of lemongrass against *Candida* species may result from a synergy of monoterpenes and other compounds such as cymene, terpinene and linalool.[11]

Anti-inflammatory activity

An in vivo study confirmed that a number of aldehydes in lemongrass oil had antioxidant activity that may have contributed to the anti-inflammatory effects observed when orally administered to rats. It has been suggested that lemongrass oil inhibits prostaglandin biosynthesis in the same way as salicylate drugs and non-steroid anti-inflammatory drugs.[11,12]

Citral, a major component of lemongrass essential oil, has been shown to inhibit the production of interleukin (IL 1β) and interleukin 6 (IL-6) in lipopolysaccharide (LPS)-stimulated alveolar macrophages of normal mice. Citral also inhibits the production of pro-inflammatory cytokines such as tumour necrosis factor-α (TNF-α).[11]

Antimicrobial activity

Many studies have confirmed that lemongrass oil has excellent antimicrobial activities.[3,13,14,15,16] It has been suggested that lemongrass and other essential oils rich in oxygenated compounds such as aldehydes and monoterpene alcohols are more active, whereas those essential oils containing larger amounts of monoterpene hydrocarbons or sesquiterpenes had lower antimicrobial activity.[13]

Another study demonstrated that lemongrass oil exhibited excellent antimicrobial activity in the vapour phase, which was significantly enhanced when used in combination with negative ions.[8]

An in vitro study confirmed that lemongrass oil exhibited significant antibacterial activity against

Streptococcus pyogenes, which plays an important role in the pathogenesis of tonsillitis. Lemongrass oil was as effective as *Cinnamomum verum*, *Thymus vulgaris* ct. thymol, *Origanum compactum* and *Satureja montana* essential oils, which are also well-known for their potent antimicrobial activity.[17]

Many cleansers used to disinfect surfaces contain harsh and irritant chemicals. In this study, surface cleansers containing essential oils and citric acid were evaluated for their disinfectant activity. A blend of lemongrass and orange oil exhibited the highest disinfectant activity when used as a surface disinfectant. It was recommended that, if it was used as a surface cleanser in hospitals and households, it may significantly reduce the spread of pathogens from environmental surfaces to healthcare workers and the general public.[18]

A study compared a topical gel containing various essential oils and evaluated their antibacterial activity against methicillin-resistant *Staphylococcus aureus* (MRSA) skin infections. The topical gel was formulated using Carbopol 940, hydroxypropylmethyl cellulose and sodium carboxymethyl cellulose. The study then compared the gel blended with thyme oil alone, the gel blended with lemongrass alone, and a blend of lemongrass and thyme oil. All the gel preparations exhibited strong antibacterial activity; however, the antibacterial activity of the gel containing the two essential oils was approximately the sum of those containing the individual oils. It was also noted that, when applied to the human skin, there was no skin irritation.[19]

Antinociceptive activity

Many studies have confirmed that lemongrass oil exhibited a significant antinociceptive activity.[3,20]

Another study confirmed that myrcene was the most potent analgesic component of lemongrass essential oil. It was reported that, unlike the central analgesic effect of morphine, myrcene did not cause tolerance on repeated injection in rats. Myrcene has a similar direct analgesic effect to peripherally acting opiates.[21]

Cardioprotective activity

An in vivo study involving mice confirmed that oral doses of lemongrass oil at a dose of 200 mg / kg of body weight exhibited cardioprotective and anti-lipid peroxidative comparable with that of vitamin E.[22]

Cholesterol lowing activity

A capsule containing 140 mg lemongrass oil was given daily to 22 individuals with high cholesterol levels for 90 days. The study demonstrated that lemongrass significantly lowered the cholesterol levels of 36% of the participants. It was suggested that lemongrass oil suppressed the activity of HMG-CoA (3-hydroxy-3-methylglutaryl coenzyme A) reductase.[23]

Insecticidal activity

C. citratus and *C. flexuosus* oils were found to give almost complete protection against *Anopheles culicifacies* (a principal malaria carrier) for up to 11 hours. The oils were considered comparable to synthetic repellents of dimethyl and dibutyl phthalate.[24]

An in vivo study investigated the topical application of 1.73 g of lemongrass oil in 22.73 g of petroleum jelly-based cream. The results of the study showed that lemongrass essential oil can provide substantial protection against mosquitos and insect bites similar to that of synthetic DEET-based products. It was stated to be the only essential oil to provide 80 to 90% protection. The authors of the study recommended blending lemongrass with other essential oils to provide longer protection of up to six hours. They also stated that concentrations above 3% could provide protection for about three to four hours without causing any skin irritation.[25]

Another study also confirmed that lemongrass oil exhibited protection against biting from two mosquito species *Anopheles aegypti* (98.66 minutes protection and 0.97% biting rate) and for *Anopheles dirus* (210 minutes protection and 0.93% biting rate). A blend of lemongrass and basil provided the most effective repellency activity.[26]

Oral health

A study reviewed the role of lemongrass in improving dental health. Lemongrass oil is recommended for the prevention and treatment of periodontitis. It has also been recommended in mouthwash or toothpaste to prevent plaque formation.[27]

Sedative activity

Lemongrass oil was found to have sedative and hypnotic activity through pentobarbital sleeping time, when orally administered to mice. The oil was also found to have anxiolytic activity and anticonvulsant activity.[28]

The aim of another study was to examine the anxiolytic effect of lemongrass oil aroma on healthy human volunteers who were subjected to an anxiogenic situation. 40 male volunteers were allocated to different groups. One group inhaled lemongrass essential oil, another group inhaled tea tree oil and another was the non-aromatic control group. Although the researchers concluded more investigations were necessary to clarify the clinical relevance of lemongrass oil as an anxiety treatment, this study showed that a very brief exposure to lemongrass oil has a perceived anxiolytic effect.[29]

Actions

Actions commonly cited in aromatherapy

Analgesic, antidepressant, antimicrobial, antiseptic, astringent, bactericidal, carminative, deodorant, febrifuge, fungicidal, galactagogue, insecticidal, nervine, sedative (nervous system), tonic[30,31,32]

Actions supported by clinical studies

Analgesic, antimicrobial, antiseptic, insecticidal, nervine

Comment

Many studies have confirmed that lemongrass oil has potent antifungal and antimicrobial activities. However, it does present a high risk of skin irritancy and sensitising activity on the skin. It is interesting to note that some studies have confirmed the efficacy of lemongrass oil as an antimicrobial agent when vaporised.

Lemongrass oil has a fresh, green and strong citrus aroma, which is enlivening and uplifting. Holmes states that when it is inhaled in low amounts it induces feelings of renewal and transformation, and helps to resolve day-to-day distressing feelings and emotions.[33]

While numerous studies have demonstrated that lemongrass oil potentially has many pharmacological activities, I would like to see more studies to examine safe ways of administering the essential oil to ensure there is no risk of dermal irritation and sensitisation.

While lemongrass oil has potent antifungal activity, I would never recommend using lemongrass oil neat on the skin to treat fungal infection because of the high risk associated with dermal irritation and sensitisation.

Aromatherapy Uses

Clinical aromatherapy

Antimicrobial

The antimicrobial activity of lemongrass oil indicates that it would be excellent in a vaporiser to disinfect the air.[34]

Lemongrass oil is often recommended for a broad range of fungal infections including athlete's foot, candidiasis, oral thrush, nail-bed infections, tinea and jock itch. Holmes recommends lemongrass oil for the treatment of cold sores and shingles.[33]

Digestive system

Lemongrass oil is considered a stimulant of the digestive system and is recommended for colitis, indigestion and gastroenteritis.[30,31,34]

Musculoskeletal system

Lemongrass oil is referred to as the connective tissue oil. Lemongrass tightens the elastin fibres in the epidermis and in the subcutis. The oil is recommended in the after-care of sports injuries, sprains, bruises and dislocations.[35]

Holmes recommends lemongrass for muscular tension and pain, acute arthritis, rheumatic pain and tendinitis.[33]

Psychological

Holmes states that the scent of lemongrass oil promotes emotional and mental renewal. He recommends lemongrass whenever we are overcome by negative and distressed feelings, and whenever we experience mental fatigue, poor concentration, mental and emotional confusion, and negative thinking and pessimism.[33]

The refreshing scent of lemongrass oil is uplifting and energising. It aids our logical thinking and is ideal to use at home or work or wherever clear, fresh thinking and good concentration are needed.[34]

Lemongrass is considered a secret aid for people who have trouble starting in the morning. Fischer-Rizzi describes the effect of the scent of lemongrass as taking a refreshing, cool morning shower.[34]

Skin care

Lemongrass oil is often recommended as a skin tonic and it is used in cleansing lotions and creams for its astringent properties.[30,33,34]

One study found that a hair tonic with 10% lemongrass oil was very effective for treating dandruff.[36] However, this is a rather high concentration, and the risk of irritation and sensitisation to the scalp would be very high. I would be very cautious in the use of lemongrass oil for skin care as it may cause dermal irritation or sensitisation.

Energetics, psyche & subtle uses

Energetics

Holmes states that lemongrass oil regulates the *Qi* and harmonises the *Shen*. It is recommended for conditions associated with irritability, moodiness, anger and agitated depression.[33]

According to the principles of the Five Elements, lemongrass oil strenghtens the Wood Element.

Subtle

Worwood states that the scent of lemongrass oil helps to clear regrets and shame. It encourages us to forgive those who have dishonoured and discredited us.[37]

Holmes states that the green and lemony scent of lemongrass oil helps to promote emotional renewal. He explains that it dispels pessimism and mental depression and helps to open the door to new positive experiences.[33]

Zeck explains that the intense radiant energy of lemongrass oil inspires expansion on all levels. She recommends it whenever there is a sense of restriction or limitation in life. It lifts the spirits and gets things moving again. Lemongrass encourages us to embark on a glorious journey of discovery.[38]

Dosage and Administration

Blending

Aromatherapy

To alleviate mental fatigue and poor concentration, consider blending lemongrass oil with essential oils such as basil, bergamot, black pepper, ginger, lemon, cold-pressed lime, peppermint or rosemary.

To make an disinfectant blend that can be added to a vaporiser, consider blending lemongrass oil with essential oils such as cinnamon bark, fragonia, kunzea, lemon, manuka, sweet orange, tea tree or thyme.

For the relief of muscular aches and pains, consider blending lemongrass oil with essential oils such as cajeput, ginger, kunzea, lemon-scented eucalyptus, spike lavender, peppermint or rosemary.

When lemongrass oil is blended with essential oils such as clove bud, cinnamon bark or tea tree, it becomes a very effective antifungal blend.

To promote mental and emotional clarity and a sense of optimism, consider blending lemongrass oil with essential oils such as bergamot, cold-pressed lime, petitgrain or sweet orange.

As a natural insect repellent, consider blending lemongrass oil with essential oils such as cajeput, Atlas cedarwood, Virginian cedarwood, Buddha wood, citronella, 1,8-cineole-rich eucalypts, peppermint eucalyptus, niaouli, spike lavender, peppermint or tea tree.

Perfumery

Lemongrass oil is not commonly used in perfumery.[2]

Mode of administration

Bath

Lemongrass oil is not recommended for use in a bath.

Topical

Massage

Inhalation

Direct inhalation, diffuser, oil vaporiser

Safety Profile

General safety

Lemongrass oil is not considered toxic. Lis-Balchin cites studies that show there was no irritation or sensitisation at 4% on humans; however, it is regarded as a very sensitising essential oil.[4]

Tisserand & Young recommend a dermal maximum of 0.7% to avoid skin sensitisation. They recommend not using on people with hypersensitive, diseased or damaged skin, and not to use topically on children under 2 years of age.[39]

Contraindications

Tisserand & Young recommend caution for oral use of lemongrass oil for individuals on diabetes medication and during pregnancy.[39]

Lis-Balchin recommends not using topically during pregnancy and lactation due to the possibility of sensitisation. She also states that the use of the essential oil in a diffuser should not prove hazardous if used in moderation.[4]

Regulatory guidelines

Lemongrass oil has GRAS status.

L

References

1. Weiss EA. *Essential oil crops.* CAB International, Wallingford, 1997.
2. Arctander S. *Perfume and flavor materials of natural origin.* Allured Publishing, Carol Stream, 1994.
3. Shah G et al. *Scientific basis for the therapeutic use of Cymbopogon citratus, Stapf (lemongrass).* Journal of Advanced Pharmaceutical Technology & Research, 2011; 2(1): 3-8. doi: 10.4103/2231-4040.79796.
4. Lis-Balchin M. *Aromatherapy science – a guide for healthcare professionals.* Pharmaceutical Press, London, 2006.
5. Khan I, Abourashed E. *Leung's encyclopedia of common natural ingredients used in food, drugs and cosmetics.* 3rd edn. John Wiley & Sons, New Jersey, 2010.
6. Blumenthal M et al. *The complete German commission E monographs: therapeutic guide to herbal medicine.* American Botanical Council, Austin, 1998.
7. de Bona da Silva C et al. *Antifungal activity of lemongrass oil and citral against Candida spp.*

The Brazilian Journal of Infectious Diseases, 2008; 12(1): 63-66.
8. Tyagi AK et al. *Liquid and vapour-phase antifungal activities of selected essential oils against Candida albicans: microscopic observations and chemical characterisation of Cymbopogon citratus*. BMC Complementary and Alternative Medicine, 2010; 10: 65. doi: 10.1186/1472-6882-10-65.
9. Qamar S et al. *Antifungal activity of lemongrass essential oils*. Pakistan Journal of Science and Industrial Research, 1992; 35(6): 246-248. Cited in Quintessential Aromatics database, 2013.
10. Taweechaisupapong S et al. *Inhibitory effect of lemongrass oil and its major constituents on Candida biofilm and germ tube formation*. South African Journal of Botany, 2012; 81: 95-102. Cited in Quintessential Aromatics database, 2013.
11. Boukhatem MN et al. *Lemon grass (Cymbopogon citratus) essential oil as a potent anti-inflammatory and antifungal drugs*. Libyan Journal of Medicine, 2014; 9(1): 25431. doi: 10.3402/ljm.v9.25431.
12. Gbenou JD et al. *Phytochemical composition of Cymbopogon citratus and Eucalyptus citriodora essential oils and their anti-inflammatory and analgesic properties on Wistar rats*. Molecular Biology Reports, 2013; 40(2): 1127–1134. doi: 10.1007/s11033-012-2155-1.
13. Chalchat JC et al. *Correlation between chemical composition and antimicrobial activity. VI Activity of some African essential oils*. Journal of Essential Oil Research, 1997; 9(1): 67-75. Cited in Quintessential Aromatics database, 2013.
14. Onawunmi GO. *Evaluation of the antifungal activity of lemongrass oil*. International Journal of Crude Drug Research, 1989; 27(2): 121-126. Cited in the Aromatherapy Database, by Bob Harris, Essential Oil Resource Consultants, UK, 2000.
15. Onawunmi GO et al. *Antibacterial constituents in the essential oil of Cymbopogon citratus (DC.) Stapf*. Journal of Ethnopharmacology, 1984; 12(3): 279-286. Cited in the Aromatherapy Database, by Bob Harris, Essential Oil Resource Consultants, UK, 2000.
16. Onawunmi GO, Ogunlana EO. *A study of the antibacterial activity of the essential oil of lemongrass (Cymbopogon citratus (DC.) Stapf)*. International Journal of Crude Drug Research, 1986; 24(2): 64-68. Cited in the Aromatherapy Database, by Bob Harris, Essential Oil Resource Consultants, UK, 2000.
17. Sfeir J et al. *In vitro antibacterial activity of essential oils against Streptococcus pyogenes*. Evidence-Based Complementary and Alternative Medicine, 2013; 2013: 269161. doi: 10.1155/2013/269161.
18. Baiju N et al. *Development of a novel surface disinfectant composition containing essential oils and a fruit acid against nosocomial pathogens commonly associated with environmental surfaces*. International Journal of Essential Oil Therapeutics, 2008; 2(1): 9-14. Cited in Quintessential Aromatics database, 2013.
19. Shukr MH, Metwally GF. *Evaluation of topical gel bases formulated with various essential oils for antibacterial activity against methicillin-resistant Staphylococcus aureus*. Tropical Journal of pharmaceutical Research, 2013; 12(6): 877-884. Cited in Quintessential Aromatics database, 2013.
20. Chandrashekar KS, Prasanna KS. *Analgesic and anti-inflammatory activities of the essential oil from Cymbopogon flexuosus*. Pharmacognosy Journal, 2010; 2(14): 23-25. Cited in Quintessential Aromatics database, 2013.
21. Lorenzetti BB et al. *Myrcene mimics the peripheral analgesic activity of lemongrass tea*. Journal of Ethnopharmacology, 1991; 34(1): 43-48. Cited in Quintessential Aromatics database, 2013.
22. Gayathri K et al. *Cardioprotective effect of lemon grass as evidenced by biochemical and histopathological changes in experimentally induced cardiotoxicity*. Human and Experimental Toxicology, 2010; 30(8): 1073-1082. doi : 10.1177/0960327110386391.
23. Elson CE et al. *Impact of lemongrass oil, an essential oil, on serum cholesterol*. Lipids, 1989; 24(8): 677-679. Cited in Quintessential Aromatics database, 2013.
24. Ansari MA, Razdan RK. *Relative efficacy of various oils in repelling mosquitoes*. Indian Journal of Malariology, 32(3): 104-111. Cited in the Aromatherapy Database, by Bob Harris, Essential Oil Resource Consultants, UK, 2000.
25. Adeniran OI, Fabiyi E. *A cream formulation of an effective mosquito repellent: a topical product from lemongrass oil (Cymbopogon citratus) Stapf*. Journal of Natural Products and Plant Resources, 2002; 2(2): 322-327.
26. Sritabutra D et al. *Evaluation of herbal essential oil as repellents against Aedes aegypti (L.) and Anopheles dirus Peyton & Harrion*. Asian Pacific Journal of Tropical Biomedicine, 2011; 1(1): S124-S128. Cited in Quintessential Aromatics database, 2013.
27. Rajesvari R, Lakshmi T. *Lemon grass oil for improvement of oral health*. Dental Hypotheses, 2013; 4(4): 115-117. doi: 10.4103/2155-8213.122671.
28. Blanco MM et al. *Neurobehavioural effect of essential oil of Cymbopogon citratus in mice*. Phytomedicine, 2009; 16(2/3): 265-270. Cited in Quintessential Aromatics database, 2013.
29. Goes TC et al. *Effect of lemongrass aroma on experimental anxiety in humans*. Journal of

L

Alternative and Complementary Medicine, 2015; 21(12): 766-773. Cited in Quintessential Aromatics database, 2013.
30. Lawless J. *The encyclopaedia of essential oils.* Element Books, Shaftesbury, 1992.
31. Lavabre M. *Aromatherapy workbook.* Healing Arts Press, Rochester, 1997.
32. Davis P. *Aromatherapy: an A-Z.* 2nd edn. C.W. Daniel Company, Saffron Walden, 1999.
33. Holmes P. *Aromatica: a clinical guide to essential oil therapeutics – Vol. I.* Singing Dragon, London, 2016.
34. Fischer-Rizzi S. *Complete aromatherapy handbook.* Sterling Publishing, New York, 1990.
35. Gumbel D. *Principles of holistic skin therapy with herbal essences.* Karl F Haug Publishers, Heidelberg, 1986.
36. Chaisripipat W et al. *Anti-dandruff hair tonic containing lemongrass (Cymbopogon flexuosus) oil.* Forschende Komplementarmedizin, 2015; 22(4): 226-229. Cited in Quintessential Aromatics database, 2013.
37. Worwood VA. *The fragrant heavens.* Transworld Publishers, London, 1999.
38. Zeck R. *The blossoming heart – aromatherapy for healing and transformation.* Aroma Tours, East Ivanhoe, 2004.
39. Tisserand R, Young R. *Essential oil safety.* 2nd edn. Churchill Livingstone, Edinburgh, 2014.

Lemon myrtle

Identification

Botanical name

Backhousia citriodora F. Muell.

Synonyms

Lemon-scented myrtle, lemon ironwood

Family

Myrtaceae

Botany and origins

The plant is native to Australia; it is considered a rare plant and typically restricted to South East Queensland. The genus *Backhousia* is named after a British botanist, James Backhouse (1794-1869). The species name *citriodora*, which means 'lemon-scented', is a neo-Latin formation (citrus and odour).[1]

Lemon myrtle is an evergreen native tree, with glassy, green, aromatic leaves, which grows up to a height of 30 m. The leaves are lanceolate and strongly lemon-scented. In early summer, the trees look spectacular with clusters of tiny white four-petalled flowers.[2]

There are two chemotypes: a citral chemotype and a laevo-citronellal chemotype.[3] The citral chemotype is the most common one used in food, cosmetics, personal care and aromatherapy, and is grown commercially in Queensland and northern New South Wales.[4]

Method of extraction

Lemon myrtle essential oil is steam-distilled from the leaves of *B. citriodora.*

Characteristics

Lemon myrtle oil has an intensely fresh lemon-like odour with a sweet undertone. Kerr compares it to lemongrass due to the high citral content; however, there are no grassy or fatty notes.[5]

Chemical composition

The two principal compounds that are responsible for the strong lemony aroma of lemon myrtle essential oil are aldehydes: citral and citronellal. Citral is a collective name used to describe the optical isomer aldehydes — neral and geranial.[2]

The chemical composition of *B. citriodora* essential oil was reported as follows:

myrcene (0.1-0.7 %), 6-methyl-5-hepten-2-one (0.1-2.5%), linalool (0.3-1.0%), citronellal (0.1-0.9%), isoneral (0.6-2.7%), isogeranial (1.0-4.2%), neral (32.0-40.2%), geranial (46.1-60.7%), *trans*-geraniol (0.4-0.7%).[4]

The Australian standard for lemon myrtle essential oil states that the minimum neral content must be 32% and the minimum geranial be 44%.[3]

Adulteration

In 2009, several batches of lemon myrtle had been adulterated with three aldehydes: caprylic aldehyde (n-octyl aldehyde), pelargonic aldehyde (n-nonyl aldehyde) and caprinic aldehyde (n-decyl aldehyde). While these aldehydes are naturally occurring in some citrus oils, none of these aldehydes have ever been found in lemon myrtle essential oil. To prevent future adulteration, the Australian standard is under revision to clearly specify that these three aldehydes should not be present in lemon myrtle essential oil.[3]

Tisserand & Young state that lemon myrtle oil may be adulterated with synthetic citral.[6]

Pharmacopoeias and standards

The purity, composition and physico-chemical

properties of lemon myrtle essential oil are defined in AS 4941-2001 Oil of *Backhousia citriodora*, Citral Type (Lemon Myrtle).

History and Traditional Uses

History

Lemon myrtle oil was first distilled in 1853 by a German Botanist Baron Ferdinand von Mueller (1825-1896), who sent a sample back to Germany to be used in the essential oil industry. Joseph H Maiden reported on the potential use of lemon myrtle for commercial production in 1889, and the German company Schimmel & Co. was the first to identify the primary ingredient, citral, which gives the oil the distinctive lemon fragrance and flavour.[7]

In the early 1900s, lemon myrtle was used as lemon flavouring and fragrance in Australia. However, less expensive high citral essential oils such as lemongrass and *Litsea* soon became more popular.[9]

During World War II, lemon myrtle essential oil was used to flavour soft drinks due to a shortage of lemon essence.[8]

The lemon myrtle industry was given a boost by its rediscovery in the 1990s as a promising culinary herb in Australian cuisine, fusing native flavours into a number of dishes.[8]

L

Traditional medicine

Indigenous Australians have long used lemon myrtle for cooking and healing purposes.[4]

Food, perfumery and flavouring

Lemon myrtle leaves are used in food applications as a fresh or dried herb. It has become popular in many countries as a herbal tea.

Lemon myrtle leaves have now become very popular in Australian cuisine. It imparts an exquisite lemon tang to seafood and chicken dishes. It has replaced the traditional kaffir lime leaves often used in South East Asian dishes.[1]

Citral is extensively used within the food and flavouring industry as a lemon flavour. It is also used as a raw material in the production of vitamin A.[5]

Therapeutics

Pharmacology and clinical studies

Antimicrobial activity

Many studies have been done confirming lemon myrtle's antibacterial and antifungal properties.[4,5]

The antimicrobial activity of lemon myrtle oil is believed to be directly related to the high citral content; however, the importance of some of the minor components such as linalool, citronellal and β-myrcene in combination with citral for enhanced antimicrobial activity have also been reported.[4]

An in vitro study confirmed that lemon myrtle essential oil was effective in inhibiting all methicillin-resistant *Staphylococcus aureus* (MRSA) growth.[9]

The antimicrobial activity of lemon myrtle oil has also been used in the treatment of *Molluscum contagiosum* in children. A 10% v/v in olive oil as a topical application had shown a reduction of greater than 90% in the number of lesions in children. It was noted that no child had any adverse reaction or displayed signs of discomfort from the application of lemon myrtle. It was concluded due to the lack of cytotoxic effects that lemon myrtle oil was acting directly on viral propagation.[10]

An in vitro study investigated and compared the antimicrobial activity of lemon myrtle oil, citral and tea tree oil against *Staphylococcus aureus, Propionibacterium acnes, Escherichia coli, Pseudomonas aeruginosa, Klebsiella pneumoniae, Candida albicans* and *Aspergillus niger*. The oils and citral were tested in the concentration range of 0.03 to 2.0% v/v using agar dilution and agar diffusion assays. The minimum inhibitory concentration (MIC) results found that lemon myrtle and citral had comparable activity against all the microorganisms, with only *S. aureus* exhibiting greater sensitivity to citral. Both lemon myrtle and citral inhibited *P. aeruginosa* at 2.0% v/v, whereas tea tree oil had no effect.[11]

Actions

Actions commonly cited in aromatherapy

Antimicrobial, carminative, uplifting[2]

Actions supported by clinical studies

Antimicrobial

Comment

Lemon myrtle oil has broad-spectrum antimicrobial activity; however, it must be used with care in any topical aromatherapy treatment as the high citral may be a potent skin sensitiser. Hayes & Markovic state that both lemon myrtle oil and citral are highly toxic to human skin cells, and high concentrations should not be applied to the skin.[11] However, Tisserand & Young recommend that the maximum permissible dermal amount used is 0.7%.[6]

Aromatherapy Uses

Clinical aromatherapy

Antimicrobial

Lemon myrtle oil's antimicrobial activity indicates that it is beneficial for conditions such as influenza, bronchitis and *Herpes simplex* infections.[1]

Immune system

Kerr states that lemon myrtle oil may support and strengthen the immune system.[5]

Psychological

Webb states that lemon myrtle oil could be used in an anti-stress blend – providing mental rejuvenation. He also recommends lemon myrtle for improving concentration, as well as being relaxing and emotionally uplifting.[2]

The aroma of lemon myrtle oil is vibrant, fresh and lemony. It is intensely invigorating and I believe that its psychological properties would be similar to that of the very expensive melissa essential oil.

Dosage and Administration

Blending

Aromatherapy

For the relief of symptoms associated with colds and flu, consider blending lemon myrtle oil with essential oils such as cajeput, 1,8-cineole-rich eucalypts, peppermint eucalyptus, fragonia, peppermint, pine or tea tree.

An air purifying blend for a diffuser can be made by blending lemon myrtle oil with essential oils such as lemon, lime, sweet orange, pine or spruce.

To alleviate mental fatigue, consider blending lemon myrtle oil with essential oils such as basil, black pepper, clove, cinnamon bark, geranium, ginger, lemon, peppermint or rosemary.

A topical antimicrobial blend can be made by blending lemon myrtle oil and tea tree oil (ratio 4:1). This would improve the antimicrobial activity of tea tree and potentially reduce the sensitising effect of lemon myrtle oil via a quenching effect.[11]

Kerr recommends adding lemon myrtle with lavender to alleviate depression; and with ylang ylang and vetiver to alleviate fear, anxiety and other negative mental states.[5]

Perfumery

Lemon myrtle is not commonly used in perfumery.

Mode of administration

Bath

Due to the high citral content, lemon myrtle oil is not recommended in a bath.

Topical

Massage. To avoid dermal irritation or sensitisation, Tisserand & Young recommend that the maximum of 0.7% be used in any dermal preparation. This is equivalent to no more than seven drops to 50 mL of carrier oil.[7]

Inhalation

Direct inhalation, diffuser, oil vaporiser

Safety Profile

General safety

Lemon myrtle is non-toxic; however, it has a high citral content indicating that it may be a dermal irritant and dermal sensitiser.

An in vitro toxicity test revealed that products containing 1% lemon myrtle oil were found to be low in toxicity and could potentially be used in the formulation of topical antimicrobial products.[4]

Contraindications

No contraindications known.

Regulatory guidelines

Lemon myrtle oil is not defined in any regulatory guideline.

References

1. Taylor R. *Lemon myrtle the essential oil.* CSIRO Rural Research, 1996: 172: 18-19.
2. Webb M. *Bush sense.* Self-published, Australia, 2000.
3. Lassak EV. *Revision of Backhousia citriodora essential oil standard.* RIRDC Publication No.11/137, Rural Industries Research and Development Corporation, Barton, 2012.
4. Sultanbawa Y. *Lemon myrtle (Backhousia citriodora) oils.* In Preedy VR. ed. *Essential oils in food preservation, flavor and safety.* Academic Press, London, 2016: 517-521.
5. Kerr J. *Lemon myrtle.* Aromatherapy Today, 2000; 16: 12-15.
6. Tisserand R, Young R. *Essential oil safety.* 2nd edn. Churchill Livingstone, Edinburgh, 2014.
7. RIRDC. *Focus on lemon myrtle.* Research & Development Corporation Industry Overview. 2014. Pub. No. 14/117. Retrieved from http://www.agrifutures.com.au/publications/focus-on-lemon-myrtle/
8. Guba R. *Lemon myrtle.* Essential News, Vol.16, 2005.
9. Zouhir A et al. *Inhibition of methicillin-resistant Staphylococcus aureus (MRSA) by antimicrobial peptides (AMPs) and plant essential oils.* Pharmaceutical Biology, 2016; 54(12): 3136-3150. doi: 10.1080/13880209.2016.1190763.

10. Burke BE et al. *Essential oil of Australian lemon myrtle (Backhousia citriodora) in the treatment of Molluscum contagiosum.* Biomedicine & Pharmacotherapy, 2004; 58(4): 245-247. Cited in Quintessential Aromatics database, 2013.

11. Hayes AJ, Markovic B. *Toxicity of Australian essential oil of Backhousia citriodora (lemon myrtle). Part 1. Antimicrobial activity and in vitro cytotoxicity.* Food and Chemistry Toxicology, 2002; 40(4): 535-543. Cited in Quintessential Aromatics database, 2013.

Lime

Identification

Botanical name

Citrus x *aurantifolia* (Christm.) Swingle

Synonyms

Citrus medica var. *acida*, West Indian lime, Key lime, Mexican lime, cold-pressed lime, distilled lime, sour lime

Family

Rutaceae

Botany and origins

Lime is a small spreading evergreen tree usually to 4-6 m, a canopy diameter to 7 m, with many irregular spaced often drooping branches, which usually have many short, stiff, very sharp spines, although some cultivars are spineless.[1]

Lime is believed to have originated from northern India and adjacent areas of Burma. Guenther suggests that lime reached the west coast of Central and South America via the Pacific Islands, carried by the Polynesians. This accounts for the great abundance of wild limes in the jungles and little-known areas of tropical central and northern South America.[2]

Limes were brought from India to Persia, Palestine, Egypt and Europe by the Arabs at about the same time as the sour orange and the lemon.[1]

There are two main types of limes. The first is the Key, West Indian and Mexican cultivars, whose fruit is small, round, moderately seedy with thin peel, smooth and a greenish flesh. This is referred to as the 'acid lime'. The other is the Tahitian or Persian types, whose fruit is larger, seedless and mainly sold as fresh limes or lime juice. This is referred to as the 'sweet lime'.[3]

Certain authorities consider *Citrus aurantifolia* as the Key lime group and the Persian group as *C. latifolia*.[1]

Persian lime oils are considered to have a flatter and weaker scent than the Key lime oils, although both are offered indiscriminately as lime oil.[1] The odour of the sweet lime resembles that of the Mexican fruit; however, it does not have the same pronounced lime bouquet characteristics.[3]

Method of extraction

There are two types of lime oil:

- expressed lime oil
- distilled lime oil.

Weiss states that distilled lime oil is obtained by two methods: steam distillation of a slurry of crushed whole limes and freshly chopped peel, or distilling the juice from the fruit pressing.[1]

Expressed lime oil is cold-pressed from the fruit rind of green limes.[3]

Characteristics

Distilled lime oil is a pale yellow to almost clear mobile liquid with a fresh, sharp, fruity citrus-type odour. Prolonged storage affects the pleasant fresh aroma of distilled lime oil. With age, the oil develops a rather harsh, terpene-like odour.[3]

Cold-pressed lime oil is a yellowish-green to olive-green mobile liquid with an intensely fresh citrus, rich and sweet odour.[3]

Chemical composition

The chemical composition of distilled Key lime oil was reported as follows:

α-pinene (1.19%), β-pinene (2.23%), myrcene (1.28%), α-terpinene (2.52%), limonene + 1,8-cineole (48.85%), γ-terpinene (10.91%), terpinolene + nonanal (7.76%), linalool (0.05%), terpinen-4-ol (0.79%), α-terpineol (6.26%), neral (0.02%), geranial (0.04%), geranyl acetate (0.08%), α-bergamotene (0.83%), β-sesquiphellandrene (1.11%), β-bisabolene (1.42%).[4]

The chemical composition of cold-pressed Key lime oil from Mexico was reported as follows:

α-pinene (2.23%), β-pinene (19.95%), sabinene (3.04%), myrcene + octanal (1.17%), limonene + 1,8-cineole (50.01%), γ-terpinene + octanol (7.10%), terpinolene + nonanal (0.41%), linalool (0.15%), terpinen-4-ol (0.22%), α-terpineol (0.26%), neral (1.43%), geranial (2.36%), geranyl acetate (0.27%), α-bergamotene (1.27%), β-sesquiphellandrene (1.55%), β-bisabolene (2.11%).[4]

L

The oil composition can vary seasonally, and the oil from the early and late harvested fruit may differ significantly. For example, the bergapten content of Persian lime peel from fully mature fruit when the fruit became yellow decreased from 350 ppm to below 50 ppm at picking.[1]

Adulteration

Expressed lime oil is adulterated with the addition of distilled lime oil, lemon oil, terpenes from lime oil or other citrus oils.[3] Weiss states that the distilled lime oil is seldom adulterated since it is relatively inexpensive and easily available; however, he states that it is frequently extended.[1]

Pharmacopoeias and standards

The purity, composition and physico-chemical properties of distilled and cold-pressed lime essential oils are defined in ISO 3519:2005 Oil of Lime Distilled, Mexican Type (*Citrus aurantifolia* (Christm.) Swingle) and ISO 3809:2004 Oil of Lime (Cold Pressed), Mexican Type (*Citrus aurantifolia* (Christm.) Swingle), Obtained by Mechanical Means.

History and Traditional Uses

History

Limes were introduced into Europe by the Moors and subsequently brought to America by the Spanish and Portuguese explorers around the sixteenth century.[1]

Traditional medicine

Guenther states that, in the days of sailing ships, no British vessel would have ventured on a long cruise without ample supplies of concentrated lime juice. Vitamins were unknown back then; however, it was known that lime juice prevented outbreaks of scurvy.[2]

Food, perfumery and flavouring

Distilled lime oil is extensively used in flavouring food and beverages, especially soft drinks. Cold-pressed lime oil is used in men's high-grade toiletries and perfumery.[1]

Therapeutics

Pharmacology and clinical studies

Anticarcinogenic activity

An in vitro study using distilled lime oil showed 78% inhibition of human cancer colon cells with a 100 μg/mL concentration at 48 hours. The *d*-limonene content of the lime oil was 30.13% and *d*-dihydrocarvone was 30.47%. The researchers suggest that lime essential oil has potential benefit in colon cancer prevention.[5]

A review article on the role of *d*-limonene confirms that it has well-established chemoprotective activity against many types of cancer. Evidence from a phase I clinical trial shows a partial response in a patient with breast cancer, and stable disease for more than six months in three patients with colorectal cancer. The author states that *d*-limonene induces phase I and phase II carcinogen metabolising enzymes (cytochrome P450), which metabolises carcinogens to less toxic forms and prevents the interaction of chemical carcinogens with DNA.[6]

Antimicrobial activity

An in vitro study confirmed that lime oil had good antimicrobial activity on a representative range of gram-positive bacteria, gram-negative bacteria and yeasts.[7]

Anticholinergic activity

Lime oil was found to inhibit acetylcholinesterase activity. Acetylcholinesterase activity is associated with Alzheimer's disease.[8]

Stress reduction activity

Forty women volunteers were randomly divided into a lime essential oil massage group and a control (plain carrier oil) group. Before and after the treatment, the physical parameters associated with stress were examined. The lime oil massage group had a significant decrease in systolic blood pressure compared to the control group.[9]

Weight reduction

An in vivo study investigated the effects of lime oil in reducing body weight using mice. One group was administered lime essential oil, in another lime was co-administered with ketotifen, an antihistamine drug that causes weight gain, and a third group was administered ketotifen.

The mice that received ketotifen demonstrated an increase in body weight and food intake compared with the control group. The group treated with lime oil displayed a reduction in weight and food consumption. The group that was co-administered lime with ketotifen displayed significant suppression in gaining weight, as well as decreased body weight. The researchers suggested that lime oil could play an important role in weight loss and could be useful in the treatment of drug-induced obesity and related diseases.[10]

Actions

Actions commonly cited in aromatherapy

Antidepressant, antiseptic, antiviral, astringent, bactericide, carminative, digestive, disinfectant, febrifuge, haemostatic, hepatobiliary stimulant, insecticide, lymphatic stimulant, tonic[11,12]

Actions supported by clinical studies

Antimicrobial, antiseptic, chemoprotective, digestive

Comment

The indications for cold-pressed lime are considered to be similar to those of lemon oil.[11] Lavabre states that the refreshing quality of lime oil is more pronounced than lemon oil.[12]

Aromatherapy Uses

Clinical aromatherapy

Antimicrobial

Lime oil has antimicrobial properties and is recommended for treating throat infections and influenza.[12]

Detoxification

Cold-pressed lime oil is a mild detoxifier and may be used for the treatment of fluid retention and cellulite.[11,12]

The high limonene content of lime oil means that it can be blended with other essential oils to support liver regeneration and detoxification.

Digestive system

As with most citrus oils, lime oil is considered a digestive tonic and is recommended for digestive problems.[12]

Psychological

Both cold-pressed and distilled lime oils are refreshing and uplifting.[12]

Lime oil is ideal to alleviate mental fogginess and mental fatigue with poor concentration. It is beneficial for those who wake up in the morning feeling low energy and for eliminating negative thinking, pessimism and depression.

Skin care

Cold-pressed lime oil acts as an astringent counteracting overproduction of sebum, and is especially useful for oily skin. Its antibacterial property is useful for the treatment of acne.[11,12]

Energetics, psyche and subtle uses

Energetics

Lime oil is *cooling* and *drying*. It is recommended to eliminate *heat*, *damp* and phlegm. For this reason, it is considered an excellent digestive and detoxifying essential oil. *Damp* conditions are often associated with chronic indigestion, abdominal bloating, lethargy, heaviness of the body and water retention.

Lime oil helps to calm and strengthen the *Shen*. Whenever the *Shen* is weak, we feel mental fatigue, lack focus, and may experience headaches. Whenever the *Shen* is feeling agitated, we suffer from anxiety, irritability and restlessness.

According to the principles of the Five Elements, lime oil tonifies the Wood Element and helps to reduce excess *damp* associated with the Earth Element.

According to Ayurveda, lime oil would strengthen *Vata* and *Pitta* and help to reduce *Kapha*.

Personality

Lime personalities are like a breath of fresh air, positively wonderful to have around. They are not too bothered by the struggles and strains of living and able to take everything quite calmly. They have a very positive approach and an unshakeable confidence in everything that they do.

According to Myers-Briggs personality types, the lime personality is likely to be an ENTP. ENTPs are energetic, enthusiast and confident. Many are nonconformists. They are innovative, have excellent analytical ability and are resourceful in solving problems. They like variety and change. Because they have so many interests, they feel that life is too short. They feel relaxed when they do new things. They enjoy travelling to exotic places. They can be inspirational and rise to leadership positions because of their quick mind. They work best when interacting with many people. They are optimistic, charming and quick-witted. They value their freedom and independence. They seek growth, excitement, and continuous improvement in their relationships. They enjoy debating and they like to have the last say. They may deny emotional pain and keep busy to avoid dealing with their feelings. They can be arrogant, argumentative and insensitive.

Subtle

Keim Loughran & Bull state that the scent of lime clears and cleanses the room and promotes psychic protection.[13]

Zeck recommends lime oil whenever you are feeling agitated or dealing with stressful situations. She explains that it helps to clear any heated emotion and helps you feel calm. The fresh, tangy scent of lime also refreshes the emotions, allowing your feelings to be explored and released constructively.[14]

Dosage and Administration

Blending

Aromatherapy

For the relief of stress, anxiety and nervous

L

tension, consider blending cold-pressed lime with essential oils such as bergamot, geranium, lavender, frankincense, neroli, sweet orange, sandalwood or ylang ylang.

To alleviate stress, anxiety and nervous tension, consider blending cold-pressed lime with essential oils such as bergamot, lemon, neroli or sweet orange.

To alleviate mental fatigue, consider blending cold-pressed lime oil with essential oils such as basil, ginger, lemon, rosemary or peppermint.

For the relief of indigestion, consider blending cold-pressed lime with essential oils such as black pepper, cardamom, coriander seed, sweet fennel, ginger, sweet orange or peppermint.

Perfumery

In perfumery, the expressed lime oil is preferred, as the terpene-like note of the distilled oil is rarely required in perfumery. The freshness of the expressed lime oil blends very well with neroli to create a delightful top note. It also blends well with clary sage, lavender, rosemary and sage. Arctander states that the tenacity of cold-pressed lime is outstanding.[3]

Mode of administration

Bath

Full body bath, foot bath

Topical

Compress, massage, ointment, skin care

Inhalation

Direct inhalation, diffuser, oil vaporiser

Safety Profile

General safety

Distilled lime oil is non-toxic, non-irritating and non-sensitising. However, cold-pressed lime oil is phototoxic. No phototoxic effects are reported for distilled lime oil.[15]

Both distilled and cold-pressed lime oils can be sensitising if oxidised. IFRA recommends that essential oils rich in limonene should only be used when the level of peroxides are kept to the lowest practical level. To avoid oxidation, it is recommended to store citrus oils in a dark, airtight container in a refrigerator.[16]

Contraindications

In order to prevent phototoxicity, IFRA recommends cold-pressed lime oil be limited to a maximum of 0.7% in topical leave-on products. If applied to the skin, Tisserand & Young recommend that the skin not be exposed to sunlight or sunbed rays for 12 hours.[16]

Regulatory guidelines

Distilled and cold-pressed lime essential oils both have GRAS status.

References

1. Weiss EA. *Essential oil crops*. CAB International, Wallingford, 1997.
2. Guenther E. *The essential oils – Vol. III*. Robert E Krieger Publishing, Malabar, 1949.
3. Arctander S. *Perfume and flavor materials of natural origin*. Allured Publishing, Carol Stream, 1994.
4. Haro L et al. *Comparative study of the essential oils of Key and Persian limes*. Perfumer & Flavorists, 1985; 10: 67-72.
5. Patil JR et al. *Apoptosis-mediated proliferation inhibition of human colon cancer cells by volatile principles of Citrus aurantifolia*. Food Chemistry, 2009; 114(4): 1351-1358.
6. Sun J. *D-limonene: safety and clinical applications*. Alternative Medicine Review, 2007; 12(3): 259-264.
7. Costa R et al. *Antimicrobial activity and chemical composition of Citrus aurantifolia (Christm.) Swingle essential oil from Italian organic crops*. Journal of Essential Oil Research, 2014; 26(6): 400-408. Cited in Quintessential Aromatics database, 2013.
8. Tundis R et al. *Comparative study on the antioxidant capacity and cholinesterase inhibitory activity of Citrus aurantifolia Swingle, C. aurantium L., and C. bergamia Risso and Poit. peel essential oils*. Journal of Food Science, 2012; 77(1): H40-H46. Cited in Quintessential Aromatics database, 2013.
9. Saiyudthong S et al. *Effect of aromatherapy massage with lime essential oil on stress*. International Journal of Essential Oil Therapeutics, 2009; 3(2/3): 76-80. Cited in Quintessential Aromatics database, 2013.
10. Asnaashari S et al. *Essential oil from Citrus aurantifolia prevents ketotifen-induced weight-gain in mice*. Phytotherapy Research, 2010; 24(12): 1893-1897. Cited in Quintessential Aromatics database, 2013.
11. Lawless J. *The encyclopaedia of essential oils*. Element Books, Shaftesbury, 1992.
12. Lavabre M. *Aromatherapy workbook*. Healing Arts Press, Rochester, 1997.
13. Keim Loughran J, Bull R. *Aromatherapy and subtle energy techniques*. Frog, Berkeley, 2000.
14. Zeck R. *The blossoming heart – aromatherapy for healing and transformation*. Aroma Tours, East Ivanhoe, 2004.
15. Opdyke DLJ. *Monographs on fragrance raw materials*. Pergamon Press, Oxford, 1979.
16. Tisserand R, Young R. *Essential oil safety*. 2nd edn. Churchill Livingstone, Edinburgh, 2014.

L

Mandarin

Identification

Botanical name

Citrus reticulata Blanco

Synonyms

Common mandarin, *Citrus nobilis* var. *deliciosa*

Family

Rutaceae

Botany and origins

Mandarin is a small evergreen tree to 4 m, with a single trunk, and many rather thin drooping branches which may be either spined or spineless. The fruit is a flattened globoid, approximately 5-10 cm in diameter. The peel colour varies from yellow to deep orange-red when ripe.[1]

Mandarin is normally divided into four groups, each suited to certain climatic and environmental conditions. The four groups are – common, king, willowleaf and satsuma.[1]

Mandarin is native to China and Indo-China and has spread to other countries of the Far East, where it is extensively grown for domestic purposes. It was first introduced to Europe in the eighteenth century. It rapidly became popular and was commercially cultivated in southern Europe and north Africa. It was then introduced to the Americas, southern Africa and Australia.[1]

Mandarin and tangerine fruits have been given the same species status. The name tangerine is used in English-speaking countries, but mandarin elsewhere.[1]

Mandarins are adaptable to a wide range of climates – from the desert, to semitropical and subtropical regions of the world. Unlike other citrus varieties, mandarins are capable of withstanding cold conditions. As a result, we can find them growing in cooler regions of the world such as Russia, Japan and New Zealand.[2]

There are three types of mandarin oil available from the same fruit – green, yellow and red mandarin oil. These are graded according to the stage of maturity of the fruits at the time of picking. The green mandarin oil produced in Europe and South America is highly regarded in the perfume industry. The yellow mandarin is the next stage of maturation after the green and is often used for both for its flavour and fragrance. Finally, the mature red mandarin fruit provides the commonly used cold-pressed red mandarin oil, which tends to be used more frequently in the flavour industry rather than the fragrance industry.[2]

Characteristics

Mandarin oil is an orange-brown to dark yellowish-brown or olive-brown coloured mobile oil with an intensely sweet, not necessarily fresh odour, and an amine-like, 'fishy' top note. This odour is due to the presence of methyl N-methylanthranilate.[3]

Method of extraction

Mandarin oil is expressed from the fruit rind of *Citrus reticulata.* Mandarin peel oil content is one of the highest of all the citrus. It can reach 17% in some seasons, and in the fruit of selected trees it can be as high as 22%.[1]

Chemical composition

The chemical composition of mandarin oil from Sicily was reported as follows:

α-thujone (0.7%), α-pinene (1.8%), camphene (0.01%), sabinene (0.22%), β-pinene (1.36%), myrcene (1.73%), limonene (73.58%), γ-terpinolene (16.7%), linalool (0.19%), citronellal (0.04%), terpinen-4-ol (0.2%), α-terpineol (0.38%), nerol (0.04%), neral (trace), geranial (0.07%), thymol (0.11%), octanal (0.08%), nonanal (0.01%), decanal (0.11%), methyl N-methylanthranilate (0.48%), β-caryophyllene (0.06%).[4]

Weiss states that up to 80 components have been detected in mandarin oil, including limonene up to 95%, γ-terpinolene up to 20%, and myrcene and *p*-cymene up to 8% each. The main components influencing the unique aroma and flavour are thymol and methyl N-methylanthranilate.[1]

Adulteration

Holmes states that there is a moderate chance of adulteration, typically with other less expensive citrus such as orange, tangerine and clementine oils.[5]

Pharmacopoeias and standards

The purity, composition and physico-chemical properties of mandarin essential oil are defined in ISO 3528:2012 Essential Oil of Mandarin, Italian Type (*Citrus reticulata* Blanco)

History and Traditional Uses

History

Arctander states that the mandarin arrived in Europe in 1805, and in the USA about 40 years later. In Europe, the fruit developed into the small ellipsoidic mandarin fruit. In the USA, the fruit

M

remained similar to the original fruit from China and it was renamed tangerine.[3]

Traditional medicine

In France, mandarin oil is considered a children's remedy, and is used to relieve tummy upsets of babies and children.[6]

In China, dried mandarin peel is called *chenpi* and is used in TCM and in Chinese cuisine. In TCM, it is used to help regulate *Qi*, strengthen the *Spleen*, assist in the elimination of *damp*, alleviate abdominal distension and enhance digestion.[7]

Food, perfumery and flavouring

Mandarin oil is extensively used in flavouring, where it is blended with other citrus oils to create interesting flavour compositions for soft drinks, candy and liqueurs.[3]

Therapeutics

Pharmacology and clinical studies

Antifungal activity

An in vitro study demonstrated that mandarin oil had antifungal activity against a wide range of moulds commonly associated with food spoilage such as *Aspergillus niger, Aspergillus flavus, Penicillium chrysogenum* and *Penicillium verrucosum*.[8]

Anti-inflammatory activity

Mandarin oil had antioxidant and anti-inflammatory activities in indomethacin-induced enterocolitis in rats.[9]

Antimicrobial activity

A study examining the antimicrobial activity against spoiling and pathogenic microorganisms indicated that mandarin oil had the best growth inhibition. However, a blend of low concentrations of sweet orange, lemon and mandarin oil displayed synergistic lethal effects, suggesting their potential use for food preservation.[10]

In vitro studies have demonstrated that mandarin oil has activity against *Escherichia coli, Staphylococcus aureus, Aspergillus flavus, Aspergillus niger, Aspergillus fumigatus* and *Candida albicans*.[11,12,13]

Antitumour activity

An in vitro study found that mandarin oil and limonene had strong dose-dependent chemoprotective effects against two human tumour cell lines. It was interesting to note that the essential oil was more effective than limonene on its own.[14]

Sedative activity

Mandarin oil was found to reduce generalised anxiety and obsessive-compulsive disorders, as well as enhance sleep time, in a study involving mice.[15]

Actions

Actions commonly cited in aromatherapy

Antidepressant, antiseptic, antispasmodic, carminative, cholagogue, depurative, digestive, diuretic, sedative[2,16,17]

Actions supported by clinical studies

Antimicrobial, sedative

Comment

Mandarin's high limonene content suggests that it may have a hepatoprotective and chemoprotective role.

Whilst many clinical studies on mandarin oil have focused on its antimicrobial activities, I would like to see studies on the oil's effect on our emotional and psychological wellbeing. Davis best describes the influence of mandarin on our psyche when she explains that the scent of mandarin breathes a message of happiness, especially to children and the child within each of us. It helps us to get in touch with our inner child.[6]

Aromatherapy Uses

Clinical aromatherapy

Digestive system

Mandarin oil has a tonic effect on the digestive system, helping to regulate metabolic processes and aiding the secretion of bile and breaking down of fats. It is beneficial for calming the intestines and relieving flatulence.[16]

Nervous system

Mandarin oil is recommended for soothing restlessness, especially in hyperactive children. It calms the activity of the sympathetic nervous system and alleviates insomnia in combination with orange oil.[18]

Pregnancy

Mandarin oil is recommended in a massage blend to prevent stretch marks during pregnancy. It should be blended with essential oils such as lavender and neroli, and wheatgerm and apricot kernel cold-pressed vegetable oils should be used as the carrier. To be effective, the massage oil should be used daily from about the fifth month of pregnancy.[6]

Psychological

Holmes states that mandarin oil promotes emotional stability and can be used to alleviate irritability, moodiness, frustration and emotional instability. The oil promotes optimism and joy. He explains that mandarin's uplifting playful energy can help to lift dark, negative and morbid feelings, especially in individuals who are feeling guilt and self-deprecation.[5]

Skin care

Mandarin oil is often used in combination with lavender, neroli and wheatgerm oil to help prevent stretch marks during pregnancy.[6,16]

Mandarin oil is recommended for acne, congested skin and oily skin.[16]

Energetics, psyche and subtle uses

Energetics

Holmes recommends mandarin oil for helping spread *Liver Qi* and harmonising the *Shen*. Whenever the *Liver Qi* is constrained and we have *Shen* disharmony, we are likely to experience nervous tension and irritability, mood swings and insomnia.[5]

Mandarin also helps to strengthen the *Spleen Qi* and assist in the elimination of excess *damp*, which is associated with abdominal distension and indigestion. According to the principles of the Five Elements, mandarin oil has an affinity with the Wood, Fire and Earth Elements.

M

Personality

The mandarin personality is described as one of the softer personalities. They are sweet, gentle, kind and loving. They are very uplifting people, may be childlike in that they need love and protection, and tend to attract protectiveness in others.[19]

Worwood explains that mandarin personalities can spend most of their life caring for other people. They love children and will do anything to protect them.

According to Myers-Briggs personality types, the mandarin personality is likely to be an ENFP. ENFPs are outgoing, lively and spontaneous. They are very enthusiastic and their joy for life can be contagious. They have a rich imagination and active mind. Their thoughts are always wandering and their mood constantly changing. They are always involved, or in love, with someone or something new. They know how to establish instant rapport and make people feel comfortable. They love emotional intensity and enjoy expressing their feelings. They can be charming and flirtatious. They relate with warmth to many people and can appear overly enthusiastic, positive and optimistic.

Subtle

Holmes states that the unique gift of mandarin oil is its ability to lighten, open and soften the emotional heart and reveal the joy buried within.[5]

Worwood beautifully describes the subtle qualities of mandarin when she states that the gentleness and sweetness of spirit is gathered in the arms of the scent of mandarin. She explains that, however gentle it may be, there is a vigour and sprightliness in how mandarin stirs the heart.[20]

Davis states that the delicate aroma of mandarin breathes a message of happiness, especially to children and the child within each of us. It helps us get in touch with our inner child.[21]

Keim Loughran & Bull explain that it is not unusual for spiritual work and development to involve psychological issues. Wounds in the personality need to be tended so the personality can be more thoroughly infused with the Divine. They state that mandarin assists in connecting us with our inner child – the part of our character that developed early in life. Mandarin will also help us access happiness, and inspires and encourages our rediscovery of the innocence and radiant joy within all of us.[22]

Dosage and Administration

Blending

Aromatherapy

To alleviate anxiety, nervous tension and stress-related conditions, consider blending mandarin oil with essential oils such as bergamot, geranium, lavender, neroli, petitgrain, sandalwood or ylang ylang.

To alleviate depression, consider blending mandarin oil with essential oils such a bergamot, geranium, jasmine absolute, lavender, neroli, sweet orange, patchouli, rose absolute, sandalwood or ylang ylang.

To alleviate fatigue, consider blending mandarin oil with essential oils such as black pepper, coriander seed, ginger, grapefruit, lemon, petitgrain or rosemary.

To alleviate indigestion, consider blending mandarin oil with essential oils such as black pepper, coriander seed, ginger, sweet fennel, peppermint or spearmint.

Perfumery

In perfumery, mandarin oil is used sparingly in colognes and as a modifier for other citrus oils. Arctander states that it enhances sweet rich floral notes such as rose, jasmine or ylang ylang, and blends well with the sweet resin and earthy oils such as benzoin or patchouli. The oil also complements spicy oils such as coriander seed, clove bud, black pepper and nutmeg.[3]

Mode of administration

Bath

Full body bath, foot bath

Topical

Compress, massage, ointment, skin care

Inhalation

Direct inhalation, diffuser, oil vaporiser

Safety Profile

General safety

Mandarin oil is non-toxic, non-irritating and non-sensitising.[16] Tisserand & Young state that skin sensitisation can occur if the essential oil is oxidised. The furanocoumarin content of mandarin peel oil is not sufficient to cause phototoxic reaction.[23]

Contraindications

No contraindications known.

Regulatory guidelines

Mandarin essential oil has GRAS status.

References

1. Weiss EA. *Essential oil crops.* CAB International, Wallingford, 1997.
2. Reeve D et al. *Riding the citrus trail: when is a mandarin a tangerine?* Perfumer & Flavorist, 2002; 27: 20-23.
3. Arctander S. *Perfume and flavor materials of natural origin.* Allured Publishing, Carol Stream, 1994.
4. Lawrence BM. *Progress in essential oils – mandarin oil.* Perfumer & Flavorist, 2001; 26: 36-43.
5. Holmes P. *Aromatica – a clinical guide to essential oil therapeutics.* Singing Dragon, London, 2016.
6. Davis P. *Aromatherapy: an A-Z.* 2nd edn. C.W. Daniel Company, Saffron Walden, 1999.
7. Liu Y et al. eds. *Dietary Chinese herbs.* Springer Science + Business Media, New York, 2015.
8. Viuda-Martos M et al. *Antifungal activity of lemon (Citrus lemon L.), mandarin (Citrus reticulata L.), grapefruit (Citrus paradisi L.) and orange (Citrus sinensis L.) essential oils.* Food Control, 2008; 19(12): 1130-1138. Cited in Quintessential Aromatics database, 2013.
9. Patil NR et al. *Screening of mandarin oil on indomethacin induced inflammatory bowel disease in Wistar rats.* Indian Journal of Pharmaceutical Education and Research, 2014; 48(Suppl.): 1-6. Cited in Quintessential Aromatics database, 2013.
10. Espina L et al. *Chemical composition of commercial citrus fruit essential oils and evaluation of their antimicrobial activity acting alone or in combined processes.* Food Control, 2001; 22(6): 896-902. Cited in Quintessential Aromatics database, 2013.
11. Sultana HS et al. *Influence of volatile constituents of fruit peels of Citrus reticulata Blanco on clinically isolated pathogenic microorganisms under in-vitro.* Asian Pacific Journal of Tropical Biomedicine, 2012; 2 (Suppl. 3): S1299-S1302. Cited in Quintessential Aromatics database, 2013.
12. Tao NG et al. *Essential oil composition and antimicrobial activity.* Chemistry of Natural Compounds, 2009; 45(3): 437-438. Cited in Quintessential Aromatics database, 2013.
13. Frassinetti S et al. *Antibacterial and antioxidant activity of essential oils from Citrus spp.* Journal of Essential Oil Research, 2011; 23(1): 27-31. Cited in Quintessential Aromatics database, 2013.
14. Manassero CA et al. *In vitro comparative analysis of antiproliferative activity of essential oil from mandarin peel and its principal component limonene.* Natural Product Research, 2013; 27(16): 1475-1478. Cited in Quintessential Aromatics database, 2013.
15. Gargano AC et al. *Essential oils from Citrus latifolia and Citrus reticulata reduce anxiety and prolong ether sleeping time in mice.* Tree and Forestry Science and Biotechnology, 2008; 2(Special 1): 1-4. Cited in Quintessential Aromatics database, 2013.
16. Lawless J. *The encyclopaedia of essential oils.* Element Books, Shaftesbury, 1992.
17. Lavabre M. *Aromatherapy workbook.* Healing Arts Press, Rochester, 1997.
18. Schnaubelt K. *Medical aromatherapy.* Frog, Berkeley, 1999.
19. Worwood VA. *The fragrant mind.* Transworld Publishers, London, 1995.
20. Worwood VA. *The fragrant heavens.* Transworld Publishers, London, 1999.
21. Davis P. *Subtle aromatherapy.* C.W. Daniel Company, Saffron Walden, 1991.
22. Keim-Loughran J, Bull R. *Aromatherapy anointing oils.* Frog, Berkeley, 2001.
23. Tisserand R, Young R. *Essential oil safety.* 2nd edn. Churchill Livingstone, Edinburgh, 2014.

Manuka

Identification

Botanical name

Leptospermum scoparium JR Forster & G Forster

Synonyms

Manex, New Zealand tea tree

Family

Myrtaceae

Botany and origins

Manuka is a small tree which is native to New Zealand. In favourable open conditions, it is a fast growing, conical-shaped bush that reaches about 4 m high.[1]

Most manuka is harvested from wild plants as very little commercial cultivation is yet carried out. Regrowth is rapid after harvesting, therefore, there are no risks of damage to the wild plants. However, it has been suggested that, in future, plantations may specialise in a particular chemotype.[2]

Method of extraction

Manuka oil is steam-distilled from the leaves and twigs of *L. scoparium.*

Characteristics

Manuka oil is a clear yellow liquid with a distinctive spicy, herbaceous and fresh aroma.

Chemical composition

An analysis of 16 commercial samples of manuka oil revealed 100 constituents, of which 51 were identified and made up about 95% of the content. The typical chemical composition of the oil is triketones (approximately 20%), sesquiterpene hydrocarbons (60-70%) and monoterpene hydrocarbons (approximately 5%).[1]

A detailed field study of manuka oil in New Zealand confirmed the presence of three chemotypes:

- monoterpene rich oil from the Northlands and the West Coast
- triketones rich oil from the East Cape and Marlborough
- sesquiterpene rich oil throughout the rest of New Zealand.[1]

L. scoparium populations from Australia in Victoria and Tasmania had different chemical profiles from the New Zealand populations. In particular, the triketones were not present in the Australian oils.[3]

Oil Component	Location		
	North	East Cape	Southern
monoterpenes	40%	3%	12%
sesquiterpenes	42%	54%	65%
triketones	1%	33%	2%

The ratio of chemical components in the three regional types of manuka oil.[1]

Variances in the composition have been noted depending on the age of the plant. For example, the percentage of monoterpenes (α-pinene, β-pinene and myrcene) increases from less than 1% in young trees to between 17% and 34% in trees that are three years older.[2]

There are also seasonal variations. The pinene levels are highest in spring and summer when the foliage is growing.[2]

The chemical composition of manuka oil obtained from a distinct chemotype found in the East Cape area of the North Island of New Zealand was reported as follows:

α-thujene (0.03%), α-pinene (1.31%), β-pinene (0.12%), myrcene (0.24%), *p*-cymene (0.16%), 1,8-cineole (0.22%), limonene (0.1%), terpinen-4-ol (0.04%), α-terpineol (0.09%), α-cubebene (3.95%), α-copaene (5.86%), β-elemene (0.55%), α-gurjunene (1.02%), β-caryophyllene (2.63%), aromadendrene (2.09%), cadina-3,5-diene (4.88%), δ-amorphene (3.81%), β-selinene (3.67%), α-selinene + viridiflorene (4.35%), flavesone (4.91%), cadina-1,4-diene (5.94%), isoleptospermone (4.62%), leptospermone (15.54%).[4]

Adulteration

Lis-Balchin states that the admixing of different trees and shrubs would give the oil variable chemical composition, which may compromise the therapeutic efficacy of the oil.[5]

Pharmacopoeias and standards

At the time of writing, the purity, composition, physico-chemical properties and therapeutic use of manuka essential oil are not defined in any pharmacopoeia monograph or standard.

History and Traditional Uses

History

Maori folklore attributes the kanuka as the 'male' tree and manuka the 'female.'[2] Other traditional uses include infusions for urinary and intestinal complaints, and as a febrifuge, sucking the gum for coughs, vapour inhalations for colds, and poultices for back pain and skin conditions, inflamed breasts, burns and scalds.[2]

The leaves of manuka were also used as topical applications for wounds, cuts, sores and skin diseases. Topical use of the various parts of manuka was common among Maori.[6]

Traditional medicine

The therapeutic properties of manuka honey are well established. It is used for slow healing ulcers and wound healing.[7] The antibacterial activity of manuka honey was shown to be active against *Staphylococcus aureus* and *Helicobacter pylori*.[5]

The antibacterial activity of many honey products are associated with hydrogen peroxide; however, those of manuka honey are derived through other mechanisms. The antibacterial activity of manuka honey is now standardised in terms of phenol concentration equivalent, which is expressed as the unique manuka factor value (UMF).[7]

The UMF rating is set by the Active Manuka Honey Association (AMHA). Maggie Tisserand explains that the manuka honey is challenged with *Staphylococcus aureus*, and the results are compared with the same test using phenol, a carbolic acid once used as a disinfectant. The number that follows the trademark UMF is equal to the concentration of phenol used. Therefore, a manuka honey with a UMF 10 rating is equal to a 10% dilution of phenol, whereas a UMF 20 rating is equivalent to a 20% dilution of phenol, making it twice as strong. She states that the high potency manuka honeys are often used for the treatment of MRSA- infected wounds. Honey that has a UMF 5 is not considered effective enough to treat MRSA.[7]

Therapeutics

Pharmacology and clinical studies

Many pharmacological studies involving manuka essential oil have been published. A systemic review of these studies will not be attempted. Rather, I have chosen a selection of studies that support the traditional and clinical uses.

Antimicrobial activity

The comparative antimicrobial activity showed greater differences between different samples of manuka and kanuka than that of tea tree. The antifungal activity of kanuka was inversely proportional to its strong antibacterial activity, whilst manuka displayed a stronger antifungal effect, though not as potent as tea tree.[8]

The antimicrobial activity of standard tea tree compared with manuka obtained from the East Cape region of New Zealand is reported in the table below.[8]

Oil Sample	Zone of inhibition (mm)	
	Candida albicans	Staphylococcus aureus
tea tree	9.0	8.5
Aust. lavender	8.0	7.0
NZ manuka	2.0	8.0
lemongrass	30.0	38.0
eucalyptus	2.0	2.5

Comparative antimicrobial activity for some essential oils

A comparative study examining the antibacterial activity of tea tree, kanuka, manuka and eucalyptus oils reported that tea tree oil had the highest antibacterial activity, with minimum inhibitory concentration (MIC) values of 0.25%. However, it was reported that manuka oil exhibited a higher activity than tea tree oil against gram-positive bacteria with MIC values of 0.12%. Both tea tree oil and manuka oil demonstrated a very good antimicrobial efficacy against various antibiotic-resistant *Staphylococcus* species. *Pseudomonas aeruginosa* was resistant to all the essential oils tested, even at high concentrations of 4%.[9]

An in vitro study confirmed that kanuka and manuka oils significantly inhibited a range of fungi and bacteria. The fungicidal properties of the oil were confirmed with an MIC ranging from 0.78% to 3.13%. The oils also displayed excellent bactericidal activity with 100% inhibition of the examined bacteria.[10]

M

A comparative study examined the use of a range of essential oils against plaque-causing bacteria and the production of plaque. Manuka oil was found to be the most effective, inhibiting all the bacteria with MICs of 0.25% and 0.13% for *Streptococci* and 0.03% for the gram-negative bacteria.[11]

The adhesive ability of the bacteria is a significant pathogenic factor in the formation of plaque. The study confirmed the inhibitory effect of the tea tree and manuka essential oils on the adhesion of *Porphyromonas gingivalis* and *Streptococcus mutans*. It was concluded that manuka and tea tree oils exhibit growth-inhibiting and bactericidal effects on periodontopathic and cariogenic bacteria, and also anti-adhesion effects on some species. The authors state that the oils are promising antibacterial agents for oral care at concentrations of 0.25 or lower.[11]

Lis-Balchin suggests that higher levels of flavescone and leptospermone give the oil a higher level of antimicrobial activity, particularly against gram-positive organisms such as *Staphylococcus* and *Streptococcus*.[5]

Antiphotoaging activity

An in vivo study investigated manuka oil for its

effects against photoaging in UV-B irradiated hairless mice. The study found that an application of 10% manuka oil significantly reduced the average length and depth of wrinkles. This was correlated with the inhibition of loss of collagen fibre content and epidermal hyperplasia. It was also reported that manuka oil could suppress UV-B induced skin inflammation by inhibiting the production of inflammatory cytokines. It was suggested that this study provides evidence that manuka oil possess antiphotoaging activity that is associated with its inhibitory activity against skin inflammation induced by UV irradiation.[12]

Antispasmodic activity

Studies using field-stimulated guinea pig ileum have confirmed that both manuka and kanuka oils induced a spasmolytic effect; however, kanuka produced an initial contraction. It was reported that there was some evidence that manuka oil acts through cAMP, whereas the mode of action of kanuka was not yet determined.[13]

Antiviral activity

An in vitro study found that *Herpes simplex* virus type 1 (HSV-1) and *Herpes simplex* virus type 2 (HSV-2) were significantly inhibited when the viruses were pretreated with manuka oil, one hour prior to cell infection. After virus penetration into the host cells, only replication of HSV-1 particle was significantly inhibited to about 41% by manuka oil. Flavesone and leptospermone, two β-triketones found in manuka oil, inhibited the virulence of HSV-1 in the same manner as the essential oil itself.[14]

Kanuka and manuka were more cytotoxic, with a maximum noncytotoxic concentration of 0.001% compared with a maximum noncytotoxic concentration of 0.006% for cajeput and clove oils. Manuka oil also reported the highest virucidal activity against HSV-1 and drug-resistant HSV-1 isolates.[15]

Mucositis activity

A study examined the effects of an essential oil mouthwash on radiation-induced mucositis of the oropharyngeal area during treatment for head and neck cancers. Patients participated in the randomised, placebo-controlled study, involving the use of a gargle containing two drops of a 1:1 mix of manuka and kanuka in water, which reported delayed onset of mucositis and reduced pain and oral symptoms relative to the placebo (gargling with water). The study confirmed that manuka and kanuka oils used in a gargle can provide relief on the development of radiation-induced mucositis.[16]

M

Actions

Actions commonly cited in aromatherapy

Analgesic, antibacterial, antifungal, anti-inflammatory, deodorant, expectorant, immune stimulant, insecticide, sedative[5,6,17]

Actions supported by clinical studies

Analgesic, antibacterial, antifungal, antiviral

Comments

Given the presence of several chemotypes, it would appear that the manuka oils with a higher sesquiterpene and β-triketone content would be most suitable for use in aromatherapy.

Aromatherapy Uses

Clinical aromatherapy

Integumentary system

It has been suggested that the sesquiterpenes found in manuka oil are responsible for manuka's ability to reduce skin irritation and promote wound healing.[17] Manuka oil is recommended for treating ringworm, insect bites, athlete's foot, acne, skin eruptions, stubborn ulcers and wounds, cuts and abrasions.[18]

Musculoskeletal system

Manuka oil has a good analgesic effect and is recommended for the relief of muscular aches and pains.[18]

Respiratory system

Manuka oil is beneficial for all types of respiratory tract infections and can be used to relieve coughs, colds and flu.[7]

Energetics, psyche and subtle uses

Energetics

Manuka oil is recommended for dispersing *wind cold* conditions. *Wind cold* is characterised as the onset of respiratory tract infections with aches and pains, chills and a dislike for cold. Manuka oil tonifies the *Qi* and strengthens the *Shen*. Whenever we experience *Qi* deficiency and our *Shen* is weak, we experience fatigue, lethargy, poor focus and depression.

Subtle

Von Braunschweig states that manuka oil is a protective oil similar to myrrh and cedarwood. She says that old psychic scars get smoothened and that the sesquiterpenes stabilise and protect the nervous system and balance the sympathetic and parasympathetic nerves. Manuka's vitalising scent is well suited to gentle souls who express themselves through sensitive skin or frequent digestive upsets.[17]

Dosage and Administration

Blending

Aromatherapy

For the relief of pain and inflammation in conditions such as rheumatoid arthritis, consider blending manuka oil with essential oils such as German chamomile, everlasting, fragonia, kunzea or lavender.

For the relief of muscular aches and pains, consider blending manuka oil with essential oils such as black pepper, cajeput, ginger, kunzea, spike lavender, rosemary or pine.

For treating fungal skin infections, consider blending manuka oil with patchouli or tea tree oil.

For the relief of the symptoms associated with colds and flu, consider blending manuka oil with essential oils such as cajeput, 1,8-cineole-rich eucalypts, fragonia, ginger, lemon, lemon myrtle, pine, tea tree or thyme.

For the relief of stress, nervous tension and anxiety, consider blending manuka oil with essential oils such as bergamot, Atlas cedarwood, geranium, lavender, mandarin, neroli, sweet orange or sandalwood.

Perfumery

Manuka oil is not commonly used in perfumery; however, it would blend well with essential oils such as bay laurel, bergamot, black pepper, Atlas cedarwood, cinnamon bark, clove bud, elemi, ginger, lavender, nutmeg, sandalwood, vetiver and ylang ylang.

Mode of administration

Bath

Full body bath, foot bath

Topical

Compress, massage, ointment, skin care

Inhalation

Direct inhalation, diffuser, oil vaporiser

Safety Profile

General safety

Lis-Balchin states that there have been no safety / toxicological evaluations performed on manuka oil, therefore, it cannot be condoned for general aromatherapy use.[5]

However, the chemistry of the oil and all the studies to date indicate that manuka oil is non-toxic, non-irritating and non-sensitising.

Contraindications

No contraindications known.

Regulatory guidelines

Manuka oil is not defined in any regulatory guideline.

References

1. *Essential oil production from manuka and kanuka*. Crop & Food Research Broadsheet, No. 116, 2000.
2. Maddocks-Jennings W et al. *A fresh look at manuka and kanuka essential oils from New Zealand*. The International Journal of Aromatherapy, 2005; 15(3): 141-146.
3. Stephens JMC. *The factors responsible for the varying levels of UMF in manuka (Leptospermum scoparium) honey*. University of Waikato, Hamilton, 2006.
4. Porter NG, Wilkins AL. *Chemical, physical and antimicrobial properties of essential oils of Leptospermum scoparium and Kunzea ericoides*. Phytochemistry, 1998; 50(3): 407-415. Cited in the Aromatherapy Database, by Bob Harris, Essential Oil Resource Consultants, UK, 2000.
5. Lis-Balchin M. *Aromatherapy science – a guide for healthcare professionals*. Pharmaceutical Press, London, 2006.
6. Anthony C. *Aromatherapy in New Zealand: indigenous use of essential oils from native plants, manuka and kanuka essential oils*. Proceedings of the Australasian Aromatherapy Conference, Sydney, 1996.
7. Tisserand M. *Aromatherapy vs. MRSA*. Singing Dragon, London, 2015.
8. Williams LR et al. *Essential oils with high antimicrobial activity for therapeutic use*. The International Journal of Aromatherapy, 1998; 8(4): 30-39.
9. Harkenthal M et al. *Comparative study on the in vitro antibacterial activity of Australian tea tree oil, cajeput oil, niaouli oil, manuka oil, kanuka oil, and eucalyptus oil*. Pharmazie, 1999; 54(6): 460-463. Cited in Quintessential Aromatics database, 2013.
10. Chen CC et al. *Investigations of kanuka and manuka essential oils for in vitro treatment of disease and cellular inflammation caused by infectious microorganisms*. Journal of Microbiology, Immunology and Infection, 2016; 49(1): 104-111. Cited in Quintessential Aromatics database, 2013.
11. Takarada K et al. *A comparison of the antibacterial efficacies of essential oils against oral pathogens*. Oral Microbiology & Immunology,

2004; 19(1): 61-64. Cited in Quintessential Aromatics database, 2013.
12. Kwon OS et al. *Topical administration of manuka oil prevents UV-B irradiation-induced cutaneous photoaging in mice.* Evidence-Based Complementary and Alternative Medicine, 2013; doi: 10.1155/2013/930857. Cited in Quintessential Aromatics database, 2013.
13. Lis-Balchin M, Hart SL. *An investigation of the actions of the essential oils of manuka (Leptospermum scoparium) and kanuka (kunzea ericoides), Myrtaceae on guinea-pig smooth muscle.* The Journal of Pharmacy and Pharmacology, 1998, 50(7): 809-811. doi: 10.1111/j.2042-7158.1998.tb07144.x
14. Reichling J et al. *Virucidal activity of a b-triketone-rich essential oil of Leptospermum scoparium (manuka oil) against HSV-1 and HSV-2 in cell culture.* Planta Medica, 2005; 71(12): 1123-1127. Cited in Quintessential Aromatics database, 2013.
15. Schnitzler P et al. *Comparative study on the cytotoxicity of different Myrtaceae essential oils on cultured Vero and RC-37 cells.* Pharmazie, 2008; 63(11): 830-835. Cited in Quintessential Aromatics database, 2013.
16. Maddocks-Jennings W et al. *Evaluating the effects of the essential oils Leptospermum scoparium (manuka) and Kunzea ericoides (kanuka) on radiotherapy induced mucositis: a randomized, placebo controlled feasibility study.* European Journal of Oncology Nursing, 2009; 13(2): 87-93. Cited in Quintessential Aromatics database, 2013.
17. von Braunschweig R. *Manuka, kanuka and tea tree oil – 3 essential oils with interesting effects on the psyche.* Proceedings of the Australasian Aromatherapy Conference, Sydney, 1998.
18. Davis P. *Aromatherapy: an A-Z.* 2nd edn. C.W. Daniel Company, Saffron Walden, 1999.

Marjoram, sweet

M

Identification

Botanical name

Origanum majorana L.

Synonyms

Majorana hortensis, knotted marjoram

Family

Lamiaceae (Labiatae)

Botany and origins

There is much confusion regarding the various species of marjoram. Sweet marjoram should not be confused with Spanish marjoram *(Thymus mastichina)* which belongs to the thyme species, or oregano *(Origanum vulgare)* which is used to produce oregano oil, and pot marjoram *(Origanum onites)*.[1]

Sweet marjoram is a tender, bushy perennial herb with woolly, hairy leaves, growing up to 0.6 m high. It is native to the Mediterranean region and is cultivated in France, Tunisia, Morocco, Italy, Hungary, Bulgaria, Poland, Germany and Turkey.[1]

The name *origanum* is derived from the Greek word *oros* meaning mountain and *ganos* meaning joy, thus 'joy of the mountains', referring to the colour and scent of their flower and leaves, and the hills they originally came from.[2]

Method of extraction

Sweet marjoram oil is steam-distilled from the dried leaves and flowering tops of the well-known culinary herb, *O. majorana.*

Characteristics

Sweet marjoram oil is a pale-yellow or pale-amber-coloured, mobile liquid with a warm-spicy, aromatic-camphoraceous and woody odour, reminiscent of nutmeg and cardamom.[3]

Chemical composition

The chemical composition of sweet marjoram essential oil from Egypt was reported as follows:

α-thujene (4.05%), tricyclene (0.95%), α-pinene (10.23%), myrcene (1.34%), β-pinene (2.79%), δ-2-carene (8.58%), *p*-cymene (2.0%), limonene (2.81%), α-phellandrene (1.46%), 1,8-cineole (1.41%), γ-terpinene (14.13%), *cis*-sabinene hydrate (4.0%), terpinolene (4.57%), *trans*-sabinene hydrate (5.25%), linalool (3.75%), terpinen-4-ol (20.39%), α-terpineol (11.06%), isobornyl acetate (0.49%), thymol (0.33%).[4]

The major constituents found in *O. majorana* var. *majorana* L. oil from France was reported as follows:

α-thujene (0.25%), α-pinene (0.5%), sabinene (4.9%), myrcene (1.1%), β-pinene (trace), *p*-cymene (0.2%), limonene (14.3%), β-phellandrene (1.8%), γ-terpinene (0.5%), terpinolene (trace), linalool (2.3%), terpinen-4-ol (47.1%), carvacrol (2.7%), α-terpineol (4.6%), linalyl acetate (2.2%), thymol (1.6%), β-caryophyllene (1.8%).[4]

Adulteration

According to Arctander, sweet marjoram oil is often adulterated with terpineol and fractions from the production of turpentine-terpineol or with the oil of *Melaleuca alternifolia*. He states that mislabelling is a common problem. Spanish marjoram, wild marjoram or blends of these oils are often labelled as 'oil of sweet marjoram'.[3] Lis-Balchin states that sweet marjoram oil is adulterated with many essential oils such as tea tree, ajowan, savory, origanum or thyme oils.[5]

Pharmacopoeias and standards

At the time of writing, an ISO standard for the purity, composition and physico-chemical properties of sweet marjoram oil was not available. However, a standard does exist for Spanish wild marjoram:

ISO 4728:2003 – Oil of Spanish Wild Marjoram (*Thymus mastichina* L.)

History and Traditional Uses

History

The herb has been used since antiquity for its medicinal and culinary purposes. The Greeks referred to marjoram as the funeral herb. It was planted on graves to bring spiritual peace to the dead.[6]

Culpeper writes of marjoram's therapeutic properties:

> *Our common sweet marjoram is warming and comforting in cold diseases of the head, stomach, sinews and other parts, taken inwardly or outwardly applied.*[6]

Culpeper recommended marjoram for diseases of the chest, obstructions of the liver and spleen, old griefs of the womb, and the windiness thereof.[6]

Herbal

Sweet marjoram is used in European herbal medicine for the treatment of respiratory ailments and bronchitis, and as an antispasmodic and an expectorant.[1] The leaves have also been used as an emmenagogue and are useful for treating gastrointestinal problems.[7]

The German Commission E states that marjoram herb and marjoram oil are used in combinations for the stimulation of appetite, for promoting digestion, for strengthening the stomach, for acute and chronic gastritis, as an antispasmodic, for flatulence, for colic-like nervous gastrointestinal disorders, for the support of intestinal activity and for functional regulation of diseases involving gallstones. However, the effectiveness for the claimed uses has not been sufficiently documented.[8]

Food, perfumery and flavouring

Sweet marjoram oil is used as a flavouring ingredient in many food products.[1]

Therapeutics

Pharmacology and clinical studies

Anti-inflammatory activity

cis-sabinene hydrate and terpineol in sweet marjoram essential oil suppressed the production of tumour necrosis factor-α (TNF-α), interleukin 1β (IL-1β), IL-6, and IL-10. They also inhibited cyclooxygenase 2 (COX2) and NFkB gene expression.[7]

Antimicrobial activity

Sweet marjoram oil has demonstrated antimicrobial activity against various pathogenic bacteria and fungi.[7,9] In one in vitro study, the antimicrobial activity of sweet marjoram was higher than eucalyptus oil.[10] Sweet marjoram oil exhibited considerable antifungal activity against a range of spoilage fungus *Aspergillus niger*.[11]

Antispasmodic activity

In vitro studies confirmed that both sweet marjoram and Spanish marjoram oils had a spasmolytic effect on electrically stimulated smooth muscle of guinea-pig ilium.[5]

Antiviral activity

An aqueous extract of sweet marjoram has been reported to have antiviral activities against *Herpes simplex* in vitro.[1]

Actions

Actions commonly cited in aromatherapy

Analgesic, anaphrodisiac, antiseptic, antispasmodic, antiviral, bactericidal, carminative, cordial, diaphoretic, digestive, diuretic, emmenagogue, expectorant, fungicidal, hypotensive, nervine, sedative, stomachic, vasodilator, vulnerary[2,12,13]

Actions supported by clinical studies

Antifungal, antimicrobial, antiseptic

Comment

Sweet marjoram has a warm, fresh herbaceous aroma, with an interesting blend of monoterpene alcohols and esters, which are likely to give the oil its antimicrobial activity and balancing effect on the nervous system.

Most of the pharmacological and clinical studies focus on sweet marjoram oil's antimicrobial activity. It would be good to see more studies investigating the use of sweet marjoram oil for strengthening and relaxing the nerves.

Aromatherapy Uses

Clinical aromatherapy

Anaphrodisiac

Sweet marjoram is considered an anaphrodisiac; it is reputed to diminish the desire for sexual contact. This property may be associated with the fact that marjoram has a long association with celibacy.[12,14]

Davis warns against excessive use of marjoram unless you are committed to lifelong celibacy as it will diminish normal sexual response.[15]

Circulatory system

Its warming properties make it useful for treating chilblains and it helps disperse bruises.[12]

Sweet marjoram oil is recommended for alleviating high blood pressure.[12,13,14,15]

Digestive system

Sweet marjoram oil stimulates and strengthens intestinal peristalsis. It is recommended as a digestive and carminative for relieving constipation, colic, flatulence and spasmodic indigestion.[12]

Musculoskeletal system

Sweet marjoram oil is warming and analgesic, making it useful for muscular spasm, rheumatic pains, sprains and strains.[12,13,14,15]

M

Nervous system

Sweet marjoram oil has the ability to strengthen and relax the nerves. It is recommended for conditions in which tiredness alternates with nervous tension, stress-related conditions characterised by anxiety or insomnia.[15]

Davis recommends not abusing the sedative properties of marjoram as it can dull the senses and cause drowsiness, and in large amounts it is stupefying.[15]

According to Tisserand, sweet marjoram oil stimulates the parasympathetic nervous system and lowers the sympathetic function.[14] Sweet marjoram oil may be rubbed into the temple for relief of headaches and migraines.[13,14]

Sweet marjoram oil is comforting for people who are lonely or suffering grief. However, it should only be used for a short period as extended use may have a deadening effect on the emotions.[16]

Holmes describes sweet marjoram oil as a primary restorative and stimulant, and recommends it for neurasthenia, nervous breakdown, chronic stress-related conditions, agitated depression, and mental or emotional burnout.[17]

Psychological

Holmes states that marjoram oil is one of the best essential oils to help us release and resolve stuck, festering emotions. He explains that marjoram is capable of profound emotional transformation that gives one renewed emotional strength and stability. He compares sweet marjoram with everlasting in its ability to address deep-seated emotional trauma and conflict.[17]

Reproductive system

Sweet marjoram oil's antispasmodic and emmenagogue properties are valued for its action on the uterine muscles. Used as a massage or hot compress over the lower abdomen, it will ease menstrual cramps.[14] Mailhebiau recommends using sweet marjoram in conjunction with clary sage for females who experience uterine and nerve spasms during their period.[16]

Respiratory system

Sweet marjoram oil can be used as an inhalation or a chest rub for the treatment of colds and flu. The oil has antibacterial and antispasmodic properties, which make it effective for nervous cough and asthma.[2] Schnaubelt recommends using it for whooping cough.[18]

Energetics, psyche and subtle uses

Energetics

Sweet marjoram oil circulates *Qi*, clears *cold phlegm* and calms the mind. This means that the oil has excellent antispasmodic properties.[2,19] It may be used for conditions such as muscular stiffness and pain, nervous spasm, intestinal colic and osteoarthritis.

Its ability to smooth the flow of *Qi* in the chest indicates that it can be used to calm and regulate the *Heart*, making it useful for palpitations, tachycardia and hypertension.[2,17]

Mojay states that sweet marjoram restores the *Qi* of the *Spleen* and has a calming effect on the nerves. This makes marjoram oil 'balancing'. The sweet, nourishing and balancing qualities of marjoram mean that it has an affinity with the Earth Element and helps to regulate the *Yi*, which is referred to as our intellect. Whenever our *Yi* is weak, we may become prone to too much worry and overthinking. This may then make us feel isolated, lonely or unsupported. Marjoram will help to calm this obsessive worry and overthinking and help restore our inner self-nurturing.[2]

On the other hand, Holmes states that sweet marjoram oil is associated with the Wood and Fire Elements. He explains this is because it helps to calm the *Liver*, activates the *Qi* and harmonises the *Shen*.[17] Whenever the *Liver* is agitated, we may experience muscle spasms, headaches, tinnitus, muscle tension and seizures. Whenever the *Shen* is agitated, we may experience anxiety, insomnia, overstimulation and palpitations.

Personality

Worwood describes the marjoram personality as a warm and friendly person who is always ready to offer comfort and solace to those in need. Marjoram personalities prefer to keep to themselves and will not intrude upon another person's privacy unless asked to. They are very generous and kind people who are always helping out friends and family. They do not expect any reward for their generosity and kindness; however, the fact that they can be taken advantage of and often don't even receive a 'thank you' means that they can become depressed, withdrawn and emotionally cold.[20]

Marjoram personalities are not out to change the world; however, they provide much needed stability and grounding to more flamboyant personality types. They are considered to be sincere, and to have great courage, stamina and perseverance.[20]

According to Myers-Briggs personality types, the sweet marjoram personality is likely to be an INTP.

INTPs are quiet, reserved and highly independent. They like to be precise. They have a natural curiosity to understand the universe and to examine its universal truths and principles. They may be good at developing complex systems and conceptual models, but prefer to leave the implementation to others. They have high standards of intellectual and professional competence. They can have difficulty explaining their deep thoughts so that others can understand. They dislike supervising others or resolving conflict. They appear to be concerned with their thoughts, interests and work, and can neglect their relationships. They prefer a calm, conflict-free atmosphere. They can appear to be formal and distant with strangers and acquaintances, but are generally open-minded and accepting of people once they know them.

Subtle

Mojay suggests that sweet marjoram oil helps to calm obsessive thinking, ease emotional craving and promote the capacity for inner self-nurturing.[2]

Holmes explains why sweet marjoram has often been referred to as the grieving herb:

> *Marjoram was associated with Osiris, the god of constant death and rebirth inherent in all of life. Significantly, emotional rejuvenation results mainly from one's ability to let go of long-held distressed emotions. The process of grieving for personal loss, for instance, is traditionally often supported with marjoram.*[17]

Zeck recommends sweet marjoram oil whenever work, stress and emotional upheaval overwhelm us. The warm herbal aroma of sweet marjoram oil will strengthen our nervous system and invigorate our spirit and reduce obsessive thinking.[21]

Dosage and Administration

Blending

Aromatherapy

To alleviate stress-related conditions associated with anxiety, insomnia and agitation, consider blending sweet marjoram oil with essential oils such as bergamot, Roman chamomile, clary sage, fragonia, geranium, lavender, neroli, patchouli, sandalwood or vetiver.

For the temporary relief of hypertension or tachycardia, consider blending sweet marjoram with essential oils such as lavender, may chang, melissa, neroli or ylang ylang.

For the relief of acute, painful, spasmodic dysmenorrhoea and acute PMS, consider blending sweet marjoram oil with essential oils such as Roman chamomile, clary sage, lavender or geranium.

For the relief of gastrointestinal spasms and colic, consider blending sweet marjoram oil with essential oils such as black pepper, cardamom, ginger, mandarin, sweet orange or peppermint.

Perfumery

Sweet marjoram is occasionally used in perfumery to introduce a fresh, slightly medicinal-aromatic warm note in fougères, colognes and oriental style perfumes.[3]

Mode of administration

Bath

Full body bath, foot bath

Topical

Compress, massage, ointment

Inhalation

Direct inhalation, diffuser, oil vaporiser

Safety Profile

General safety

Sweet marjoram oil is non-toxic, non-irritating and non-sensitising.[12]

Tisserand & Young state that there are no known hazards or contraindications for sweet marjoram essential oil.[22]

Contraindications

Sweet marjoram oil is contraindicated during pregnancy.[12,14,15,17]

While marjoram herb has been classified as an emmenagogue, none of the herbal texts that I reviewed indicated that marjoram was contraindicated during pregnancy.

No other contraindications known.

Regulatory guidelines

Sweet marjoram essential oil has GRAS status.

References

1. Khan I, Abourashed E. *Leung's encyclopedia of common natural ingredients used in food, drugs and cosmetics*. 3rd edn. John Wiley & Sons, New Jersey, 2010.
2. Mojay G. *Aromatherapy for healing the spirit*. Healing Arts Press, Rochester, 1997.
3. Arctander S. *Perfume and flavor materials of natural origin*. Allured Publishing, Carol Stream, 1994.
4. Lawrence BM. *Progress in essential oils – marjoram oil and extract*. Perfumer & Flavorist, 2007; 32: 32-37.
5. Lis-Balchin M. *Aromatherapy science – a guide for healthcare professionals*. Pharmaceutical Press, London, 2006.
6. Le Strange R. *A history of herbal plants*. Angus and Robertson, United Kingdom, 1977.
7. Bina F et al. *Sweet marjoram: a review of ethnopharmacology, phytochemistry and biological activities*. Journal of Evidence-Based Complementary & Alternative Medicine, 2017; 22(1): 175-185. doi: 10.1177/2156587216650793.
8. Blumenthal M et al. *The complete German commission E monographs: therapeutic guide to herbal medicine*. American Botanical Council, Austin, 1998.
9. Stefanakis MK et al. *Antibacterial activity of essential oils from plants of genus Origanum*. Food Control, 2013; 34(2): 539-546. Cited in Quintessential Aromatics database, 2013.
10. Mahboubi M, Feizabadi MM. *The antimicrobial activity of thyme, sweet marjoram, savory and eucalyptus oils on Escherichia coli, Salmonella typhimurium, Aspergillus niger and Aspergillus flavus*. Journal of Herbal Medicine, 2009; 8(30): 36-43.
11. Baratta MT et al. *Antimicrobial and antioxidant properties of some commercial essential oils*. Flavour and Fragrance Journal, 1998; 13(4): 235-244. Cited in Quintessential Aromatics database, 2013.
12. Lawless J. *The encyclopaedia of essential oils*. Element Books, Shaftesbury, 1992.
13. Lavabre M. *Aromatherapy workbook*. Healing Arts Press, Rochester, 1997.
14. Tisserand R. *The art of aromatherapy*. C.W. Daniel Company, Saffron Walden, 1977.
15. Davis P. *Aromatherapy: an A-Z*. 2nd edn. C.W. Daniel Company, Saffron Walden, 1999.
16. 16. Mailhebiau P. *Portraits in oils*. C.W. Daniel Company, Saffron Walden, 1995
17. Holmes P. *Aromatica: a clinical guide to essential oil therapeutics – Vol. I*. Singing Dragon, London, 2016.
18. Schnaubelt K. *Medical aromatherapy*. Frog, Berkeley, 1999.
19. Holmes P. *The energetics of Western herbs – Vol. I*. Artemis Press, Boulder, 1986.
20. Worwood VA. *The fragrant mind*. Transworld Publishing, London, 1995.
21. Zeck R. *The blossoming heart – aromatherapy for healing and transformation*. Aroma Tours, East Ivanhoe, 2004.
22. Tisserand R, Young R. *Essential oil safety*. 2nd edn. Churchill Livingstone, Edinburgh, 2014.

May chang

Identification

Botanical name

Litsea cubeba (Lour.) Pers.

Synonyms

The essential oil is often referred to by its botanical name *Litsea cubeba.*

Family

Lauraceae

Botany and origins

It has been known for its fragrant flowers, fruit and leaves for a long time. The small fruit resembles cubeb pepper, hence its name.[1]

May chang is a small fragrant tropical tree which grows in eastern Asia. China is the largest producer of may chang oil. In Taiwan and other parts of South East Asia, it is called 'mountain pepper'.[2]

Although *L. cubeba* is normally associated with China, it can be found growing in its natural environment in the eastern Himalayan areas of Assam, Manipur and other autonomous regions of northeastern India.[3]

An oil can also be distilled from the bark whose

main constituent is citronellal, and from the leaves with the main constituent, 1,8-cineole, but both are of no commercial importance.[2]

Method of extraction

May chang essential oil is steam-distilled from the small, pepper-like fruits of *L. cubeba.*

Characteristics

While it is often compared with lemongrass, its odour is considered to be finer, more lemon-like and less fatty. May chang oil is a pale yellow, mobile oil with an intensely lemon-like, fresh and sweet aroma and a soft and sweet-fruity dryout. Arctander states that lemongrass has superior odour tenacity due to its heavy sesquiterpene constituents.[1]

Chemical composition

May chang is chemically similar to lemongrass, melissa and other essential oils rich in citral. Citral, which comprises around 75% of may chang oil, has two isomers, neral and geranial. The chemical composition of may chang oil from dried fruits of *L. cubeba* from Jiangxi Province (China) was reported as follows:

α-pinene (3.8%), sabinene (4.5%), β-pinene (6.2%), limonene (26.3%), 1,8-cineole (1.6%), linalool (1.4%), citronellal (0.5%), neral (21.9%), geranial (26.0%), nerol (0.5%), geraniol (0.6%), β-caryophyllene (0.8%).[3]

The ISO standard 3214:2000 for *Litsea cubeba* specifies the following chemical composition:

α-pinene (<1.5%), limonene (9-15%), 2-methyl-2-heptene-6-one (1.8-3%), citronellal (<1.5%), linalool (1.5-3.0%), neral (25-33%), geranial (38-45%), citronellol (0.5-1.5%), nerol (0.2-1.2%), geraniol (0.5-1.5%).[4]

Adulteration

Lis-Balchin states that *L. cubeba* oil is not an expensive oil, therefore, substitution with citral is not considered economical. However, she states that it may be blended or substituted with lemongrass. It may also be substituted with *L. citrata*, another plant that grows in China. However, this plant has a lower citral content.[5]

Pharmacopoeias and standards

The purity, composition and physico-chemical properties of *Litsea cubeba* are defined in ISO 3214:2000 Oil of Litsea cubeba (*Litsea cubeba* Pers.).

History and Traditional Uses

History

The English name 'may chang' is a derivative of its Cantonese name *Myu Tsam Fa*, which literally means '*May* (the month) *Tsam* (a surname) flower.'[6]

Arctander states that it was not until the 1950s that may chang oil was first steam distilled.[1]

Traditional medicine

In TCM, may chang is used to treat dysmenorrhoea that is alleviated with heat or pressure, stomach aches, lower back pain, chills, headaches and muscular aches from external conditions. May chang fruits are reputed to alleviate chronic asthma, as well as being a treatment for coronary heart disease and high blood pressure.[7]

Herbal

The berries are traditionally brewed into a decoction for gastric and abdominal pain.[6]

Food, perfumery and flavouring

May chang oil is used as a flavour enhancer in foods and cosmetics; as a raw material in the manufacture of citral, vitamins A, E and K, ionone and methyl ionone; and as an insecticide.[8]

Therapeutics

Pharmacology and clinical studies

Many pharmacological studies involving may chang essential oil have been published. A systemic review of these studies will not be attempted. Rather, I have chosen a selection of studies that support the traditional and clinical uses.

M

Antimicrobial activity

An in vitro study confirmed that *L. cubeba* oil had high antibacterial activity against the cariogenic bacteria – *Streptococcus mutans, S. sobrinus* and *S. sanguinis.*[9]

An in vitro study examined the antibacterial activity of may chang essential oil against *Escherichia coli.* The minimum inhibitory concentration (MIC) and minimum bactericidal concentration (MBC) were both 0.125% (v/v). Damage to the cell wall of *E. coli* was observed, indicating that the oil might be able to penetrate and destroy the outer and inner membranes of *E. coli* cells.[10]

The oil from *L. cubeba* grown in Tibet displayed high fungicidal activity against a range of fungal organisms.[11]

Another study confirmed the antifungal activities of the distilled oil from the ripe fruits of *L. cubeba* harvested in India against *Fusarium moniliforme, F. solani, Alternaria alternate* and *Aspergillus niger.* The antifungal activity of the oil improved with an increase in concentration. The antifungal activity was attributed to citral.[12]

The minimum inhibitory and bactericidal concentrations were determined under nutritive and non-nutritive conditions for 30 essential oils reputed to have good antimicrobial activity. May chang oil was one of 10 essential oils that was effective at 0.2% (v/v) concentration in nutritive conditions. The antibacterial efficacy of the essential oils was more significant in non-nutritive conditions. May chang oil also had a powerful antimicrobial effect against multi-resistant bacterial strains.[13]

Cardiovascular activity

It is believed that citral is the main constituent responsible for the beneficial effects seen in the experiments involving experimentally induced cardiac arrhythmia. Experiments have found that citral increases blood flow in the rabbit heart, and improved the ECG profile in rabbits with experimentally induced cardiac arrhythmia and in rats with isoprenaline-induced cardiac ischaemia.[7]

Cosmetic applications

L. cubeba oil exhibited a potent inhibitory effect on tyrosinase and a protective effect against UV-TiO_2-NO_2 induced protein oxidation at 0.01 mg/mL. The results suggest that the oil could serve as a new natural skin-whitening agent.[14]

M

Hypotensive activity

Tisserand & Balacs cite clinical trials using may chang for the treatment of experimentally induced cardiac arrhythmias. It was compared with propranolol (a beta-blocker, antihypertensive and anti-anginal drug). The test results confirmed may chang's ability to reduce arrhythmias was from 15 minutes to 6.5 minutes, while propranolol reduced the arrhythmia time from 15 minutes to 0.6 minutes.[7]

Immunosuppressive activity

May chang oil decreased the production of TNF-α and cytokine IL-12 in a dose-dependent manner in lipopolysaccharide-stimulated dendritic cells. The contact hypersensitivity response was also inhibited in mice treated with *L. cubeba* oil. It was suggested that *L. cubeba* oil could be applied in the treatment of contact hypersensitivity, inflammatory diseases and autoimmune diseases.[15]

Neuropharmacological activity

Oral administration of 100, 300 and 500 mg/kg of *L. cubeba* fruit oil significantly prolonged pentobarbitone-induced mouse sleeping time by 20, 110.8 and 159.6% respectively. The same study using mice in a maze test suggested that *L. cubeba* oil had anxiolytic activity on mice.[16]

Actions

Actions commonly cited in aromatherapy

Antidepressant, anti-inflammatory, antiseptic, astringent, calming, carminative, deodorant, galactagogue, insecticide, stimulant, tonic[17,18,19]

Actions supported by clinical studies

Antimicrobial, antiseptic

Comment

Many studies have confirmed the potent antimicrobial activity of essential oils high in citral such as may chang. However, *L. cubeba* oil and other oils high in citral need to be used cautiously in topical preparations, as there is always a risk of dermal irritation on people with hypersensitive skin or children under the age of two.

Holmes explains that the scent of may chang oil promotes emotional renewal. The oil can also be used as a stimulant to promote alertness and focus, and eliminate negative thinking.[6]

Aromatherapy Uses

Clinical aromatherapy

Antimicrobial

Holmes recommends using may chang oil whenever infections are present with high fever and pain. The oil is also invaluable for its ability to clear heat and reduce pain.[6]

Cardiovascular system

May chang oil has been used as a treatment for coronary heart disease and high blood pressure.[7]

Digestive system

May chang oil is recommended as a digestive stimulant and for upper gastric deficiency with dyspepsia, flatulence and appetite loss.[6]

Musculoskeletal system

May chang oil is recommended for the relief of muscular tension and pain, acute arthritic and rheumatic pain, inflammation and tendinitis.[6]

Psychological

The pleasant, refreshing citrus aroma of may chang oil can be used to alleviate stress and anxiety which may lead to depression. May chang oil promotes alertness and optimism. Holmes calls may chang oil an 'emotional detoxifier', describing its effect on the psyche as expansive and clarifying. He recommends it for conditions associated with lack of focus and attention, poor short-term memory, mental fogginess, confusion, negative thinking, pessimism and depression.[6]

Holmes states that the lemon-green aromatic quality of may chang promotes the opportunity for emotional transformation.[6]

Skin care

May chang oil is recommended for the treatment of oily skin and acne. It is also reputed to reduce excess perspiration and is a deodorant.[17,20] However, do not use on people with hypersensitive, diseased or damaged skin.

Energetics, psyche and subtle uses

Energetics

According to the principles of the Five Elements, may chang oil helps to balance the Wood Element. The oil regulates the *Qi*, clears *heat* and balances the *Shen*. It helps to disperse the *Liver Qi* and calms the *Shen*. Whenever the *Liver Qi* is constrained and the *Shen* is agitated, we may feel irritable, anxious and over-talkative, and suffer from insomnia. Holmes also recommends may chang oil for *Stomach-Spleen Qi* stagnation which may be associated with indigestion, flatulence, bloating, nausea and appetite loss.[6]

Subtle

May chang oil helps to promote optimism, vision and foresight whenever there is pessimism, negative thinking and loss of vision.[6]

Dosage and Administration

Blending

Aromatherapy

Lavabre describes may chang oil as a blend enhancer. This means that the oil would have enough personality to modify your blend without overpowering it, as long as you do not go overboard using it.[18]

For the relief of palpitations, tachycardia and arrhythmia, consider blending may chang oil with essential oils such as melissa, neroli, lavender, sweet marjoram or ylang ylang.

For the relief of muscular aches and pain, consider blending may chang oil with essential oils such as black pepper, cajeput, ginger, kunzea, spike lavender, pine or rosemary.

Perfumery

Arctander states that *L. cubeba* oil has a pleasant taste, and that the oil is used in flavour work as a modifier for lemon and lime flavours. In perfumery, it could replace lemongrass. It blends very well with all citrus oils, petitgrain oil, rosemary oil and lavender oil. Unfortunately, may chang oil does not have a strong fixative power, and needs clever blending for successful use in soap perfumes.[1]

Mode of administration

Bath

Due to the high citral content, I would not recommend using may chang oil in a bath as it will cause skin irritation and sensitisation.

Topical

Compress, massage, ointment

Inhalation

Direct inhalation, diffuser, oil vaporiser

Safety Profile

General safety

May chang oil is non-toxic, non-irritating, but possibly sensitising in some individuals. Tisserand & Young caution the use of may chang oil on people with hypersensitive, diseased, or damaged skin and for children under two years of age.[21]

Based on the high percentage of citral in may chang oil and the IFRA maximum limits for citral, Tisserand & Young suggest that a maximum of 0.8% may chang oil be allowed for topical use.[21]

Contraindications

No contraindications known.

Regulatory guidelines

May chang essential oil is not defined in any regulatory guideline.

References

1. Arctander S. *Perfume and flavor materials of natural origin*. Allured Publishing, Carol Stream, 1994.
2. Weiss EA. *Essential oil crops*. CAB International, Wallingford, 1997.
3. Lawrence BM. *Progress in essential oils – Litsea cubeba*. Perfumer & Flavorist, 2013; 38: 46-47.
4. *ISO 3214 – Oil of Litsea cubeba (Litsea cubeba Pers.)*. International Organization for Standardization, Geneva, 2000.
5. Lis-Balchin M. *Aromatherapy science – a guide for healthcare professionals*. Pharmaceutical Press, London, 2006.
6. Holmes P. *Aromatica: a clinical guide to essential oil therapeutics – Vol. I*. Singing Dragon, London, 2016.
7. Tisserand R, Balacs T. *May chang*. The International Journal of Aromatherapy, 1992; 4(3): 25-27.
8. Luo M et al. *Acute and genetic toxicity of essential oil extracted from Litsea cubeba (Lour.)*

Pers. Journal of Food Protection, 2005; 68(3): 581-588. Cited in Quintessential Aromatics database, 2013.
9. Yang TS et al. *Antimicrobial activity of the essential oil of Litsea cubeba on cariogenic bacteria.* Journal of Essential Oil Research, 2013; 25(2): 120-128. doi: 10.1080/10412905.2012.758602.
10. Li WR et al. *Antibacterial activity and kinetics of Litsea cubeba oil on Escherichia coli.* PLoS ONE, 2014; 9(11): e110983. doi: 10.1371/journal.pone.0110983.
11. Yang Y et al. *The fungicidal terpenoids and essential oil from Litsea cubeba in Tibet.* Molecules, 2010; 15: 7075- 7082. doi: 10.3390/molecules15107075.
12. Gogoi P et al. *Antifungal activity of the essential oil of Litsea cubeba Pers.* Journal of Essential Oil Research, 1997; 9(2): 213-215. Cited in Quintessential Aromatics database, 2013.
13. Ezzaouia S et al. *Investigation of essential oils to fight multiresistant bacteria in hygienic and therapeutic applications.* International Journal of Essential Oil Therapeutics, 2007; 1(2): 51-55. Cited in Quintessential Aromatics database, 2013.
14. Huang XW et al. *Potential cosmetic application of essential oil extracted from Litsea cubeba fruits from China.* Journal of Essential Oil Research, 2013; 25(2): 112-119. Cited in Quintessential Aromatics database, 2013.
15. Chen HC et al. *Immunosupressive effect of Litsea cubeba L essential oil on dendritic cell and contact hypersensitivity responses.* International Journal of Molecular Sciences, 2016; 17: 1319. doi: 10.3390/ijms17081319.
16. Chen CJ et al. *Neuropharmacological activities of fruit essential oil from Litsea cubeba Persoon.* Journal of Wood Science, 2012; 58(6): 538-543.
17. Lawless J. *The encyclopaedia of essential oils.* Element Books, Shaftesbury, 1992.
18. Lavabre M. *Aromatherapy workbook.* Healing Arts Press, Rochester, 1997.
19. Schnaubelt K. *Advanced aromatherapy.* Healing Arts Press, Rochester, 1995.
20. Davis P. *Aromatherapy: an A-Z.* 2nd edn. C.W. Daniel Company, Saffron Walden, 1999.
21. Tisserand R, Young R. *Essential oil safety.* 2nd edn. Churchill Livingstone, Edinburgh, 2014.

M

Melissa

Identification

Botanical name

Melissa officinalis L.

Synonyms

Lemon balm, balm, common balm, bee balm

Family

Lamiaceae (Labiatae)

Botany and origins

Melissa is a sweet-scented perennial herb which grows up to 0.9 m high, with serrated leaves and tiny white or pink flowers. Melissa is distilled in the south of France, Germany, Italy and Spain; however, the total production of genuine melissa oil is only a fraction of the quantity commercially offered.[1]

The name is from the Greek word signifying *bee*, indicative of the attraction the plant has for bees, and the word *balm*, an abbreviation of the term *balsam*.[2]

Method of extraction

Melissa oil is steam-distilled from the leaves and flowering tops of *M. officinalis.*

Characteristics

Melissa oil is a pale-yellow or pale-amber-coloured, mobile liquid with an intensely fresh and sweet citrus and herbaceous odour.[1]

Chemical composition

The chemical composition of melissa oil from Turkey was reported as follows:

α-pinene (0-1.0%), β-pinene (0-10.7%), citronellal (0-20.3%), linalool (0-4.2%), neral (3.2-32.1%), geranial (37.7-84.6%), geraniol (0-19.7%).[3]

The chemical composition of melissa oil from Germany was reported as follows:

ocimene (1.7%), citronellal (6.6%), neral (26.2%), geranial (37.3%), neryl acetate (4.8%), β-caryophyllene (11.2%), α-humulene (0.6%), caryophyllene oxide (0.7%).[4]

Adulteration

Arctander states that melissa oil enjoys the reputation of being the most frequently adulterated essential oil. The herb may be distilled with lemon oil, Spanish verbena oil, lemongrass oil, citronella oil and various mixtures or fractions thereof.[1]

Pharmacopoeias and standards

At the time of writing, the purity, composition,

physico-chemical properties and therapeutic use of melissa essential oil are not defined in any pharmacopoeia monograph or standard.

History and Traditional Uses

History

Melissa herb was highly esteemed by Paracelsus, who believed it could completely revivify a man. Herbalist John Evelyn (1620-1706) described melissa as the ruler of the brain, strengthening the memory and removing melancholy.[2]

Avicenna recommended melissa for strengthening the heart. A spirit of balm made by combining melissa with lemon peel, nutmeg, angelica root and other herbs and spices enjoyed a great reputation under the name of Carmelite water. This was considered beneficial for the treatment of nervous headaches, digestive problems and neuralgic affections.[2]

Traditional medicine

In traditional European medicine, melissa herb was used for the treatment of melancholy and for enhancing the memory. Greek physicians used melissa to treat wounds.[5]

Herbal

Melissa herb is used in numerous European herbal pharmaceutical preparations as a carminative and mild relaxant.[5] The herb is listed in the German Commission E Monographs for the treatment of nervous sleeping disorders and functional gastrointestinal complaints.[6]

Food, perfumery and flavouring

Melissa extract and essential oil are extensively used in cosmetics and food products as a flavouring.[5]

Therapeutics

Pharmacology and clinical studies

Many pharmacological studies involving melissa essential oil have been published. A systemic review of these studies will not be attempted. Rather, I have chosen a selection of studies that support the traditional and clinical uses.

Antibacterial activity

An in vitro study confirmed that melissa oil had excellent antibacterial activity when used on its own and when used with standard antibiotics. The results suggest that, in some cases, essential oils could be used in synergy with antibiotic in some bacteria; however, an antagonistic effect was observed in some bacteria.[7]

Melissa oil displayed very high antibacterial activity against four bacterial strains responsible for nosocomial infections – *Pseudomonas aeruginosa, Klebsiella pneumonia, Staphylococcus aureus* and *Citrobacter koseri*. Melissa oil displayed stronger antibacterial activity when compared to standard antibiotics used as controls – cefaclor, oxacillin and vancomycin. However, the antibacterial effect of melissa was lower when compared to imipenem standard antibiotic.[8]

Anticarcinogenic activity

The anticarcinogenic activity of melissa oil was investigated and compared with the anticarcinogenic effects of methotrexate and Vepesid. The results confirmed that melissa oil has anticarcinogenic activity.[9]

An in vitro study examined the cytotoxicity of melissa oil against a range of human cancer cell lines. At dilutions between 1:50,000 and 1:2,000, the essential oil induced a significant dose-dependent inhibitory effect on all the cancer cell lines.[10]

Antidiabetic activity

An in vitro study found that melissa oil may play an important role on the effect of antidiabetes.[11]

Mice administered with melissa oil for 6 weeks showed significantly reduced blood glucose improved glucose tolerance and significantly higher serum insulin levels compared to the control group. It was suggested that the hypoglycaemic mechanism of melissa oil was due to the enhanced glucose uptake and metabolism in the liver and adipose tissue, and the inhibition of gluconeogenesis in the liver.[12]

Anti-inflammatory activity

An in vivo study using mice confirmed that melissa oil showed significant reduction and inhibition of oedema when compared with the control and standard drug – indomethacin. It was concluded that melissa oil possesses potential anti-inflammatory activities.[13]

An in vitro study confirmed that melissa essential oil demonstrated good to moderate activity in inhibiting the enzyme 5-lipoxygenase. The mechanisms of inflammation involve the metabolism of arachidonic acid which begins with its oxidation by 5-lipoxygenase.[14]

Antioxidant activity

An in vitro study confirmed that melissa oil exhibited very strong free radical scavenging capacity and very strong inhibition of lipid peroxidation.[15]

Antispasmodic activity

An in vitro study confirmed that melissa oil

exhibited strong antispasmodic activity on isolated rat ileum.[16]

Antiviral activity

Hot water extracts of melissa have strong antiviral properties against mumps, *Herpes simplex*, and other viruses. Polyphenols and the tannin present have been identified as responsible for these antiviral properties.[6]

An in vitro study confirmed that melissa oil was able to reduce the viral infectivity of three different infective doses of herpes simplex virus (HSV) type 2. The antiviral effect of melissa oil was not statistically different from that of acyclovir, which was used as a control.[17]

The results of an in vitro study indicate that melissa oil affects the *herpes simplex* virus before adsorption, but not after penetration into the host cell. It was suggested that, considering the lipophilic nature of melissa oil, which is able to penetrate the skin, it may be suitable for a topical treatment of herpes infections.[18]

Clinical studies indicate that melissa oil reduces the infectivity of acyclovir-resistant herpes viruses.[19]

Dementia

A double-blind, placebo-controlled trial confirmed that topical application of melissa oil significantly reduced agitation in severe dementia patients. It was concluded that aromatherapy with melissa oil is a safe and effective treatment for clinically significant agitation in people with severe dementia.[20]

Another study confirmed that both lavender and melissa oils reduced agitation in dementia patients. The researchers were able to determine the receptor binding properties at a number of ligand-gated and G-protein coupled receptors implicated in agitation. It was also reported that melissa oil demonstrated greater potency than lavender oil.[21]

Melissa oil demonstrated high acetylcholinesterase inhibitory activity. Recent research indicates that inhibition of cholinesterase may be effective for treating Alzheimer's disease.[22]

Sedative activity

A placebo-controlled, double-blind study found that a 600 mg dose of encapsulated extract of lemon balm in healthy adults significantly improved accuracy of attention and memory functions, and increased calmness.[6]

The hydroalcoholic extract of melissa is a CNS sedative (in mouse); however, recent studies indicate that the essential oil does not appear to play a role in this activity.[23]

A 50:50 blend of melissa oil and lavender oil inhibited [^{3}H] flunitrazepam binding, whereas the individual essential oils had no effect. The data suggests that the two oils had anti-agitation effects.[24]

A double-blind, placebo-controlled, randomised, balanced crossover experiment using 18 healthy human volunteers receiving two separate single doses of a standardised melissa extract (300 mg, 600 mg) showed that the 600 mg dose reduced the negative mood effects of the Defined Intensity Stress Simulation battery. Significantly increased self-ratings of calmness and reduced self-ratings of alertness were also reported. The results suggest that the ability of melissa extract to reduce the effects of stress deserves further investigation.[25]

Actions

Actions commonly cited in aromatherapy

Analgesic, antidepressant, antiseptic, antispasmodic, antiviral, bactericidal, carminative, cordial, diaphoretic, febrifuge, hypotensive, insect repellent, nervine, sedative, sudorific, tonic [26,27,28]

Actions supported by clinical studies

Anti-inflammatory, antiviral, bactericidal, sedative

Comment

Melissa is a herb native to the eastern Mediterranean region and western Asia that has a long traditional use for a range of therapeutic purposes, such as an antispasmodic, carminative, sedative/hypnotic, and for strengthening the memory and relief of stress-induced headaches.

However, Sorensen states that, in order to evaluate the different claims made for melissa oil, we should differentiate between studies using melissa alcoholic extract or melissa essential oil.[29] Many studies involving melissa use hydroalcoholic extracts.

Review of traditional uses and clinical data support the use of melissa oil for modulation of mood and cognitive performance.

There is no doubt that melissa oil has great therapeutic potential in aromatherapy. However, the adulteration of the oil being the rule rather than the exception really concerns me; therefore, extreme care must be taken to use the genuine oil.

Aromatherapy Uses

Clinical aromatherapy

Cardiovascular system

Melissa oil is reputed to lower high blood pressure, and it has a calming effect on over-rapid breathing and heartbeat.[30] Tisserand suggests that melissa is a tonic of the heart. He recommends it for all heart conditions where there is overstimulation or heat, leading to weakness of the heart.[31]

Digestive system

Melissa oil is reputed to regulate the digestive system, relieve cramps, reduce flatulence and stimulate the gall bladder and liver.[32] The action of melissa oil has been compared with that of peppermint and sweet fennel. It is a tonic and is recommended for nausea, vomiting and indigestion, especially of nervous origins.[33]

Immune system

Studies in Germany have found melissa oil to possess antiviral properties against *herpes simplex* and *herpes zoster*. Dr Wabner suggests using an undiluted blend of rose and melissa oil directly onto the herpes lesions. He states that the herpes lesions often disappear within one or two days.[34] Care should be taken to apply the oil to the blisters only and not the surrounding skin, to minimise irritation.

Psychological

Fischer-Rizzi describes melissa oil as a gift from heaven and recommends using the oil for overstimulation of the nervous system that causes stress, anxiety, insomnia, depression and lost inner direction.[32]

Melissa oil is considered a sedative and is recommended for reducing anger in times of crisis or trauma.[35] The oil is well known for its uplifting and antidepressant qualities.[27]

Skin care

Melissa oil is often recommended for the treatment of oily skin and acne.[26,32] However, there is a high risk of skin irritation or skin sensitisation, and for this reason, I prefer using essential oils which are less likely to cause an irritation.

Energetics, psyche and subtle uses

Energetics

Energetically, melissa is *cooling* and *drying*. It is indicated for stagnation of *Qi* and for reducing *heat* in the Liver and Heart. Melissa's *cooling*, soothing influence on the Heart and nervous system makes it effective for alleviating restlessness, insomnia and nervous tension.[28]

According to the principles of the Five Elements, melissa oil helps to balance the Wood and Fire Elements.

Mojay explains that melissa oil strengthens and balances the *Shen* and the *Hun*.[28] Whenever the *Shen* is feeling agitated, we suffer from anxiety, restless and insomnia. The *Hun*, otherwise known as the 'Ethereal Soul', is responsible for our ability to make decisions and to have a good sense of direction in life. Whenever the *Hun* is weak, we always feel like we are running into brick walls, we do not respond well to pressure, and we feel as if we have no sense of purpose or direction in our life.

Personality

Worwood describes the melissa personality as full of energy and delightful. She states that their youthfulness has a revitalising effect on everyone they meet. They consider life to be too precious to be wasted, so they are always busy doing exciting and interesting activities. They are considered to be very organised individuals. Melissa personalities are very enthusiastic and like to try new and exciting things. Their enthusiasm and energy may make it difficult for them to meditate or participate in solitary practices.[36]

Worwood explains that melissa personalities are likely to attract jealousy and envy from people who admire their vivacious, outgoing nature and their incredible sense of control. Such people may wish to control melissa personality types by making them behave more like themselves. However, melissa personality types will always see the good side of people, despite the attempts of negative people to drag them down.[36]

According to Myers-Briggs personality types, the melissa personality is likely to be an ESFJ. ESFJs are warm-hearted, outgoing and friendly. They are highly sociable and they become restless when separated from others. They thrive on being needed and appreciated. They are more attuned to the needs of others than their own. ESFJs enjoy busy lives. They like to be involved in community service organisations and volunteer activities. They enjoy spending time with their friends and family. They are service oriented and want to provide practical help to others. They tend to be talkative and are comfortable chatting with just about anyone. They value harmony and try not to offend or disappoint anyone.

Subtle

Davis states that melissa oil is of great comfort during bereavement. She explains that the sweet fresh fragrance seems to dispel fear and regret and bring acceptance and understanding as the time of death approaches.[37]

Melissa oil is recommended for the heart chakra. Davis suggests using it to expand feelings of love from the individual towards total acceptance of unconditional love.[37]

Mojay recommends melissa for people who are

easily traumatised by confrontation. They often manifest their strength by attempting to contain, rather than respond to and express, their feelings of hurt and anger.[28]

Melissa oil promotes sensitivity and intuition, helps us find inner contentment and strengthens the 'wisdom of the heart'.[32]

Keim Loughran & Bull explain that melissa oil helps us release emotional blocks and heal the wounds caused by the death of a loved one. It teaches us that death is a part of life, without interfering in the natural grief process.[38]

Worwood explains that melissa oil is a spiritual conduit. She describes the oil as encouraging strength and having a revitalising effect that is especially appreciated before meditation or prayer.[39]

Zeck states that melissa oil softens extreme emotions and soothes resentment. It allows us to reflect on all that we have to be grateful for.[40]

Dosage and Administration

Blending

Aromatherapy

For the relief of nervous tension, stress and irritability, consider blending melissa oil with essential oils such as bergamot, frankincense, geranium, lavender, neroli, sweet orange or sandalwood.

For the relief of insomnia, consider blending melissa oil with essential oils such as lavender, neroli, sweet marjoram or sandalwood.

To promote mental alertness, consider blending melissa oil with essential oils such as bergamot, basil, ginger, grapefruit, lemon, cold-pressed lime, myrtle, pine or peppermint.

For the topical treatment of cold sores, consider blending melissa oil with essential oils such as bergamot, rose otto or tea tree.

To dispel melancholy and alleviate depression, consider blending melissa oil with essential oils such as bergamot, geranium, jasmine absolute, lavender, neroli, sweet orange, sandalwood or ylang ylang.

Perfumery

In describing the role of melissa in perfumery, Arctander refers to the French perfume of the late 1930s created by Nina Ricci, 'Coeur-Joie', which means 'heart's delight'. He explains that the perfume had a melissa-like, fresh top note and lightness of floral fragrance.[1]

Mode of administration

Bath

Melissa oil can be sensitising; therefore, I would not recommend it in a bath.

Topical

Massage, ointment, skin care

Inhalation

Direct inhalation, diffuser, oil vaporiser

Safety Profile

General safety

Melissa oil is non-toxic. However, care must be taken as the oil is a possible sensitiser and dermal irritant.[26] Melissa oil is one of the most frequently adulterated essential oils.

Contraindications

No contraindications known.

Regulatory guidelines

Melissa oil has GRAS status.

References

1. Arctander S. *Perfume and flavor materials of natural origin*. Allured Publishing, Carol Stream, 1994.
2. Grieve M. *A modern herbal – Vol. II*. Dover Publications, New York, 1971.
3. Lawrence BM. *Progress in essential oils – melissa or lemon balm oil*. Perfumer & Flavorist, 2008; 33: 66-70.
4. Lawrence BM. *Progress in essential oils – melissa oil, or lemon balm oil*. Perfumer & Flavorist, 2011; 36: 57-59.
5. Khan I, Abourashed E. *Leung's encyclopedia of common natural ingredients used in food, drugs and cosmetics*. 3rd edn. John Wiley & Sons, New Jersey, 2010.
6. Blumenthal M et al. *The complete German commission E monographs: therapeutic guide to herbal medicine*. American Botanical Council, Austin, 1998.
7. Moussaoui F, Alaoui T. *Evaluation of antibacterial activity and synergistic effect between antibiotic and the essential oils of some medicinal plants*. Asian Pacific Journal of Tropical Biomedicine, 2016; 6(1): 32-37. Cited in Quintessential Aromatics database, 2013.
8. Jalal Z et al. *Phytochemistry of the essential oil of Melissa officinalis L. growing wild in Morocco: preventive approach against nosocomial infections*. Asian Pacific Journal of Tropical Biomedicine. 2015;5(6):459-461. doi:10.1016/j.apjtb.2015.03.003.
9. Allahverdiyev A et al. *Investigation of the anticancerogenic effect of the essential oil*

M

of Melissa officinalis L. Pharmaceutical & Pharmacological Letters, 2001; 1(1): 26-29. Cited in Quintessential Aromatics database, 2013.

10. de Sousa AC et al. *Melissa officinalis L. essential oil: antitumoral and antioxidant activities.* Journal of Pharmacy and Pharmacology, 2004; 54(5): 677-681. Cited in Quintessential Aromatics database, 2013.
11. Yen HF et al. *In vitro anti-diabetic effect and chemical component analysis of 29 essential oils products.* Journal of Food and Drug Analysis, 2015; 23(1): 124-129. Cited in Quintessential Aromatics database, 2013.
12. Chung MJ et al. *Anti-diabetic effects of lemon balm (Melissa officinalis) essential oil on glucose- and lipid-regulating enzymes in type 2 diabetic mice.* British Journal of Nutrition, 2010; 104(2): 180-188. Cited in Quintessential Aromatics database, 2013.
13. Bounihi A et al. *In vivo potential anti-inflammatory activity of Melissa officinalis L. essential oil.* Advances in Pharmacological Sciences, 2013; 2013: 101759. doi: 10.1155/2013/101759.
14. Baylac S, Racine P. *Inhibition of 5-lipoxygenase by essential oils and other natural fragrance extracts.* International Journal of Aromatherapy. 2003; 13(2/3): 138-142.
15. Mimica-Dukic N et al. *Antimicrobial and antioxidant activities of Melissa officinalis L. (Lamiaceae) essential oil.* Journal of Agricultural and Food Chemistry, 2004; 52(9): 2485-2489. Cited in Quintessential Aromatics database, 2013.
16. Sadraei H et al. *Relaxant effect of essential oil of Melissa officinalis and citral on rat ileum contractions.* Fitoterapia, 2003; 74(5): 445-452. Cited in Quintessential Aromatics database, 2013.
17. Allahverdiyev A et al. *Antiviral activity of the volatile oils of Melissa officinalis L. against Herpes simplex virus type-2.* Phytomedicine, 2004; 11(7/8): 657-661. Cited in Quintessential Aromatics database, 2013.
18. Schnitzler P et al. *Melissa officinalis oil affects infectivity of enveloped herpes viruses.* Phytomedicine, 2008; 15(9): 734-740. Cited in Quintessential Aromatics database, 2013.
19. Reichling J, Schnitzler P. *Phyto-antiviral agents for the topic treatment of recurrent herpes labialis episodes.* Zeitschrift fur Phytotherapie, 2011; 32(6): 260-265. Cited in Quintessential Aromatics database, 2013.
20. Ballard CG et al. *Aromatherapy as a safe and effective treatment for the management of agitation in severe dementia: the results of a double-blind placebo-controlled trial with melissa.* Journal of Clinical Psychiatry, 2002; 63(7): 553-558. Cited in Quintessential Aromatics database, 2013.
21. Elliott MSJ et al. *The essential oils from Melissa officinalis L. and Lavandula angustifolia Mill. as potential treatment for agitation in people with severe dementia.* International Journal of Essential Oil Therapeutics, 2007;1(4):143-152. Cited in Quintessential Aromatics database, 2013.
22. Chaiyana W, Okonogi S. *Inhibition of cholinesterase by essential oil from food plant.* Phytomedicine, 2012; 19(8/9): 836-839. Cited in Quintessential Aromatics database, 2013.
23. Bruneton J. *Pharmacognosy.* 2nd edn. Lavoisier Publishing, Paris, 1999.
24. Huang L et al. *Pharmacological profile of essential oils derived from Lavandula angustifolia and Melissa officinalis with anti-agitation properties: focus on ligand-gated channels.* Journal of Pharmacy and Pharmacology, 2008; 60(11): 1515-1522. doi: 10.1211/jpp/60.11.0013.
25. Kennedy DO et al. *Attenuation of laboratory-induced stress in humans after acute administration of Melissa officinalis (lemon balm).* Psychosomatic Medicine, 2004; 66(4): 607-613. Cited in Quintessential Aromatics database, 2013.
26. Lawless J. *The encyclopaedia of essential oils.* Element Books, Shaftesbury, 1992.
27. Lavabre, M. *Aromatherapy workbook.* Healing Arts Press, Rochester, 1997.
28. Mojay G. *Aromatherapy for healing the spirit.* Healing Arts Press, Rochester, 1999.
29. Sorensen J. *Melissa officinalis.* The International Journal of Aromatherapy, 2000; 10(1/2): 7-15.
30. Davis P. *Aromatherapy: an A-Z.* 2nd edn. C.W. Daniel Company, Saffron Walden, 1999.
31. Tisserand R. *The art of aromatherapy.* C.W. Daniel Company, Saffron Walden, 1977.
32. Fischer-Rizzi S. *Complete aromatherapy handbook.* Sterling Publishing, New York, 1990.
33. Tisserand R. *In praise of melissa.* The International Journal of Aromatherapy, 1989; 1(4): 10-11.
34. Wabner D, Wurdack I. *Rose oil: its use in therapy and cosmetics.* International Journal of Aromatherapy. 1989; 2(1):28-11.
35. Schnaubelt K. *Medical aromatherapy.* Frog, Berkeley, 1999.
36. Worwood VA. *The fragrant mind.* Transworld Publishers, London, 1995.
37. Davis P. *Subtle aromatherapy.* C.W. Daniel Company, Saffron Walden, 1991.
38. Keim Loughran J, Bull R. *Aromatherapy anointing oils.* Frog, Berkeley, 2001.
39. Worwood VA. *The fragrant heavens.* Transworld Publishers, London, 1999.
40. Zeck R. *The blossoming heart – aromatherapy for healing and transformation.* Aroma Tours, East Ivanhoe, 2004.

Myrrh

Identification

Botanical name

Commiphora myrrha (Nees) Engl.

Synonyms

Commiphora molmol, Commiphora madagascariensis, gum myrrh, myrrha, Somali myrrh

Family

Burseraceae

Botany and origins

The name myrrh is derived from the Arabic and Hebrew word *mur*, which means bitter.[1]

Myrrh is the resinous exudation, or gum, collected from the myrrh bush, botanically known as *C. myrrha*, either when it is wounded or from natural fissures. There are several *Commiphora* species from which the myrrh resin is produced.

The resin flows out as a thick pale-yellow liquid and turns reddish-brown as it dries and hardens. The bush which is a native of northeastern Africa and southern Arabia has sturdy knotted branches, trifoliate leaves and small white flowers.[2]

To increase the yield and production, incisions are made into the bark. Lumps of the gum often fall to the ground and become contaminated with sand, other lumps are peeled off the trunk, and these usually make a better grade of myrrh. However, myrrh cannot be evaluated just by its appearance. Lumps of high odour value may have poor appearance because they have fallen to the ground.[2]

Myrrh resin consists of rounded or irregular tears or agglutinated masses of smaller and larger tears of a moderate yellow to dark or reddish brown colour. The lumps are usually covered with a lighter-coloured or yellowish dust.[2]

Method of extraction

Myrrh essential oil is steam-distilled from the myrrh resin. A myrrh absolute is prepared from myrrh resinoid. The resinoid is a very dark, reddish-orange-brown, viscous mass and is very difficult to pour at room temperature.[2]

Characteristics

Myrrh oil is a pale yellow to pale orange coloured liquid. It has a warm-spicy odour with a sharp-balsamic, slightly medicinal top note. Arctander states that the sweetness increases to a deep, warm-spicy and aromatic dryout, which is unique and difficult to replicate. However, the oil lacks tenacity.[2]

Chemical composition

The composition of myrrh essential oil produced from resin collected from the Ogaden region in Ethiopia was as follows:[3]

δ-elemene (2.1%), α-copaene (0.2%), β-bourbonene (1.2%), β-ylangene (0.3%), β-elemene (8.7%), β-caryophyllene (1.3%), γ-elemene (1.1%), *allo*-aromadendrene (0.25%), α-humulene (0.6%), γ-muurolene (0.2%), germacrene D (3.2%), β-selinene (0.6%), α-selinene (0.5%), bicyclogermacrene (0.2%), δ-cadinene (0.4%), γ-cadinene (1.2%), germacrene B (4.3%), furanodiene (19.7%), elemol (0.2%), furanoeudesma-1,4-diene (1.2%), furanoeudesma-1,3-diene (34.0%), lindestrene (12.0%), T-cadinol (1.6%), 2-methoxyfuranodiene (2.1%).

Adulteration

The resin from opopanax and other *Commiphora* species are blended with myrrh resin to extract the essential oil.[2]

Pharmacopoeias and standards

The purity, composition and physico-chemical properties of myrrh are defined in several standards and monographs.

- ESCOP 2003 Monographs
- European Pharmacopoeia
- Assessment Report on *Commiphora molmol* Engler, gummi-resina. European Medicines Agency.

History and Traditional Uses

History

Myrrh is one of the oldest known aromatic substances, mentioned as far back as 4,000 years. It was an ingredient of incense used for religious ceremonies and fumigations by the ancient Egyptians. It is also used in the famous Egyptian perfume 'kyphi' and was an important ingredient in embalming.[4]

It was reputed to reduce wrinkles and preserve a youthful complexion. Egyptian women used myrrh in their facial preparations. It has a slightly cooling effect on the skin, and so would be especially useful in a hot, dry climate.[5]

Myrrh never enjoyed the same level of popularity as frankincense throughout the Roman Empire; however, the price of myrrh was always much higher than frankincense.[6]

Myrrh's therapeutic properties are frequently mentioned in the old and new testaments, the Koran, and in Greek and Roman texts.

In the Song of Solomon, a love poem, the constant reference to myrrh suggests that it was for the incomparable financial value of myrrh that the writer used it to compare with the beauty of the maiden.[7]

> *A bundle of myrrh is my beloved to me, he shall lie all night betwixt my breasts.*[8]
>
> Song of Solomon 4:13 (King James Version)
>
> *Thy two breasts are like two young roes that are twins, which feed among the lilies.*
>
> *Until the day break, and the shadows flee away, I will get me to the mountain of myrrh, and to the hill of frankincense.*[8]
>
> Song of Solomon 4:5-4:6 (King James Version)

Myrrh was one of the gifts presented to the infant Jesus:

> *And when they came into the house, they saw the young child with Mary his mother, and fell down, and worshipped him: and when they opened their treasures, they presented unto him gifts; gold and frankincense and myrrh.*[8]
>
> Matthew 2:11 (King James Version)

It was presented at the death of Christ:

> *... and brought a mixture of myrrh and aloes, about hundred pound. Then took they the body of Jesus, and wound it in linen clothes with spices, as the manner of the Jews is to bury.*[8]
>
> John 19:39-40 (King James Version)

Frankincense has been associated with Christ's divinity, and myrrh with his persecution and death.[6]

English herbalist Joseph Miller gives us a detailed account of the therapeutic applications of myrrh:

> *Myrrh is of an opening, heating, drying nature, resists putrefaction, and is of great service in uterine disorders, opens the obstruction of the womb, procuring the menses, expediting the birth, and expelling the secundines. It is good likewise for old coughs and hoarseness, and the loss of voice, and is very useful against pestilential and infectious distempers, both taken inwardly, and flung upon burning coals and the fume received. Outwardly applied it cures wounds and ulcers, and prevents gangrene and mortifications.*[5]

Traditional medicine

Myrrh has been used since ancient times as a stimulant, antiseptic, expectorant, antispasmodic, emmenagogue and stomachic. It has also been used for the treatment of cancers, leprosy, syphilitic ulcers, sores, sore throats, asthma, coughs, weak gums, gingivitis and loose teeth.[1]

Myrrh was introduced in Chinese medicine in the seventh century, and was used for treating conditions involving bleeding, pain and wounds.[9]

In Egypt, myrrh is used for the treatment of schistosomiasis. Several Egyptian investigations have demonstrated antischistosomal activity of oral preparations of myrrh. However, this activity could not be confirmed by other investigators. The EMA report for myrrh suggests that the potential antischistosomal activity of myrrh remains controversial.[10]

Herbal

Myrrh is commonly used as a tincture [1:5 (g/ mL) in 90% ethanol] for stomach problems, alleviating mild gastrointestinal complaints, as a local astringent, and as an anaesthetic for gingivitis and mouth infections. The tincture is also used topically for the treatment of minor wounds, abrasions, furuncles and skin inflammations.[10]

Food, perfumery and flavouring

Myrrh oil is used as a flavour component in many food products, including alcoholic and non-alcoholic beverages, frozen dairy desserts, candy, baked goods, gelatins and puddings, and meat and meat products.[1]

Therapeutics

Pharmacology and clinical studies

While the chemistry, pharmacology and uses of myrrh have been extensively reviewed, many of the studies involve the use of the resin or the tincture and not the essential oil. It is for this reason that Lis-Balchin states that there is lack of scientific data to prove that myrrh essential oil alleviates any of the conditions often attributed to the resin.[11]

The EMA report states that myrrh is a gum-resin with a complicated chemistry. Most of the studies have investigated the components of the volatile oil, which is dominated by furano-sesquiterpenes, some of which have pharmacological activity.[10]

Analgesic activity

Two sesquiterpenes (furanoeudesma-1,3-diene and curzarene) in the resin of myrrh have analgesic effects blocked by naloxone. This indicates that it may have an interaction with brain opioid mechanisms.[6]

Ethanolic extracts of *C. myrrha* demonstrated analgesic and anti-inflammatory activities in mice studies, providing evidence to support the traditional use of myrrh for inflammatory pain.[12]

Anticarcinogenic activity

A study found that myrrh and frankincense essential oils exhibited an inhibitory effect on five tumour cell lines: MCF-7, HS-1, HepG2, HeLa and A549. A significant inhibitory effect was noted on cell lines MCF-7 and HS-1 from both myrrh and frankincense essential oil. The anticancer effects of myrrh were markedly increased compared to those of frankincense. In addition, the researchers stated that the results indicate that the breast cancer cell line exhibited increased sensitivity to the myrrh essential oil. It was also noted that cell lines were more sensitive to β-elemene compared with frankincense and myrrh. This may suggest that β-elemene is important for the antitumour activity of frankincense and myrrh.[13]

Anti-inflammatory activity

The anti-inflammatory effect of myrrh was observed in a study in which the oil inhibited interleukin (IL)-6 due to down-regulating PGE2 production, but not via nuclear factor kappaB (κB) inhibition in human gingival fibroblasts.[14]

Myrrh inhibited LPS-induced productions of inflammatory mediators such as nitric oxide, prostaglandin E2, and tumour necrosis factor-α (TNF-α), but not of (IL)-1β and IL-6, in peritoneal macrophages. The researchers also found that myrrh inhibited LPS-induced activation of c-jun NH2-terminal kinase (JNK), but not of extracellular signal-regulated kinase (ERK) and nuclear factor κB. Myrrh also reduced cecal ligation and puncture (CLP) induced mortality, and inhibited CLP-induced production of IL-1β, IL-6 and TNF-α in serum and liver. These results suggest that myrrh may be beneficial in inflammatory diseases such as sepsis.[15]

Another study confirmed the efficacy of frankincense and myrrh in the treatment of inflammatory diseases. The study evaluated the effects on adjuvant-induced arthritis to explore the underlying mechanisms by analysing the signal pathways evaluated by expression of inflammatory cytokines, c-jun and c-fos and corresponding phosphorylation levels. The researchers concluded that administration of combined frankincense and myrrh suppressed arthritic progression in rats more effectively than single drug treatment.[16]

Antimicrobial activity

Lis-Balchin states that the antibacterial and antifungal activities of myrrh essential oil were very low.[15]

Another study stated that eight sesquiterpene fractions extracted from myrrh showed activity against *Escherichia coli, Staphylococcus aureus, Pseudomonas aeruginosa* and *C. albicans,* with minimum inhibitory concentrations ranging from 0.18 to 2.8ug/mL.[17]

Hepatoprotective activity

The oleo-gum-resin of myrrh was found to alleviate the adverse effect of ethanol ingestion in mice studies by enhancing the lipid metabolism and the hepatic antioxidant defence system.[18]

Wound-healing activity

C. myrrha demonstrated wound-healing activities in mice studies. The leukocyte count was used to monitor the healing progress. Myrrh was found to enhance white blood cell proliferation throughout the healing period, providing evidence to support the traditional use of myrrh for wound healing.[19]

Actions

Actions commonly cited in aromatherapy

Anticatarrhal, anti-inflammatory, antimicrobial, antiseptic, astringent, balsamic, carminative, cicatrisant, emmenagogue, expectorant, fungicidal, sedative, stimulant, stomachic, tonic, uterine, vulnerary[20,21,22,23]

Actions supported by clinical studies

Antimicrobial, antiseptic, cicatrisant, expectorant, vulnerary

Comment

There is no doubt that myrrh has a long history of therapeutic use. Myrrh was used in the treatment of wounds and mouth infections as far back as the ancient Greeks and Romans. Myrrh has been included, and remains, in many pharmacopoeias over the centuries. On the basis of myrrh's long-standing use and experience, we can confirm that myrrh is effective for the treatment of minor ulcers and inflammation in the mouth (stomatitis and gingivitis), and for the treatment of minor wounds and furuncles.[10]

Clinical studies demonstrating the antibacterial, local anaesthetic and anti-inflammatory activity of myrrh tincture support the use of myrrh for the treatment of wounds and skin inflammations.[10]

Aromatherapy Uses

Clinical aromatherapy

Antimicrobial

Myrrh is well known for its antibacterial, antifungal and anti-inflammatory actions. The tincture can be used in the treatment of mouth, gum and throat infections.[21] The oil can be incorporated into an ointment which is applied externally for the treatment of haemorrhoids, bed sores and wounds.[23]

Digestive system

Myrrh oil is reputed to stimulate the stomach

and digestive system, and is a useful remedy for treating diarrhoea, dyspepsia and loss of appetite.[21,22]

The German Commission E recommends using five to 10 drops of myrrh tincture in a glass of water as a gargle for oral and pharyngeal mucosa.[9]

Integumentary system

Myrrh oil is used for the treatment of chronic wounds and ulcers. This is due to its antiseptic, astringent and anti-inflammatory properties. It is beneficial for mature skin, wounds that are slow to heal, and for weepy eczema and athlete's foot.[21,22,23] It heals cracked and chapped skin and can be added to skin care creams.[21,22]

Nervous system

Myrrh oil instils a deep sense of calm and tranquillity on the mind.[24]

Reproductive system

Myrrh oil is a uterine stimulant and promotes menstruation, thus relieving painful periods.[22] Holmes says that it stimulates the uterus and promotes the menses and childbirth.[24]

Respiratory system

Myrrh oil is an excellent expectorant, and as such is beneficial in the treatment of coughs, bronchitis and colds.[21,22,23]

Energetics, psyche and subtle uses

Energetics

According to TCM, myrrh is *warming* and *drying*.[23,24] It is recommended for conditions associated with *excess damp* such as chronic ulcers and wounds, respiratory tract infections with phlegm and mucus, and diarrhoea.[24]

Mojay compares myrrh with frankincense. He explains that the sweet, resinous and earthy base note aroma of myrrh is associated with the Earth Element. It therefore helps to clear and ground the *Yi*. Disharmony of the *Yi* leads to overthinking, worry and mental distraction.[23]

According to the principals of Ayurveda, myrrh essential oil may aggravate *Pitta* and help balance excess *Kapha*. The oil is excellent for *Kapha* emotions and for people afraid to speak out.[25]

Personality

Myrrh oil should be considered for someone who is prone to overthinking, worry and mental distraction.[23]

According to Myers-Briggs personality types, the myrrh personality is likely to be an INFJ. INFJs are quiet, compassionate, concerned and tender-hearted. They often have complex personalities. They have a rich imagination and are very aware of other people's emotions. They are very committed to their inspirations and ideals and inspire insight and growth in others. INFJs like balance between time alone for their many creative projects, and time with friends and family. They prefer to spend more time with mental and emotional pursuits rather than physical ones. They can be highly demanding of themselves and others. They are often perfectionists. They like to make significant contributions to the welfare of humankind. They like to think things through carefully and are good at concentrating. They are tender and gentle in their relationships. They are very good listeners and communicate clearly when they feel comfortable. They share their feelings and emotions in private and only with a small number of friends. They often feel responsibility for other people's feelings. They can be moody and melancholic. They are very sensitive to criticism and rejection and feel deeply hurt when they are not understood. They have a strong need for harmony – they can feel tense, frustrated and even become ill when they are not able to attain it.

Subtle

Myrrh's effect on the spirit is like that of frankincense – one of inner stillness and peace, of an awareness free from restlessness and the mundane. Myrrh unites the spiritual with the physical.[24]

Myrrh is thought to enhance spirituality. It should be used as a meditation aid or before any healing session.[19] It can be used to strengthen the base chakra and is particularly valuable for people who feel emotionally or spiritually stuck and want to move forward in their lives.[20]

Mojay states that myrrh promotes inner stillness and peace. Myrrh strengthens the link between our base chakra and crown chakra. In doing so Mojay explains:

> *... the dreams and visions of the soul can find a channel for earthly expression, and tap the force they need for their 'magical' realization.*[23]

Myrrh helps us get through the challenges in life. It helps us to understand and cope with our physical, emotional and spiritual wounds. It will provide support and protect us. It gives us strength and allows us to connect with our spirituality.[26]

Keim Loughran & Bull recommend using myrrh whenever we feel exhausted and overwhelmed by our own troubles or the suffering of others, or to help us understand, from a spiritual perspective, the meaning of emotional challenges.[27]

Dosage and Administration

Blending

Aromatherapy

To promote wound healing, consider blending myrrh oil with essential oils such as German chamomile, everlasting, frankincense or lavender.

To help alleviate catarrhal conditions associated with bronchitis or asthma, consider blending myrrh oil with essential oils such as aniseed, Atlas cedarwood, cajeput, 1,8-cineole-rich eucalypts, fragonia, spike lavender, myrtle, pine or spruce.

To balance the base chakra and to help strengthen the link between the base and crown chakras, you may consider blending myrrh oil with essential oils such patchouli, frankincense, sandalwood and Atlas cedarwood.

Perfumery

The sweet, warm balsamic note of myrrh is used in oriental spicy style perfumes. It is also often blended with geranium, patchouli and other heavy floral bases.[1]

Arctander states that it may be used in small amounts to create heavy-floral, heavy oriental or woody style perfumes. He also states that it is excellent in high-class forest notes and moss notes. He recommends blending it with cypress, juniper berry and petitgrain.[2]

Guenther states that myrrh oil is most valuable in oriental style perfumes. He explains that its suave, balsamic, heavy odour blends well with essential oils such as opopanax, sandalwood, frankincense, vetiver, patchouli and geranium.[28]

Mode of administration

Bath

Full body bath, foot bath

Topical

Compress, massage, ointment, skin care

Inhalation

Direct inhalation, diffuser, oil vaporiser

Mouth wash

As a rinse or gargle, the recommended dose for the treatment of mild inflammations of the oral and pharyngeal mucosa is 5-10 drops of myrrh tincture in a glass of water.[9]

Safety Profile

General safety

Myrrh oil is non-toxic, non-irritating and non-sensitising.[21]

Contraindications

Many ancient physicians classified myrrh as an abortifacient. Myrrh oil is contraindicated during pregnancy.[20,21,22] Riddle states that there has been no scientific evidence to confirm this.[29]

However, Tisserand & Young state that myrrh may be fetotoxic due to β-elemene and the furanodiene content. They also state that myrrh is contraindicated (for all routes) during pregnancy and lactation.[30]

Braun & Cohen also state that the safety of myrrh during pregnancy is unknown, and until safety is confirmed, it should not be used during pregnancy.[12]

Regulatory guidelines

Myrrh essential oil has GRAS status.

References

1. Khan I, Abourashed E. *Leung's encyclopedia of common natural ingredients used in food, drugs and cosmetics*. 3rd edn. John Wiley and Sons, New Jersey, 2010.
2. Arctander S. *Perfume and flavor materials of natural origin*. Allured Publishing, Carol Stream, 1994.
3. Lawrence BM. *Progress in essential oils – myrrh*. Perfumer & Flavorist. 29; 2004: 91-95.
4. Grieve M. *A modern herbal – Vol. II*. Dover Publications, New York, 1971.
5. Tisserand R. *The art of aromatherapy*. C.W. Daniel Company, Saffron Walden, 1977.
6. Langenheim JH, *Plant resins – chemistry, evolution, ecology, and ethnobotany*. Timber Press, Portland, 2003.
7. Stoddart M. *The scented ape*. Cambridge University Press, Cambridge, 1990.
8. https://www.kingjamesbibleonline.org
9. Blumenthal M et al. *The complete German commission E monographs: therapeutic guide to herbal medicines*. American Botanical Council, Austin, 1998.
10. Committee on Herbal Medicinal Products (HMPC). *Assessment report on Commiphora molmol Engler, gummi-resina*. European Medicines Agency, London, 2011. Doc ref. EMA/HMPC/96910/2010.
11. Lis-Balchin M. *Aromatherapy science – a guide for healthcare professionals*. Pharmaceutical Press, London, 2006.
12. Braun L, Cohen M. *Herbs & natural supplements: an evidence-based guide – Vol. 2*. 4th edn. Elsevier, Chatswood, 2015.
13. Chen Y et al. *Composition and potential anticancer activities of essential oils obtained from myrrh and frankincense*. Oncology Letters, 2013; 6(4): 1140-1146. doi: 10.3892/ol.2013.1520.

M

14. Tipton D et al. *Effect of myrrh oil on IL-1β stimulation of NF-κB activiation and PGE2 production in human gingival fibroblasts and epithelial cells.* Toxicology in Vitro. 2006; 20(2): 248-255. Cited in Quintessential Aromatics database, 2013.
15. Kim MS et al. *Myrrh inhibits LPS-induced inflammatory response and protects from cecal ligation and puncture-induced sepsis.* Evidence-Based Complementary and Alternative Medicine, 2012; 2012: 278718. doi: 10.1155/2012/278718.
16. Su S et al. *Frankincense and myrrh suppress inflammation via regulation of the metabolic profiling and the MAPK signaling pathway.* Scientific Reports, 2015; 5: 13668. doi: 10.1038/srep13668.
17. Dolara P et al. *Local anaesthetic, antibacterial and antifungal properties of sesquiterpenes from myrrh.* Planta Medica, 2000; 66(4): 356-358. Cited in Quintessential Aromatics database, 2013.
18. Al-Rejaie SS. *Effect of oleo-gum-resin on ethanol-induced hepatoxicity in rats.* Journal of Medicinal Science, 2012; 12(1): 1-9. Cited in Quintessential Aromatics database, 2013.
19. Haffor A-SA. *Effect of Commiphora molmol on leukocytes proliferation in relation to histological alterations before and during healing from injury.* Saudi Journal of Biological Sciences, 2010; 17(2): 139-146. Cited in Quintessential Aromatics database, 2013.
20. Davis P. *Aromatherapy: an A-Z.* 2nd edn. C.W. Daniel Company, Saffron Walden, 1999.
21. Lawless J. *The encyclopaedia of essential oils.* Element Books, Shaftesbury, 1992.
22. Lavabre M. *Aromatherapy workbook.* Healing Arts Press, Rochester, 1997.
23. Mojay G. *Aromatherapy for healing the spirit.* Healing Arts Press, Rochester, 1999.
24. Holmes P. *The energetics of Western herbs – Vol II.* Artemis Press, Boulder, 1989.
25. Miller L, Miller B. *Ayurveda and aromatherapy.* Lotus Press, Twin Lakes, 1995.
26. Davis P. *Subtle aromatherapy.* C.W. Daniel Company, Saffron Walden, 1991.
27. Keim Loughran J, Bull R. *Aromatherapy and subtle energy techniques.* Frog, Berkeley, 2000.
28. Guenther E. *The essential oils – Vol IV.* Robert E Krieger Publishing, Malabar, 1948.
29. Riddle J. *Eve's herbs.* Harvard University Press, Cambridge, Massachusetts, 1997.
30. Tisserand R, Young R. *Essential oil safety.* 2nd edn. Churchill Livingstone, Edinburgh, 2014.

Myrtle

Identification

Botanical name

Myrtus communis L.

Synonyms

Corsican pepper

Family

Myrtaceae

Botany and origins

Myrtle is an evergreen shrub or small tree, 3-7 m high, with many branches, a brownish red bark and small sharp-pointed leaves. It has fragrant white or pinkish flowers.[1]

It is native to the Mediterranean region and western Asia. The oil is produced in Tunisia, France, Corsica, Spain, Morocco and Italy.[2] It is also found in South America, northwestern Himalaya and Australia. It grows in Turkey, Iran, Greece, Algeria, Croatia and Montenegro.[3]

Myrtle should not be confused with the wax myrtle (*Myrica cerifera*) or bog myrtle (*Myrica gale*), whose essential oils are toxic.[1]

Method of extraction

Myrtle essential oil is produced by steam distillation of the leaves and twigs of *M. communis*, and in some places, the flowers, which are highly fragrant, are also included. This may explain the significant difference between the myrtle oils from various regions.[2]

Characteristics

Myrtle oil is a pale yellow to orange-yellow mobile liquid with a fresh, camphoraceous, spicy and floral-herbaceous odour. Arctander states that the Tunisian and Corsican myrtle oils are very fresh, have a strong top note, and display a sweet-herbaceous and fresh middle note.[2]

Chemical composition

There is considerable variability in the composition of myrtle oil depending on many environmental and genetic factors. The most important constituents of myrtle oil are the terpenoids – myrtenol, myrtenol acetate, limonene, linalool, α-pinene, 1,8-cineole, α-caryophyllene, *p*-cymene, geraniol, nerol and methyl eugenol.[3]

There are different essential oil chemotypes that can distinguish myrtle oil from different origins.

Bradesi et al. proposed a classification of *M. communis* essential oil on the basis of myrtenyl acetate content into two chemotypes. Each chemotype group can be further divided into two subgroups, according to the ratio of α-pinene to myrtenyl acetate or α-pinene to 1,8-cineole.[3]

The composition of myrtle oil from Algeria was reported as follows:

α-pinene (46.9 ± 3.4%), β-pinene (0.4 ± 0.1%), myrcene (1.7 ± 0.4%), *p*-cymene (0.6 ± 0.2%), 1,8-cineole (25.2 ± 2.3%), (*Z*)-β-ocimene (0.8 ± 0.1%), (*E*)-β-ocimene (0.6 ± 0.1%), linalool (5.6 ± 0.9%), alloocimene (0.2 ± 0.1%), terpinen-4-ol (trace), α-terpineol (1.3 ± 0.7%), estragole (0.4 ± 0.1%), linalyl acetate (4.2 ± 0.8%), α-terpenyl acetate (1.1 ± 0.6%), geranyl acetate (4.2 ± 1.2%), methyl eugenol (0.5 ± 0.2%).[4]

Interestingly no myrtenol was listed in this oil.

The chemical composition of myrtle oil from Italy was reported as follows:

α-pinene (41.0%), camphene (1.2%), β-pinene (0.2%), δ-3-carene (0.7%), myrcene (0.6%), α-phellandrene (0.5%), limonene (6.2%), 1,8-cineole (13.8%), γ-terpinene (1.3%), *p*-cymene (0.7%), 3-octanol (1.6%), decanal (0.4%), linalool (2.1%), methyl chavicol (0.8%), β-caryophyllene (1.1%), geranyl acetate (1.0%), α-terpineol (2.2%), citronellol (1.0%), myrtenol and nerol (2.0%), geraniol (1.2%), eugenol (1.1%).[5]

M

Adulteration

Arctander states that myrtle oil is frequently adulterated. It is adulterated with 1,8-cineole, camphene, and fractions from the production of linalyl acetate have been used.[2] Lis-Balchin states that myrtle oils from different countries are often blended together.[6]

Pharmacopoeias and standards

At the time of writing, the purity, composition, physico-chemical properties and therapeutic use of myrtle essential oil are not defined in any pharmacopoeia monograph or standard.

History and Traditional Uses

History

The ancient Persians regarded myrtle as a holy plant. Myrtle was a symbol of love and peace to the Jews, and the Greeks regarded it as sacred. Dioscorides prescribed extracts of the leaves for lung and bladder infections.[1]

In the sixteenth century, the leaves and flowers were the major ingredients of a skin lotion known as 'angels water'. The berries are used in bitters and certain liqueurs.[1]

Traditional medicine

In traditional medicine, the leaves and fruits of myrtle are frequently used as an infusion and decoction for the treatment of stomach aches, hypoglycaemia, cough, constipation, poor appetite, as well as externally for wound healing. In Italian folk medicine, the fruits are used for treating infectious conditions including diarrhoea and dysentery, and the leaves are used as an antiseptic and anti-inflammatory agent, as well as a mouthwash for treating candidiasis.[3]

Herbal

Infusions made from the leaves and young branches of myrtle are considered stimulant, antiseptic, astringent and hypoglycaemic. Myrtle leaves are also used as a remedy for asthma, eczema, psoriasis, diarrhoea, gastrointestinal disorders and urinary infections.[3]

Food, perfumery and flavouring

Myrtle as a spice finds very little application because of its bitterness, despite its pleasant aroma. The taste is very intense, unpleasant and strongly bitter, so its culinary application is limited to Sardinia, where the berries and leaves are used to produce two well-known liquors, *mirto rosso* and *mirto bianco*, respectively.[3]

Foods flavoured with the smoke of myrtle are common in some rural areas of Italy and Sardinia.[3]

A constituent of myrtle oil, myrtenol, has a warm woody odour and is used in perfumery.[1]

Therapeutics

Pharmacology and clinical studies

Many pharmacological studies involving myrtle oil have been published. A systemic review of these studies will not be attempted. Rather, I have chosen a selection of studies with an emphasis on those studies that support the traditional and clinical uses.

Antifungal activity

An in vitro study demonstrated that myrtle essential oil displayed antifungal activity against 12 strains of *Candida albicans*. All strains had MICs of 0.35% to 1.4%, and the majority were resistant to fluconazole.[7]

Myrtle oil inhibited the growth of all tested yeasts at a concentration ranging from 0.06-4 uL/mL.[8]

In another study, ethanolic extracts of *M. communis* leaves were found to have antifungal activity against 24 clinical isolates of *Candida*.[9]

A study found that myrtle oil showed significant antifungal activity when combined with antifungal pharmaceutical drug, amphotericin B.[10]

Anti-inflammatory activity

In vitro experimental results confirmed the ability of myrtle essential oil to exert anti-inflammatory and mucolytic actions on the upper airway epithelium.[11]

Antimicrobial activity

Myrtle oil exhibited antimicrobial activities against a wide number of microorganisms, particularly those antibiotic resistant strains responsible for nosocomial infections. Consistent with previous studies, myrtle essential oil was active against both methicillin-resistant and methicillin-sensitive *Staphylococcus aureus* at concentrations from 4-8 μL/mL.[8]

A study examined the antimicrobial effectiveness of myrtle oil, when used alone and in combination with conventional antibiotics, against multidrug-resistant *Acinetobacter baumannii* wound isolates. The results confirmed a good antimicrobial effect of myrtle oil when used on its own; however, it was even better when used in combination with the drugs.

This confirms a synergist effect with myrtle oil and the antibiotics such as polymyxin B and ciprofloxacine against *A. baumannii*. This synergy provides an opportunity for future development of treatment strategies for lethal wound infections caused by multidrug-resistant *A. baumannii*.[12]

The antimicrobial activity of myrtle leaf oil was tested against nalidixic acid-resistant strain of *Salmonella typhimurium* on tomatoes and iceberg lettuce. The results show that the use of myrtle leaf oil caused a significant reduction on the *S. typhimurium* population. It was suggested that myrtle oil could be a useful tool as an alternative to the use of chlorine or other synthetic disinfectants in fruit and vegetables, especially for organic products.[13]

Iranian myrtle oil had excellent antimicrobial activity against *E. coli, S. aureus* and *C. albicans*.[14]

An in vitro study of Sardinian *M. communis* essential oil confirmed that the oil had strong antimicrobial activity against 10 clinical isolates of *Helicobacter pylori* that had resisted two courses of triple-drug therapy.[15]

Antioxidant activity

Myrtle oil did not exhibit very strong DPPH scavenging activity, especially compared to synthetic antioxidants.[16] Another study found that the methanolic extracts of myrtle showed better antioxidant activity than the essential oil.[17]

Antiviral activity

A double-blind, randomised, placebo-controlled study examined the topical application of myrtle ointment in 80 patients with HSV-1 infection. Patients were instructed to apply the ointment 3 to 5 times a day for up to 5 days. The total duration and severity of the clinical symptoms in all the patients using the myrtle ointment were significantly reduced by day 2 compared with the placebo group.[18]

Hypoglycaemic activity

An in vivo study showed that myrtle oil exerts hypoglycaemic as well as mild hypotriglyceridemic activity in diabetic rabbits. It was stated that the reduction in blood glucose level may be due to the reversible inhibition of α-glucosidases present in the brush-border of the small intestinal mucosa, the higher rate of glycolysis as envisaged by the higher activity of glucokinase, one of the key enzymes of glycolysis, and the enhanced rate of glycogenesis, as evidenced by the higher amount of liver glycogen present after myrtle oil administration.[19]

Insecticidal activity

A study found that the protection time against *Anopheles stephensi* mosquito of complete bites provided by 25% DEET was 6.23 hours, contrastable with the results of 50% myrtle oil providing protection time of 4.26 hours. It was concluded that myrtle essential oil can be useful and safe in preventing mosquito bites, and has potential use as a botanical repellent.[20]

Laboratory tests found that Iranian myrtle oil displayed insect repellency activity against the sandfly – *Phlebotomus papatasi*.[21]

The insecticidal oil of 54 plant oils, including myrtle, were tested for their insecticidal activity against *Pediculus humanus capitis* using direct contact and fumigation methods. At 0.125 mg/cm^2, the pediculicidal activity of myrtle was comparable with that of d-phenothrin and pyrethrum, two commonly used pediculicides. It was concluded that essential oils such as myrtle and others tested merit further study as potential control agents for *P. humanus capitis*.[22]

Actions

Actions commonly cited in aromatherapy

Anticatarrhal, antiseptic, astringent, bactericidal, balsamic, expectorant, slightly sedative[23,24]

Actions supported by clinical studies

Antibacterial, antifungal, antiviral, insecticidal, expectorant

Comment

Lis-Balchin states that there is little data for the bioactivity of myrtle essential oil, although its

M

use in herbal medicine has been extensively researched.[6]

There is considerable variability in the composition of myrtle oil. It is, therefore, very important to know the origin of myrtle oil and the chemical composition, as it may influence the bioactivity of the oil. Schnaubelt recommends using the Corsican variety of *M. communis*. This oil has a brilliant green colour and has a high 1,8-cineole content.[25]

Aromatherapy Uses

Clinical aromatherapy

Psychological

Fischer-Rizzi states that myrtle oil is recommended for people with addictive or self-destructive behaviour:

> *Myrtle is helpful for people whose body seems draped in a gray brown veil from smoking, drug abuse, or emotions like anger, greed, envy or fear. In such cases myrtle oil helps to cleanse the person's delicate inner being to dissolve disharmony.*[26]

Respiratory system

Myrtle oil is beneficial for chronic conditions of the respiratory system such as bronchitis, catarrhal conditions and chronic coughs.[23,24,26,27]

It has an unobtrusive odour and is well tolerated by young children. It is slightly sedative, unlike eucalyptus oil which has a stimulating odour, and is recommended as a chest rub, inhalation or oil burner at night.[27]

Skin care

Myrtle oil may be used for the treatment of acne, oily skin and open pores.[22,27] Schnaubelt describes green myrtle as a gentle oil which is regenerating, astringent and antiallergenic.[28] Myrtle oil is astringent and has been used to reduce haemorrhoids.[25,27]

Urinary system

Myrtle oil has been used as an antiseptic for the treatment of urinary tract infections. For bladder infections or infections of the ureter, a sitz bath is recommended.[26]

Energetics, psyche and subtle uses

Energetics

Energetically, myrtle's principal actions are to circulate and regulate *Qi* and to clear *cold phlegm*.

Subtle

Myrtle carries a deep inner wisdom and may serve as a companion for the dying.[26]

Keim Loughran & Bull state that myrtle provides protection during major life transitions and that it promotes harmony, love and respect.[29]

Worwood states that the spirit of myrtle is energetic truth and forgiveness, giving support to the unsupported and teaching us that divine love embraces all living beings.[30]

Zeck suggests using myrtle whenever you are in pain, struggling or feeling disheartened. She explains that myrtle is like a shining beacon, touching the soul with a refreshing innocence and radiating the beauty of life.[31]

Dosage and Administration

Blending

Aromatherapy

For the relief of symptoms associated with colds and flu, consider blending myrtle oil with essential oils such as bay laurel, cajeput, peppermint eucalyptus, 1,8-cineole-rich eucalypts, fragonia, ginger, manuka, niaouli, spike lavender or tea tree.

For the relief of bronchial catarrh, consider blending myrtle oil with essential oils such as Atlas cedarwood, cypress, peppermint eucalyptus, 1,8-cineole-rich eucalypts, ginger, ravintsara and pine.

For acne and congested skin, consider blending myrtle oil with essential oils such as cypress, lavender, juniper berry, palmarosa or tea tree.

Perfumery

Arctander states that myrtle oil blends excellently with bay laurel, bergamot, clary sage, lavender, and rosemary oil. In flavouring, he also explains that it blends well with spice oils such as clove bud, cinnamon bark or leaf oil, cardamom, ginger and nutmeg oils.[2]

Mode of administration

Bath

Full body bath, foot bath, sitz bath

Topical

Compress, massage, ointment, skin care

Inhalation

Direct inhalation, diffuser, oil vaporiser

Safety Profile

General safety

Myrtle oil is non-toxic, non-irritating and non-sensitising.[23]

Contraindications

No contraindications known.

Toxicity

Based on the estragole and methyl eugenol content of myrtle oil, Tisserand & Young suggest that myrtle oil may be potentially carcinogenic. However, they go on to recommend a maximum dermal dose of 1.9% based on a myrtle oil containing 1.4% estragole and 0.8% methyl eugenol. Oral ingestion of myrtle oil is contraindicated for individuals taking antidiabetic medication.[32]

Regulatory guidelines

Myrtle oil is not defined in any regulatory guideline.

References

1. Weiss EA. *Essential oil crops.* CAB International, Wallingford, 1997.
2. Arctander S. *Perfume and flavor materials of natural origin.* Allured Publishing, Carol Stream, 1994.
3. Aleksic V, Knezevic P. *Antimicrobial and antioxidative activity of extracts and essential oils of Myrtus communis L.* Microbiological Research, 2014; 169(14): 240-254. doi: 10.1016/j.micres.2013.10.003.
4. Brada M et al. *Composition of the essential oil of leaves and berries of Algerian myrtle (Myrtus communis L.)* Journal of Essential Oil Research, 2012; 24(1): 1-3. doi: 10.1080/10412905.2012.645299.
5. Lawrence BM. *Progress in essential oils – myrtle oil.* Perfumer & Flavorist, 2007; 32: 54-62.
6. Lis-Balchin M. *Aromatherapy science – a guide for healthcare professionals.* Pharmaceutical Press, London, 2006.
7. Ragno R et al. *In vitro activity of essential oil of Myrtus communis L. against Candida albicans (letter).* International Journal of Essential Oil Therapeutics, 2008; 2(4): 156-157. Cited in Quintessential Aromatics database, 2013.
8. Zomorodian K et al. *Chemical composition and antimicrobial activities of the essential oil from Myrtus communis leaves.* Journal of Essential Oil Bearing Plants, 2013; 16(1): 76-84. doi: 10.1080/0972060X.2013.764183.
9. Nejad BS et al. *Antifungal efficacy of Myrtus communis Linn.* Jentashapir Journal of Health Research, 2014; 5(4): e21879. doi: 10.5812/jjhr.21879.
10. Mahboubi M, Ghazian Bidgoli F. *In vitro synergistic efficacy of combination of amphotericin B with Myrtus communis essential oil against clinical isolates of Candida albicans.* Phytomedicine, 2010; 17(10): 771-774. Cited in Quintessential Aromatics database, 2013.
11. Fenu G et al. *Therapeutic properties of myrtle essential oil: an in vitro study on human nasal mucosa cells.* International Journal of Essential Oil Therapeutics, 2008; 2(1): 21-25. Cited in Quintessential Aromatics database, 2013.
12. Aleksic V et al. *Synergistic effect of Myrtus communis L. essential oils and conventional antibiotics against multi-drug resistant Acinetobacter baumannii wound isolates.* Phytomedicine, 2014; 21(12): 1666-1674. Cited in Quintessential Aromatics database, 2013.
13. Gündüz GT et al. *Efficacy of myrtle oil against Salmonella typhimurium on fresh produce.* International Journal of Food Microbiology, 2009; 130(2): 147-150. doi: 10.1016/j.ijfoodmicro.2009.01.010.
14. Yadegarinia D et al. *Biochemical activities of Iranian Mentha piperita L. and Myrtus communis L. essential oils.* Phytochemistry, 2006; 67(12): 1249-1255. Cited in Quintessential Aromatics database, 2013.
15. Deriu A et al. *In vitro activity of essential oil of Myrtus communis L. against Helicobacter pylori.* International Journal of Antimicrobial Agents, 2007; 30(6): 562-563. Cited in Quintessential Aromatics database, 2013.
16. Mimica-Dukić N et al. *Essential oil of Myrtus communis L. as a potential antioxidant and antimutagenic agents.* Molecules, 2010; 15; 2759-2770. doi: 10.3390/molecules15042759.
17. Aidi Wannes W et al. *Antioxidant activities of the essential oils and methanol extracts from myrtle (Myrtus communis var. italica L.) leaf, stem and flower.* Food and Chemical Toxicology, 2010; 48(5): 1362-1370. Cited in Quintessential Aromatics database, 2013.
18. Zolfaghari ME et al. *Clinical trial of efficacy of myrtle oil in the treatment of Herpes simplex.* Iranian Journal of Medical Sciences, 1997; 22(3/4): 134-137. Cited in Quintessential Aromatics database, 2013.
19. Sepici A et al. *Hypoglycaemic effects of myrtle oil in normal and alloxan-diabetic rabbits.* Journal of Ethnopharmacology, 2004; 93(2/3): 311-318. doi: 10.1016/j.jep.2004.03.049.
20. Tavassoli M et al. *Repellency effects of essential oils of myrtle (Myrtus communis), marigold (Calendula officinalis) compared with DEET against Anopheles stephensi on human volunteers.* Journal of Arthropod-Bourne Diseases, 2011; 5(2): 10-22.
21. Yabhoobi-Ershadi MR et al. *Repellency effect of myrtle essential oil and DEET against Phlebotomus papatasi, under laboratory conditions.* Iranian Journal of Public Health, 2006; 35(3): 7-13. Cited in Quintessential Aromatics database, 2013.
22. Yang YC et al. *Insecticidal activity of plant essential oils against Pediculus humanus capitis (Anoplura: Pediculidae).* Journal of Medical Entomology, 2004; 41(4): 699-704. Cited in Quintessential Aromatics database, 2013.
23. Lawless J. *The encyclopaedia of essential oils.* Element Books, Shaftesbury, 1992.
24. Lavabre M. *Aromatherapy workbook.* Healing Arts Press, Rochester, 1997.

25. Schnaubelt K. *The healing intelligence of essential oils*. Healing Arts Press, Rochester, 2011.
26. Fischer-Rizzi S. *Complete aromatherapy handbook*. Sterling Publishing, New York, 1990.
27. Davis P. *Aromatherapy: an A-Z*. 2nd edn. C.W. Daniel Company, Saffron Walden, 1999.
28. Schnaubelt K. *Advanced aromatherapy*. Healing Arts Press, Rochester, 1995.
29. Keim Loughran J, Bull R. *Aromatherapy and subtle energy techniques*. Frog, Berkeley, 2000.
30. Worwood VA. *The fragrant heavens*. Transworld Publishing, London, 1999.
31. Zeck R. *The blossoming heart – aromatherapy for healing and transformation*. Aroma Tours, East Ivanhoe, 2004.
32. Tisserand R, Young R. *Essential oil safety*. 2nd edn. Churchill Livingstone, Edinburgh, 2014.

Neroli

Identification

Botanical name

Citrus x aurantium L.

Synonyms

Orange flower, orange blossom, neroli bigarade

Family

Rutaceae

Botany and origins

Bitter orange is an evergreen tree with long but not very sharp spines and very fragrant flowers. It is a native of southern China and India.[1]

Neroli oil is produced from the flowers of several citrus species: the oil obtained from bitter orange is called neroli bigarade oil or orange flower oil, the oil from sweet orange flowers is called neroli Portugal, and the oil from lemon flowers is called neroli citronier.[2]

Neroli bigarade is produced in the south of France, Italy, Tunisia, Morocco, Haiti, Guinea, Comoro Islands and Algeria. Orange flowers must be distilled immediately after being picked in order to avoid decay and any unpleasant off-notes due to decay processes. After the processing of the flowers, the distillers usually distill the leaves, since the trees are trimmed in the process of harvesting the flowers.[3]

As neroli oil is slightly water soluble, the water remaining after the distillation of neroli essential oil contains traces of neroli oil. This is sold as orange flower water, which is used in cosmetics and in food flavouring. Orange flower water is often solvent extracted to recover the oil, which is known as orange flower water absolute. This oil has a dark to brownish yellow colour with an intense floral odour. It is used in perfumery.[2]

Method of extraction

Neroli essential oil is obtained from the freshly picked flowers of *C. aurantium* var. *amara* by steam distillation.

Characteristics

Neroli oil is a pale yellow mobile oil which tends to become darker and more viscous with age. It has a powerful, light and refreshing floral top note with very little tenacity. Arctander states that the keeping qualities of neroli are very poor, and its odour loses its freshness after a few months if the oil is not stored correctly.[2]

Chemical composition

The chemical composition of neroli from Egypt was reported as follows:

α-pinene (4.26%), camphene (5.5%), sabinene (2.55%), β-pinene (8.67%), myrcene (2.15%), δ-3-carene (2.46%), limonene (22.43%), terpinene (4.14%), α-terpineol (1.87%), linalool (2.52%), linalyl acetate (0.87%), geraniol (1.02%), nerol (6.97%), citronellol (1.87%), citral (2.41%), β-citral (1.87%), methyl anthranilate (1.89%).[3]

Adulteration

Arctander states that artificial neroli oils are very common. They may be composed of terpeneless petitgrain oil, bitter orange oil, indole, linalyl acetate, linalool, methyl-beta-naphthyl ketone, decanal, nonanal, decanol, nonanol, nerol, nerolidol, isojasmone, hydroxycitronellal-methyl-anthranilate, phenylethyl alcohol, menthanyl ketone, nopyl acetate, expressed or terpeneless lime.[2]

Lis-Balchin states that it is seldom possible to find a decent neroli oil due to the high cost of production and the fact that it is so commonly adulterated.[4]

Neroli is commonly adulterated with geraniol from palmarosa, linalool from rosewood, sweet orange oil, citral from *Litsea cubeba* oil and Paraguay petitgrain. It is also blended with methyl-*n*-methyl anthranilate, methyl anthranilate, synthetic phenyl ethyl alcohol and synthetic indole.[5]

Pharmacopoeias and standards

The purity, composition and physico-chemical properties of neroli essential oil are defined in ISO 3517:2012 Essential Oil of Neroli (*Citrus aurantium* L., syn. *Citrus amara* Link, syn. *Citrus bigaradia* Loisel, syn. *Citrus vulgaris* Risso).

It is also listed in the European Pharmacopoeia.

History and Traditional Uses

History

The bitter orange was first cultivated in the Mediterranean by Arabs in the tenth and eleventh centuries. The oil was first distilled in the early sixteenth century.[2] Neroli is named after the seventeenth century Italian Princess of Nerola, Anna Maria de La Tremoille, who wore the oil in her gloves.[6]

Herbal

The flowers and the oil have been traditionally used for gastrointestinal complaints, nervous conditions, gout, sore throat, as a sedative and for sleeplessness.[1]

Food, perfumery and flavouring

Neroli oil is one of the key essential oils in the classic eau de cologne, along with lavender, bergamot, lemon and rosemary oils. This cologne was valued as a gentle tonic to the nervous system.[7]

Orange blossom water has traditionally been used in Europe in cooking and in skin care preparations. It is especially soothing and anti-inflammatory, and has a calming and uplifting effect similar to the essential oil.[7]

Therapeutics

Pharmacology and clinical studies

Many pharmacological studies involving neroli essential oil have been published. A systemic review of these studies will not be attempted. Rather, I have chosen a selection of studies that support the traditional and clinical uses.

Anticonvulsant activity

Neroli oil possessed biologically active constituents that had anticonvulsant activity in mice.[8]

Antifungal activity

The essential oils from the peel, leaves and flowers of *C. aurantium* var. *amara* were tested for their antifungal activity against two plant pathogenic fungi *Penicillium digitatum* and *Penicillium italicum*. The oil that showed the best activity was neroli oil.[9]

Antimicrobial activity

Neroli oil exhibited strong antibacterial activity against *Pseudomonas aeruginosa*. It also exhibited a very strong antifungal activity compared with the standard antibiotic (Nystatin).[10]

Anxiolytic activity

A study examined the effects of an aromatherapy blend of lavender, Roman chamomile and neroli with a 6:2:0.5 ratio on the anxiety, sleep and blood pressure of percutaneous coronary intervention patients in intensive care nursing. Participants received 10 treatments before their medical intervention, and the same essential oils were used another 10 times after the medical intervention. The results confirmed that aromatherapy effectively reduced the anxiety levels and increased the sleep time of the patients admitted to the ICU.[11]

A randomised clinical trial examined the role of neroli oil to alleviate anxiety during the first stage of pregnancy. The results of the trial confirmed that neroli was able to significantly lower anxiety.[12]

The inhalation of neroli oil was compared with Xanax, an anxiolytic drug. The in vivo study involving animals confirmed that neroli oil had a similar anxiolytic affect to Xanax.[13]

Cardiovascular system

Neroli was effective in diminishing the amplitude of heart muscle contractions, benefiting people who suffer from palpitations or other types of cardiac spasms. The oil was found to reduce the symptoms associated with post-cardiac surgery patients.[14]

Hypotensive activity

A study examined the effects of an aromatherapy blend of lavender, ylang ylang, marjoram and neroli (20:15:10:2) in prehypertensive and hypertensive subjects. The placebo group was asked to inhale an artificial fragrance for 24 hours and a control group received no treatment. The daytime systolic blood pressure during the 24-hour ambulatory blood pressure measurements of the aromatherapy group had significant decreases compared with the measurements of the placebo group and the control group. There was no significant difference in the night time diastolic blood pressure.[15]

Menopausal symptoms

Sixty-three healthy postmenopausal women

participated in a randomised controlled trial which investigated the effects of inhalation of neroli oil on menopausal symptoms, stress and oestrogen. Compared with the control group, the neroli group showed significant improvements. Systolic blood pressure was significantly lower in the group inhaling 0.5% neroli oil than in the control group. The neroli group also had significantly lower diastolic blood pressure, and improved serum cortisol and oestrogen concentrations. It was concluded that inhalation of neroli oil helps relieve menopausal symptoms, increase sexual desire and reduce blood pressure in postmenopausal women.[16]

Sedative activity

A randomised controlled trial was conducted in an intensive care unit using neroli oil. 100 post-cardiac surgery patients were split into four groups. Group one was the control group with no intervention; group two received a talk; group three had a 20-minute foot massage with plain vegetable oil; and group four had a foot massage with a 2.5% neroli in a massage oil. The study confirmed that a significant psychological benefit was found in both massage groups. A five-day follow up questionnaire confirmed that the patients perceived more psychological benefit from neroli massage than the massage with plain vegetable oils.[17]

N

The effects of the ambient odour of lavender, neroli and placebo were examined for their relaxing, stimulating or no effect on mood. Relaxing odours decreased heart rate and skin conductance, while stimulating odours had the reverse effects.[18]

Actions

Actions commonly cited in aromatherapy

Antidepressant, antiseptic, antispasmodic, bactericidal, carminative, cicatrisant, cordial, deodorant, digestive, nervine[7,19,20,21]

Actions supported by clinical studies

Antifungal, antimicrobial, anxiolytic, nervine

Comment

Review of traditional uses and clinical data support the use of neroli oil for improving the mood and reducing symptoms of stress-induced disorders such as anxiety and depression.

Lis-Balchin states that, because the aroma of neroli oil is considered very pleasant for many people, it may have a relaxing effect on a person.[4]

Aromatherapy Uses

Clinical aromatherapy

Baby remedy

Holmes recommends using orange flower water for babies and infants. It may be used in a humidifier, in their bath water or by adding a teaspoon to the feeding bottle. It makes a very soothing, digestive, carminative remedy for infant colic and its sedative action will help them sleep.[22]

Cardiovascular system

Neroli oil is beneficial for the heart since it regulates heart rhythm and helps to reduce cramp-like nervous heart conditions.[6] The oil is indicated for the treatment of hypertension and palpitations.[11,20]

Digestive system

Neroli oil may be used to relieve spasms of the smooth muscles of the digestive system. It is beneficial in the treatment of chronic diarrhoea, especially when it arises from nervous tension.[19]

Nervous system

Neroli oil is regarded as one of the most effective sedative and antidepressant remedies, and is recommended for the treatment of insomnia and states of anxiety and depression.[7,19]

Davis states that it can be very effective to reduce anxiety before any stressful event, such as an interview, examination or public appearance.[19] Schnaubelt recommends neroli oil for nervous individuals who are exhausted.[23]

Psychological

Fischer-Rizzi refers to neroli as a 'rescue remedy' of essential oils:

> *The sweet scent reaches deep into the soul to stabilize and regenerate. For long standing psychological tension, exhaustion and seemingly hopeless situations, the oil strengthens and brings relief. For people who are thin skinned, neroli can strengthen their inner being and build a protective shield. Neroli offers the gift of strength and courage that helps us see life's beauty.*[6]

Mojay recommends neroli oil for individuals who are emotionally intense, and who are sometimes unstable and easily alarmed and agitated.[21] Holmes describes neroli as promoting clarity, sensitivity and space, and describes it as enhancing the 'lightness of being'.[22]

Skin care

In skin care, neroli oil is regarded as being non-allergenic and is recommended to reduce redness and irritation. It is beneficial for all skin types, especially dry sensitive skin with broken capillaries.[19,20]

The oil is reputed to have a rejuvenating effect on the skin as it has an ability to stimulate the growth of healthy new cells.[19]

Energetics, psyche and subtle uses

Energetics

Neroli oil clears *heat*, relaxes the nerves and uplifts the spirits.[21,22] Mojay describes neroli oil as one of the best oils to calm and stabilise the *Heart* and mind. He explains that neroli is particularly beneficial for *hot*, agitated conditions of the *Heart* characterised by restlessness, insomnia and palpitations.[21]

Neroli oil has a calming effect on the *Heart* and *Shen*, which are associated with the Fire Element. It essentially has a *cooling* and calming effect on excess Fire.[21]

Personality

The neroli personality is described as being one of the most spiritual personalities. Worwood states that, whatever their age, there is a built-in wisdom that extends far beyond that of worldly knowledge. She describes neroli as a personality that seems to have found a way to be ageless, forever young in a spring-like way.[24]

They are always able to find happiness in everything. They acknowledge the imperfections in people, but always focus and look for the good in people. Neroli personality's good intentions mean that they can easily be taken advantage of by the people they love. Their friends and family get so used to being put first that they neglect their own needs.[24]

Worwood explains that neroli personality types are happiest when they are searching the mysteries of life. They can become saddened by the lack of understanding in the world today and can become very sensitive souls. They have very high morals. They believe that no one has the right to dictate how one should think, feel or act.[24]

According to Myers-Briggs personality types, the neroli personality as likely to be an ENFP. ENFPs are outgoing, lively and spontaneous. They are very enthusiastic and their joy for life can be contagious. They have a rich imagination and active mind. Their thoughts are always wandering and their mood constantly changing. They can be inspiring and charismatic leaders. They are always involved, or in love, with someone or something new. They know how to establish instant rapport and make people feel comfortable. They love emotional intensity and enjoy expressing their feelings. They can be charming and flirtatious. They relate with warmth to many people and can appear overly enthusiastic, positive and optimistic.

Subtle

Neroli oil is associated with purity. It brings us in touch with our higher selves. It facilitates all spiritual work and is recommended for enhancing creativity.[25]

Keim Loughran & Bull state that neroli is the essential oil that assists the subconscious mind to reveal itself and unite with the conscious mind, bringing awareness to the present moment and helping to resolve blocks. This releases a flood of positive energy that becomes available to the super-conscious. They state that, as this energy flows from self to soul to spirit, we are in direct communication with the world of manifestation. Neroli helps us manifest our deepest and highest aspiration.[26]

Worwood explains that neroli touches the realms of the angels, and anyone who uses it is brushed with the light of angels' wings. She describes neroli as pure spirit, representing the purity in all things, always loving and peaceful. It also has another purpose – to bring self-recognition and relief.[27]

Mojay describes neroli oil as both sensual and spiritual. It helps to re-establish the links between a disconnected body and mind.[21]

Dosage and Administration

Blending

Aromatherapy

For the relief of symptoms associated with depression, consider blending neroli oil with essential oils such as bergamot, geranium, fragonia, lavender, jasmine absolute, rose otto, sweet orange, sandalwood or ylang ylang.

For the relief of anxiety, nervous tension and stress-related conditions, consider blending neroli oil with essential oils such as bergamot, clary sage, geranium, lavender, mandarin, sweet orange, petitgrain, rosemary or sandalwood.

To assist in the management of hypertension, consider blending neroli oil with essential oils such as lavender, may chang, sweet marjoram or ylang ylang.

For sensitive skin, consider blending neroli oil with essential oils such as German chamomile, everlasting, lavender or sandalwood.

Perfumery

Neroli is considered the perfect starting material for the classic eau de cologne style perfume.

Arctander states that it blends well with all the citrus oils and numerous floral absolutes.[2]

Mode of administration

Bath

Full body bath, foot bath

Topical

Compress, massage, ointment, skin care

Inhalation

Direct inhalation, diffuser, oil vaporiser

Safety Profile

General safety

Neroli oil is non-toxic, non-irritating and non-sensitising.[7] Lis-Balchin states that, due to widespread adulteration, there is a high sensitisation potential.[4]

Contraindications

No contraindications known.

Regulatory guidelines

Neroli oil has been granted GRAS status.

References

1. Khan I, Abourashed E. *Leung's encyclopedia of common natural ingredients used in food, drugs and cosmetics*. 3rd edn. John Wiley & Sons, New Jersey, 2010.
2. Arctander S. *Perfume and flavor materials of natural origin*. Allured Publishing, Carol Stream, 1994.
3. Weiss EA. *Essential oil crops*. CAB International, Wallingford, 1997.
4. Lis-Balchin M. *Aromatherapy science – a guide for healthcare professionals*. Pharmaceutical Press, London, 2006.
5. Schmidt E, Wanner J. *Adulteration of essential oils*. In Baser KHC, Buchbauer G. eds. *Handbook of essential oils – science, technology and applications*. 2nd edn. CRC Press, Boca Raton, 2016: 707-745.
6. Fischer-Rizzi S. *Complete aromatherapy handbook*. Sterling Publishing, New York, 1990.
7. Lawless J. *The encyclopaedia of essential oils*. Element Books, Shaftesbury, 1992.
8. Azanchi T et al. *Anticonvulsant activity of Citrus aurantium blossom essential oil (neroli): involvement of the GABAergic system*. Natural Product Communications, 2014; 9(11): 1615-1618.
9. Trabelsi D et al. *Chemical composition and antifungal activity of essential oils from flowers, leaves and peels of Tunisian Citrus aurantium against Penicillium digitatum and Penicillium italicum*. Journal of Essential Oil Bearing Plants, 2016; 19(7): 1660-1674. doi: 10.1080/0972060X.2016.1141069.
10. Haj Ammar A et al. *Chemical composition and in vitro antimicrobial and antioxidant activities of Citrus aurantium L. flowers essential oil (neroli oil)*. Pakistan Journal of Biological Sciences, 15(21): 1034-1040. doi: 10.3923/pjbs.2012.1034.1040.
11. Cho MY et al. *Effects of aromatherapy on the anxiety, vital signs and sleep quality of percutaneous coronary intervention patients in intensive care units*. Evidence-Based Complementary and Alternative Medicine, 2013; 2013: 381381. doi: 10.1155/2013/381381. Cited in Quintessential Aromatics database, 2013.
12. Namazi M et al. *Aromatherapy with Citrus aurantium oil and anxiety during the first stage of labor*. Iranian Red Crescent Medical Journal, 2014; 16(6): e18371. doi: 0.5812/ircmj.18371. Cited in Quintessential Aromatics database, 2013.
13. Chen YJ et al. *Inhalation of neroli essential oil and its anxiolytic effects*. Journal of Complementary and Integrative Medicine, 2008; 5(1). doi: 10.2202/1553-3840.1143.
14. Stevenson C. *Orange blossom evaluation*. The International Journal of Aromatherapy, 1992; 4(3): 22-24.
15. Kim IH et al. *Essential oil inhalation on blood pressure and salivary cortisol levels in prehypertensive and hypertensive subjects*. Evidence-Based Complementary and Alternative Medicine, 2012; 2012: 984203. doi 10.1155/2012/984203.
16. Choi SY et al. *Effects of inhalation of essential oil of Citrus aurantium L. var. amara on menopausal symptoms, stress, and estrogen in postmenopausal women: a randomized controlled trial*. Evidence-Based Complementary and Alternative Medicine, 2014; 2014: 796518. doi: 10.1155/2014/796518.
17. Stevenson C. *The psychophysiological effects of aromatherapy massage following cardiac surgery*. Complementary Therapies in Medicine, 1994; 2(1): 27-35. Cited in Quintessential Aromatics database, 2013.
18. Campenni CE et al. *Role of suggestion in odor-induced mood change*. Psychological Reports, 2004; 94(3): 1127-1136. Cited in Quintessential Aromatics database, 2013.
19. Davis P. *Aromatherapy: an A-Z*. 2nd edn. C.W. Daniel Company, Saffron Walden, 1999.
20. Lavabre M. *Aromatherapy workbook*. Healing Arts Press, Rochester, 1997.
21. Mojay G. *Aromatherapy for healing the spirit*. Healing Arts Press, Rochester, 1999.
22. Holmes P. *Neroli – the lightness of being*. The International Journal of Aromatherapy, 1995; 7(2): 14-17.

N

23. Schnaubelt K. *Medical aromatherapy*. Frog, Berkeley, 1999.
24. Worwood VA. *The fragrant mind*. Transworld Publishers, London, 1995.
25. Davis P. *Subtle aromatherapy*. C.W. Daniel Company, Saffron Walden, 1991.
26. Keim Loughran J, Bull R. *Aromatherapy anointing oils*. Frog, Berkeley, 2001.
27. Worwood VA. *The fragrant heavens*. Transworld Publishers, London, 1999.

Niaouli

Identification

Botanical name

Melaleuca quinquenervia (Cav.) S.T. Blake

Synonyms

Broad-leaf paperbark, broad-leaf tea tree, paperbark

Arctander states that niaouli is steam-distilled from the leaves of *M. viridiflora*; however, Lassak states that the names *M. leucadendron* var. *viridiflora* and *M. viridflora* have been misapplied to this species.[1,2] Weiss also confirms this and states that the source of confusion is because *M. quinquenervia* has several cultivars which produce oils of differing composition.[3]

1,8-cineole-rich *M. quinquenervia* oil is referred to as niaouli, while the nerolidol/linalool-rich *M. quinquenervia* oil is referred to as nerolina.[4]

Family

Myrtaceae

Botany and origins

M. quinquenervia is an evergreen tree, up to 8 to 12 m in height, with a papery bark. It grows well in swampy ground. In Australia, it is commonly found growing wild along the coastal strip of New South Wales, and all the way up to the northern tip of Queensland.[2]

It can also be found growing in its wild habitat in southern Papua New Guinea and in New Caledonia. New Caledonia has always been the main producer of niaouli oil. The centre of production is located around the Gomen region, which is why niaouli oil is known in France as gomenol.[5]

M. quinquenervia has also been introduced to Madagascar.[5] The oil from Madagascar is preferred in aromatherapy, as the oil from New Caledonia is often obtained by fractional distillation and is cut.[6,7]

The *M. quinquenervia* tree has been regarded as a weed in the USA. It was introduced to southern Florida from Australia in the early twentieth century and it has now become the world's worst woody weed.[8]

Method of extraction

Niaouli essential oil is produced by steam distillation of the leaves and twigs of *M. quinquenervia*.

Characteristics

Arctander describes niaouli oil as a pale yellow to greenish or almost colourless oil, with a strong, fresh, sweet-camphoraceous odour reminiscent of eucalyptus and cardamom.[1]

The 1,8-cineole chemotype has an odour similar to that of eucalyptus, while the nerolidol/linalool chemotype (nerolina) has a pleasant floral green citrus aroma with a woody waxy nuance. Webb states that nerolina has the most pleasant aroma of all the *Melaleuca* species because of the nerolidol and linalool content, which gives it a fresh, green fruity aroma.[4]

Chemical composition

A study of *M. quinquenervia* leaf oils over its geographical range in Australia and Papua New Guinea has shown a wide variation in chemical composition and has identified two chemotypes.[9]

- chemotype 1 is comprised of (*E*)-nerolidol (74-95%) and linalool (14-30%). Two divisions occur in this chemotype, which are based on the presence or absence of significant proportions of linalool (14-40%).
- chemotype 2 contains 1,8-cineole (10-75%), viridiflorol (13-66%), α-terpineol (0.5-14%), and β-caryophyllene (0.5-28%) in varying proportions and in order of dominance in the oils.

Lawrence reports that there are four chemotypes of the *M. quinquenervia* species:

- chemotype 1 – oils rich in 1,8-cineole with varying amounts of α-terpineol
- chemotype 2 – oils rich in viridiflorol with varying amounts of 1,8-cineole and α-terpineol
- chemotype 3 – oils rich in (*E*)-nerolidol with varying amounts of linalool
- chemotype 4 – oils rich in 1,8-cineole with

N

varying amounts of monoterpene hydrocarbons.[5]

Webb states that within the nerolidol/linalool chemotype there is much variation in the percentage of the main constituents. He states that there have been plants discovered with extremely high nerolidol content (>95%) and trace linalool, as well as plants with a higher ratio of linalool to nerolidol.[10]

The nerolidol/linalool chemotype is more common around northern NSW, while the 1,8-cineole chemotype is more prevalent in the southern regions.[1] The nerolidol/linalool chemotype has been known since 1935, but it was not commercially harvested and an oil was not produced until 1997.[10]

The 1,8-cineole and (*E*)-nerolidol chemotype variants represent 70% of the *M. quinquenervia* tree population.[11]

Niaouli oil from New Caledonia is classified into three chemotypes:

- chemotype 1 is rich in terpinene derivatives
- chemotype 2 is rich in 1,8-cineole
- chemotype 3 is rich in α-pinene and viridiflorol.[12]

The main component range of the niaouli chemotypes from New Caledonia are as follows:[12]

Component	Chemotype 1	Chemotype 2	Chemotype 3
α-pinene	0-17%	1.0-25.0%	5.0-27.7%
β-pinene	0.1-2.0%	0.5-5.0%	0.4-5.0%
p-cymene	0.4-40.0%	0-10.0%	0-1.0%
limonene	1.0-6.0%	0.5-15.0%	1.0-10.0%
1,8-cineole	0.1-47.0%	20-76.3%	2.0-40.0%
γ-terpinene	0-32.4%	0.1-2.0%	0.1-3.0%
terpinolene	0.05-19.2%	0.05-1.0%	0.01-1.0%
terpinen-4-ol	0.5-5.0%	0-3.0%	0.05-1.0%
α-terpineol	0.5-24.5%	0-15.0%	0-5.0%
α-terpinyl acetate	0-5.0%	0-11.4%	0-0.5%
$C_{15}H_{26}O$	0-10.8%	0-5.0%	0-10.0%
viridiflorol	4.0-50.0%	0-45.0%	10.0-67.4%

$C_{15}H_{26}O$ is most likely to be nerolidol.

Adulteration

Arctander states that the oil is frequently adulterated in countries where it is not readily available. Eucalyptus oil blended with trace amounts of terpinyl esters, aldehydes, terpineol and terpinolene are often sold as niaouli oil.[1]

Pharmacopoeias and standards

At the time of writing, the purity, composition, physico-chemical properties and therapeutic use of niaouli essential oil are not defined in any pharmacopoeia monograph or standard.

History and Traditional Uses

History

Lassak states that the young leaves were bruised in water as a liquid drunk to relieve headaches and colds and during general sickness. The oil is used for coughs and colds and applied externally for neuralgia and rheumatism. The oil was used as a vermifuge.[2]

Niaouli oil has been produced by steam distillation since 1893 in the Gomen-Ouaco area, located in the northern part of New Caledonia. The oil has been available and distributed by Gomenol Co. (France) in aromatherapy preparations for all of the last century.[12]

Traditional medicine

In France, numerous pharmaceuticals containing niaouli were made up to the 1980s, such as a syrup for respiratory tract infections and suppositories for vaginal infections.[6]

Herbal

The German Commission E recommends niaouli oil for catarrh of the upper respiratory tract.[13] Unless otherwise prescribed, it recommends a daily dose 0.2 g of the oil internally. However, I agree with Tisserand & Young, who state that this dosage may be considered unsafe considering the oral toxicity of eucalyptus oil in humans.[14]

Food, perfumery and flavouring

Niaouli oil is used in medicinal preparations, in cough drops, vaporiser liquids, mouth sprays and gargles, and to flavour toothpaste.[1]

Therapeutics

Pharmacology and clinical studies

Anthelmintic activity

Niaouli oil was found to be an effective anthelmintic activity on *Haemonchus contortus* eggs. It was suggested that the oil could be a good candidate for nematode control; however, more studies are required to confirm that it is safe to use.[15]

Antifungal activity

Studies have reported that niaouli oil has moderate antifungal activity.[8]

Antimicrobial activity

Niaouli oil displayed strong antimicrobial activity against pathogenic microorganisms, which are the main causative agents of dental caries and infectious diseases. The results of a study indicated the efficacy of niaouli oil against *Streptococcus mutans* by displaying complete inhibition, as it is the main organism to initiate dental plaque.[11]

Immunomodulatory activity

The in vivo immunomodulatory effect of niaouli oil was investigated using a mouse model. Niaouli oil potentiates T cell-mediated cellular immunity and macrophage activity, but not humoral immunity. It was suggested that the study provides a rationale for clinical application of niaouli oil to control infectious diseases.[16]

Actions

Actions commonly cited in aromatherapy

Analgesic, antibacterial, anticatarrhal, anti-inflammatory, antirheumatic, antiseptic, antiviral, decongestant, febrifuge, insecticide, stimulant, vermifuge, vulnerary[17,18,19,20]

Actions supported by clinical studies

Antibacterial, antiviral

Comment

As there are three niaouli chemotypes, it is important to know which one you are using, as this will have a significant impact on the therapeutic outcome.

All the *M. quinquenervia* oils have promising antimicrobial activity. Linalool, nerolidol and viridiflorol make niaouli oil one of the most pleasant and agreeable melaleucas to smell. It also provides the oil with a diverse range of aromatherapy applications from skin care to stress-related conditions.

Schnaubelt states that the oil helps us avoid catching a cold when other members of the household are already sneezing or are sick with the flu. He explains that the unfamiliar scent of the oil becomes more and more agreeable as we become aware of its benefits.[21]

Aromatherapy Uses

Clinical aromatherapy

Antimicrobial

Webb cites Pénoël, who recommends using niaouli oil as an antiviral to assist in the treatment of shingles and cold sores.[4]

Dental hygiene

Niaouli oil displayed promising antimicrobial activity against pathogenic microorganisms responsible for dental caries and infectious diseases of the gums. Results of a study indicated that niaouli oil showed complete inhibition against *S. mutans*, the prime organism involved in the formation of dental plaque.[11]

Schnaubelt recommends rubbing niaouli oil on the gums to strengthen them and to reduce inflammation. He also recommends using the oil on dental floss to protect the teeth and improve gum health.[20]

Integumentary system

Niaouli oil is recommended for cleaning minor wounds and burns. Davis recommends using 5-6 drops of niaouli in 250 mL of boiled and cooled water to wash and clean a wound or burn. It is antiseptic and a vulnerary and will help healing.[17]

Musculoskeletal system

Niaouli oil is recommended for muscular aches and pains and for the relief of arthritis.[18]

Nervous system

Webb cites Pénoël, who recommends using niaouli oil for fatigue and stress-related conditions because it has hormone-like activity as an adrenal tonic.[4]

Reproductive system

Niaouli oil is well tolerated by the skin and mucous membranes, which makes it suitable as a vaginal douche for the treatment of cystitis and other urinary tract infections.[7,17,18]

Respiratory system

Niaouli oil is recommended for acute and chronic bronchitis and sinusitis.[6] Niaouli is an excellent expectorant and it also has antiallergenic and antiasthmatic properties.[7,20]

Skin care

Davis says that, because niaouli oil is non-irritant, it is well suited to skin care application. It is recommended for the treatment of acne and boils.[17]

Energetics, psyche and subtle uses

Energetics

Niaouli oil warms the *Lungs*, expels phlegm and relieves coughing. It is used to eliminate *Lung phlegm-cold* and *damp*, which is associated with coughing, wheezing and mucous congestion. I recommend using niaouli oil to tonify *Qi*. It helps to alleviate mental fatigue and confusion, poor focus and headaches. According to the principles of the Five Elements, niaouli oil has strong affinity with the Metal Element.

Dosage and Administration

Blending

Aromatherapy

For the relief of symptoms associated with colds

and flu, consider blending niaouli oil with essential oils such as 1,8-cineole-rich eucalypts, lemon-scented eucalyptus, peppermint eucalyptus, cajeput, fragonia, kunzea, lemon, pine or tea tree.

For the treatment of minor wounds, consider blending niaouli oil with essential oils such as everlasting, lavender, frankincense, myrrh or tea tree.

For the relief of sinusitis, consider blending niaouli oil with essential oils such as cajeput, 1,8-cineole-rich eucalypts, fragonia, peppermint or pine.

For the relief of muscular aches and pains, consider blending niaouli oil with essential oils such a cajeput, peppermint eucalyptus, ginger, kunzea, spike lavender, pine or rosemary.

For the relief of anxiety, stress and mental exhaustion, consider blending niaouli oil with essential oils such as bergamot, lavender, sweet orange, neroli or sandalwood.

Perfumery

Niaouli oil is not commonly used in perfumery.

Mode of administration

Bath

Full body bath, foot bath. Schnaubelt suggests using niaouli oil in a shower. He recommends anywhere from 5 to 20 drops using a loofah glove along the energy meridians while in the shower. It is a fast-acting treatment and leaves you feeling invigorated and refreshed.[20]

Topical

Compress, massage, ointment, skin care

Inhalation

Direct inhalation, diffuser, oil vaporiser

Safety Profile

General safety

The chemical profile of all the *M. quinquenervia* chemotypes suggests that the oils are non-toxic, non-irritant and non-sensitising.[10,14]

Contraindications

No contraindications known.[14]

Regulatory guidelines

M. quinquenervia oil is not defined in any regulatory guideline.

N

References

1. Arctander S. *Perfume and flavor materials of natural origin.* Allured Publishing, Carol Stream, 1994.
2. Lassak E, McCarthy T. *Australian medicinal plants.* Methuen Australia, North Ryde, 1983.
3. Weiss EA. *Essential oil crops.* CAB International, Wallingford, 1997.
4. Webb M. *Bush sense.* Self-published, Australia, 2000.
5. Lawrence BM. *Progress in essential oils – niaouli oil.* Perfumer & Flavorist, 2013; 38: 44-48.
6. Collin P, Price L, *Niaouli.* The Aromatherapist, 1997; 4(2): 15-19.
7. Schnaubelt K. *Medical aromatherapy.* Frog, Berkeley, 1999.
8. Barbosa LCA et al. *Chemistry and biological activities essential oils from Melaleuca L. species.* Agriculturae Conspectus Scientificus, 2013; 78(1): 11-23.
9. Ireland BF et al. *Chemical variation in the leaf essential oil of Melaleuca quinquenervia (Cav.) S.T. Blake.* Biochemical systematics and Ecology, 2002; 30(5): 457-470. doi: 10.1016/S0305-1978(01)00112-0.
10. Webb M. *Australian essential oil profile – nerolina.* Aromatherapy Today, 2001, 18: 24-36.
11. Vasundhara M et al. *Chemovariant of Melaleuca quinquenervia (Cav.) S.T. Blake and its antipathogen activity.* European Journal of Pharmaceutical and Medical Research, 2016; 3(6): 482-487.
12. Trilles BL et al. *Occurrence of various chemotypes in niaouli [Melaleuca quinquenervia (Cav.) S.T. Blake] essential oil from New Caledonia.* Flavour and Fragrance Journal, 2006; 21(4): 677-682.
13. Blumenthal M. et al. *The complete German commission E monographs: therapeutic guide to herbal medicine.* American Botanical Council, Austin, 1998.
14. Tisserand R, Young R. *Essential oil safety.* 2nd edn. Churchill Livingstone, Edinburgh, 2014.
15. Gaínza, YA et al. *Anthelmintic activity in vitro of Citrus sinensis and Melaleuca quinquenervia essential oil from Cuba on Haemonchus contortus.* Industrial Crops and Products, 2015; 76: 647-652. doi: 10.1016/j.indcrop.2015.07.056.
16. Nam SY et al. *Essential oil of niaouli preferentially potentiates antigen-specific cellular immunity and cytokine production by macrophages.* Immunopharmacology and Immunotoxicology, 2008; 30(3): 459-474. doi: 10.1080/08923970802135187.
17. Davis P. *Aromatherapy: an A-Z.* 2nd edn. C.W. Daniel Company, Saffron Walden, 1999.
18. Lawless J. *The encyclopaedia of essential oils.* Element Books, Shaftesbury, 1992.
19. Lavabre M. *Aromatherapy workbook.* Healing Arts Press, Rochester, 1997.
20. Schnaubelt K. *Advanced aromatherapy.* Healing Arts Press, Rochester, 1995.
21. Schnaubelt K. *The healing intelligence of essential oils.* Healing Arts Press, Rochester, 2011.

Nutmeg

Identification

Botanical name

Myristica fragrans Houtt.

Synonyms

Myristica officinalis, Myristica moschata, Myristica aromatica, Myristica amboinensis

Family

Myristicaceae

Botany and origins

Nutmegs are the dried kernels of the seeds of *Myristica fragrans*, an evergreen tree to 15 m with dark green leaves, yellow flowers without petals, and large yellowish fruit. All parts of the tree are aromatic.[1]

Nutmeg is native to Banda and Amboina islands in the Moluccas, Indonesia, and is seldom found as a wild plant because of its popularity as a spice. Nutmeg is commercially cultivated in Indonesia, Grenada and Sri Lanka.[1]

The dried, finger-like husk which surrounds the nutmeg seed inside the shell of the fruit is known commercially as mace. Dried, pulverised mace is a well-known household spice.[2]

Nutmeg also contain 24-40% fixed oil obtained by expressing crushed nuts between heated plates in the presence of steam or by solvent extraction. The expressed oil or nutmeg butter is a highly aromatic, orange-coloured fat with the consistency of butter at ambient room temperature. It consists mainly of trimyristin and volatile oils.[1]

Method of extraction

Nutmeg oil is produced by steam distillation or steam-and-water distillation of the freshly comminuted, dried nutmegs.[2]

Characteristics

Nutmeg oil is a pale yellow mobile liquid with a light, fresh, warm-spicy and aromatic odour. The undertone and dry out is warm and sweet with a slightly woody aroma.[2]

Chemical composition

A comparison of chemical composition of the East Indian and West Indian nutmeg oil was reported as follows:[3]

Constituent	East Indian nutmeg	West Indian nutmeg
α-pinene	18.0-26.5%	10.6-13.2%
camphene	0.3-0.4%	0.2%
β-pinene	9.7-17.7%	7.8-12.1%
sabinene	15.4-36.3%	42.0-50.7%
myrcene	2.2-3.7%	2.5-3.4%
α-phellandrene	0.4-1.0%	0.4-0.7%
α-terpinene	0.8-4.0%	0.8-4.2%
limonene	2.7-3.6%	3.1-4.4%
1,8-cineole	1.5-3.2%	2.5-4.2%
γ-terpinene	1.3-6.8%	1.9-4.7%
linalool	0.2-0.9%	0.3-0.9%
terpinen-4-ol	2.0-10.9%	3.5-6.1%
safrole	0.6-3.2%	0.1-0.2%
methyl eugenol	trace-1.2%	0.1-0.2%
myristicin	3.3-13.5%	0.5-0.9%

Lis-Balchin states that myristicin is usually lower in the West Indian nutmeg oil; however, the West Indian and East Indian oils are often blended. She explains that perfumers prefer the East Indian nutmeg.[4]

ISO standards have set minimum and maximum limits for a typical chemical profile of nutmeg oil:

α-pinene (15-28%), β-pinene (13-18%), sabinene (14-29%), δ-3-carene (0.5-2%), limonene (2-7%), γ-terpinene (2-6%), terpinen-4-ol (2-6%), safrole (1-2.5%), myristicin (5 to 12%).[1]

N

Adulteration

Nutmeg oil is often adulterated with *Melaleuca alternifolia* essential oil, and monoterpenes such as α-pinene, β-pinene, camphene, sabinene, myrcene, α-phellandrene and β-phellandrene, as well as synthetic linalool, terpinene-4-ol and α-terpineol.[2,5]

Pharmacopoeias and standards

The purity, composition and physico-chemical properties of nutmeg essential oil are defined in ISO 3215:1988 – Oil of Nutmeg, Indonesian Type (*Myristica fragrans* Houtt.).

History and Traditional Uses

History

The use of nutmeg as a food flavouring and a medicine has a long history. It was recorded in the Sanskrit as *jai phal* and probably arrived by trade from the Hindu colonists of Java.[1]

Nutmeg was not known to the Greeks or Romans. The first recorded use of nutmeg in Europe was in 540 AD by Actius of Constantinople. It is believed that Arab traders brought it to Europe from the Moluccas via Java and India and, as with other spices, the Arabs hid the true source to avoid competition.[1]

By the twelfth century it was well known in Europe, and in 1191, when Emperor Henry VI entered Rome for his coronation, the streets were fumigated with nutmegs and other strewing aromatics.[1]

In search for a route to the spice islands, Vasco da Gama reached the Moluccas, the source of the nutmeg trade. The Portuguese dominated the nutmeg trade for nearly a century. Then the Dutch controlled the trade of nutmegs in the seventeenth century for another 200 years.[1]

In 1650, the Dutch attempted to limit nutmeg production to Banda and Amboina by forcible destruction of all other trees. During the British occupation of the Moluccas (1796-1802), the East India Company sent its botanist, Christopher Smith, to collect seedlings of nutmeg and cloves to establish the spices in Penang and other countries under the control of the British. Nutmeg was introduced to Sri Lanka in 1804 where it flourished and continues to do so as a minor crop. Nutmeg was also taken to the Caribbean island of St Vincent in 1802 and to Trinidad in 1824.[1]

Nutmegs have long been known for their narcotic effect. The first recorded hallucinogenic effect was by Lobelius in 1576. The physiologist JE Purkinje in 1829 ate three nutmegs and described the effects as similar to cannabis intoxication, including disorientation, hallucinations and later a deep sleep. The response to nutmeg intoxication is extremely varied. It appears that freshly grated nutmegs produce the most profound intoxication.[1]

N

Traditional medicine

The Ayurvedic name for nutmeg is *made shaunda*, narcotic fruit. Nutmeg powder is mixed with betel nut and snuff in certain parts of southern India. Powdered nutmeg is also used as snuff in Indonesia. Weiss states that in Zanzibar local people chewed nutmegs as an alternative to smoking the local *bhang* (marijuana), with almost the same effects.[1]

The pericarps of nutmeg are made into a sweet snack called *pala manis* or *pala gulu* by repeated soaking in a sugar solution. Indigenous Malukans topically apply nutmeg oil to give a warm invigorating sensation, to relieve headaches, stomach aches, diarrhoea and flu symptoms.[6]

Nutmegs have been used in Western and Chinese herbal medicine as a muscle relaxant, to alleviate digestive discomfort and abdominal pain, and as a sedative and muscle relaxant. In Vietnam, powdered nutmeg is used in boiled rice as a remedy against dysentery, anorexia and colic, and to treat malarial debility.

Nutmeg is traditionally used for inflammatory conditions and to treat joint and muscle pain as well as liver disease. Nutmeg oil is helpful to dissolve kidney stones and alleviate infections of the kidney.[7]

Herbal

The German Commission E recommends nutmeg for gastrointestinal ailments such as diarrhoea, gastric spasms and flatulence.[8] Mace has been used as an anti-parasitic, and is externally used for the treatment of rheumatism.[9]

Food, perfumery and flavouring

Nutmeg is extensively used as a domestic spice in cooking, in cakes, drinks and other foods.[9]

The oil is used as a flavour ingredient in many food products and in non-alcoholic and alcoholic beverages. Nutmeg oil is used in many foods and beverages. Nutmeg oil is used in the food industry to mask the smell of boiled cabbage.[4]

Therapeutics

Pharmacology and clinical studies

Many pharmacological studies involving nutmeg essential oil have been published. A systemic review of these studies will not be attempted. Rather, I have chosen a selection of studies that support the traditional and clinical uses.

Antiangiogenic activity

An in vivo study confirmed that nutmeg oil had significant antiangiogenic activity in mice. It was suggested that nutmeg essential oil could be developed as an antiangiogenic drug. Antiangiogenic drugs inhibit the growth of new blood cells. They are often used for the treatment of cancer, and for macular degeneration of the eye and other diseases involving proliferation of blood vessels.[10]

Anticonvulsant activity

An in vivo test investigated the anticonvulsant activity of nutmeg oil, using well-established animal seizure models. The results of the study indicated that nutmeg oil may be effective against grand mal and partial seizures as it prevented seizure spread in animal studies. However, it was also stated that slight potentiation of clonic seizure activity limits its use for the treatment of myoclonic and absence seizures.[11]

Anti-inflammatory activity

Nutmeg oil exhibited an anti-inflammatory effect

on acute inflammation in animal studies. The data from this study indicated that nutmeg oil showed pharmacological activities similar to those of non-steroidal anti-inflammatory drugs.[12]

Nutmeg extracts have been found to inhibit the biosynthesis of prostaglandins in animal studies. The anti-inflammatory activity of mace was confirmed in carrageenan-induced oedema in rats.[9]

Myristicin was found to have anti-inflammatory properties related to its inhibition of nitric oxide, cytokines, chemokines and growth factors in double-stranded RNA (dsRNA)-stimulated macrophages via the calcium pathway.[13]

Another report suggests that the anti-inflammatory action of myristicin might be due to the inhibition of chemokines, cytokines, nitrous oxide and growth factors in dsRNA-stimulated macrophages via the calcium pathway.[6]

In an in vivo study, it was demonstrated that nutmeg oil could alleviate the CFA-injection induced joint swelling, mechanical allodynia and heat hyper-analgesia of rats through inhibition of COX-2 expression and blood substance P level. It was suggested that nutmeg oil could be used as a potential chronic pain reliever.[14]

Antimicrobial activity

The antibacterial activity of nutmeg oil was tested in a study on 25 different bacterial strains, and it was observed to be equally effective against the majority of gram-positive and gram-negative microbes.[6]

In another study, several commonly used spices were evaluated for their antifungal activity. Turmeric and nutmeg were found to be most active.[6]

An in vitro study confirmed that nutmeg oil showed antimicrobial activity against a range of microorganisms, except for *Pseudomonas aeruginosa* and *Candida albicans*.[15]

In one in vitro study, nutmeg essential oil exhibited the strongest antibacterial activity against *Shigella dysenteriae* with low cytotoxic effects. The MIC values of nutmeg oil ranged from 0.31 to 1 mg/ mL.[1 16]

Antioxidant activity

Oxidation of lipids is one of the main causes of rancidity in food products. A study investigated the antioxidant activity of a number of essential oils including nutmeg. When maintained at room temperature, all the oils tested had good radical-scavenger properties. When heated up to 180°C, nutmeg oil was the only oil that had significantly higher free radical-scavenger activity. All the essential oils tested were able to protect α-tocopherol, contained in virgin olive oil, against thermal oxidative degradation. It was suggested that nutmeg and other essential oils tested exhibited good antioxidant activity and might be efficiently used to control lipid oxidation during food processing.[17]

Nutmeg oil showed better antioxidant activity compared to other tested oleoresins and synthetic antioxidants, butylated hydroxy anisole and butylated hydroxy toluene. It was suggested that nutmeg oil should be considered as a natural food preservative.[18]

Antiparasitic activity

An in vitro study investigated nutmeg essential oil cytotoxicity on Vero cell line and antiparasitic activity against *Toxoplasma gondii* parasite. It displayed a very low cytotoxic activity against Vero cells and inhibition against *T. gondii*, which was similar to clindamycin, a standard pharmaceutical often used.[19]

Chemoprotective activity

An in vitro study tested essential oils from common spices such as nutmeg, ginger, cardamom, celery seed, black pepper, cumin and coriander for their ability to suppress the formation of DNA adducts by aflatoxin B1 in a microsomal enzyme-mediated reaction. All the oils significantly inhibited adduct formation in a dose-dependent manner. It was suggested that the enzymatic modulation is due to the chemical constituents of the oils, and that this means that the oils could be used as potential anticarcinogenic agents.[20]

An in vivo study examined the influence of cardamom, dill seed, coriander seed, cumin seed, ginger and nutmeg oil on the activity of hepatic carcinogen metabolising enzymes of cytochrome P450 and glutathione S-transferase (GST) in mice. The oils were administered by gavage for 10 days. All the essential oils significantly elevated GST activity, which indicated their potential as 'blocking agents' in chemoprotective strategies. The results indicated that the intake of essential oils affected host enzymes associated with activation and detoxification of xenobiotic compounds, including chemical mutagens and carcinogens.[21]

Nutmeg oil showed significant inhibition on the expansion of a colon cancer cell line in an in vitro study.[6]

Ethanolic extract of nutmeg was used to test anticancer activity against human cancer cell lines, and it showed more than 70% growth inhibition at a concentration of 100 μg/ mL.[6]

Hepatoprotective activity

Myristicin, one of the major essential oil components in nutmeg oil, was found to have significant hepatoprotective activity. A study found that nutmeg oil showed significant effect on lipopolysaccharide-induced hepatic injury in D-galactosamine sensitised rats.[22]

Another study found that aqueous extract of nutmeg had a significant hepatoprotective and antioxidant activity against isoproterenol-induced hepatotoxicity and oxidative stress.[6]

Psychotropic activity

Nutmeg is reported to have psychotropic properties.[9,23]

Weiss states that the aromatic ethers are the most likely source of hallucinations, but the mode of action remains obscure. Myristicin constitutes about 4% of nutmeg oil, and 25% of this fraction is elemicin, which degrades to two potent hallucinogens, TMA (trimethoxyamphetamine) and MMDA (3-methoxy-4,5-methylenedioxy amphetamine) by becoming ammoniated in the body. Crude nutmeg produces a degree of monoamine oxidase inhibition in vivo and in vitro studies.[1]

A report states that several intoxications have been reported after ingestion of approximately 5 g of nutmeg which corresponds to approximately 1-2 mg of myristicin per kg body weight. It was stated that, while the intoxication may be ascribed to the actions of myristicin, it is likely that other components of nutmeg may be involved.[24]

Another study confirmed that nutmeg oil had an antidepressant effect in mice. The effect of nutmeg extract on memory and learning was also noted in a study involving mice by administering 5-20 mg/kg orally. A significant enhancement was observed in the elevated plus-maze and passive avoidance tests.[9]

Sedative activity

Tisserand & Balacs cite a study confirming that hexane extracts of nutmeg significantly inhibited liver drug-metabolising enzyme activity, as shown by a prolonged hexobarbital sleeping time in rats. It has been reported that myristicin and licarin-B provoked sleep at sub-hypnotic doses of hexobarbital, suggesting that it is a CNS depressant. Licarin-B is found in the whole nutmeg.[25]

Actions

Actions commonly cited in aromatherapy

Analgesic, anti-inflammatory, antipyretic, anti-rheumatic, antiseptic, antispasmodic, antithrombotic, carminative, digestive, emmenagogue, prostaglandin inhibitor, stimulant, tonic[6,14,26,27]

Actions supported by clinical studies

Anti-inflammatory, carminative, hepatoprotective, nervine

Comment

Nutmeg presents us with an interesting dilemma. On one hand, nutmeg extracts have a such a diverse range of important pharmacological activities; however, on the other hand, the therapeutic dosage required might induce psychotropic effects. Then we have the challenge that it has both chemoprotective activity and has contains components such as safrole and methyl eugenol, which may have potential carcinogenic activity.

Tisserand & Young state that nutmeg oil was not mutagenic in the Ames test, and that the oil significantly induced GST in mouse liver studies. It is therefore likely that the oil is not carcinogenic.[28]

It is believed that myristicin is the important pharmacological component in nutmeg. It is likely that the West Indian nutmeg is therapeutically more potent than the East Indian nutmeg because of the higher myristicin content.[28]

Tisserand & Balacs state it would be ideal if we could find a nutmeg oil high in myristicin and low in safrole and methyl eugenol – the two components responsible for the carcinogenic activity.[25]

More efforts are needed to study the traditional uses of nutmeg, and for subsequent validation of the mechanism of action.

Aromatherapy Uses

Clinical aromatherapy

Digestive system

Nutmeg oil is useful as a digestive stimulant, helping people who cannot assimilate food. It may be useful for the treatment of flatulence, nausea, chronic vomiting and diarrhoea.[26,27,29]

Musculoskeletal system

Nutmeg oil can be used topically to alleviate muscular aches and pains as well as rheumatism.[26,27,29]

Nervous system

Nutmeg oil is a tonic and stimulant and assists in alleviating general fatigue.[26,27,29]

Energetics, psyche and subtle uses

Energetics

The *warming* qualities of nutmeg indicate that it is the ideal essential oil to use to dispel *cold*. In TCM, *cold* is associated with poor digestive function, the onset of an infection with headaches, chills and fatigue, fluid congestion, and general aches and pains.

According to the Five Elements, nutmeg oil has a strong affinity with the Earth and Water Elements. It helps to eliminate *damp*, which weakens the Earth Element, and eliminates excess *cold*, which weakens the Water Element.

Subtle

Worwood states that nutmeg oil can be used to encourage calm, peace and comfort. She recommends using nutmeg oil when our ego has received many life-blows and is depressed or unable to connect with the higher realms.[30]

Zeck recommends using nutmeg oil whenever our physical energy has been drained due to illness, accident or long-standing stress. She states that nutmeg oil will rekindle the flame of your life force that will help you feel spiritually cleansed and physically rejuvenated.[31]

Dosage and Administration

Blending

Aromatherapy

For the relief of musculoskeletal aches and pains and joint inflammation, consider blending nutmeg oil with essential oils such as black pepper, cajeput, clove bud, ginger, kunzea, juniper berry, spike lavender or rosemary.

For the relief of anxiety, stress and nervous tension, consider blending nutmeg oil with essential oils such as Atlas cedarwood, bergamot, fragonia, frankincense, geranium, lavender, sweet orange, mandarin, patchouli, palmarosa, rose otto, sandalwood or vetiver.

To make an energising blend that promotes wellbeing, consider blending nutmeg oil with essential oils such as basil, cardamom, clove bud, ginger, lemon, lime, lemongrass or rosemary.

For the relief of indigestion, consider blending nutmeg oil with essential oils such as basil, coriander seed, sweet fennel, ginger, sweet orange, sweet marjoram or peppermint.

Perfumery

Nutmeg oil is used in perfumery for modern spicy style perfumes. It is used in men's fragrances and aftershaves. Arctander states that it blends well with bay laurel oil, clary sage, geranium, lavender, sweet orange, oakmoss absolute and rosemary.[2]

Mode of administration

Bath

Full body bath, foot bath

Topical

Compress, massage, ointment, skin care

Inhalation

Direct inhalation, diffuser, oil vaporiser

Safety Profile

General safety

Nutmeg oil is non-toxic, non-irritating and non-sensitising.[26]

The psychotropic effects associated with nutmeg are believed to be due to the myristicin and elemicin found in the nutmeg. It is believed that myristicin and elemicin are metabolised to TMA and MMDA, both of which are hallucinogenic substances.[32]

However, closer investigation has revealed the following:[32]

Component	Psychotropic effect
whole nutmeg	highly active
whole nutmeg less the essential oil	no activity
nutmeg oil	weakly active
myristicin on its own	no activity

Nutmeg deprived of its essential oil has no psychotropic effect. It appears that the psychotropic properties are due not only to the myristicin and elemicin, but to other constituents found in nutmeg. While ground nutmeg is moderately to strongly psychotropic when taken in high oral doses, the effect of the essential oil is very weak, and it appears that non-oral doses will not have any affect at all.

Tisserand & Young state that the maximum dermal use level is 0.8% for the East Indian nutmeg oil because of its safrole content and 5% for the West Indian nutmeg oil.[28]

It has been reported that the metabolism of myristicin resembles that of safrole; however, it was found that the acute toxicology of myristicin appears to be low. Hallström & Thuvander state that it is likely from all the available data that the intake of myristicin from nutmeg oil and other spices in food, which may be estimated as a few mg per person per day, would not cause any adverse effects on humans.[24]

Contraindications

No contraindications known.[28]

N

Toxicity

Lis-Balchin cites studies that found that myristicin caused ataxia and disorientation in monkeys. She states that it is converted in the body to amphetamine and is structurally similar to sympathomimetic amines.[4]

She states that several intoxications after ingestion of approximately 5 g of nutmeg have been reported. However, she does point out that, while these intoxications may be ascribed to the actions of myristicin, it is likely that other components of nutmeg may be involved.[4]

Tisserand & Young explain that nutmeg oil contains both carcinogens and anticarcinogens. However, they then explain that existing data suggests that the oil is not carcinogenic.[28]

Regulatory guidelines

Nutmeg oil has GRAS status.

References

1. Weiss EA. *Essential oil crops.* CAB International, Wallingford, 1997.
2. Arctander S. *Perfume and flavor materials of natural origin.* Allured Publishing, Carol Stream, 1994.
3. Lawrence BM. *Essential oils 1976-1978.* Allured Publishing, Carol Stream, 1979.
4. Lis-Balchin M. *Aromatherapy science – a guide for healthcare professionals.* Pharmaceutical Press, London, 2006.
5. Schmidt E, Wanner J. *Adulteration of essential oils.* In Baser KHC, Buchbauer G. eds. *Handbook of essential oils – science, technology and applications.* 2nd edn. CRC Press, Boca Raton, 2016: 707-745.
6. Nagja T et al. *Myristica fragrance: a comprehensive review.* International Journal of Pharmacy and Pharmaceutical Sciences, 2016; 8(2): 27-30.
7. Periasamy G et al. *Nutmeg (Myristica fragrans Houtt.) oils.* In Preedy VR. ed. *Essential oils in food preservation, flavor and safety.* Academic Press, London, 2016: 607-616.
8. Blumenthal M et al. *The complete German commission E monographs: therapeutic guide to herbal medicine.* American Botanical Council, Austin, 1998.
9. Khan I, Abourashed E. *Leung's encyclopedia of common natural ingredients used in food, drugs and cosmetics.* 3rd edn. John Wiley & Sons, New Jersey, 2010.
10. Piaru SP et al. *Antioxidant and antiangiogenic activities of the essential oils of Myristica fragrance and Morinda citrifolia.* Asian Pacific Journal of Tropical Medicine, 2012; 5(4): 294-298. Cited in Quintessential Aromatics database, 2013.
11. Wahab A et al. *Anticonvulsant activities of nutmeg of Myristica fragrans.* Phytotherapy Research, 2009; 23(2): 153-158. Cited in Quintessential Aromatics database, 2013.
12. Olajide OA et al. *Evaluation of the pharmacological properties of nutmeg oil in rats and mice.* Pharmacological Biology, 2000; 38(5): 385-390. Cited in Quintessential Aromatics database, 2013.
13. Lee JY, Park W. *Anti-inflammatory effect of myristicin on RAW 264.7 macrophages stimulated with polyinosinic-polycytidylic acid.* Molecules; 2011; 16(8): 7132-7142. doi: 10.3390/molecules16087132.
14. Zhang WK et al. *Nutmeg oil alleviates chronic inflammatory pain through inhibition of COX-2 expression and substance P release in vivo.* Food & Nutrition Research, 2016; 60(1): 30849. doi: 10.3402/fr.v60.30849.
15. Pal M et al. *Composition and anti-microbial activity of essential oil of Myristica fragrans from Andaman Nicobar Island.* International Journal of Pharmacy and Life Sciences, 2011; 2(10): 1115-1117.
16. Piaru SP et al. *Determination of antibacterial activity of essential oil of Myristica fragrans Houtt. using tetrazolium microplate assay and its cytotoxic activity against Vero cell line.* International Journal of Pharmacology, 2012; 8(6): 572-576. doi: 10.3923/ijp.2012.572.576.
17. Tomaino A et al. *Influence of heating on antioxidant activity and the chemical composition of some spice essential oils.* Food Chemistry, 2005; 89(4): 549-554. Cited in Quintessential Aromatics database, 2013.
18. Kapoor IPS et al. *Chemical composition and antioxidant activity of essential oil and oleoresins of nutmeg (Myristica fragrans Houtt.) fruits.* International Journal of Food Properties, 2013; 16(5): 1059-1070. doi: 10.1080/10942912.2011.576357.
19. Pillai S et al. *Anti-parasitic activity of Myristica fragrans Houtt. essential oil against Toxoplasma Gondii parasite.* Procedia APCBEE, 2012; 92-96. doi: 10.1016/j.apcbee.2012.06.017.
20. Hashim S et al. *Modulatory effects of essential oils from spices on the formation of DNA adduct by aflatoxin B1 in vitro.* Nutrition and Cancer, 1994; 21(2): 169-175. Cited in Quintessential Aromatics database, 2013.
21. Banerjee S et al. *Influence of certain essential oils on carcinogen-metabolising enzymes and acid-soluble sulphydryls in mouse liver.* Nutrition and Cancer, 1994; 21(3): 263-269. Cited in Quintessential Aromatics database, 2013.
22. Morita T, Sugiyama K. *A newly found physiological effect of myristicin, an essential oil from nutmeg: with reference to a hepatoprotective effect.* Aroma Research, 2004; 5(1): 23-27.
23. Bruneton J. *Pharmacognosy.* 2nd edn. Lavoisier Publishing, Paris, 1999.

24. Hallström H, Thuvander A. *Toxicological evaluation of myristicin*. Natural Toxins, 1997; 5(5): 186-192. Cited in Quintessential Aromatics database, 2013.
25. Tisserand R, Balac T. *Nutmeg – a review of the toxicology and pharmacology of nutmeg and its essential oil*. The International Journal of Aromatherapy, 1994; 6(4): 28-37.
26. Lawless J. *The encyclopaedia of essential oils*. Element Books, Shaftesbury, 1992.
27. Lavabre M. *Aromatherapy workbook*. Healing Arts Press, Vermont, 1997.
28. Tisserand R, Young R. *Essential oil safety*. 2nd edn, Churchill Livingstone, Edinburgh, 2014.
29. Valnet J. *The practice of aromatherapy*. C.W. Daniel Company, Saffron Walden, 1980.
30. Worwood VA. *The fragrant heavens*. Transworld Publishers, London, 1999.
31. Zeck R. *The blossoming heart – aromatherapy for healing and transformation*. Aroma Tours, East Ivanhoe, 2004.
32. Tisserand R, Balacs T. *Essential oil safety*. Churchill Livingstone, Edinburgh, 1995.

Oakmoss absolute

Identification

Botanical name

Evernia prunastri L.

Family

Usneaceae

Botany and origins

Oakmoss is a light green lichen found growing primarily on oak trees. The oak tree is indigenous to Europe and North America; the lichen is collected all over central and southern Europe, especially France, the Balkan states and Hungary, as well as in Morocco and Algeria.[1]

Besides true oakmoss, *E. prunastri*, so-called 'tree moss' or 'fir moss' is obtained from two related lichens, *E. furfuracea* and *Usnea barbata*. Both of them grow on spruces and pines in the humid forests of central and southern Europe.[2]

Method of extraction

Freshly harvested oakmoss has no scent. Oakmoss contains depsides which are odourless. The characteristic oakmoss absolute scent only develops after hydrolytic cleavage of the depsides. This hydrolysis can only be performed in an enzymatic way or by treatment with hot water or steam. During this reaction, a part of the potential odorants are lost in the form of free acids, which after esterification give the characteristic compounds.[3]

Oakmoss concrete is obtained by solvent extraction of lichen, *E. prunastri*, with a hydrocarbon. The concrete is then either vacuum-distilled to yield an absolute oil or subjected to further extraction with alcohol to yield an absolute.[1]

Characteristics

The absolute is a dark green or brown-coloured, very viscous liquid with an extremely tenacious, earthy-mossy odour and a leather-like undertone.[1] Perfumer Roja Dove states that oakmoss absolute has an earthy, damp, animalic, leather-like quality reminiscent of the forest.[4]

Chemical composition

The chemical composition of oakmoss absolute was reported as follows: limonene, longifolene, β-elemene, *cis*-heptadeca-1,8-diene, *cis*-heptadeca-1,8,11-triene and 4,6-dimethyl-dec-4-en-3-one.[5]

Adulteration

Arctander points out that very few commercially available oakmoss extracts are 'true and genuine'. Several different botanical sources are often used to create oakmoss absolute. *E. furfuracea* and *U. barbata*, referred to as 'tree moss' and 'fir moss', are much darker in colour and the odour is much less refined than that of the true oakmoss extract. Other lichens and algae are used in the production of so-called oakmoss products.[1]

Lawrence states that one of the problems with oakmoss extracts is that they can vary considerably from one supplier to another. He explains that there are a number of reasons for this such as the origin of the raw material, the blending of raw materials from different origins and the processing conditions. He claims that oakmoss is probably one of the most 'compounded' natural fragrance materials available.[5]

Pharmacopoeias and standards

At the time of writing, the purity, composition, physico-chemical properties and therapeutic use of oakmoss absolute are not defined in any pharmacopoeia monograph or standard.

O

History and Traditional Uses

History

It has been used in perfumery since the sixteenth century and was well known in ancient Egypt.[4]

Herbal

A lichen *Lobaria pulmonaria*, which is similar to oakmoss, is listed in the British Herbal Pharmacopoeia for the treatment of bronchitis and asthma.[6]

Food, perfumery and flavouring

The absolute is generally used as a fixative in perfumes and the concrete is used primarily in soaps.[1]

Therapeutics

Pharmacology and clinical studies

There is no information regarding pharmacological or clinical studies of oakmoss absolute.

Actions

Actions commonly cited in aromatherapy

Antiseptic, demulcent, expectorant, fixative[7]

Actions supported by clinical studies

None of the actions commonly cited in aromatherapy can be supported by clinical studies.

Comment

Review of traditional uses and clinical data cannot confirm any clinical applications for oakmoss absolute in aromatherapy. Oakmoss absolute has a pleasant fresh green note that may be beneficial for improving mood and reducing the symptoms of stress-induced disorders such as anxiety and depression.

Aromatherapy Uses

Clinical aromatherapy

Oakmoss absolute is not commonly used in aromatherapy.

Energetics, psyche and subtle uses

Subtle

Keim Loughran & Bull explain that oakmoss absolute helps to ground us, while healing past traumas that prevent us from being fully present. It gently allows us to release fears and mistrust, opening our heart to embrace physical experience – its joys as well as sorrows. When we are fully in the here and now, we are open to receiving the generosity and abundance of the earthly experience. For some people, this will be in the form of monetary wealth, for others it will reveal itself as emotional, creative, resourceful or inspirational abundance.[8]

Oakmoss absolute will promote the types of abundance that will be most spiritually profound for the individual. It is also said to help integrate the experience of true security that is not associated with money or accomplishments – one that is founded on trusting the generosity and ultimate safety of the universe.[8]

Dosage and Administration

Blending

Perfumery

Oakmoss absolute imparts richness and depth to chypre and fougère style perfumes. Oakmoss can also be used in conifer-type and woody-type perfumes.[9]

Oakmoss absolute can lend body and naturalness, with rich pleasant undertones and excellent fixative value, in floral fragrances.[1]

Mode of administration

Topical

Massage, ointment

Inhalation

Direct inhalation, diffuser, oil vaporiser

Safety Profile

General safety

The IFRA recommendation for tree moss and oakmoss extracts obtained from the *Usnea* and *Evernia* species is that they should not be used individually or in combination such that the level exceeds 0.1% in consumer products.[10]

Tisserand & Young cite studies that suggest that the high risk of skin sensitisation that occurs with oakmoss absolute is due to the contamination of the oil with resin acids that are naturally found in the oakmoss resin and are known to be highly allergenic.[10]

IFRA warns that oakmoss absolute should contain minimal traces of resin acids and that oxidised products of resin acids are sensitising.[10]

The European Commission's Scientific Committee on Consumer Products report on oakmoss/tree moss sensitisation states that a reduction in the level of chloroatranol and atranol (the main allergens) to <2 ppm each in the oil would reduce the risk of any sensitising potential.[11]

Contraindications

No contraindications known.

Regulatory guidelines

Oakmoss absolute is not defined in any regulatory guideline.

References

1. Arctander S. *Perfume and flavor materials of natural origin*. Allured Publishing, Carol Stream, 1994.
2. Ding D. *Oakmoss and treemoss in China*. Perfumer & Flavorist, 1988; 13; 13-16.
3. Boelens M. *Formation of volatile compounds from oakmoss*. Perfumer & Flavorist, 1993; 18: 27-30.
4. Dove R. *The essence of perfume – the master perfumer's definitive guide*. Black Dog, London, 2014.
5. Lawrence BM. *Essential oils 1976-1978*. Allured Publishing, Wheaton, 1979.
6. *British herbal pharmacopoeia*. British Herbal Medicine Association, Bournemouth, 1983.
7. Lawless J. *The encyclopaedia of essential oils*. Element Books, Shaftesbury, 1992.
8. Keim Loughran J, Bull R. *Aromatherapy and subtle energy techniques*. Frog, Berkeley, 2000.
9. Curtis T, Williams DG. *Introduction to perfumery*. Ellis Horwood, Hertfordshire, 1994.
10. Tisserand R, Young R. *Essential oil safety*. 2nd edn. Churchill Livingstone, Edinburgh, 2014.
11. *Opinion on oakmoss/treemoss (sensitisation only)*. European Commission Health & Consumer Protection Directorate-General, Brussels, 2008. Retrieved from https://ec.europa.eu/health/ph_risk/committees/04_sccp/docs/sccp_o_131.pdf

Opopanax

Identification

Botanical name

Commiphora guidottii Chiov.

Synonyms

Scented myrrh, sweet myrrh, bisabol myrrh

Family

Burseraceae

Botany and origins

Opopanax oleoresin is extracted from a tall tropical tree that is closely related to myrrh, which contains a natural oleoresin. The tree grows wild in Somalia and Ethiopia.[1]

According to Guenther, opopanax gum was originally extracted from *Opopanax chironium* Koch., but in the 1950s, the source of the gum was *Commiphora erythraea* Ehrenb.[2] This had been regarded as the principal source of the gum by most authorities; however, Tisserand & Young state that the principal source is now *Commiphora guidottii*.[3]

In 1998, *Commiphora guidottii* was listed by IUCN Red List of Threatened Species as low risk/near threatened. The threat reported that the habitat is being degraded in places where there is overcutting from charcoal production and the expansion of agricultural activities.[4]

Method of extraction

Opopanax essential oil is obtained from steam or water distillation of the oleoresin.

Characteristics

Opopanax oil is an orange-coloured, pale yellow or olive-yellowish to dark amber-greenish liquid with a sweet-balsamic, spicy, warm, animal-like odour. It resinifies on exposure to air.[1]

The scent of opopanax is often compared with myrrh; however, Arctander states that they are quite distinct:

> *... the difference between the two oils is obvious: the vegetable-soup-like, slightly animal-sweet odour of opopanax is entirely different from the medicinal-sharp freshness of myrrh oil.*[1]

Arctander explains that opopanax has a richer, deeper balsamic note, while myrrh oil has a light, fresh top note with little tenacity.[1]

Chemical composition

The chemical composition of opopanax oil obtained from *C. erythraea* was reported as follows:

(*Z*)-β-ocimene (0.4%), (*E*)-β-ocimene (26.2%), *cis*-α-bergamotene (0.9%), α-santalene (20.1%), *trans*-α-bergamotene (5.2%), *epi*-β-santalene (0.8%), (*E*)-β-farnesene (0.6%), β-santelene (0.5%), *ar*-curcumene (1.1%), curzerene (0.6%), (*Z*)-α-bisabolene + (*E*)-α-bisabolene (14.2%), γ-bisabolene (1.3%). It was noted that the oil contained an additional 215 constituents (26.5% of the oil), but these were not identified.[5]

Adulteration

Opopanax is occasionally adulterated with myrrh

oil, copaiba balsam, traces of lovage oil and certain fractions of Siberian pine needle oil.[1]

Pharmacopoeias and standards

At the time of writing, the purity, composition, physico-chemical properties and therapeutic use of opopanax essential oil are not defined in any pharmacopoeia monograph or standard.

History and Traditional Uses

History

Opopanax gum has traditionally been used as an ingredient in incense.[6]

Traditional medicine

Opopanax is used in Somali traditional medicine for the treatment of diarrhoea. It is also used for its wound healing properties.[7]

Food, perfumery and flavouring

Opopanax is used as a fixative and fragrance component in high-class perfumery as a base for woody, heavy floral, leather, oriental, chypre, fougère and fantasy type perfumes. It is also used in liqueurs to give body and wine-like notes.[1]

Therapeutics

Pharmacology and clinical studies

Antispasmodic activity

The major component, T-cadinol, in the resin of opopanax from Ethiopia and Somalia had smooth-muscle-relaxing properties in an in vivo study on rats.[8]

Actions

Actions commonly cited in aromatherapy

Antiseptic, antispasmodic, balsamic, expectorant[6]

Actions supported by clinical studies

Antispasmodic, balsamic

Comment

There are no clinical or pharmacological studies to confirm any of the therapeutic properties of opopanax essential oil; however, Lawless suggests that opopanax oil has similar properties to myrrh.[6]

Aromatherapy Uses

Clinical aromatherapy

Opopanax oil is not commonly used in aromatherapy; however, it has been compared to myrrh.

Energetics, psyche and subtle uses

Energetics

According to the principles of TCM, opopanax oil would be *warming* and *drying*. It is recommended for conditions associated with excess *damp* such as chronic ulcers and wounds, respiratory tract infections with phlegm and mucus, and diarrhoea.

Subtle

Opopanax oil helps to heal physical, emotional, mental and spiritual wounds, and also provides physical and psychic protection.[9]

Dosage and Administration

Blending

Aromatherapy

To promote wound healing, consider blending opopanax oil with essential oils such as everlasting, frankincense or lavender.

For the relief of catarrhal conditions associated with bronchitis or asthma, consider blending opopanax oil with essential oils such as aniseed, Atlas cedarwood, cajeput, 1,8-cineole-rich eucalypts, fragonia, spike lavender, myrtle, pine or spruce.

To balance the base chakra and to help strengthen the link between the base and crown chakra, consider blending opopanax oil with essential oils such as patchouli, frankincense, sandalwood and Atlas cedarwood.

Perfumery

Arctander states that opopanax oil prefers heavy-sweet floral blends. It blends well with clary sage, coriander seed, cistus, patchouli and other woody and heavy floral oils. It is used to create chypre, fougère, leather-based and oriental compositions.[1]

However, Arctander warns us that opopanax has the tendency of 'showing up' in a rather unattractive manner after a short aging period of the perfume. He states that it is the perfumer's responsibility to utilise the effects of the oil without permitting the strong opopanax notes to overpower the perfume.[1]

Mode of administration

Bath

Full body bath, foot bath

Topical

Massage, ointment, skin care

Inhalation

Direct inhalation, diffuser, oil vaporiser

Safety Profile

General safety

Opopanax oil is non-toxic, non-irritant and non-sensitising.[6]

Tisserand & Young state that there is a moderate risk of skin sensitisation. IFRA recommends that opopanax oil should not be used at levels over 0.6%. Tisserand & Young challenge this as no allergens have ever been identified in opopanax oil, and state that the IFRA decision is based on poor data. The oil was previously believed to be phototoxic; however, this has now been confirmed not to be true.[3]

Contraindications

No contraindications known.

Regulatory guidelines

Opopanax essential oil is not defined in any regulatory guideline.

References

1. Arctander S. *Perfume and flavor materials of natural origin.* Allured Publishing, Carol Stream, 1994.
2. Guenther E. *The essential oils – Vol. IV.* Robert E Krieger Publishing, Malabar, 1952.
3. Tisserand R. Young R, *Essential oil safety*. 2nd edn. Churchill Livingstone, Edinburgh, 2014.
4. Thulin M. *Commiphora guidottii.* The IUCN Red List of Threatened Species 1998: e.T35815A9959165. doi: 10.2305/IUCN.UK.1998.RLTS.T35815A9959165.
5. Lawrence BM. *Progress in essential oils – opopanax oil.* Perfumer & Flavorist, 2004; 29: 95.
6. Lawless J. *The encyclopaedia of essential oils.* Element Books, Shaftesbury, 1992.
7. Burfield T. *Updated list of threatened aromatic plants used in the aroma & cosmetics industries.* v1.21, Cropwatch, March 2010.
8. Langenheim JH. *Plant resins – chemistry, evolution, ecology, ethnobotany.* Timber Press, Portland, 2003.
9. Keim Loughran J, Bull R. *Aromatherapy and subtle energy techniques.* Frog, Berkeley, 2000.

Orange, sweet

Identification

Botanical name

Citrus sinensis L. Osbeck

Synonyms

Orange oil, *Citrus aurantium* var. *dulcis, C. vulgaris* Risso

Family

Rutaceae

Botany and origins

Within the species *Citrus sinensis* there are many different cultivars. The three most common cultivars are navel, Jaffa and Valencia. It is a smaller tree than the bitter orange tree, less hardy and with few or no spines, and the fruits are smaller with a sweet pulp and non-bitter membrane.[1]

The navel orange is named because of its shape; segmented skin looks like a human navel. The navel orange originated as a single mutation in a Brazilian monastery in 1920. Every single navel orange originates from it because they do not produce seeds and propagation is by graft cuttings.[2]

The Valencia orange was named by William Wolfkill, an agronomist, after the Spanish city of Valencia, known for its orange production.[2]

Method of extraction

Sweet orange essential oil is cold-pressed from the ripe or almost ripe outer peel of the orange fruit. Machine expression usually yields oils with high evaporation residue, while the various hand-expression methods lead to oils with low residue. Arctander states that the amount of residue in an orange oil has no direct relation to the quality of the oil. It may affect the tenacity, but not the odour or the flavour. The higher content of oxygenated compounds in an orange oil is probably due to the fact that the oil has been expressed from not fully ripe fruits.[3]

Orange essential oil is produced in much larger volumes than any other essential oil. Most of this production is used in foods and beverages.[4]

Characteristics

Expressed sweet orange oil is a yellow-orange to dark orange-coloured mobile liquid with a sweet, fresh citrus odour, distinctly reminiscent of the odour from a scratched orange peel. Machine-expressed sweet orange oils are generally lighter in colour, whereas hand-pressed oils are generally darker.[3]

Chemical composition

The major constituent of orange oil is limonene, a monoterpene hydrocarbon. The chemical composition of sweet orange was reported as follows:

α-pinene (0.54%), myrcene (2.08%), linalool (0.25%), limonene (95.37%), neral (0.06%), citronellal (0.10%), decanal (0.06%), geranial (0.12%).[5]

Adulteration

Expressed sweet orange oil is frequently adulterated with *d*-limonene – isolated or synthetic – or with other citrus oils, or with a mixture of monoterpenes or distilled oils from the citrus fruit juice manufacturers.[3]

Pharmacopoeias and standards

The purity, composition and physico-chemical properties of sweet orange oil are defined in ISO 3140:2011 Oil of Sweet Orange [*Citrus sinensis* (L.) Osbeck], Obtained by Physical Extraction of the Peel.

History and Traditional Uses

History

O

The orange tree is believed to be native to the region between the Himalayas and southwestern China. It was not until the early sixteenth century that the Portuguese explorers introduced the fruit to Europe. It was introduced to the Americas by Columbus and was primarily grown in the West Indies and Florida. Most of the essential oil produced today comes from Israel, Brazil, North America and Australia.[5]

Traditional medicine

The therapeutic properties of orange were first recognised in ancient China, where the dried peel had been used for centuries to treat coughs, colds and anorexia.[1]

Food, perfumery and flavouring

Sweet orange oil is extensively used in food flavouring.[1] *d*-limonene serves as an important starting material for the synthesis of *l*-carvone, an important source of synthetic spearmint flavour. The price of *l*-carvone from sweet orange oil is usually two-thirds the cost of spearmint.[5]

Other uses

A number of other products are derived from sweet orange oil. For example, the carotenoids which are extracted from the orange oil processing waste are used to create natural colours for use in food and drinks.[5]

The orange wax, another by-product of orange oil processing, is used in perfumery. *d*-limonene, which is redistilled from orange oil, is used in the plastics industry, pressure sensitive adhesives and quick drying inks. Weiss states that orange oil is so important to the plastics industry that a very large portion of the mid-season orange oil from the USA is solely produced for the production of *d*-limonene.[5]

Therapeutics

Pharmacology and clinical studies

Many pharmacological studies involving sweet orange essential oil have been published. A systemic review of these studies will not be attempted. Rather, I have chosen a selection of studies that support the traditional and clinical uses.

Alzheimer's disease

The role of essential oils for the management of Alzheimer's disease (AD) has been extensively researched. One study used a range of psychometric tools to measure the cognitive function and concentration of AD patients exposed to a blend of lavender, sweet orange, lemon and rosemary. Sweet orange and lavender oils activate the parasympathetic nervous system, while rosemary and lemon are known to relieve depression and improve concentration. The study concluded that aromatherapy can improve cognitive function in AD patients.[6]

Another study found that aromatherapy does not reduce combative, resistive behaviours in individuals with dementia. However, it was stated that research with a larger sample in future studies may provide other results.[7]

Antidepressant activity

Twenty depressed male inpatients receiving antidepressant medication were divided into two groups. One group was given antidepressants alone and the other group was exposed to the fragrance of a blend of lemon, sweet orange and bergamot essential oils, while continuously having their medication reduced weekly until their depression remitted, usually within four to 11 weeks. The Hamilton Rating Scale for Depression and Self-Rating Depression Scale were used to evaluate psychiatric states. The researchers confirmed that both scores improved in both groups.[8]

By the end of 11 weeks, nine of the 12 patients in the aromatherapy group had reduced their antidepressant drug intake to zero, whilst the other three had reduced their dosage by 50-75%. On the other hand, all subjects in the antidepressant group still needed their usual doses of antidepressant at remission.[8]

Urinary cortisol and dopamine levels were significantly high in both groups before treatment, and both were reduced by treatment. However, the levels were significantly lower in the aromatherapy group compared to the antidepressant group after treatment. The aromatherapy group also had higher values of natural killer cell activity return to almost the normal range. It was suggested that the results support the concept that depression may be based on homeostatic dysregulation, and that the citrus blend may improve the homeostatic balance more effectively than treatment with antidepressants. However, the researchers stated that caution was recommended in interpreting the results due to the small size of the study.[8]

Antifungal activity

The antifungal activity of sweet orange oil was evaluated using the agar dilution method. The results of the in vitro study confirmed that sweet orange oil and other citrus oils had significant antifungal activity.[9]

Another in vitro study confirmed that citrus oils – sweet orange, mandarin and grapefruit – displayed strong antifungal activity against a range of moulds commonly associated with food spoilage. Sweet orange oil was the most effective against *Aspergillus niger*. Mandarin oil was most effective at reducing the growth of *Aspergillus flavus* and grapefruit was the best inhibitor of the moulds *Penicillium chrysogenum* and *P. verrucosum*.[10]

Antimicrobial activity

Sweet orange oil has been reported to exhibit excellent antimicrobial properties.[11,12,13]

Essential oil vapours of orange and bergamot, blended 1:1 ratio, were found to be effective at removing methicillin-resistant *Staphylococcus aureus* (MRSA) and vancomycin-resistant *Enterococcus* sp. (VRE) from a stainless-steel bench surface and reducing the formation of biofilm. It was suggested that citrus vapours have the potential for application in a clinical environment as a secondary disinfectant to reduce surface contamination by VRE and MRSA.[14]

Anxiolytic activity

A plethora of clinical studies were found to highlight the benefits of sweet orange oil for patients suffering from anxiety.

Seventy-two patients took part in a study to investigate the efficacy of the ambient odour of sweet orange oil to reduce anxiety in a dental office. Twice a day, morning and noon, 0.25 mL of sweet orange oil was added to a hidden electrical diffuser in a dental waiting room. No orange oil was diffused for the control group. The results of the study demonstrated that the exposure to ambient odours of sweet orange oil had a relaxation effect when compared to the non-odour control group. It was also found that women who were exposed to the sweet orange odour had a lower level of anxiety, a more positive mood and a higher level of calmness compared to the men in the test group. It was reported that the effect of the odour played a minor role for men, possibly due to their lesser olfactory sensitivity; however, it was stated that the experimental design did not take into account the different baseline anxieties for different dental procedures, and more females may have entered the room when the odour was at its maximum.[15]

Forty healthy male volunteers were submitted to an anxiogenic situation. Psychologic parameters such as state-anxiety, subjective tension, sedation, and physiologic parameters such as heart rate and gastrocnemius electromyogram were evaluated before inhalation of sweet orange, during inhalation and after the anxiogenic situation. The results of the study confirmed an anxiolytic activity of sweet orange oil.[16]

A clinical trial involving 200 patients between the ages of 18 and 77 years (half men, half women) revealed that, compared to the control group, both ambient odours of sweet orange and lavender reduced anxiety and improved mood in patients waiting for dental treatment. It was reported that odours are capable of altering emotional states and may be helpful in reducing anxiety in dental patients.[17]

Autonomic nervous system activity

Inhalation of sweet orange oil increased the activity of the parasympathetic nervous system by 12% and decreased sympathetic nervous system activity by 16%. The study concluded that changes in mood caused by inhalation of essential oils could be detected using the light reflex of the pupil.[18]

Anticarcinogenesis activity

Oral doses of sweet orange oil and lemon oil inhibited tumour formation and growth in a study involving chemically induced tumours in mice. The researchers stated that the two citrus oils inhibited the tumour formation due to their high *d*-limonene content.[19]

The results of an in vitro study provided conclusive evidence of the apoptotic and antiangiogenesis potential of sweet orange oil in colon cancer cells.[20]

Sedative activity

A blind, randomised clinical trial involving 120 children undergoing dental extraction under sevoflurane anaesthesia investigated the effects of sweet orange oil on induction and in recovery. It was found that the children exposed to sweet orange oil were more relaxed and cooperative during induction.[21]

39 healthy volunteers participated in a study to investigate the effect of sweet orange oil on human autonomic parameters and emotional responses in healthy subjects after transdermal absorption. In order to exclude olfactory stimulation, the inhalation of the scent of the oils was prevented by breathing masks. Four autonomic parameters – blood pressure, breathing rate, pulse rate and skin temperature – were recorded. Emotional responses were assessed by means of rates scales. Compared with the placebo, the results found that sweet orange oil caused significant decrease in breathing rate and pulse rate, which indicated a decrease of autonomic arousal. At an emotional level, the sweet orange group rated themselves more cheerful and more vigorous than subjects in the control group.[22]

O

Actions

Actions commonly cited in aromatherapy

Antidepressant, antiseptic, antispasmodic, carminative, cholagogue, digestive, lymphatic stimulant, sedative, stomachic[23,24,25]

Actions supported by clinical studies

Antidepressant, antimicrobial, antiseptic, anxiolytic

Comment

Sweet orange oil is usually one of the first essential oils I introduce to a child or an adult who is not familiar with aromatherapy. I have never had a negative response to the delightful, sweet, cheerful scent of sweet orange oil. It is not surprising that Worwood describes sweet orange oil as follows:

> *There can be very few people who dislike the smell and taste of the orange fruit, and there are very few people who wouldn't fall under the spell of the cheerful, optimistic orange personality. These sunny people are a joy to be with.*[26]

Evidence supports that essential oils with high *d*-limonene content have a strong chemoprotective and hepatoprotective activity.[6]

Review of traditional uses and clinical data also support the role of sweet orange oil for its gastroprotective activity and as an effective antimicrobial agent. Many studies also confirm that citrus aromas are uplifting and can be helpful to alleviate stress, anxiety and depression.

Aromatherapy Uses

Clinical aromatherapy

Digestive system

Sweet orange oil helps to settle the digestive system; it prevents and eases spasms and relieves cramps. It is excellent for treating constipation, flatulence and irritable bowel.[23,25] It appears to have a normalising effect on the peristaltic action of the intestines and is recommended for constipation or diarrhoea.[27]

Sweet orange oil is known as a hepatic and cholagogue, and may be used to improve the flow of bile and improve the metabolism of fats.[25]

Lymphatic system

Sweet orange oil is known to stimulate lymph fluids, which assists in treating swollen tissue.[23,24,28] This makes it useful in blends for the treatment of cellulite.

Nervous system

Davis states that the properties of sweet orange oil overlap with those of neroli. It is considered to have a mildly sedative and antidepressant effect.[27]

It is recommended in the treatment of anxiety, nervousness and insomnia, and may be used with similarly relaxing oils such as bergamot, geranium, lavender, neroli and sandalwood.

Psychological

Fischer-Rizzi describes the influence of sweet orange on the mood as positive and joyful. Orange oil harmonises feelings and awakens creativity. The oil is ideal to use whenever we are taking everything too seriously and have forgotten how to laugh, or whenever we feel tense, nervous or withdrawn. It helps to reduce our fears of the unknown and helps us greet new adventures.[28]

Skin care

Sweet orange oil is beneficial for soothing dry, irritated or acne-prone skin. It is considered to have regenerative properties and can be used for treating aging skin and rough or calloused skin.[28]

Energetics, psyche and subtle uses

Energetics

According to the principles of TCM, sweet orange oil helps to circulate stagnant *Qi*, especially when it accumulates in the *Liver*, *Stomach* and intestines. It is considered to be one of the best all-round oils for the digestive system.[25]

Mojay states that this makes it suitable for abdominal distention and pain, poor appetite, indigestion, flatulence, nausea and vomiting.[25]

In TCM, the main organ responsible for ensuring the smooth flow of *Qi* throughout the body is the *Liver*. Whenever our *Qi* stagnates, we experience tension, frustration, moodiness and irritability. The sweet, vibrant, warm aroma of sweet orange will help to alleviate these conditions.[25]

According to the principles of the Five Elements, sweet orange oil helps to balance the Wood Element. From an energetic perspective, sweet orange assists the *Liver*, the *Yin* organ associated with the Wood Element, to ensure the smooth flow of *Qi*. The internal condition associated with the Wood Element is anger. Sweet orange also helps us to be more relaxed whenever we feel frustration, irritability and anger.

Personality

The refreshing, cheerful and sensual nature of sweet orange gives warmth and joy to all who are around it, both adults and children alike.[28]

Worwood states that orange personalities are cheerful and optimistic, openhearted, witty and honest. They embrace ideas and suggestions as easily as they embrace people. They have a carefree, friendly smile and joy in their eyes, with faith and understanding which seems to exude from every pore in their body. This is why it is common for people to love being around an orange personality.[26]

Mojay recommends sweet orange for the person who is hard working, a high achiever and is always striving for perfection. He explains that they may find it difficult to delegate and they can become tense and irritable because they 'try too hard'. He says that sweet orange oil will help us to take a more relaxed approach, instilling a more positive attitude and encouraging one to be more adaptable and adopt a more easygoing approach to life.[25]

According to Myers-Briggs personality types, the sweet orange personality is likely to be an ENFP. ENFPs are outgoing, lively and spontaneous. They are very enthusiastic and their joy for life can be contagious. They have a rich imagination and active mind. Their thoughts are always wandering and their mood constantly changing. They can be inspiring and charismatic leaders. They are always involved, or in love, with someone or something new. They know how to establish instant rapport and make people feel comfortable. They love emotional intensity and enjoy expressing their feelings. They can be charming and flirtatious. They relate with warmth to many people and can appear overly enthusiastic, positive and optimistic.

Subtle

Worwood explains that the scent of sweet orange is bursting with vitality, bringing happiness to the heavy heart and to those who seem lost. She explains that the scent of orange is so adaptable, at times it seems so gentle and at other times it gives us the determination required to invigorate our sense of being.[29]

Keim Loughran & Bull have personified the qualities of sweet orange perfectly:

> *People who meet the Dalai Lama often comment on the extraordinary joy that he radiates. His eyes are surrounded by fine laugh lines, his giggle is infectious, and even though he has experienced incredible suffering, his strength, compassion, serenity and faith inspire all who have met him.*[30]

Sweet orange oil will nourish our soul, helping us to become more confident and loving.[30]

Zeck recommends using sweet orange oil when you are feeling gloomy and unable to see the light at the end of the tunnel. Sweet orange will help you access a bubbling light-heartedness and radiant inner warmth that will help you loosen up and find your sense of humour. She also recommends using sweet orange if you are taking life too seriously and you need to lighten up.[31]

O

Dosage and Administration

Blending

Aromatherapy

Sweet orange oil is referred to as a blend equaliser. It helps your blend to flow harmoniously and controls the intensity of the most active ingredients in your blend.[24]

Fischer-Rizzi states that blending with sweet orange oil is virtually foolproof as it blends so easily with so many essential oils. She also explains that lemon and orange oil work in harmony together. Lemon represents the masculine or *Yang* energy, providing energy and energising the spirit, while sweet orange oil represents the feminine or *Yin* energy, which strengthens the heart and soul, making us feel as though we want to hug the world – such a beautiful and simple combination.[28]

For the relief of anxiety, irritability, stress and nervous tension, consider blending sweet orange oil with essential oils such as bergamot, frankincense, geranium, lavender, neroli, patchouli, sandalwood or ylang ylang.

To alleviate the symptoms of depression, consider blending sweet orange oil with essential oils such as bergamot, geranium, jasmine absolute, lavender, lemon, neroli, rose absolute or otto, sandalwood or ylang ylang.

To alleviate insomnia, consider blending sweet orange oil with essential oils such as clary sage, lavender, neroli, petitgrain, sandalwood or vetiver.

To alleviate the symptoms of indigestion, consider blending sweet orange oil with essential oils such as black pepper, cardamom, coriander seed, sweet fennel, ginger, spearmint or peppermint.

Perfumery

In perfumery, sweet orange essential oil is used in eau de colognes, fougère, chypre, aldehydic and fruity based perfumes.[3]

Mode of administration

Bath

Full body bath, foot bath

Topical

Compress, massage, ointment, skin care

Inhalation

Direct inhalation, diffuser, oil vaporiser

Safety Profile

General safety

Sweet orange oil is non-toxic, non-irritating and non-sensitising. The oil is not considered to be phototoxic. However, IFRA recommends that essential oils rich in limonene should only be used when the levels of peroxides are kept to the lowest practical level. This can be achieved by the addition of antioxidants.[4]

Contraindications

No contraindications known.

Regulatory guidelines

Sweet orange essential oil has GRAS status.

References

1. Khan I, Abourashed E. *Leung's encyclopedia of common natural ingredients used in food, drugs and cosmetics*. 3rd edn. John Wiley & Sons, New Jersey, 2010.
2. Etebu E, Nwauzoma AB. *A review on sweet orange (Citrus sinensis L Osbeck): health, diseases and management*. American Journal of Research Communication, 2014; 2(2): 33-70.
3. Arctander S. *Perfume and flavor materials of natural origin*. Allured Publishing, Carol Stream, 1994.
4. Tisserand R, Young R. *Essential oil safety*. 2nd edn. Churchill Livingstone, Edinburgh, 2014.
5. Weiss EA. *Essential oil crops*. CAB International, Wallingford, 1997.
6. Jimbo D et al. *Effect of aromatherapy on patients with Alzheimer's disease*. Psychogeriatrics, 2009; 9(4): 173-179. Cited in Quintessential Aromatics database, 2013.
7. Gray SG, Clair AAC. *Influence of aromatherapy on medication administration to residential-care residents with dementia and behavioural challenges*. American Journal of Alzheimer's Disease and Other Dementias, 2002; 17(3): 169-174. Cited in Quintessential Aromatics database, 2013.
8. Komori T et al. *Effects of citrus fragrance on immune function and depressive states*. Neuroimmunomodulation, 1995: 2(3); 174-180. Cited in Quintessential Aromatics database, 2013.
9. Van Hung P et al. *Comparison of antifungal activities of Vietnamese citrus essential oils*. Natural Product Research, 2013; 27(4/5): 506-508. Cited in Quintessential Aromatics database, 2013.
10. Viuda-Martos M et al. *Antifungal activity of lemon (Citrus lemon L.), mandarin (Citrus reticulata L.), grapefruit (Citrus paradisi L.) and orange (Citrus sinensis L.) essential oils*. Food Control, 2008; 19(12): 1130-1138. Cited in Quintessential Aromatics database, 2013.
11. Singh G et al. *Chemical and fungitoxic investigations on the essential oil of Citrus sinesis (L.) Pers*. Journal of Plant Diseases & Protection, 1993; 100(10): 69-74. Cited in the Aromatherapy Database, by Bob Harris, Essential Oil Resource Consultants, UK, 2000.
12. Tao NG et al. *Chemical composition and antimicrobial activities of essential oil from the peel of bingtang sweet orange (Citrus sinensis Osbeck)*. International Journal of Rood Science and Technology, 2009; 44(7): 1281-1285. Cited in Quintessential Aromatics database, 2013.
13. Frassinetti S et al. *Antibacterial and antioxidant activity of essential oils from Citrus spp*. Journal of Essential Oil Research, 2011; 23(1): 27-31. Cited in Quintessential Aromatics database, 2013.
14. Laird K et al. *Reduction of surface contamination and biofilms of Enterococcus sp. and Staphylococcus aureus using a citrus-based vapour*. Journal of Hospital Infection, 2012; 80(1): 61-66. Cited in Quintessential Aromatics database, 2013.
15. Lehrner J et al. *Ambient odour of orange in a dental office reduces anxiety and improves mood in female patients*. Physiology and Behavior, 2000; 71(1/2): 83-86. Cited in Quintessential Aromatics database, 2013.
16. Goes TC et al. *Effect of sweet orange aroma on experimental anxiety in humans*. Journal of Alternative and Complementary Medicine, 2012; 18(8): 798-804. Cited in Quintessential Aromatics database, 2013.

17. Lehrner J et al. *Ambient odors of orange and lavender reduce anxiety and improve mood in a dental office.* Physiology and Behavior, 2005; 86(1/2): 92-95. Cited in Quintessential Aromatics database, 2013.
18. Miyazaki Y et al. *The effect of essential oils on mood in humans.* Chemical Senses, 1991; 16(2): 184. Cited in Quintessential Aromatics database, 2013.
19. Wattenberg LW, Coccia JB. *Inhibition of 4-(methylnitrosamino)-1-(3-pyridyl)-1-butanone carcinogenesis in mice by d-limonene and citrus fruit oils.* Carcinogenesis, 1991; 12(1): 115-117. Cited in Quintessential Aromatics database, 2013.
20. Chidambara Murthy K et al. *D-limonene rich volatile oil from blood oranges inhibits angiogenesis, metastasis and cell death in human colon cancer cells.* Life Sciences, 2012; 91(11/12): 429-439. Cited in Quintessential Aromatics database, 2013.
21. Mehta S, Stone DN, Whitehead HF. *Use of essential oils to promote induction of anaesthesia in children.* Anaesthesia, 1998; 53(7): 711. Cited in the Aromatherapy Database, by Bob Harris, Essential oil Resource Consultants, UK, 2000.
22. Hongratanaworakit T, Buchbauer G. *Autonomic and emotional responses after transdermal absorption of sweet orange oil in humans: placebo controlled trial.* International Journal of Essential Oil Therapeutics, 2007; 1(1): 29-34. Cited in Quintessential Aromatics database, 2013.
23. Lawless J. *The encyclopaedia of essential oils.* Element Books, Shaftesbury, 1992.
24. Lavabre M. *Aromatherapy workbook.* Healing Arts Press, Rochester, 1997.
25. Mojay G. *Aromatherapy for healing the spirit.* Healing Arts Press, Rochester, 1999.
26. Worwood VA. *The fragrant mind.* Transworld Publishers, London, 1995.
27. Davis P. *Aromatherapy: an A-Z.* 2nd edn. C.W. Daniel Company, Saffron Walden, 1999.
28. Fischer-Rizzi S. *Complete aromatherapy handbook.* Sterling Publishing, New York, 1990.
29. Worwood VA. *The fragrant heavens.* Transworld Publishers, London, 1999.
30. Keim Loughran J, Bull R. *Aromatherapy anointing oils.* Frog, Berkeley, 2001.
31. Zeck R. *The blossoming heart – aromatherapy for healing and transformation.* Aroma Tours, East Ivanhoe, 2004.

Oregano

Identification

Botanical name

Oils from many origins are often offered as oregano oil. Some of the commonly used plants include *Origanum onites* L., *Origanum vulgare* L. subsp. *hirtum* (Link) letswaart and *Thymus capitatus* L.[1]

Synonyms

European oregano, wild marjoram, common marjoram, origanum oil

Family

Lamiaceae (Labiatae)

Botany and origins

Oregano is a hardy, bushy perennial herb that grows up to 90 cm and is native to Europe, but is cultivated all over the world.[2]

Oregano is a common name for a herb which is derived from more than 60 plant species. The taxonomy of the genus is very complicated. *Origanum* species is characterised by a very large morphological and chemical diversity, resulting in the distinction of 49 taxa and 42 species.[1]

The majority of species are distributed within the Mediterranean region, with nine species located in Greece and 21 in Turkey. 60% of all *Origanum* species are recorded to grow in Turkey.[1]

The four main groups commonly used for culinary purposes can be distinguished as:

- Greek oregano – *Origanum vulgare* L. subsp. *hirtum* (Link) letswaart
- Spanish oregano – *Coridothymus capitatus* L. Hoffmanns & Link
- Turkish oregano – *Origanum onites* L.
- Mexican *oregano – Lippia graveolens HBK.*[3]

The genus *Lippia* (family Verbenaceae) is the most well known of several plants in Mexico that is similar to the Mediterranean oregano in terms of flavour and aroma.[1]

Method of extraction

Oregano oil is steam-distilled from the dried, flowering herb of several plant species native to Europe.

Characteristics

Oregano oil has a strong herbaceous, camphoraceous odour with a dry-woody and phenolic dry out.[4]

Chemical composition

Because there are so many species of *Origanum* used around the world, it is not surprising that there is so much variation in the chemical constituents of the oils. Carvacrol and thymol are considered the major components of oregano essential oils.[5]

The composition of three essential oils of *O. vulgare* L. subsp. *hirtum* populations growing wild in southern Italy appeared to be quite different. Three different chemotypes were identified:

- **carvacrol/thymol chemotype:** *p*-cymene (2.81±0.2%), γ-terpinene (2.38±0.40%), linalool (2.87±0.3%), α-terpineol (0.22±0.03%), thymol (18.21±0.8%), carvacrol (21.89±0.7%), (*E*)-β-caryophyllene (3.72±0.51%), γ-muurolene (4.48±0.58%), β-bisabolene (4.13±0.42%), δ-cadinene (3.17±0.51%), spathulenol (3.9±0.4%).[3]
- **thymol/α-terpineol chemotype:** *p*-cymene (1.25±0.3%), γ-terpinene (4.59±0.80%), linalool (4.10±0.2%), α-terpineol (15.1±0.6%), thymol (26.75±0.7%), carvacrol (6.45±0.65%), (*E*)-β-caryophyllene (2.11±0.1%), γ-muurolene (2.59±0.2%), β-bisabolene (2.81±0.2%), δ-cadinene (0.99±0.1%), spathulenol (1.2±0.2%).[3]
- **linalyl acetate/linalool chemotype:** *p*-cymene (2.01±0.1%), γ-terpinene (4.9±0.10%), linalool (12.5±0.7%), α-terpineol (3.9±0.1%), linalyl acetate (15.9±0.5%), thymol (3.24±0.3%), carvacrol (0.46±0.02%), (*E*)-β-caryophyllene (4.29±0.3%), γ-muurolene (3.61±0.2%), β-bisabolene (2.51±0.2%), δ-cadinene (2.09±0.3%), spathulenol (1.2±0.01%).[3]

The majority of oregano oils belong to the carvacrol/thymol chemotype.[3]

The time of the day of harvesting and the stage of the plant's development were found to influence the chemical composition of *O. onites* oil. The highest carvacrol content (52.58%) was obtained from pre-flowering period at 10:00 h and the lowest (24.66%) at the same stage but at 06:00 h. Carvacrol generally showed higher percentage at post-flowering stages, while the thymol content of oregano oil was highest at pre-flowering at 12:00 h (23.76%) and at its lowest post-flowering at 20:00 h (2.79%).[6]

In general, the carvacrol percentage of oregano oil was high in the mornings whereas the thymol content was low at the same time.[6]

For γ-terpinene, the highest content (11.16%) was obtained from 12:00 h at post-flowering stage and the lowest content (7.02%) was obtained from 10:00 h at pre-flowering. The highest *p*-cymene content (7.97%) was obtained from 10:00 h at pre-flowering, while 16:00 h at pre-flowering had the lowest *p*-cymene content (5.24%). The linalool showed significant changes in concentration during the development stages, and in terms of the time of the day the plant is harvested. The highest linalool content (13.93%) was observed at 06:00 h from full-flowering; the lowest content of linalool (0.14%) was obtained at 10:00 h from pre-flowering.[6]

Adulteration

Oregano oil is commonly adulterated with synthetic thymol and carvacrol, or with limonene from other sources.[7] Arctander states that oregano oil is often subject to adulteration with thyme oil.[4]

Pharmacopoeias and standards

The purity, composition and physico-chemical properties of oregano oil are defined in ISO 13171:2016 Essential Oil of Oregano [*Origanum vulgare* L. subsp. *hirtum* (Link) letsw]

History and Traditional Uses

History

The name *Origanum* is derived from two Greek words, *oros* (mountain) and *ganos* (joy), referring to the appearance the oregano plants give the hillsides on which they grow. The ancient Greeks used oregano extensively. It was a remedy for narcotic poisons, convulsion and dropsy. If oregano grew on a grave, it foretold the happiness of the departed.[8]

Traditional medicine

Oregano has been used as a folk remedy to treat respiratory disorders, whooping and convulsive coughs, dyspepsia, headaches, nervousness, rheumatoid arthritis, toothaches, and irregular and painful menstruation.[1,9]

Turkish villagers have traditionally used *kekik* water, the water obtained from the distillation of the oil from the oregano herb.[1]

Herbal

Oregano herb is listed in the German Commission E Monographs for ailments and difficulties of the respiratory tract, coughing, bronchial catarrh, as an expectorant, and for antispasmodic relief of coughing. It is also used for disturbances of the gastrointestinal tract, bloating, stimulation of gallbladder excretion and digestion, and an appetite stimulant. However, the German Commission E states that the efficacy has not been documented.[10]

O. vulgare has been used as a stimulant, carminative, diaphoretic and nerve tonic, and as a cure for asthma, coughs, indigestion, rheumatism, toothaches, headaches, spider bites and coronary conditions.[2]

Food, perfumery and flavouring

The oregano herb is mainly used as flavouring or seasoning in some of the most accepted cuisines of the world such as Italian, Greek and Mexican dishes. The flowering tops are used in beers and ales, and the fresh and dried leaves are added to soups, casseroles, sauces, stews, stuffing, eggs, olives, tea and tomato-based dishes.[9]

Therapeutics

Pharmacology and clinical studies

Many pharmacological studies involving oregano essential oil have been published. A systemic review of these studies will not be attempted. Rather, I have chosen a selection of studies that support the traditional and clinical uses.

Analgesic activity

O. onites essential oil from Turkey was found to have significant analgesic activity in animal studies. When applied at 0.33 mL/kg, the activity of the oil was comparable to that of morphine (applied at 1 g/kg) but at 0.03 mL/kg it was more potent than the analgesic activity of fenoprofen (at 8 mg/kg).[1]

Antibacterial activity

The antimicrobial activity of oregano oil is primarily attributed to the action of its principal phenol compounds – carvacrol and thymol – which, when tested separately, exhibit significant bactericidal activity.

Due to their hydrophobic nature, carvacrol and thymol interact with the lipid bilayer of the cytoplasmic membranes of the bacteria causing loss of integrity and leakage of cellular material such as ions, ATP and nucleic acid.[11]

O. vulgare oil exhibited a high antibacterial activity against *Escherichia coli, Pseudomonas aeruginosa, Staphylococcus aureus, Salmonella typhimurium* and *Bacillus subtilis*. The oil had good bactericidal activity at a dilution as high as 1/50,000.[12]

Another study examined the antibacterial effect of oregano oil when combined with antibiotics. The combination of oregano oil and amoxicillin, polymycin, lincomycin and maquindox florfenicol displayed synergism against *E. coli*.[13]

E. coli, Enterococcus faecalis and MRSA were inhibited by oregano essential oil at a concentration of 0.125%.[14]

Oregano oil was found to possess strong antibacterial activity compared with the antibiotic ampicillin on a range of bacteria. Gram-positive bacteria were more sensitive to oregano oil than gram-negative bacteria.[15]

Antifungal activity

The antifungal activity of oregano oil at a concentration of 1 ul/mL against *Aspergillus niger* has been observed. Numerous studies have confirmed the antifungal activity of the carvacrol/thymol chemotypes of oregano oil against fungal growths.[1]

Antiviral activity

The results of an in vitro study demonstrated that oregano oil has effective antiviral activity in inactivating nonenveloped murine norovirus, a human norovirus surrogate.[16]

Insecticidal activity

Oregano oil with high carvacrol content displayed strong insecticidal activity against *Drosophila melanogaster* and strong ovicidal activity against the eggs of stored product insects *Tribolium confusum* and *Ephestia cautella* at low concentrations.[1]

Actions

Actions commonly cited in aromatherapy

Analgesic, antirheumatic, antiseptic, antispasmodic, antiviral, bactericidal, carminative, choleretic, diaphoretic, emmenagogue, expectorant, febrifuge, fungicidal, parasiticide, rubefacient, stimulant, tonic[17,18,19]

Actions supported by clinical studies

Analgesic, antibacterial, antifungal, antiviral

Comment

Lawless states that oregano oil should not be used on the skin as it is a dermal toxin, skin irritant and mucous membrane irritant.[17]

I agree with Lawless, who suggests that oregano should not be used in aromatherapy. The oil has such potent antimicrobial activity. It must, therefore, be used with extreme care, as topical use often leads to irritation of the skin.

Schnaubelt and Lavabre recommend the best way to take oregano internally is in a capsule form.[18,20] Lavabre highly recommends it for the treatment of viral diseases, bronchitis and catarrhal conditions. He suggests that it be used to improve circulation and for muscular pain.[18]

Aromatherapy Uses

Clinical aromatherapy

Antimicrobial

Schnaubelt states that, when it comes to combating bacterial infections, oregano is 'aromatherapy's

O

heavy artillery'. He actually suggests that it is safer to use internally. He explains that oregano oil is best suited for treating acute bacterial infections of the gastrointestinal tract and the respiratory system. He explains that just taking 1 drop in a carrier oil per day or in a capsule will be very effective. However, he advises against long-term use as essential oils with high level of phenols can be hepatotoxic.[21]

Dosage and Administration

Blending

Aromatherapy

As oregano oil is a strong dermal irritant and mucous membrane irritant, no aromatherapy blends are provided.

Perfumery

Oregano oil is used in perfumery for its powerful refreshing note and its spicy-herbaceous effect. It is often used in soap perfumes where a 'medicinal' aroma is required. Traces of oregano oil can be useful for top note effects in citrus colognes, fougères, forest notes, chypres, lavender colognes and spicy herbaceous aftershaves.[4]

It blends well with cedarwoods, citronella, lavender, oakmoss absolute, pine needle oils, spike lavender and rosemary.[4]

O

Mode of administration

Bath

Oregano oil is not recommended for use in a bath.

Topical

Oregano oil is not recommended for topical application.

Inhalation

Direct inhalation, diffuser, oil vaporiser

Ingestion

There is a high risk of irritation to the mucous membrane, therefore, as Schnaubelt recommends, the best way to take oregano internally is in a capsule form.[21]

Safety Profile

General safety

The main constituents in oregano oil are carvacrol and thymol. Both constituents are phenols that contribute to oregano's skin irritant and mucous membrane irritant properties.

Oregano oil is not recommended for use on people with hypersensitive skin, diseased or damaged skin, or children under two years of age. Tisserand & Young recommend a maximum dermal use level of 1.1% based on an average total content of thymol and carvacrol of 87.8%.[22]

Contraindications

Tisserand & Young state that oregano oil is contraindicated during pregnancy and breastfeeding.[22]

Regulatory guidelines

Oregano oil has GRAS status.

References

1. Kintzios SE. *Oregano – the genera Origanum and Lippia*. Taylor & Francis, London, 2002. (Medical and Aromatic Plants – Industrial Profiles; 25).
2. Khan I, Abourashed E. *Leung's encyclopedia of common natural ingredients used in food, drugs and cosmetics*. 3rd edn. John Wiley & Sons, New Jersey, 2010.
3. de Martino L et al. *Chemical composition and antimicrobial activity of the essential oils from three chemotypes of Origanum vulgare L. ssp. hirtum (Link) letswaart growing wild in Campania (Southern Italy)*. Molecules, 2009; 14(8): 2735-2746. doi: 10.3390/molecules14082735.
4. Arctander S. *Perfume and flavor materials of natural origin*. Allured Publishing, Carol Stream, 1994.
5. Singletary K. *Oregano: overview of literature on health benefits*. Nutrition Today, 2010;45(3):129-138. doi: 10.1097/NT.0b013e3181dec789.
6. Toncer O et al. *Changes in essential oil composition of oregano (Origanum onites L.) due to diurnal variation at different development stages*. Notulae Botanicae Horti Agrobotanici Cluj-Napoca, 2009; 37(2): 177-181.
7. Schmidt E, Wanner J. *Adulteration of essential oils*. In Baser KHC, Buchbauer G. eds. *Handbook of essential oils – science, technology and applications*. 2nd edn. CRC Press, Boca Raton, 2016: 707-745.
8. Grieve M. *A modern herbal – Vol. II*. Dover Publications, New York, 1971.
9. Ortega-Ramirez LA et al. *Oregano (Origanum spp.) oils*. In Preedy VR. ed. *Essential oils in food preservation, flavor and safety*. Academic Press, London, 2016: 625-631.
10. Blumenthal M et al. *The complete German commission E monographs: therapeutic guide to herbal medicine*. American Botanical Council, Austin, 1998.
11. Nostro A. *Effects of oregano, carvacrol and thymol on Staphylococcus aureus and Staphylococcus epidermidis biofilms*. Journal of Medical Microbiology, 2007; 56: 519-523. doi: 10.1099/jmm.0.46804-0.

12. Sivropoulou A et al. *Antimicrobial and cytotoxic activities of Origanum essential oils.* Journal of Agricultural and Food Chemistry, 1996; 44(5): 1202-1205. Cited in Quintessential Aromatics database, 2013.
13. Si H et al. *Antibacterial effect of oregano essential oil alone and in combination with antibiotics against extended-spectrum B-lactamase-producing Escherichia coli.* FEMS Immunology and Medical Microbiology, 2008; 53(2): 190-194. Cited in Quintessential Aromatics database, 2013.
14. Da Costa AC et al. *Antibacterial activity of the essential oil of Origanum vulgare L. (Lamiaceae) against bacterial multiresistant strains isolated from nosocomial patients.* Brazilian Journal of Pharmacognosy, 2009; 19(1B): 236-241. Cited in Quintessential Aromatics database, 2013.
15. Ozkalp B. et al. *The antibacterial activity of essential oil of oregano (Origanum vulgare l.)* Journal of Food, Agriculture & Environment, 2010; 8(2): 272-274.
16. Gilling DH et al. *Antiviral efficacy and mechanism of action of oregano essential oil and its primary component against murine norovirus.* Journal of Applied Microbiology, 2014; 116(5): 1149-1163. doi: 10.1111/jam.12453.
17. Lawless J. *The encyclopaedia of essential oils.* Element Books, Shaftesbury, 1992.
18. Lavabre M. *Aromatherapy workbook.* Healing Arts Press, Rochester, 1997.
19. Valnet J. *The practice of aromatherapy.* C.W Daniel Company, Saffron Walden, 1980.
20. Schnaubelt K. *Medical aromatherapy.* Frog, Berkeley, 1999.
21. Schnaubelt K. *Advanced aromatherapy.* Healing Arts Press, Rochester, 1995.
22. Tisserand R, Young R. *Essential oil safety.* 2nd edn. Churchill Livingstone, Edinburgh, 2014.

Palmarosa

Identification

Botanical name

Cymbopogon martinii Roxb. var. *martinii*

Synonyms

Motia, rosha grass, *Andropogon martinii* Roxb. var. *martinii*

Family

Poaceae (Gramineae)

Botany and origins

Palmarosa is a tufted perennial grass with numerous stiff stems. The grass grows wild in India, particularly northeast of Bombay towards the Himalaya Mountains. The Dutch introduced palmarosa to Java in the 1930s. The grass is also cultivated in the Seychelle Islands and the Comoro Islands.[1]

Method of extraction

Palmarosa oil is steam-distilled from wild growing, fresh or dried grass of the plant *C. martinii.*

Characteristics

Palmarosa oil is a pale-yellow or pale-olive-coloured oil with a sweet, floral-rosy odour, and various undertones or top notes according to the quality and age of the oil.[2]

Chemical composition

The chemical composition of palmarosa oil from India was reported as follows:

myrcene (1.0%), linalool (2.5%), geraniol (73.1%), geranyl acetate (15.8%), limonene (0.5%), β-caryophyllene (2.0%).[3]

Arctander states that palmarosa oil is one of the best natural sources of geraniol; however, the oil has lost its importance due to the availability of low-cost synthetic geraniols.[2]

Adulteration

Arctander states that palmarosa oil is also frequently adulterated with its close relative gingergrass.[2] Turpentine and citronella oil are often used with synthetic geraniol to adulterate palmarosa. Palmarosa oil itself is often used as a cheap substitute for rose and geranium oils.[4]

Pharmacopoeias and standards

The purity, composition and physico-chemical properties of palmarosa essential oil are defined in ISO 4727:1988 – Oil of Palmarosa (*Cymbopogon martinii* (Roxburgh) W. Watson var. *motia*)

History and Traditional Uses

History

There is no record of when palmarosa oil was first distilled in India, but bruised leaves were used to perfume bath water and provide poultices to relieve pain of neuralgia, lumbago, sciatica and rheumatic pain.[1]

P

The oil was traded between India and Persia and then shipped to Constantinople, where it became known to European traders as Turkish or Indian geranium oil; however, Arctander states that this name is a carry-over from the days when palmarosa was used as an adulterant for Turkish rose oil and it was imported into Turkey for this purpose.[2]

Traditional medicine

In India, the oil is massaged into the joints to alleviate lumbago and rheumatism, and taken internally to relieve stomach disorders.[1]

According to Ayurveda texts from the fourteenth century, palmarosa was recommended for cough, heart disease, colic, bleeding disorders, epilepsy, sinusitis, fever due to catarrh, diseases of the throat, fever, anorexia, obstinate skin diseases, lower backache, urinary disorders and scorpion bites. It is also used topically in an insect repellent.[5]

Food, perfumery and flavouring

It is extensively used in perfumery for scenting soaps.

Therapeutics

Pharmacology and clinical studies

Anthelmintic activity

An in vitro study confirmed that palmarosa oil and its main constituent geraniol has potent anthelmintic activity against nematode, *Caenorhabditis elegans*.[6]

Antifungal activity

Palmarosa oil has been reported to exhibit excellent antifungal activity.[7,8,9,10]

An in vitro study found that palmarosa essential oil exhibited strong inhibitory activity against 20 fluconazole-resistant strains *of Candida albicans*. It was very interesting to note that the researchers found that the oil exhibited significant synergy with fluconazole or amphotericin B against the test isolates. The findings suggest the possible effective use of certain essential oils in combination with fluconazole or amphotericin B.[11]

Antimicrobial activity

Palmarosa oil has been reported to exhibit significant antimicrobial activity.[7,8,9,12]

Insecticidal activity

Palmarosa oil was found to give almost complete protection against *Anopheles culicifacies* (a principal malaria carrier) for up to 11 hours. Palmarosa oil was considered comparable with synthetic repellents such as dimethyl phthalate and dibutyl phthalate.[13]

Neuroprotective activity

Palmarosa oil demonstrated potential neuroprotective activity against global cerebral ischemia/reperfusion-induced oxidative stress in rats. Palmarosa oil may have therapeutic potential in cerebrovascular diseases.[14]

Inhalation of palmarosa increased glutathione peroxidase activity in mice studies. The researchers stated that the beneficial effects of palmarosa on oxidative stress could prevent liver toxicity.[15]

Actions

Actions commonly cited in aromatherapy

Antidepressant, antifungal, antimicrobial, antiseptic, antiviral, cicatrisant, digestive, febrifuge, hydrating, insect repellent, neurotonic[16,17,18]

Actions supported by clinical studies

Antifungal, antimicrobial, insect repellent

Comment

Palmarosa oil has a long history of use in traditional Ayurveda medicine. It is relatively non-toxic and is considered a very effective and safe antimicrobial. Its unique, refreshing floral scent means that it is well suited in aromatherapy blends for use in skin care preparations and for promoting general wellbeing.

Aromatherapy Uses

Clinical aromatherapy

Antimicrobial

Palmarosa oil has strong antifungal activity and is recommended for fungal infections such as oral thrush, intestinal dysbiosis, candidiasis and tinea. It is recommended for bacterial infections such as gastroenteritis, bronchitis, cystitis, vaginitis and cervicitis.[19]

Schnaubelt describes palmarosa oil as one of the most powerful, yet gentle antiviral oils. He states that it is useful for rhinitis, sinusitis, bronchitis, viral enteritis, cystitis, vaginitis, cervicitis, acne and eczema.[20]

Cardiovascular system

Holmes recommends palmarosa oil for cardiac deficiency with palpitations, chronic stress-related heart disorders, and hypertension or hypotension.[19]

Digestive system

Palmarosa oil acts as a tonic to the digestive system and is reputed to have a beneficial effect on pathogens in the intestinal flora.[17,21] It is reputed to be a digestive stimulant and is recommended for loss of appetite and a sluggish digestion.[21]

Holmes describes palmarosa oil as a microflora restorative. He explains that its antifungal and antibacterial activity means that it is beneficial for intestinal microflora dysbiosis with diarrhoea or constipation, microbial toxicosis and chronic intestinal parasites.[19]

Palmarosa oil is also a gastrointestinal restorative and can be used for intestinal hyperpermeability with food sensitivities, gluten sensitivity, peptic ulcers, ulcerative colitis and inflammatory bowel disease.[19]

Nervous system

Palmarosa oil is as referred to as a nerve restorative and is recommended for neurasthenia, debility, burnout and depression.[19]

Psychological

Palmarosa oil has a calming yet uplifting effect on emotions and may be used to alleviate stress, restlessness and anxiety.[16,17,21]

Palmarosa oil is recommended for psychological and emotional conditions such as emotional confusion, mood swings, irritability, negative feelings, loss of insight, discouragement, feelings of insecurity and emotional disconnection.[19]

Skin care

Palmarosa oil is extensively used in skin care. It is antiseptic, has hydrating properties, helps to balance sebum production and is reputed to stimulate cellular regeneration.[17,18,21]

Holmes compares the antimicrobial activity of palmarosa with the melaleuca oils. However, he explains that it has excellent skin-regenerative and tissue-healing capacity in skin care similar to lavender. He suggests that palmarosa is better than lavender as it has excellent emollient quality, which makes it useful for treating dry, irritated skin conditions.[19]

Palmarosa oil is recommended for all skin types, especially acne, dermatitis and minor skin infections, and is also helpful for dry, undernourished skin conditions.[17,21]

Energetics, psyche and subtle uses

Energetics

Palmarosa oil is *cooling* and moistening. It clears *heat* and strengthens the *Yin Qi*. Mojay compares palmarosa oil to geranium and rose – it helps to clear *heat* and strengthens the *Yin Qi*. It also reinforces the *Heart Yin* and calms the *Shen*. It is indicated for palpitations, restlessness, insomnia and anxiety. Therefore, palmarosa has a strong affinity with the Fire Element by cooling excess *heat*.[16]

Holmes explains that its sweet aroma means that it also has an affinity with the Earth Element, therefore, palmarosa strengthens the *Spleen*. Palmarosa oil is recommended for *Spleen* deficiency symptoms such as fatigue, irregular stools, chronic digestive problems and weight loss. Palmarosa oil will also help eliminate *Spleen* toxic *damp* conditions associated with chronic indigestion, abdominal bloating, diarrhoea and mucus in the stools.[19]

According to the principles of Ayurveda, I would recommend palmarosa oil for reducing excess *Pitta*.

Subtle

Mojay explains that palmarosa oil encourages both free-flowing adaptability and a feeling of security. He recommends it for people who have suffered from nervousness and insecurity, and the frequent absence of intimate loved ones.[16]

Holmes states that palmarosa's sweet aroma is ideal whenever we feel emotionally cold and empty. It is nourishing and supportive when there is a conflict between our feelings and thoughts. He recommends using it when we become emotionally rigid, preventing us form insight or discernment into our feelings.[19]

Keim Loughran & Bull state that palmarosa oil helps facilitate the healing process of the body, mind and spirit. They explain that it will help us be patient during the healing process.[22]

Worwood explains that palmarosa oil encourages us to be kind and gentle to ourselves. By not being overcritical or judgemental, we can learn to love who we are, allowing us to love others in the same way. She also explains that the scent of palmarosa gives us direction and purpose.[23]

Dosage and Administration

Blending

Aromatherapy

For the relief of anxiety, stress-related conditions and nervous tension, consider blending palmarosa oil with essential oils such as bergamot, fragonia, frankincense, geranium, lavender, neroli, sweet orange, sandalwood or vetiver.

As an antimicrobial and antifungal treatment for a range of acute fungal, viral and bacterial infections, consider blending palmarosa oil with essential oils such as cajeput, fragonia, lemon, manuka, niaouli, tea tree, or thyme ct. linalool.

As a skin regenerator to promote healing of the skin, consider blending palmarosa oil with

P

essential oils such as carrot seed, everlasting, frankincense, lavender, myrrh, patchouli, rose otto or absolute or sandalwood.

As a natural essential oil insect repellent, consider blending palmarosa oil with essential oils such as citronella, Virginian cedarwood, kunzea, lemongrass, niaouli, spike lavender or sandalwood.

As a cardiac restorative and to cool excess heat according to TCM, consider blending palmarosa with essential oils such as bergamot, melissa, neroli, lavender or sandalwood.

Perfumery

Palmarosa oil has traditionally been used for scenting soaps and household products. It is used for its lingering rosy aroma and for the isolation of geraniol. It is an excellent extender for rose-based perfumes, especially when used in combination with patchouli; however, please use it sparingly or the grassy citrus notes will overpower the delicate floral rose notes.[2]

Mode of administration

Bath

Full body bath, foot bath, sitz bath

Topical

Compress, massage, ointment, skin care

Inhalation

Direct inhalation, diffuser, oil vaporiser

P

Safety Profile

General safety

Palmarosa oil is non-toxic, non-irritating and non-sensitising.[17] However, based on its high geraniol content, EU legislation classifies all geraniol-rich essential oils as having sensitisation potential.[4] However, Tisserand & Young state that the risk of an allergic reaction to geraniol is low.[24]

Contraindications

No contraindications known.

Regulatory guidelines

Palmarosa oil has GRAS status.

References

1. Weiss EA. *Essential oil crops.* CAB International, Wallingford, 1997.
2. Arctander S. *Perfume and flavor materials of natural origin.* Allured Publishing, Carol Stream, 1994.
3. Lawrence BM. *Progress in essential oils – palmarosa oil.* Perfumer & Flavorist, 2004; 29: 53-57.
4. Lis-Balchin M. *Aromatherapy science – a guide for healthcare professionals.* Pharmaceutical Press, London, 2006.
5. Khare CO. *Ayurvedic pharmacopoeial plant drugs.* CRC Press, Boca Raton, 2015.
6. Kumaran AM et al. *Geraniol, the putative anthelmintic principle of Cymbopogon martinii.* Phytotherapy Research, 2003; 17(8): 957. Cited in Quintessential Aromatics database, 2013.
7. Misra N, Batra S, Mishra D. *Antifungal efficacy of essential oil of Cymbopogon martinii (lemongrass) against Aspergilli.* International Journal of Crude Drug Research, 1988; 26(2): 73-76. Cited in the Aromatherapy Database, by Bob Harris, Essential Oil Resource Consultants, UK, 2000.
8. Srivastava S. Naik SN, Maheshwari RC. *In vitro studies on antifungal activities of palmarosa and eucalyptus oils.* Indian Perfumer, 1993; 37(3): 277-279. Cited in the Aromatherapy Database, by Bob Harris, Essential Oil Resource Consultants, UK, 2000.
9. Pattnaik S, Subramanyam VR, Kole CR, Sahoo S. *Antibacterial activity of essential oils from Cymbopogon: inter- and intra-specific differences.* Microbios, 1995; 84(341): 239-245. Cited in the Aromatherapy Database, by Bob Harris, Essential Oil Resource Consultants, UK, 2000.
10. Singatwadia A, Katewa SS. *In vitro studies on antifungal activity of essential oil of Cymbopogon martinii and Cymbopogon citratus.* Indian Perfumer, 2001; 45(1): 53-55. Cited in Quintessential Aromatics database, 2013.
11. Kahn MSA et al. *Anti-candidal activity of essential oils alone and in combination with amphotericin B or fluconazole against multi-drug resistant isolates of Candida albicans.* Medical Mycology, 2012; 50(1): 33-42. Cited in Quintessential Aromatics database, 2013.
12. Duarte MCT et al. *Activity of essential oils from Brazilian medicinal plants on Escherichia coli.* Journal of Ethnopharmacology, 2007; 111(2): 197-201. Cited in Quintessential Aromatics database, 2013.
13. Ansari MA, Razdan RK. *Relative efficacy of various oils in repelling mosquitoes.* Indian Journal of Malariology, 32(3): 104-111. Cited in the Aromatherapy Database, by Bob Harris, Essential Oil Resource Consultants, UK, 2000.
14. Buch P et al. *Neuroprotective activity of Cymbopogon martinii against cerebral ischemia/reperfusion-induced oxidative stress in rats.* Journal of Ethnopharmacology, 2012; 142(1): 35-40. Cited in Quintessential Aromatics

database, 2013.
15. Andrade BF et al. *Effect of inhaling Cymbopogon martinii essential oil and geraniol on serum biochemistry parameters and oxidative stress in rats.* Biochemistry Research International, 2014; 2014: 493183. doi: 10.11545/2014/493183. Cited in Quintessential Aromatics database, 2013.
16. Mojay G. *Aromatherapy for healing the spirit.* Healing Arts Press, Rochester, 1999.
17. Lawless J. *The encyclopaedia of essential oils.* Element Books, Shaftesbury, 1992.
18. Lavabre M. *Aromatherapy workbook.* Healing Arts Press, Rochester, 1997.
19. Holmes P. *Aromatica: a clinical guide to essential oil therapeutics – Vol. I.* Singing Dragon, London, 2016.
20. Schnaubelt K. *Medical aromatherapy.* Frog, Berkeley, 1999.
21. Davis P. *Aromatherapy: an A-Z.* 2nd edn. C.W. Daniel Company, Saffron Walden, 1999.
22. Keim Loughran J, Bull R. *Aromatherapy anointing oils.* Frog, Berkeley, 2001.
23. Worwood VA. *The fragrant heavens.* Transworld, London, 1999.
24. Tisserand R, Young R. *Essential oil safety.* 2nd edn. Churchill Livingstone, Edinburgh, 2014.

Parsley seed

Identification

Botanical name

Petroselinum crispum (Mill.) Fuss

Synonyms

Garden parsley, common parsley, *Petroselinum sativum* Hoffm.

Family

Apiaceae (Umbelliferae)

Botany and origins

Parsley is native to the eastern Mediterranean countries and has been used commonly in food for more than 2,000 years. The plant has been widely cultivated for so long that it is rarely found in its wild state anymore. Cultivation for the purposes of producing seed for distillation is not very common.[1]

It is a short-lived perennial with a multi-branched stem, up to 0.7 m in height. Nowadays it is extensively cultivated in Germany, France, Belgium and Hungary. The ripe fruits or seeds and the above ground leaf are commonly used.[2]

Method of extraction

This oil is produced by the steam distillation of the ripe fruit (seed) of *P. crispum*, the common garden parsley.

Characteristics

The oil is a yellowish to amber-coloured liquid with a warm-woody, spicy, somewhat sweet-herbaceous odour.[1]

Chemical composition

The chemical composition of 11 parsley seed oils from root and leaf cultivars from Poland were examined. The composition of the seed oil of the parsley leaf cultivars known as 'Festival', 'Karnaval' and 'Paramount' were as follows:

Compound	Festival oils	Karnaval oil	Paramount oils
α-thujene	0.2-0.3%	0.2%	0.2%
α-pinene	31.0-40.6%	26.7%	26.0-30.8%
camphene	0.2-0.3%	0.3%	0.2-0.6%
sabinene	0-0.7%	0.9%	0-0.4%
β-pinene	19.0-27.2%	19.7%	18.6-19.9%
Myrcene	Trace-0.2%	0.2%	0-0.5%
α-phellandrene	0.2-0.3%	0.2%	0.2-0.3%
β-phellandrene	4.9-8.8%	4.5%	4.4-4.9%
γ-terpinene	0-0.1%	-	0-0.2%
myrtenal	0.2-0.5%	0.5%	0-trace
myristicin	12.4-18.3%	31.0%	41.1-42.2%
elemicin	Trace-0.6%	0.9%	0-2.7%
allylmethoxybenzene	5.6-12.8%	5.7%	2.0-2.4%
carotol	0.1-0.3%	0.3%	trace-0.4%
apiole	3.7-10.2%	8.8%	trace-0.5%

Parsley seed oil from the root cultivar could easily be identified from parsley seed oil from the leaf cultivar because the oil has higher levels of apiole (16.6-74.9%) compared to (trace-10.2%) in the seed oil of leaf parsley.[3]

There was also a higher percentage of apiole in the seed oil from the flat leaf cultivars, where only traces of apiole could be found in the curled leaf cultivars.[4]

Adulteration

Parsley seed oil is often adulterated with turpentine oil or pure α-pinene, β-pinene or elemicin from elemi resinoid. It is also often blended with nutmeg oil and carrot seed oil.[5] Lis-Balchin states that parsley seed essential oil can be

P

grossly adulterated with other components such as benzyl benzoate.[6]

Pharmacopoeias and standards

The purity, composition and physico-chemical properties of parsley seed essential oil are defined in ISO 3527: 2016 Essential Oil of Parsley Fruits (*Petroselinum sativum* Hoffm.).

History and Traditional Uses

History

The botanical name *Petroselinum* comes from the Greek word for stone, which is *petro*. This is because parsley was found growing on the rocky hillsides in Greece. The Ancient Greeks did not use parsley in their cooking; however, it was highly revered as a symbol of death and as a funeral herb. It was also made into garlands and given to horses as fodder.[7]

It was reputed to have sprung from the blood of a Greek hero, *Archemorus*, the forerunner of death. Homer explains that chariot horses were fed the leaves.[8]

During medieval times, parsley was surrounded by many superstitions. One superstition believed that the long germination time of the seed was due to the seed having to travel to hell and back seven times before it sprouted. Superstitious farmers refused to plant parsley and were often afraid to grow it.[7]

P

Traditional medicine

The leaf, root and seed of parsley have mainly been used for their carminative and diuretic properties.[8]

Herbal

Parsley herb, seed, extract and oils have numerous pharmacological and biological properties, including laxative, hypotensive, antimicrobial and tonic. Recent studies suggest that the herb may be useful for reducing bone resorption and maintaining bone health, as well as for cancer chemoprevention.[2]

Food, perfumery and flavouring

The main use of parsley seed oil is in flavours for meat sauces, seasonings, spice blends, canned foods and pickles. The oil has even been used in tobacco flavouring.[1]

Therapeutics

Pharmacology and clinical studies

Antifungal activity

An in vitro study found that parsley seed oil was highly active against the three dermatophytes – *Epidermophyton floccosum*, *Trichophyton* var. *interdigitale* and *T. rubrum*.[9]

Antimicrobial activity

An in vitro study confirmed that parsley seed oil shows significant antimicrobial activity against *Pseudomonas aeruginosa,* and moderate antifungal activity against *Aspergillus* species.[10] However, another in vitro study using parsley seed oil from India found that the oil did not have prominent antibacterial activity.[11]

Antioxidant activity

Out of 13 essential oils examined for their antioxidant activity, parsley seed oil exhibited the strongest antioxidant activity towards malonaldehyde formation from squalene upon UV-irradiation. The main component showing antioxidant activity was myristicin.[12]

Insecticidal activity

Twelve essential oils from the Apiaceae and their components were tested for their insecticidal activity against the Asian tiger mosquito, *Aedes albopictus*. Parsley seed oil resulted in >90% larval mortality when used at 0.1 mg/mL. The individual compounds, myristicin and apiol, resulted in >80% larvae mortality when used at 0.1 mg/mL.[13]

Spasmolytic activity

An in vitro study confirmed that parsley seed oil exhibited spasmolytic activity on the electrically stimulated smooth muscle of the guinea pig. It was reported that parsley seed oil had calcium channel blocking activity.[14]

Actions

Actions commonly cited in aromatherapy

Antimicrobial, antirheumatic, antiseptic, carminative, depurative, diuretic, emmenagogue, febrifuge, hypotensive, laxative, stimulant, stomachic, uterine tonic[15]

Actions supported by clinical studies

Antimicrobial, antioxidant, insecticidal, spasmolytic

Comment

It is not surprising that very few books mention using parsley seed oil. Parsley seed essential oil has a myristicin content anywhere from 9 to 77%, and the apiole content can be from 0 to 80%.[6] This indicates that it can be a potentially hazardous essential oil. The German Commission E states that the therapeutic application for parsley seed cannot be justified because of the high risks.[16]

Aromatherapy Uses

Clinical aromatherapy

I prefer not to use parsley seed oil in aromatherapy; however, it is often recommended for the following conditions.

Circulatory system

Davis states that parsley seed oil is a tonic to the blood vessels, and can be used externally for the treatment of haemorrhoids. She also recommends using it for the treatment of bruises.[17]

Detoxification

Parsley seed oil is recommended by Lawless for its diuretic and depurative properties, and arthritis, cellulitis, rheumatism and indigestion.[15]

Reproductive system

Parsley seed oil is also recommended as a uterine tonic, and should be useful for the treatment of amenorrhoea and dysmenorrhoea.[15,17]

Urinary system

Hot compresses with parsley seed oil over the bladder are beneficial for treating cystitis and kidney problems.[17]

Dosage and Administration

Blending

Aromatherapy

Due to parsley seed's high toxicity risk, no aromatherapy blends are recommended.

Perfumery

Arctander states that parsley seed oil is used in perfumery for 'special effects'. He states that it is used in perfumes to create a warm-spicy effect for oriental, chypre and modern fantasy style perfumes. It blends well with oils such as aniseed, clary sage and oakmoss absolute.[1] Parsley seed oil would blend well with other spice oils and with citrus oils. However, the maximum use level should be 0.2%.[2]

Mode of administration

Bath

Parsley seed oil is not recommended for use in bath.

Topical

Parsley seed oil is not recommended for topical application.

Inhalation

Parsley seed oil is not recommended for use in inhalation.

Safety Profile

General safety

Lawless states that parsley seed essential oil is moderately toxic and irritant, and that it should be used in moderation.[15]

The hazardous constituent in parsley seed oil is apiol. This is believed to contribute to the oil's abortifacient properties. The oil also contains myristicin. While myristicin is known to be psychotropic, Tisserand & Young report that parsley seed oil does not exhibit any neurotoxic properties.[18]

Contraindications

Parsley seed oil is contraindicated during pregnancy and breastfeeding, and in inflammatory kidney diseases.[15,18]

Toxicity

Parsley seed oil has a high concentration of apiole, which may cause vascular congestion and increase smooth muscle contractibility in the bladder, intestines and uterus. Damage to the kidney epithelia and heart arrhythmia has been reported.[2]

Parsley seed is commonly used as an abortifacient in South America.[17] Tisserand & Young state that the hazards associated with parsley seed oil include risk of drug interaction, hepatotoxicity, nephrotoxicity and a potential abortifacient.[18]

Regulatory guidelines

Parsley seed oil has GRAS status.

References

1. Arctander S. *Perfume and flavor materials of natural origin.* Allured Publishing, Carol Stream, 1994.
2. Khan I, Abourashed E. *Leung's encyclopedia of common natural ingredients used in food, drugs and cosmetics.* 3rd edn. John Wiley & Sons, New Jersey, 2010.
3. Lawrence BM. *Progress in essential oils – parsley seed.* Perfumer & Flavorist. 2010:35:57-58
4. Franz C, Novak J. *Sources of essential oils.* in Başer HC, Buchbauer G. eds, *Handbook of essential oils – science, technology and applications.* 2nd edn, CRC Press, Boca Raton, 2010: 165-194.
5. Schmidt E, Wanner J. *Adulteration of essential oils.* In Baser KHC, Buchbauer G. eds. *Handbook of essential oils – science, technology and applications.* 2nd edn. CRC Press, Boca Raton, 2016: 707-745.
6. Lis-Balchin M. *Aromatherapy science – a guide for healthcare professionals.* Pharmaceutical Press, London, 2006.

P

7. Hemphill I. *Spice notes.* Pan Macmillan Australia, Sydney, 2000.
8. Grieve M. *A modern herbal – Vol. II.* Dover Publications, New York, 1971.
9. Janssen AM et al. *Screening of some essential oils for their activities on dermatophytes.* Pharmaceutisch Weekblad Scientific Edition (Utrecht), 1988; 10(6): 277-278. Cited in Quintessential Aromatics database, 2013.
10. Afifi NA et al. *Some pharmacological activities of essential oils of certain Umbelliferous fruits.* Veterinary Medicine Journal, Giza, 1994; 42(3): 85-92. Cited in Quintessential Aromatics database, 2013.
11. Minija J, Thoppil JE. *Studies on essential oil composition and microbicidal activities of two south Indian spices of the Apiacea.* International Journal of Aromatherapy, 2002; 12(4): 213-215.
12. Wei A, Shibamoto T. *Antioxidant activities and volatile constituents of various essential oils.* Journal of Agricultural and Food Chemistry, 2007; 55(5): 1737-1742. Cited in Quintessential Aromatics database, 2013.
13. Sea SM et al. *Larvicidal and acetylcholine esterase inhibitory activity of Apiaceae plant essential oils and their constituents against Aedes albopictus and formulation development.* Journal of Agricultural and Food Chemistry, 2015; 63(45): 9977-9986. Cited in Quintessential Aromatics database, 2013.
14. Neuhaus-Carlisle K et al. *Calcium-channel blocking activity of essential oils from Petroselinum crispum, Apium graveolens and isolated phenylpropane constituents.* Pharmaceutical & Pharmacological Letters, 1993; 3: 77-79. Cited in Quintessential Aromatics database, 2013.
15. Lawless J. *The encyclopaedia of essential oils.* Element Books, Shaftesbury, 1992.
16. Blumenthal M et al. *The complete German commission E monographs: therapeutic guide to herbal medicine.* American Botanical Council, Austin, 1998.
17. Davis P. *Aromatherapy: an A-Z.* 2nd edn. C.W. Daniel Company, Saffron Walden, 1999.
18. Tisserand R, Young R. *Essential oil safety.* 2nd edn. Churchill Livingstone, Edinburgh, 2014.

P

Patchouli

Identification

Botanical name

Pogostemon cablin (Blanco) Benth.

Synonyms

Pogostemon patchouly, Pogostemon heyneanus, patchouly oil

Family

Lamiaceae (Labiatae)

Botany and origins

Patchouli is an aromatic, perennial shrub with erect stems, large green leaves and small white-pink flowers. The common name patchouli is probably derived from the Tamil *paccilai* and the species name from the Philippine vernacular *cablin.*[1]

P. cablin is the prime source for the production of patchouli oil, but several other species, *P. commosum, P. hortensis, P. heyneasus* and *P. plectranthoides,* are cultivated for their oils, which are also referred to as patchouli oil. These are, however, considered to be inferior to the oil produced from *P. cablin.*[1]

Patchouli is a native to tropical regions of Asia, and is now extensively cultivated in Indonesia, Philippines, Malaysia, China, India, Mauritius, some Caribbean countries, West Africa and Vietnam.[2] Indonesia is the major producer of patchouli oil in the world. In 2013, Indonesia produced an estimated 550 tonnes of oil, which represented more than 80% of the world total production for the year.[3]

Method of extraction

Arctander explains that it is necessary to rupture the cell walls of the patchouli leaf before steam distillation. This is done by controlled, light fermentation, by scalding with superheated steam, or by stacking or baling the dried leaves, thus 'curing' them by fermentation. This is said to produce the best quality patchouli oil.[4]

Weiss states that fresh patchouli leaves should not be used for the distillation of patchouli oil, as the distillation process does not rupture the cells within the leaf. The leaf is dried or lightly fermented. This allows the leaf cell structure to become more permeable, allowing the oil to be liberated. However, it has also been noted that fermentation does not improve the yield of the oil, and may actually contribute to an unpleasant aroma in the oil.[1]

Traditionally patchouli oil is distilled in stills made of iron. It is known that, as the iron oxidises, it will leach into the oil, contributing to the slightly darker colour. Research has shown that this should not adversely affect the quality of the oil. However, the perfume industry considers the colouring undesirable and redistills the oil to remove the iron content.[1]

One study found that the ground dried leaves that were slowly distilled for 10 hours produced an essential oil with 47% patchouli alcohol. The higher content of patchouli alcohol is considered a sign of higher quality patchouli oil.[3]

In another study, a five and half month-old crop was harvested that had been sprayed with a combination of soil fungi isolated from the rhizomes of patchouli plant. The results found that the patchouli treated with *Aspergillus terreus* was found to be statistically superior, as the amount of patchouli alcohol was significantly higher than the untreated patchouli. It was noted that the increase in patchouli alcohol may be due to fungal enzymes such as alcohol dehydrogenase that are known to enhance the production of alcohol. The authors concluded that fungi such as *A. terreus* may be used as an effective biocatalyst to enhance the quality of patchouli oil.[5]

Characteristics

Patchouli oil is a dark orange or brownish coloured, viscous oil, with an extremely rich, sweet herbaceous, aromatic spicy and woody balsamic odour. Arctander states that an almost wine-like, ethereal-floral sweetness in the initial top note is a characteristic of a good oil. He also explains that the odour should remain sweet at all stages of evaporation. The body should display a rich root-like note with a delicate earthiness, and should not include 'mould-like' or 'musty' dry odours.[4]

Chemical composition

Patchouli oil is very complex – over 60 constituents have been detected. The typical constituents found in patchouli oil include patchouli alcohol (30-35%), α- & β-guaiene (2-15%), α-patchoulene (3-55%), pogostol (2%), and traces of valencene, elemol and farnesol.[1]

Patchouli alcohol is the main component that is characteristic of patchouli essential oils. The percentage of patchouli alcohol in patchouli oil is considered an indication of the quality of the oil. 30% is the minimum percentage of patchouli alcohol in patchouli that is acceptable in the essential oil market.[3]

The analysis of patchouli oil that had been distilled over a ten-hour period was as follows:

β-patchoulene (0.83%), α-guaiene (6.43%), β-caryophyllene (0.94%), α-patchoulene (2.73%), patchoulene (0.78%), α-caryophyllene (0.47%), α-aromadendrene (0.33%), β-chamigrene (0.19%), α-bulnesene (8.18%), β-caryophyllene oxide (2.7%), patchouli alcohol (46.55%), spathulenol (0.28%), dihydrokaranone (1.59%), 3,9-diene guaia (0.38%), cuminaldehyde (0.4%), others (27.22%).[3]

Adulteration

Arctander states that patchouli oil is occasionally adulterated with cedarwood oil, clove oil sesquiterpenes, cedarwood derivatives, methyl abietate, hydroabietic alcohols, vetiver residues and camphor residues.[4]

Holmes states that it is a commonly adulterated oil. He explains that other species and genera are often included in the plant material, or they are distilled separately and then added to the patchouli oil.[6]

The herbs commonly used include Java patchouli (*Pogostemon heyneanus* Bentham, syn. *P. patchouli.*); Chinese patchouli (*Microtoena insuavis* (Hance) Prain ex Briquet); Gurjun balsam (*Dipterocarpus turbinatus*) from India; and Caeserweed (*Urena lobata* L.).[6]

Pharmacopoeias and standards

The purity, composition and physico-chemical properties of patchouli oil are defined in ISO 3757:2002 Oil of Patchouli [*Pogostemon cablin* (Blanco) Benth.]

History and Traditional Uses

P

History

The oil is widely used in Asia for incense, body and garment perfumes, insect repellents, and sprinkled in temples. Arabs used it to perfume carpets, Indians for textiles and the Chinese produced a perfumed ink for use on scrolls.[7]

The West's fascination with patchouli began in the first decades of the nineteenth century. In the nineteenth century, there was an enormous amount of trade between India, the Middle East and Europe. Among the most popular goods from the East were the carpets, fabrics, clothes and woven accessories. Many of these, if not all, had layers of crushed or coarse-ground patchouli herb liberally sprinkled amongst them. This was not for aesthetic purposes but for commercial purposes. Patchouli had always been used in Asia as a repellent to moths and small insects. The popularity of the patchouli scent grew to a stage that domestically produced garments, if they were to sell at all, also had to carry the scent of patchouli.[8]

Patchouli became the signature scent for the hippies in the 1960s. Its scent was used to mask the tarry odour of marijuana. It has become one of the most overused social scents of the recent decades, reminding us of the psychedelic 1960s.[7]

Traditional medicine

In Asia, patchouli herb had long served as a deodorant and insect repellent. Patchouli has for centuries been part of the traditional systems of medicine in Malaysia, China and Japan.[2]

Holmes explains that patchouli is one of the very few herbal remedies that is common to all three of the world's traditional medical systems – traditional Chinese, Ayurvedic and Greek. He explains that these medical systems utilised the herb for its regenerating, disinfecting, moistening and cooling effect for topical applications on the skin.[6]

Chinese traditional formulae, such as *baoji* pill and *houdan* pill, contain patchouli herb and are used to treat inflammatory conditions.[9] In Japanese (Kampo) medicine, patchouli is referred to as *kakko* and is used for the purposes of virology and a digestive tonic.[10]

Food, perfumery and flavouring

The oil is extensively used in perfumery, cosmetics and soaps.[2]

Other uses

Dried patchouli leaves were traditionally used to ward off moths from carpets and fine woven goods such as shawls and jackets. This is a practice which dates back to the Victorian period.[8]

Weiss, Mojay and Lawless state that patchouli oil can be used as an antidote to snake bite.[1,11,12] However, I would not suggest trying this, as Australia is home to some of the most venomous snakes in the world.

There is some evidence that it works as an insect repellent and may be effective for killing mites.[10]

Patchouli oil is often used as a flavouring agent in cigarettes.[2]

Therapeutics

Pharmacology and clinical studies

Many pharmacological studies involving patchouli essential oil have been published. A systemic review of these studies will not be attempted. Rather, I have chosen a selection of studies that support the traditional and clinical uses.

Anti-inflammatory activity

A few clinical studies have confirmed that patchouli alcohol has anti-inflammatory properties. A study of the major compounds in patchouli oil found that patchouli alcohol effectively inhibits cyclooxygenase (COX-1/COX2) enzymes, which suggests that patchouli oil has anti-inflammatory activity.[13]

Antimicrobial activity

Pogostone, a constituent found in patchouli oil, is reported to having antimicrobial activities and is responsible for the oil's bactericidal properties.[2]

Among 10 essential oils studied for antimicrobial activity, patchouli oil was found to be the most effective in inhibiting 20 bacterial strains and 12 fungi.[9]

Patchouli alcohol exhibited selective antibacterial activity against *Helicobacter pylori* without affecting the normal flora of the gastrointestinal tract.[9]

A study using molecular docking technology and in vitro antimicrobial tests proved that patchouli oil had strong antimicrobial activity. 26 of the compounds found in patchouli were also tested and it was confirmed that pogostone and (-)-patchouli alcohol had the most potent antimicrobial activity.[14]

The results of the molecular docking study indicated that most of the chemical constituents found in patchouli oil had multi-target effects. They inhibited DNA replication in bacteria in the same way that ciprofloxacin does. The patchouli oil constituents also caused bacterial cell wall defects in the same way that benzylpenicillin does.[14]

Antiphotoaging activity

Patchouli oil prevented photoaging by exhibiting antioxidative activity and maintaining skin structural integrity. Similarly, the use of patchouli alcohol increased the revitalisation of UV-induced skin lesions through antioxidant and anti-inflammatory actions.[9]

Antiviral activity

The oral administration of patchouli alcohol (20 mg/kg to 80 mg/kg) in a study involving mice augmented protection against influenza virus by improving the immune response and attenuating systemic as well as pulmonary inflammatory responses.[9]

The antiviral activity of patchouli oil was studied in vitro, in vivo and in silico (using computer modelling). The results of a study suggest that the inhibition of the influenza virus by patchouli alcohol occurs much more effectively after the penetration of the virus into the cell. The researchers concluded that the function of the neuraminidase (NA) protein may be suppressed by the patchouli alcohol. The most effective antiviral drugs are NA inhibitors, which target the NA glycoproteins of influenza A and B virus.[15]

The same study also found patchouli alcohol to be more effective than oseltamivir (Tamiflu antiviral medication) in vivo using mice. An oral treatment showed that, at a dose of 5 mg/kg/day, patchouli alcohol displayed strong protection against the influenza virus. When the dose was lowered to 1 mg/kg/day, patchouli alcohol showed weaker protection.[15]

The results of the study confirmed that patchouli alcohol possesses potentially potent antiviral activity against Asian influenza (H2N2) virus and should be considered as a potential source of anti-influenza agents for the pharmaceutical industry.[15]

CNS activity

One study found that the inhalation of patchouli oil resulted in a reduction of CNS activity as assessed by systolic blood pressure. It was reported that the degree of CNS reduction relative to the control was approximately 40%. It was suggested that patchouli oil improves mood.[10]

Actions

Actions commonly cited in aromatherapy

Antidepressant, antiphlogistic, antiseptic, aphrodisiac, astringent, cicatrisant, cytophylactic, deodorant, diuretic, febrifuge, fungicide, insecticide, sedative[2,11,12]

Actions supported by clinical studies

Antidepressant, anti-inflammatory, antiseptic, antiviral, fungicide, sedative

Comment

The commercial importance of patchouli oil has been its unique fragrance, which is commonly used in perfumery. However, patchouli herb does have some very important biological activities that have been well understood in TCM and Ayurveda, but not in aromatherapy.

Much of the research on the pharmacological activities of patchouli alcohol, found in patchouli oil, is helping to validate many of the traditionally reported uses of the oil in Ayurveda and TCM.

In aromatherapy, patchouli oil is often thought of as a classic 'grounding' oil. I like the term Holmes uses to describe patchouli – 'a sensory integrator.' He means that it makes us literally come to our senses, grounding us fully in the physical experience.[6]

Aromatherapy Uses

Clinical aromatherapy

Antimicrobial

Holmes recommends using patchouli oil for fungal skin infections such as tinea, and for the treatment of ringworms. He also refers to it as an antifungal restorative, and suggests using patchouli oil for intestinal microflora dysbiosis and candidiasis.[6]

Integumentary system

It is recommended for treating conditions such as sores, fissures, injuries, scars, skin inflammations, eczema, and fungal and parasitic skin infections.[12,16,17]

Nervous system

Patchouli is beneficial for alleviating depression, anxiety, restlessness, irritability, insomnia, sexual anxiety and stress-related conditions.[6,12,16]

Psychological

Mojay says that patchouli oil calms the mind when it is stimulated with overthinking and worry.[11]

Holmes states that patchouli oil stabilises the mind, supports emotional security and promotes cognitive flexibility. Patchouli oil is recommended for feelings of disconnection, oversensitivity, worry and obsessive thoughts, inability to let go, feelings of agitation, and fearfulness. It is also recommended whenever there are sensory-emotional inhibition and sexual disinterest or inhibition, resulting in loss of libido.[6]

Patchouli oil is suited to the mentally active and tense individual who easily feels divorced from both sensual pleasure and creative expression.[11]

Skin care

Patchouli oil is best known for skin care and for topical applications because of its regenerating, disinfecting, moistening and cooling of the skin.[12,16]

Patchouli oil is suited to oily congested skin and for dandruff, acne, seborrheic and inflammatory eczema, or dermatitis.[6]

Energetics, psyche and subtle uses

Energetics

Mojay says that patchouli's most valuable therapeutic use is mainly energetic and psychological. Patchouli oil is good for those who, due to excessive mental activity and nervous strain, feel 'out of touch' with their body and their sensuality.[11]

Patchouli oil strengthens our *Spleen Qi* and helps eliminate *damp*. When our *Spleen Qi* is weak and we have excess *damp*, we suffer from lethargy and fatigue, chronic indigestion, abdominal bloating and diarrhoea.[6,11] Holmes states that patchouli oil nourishes the *Kidney Yin* and *Heart Yin* and calms the *Shen*. When the *Heart Yin* is deficient and the *Shen* agitated, we experience anxiety, fearfulness, worry, insomnia and mental agitation. When the *Kidney Yin* is deficient, we experience restlessness, fatigue and insomnia.[6]

Patchouli helps to harmonise the Earth Element and the spirit associated with the Earth Element – the *Yi*. The *Yi* is known as our intellect. According to TCM, whenever our *Yi* is not balanced, we may experience obsessive worrying thoughts and confused thinking.

Personality

Worwood states that patchouli personality types are well balanced and grounded. She says there is an elderly quality about them, no matter how old they are.[18]

Patchouli personalities epitomise the introvert characteristics. Worwood explains that patchouli personalities do not have a lot of friends. They are perfectly happy on their own and quite capable of seeking out the company of others when desired.[18]

According to Myers-Briggs personality types, the patchouli personality is likely to be an ISTP. ISTPs are quiet and they prefer to stand back and observe. They can be difficult to understand and remain a mystery to many people. They are independent and do not like to behave to the rules of society. They appear cool, dispassionate and analytical. They can be very disorganised in things where they have no interest. They dislike supervising or being supervised. They tend to ignore rules, policies and regulations when they can get in the way of results. They tend to remain calm in a crisis. They have little need for talking or socialising. They often have poor interpersonal skills and seem detached or uncaring to those who are not close to them.

P

Subtle

Patchouli oil's earthy notes are responsible for its grounding, centring and sensual effects, which are in keeping with its base note. The grounding effect can help heal negative detachment from both our body and our environment.[8]

Patchouli oil has a harmonising and stabilising effect on the mind when overthinking and worrying tend to destabilise one's self-confidence. It is recommended for 'dreamers' and people who tend to neglect or feel detached from their bodies. This may be beneficial for people who are engaged on a spiritual path and are placing an undue share of importance on their mental/psychic experiences, to the detriment of their physical wellbeing.[19]

Holmes states that patchouli has a gentle yet persistent sensual quality that seduces us into accepting our body needs and nurturing our sensuality. He also explains that patchouli helps us connect with the spirit that is immanent in all of nature.[6]

Worwood states that patchouli brings with it the sense of the sacredness of life. Patchouli will remind us that sitting quietly under a tree is good if there is purpose in it – the purpose of knowing and appreciating.[20]

Keim Loughran & Bull explain that patchouli teaches us that the physical body is sacred and that our senses are avenues to our soul and doorways to spirit. Patchouli asks us to experience our senses and sensuality as a sacred gift. It helps the mind to relax and connect with the knowledge of the body. Patchouli is grounding, yet it enlightens our mind and brings pleasure and delight.[21]

We often associate the earthy sweet aroma of patchouli oil with the base chakra, but it also helps facilitate the enjoyment of the senses and awakening of creativity. Therefore, it also helps to open and balance the sacral chakra.

Dosage and Administration

Blending

Aromatherapy

Patchouli oil can easily overpower a blend, so it is best to use with other essential oils that have a rich and heavy aroma. It is a blend modifier, so use patchouli oil sparingly in a blend.

For the relief of anxiety, nervous tension and stress-related conditions, consider blending patchouli oil with essential oils such as bergamot, Roman chamomile, geranium, fragonia, lavender, neroli, sandalwood, vetiver or ylang ylang.

To create a grounding blend to soothe agitation and lack of feeling connected, consider blending patchouli oil with essential oils such as Atlas cedarwood, angelica root, myrrh, spikenard, sandalwood or vetiver.

For the relief of insomnia, consider blending patchouli oil with essential oils such as Atlas cedarwood, lavender, sweet marjoram, neroli, sweet orange or sandalwood.

For skin regeneration of damaged skin, consider blending patchouli oil with essential oils such as German chamomile, everlasting, frankincense, myrrh, rose absolute, sandalwood or vetiver.

For the treatment of fungal infections of the skin, consider blending patchouli oil with essential oils such as cajeput, fragonia or tea tree.

Perfumery

Patchouli oil imparts strength, character, allure and lasting qualities to a blend. It is very grounding and balancing. It contributes to the rich base note of a perfume.

Arctander states that patchouli oil is extensively

used in perfumery. It blends beautifully with labdanum, vetiver, sandalwood, the cedarwoods, oakmoss absolute, geranium, clove, neroli, myrrh, opopanax, sage, clary sage and pine needle oils, just to name a few. It is used to create oriental bases, woody bases and fougères, chypres and powder-type perfumes.[4]

Mode of administration

Bath

Full body bath, foot bath

Topical

Massage, ointment, skin care

Inhalation

Direct inhalation, diffuser, oil vaporiser

Safety Profile

General safety

Patchouli oil is non-toxic, non-irritating and non-sensitising. Patchouli oil is considered one of the safest essential oil as regards to its toxicology.[22]

Contraindications

No contraindications known.

Regulatory guidelines

Patchouli oil has GRAS status.

References

1. Weiss EA. *Essential oil crops.* CAB International, Wallingford, 1997.
2. Khan I, Abourashed E. *Leung's encyclopedia of common natural ingredients used in food, drugs and cosmetics.* 3rd edn. John Wiley & Sons, New Jersey, 2010.
3. Yahya A, Yunus RM. *Influence of sample preparation and extraction time on chemical composition of steam distillation derived patchouli oil.* Procedia Engineering, 2013; (53): 1-6.
4. Arctander S. *Perfume and flavor materials of natural origin.* Allured Publishing, Carol Stream, 1994.
5. Jayaram A, Vasundhara M, Ananda S. *Fungi as a biotransformation tool in patchouli (Pogostemon patchouli Pellet) essential oil.* International Journal of Science and Research, 2014; 3(11): 1312-1317.
6. Holmes P. *Aromatica: a clinical guide to essential oil therapeutics – Vol. I.* Singing Dragon, London, 2016.
7. Morris E. *Fragrance – the story of perfume from Cleopatra to Chanel.* Products of Nature and Art, New York, 1984.
8. Holmes P. *Patchouli oil.* The International Journal of Aromatherapy, 1997; 8(1): 18.
9. Swamy MK, Sinniah UR. *A comprehensive review on the phytochemical constituents and pharmacological activities of Pogostemon cablin Benth.: an aromatic medicinal plant of industrial importance.* Molecules, 2015; 20(5); 8521-8547. doi: 10.3390/molecules20058521.
10. *Patchouli.* Retrieved Feb 2, 2016, from http://examine.com/supplements/patchouli/
11. Mojay G. *Aromatherapy for healing the spirit.* Healing Arts Press, Rochester, 1999.
12. Lawless J. *The encyclopaedia of essential oils.* Element Books, Shaftesbury, 1992.
13. Raharjo SJ, Fatchiyah F. *Virtual screening of compounds from the patchouli oil of Pogostemon herba for COX-1 inhibition.* Bioinformation, 2013; 9(6): 321-324. doi: 10.6026/97320630009321.
14. Yang X et al. *Evaluation of the antibacterial activity of patchouli oil.* Iranian Journal of Pharmaceutical Research, 2013; 12(3): 307-316.
15. Wu H et al. *Inhibitory effect and possible mechanisms of action of patchouli alcohol against influenza A (H2N2) virus.* Molecules, 2011; 16(8): 6489-6501. doi: 10.3390/molecules16086489
16. Davis P. *Aromatherapy: an A-Z.* 2nd edn. C.W. Daniel Company, Saffron Walden, 1999.
17. Lavabre M. *Aromatherapy workbook.* Healing Arts Press, Rochester, 1997.
18. Worwood VA. *The fragrant mind.* Transworld Publishers, London, 1995.
19. Davis P. *Subtle aromatherapy.* C.W. Daniel Company, Saffron Walden, 1991.
20. Worwood VA. *The fragrant heavens.* Transworld Publishers, London, 1999.
21. Keim Loughran J, Bull R. *Aromatherapy anointing oils.* Frog, Berkeley, 2001.
22. Lis-Balchin M. *Aromatherapy science – a guide for healthcare professionals.* Pharmaceutical Press, London, 2006.

Pennyroyal

Identification

Botanical name

Mentha pulegium L.

Synonyms

Pulegium, European pennyroyal

Family

Lamiaceae (Labiatae)

P

Botany and origins

Mentha pulegium can be found throughout southeast and central Europe, from Ireland and Central Poland to Ukraine. It is also found growing in the Iberian Peninsula, and North African countries that border the Mediterranean such as Algeria, Morocco and Tunisia. Lawrence states that pennyroyal oil is produced only from wild plants that are harvested when they are in full flower. The main countries where the oil is produced are Spain, Morocco and Turkey.[1]

Another plant called American pennyroyal (*Hedeoma pulegioides*) also produces an essential oil rich in pulegone.[2]

Method of extraction

Pennyroyal oil is steam-distilled from freshly harvested dried herb of *M. pulegium.*

Characteristics

The oil is a pale yellow to almost colourless mobile liquid with a very fresh, strong herbaceous-minty aroma.[2]

Chemical composition

The chemical composition of pennyroyal oil from Spain was reported as follows:

α-pinene (1.5%), camphene (0.1%), β-pinene + sabinene (0.5%), limonene + 1,8-cineole + β-ocimene (0.8%), *p*-cymene (0.1%), 3-octanol (1.2%), menthone (15.6%), isomenthone + menthofuran (2.2%), pulegone + isomenthol (72.4%), piperitone (0.5%).[1]

The chemical composition of pennyroyal oil from Algeria was reported as follows:

α-pinene (0.5%), limonene (4.3%), menthone (19.24%), isomenthone (6.06%), isopulegone (0.55%), pulegone (38.8%), piperitone (6.4%), piperitenone (16.5%).[3]

There are three chemotypes of pennyroyal oil with the following major components:

- pulegone
- piperitone
- isomenthone/neoisomenthol.[3]

Adulteration

Not reported.

Pharmacopoeias and standards

At the time of writing, the purity, composition, physico-chemical properties and therapeutic use of pennyroyal essential oil are not defined in any pharmacopoeia monograph or standard.

P

History and Traditional Uses

History

Pennyroyal derives its Latin name from *pulex*, meaning flea, alluding to its traditional use as a strewing herb to repel fleas. It was highly regarded by Pliny and Dioscorides, who described its numerous virtues.[4]

Culpepper describes the uses of pennyroyal herb:

> *Drunk with wine, it is good for venomous bites, and applied to the nostrils with vinegar revives those who faint and swoon. Dried and burnt, it strengthens the gums, helps the gout, if applied of itself to the place until it is red, and applied in a plaster, it takes away spots or marks on the face; applied with salt, it profits those who are splenetic or liver-grown.*[4]

Pennyroyal is reputed to have been used as an abortifacient since ancient times.[5]

Herbal

Pennyroyal herb is listed in the British Herbal Pharmacopoeia for the treatment of flatulence, dyspepsia, intestinal colic, the common cold, delayed menstruation and gout.[6]

Food, perfumery and flavouring

The oil is rarely used in flavours. It may be used in industrial perfumes, fragrances for detergents and household products.[2]

Other uses

Pennyroyal oil is mainly used as a starting material for the production of synthetic menthol, which is derived from pulegone.[2]

Therapeutics

Pharmacology and clinical studies

Acaricidal activity

The acaricidal activity of a range of essential oils was evaluated at different doses. Pennyroyal oil was found to be the most effective. At a dose of 0.025 $\mu l/cm^2$, at an exposure time of five minutes, more than 98% of house mites were killed. It was concluded that pennyroyal has potent acaricidal activity.[7]

Antibacterial activity

An in vitro study confirmed that pennyroyal oil displayed strong antibacterial activity against gram-positive bacteria, but not against gram-negative bacteria.[3]

Hepatotoxicity

Pennyroyal has been associated with severe hepatotoxicity and death. The main constituent of pennyroyal, R-(+)-pulegone, is biotransformed through the hepatic cytochrome P450 system to toxic intermediates, which can cause massive centrilobular hepatic necrosis.[8]

A study using mice confirmed that specific cytochrome P450 inhibitors, disulfiram and cimetidine, significantly mitigated the effects of pennyroyal toxicity, and do so more effectively than either agent alone.[8]

Insecticidal activity

Pennyroyal oil from Morocco was tested for its insecticidal activity against adult weevil, *Sitophilus oryzae* (L.). The oil tested was found to have a very high pulegone content (81.46%). The oil displayed strong fumigant effect against the adult weevils. It was reported that, at 2 μl of essential oil/ litre of air, the insects were totally decimated within four days. At lower concentrations, the entire population of the insects died within eight days of fumigation. It was concluded that the fumigant effect of pennyroyal oil against adult weevils could be explained by the high content of pulegone.[9]

Actions

Actions commonly cited in aromatherapy

Antiseptic, antispasmodic, carminative, diaphoretic, digestive, emmenagogue, insect repellent, refrigerant, stimulant[10,11]

Actions supported by clinical studies

Acaricidal, insecticidal

Comment

Considering the high percentage of ketones – pulegone and menthone – found in pennyroyal, and the well-documented cases of poisoning that have occurred from high doses, I do not recommend using pennyroyal oil in aromatherapy.

Pennyroyal oil may be considered at low dilution in pet care products as a flea repellent. However, I prefer that it be used in a wash-off product rather than a leave-on product.

Aromatherapy Uses

Clinical aromatherapy

Lavabre recommends pennyroyal oil for the treatment of dyspepsia, nausea, vomiting, amenorrhoea and dysmenorrhoea. It is also reputed to be an excellent flea and mosquito repellent.[10]

However, I recommend not using pennyroyal oil in aromatherapy.

Dosage and Administration

Blending

Aromatherapy

As pennyroyal is toxic and not recommended for use in aromatherapy, no aromatherapy blends are provided.

Perfumery

Pennyroyal oil is not used in perfumery.

Mode of administration

Bath

Pennyroyal oil is not recommended for use in a bath.

Topical

Pennyroyal oil is not recommended in topical leave-on products.

Inhalation

Pennyroyal oil is not recommended in a vaporiser or for inhalation purposes.

Safety Profile

General safety

Pennyroyal oil is considered toxic and an abortifacient. It is not recommended for use in aromatherapy.[11,13]

Tisserand & Young state that the maximum dermal use level is 1.3%.[12] This would equate to approximately 2 drops to every 10 mL of base oil.[12]

Contraindications

Tisserand & Young describe pennyroyal as a hepatotoxin and a neurotoxin. They also recommend that it is contraindicated for all routes during pregnancy and breastfeeding.[12]

Toxicity

The toxicity of pennyroyal oil is due to the pulegone content, which is toxic to the liver because it is metabolised to epoxides.[13,14]

Tisserand & Balacs report several fatalities involving the ingestion of pennyroyal.[13] One case involves that of an 18-year-old woman who died after ingesting the equivalent of 24 g of pulegone. She was alternately lethargic or agitated, suffered from nausea and abdominal pain, and developed massive hepatic necrosis and renal insufficiency.[15]

The emergency treatment for pennyroyal poisoning is the administration of N-acetylcysteine, as soon as possible after ingestion (140 mg/kg, then 70 mg/kg every four hours). N-acetylcysteine

P

is an antioxidant agent that protects against endotoxaemia.[14,15]

A pennyroyal oil dose of 500 mg/kg body weight produced extensive hepatic centrilobular necrosis, as well as pulmonary bronchiolar necrosis. The oil was then fractionated and tested. It was found that pulegone was the only fraction that was responsible for significant organ damage.[16]

Another study found that hepatic glutathione was reduced in concentration by 75% within three hours after the administration of pennyroyal and pulegone.[16]

High concentrations of pennyroyal to the skin will lead to significant absorption and result in acute toxicity of pulegone. They cite a case in which a 30 kg dog died after receiving a topical treatment for fleas of 60 mL of pure pennyroyal oil. Less than one hour after the treatment, the dog became listless and was shampooed in an attempt to remove the oil. Vomiting began two hours after the application and diarrhoea within 30 hours. Death followed seizures, even though supportive veterinary treatment was provided. Necropsy revealed haemorrhage into the thoracic cavity, congested and oedematous lungs with areas subpleural haemorrhages, and evidence of liver damage.[16]

Moderate to severe toxicity has been reported in humans from exposure to at least 10 mL of pennyroyal oil. There have been three cases of death reported as a result of ingesting pennyroyal to induce an abortion.[17]

P

Regulatory guidelines

Pennyroyal oil has GRAS status by the US Food and Drug Administration for usage in food at 0.59-22.43 ppm.[17]

References

1. Lawrence BM. *The composition of commercially important mints.* In Lawrence BM. ed. *Mint: the genus Mentha.* Taylor & Francis Group, London, 2007: 421-495.
2. Arctander S. *Perfume and flavor materials of natural origin.* Allured Publishing, Carol Stream, 1994.
3. Boukhebti H et al. *Chemical composition and antibacterial activity of Mentha pulegium L. and Mentha spicata L. essential oils.* Der Pharmacia Lettre, 2011; 3(4): 267-275.
4. Grieve M. *A modern herbal. Vol. II.* Dover Publications, New York. 1971.
5. Riddle J. *Eve's herbs.* Harvard University Press, Cambridge, 1997.
6. *British herbal pharmacopoeia.* British Herbal Medicine Association, Bournemouth, 1983.
7. Rim IS, Jee CH. *Acaricidal effects of herb essential oils against Dermatophagoides farinae and D. pteronyssinus (Acari: Pyroglyphidae) and qualitative analysis of a herb Mentha pulegium (pennyroyal).* Korean Journal of Parasitology, 2006; 44(2): 133-138.
8. Sztajnkrycer M et al. *Mitigation of pennyroyal oil hepatotoxicity in the mouse.* Academic Emergency Medicine, 10(10): 1024–1028. doi: 10.1197/S1069-6563(03)00337-3.
9. Zekri N. et al. *Phytochemical study and insecticidal activity of Mentha pulegium L. oils from Morocco against Sitophilus oryzae.* Mediterranean Journal of Chemistry, 2013; 2(4); 607-619. doi: 10.13171/mjc.2.4.2013.08.11.23.
10. Lavabre M. *Aromatherapy workbook.* Healing Arts Press, Rochester, 1997.
11. Lawless J. *The encyclopaedia of essential oils.* Element Books, Shaftesbury, 1992.
12. Tisserand R, Young R. *Essential oil safety.* 2nd edn. Churchill Livingstone, Edinburgh, 2014.
13. Tisserand R, Balacs T. *Essential oil safety.* Churchill Livingstone, Edinburgh, 1995.
14. McGuffin M et al. eds. *American herbal products association's botanical safety handbook.* CRC Press, Boca Raton, 1997.
15. Bruneton J. *Toxic plants.* Lavoisier Publishing, Paris, 1999.
16. Hayes J et al. *Biological and toxicological properties of mint oil and their major isolates: safety assessment.* In Lawrence BM. ed. *Mint: the genus Mentha.* Taylor & Francis Group, London, 2007: 421-495.
17. Tucker AO. *Mentha: economic uses.* In Lawrence BM. ed. *Mint: the genus Mentha.* Taylor & Francis Group, London, 2007: 519-527.

Peppermint

Identification

Botanical name

Mentha x *piperita* L.

Synonyms

Mitcham mint, mint

Family

Lamiaceae (Labiatae)

Botany and origins

The first botanical record of peppermint appeared in 1696 when the plant was collected in Hertfordshire (England) by Dr Eales. The plant was given the name peppermint because it resembled spearmint and it possessed a pepper-type taste. The botanical origin of peppermint is *Mentha* x *piperita* L, a natural hybrid of *Mentha aquatic* L. x *Mentha spicata* L.[1]

Peppermint is native to southern Europe and was brought to the USA in the early nineteenth century.[2] The United States is the major producer of peppermint.[2,3] Peppermint is also cultivated in Argentina, Brazil, France, Italy, Morocco, Bulgaria, The Netherlands, Spain, Germany, England, India and Australia.[2]

Peppermint is a perennial herb, growing to a height of 30 to 100 cm, and belonging to a genus consisting of some 20 varieties and hybrids.[3]

The various mints used to produce the mint oils are as follows:[4]

Name	Botanical name	Main constituent	%
peppermint	*M. x piperita*	menthol	29-46%
native spearmint	*M. spicata*	carvone	50-70%
scotch spearmint	*M. gracilis*	carvone	50-70%
cornmint	*M. arvensis*	menthol	70-95%
pennyroyal	*M. pulegium*	pulegone	60-90%
bergamot mint	*M. citrata*	linalyl acetate	57-63%

The major components of the different mints are menthol and pulegone. *M. arvensis*, also known as cornmint, Japanese mint or *hakka*, is cheaper to produce than peppermint and spearmint, and is often used as a 'blender' in mint flavours and as an adulterant in peppermint oil. Cornmint is considered more toxic than peppermint oil as it has a higher pulegone content.[4] *M. arvensis* grows wild in China and in parts of Japan. It is cultivated on a large scale in Japan, Brazil and Taiwan.[2]

Method of extraction

Peppermint oil is steam-distilled from the partially dried herb of *M.* x *piperita*.

Characteristics

Peppermint essential oil is a pale-yellow or pale-olive-coloured liquid with a fresh, strong grassy-minty odour, a deep balsamic-sweet undertone and a sweet, clean dryout note. The odour gives the impression of coolness, often due to the psychological effect of associating the known flavour with the impression of the odour.[2]

Cornmint essential oil is a pale yellow or almost colourless liquid with a strong, fresh and somewhat bittersweet aroma, very reminiscent of peppermint. The undertone is somewhat harsh-woody and the dryout is bitter herbaceous.[2]

Chemical composition

The chemical composition of peppermint oil was reported as follows:

menthol (40.0%), menthone (18.7%), 1,8-cineole (7.3%), methyl acetate (3.8%), menthofuran (3.0%), isomenthone (2.5%), limonene (2.5%), β-pinene (1.8%), α-pinene (1.4%), germacrene D (1.3%), *trans*-sabinene hydrate (1.0%), pulegone (0.8%).[5]

The European Pharmacopoeia has established the following limits for the major constituents found in peppermint oil:

menthol (30-55%), menthone (14-32%), 1,8-cineole (3.5-14%), methyl acetate (2.8-10%), menthofuran (1-9%), isomenthone (1.5-10%), limonene (1-5%), pulegone (<4%), carvone (<1%).[6]

The ratio of 1,8-cineole content to limonene content should be 2. To comply with the European Pharmacopoeia, peppermint oil must not contain more than 4% pulegone and not more than 1% carvone.[7]

Natural *M. arvensis* oil contains so much menthol that it may solidify at room temperature. By freezing the oil, about 40% menthol is recovered, leaving the so-called 'dementholised' oil, which is still liquid and still containing about 55% menthol.[2]

The chemical composition of cornmint oil from Japan was reported as follows:

menthol (76.8%-86.3%), menthone (2.8%-6.1%), menthyl acetate (2.7%-9.3%), isomenthone (0.8%-2.1%), limonene (0.7%-2.3%), β-pinene (0%-1.1%), α-pinene (0%-0.5%), pulegone (0%-0.8%), piperitone (1.4%-2.7%).[1]

Adulteration

Arctander states that peppermint oil is frequently adulterated with *M. arvensis*. He explains that modest addition of this oil can hardly be detected in chemical analysis, but an organoleptic test by an experienced flavourist will usually detect the adulteration. Menthyl acetate is also used in adulteration of peppermint. The USA has strict controls for the production of *M. arvensis* that make adulteration of true peppermint oil impossible; however, Arctander states that the adulteration of peppermint with cornmint is extremely widespread in other parts of the world.[2]

Pharmacopoeias and standards

The purity, composition and physico-chemical properties of peppermint oil are defined in several standards and monographs. The following pharmacopoeia and composition standards are

P

available:

- ISO 856:2006 – Oil of Peppermint (*Mentha* x *piperita* L.)
- WHO Monographs on Selected Medicinal Plants – Vol. 2
- German Commission E
- European Pharmacopoeia
- Community Herbal Monograph on *Mentha* x *Piperita* L., aetheroleum. European Medicines Agency.

Peppermint leaf herb is the subject of many international monographs.

History and Traditional Uses

History

The written history of mint dates back to an ancient Greek myth in which the god Pluto was said to have affections for a beautiful nymph named *Minthe*, but his jealous wife Persephone cast a spell on the nymph transforming her to a plant. When Pluto could not reverse the spell, he gave her a sweet scent associated with peppermint.[7]

Pliny tells us that the Greeks and Romans crowned themselves with peppermint at their feasts, and that peppermint was used to flavour their sauces and wines. Two species of mint were used by the ancient Greek physicians; however, neither is likely to be the *M. piperita* of today. It was only recognised as a distinct species in the seventeenth century.[8]

P

Culpeper was well aware of peppermint's excellent effect on the digestive system:

> *It is useful for complaints of the stomach, such as wind, vomiting … for which there are few remedies of greater efficacy.*[8]

The mints have been utilised for their medicinal properties for thousands of years, but the oil itself may not have been used as a medicine much before the sixteenth century when distillation reached England.[4]

Traditional medicine

The World Health Organization monograph reports that peppermint leaf herb is used in folk and traditional medicine as an emmenagogue, vermifuge, lactation enhancer and sedative. It is also used to treat bronchitis, bacillary dysentery, diabetes, diarrhoea, dysmenorrhoea, fevers, hypertension, jaundice, nausea, pain, and respiratory and urinary tract infections.[9]

Herbal

The German Commission E recommends peppermint oil internally for the treatment of spastic discomfort of the upper gastrointestinal tract and bile ducts, irritable colon, catarrhs of the respiratory system and inflammation of the oral mucosa. It is recommended externally for myalgia and neuralgia.[10]

According to the British Herbal Compendium, peppermint herb is used for the treatment of dyspepsia, flatulence, intestinal colic and biliary disorders.[11]

Bone & Mills state that the traditional therapeutic uses of peppermint include treatment of digestive disorders, flatulence, colic, cramps, nausea and vomiting, inhalation for respiratory disorders such as bronchitis, cough, colds and influenza, and topically for headaches and nervous disorders.[12]

Food, perfumery and flavouring

Peppermint oil is extensively used in food flavouring, as a fragrance component in toothpastes, mouthwashes, soaps, detergents and perfumes.[3]

Cornmint oil is extensively used in flavouring of candy, all types of toothpastes, mouthwashes and gargles.[2]

Therapeutics

Pharmacology and clinical studies

Many pharmacological studies involving peppermint essential oil have been published. A systemic review of these studies will not be attempted. Rather, I have chosen a selection of studies that support the traditional and clinical uses.

Analgesic

A randomised, double-blind, placebo-controlled crossover study examined the efficacy of a blend of eucalyptus oil and peppermint oil for the relief of headaches in 32 patients. Five different preparations were used:[13]

- 10 g peppermint oil and 5 g eucalyptus oil
- 10 g peppermint oil and traces of eucalyptus oil
- traces of peppermint oil and 5 g of eucalyptus oil
- traces of both peppermint and eucalyptus oil
- a placebo.

The preparations and the placebo were applied topically to the forehead and temples, and the neurophysiological, psychological parameters were measured. A significant analgesic effect, with a reduction in sensitivity to the headache, was produced with peppermint oil, whereas peppermint and eucalyptus together had little influence on pain sensitivity. However, it was reported that the combination had a mentally relaxing and muscle relaxing effect and improved cognitive performance.[13]

The effect of locally applied 10% peppermint oil in an ethanol solution on tension-type headaches was examined in a randomised, placebo-controlled, double-blind crossover study. Compared with the application of a placebo, the peppermint oil treatment, which was applied across the forehead and temples, significantly reduced the clinical headache intensity after 15 minutes. The reduction in pain intensity continued over a one-hour observation period. The patients all reported no adverse effects. This study confirmed that peppermint oil in a 10% ethanol solution efficiently alleviates tension-type headaches and is a well-tolerated and cost-effective alternative to other conventional therapies.[14]

Braun & Cohen cite research that indicates that menthol engages in synergistic excitation of GABA receptors and sodium ion channels, resulting in analgesia.[7]

Anti-inflammatory activity

A study examined the effectiveness of peppermint oil in reducing the symptoms of pruritis. 50 volunteers who were diagnosed with chronic pruritus were divided into two groups – group I was instructed to apply a 5% dilution of peppermint oil in a petrolatum base, and group II applied the petrolatum base without any essential oils. The results showed that there was a significant improvement for the peppermint oil users and no significant improvement among the petrolatum-only users.[15]

Antimicrobial activity

Peppermint oil and its main constituent menthol have significant antibacterial, antifungal and antiplasmid activities, and are able to potentiate the effect of some antibiotics.[7]

Lis-Balchin tested in vitro 18 different commercial samples of *M.* x *piperita* oils for antimicrobial activity against 25 bacterial species, 20 different strains of *Listeria monocytogenes* and three different filamentous fungi. Nine species of bacteria, including *Bacillus subtilis, Clostridium sporogenes, Enterobacter aerogenes, Micrococcus luteus* and *Proteus vulgaris,* were inhibited to varying degrees by all 18 samples of peppermint. *Streptococcus faecalis* and *Pseudomonas aeruginosa* were totally unaffected by any of the oils. One strain of *L. monocytogenes* was completely resistant.[16]

Peppermint oil and its components carvone, menthol and menthone were found to have strong antifungal activity against *Candida albicans, C. tropicalis* and *C. glabrate*. The average MIC of peppermint oil was 225 ug/ml. At MIC, the cell growth was completely terminated and clear zones of inhibition were observed. Peppermint oil also showed very low haemolysis in comparison to fluconazole.[17]

The antimicrobial activity of three mint species – *Mentha aquatica, Mentha piperita* and *Mentha longifolia* – were examined. All of the essential oils exhibited strong antibacterial activity, particularly against *Escherichia coli* strains, although two *P. aeruginosa* strains were completely resistant. The most effective antimicrobial oil was *M. piperita*. All oils had significant antifungal activity. All were considered more effective than the commercial fungicide, bifonazole.[18]

Antispasmodic activity

In vitro studies have confirmed the antispasmodic properties of peppermint oil.[7]

Lis-Balchin tested in vitro 18 different commercial samples of *Mentha x piperita* oils for antispasmodic activity. While the chemical composition of the oils varied – menthone (17-31%), menthol (32-49%), and menthofuran (5-12%) – the spasmolytic activity of all the samples at a 1/1000 dilution was consistent irrespective of their chemical composition. She concluded that the use of 'average' peppermint oil as an antispasmodic medicine was thus acceptable.[16]

Lis-Balchin states that the mode of action seems to be via cAMP rather than calcium or potassium channels.[19]

In one trial, peppermint oil was found to be beneficial in helping reduce colonic spasm during endoscopy.[12,20]

Antiviral activity

The inhibition of virus replication by peppermint oil was determined using a plaque reduction assay. At a concentration of 0.01%, peppermint oil reduced the herpes simplex virus type 1 (HSV-1) by 82% and HSV-2 by 92%. When peppermint oil was added to the cells prior to viral infection it had no effect, but pretreatment of the viruses or addition to the cells during adsorption reduced plaque formation by 79.8% and 72.9% respectively. The virucidal activity of peppermint oil was also found to be effective against the acyclovir-resistant strain of HSV-1. The activity of the virus was inhibited by 99%.[21]

It was concluded that peppermint oil exerts antiviral activity before or during adsorption, but not after penetration of the virus into the cells. The researchers also stated that the infectivity of the virus was reduced due to direct interaction of the oil with the viral envelope and glycoproteins.[21]

Choleretic activity

The choleretic activity of peppermint oil has been confirmed. Peppermint oil and two common essential oil constituents, limonene and geranyl acetate, were tested for their effect on bile secretion in rats. The three substances were individually administered to the animals via a cannulated bile duct, and the choleretic activity was calculated on the percentage increase in bile collected every 30 minutes for four hours. The results indicated that peppermint exhibited the strongest choleretic activity.[22]

The action of peppermint on morphine-induced contraction and blockage of Oddi's sphincter in guinea pigs was investigated. Five minutes after the blockage was induced, the oil was injected and the effect on morphine spasm was noted. Peppermint was found to exhibit a pronounced spasmolytic effect.[23]

Balacs cites research which found that peppermint oil exerts its inhibitory effect by interfering with the mobilisation of calcium ions into the tissue. Calcium was implicated in the relaxant effect of peppermint in isolated human gut, and it was discovered that menthol was responsible. Menthol reduces the calcium influx through voltage-dependent channels.[24]

Peppermint oil displayed a relaxing effect on the gall bladder and slowed intestinal transit, inhibiting gall bladder emptying and prolonging orocaecal transit time in a manner comparable to N-butylscopolamine.[25]

Braun & Cohen cite studies confirming that peppermint oil promoted bile acid secretion and decreased cholesterol levels in bile. The oil has been shown to up-regulate bile acid synthesis-related genes, suggesting that the pharmacological mechanism is related to gene expression involved in bile acid synthesis.[7]

Cooling activity

Peppermint oil often raises a contradiction concerning its warming and cooling effects. It is often listed as having a cooling action; however, Holmes clearly states that it has a warming effect.[26]

Mills attributes this contradictory effect to menthol, a monoterpene alcohol whose physical properties impart a noticeable cooling effect to the skin (vasoconstriction), later followed by pronounced vasodilation and rubefacient effect. This is also accompanied by a slight anaesthetic action (due at least in part to an excitation of cold receptors).[27]

The transient receptor potential channel melastatin 8 (TRPM8) is a non-selective cation channel on primary afferent nerve fibres activated by noxious and innocuous cool temperatures. TRPM8 is the predominant thermoreceptor for cellular and behavioural responses to cold temperatures. It is now known that TRPM8 is also activated by compounds that evoke cooling sensations such as menthol.[12]

Gastrointestinal activity

A double-blind, placebo-controlled multicentre trial involving 45 patients investigated the effects of a blend of peppermint and caraway on non-ulcer dyspepsia. A commercial product, Enteroplant, consisting of 90 mg of peppermint oil and 50 mg of caraway oil in an enteric-coated capsule, was given to patients three times daily for four weeks. By the end of the treatment, 63.2% of patients were free from pain, whereas before treatment all patients reported moderate to severe pain. Overall symptoms had improved in 89.9% of cases. Compared with the placebo, Enteroplant was superior in reducing pain frequency, medical prognosis and the severity of the disorder.[28]

Clinical trials involving patients who had just had a colostomy found that peppermint oil helped to reduce much of the distress associated with a colostomy. Patients were given oral doses of enteric-coated capsules containing peppermint. Peppermint was chosen as it not only had an odour that would mask the odour from the colostomy bag, but also because of its effect on the smooth muscle of the bowel. It was found to reduce colonic pressure and prevent foaming, all of which helped to reduce postoperative colic and the frequency of bag change.[29]

In a literature search, 16 clinical trials using 180-200 mg enteric-coated capsules of peppermint oil for the treatment of irritable bowel syndrome (IBS) involving 65 patients were identified. Nine out of the 16 studies were randomised, double-blind crossover trials. Placebo was used in 12 of the studies, and anticholinergics in three studies were used as comparator. The average response rate in terms of 'overall success' was 58% for peppermint oil and 29% for the placebo. It was concluded that enteric-coated peppermint oil may be the drug of first choice in IBS patients with non-serious constipation or diarrhoea to alleviate symptoms and to improve the quality of life.[30]

Fifty-five patients with IBS were treated with peppermint oil (two enteric-coated capsules twice per day or placebo) for four weeks in a double-blind study. The study confirmed that there was a statistically significant reduction of the symptoms associated with IBS, while no change was found with the placebo.[31]

A systemic review and meta-analysis of randomised controlled trials confirmed that peppermint oil was more effective than placebo in the treatment of IBS.[32]

A literature search up to February 2013 identified all the randomised-controlled trials that examined the efficacy and safety of enteric-coated peppermint oil capsules compared with a placebo for the treatment of active IBS. The study quality was evaluated using the Cochrane Risk of Bias Tool. Nine studies that evaluated 726 patients were identified. Peppermint oil was found to be significantly superior to the placebo for global improvement of IBS symptoms and improvement in abdominal pain. It was concluded that peppermint oil is a safe and effective short-term treatment for IBS.[33]

By reducing the calcium influx, peppermint oil is able to induce smooth muscle relaxation within the gastrointestinal (GI) tract. Peppermint oil must be formulated with a delayed release enteric coating to ensure delivery to the lower GI tract and colon. The inappropriate release of peppermint oil in the upper GI tract induces relaxation of the lower esophageal sphincter, leading to reflux and heartburn, the primary adverse effects of peppermint oil.[34]

Researchers stated that it is evident that peppermint oil has a physiological effect on gut motility through mediating calcium release and enhancing smooth muscle contraction.

Apart from the spasmolytic effects, peppermint oil also has an anti-inflammatory and antimicrobial activity. Using lipopolysaccharide (LPS)-stimulated monocytes from healthy volunteers, researchers were able to confirm the anti-inflammatory activity of *l*-menthol on the levels of arachidonic acid metabolism into LTB4 (leukotriene B4) and PGE2 (prostaglandin E2), which served as markers for lipoxygenase and cyclooxygenase pathways. Results indicated that *l*-menthol significantly reduced LTB4, PGE2 and IL-1B production at low doses and in a dose-dependent manner, thereby serving as an anti-inflammatory agent.[34]

Additionally, peppermint oil has been shown to inhibit the proliferation of *Helicobacter pylori, Salmonella enteritidis* and *Escherichia coli.* It was stated that, given the relationship between small intestinal bacterial overgrowth and IBS, the antimicrobial activity of peppermint oil in the small intestines may provide another mechanism for the symptomatic improvement of IBS.[34]

Insecticidal activity

The larvicidal and repellent potential of peppermint oil was assessed against the larval and adult stages of *Aedes aegypti*. The study confirmed that peppermint essential oil is an efficient larvicide and repellent against *Aedes aegypti*. The investigations found that peppermint oil offered 150 minutes of complete protection time with 0.1 mL of neat essential oil applied to the arms of the volunteer. After 150 minutes the repellency efficacy of the oil began to decrease. The percentage repellency decreased to 93.2% after 165 minutes and 73.1% after 180 minutes.[35]

Nausea and vomiting

The results of a study evaluating the effects of peppermint oil on nausea and vomiting during pregnancy found that there was no statistically significant difference between the peppermint group and the placebo group. The results of this study suggested that peppermint oil did not affect nausea and vomiting during pregnancy.[36]

A randomised, double-blind clinical trial examined the efficacy of *M. spicata* and *M.* x *piperita* essential oils in preventing chemotherapy-induced nausea and vomiting. The results of this study found that there was a significant reduction in the intensity and number of emetic events in the first 24 hours from both spearmint and peppermint oils when compared with the control group.[37]

A randomised trial investigated the role of aromatherapy on patients experiencing postoperative nausea. A blend of ginger, peppermint, spearmint and cardamom was used in the study. Over 300 patients participated in the trial. The number of antiemetic medications requested after aromatherapy intervention was significantly reduced.[38]

Performance enhancement

Twenty-one healthy volunteers completed a study to examine the effect of peppermint oil on sleep, alertness and mood when presented before bedtime. Peppermint oil was found to reduce fatigue and improve mood. The subjects who rated peppermint oil as very intense had more total sleep than those who rated it as moderately intense. This indicated more slow-wave sleep. It also increased the NREM sleep in women, but not in men, where the alertness was more evident than women. It was suggested that there are many individual factors influencing the results on the physiological sleep, self-rated mood and alertness.[39]

Twelve healthy male students consumed one 500 mL bottle of water each containing 0.05 mL of peppermint essential oil daily for 10 days. The blood pressure, heart rate and spirometry parameters, including forced vital capacity, peak expiratory flow rate and peak inspiratory flow, were determined one day before and then one day after the supplementation period. Participants also underwent a treadmill-based exercise test with metabolic gas analysis. The results of the experiment support the effectiveness of peppermint oil on exercise performance. It was suggested that the relaxation of the bronchial smooth muscles, increase in the ventilation and brain oxygen concentration, and decrease in the blood lactate level are the most plausible explanations.[40]

Respiratory system activity

Menthol exhibited a surfactant-like effect in an in vitro study. Menthol inhalation produced a significant reduction in cough frequency and an increase in cough latency in guinea pigs, demonstrating the efficacy of menthol as an antitussive in chemically induced coughs.[12]

Menthol is considered a nasal decongestant. This is linked to the cool sensation thought to be due to the stimulation of the nasal cavity thermoreceptors.[41]

Actions

Actions commonly cited in aromatherapy

Analgesic, antidepressant, antineuralgic, antiphlogistic, antiseptic, antispasmodic, astringent, carminative, cephalic, cholagogue, cordial, decongestant, digestive, emmenagogue, expectorant, febrifuge, hepatic, nervine, stimulant (nervous system), stomachic, sudorific, vasoconstrictor, vermifuge[42,43,44]

Actions supported by clinical studies

Analgesic, antifungal, antineuralgic, antibacterial, antiviral, carminative, cholagogue, digestive, stimulant, stomachic

Comment

Review of traditional uses and clinical data support peppermint's role in relieving digestive ailments. The EMA report for peppermint oil states that there is well-established evidence to use peppermint oil for the symptomatic relief of minor spasms of the gastrointestinal tract, flatulence and abdominal pain. Topically, it is confirmed to be effective for the symptomatic relief of mild tension-type headaches.[45]

Aromatherapy Uses

Clinical aromatherapy

Analgesic

Peppermint oil is used in liniments for the relief of muscle pain, lumbago, bruises and contusions, joint pain and insect bites. The local anaesthetic action of peppermint is significant. The oil is recommended for myalgia and neuralgia.[10,42]

The EMA recommends the topical application and inhalation of peppermint oil for the relief of localised muscle pain.[45] Schnaubelt states that peppermint oil liberally applied in a 15% dilution in rubbing alcohol to the forehead, neck and shoulders will help alleviate and treat migraine headaches.[46]

Digestive system

Peppermint is one of the most effective essential oils for the digestive system. It relieves dyspepsia, nausea, vomiting, stomach pains, diarrhoea and flatulence.[42,43,44,46,47]

The German Commission E recommends peppermint oil for obstructions of the bile ducts, gall bladder inflammations and severe liver damage.[10]

Peppermint oil enhances production of bile. The choleretic effect of peppermint oil has an antispasmodic action, decreasing abdominal distension and abdominal pain.[45]

Many studies confirm that enteric-coated peppermint oil capsules are effective for the relief of conditions such as irritable bowel syndrome. When taking capsules for gastrointestinal relief, symptoms should resolve within one to two weeks. At times when symptoms are more persistent, the intake of gastro-resistant capsules can be continued for periods of no longer than three months.[45]

Integumentary system

The EMA recommends the topical application and inhalation of peppermint oil for the relief of localised pruritic conditions in intact skin.[45]

Lymphatic system

Gumbel states that peppermint oil has a special affinity with the blood and lymph, and that peppermint's refreshing effect on all the tissues lies in the liberating influence on the lymphatic system. He explains that the oil's vasoconstrictive effect increases blood flow to the spleen, stimulating the regenerative activity of the spleen in the development of new blood corpuscles. The lymphatic system is activated in its function through accelerated lymph and tissue fluid circulation.[48]

Nervous system

Cold compresses of peppermint oil may be applied to the forehead and temples to relieve headaches and migraines.[42,43,46,47]

Psychological

Holmes states that peppermint oil promotes motivation, self-confidence and alertness. He recommends it for loss of motivation, low self-esteem and self-confidence, and distressed feelings in general.[49]

Fischer-Rizzi states that peppermint oil helps people become clear-headed and refreshes the spirits. She explains that it is beneficial for people who are unable to concentrate or who have mental fatigue and memory lapses.[50]

Respiratory system

Peppermint oil is beneficial for fevers and headaches associated with colds and influenza. It is recommended at the onset of a cold to alleviate the symptoms of cold.[17] It is beneficial for sinus congestion, infection or inflammation.[42,43,46]

The EMA recommends the topical application and inhalation of peppermint oil for the relief of symptoms of coughs and colds.[45]

Skin care

Davis recommends a steam treatment with peppermint to cleanse and decongest the skin.[17] It cools by constricting the capillaries and is a very refreshing skin tonic.[47]

Energetics, psyche and subtle uses

Energetics

Mojay states that peppermint is *cooling* and *drying*.[44] Holmes states that peppermint oil activates *Qi* and strengthens the *Shen*. He also explains that it helps to balance the *Middle Heater* and *Stomach Qi* to descend, to help alleviate indigestion, appetite loss, epigastric bloating, distension and abdominal pain.[49]

It tonifies the Wood Element and helps to balance the Earth Element. Mojay states that it strengthens the Intellect (*Yi*), the spirit associated with the Earth Element. The *Yi* helps us to assimilate new ideas and provides us with a clear mind.[44]

Personality

Worwood describes the peppermint personality as difficult to forget. Some may find them brash and overpowering. They have a fearless spirit, and are swift and quick thinkers. They are friendly people who are concerned about the fate of others. Whatever work they take on, they are always dynamic and get totally involved.[51]

Peppermint personalities are described as 'the salesmen of life'. They make excellent speakers and have a quick intellect. They require a job that is both physically and mentally challenging. It must combine mental agility and physical stamina to be truly satisfying for them.[51]

According to Myers-Briggs personality types, the peppermint personality is likely to be an ENTJ. ENTJs are dynamic, energetic, confident and competent. They naturally move into positions where they can take charge. They enjoy confrontation and they like to engage in intellectually stimulating exchanges. They like and respect people who challenge them and have little or no respect for those that don't. They have an improvement plan for everything, including their leisure. They like to set goals and provide directions. They see obstacles as challenges. They dislike inefficiency, incompetence and indecisiveness. They are competitively driven and often considered to be workaholics. They can be very honest and direct and do not hesitate to express themselves. When stressed, they can have explosive outbursts or be judgemental on themselves and others.

Subtle

Davis states that peppermint oil acts on the ego, dispelling pride. She recommends using it to help overcome feelings of inferiority. It is associated with cleanliness and assists people who wish to live an ethical life.[52]

Mojay states, that while peppermint oil enhances concentration, it works on another level to facilitate the digestion of new ideas. He explains that it is the type of oil that enhances our receptive capacities on both mental and spiritual levels, and would be beneficial for those in need of inspiration and insight.[44]

Keim Loughran & Bull state that peppermint oil helps to clarify the chakras. It promotes healthy self-esteem, integrity and ethics associated with the solar plexus chakra, and it promotes clarity of communication associated with the throat chakra. It also strengthens our third eye chakra by stimulating the conscious mind and promoting inspiration and insight.[53]

Worwood explains that peppermint oil can energise us whenever we feel lethargic and feel that all is lost. She also explains that it can stimulate our dream time. It increases sensitivity, awareness and perception of our dreams so that we can remember them and take on the wisdom of other worlds.[54]

Zeck explains that the stimulating qualities of peppermint oil help you sustain the energy you require to maintain focus and balance. She explains that peppermint will help you connect with your passion and live life with purpose.[55]

Dosage and Administration

Blending

Aromatherapy

For the relief of indigestion, spasms, and irritable bowel, consider blending peppermint oil with essential oils such as aniseed, caraway seed, coriander seed, sweet fennel, ginger, sweet orange or spearmint.

For the relief of nausea, consider blending peppermint oil with ginger essential oil.

For the relief of sinus and bronchial congestion, consider blending peppermint oil with essential oils such as cajeput, 1,8-cineole-rich eucalypts, peppermint eucalyptus, fir, hyssop, niaouli, pine or spruce.

For the relief of muscular aches and pains and arthritis, consider blending peppermint oil with essential oils such as black pepper, cajeput, ginger, kunzea, spike lavender, rosemary or wintergreen.

For the relief of mental fatigue, consider blending peppermint oil with essential oils such as basil, black pepper, ginger, lemon, pine or rosemary.

Perfumery

Peppermint oil is occasionally used in perfumes for its general lifting effect at low concentrations. It is typically used in lavender colognes, fougères and geranium bases.[2]

To the perfumer, anything that smells cool and fresh would be classified as minty. Peppermint is definitely minty and can be used in perfumery to provide a cool, fresh, mint top note. The minty scent can be used to convey freshness and a natural outdoors impression.[56]

Mode of administration

Bath

Full body bath, foot bath

Topical

Compress, massage, ointment, skin care

Inhalation

Direct inhalation, diffuser, oil vaporiser

Ingestion

For irritable colon, the German Commission E monograph for peppermint oil recommends internal daily dose of 0.6 mL in an enteric-coated capsule.[10]

The capsules should be swallowed whole. If broken or chewed, this will release the peppermint oil prematurely causing local irritation of the mouth and oesophagus and possibly causing heartburn.[45] The EMA states that oral use of enteric-coated peppermint oil capsules is not recommended for children under eight years of age as there is insufficient research available.

Safety Profile

General safety

Peppermint oil is non-toxic, non-irritant and may occasionally be sensitising.[43]

Menthol vapours inhibit respiration and may cause very transient apnoea in very young children. The risk is said to be minimal, yet direct application of peppermint oil or menthol on the nasal mucosa of very young children is discouraged.[12,39]

The German Commission E recommends that preparations containing peppermint oil should not be used on the face, particularly the nose, of infants and small children.[10]

The only concern regarding the use of peppermint oil is to select peppermint oils with a lower percentage of menthone and pulegone. Tisserand suggests that levels of both these two constituents in peppermint oil is unlikely to produce any toxic effects when the oil is used externally, but caution may be required regarding oral use.[4]

Lawless recommends using peppermint oil instead of cornmint. She explains that cornmint is often fractionated as it is more commonly used for flavouring. She states that cornmint is non-toxic, non-irritant, but may cause sensitisation in some individuals.[43]

Contraindications

Tisserand & Young state that peppermint oil should be avoided altogether in cases of cardiac fibrillation and individuals with G6PD deficiency. They explain that this is an inherited enzyme deficiency that can be found in people of Chinese, West African, Mediterranean or Middle Eastern origin. People with G6PD deficiency will typically have abnormal blood reactions to drugs such as antimalarials, sulfonamides, chloramphenicol, streptomycin and aspirin.[57]

Regulatory guidelines

Peppermint essential oil has GRAS status.

References

1. Lawrence BM. *The composition of commercially important mints.* In Lawrence BM. ed. *Mint: the genus Mentha.* Taylor & Francis Group, London, 2007: 217-323.
2. Arctander S. *Perfume and flavor materials of natural origin.* Allured Publishing, Carol Stream, 1994.
3. Khan I, Abourashed E. *Leung's Encyclopedia of common natural ingredients used in food, drugs and cosmetics.* 3rd edn. John Wiley & Sons, New Jersey, 2010.
4. Tisserand R. *Mint family matters.* The International Journal of Aromatherapy, 1992; 4(1): 20.
5. Lawrence BM. *Essential oils 1981-1987.* Allured Publishing, Wheaton, 1989
6. *European pharmacopoeia.* 3rd edn. Council of Europe, Strasbourg, 1996.
7. Braun L, Cohen M. *Herbs & natural supplements: an evidence-based guide – Vol. 2.* 4th edn. Elsevier, Chatswood, 2015.

8. Le Strange R. *A history of herbal plants*. Angus and Robertson, United Kingdom, 1977.
9. *WHO monographs on selected medicinal plants – Vol. 2*. World Health Organization, Geneva, 2004.
10. Blumenthal M et al. *The complete German commission E monographs: therapeutic guide to herbal medicine*. American Botanical Council, Austin, 1998.
11. British Herbal Medicine Association Scientific Committee. *British Herbal Pharmacopoeia*. BHMA, Bournemouth, 1983.
12. Bone K, Mills S. *Principles and practice of phytotherapy*. 2nd edn. Churchill Livingstone, Edinburgh, 2013.
13. Göbel H et al. *Effect of peppermint and eucalyptus oil preparations on neurophysiological and experimental algesimetric headache parameters*. Cephalalgia, 1994; 14(3): 228-234. doi: 10.1046/j.1468-2982.1994.014003228.x.
14. Göbel H et al. *Effectiveness of Oleum menthae piperitae and paracetamol in therapy of headache of the tension type*. Nervenarzt, 1996; 67(8): 672-681. Cited in Quintessential Aromatics database, 2013.
15. Elsaie LT et al. *Effectiveness of topical peppermint oil on symptomatic treatment of chronic pruritus*. Clinical, Cosmetic and Investigational Dermatology, 2016; 9: 333-338. doi: 10.2147/CCID.S116995.
16. Lis-Balchin M et al. *A study of the variability of commercial peppermint oils using antimicrobial and pharmacological parameters*. Medical Science Research, 1997; 25(3): 151-152. Cited in Quintessential Aromatics database, 2013.
17. Samber N et al. *Evaluation of Mentha piperita essential oil and its major constituents for antifungal activity in Candida ssp.* International Journal of Innovative Research in Science, Engineering and Technology, 2014; 3(2): 9404-9411.
18. Mimica-Dukic N et al. *Antimicrobial and antioxidant activities of three Mentha species essential oils*. Planta Medica, 2003; 69(5): 413-419. Cited in Quintessential Aromatics database, 2013.
19. Lis-Balchin M. *Aromatherapy science – a guide for healthcare professionals*. Pharmaceutical Press, London, 2006.
20. Leicester R et al. *Peppermint oil to reduce colonic spasm during endoscopy*. Lancet, 1983; 2(8395): 989.
21. Schumacher A et al. *Virucidal effect of peppermint oil on the enveloped viruses Herpes simplex virus type 1 and type 2 in vitro*. Phytomedicine, 2003; 10(6/7): 504-510. Cited in Quintessential Aromatics database, 2013.
22. Trabace L et al. *Choleretic activity of some typical components of essential oils*. Planta Medica, 1992; 58(Suppl 1): a650-651. Cited in the Aromatherapy Database, by Bob Harris, Essential Oil Resource Consultants, 2000.
23. Giachetti D, et al. *Pharmacological activity of essential oils on Oddi's sphincter*. Planta Medica, 1988; 54(5): 389-392. Cited in the Aromatherapy Database, by Bob Harris, Essential Oil Resource Consultants, 2000.
24. Balacs T. *Peppermint pharmacology*. The International Journal of Aromatherapy, 1992; 4(1): 22.
25. Goerg KJ, Spilker TH. *Effect of peppermint oil and caraway oil on gastrointestinal motility in healthy volunteers: a pharmacodynamic study using simultaneous determination of gastric and gall-bladder emptying and orocaecal transit time*. Alimentary Pharmacology and Therapeutics, 2003; 17: 445-451. doi: 10.1046/j.0269-2813.2003.01421.x.
26. Holmes P. *The energetics of Western herbs – Vol. I*. Artemis Press, Boulder, 1989.
27. Mills S. *The essential book of herbal medicine*. Arkana Penguin Books, England, 1991.
28. May B et al. *Efficacy of a fixed peppermint oil/caraway combination in non-ulcer dyspepsia*. Azneimittel-Forschung, 1996; 46(12): 1149-1153. Cited in Quintessential Aromatics database, 2013.
29. Gallacher M et al. *A sweet smell of success*. Nursing Times, July 5, 1989; 85(27): 48.
30. Grigoleit HG, Grigoleit P. *Peppermint oil in irritable bowel syndrome*. Phytomedicine, 2005; 12(8): 601-606. Cited in Quintessential Aromatics database, 2013.
31. Cappello G et al. *Peppermint oil (Mintoil ®) in the treatment of irritable bowel syndrome: a prospective double blind placebo-controlled randomized trial*. Digestive and Liver Disease, 2007; 39(6): 530-536. Cited in Quintessential Aromatics database, 2013.
32. Ford AC et al. *Effect of fibre, antispasmodics and peppermint oil in the treatment of irritable bowel syndrome: systematic review and meta-analysis*. BMJ, 2008; 337: a2313. doi: 10.1136/bmj.a2313.
33. Khanna R et al. *Peppermint oil for the treatment of irritable bowel syndrome: a systematic review and meta-analysis.* Journal of Clinical Gastroenterology, 2014; 48(6): 505-512. doi: 10.1097/MCG.0b013e3182a88357.
34. Shams R et al. *Peppermint oil: clinical uses in the treatment of gastrointestinal diseases*. JSM Gastroenterology and Hepatology, 2015; 3(1): 1036.
35. Kumar S et al. *Bioefficacy of Mentha piperita essential oil against dengue fever mosquito Aedes aegypti L*. Asian Pacific Journal of Tropical Biomedicine, 2011; 1(2): 85-88. doi: 10.1016/S2221-1691(11)60001-4.
36. Pasha H et al. *Study of the effect of mint oil on nausea and vomiting during pregnancy*. Iranian Red Crescent Medical Journal, 2012; 14(11): 744-747. Cited in Quintessential Aromatics database, 2013.

37. Tayarani-Najaran Z et al. *Antiemetic activity of volatile oil from Mentha spicata and Mentha x piperita in chemotherapy-induced nausea and vomiting*. Ecancermedicalscience, 2013; 7: 290. doi: 10.3332/ecancer.2013.290. Cited in Quintessential Aromatics database, 2013.
38. Hunt R et al. *Aromatherapy as treatment for postoperative nausea: a randomized trial*. Anesthesia and Analgesia, 2013; 117(3): 597-604. Cited in Quintessential Aromatics database, 2013.
39. *Mentha – peppermint oil (Menthae piperitae aetheroleum)*. Retrieved Oct 5, 2017, from https://herbalref.com/mentha-peppermint-oil-menthae-piperitae-aetheroleum/
40. Meamarbashi A, Rajabi A. *The effects of peppermint on exercise performance*. Journal of the International Society of Sports Nutrition, 2013; 10: 15.
41. Bruneton J. *Pharmacognosy*. 2nd edn. Lavoisier Publishing, Paris, 1999.
42. Lavabre M. *Aromatherapy workbook*. Healing Arts Press, Rochester, 1997.
43. Lawless J. *The encyclopaedia of essential oils*. Element Books, Shaftesbury, 1992.
44. Mojay G. *Aromatherapy for healing the spirit*. Healing Arts Press, Rochester, 1999.
45. Committee on Herbal Medicinal Products (HMPC). *Community herbal monograph on Mentha x Piperita L. aetheroleum*. European Medicines Agency, London, 2007. EMEA/HMPC/349466/2006
46. Schnaubelt K. *Medical aromatherapy*. Frog, Berkeley, 1999.
47. Davis P. *Aromatherapy: an A-Z*. 2nd edn. C.W. Daniel Company, Saffron Walden, 1999.
48. Gumbel D. *Principles of holistic skin therapy with herbal essences*. Karl F Haug Publishers, Heidelberg, 1986.
49. Holmes P. *Aromatica: a clinical guide to essential oil therapeutics – Vol. I*. Singing Dragon, London, 2016.
50. Fischer-Rizzi S. *Complete aromatherapy handbook*. Stirling Publishing, New York, 1989.
51. Worwood VA. *The fragrant mind*. Transworld Publishers, London, 1995.
52. Davis P. *Subtle aromatherapy*. C.W. Daniel Company, Saffron Walden, 1991.
53. Keim Loughran J, Bull R. *Aromatherapy and subtle energy techniques*. Frog, Berkeley, 2000.
54. Worwood VA. *The fragrant heavens*. Transworld Publishers, London, 1999.
55. Zeck R. *The blossoming heart – aromatherapy for healing and transformation*. Aroma Tours, East Ivanhoe, 2004.
56. Doyle J. *The mint note in perfumery*. Perfumer & Flavorist, 1998; 23: 13-18.
57. Tisserand R, Young R. *Essential oil safety*. 2nd edn. Churchill Livingstone, Edinburgh, 2014.

Petitgrain

Identification

Botanical name

Citrus x aurantium L.

Synonyms

Citrus bigaradia, petitgrain bigarade

Family

Rutaceae

Botany and origins

Petitgrain oil is produced from the leaves of the bitter orange. It is an evergreen tree with long but not very sharp spines and very fragrant flowers. It is a native of southern China and northeastern India.[1] The tree is cultivated in mild-temperate, semitropical and tropical areas of the world such as the south of France, Italy, Algeria, Tunisia, Morocco, Spain, West Africa and Paraguay. Haiti has become the largest producer of petitgrain oil; however, it has a cruder odour than the French oil because of the poorer distillation techniques.[2]

The word petitgrain is derived from the French word meaning 'little seed', referring to the small unripe fruits from which the oil was originally obtained. The name was retained when the leaves and twigs became the main source.[3] Oils obtained from the leaves of other citrus species such as lemon, bergamot and mandarin may also be labelled petitgrain.[3]

The oil produced from Paraguay is referred to as 'petitgrain Paraguay', while the oil from France is referred to as 'petitgrain bigarade'.[2]

It has been suggested that the oil from France is of a superior quality. This is because the French producers are careful to only use the leaf and not include any of the wooden branches, nor any small unripe fruit.[4]

During the distillation, it is important to ensure that the leaf matter is distilled rapidly with wet steam to prevent hydrolysis of linalyl acetate, the most important constituent of petitgrain.[4]

Method of extraction

Petitgrain is steam-distilled from the leaves of

C. aurantium.

Characteristics

Bigarade petitgrain oil is a pale yellow or amber-coloured liquid of pleasant, fresh-floral, sweet odour, reminiscent of orange flowers, with a slightly woody-herbaceous undertone and very faint but sweet-floral dryout.[2]

Paraguay petitgrain oil is very similar to bigarade petitgrain oil, although its top note is slightly harsh, quickly giving way to a heavy and sweet body note of a typical petitgrain character.[2]

Chemical composition

There can be a wide variation in the chemistry of petitgrain oils from country to country and region to region. For example, the percentage of linalyl acetate was as follows: France (64-68%), Paraguay (35-55%), Brazil (50-80%), Sicily (50-75%) and Algeria (25-35%), and the percentage of linalool was as follows: Paraguay (min 54%), Brazil (5-10%), Sicily (10-20%) and Algeria (30-40%).[3]

The most important constituent that defines the quality of petitgrain is linalyl acetate.[2]

The major constituents found in five samples of petitgrain oil from Italy was reported as follows:

β-pinene (0.65-1.15%), limonene (0.44-2.17%), myrcene (0.56-1.24%), linalool (21.7-32.55%), α-terpineol (3.09-5.63%), nerol (0.75-0.99%), neral (0.21-0.43%), geraniol (0.71-0.95%), linalyl acetate (50.68-62.57%), geranial (0.38-0.64%), neryl acetate (1.04-1.73%), geranyl acetate (1.9-3.16%).[5]

Adulteration

Arctander states that petitgrain oil is often adulterated with synthetic chemicals such as nerone, a methanyl ketone, which has a similar 'petitgrain note'; however, it is not present in the natural oil.[2] Petitgrain essential oil is subject to adulteration by the addition of limonene and rectified orange terpenes.[6] Lis-Balchin states that lemongrass, citral, lemon oil, *Leptospermum citratum* and orange oil fractions can all be used to adulterate petitgrain. Petitgrain oil is used as an adulterant for the expensive neroli oil.[7]

Pharmacopoeias and standards

The purity, composition and physiochemical properties of petitgrain essential oil from Paraguay are defined in ISO 3064:2014 Essential Oil of Petitgrain, Paraguayan Type [*Citrus aurantium* L. var. Paraguay (syn. *Citrus aurantium* L. var. *bigaradia* Hook f.)].

History and Traditional Uses

History

Most of the petitgrain oil available today comes from Paraguay. The plant was introduced to Paraguay in the eighteenth century by Spanish Jesuits.[3]

Herbal

As petitgrain oil is produced for the perfume and fragrance industry, there are no herbal uses.

Food, perfumery and flavouring

Petitgrain is an important raw material for perfumery, especially for eau de cologne and for scenting soaps. The oil is also widely used as a flavour component in most food products, including alcoholic and non-alcoholic beverages.[1,2]

Therapeutics

Pharmacology and clinical studies

Antibacterial activity

Lis-Balchin cites several studies that confirm that petitgrain oil has strong antibacterial activity.[7]

Antifungal activity

Lis-Balchin cites several studies that confirm that petitgrain oil has moderate antifungal activity.[7] However, another study confirmed that petitgrain oil had strong antifungal activity against a range of pathogenic fungi. The researchers recommended that petitgrain oil was particularly effective for its action against yeasts.[8]

Antispasmodic activity

Petitgrain oil has spasmogenic effect on electrically stimulated smooth muscle guinea pig ileum in vitro followed by spasmolysis.[7]

Actions

Actions commonly cited in aromatherapy

Antidepressant, antispasmodic, deodorant, digestive, sedative, stomachic[9,10,11]

Actions supported by clinical studies

Antibacterial, antifungal, antispasmodic

Comment

Petitgrain has a pleasant, citrus-like aroma with a diverse chemical composition of monoterpene hydrocarbons, monoterpene alcohols and esters, which gives the oil its antimicrobial, uplifting and sedative properties and balancing effect on the nervous system.

While more studies are required, I would suggest the use of petitgrain oil for improving mood and reducing symptoms of stress-induced disorders such as anxiety and depression.

Aromatherapy Uses

Clinical aromatherapy

Digestive system

Petitgrain oil is a digestive and antispasmodic and is recommended for the treatment of dyspepsia.[10,11]

Nervous system

Petitgrain oil has a stabilising effect on the nervous system.[12] It is uplifting and refreshing and is recommended for nervous exhaustion and stress-related conditions.[11,12] It is similar to neroli in its action, though the latter is considered more effective with serious states of depression.[9,10] It is relaxing and may be used for the treatment of insomnia.[9,10,11]

Petitgrain oil is recommended for people with insomnia stemming from anguish due to solitude, and from emotional shortcomings that generate increasing troubles.[13]

Mailhebiau refers to petitgrain oil as a 'rhythmic essence'. He explains that it can alleviate psychophysiological tension.[13]

Respiratory system

Petitgrain oil is recommended for the control of asthma in people with irritability, anxiety and depression.[13]

Skin care

Petitgrain oil has a tonic effect on the skin. It is helpful for acne and skin blemishes, and helps to reduce overactive sebaceous glands.[9,13] It is used in bath preparations and has deodorising properties.[9]

Mailhebiau recommends blending petitgrain with carrot seed and lavender as a cellular regenerator and for acne.[13]

Energetics, psyche and subtle uses

Energetics

Petitgrain oil would be beneficial for reducing *hot*, agitated conditions of the *Heart* characterised by restlessness, insomnia and palpitations. The oil has a calming effect on the *Heart* and *Shen*, which are associated with the Fire Element. It essentially has a *cooling* and calming effect on excess the Fire Element.

Personality

The petitgrain personality is closely associated with neroli, and to a lesser extent, the orange personality. The qualities associated with a petitgrain personality are revitalising, balancing, restoring and clarifying. Worwood describes petitgrain personalities as the providers of comfort and emotional nourishment.[14]

In relationships, petitgrain personalities may have difficulty in expressing their feelings about a person. Because they do not like to take risks, a long-term romantic relationship may often elude them. Negative petitgrain personalities will become very disillusioned with the apathy for life in this world, and often try to alleviate these feelings by doing something positive, no matter how small it may be.[14]

Mailhebiau explains that petitgrain personalities have an altruistic nature that drives them to pursue a social or humanitarian vocation – as a nurse, social worker or teacher. However, this only enables them to conceal the inner conflict that they may have. He states that they will suffer as long as they fail to admit their soul is suffocating and the love they seek cannot be found in the people with whom they associate.[13]

Subtle

Davis suggests that, while neroli activates the highest psychic or spiritual levels of the mind, petitgrain relates to the conscious, intellectual aspect of the mind.[15]

Worwood states that the spirit of petitgrain is embodied in gentle strength, assisting us when we are feeling most vulnerable or fragile, and taking everything a little too personally and emotionally. It will give us the strength and courage to move forward, encouraging positive outcomes during difficult and challenging times.[16]

Zeck explains that the fresh, stimulating aroma of petitgrain awakens our conscious mind and our memories. This leads us to a deeper awakening that can bring new insights that will guide us through life.[17]

Dosage and Administration

Blending

Aromatherapy

Davis states that petitgrain oil resembles neroli, though it is less sedative.[9] It can be used as an extender for neroli oil in an aromatherapy blend.

To alleviate stress, anxiety and nervous tension, consider blending petitgrain oil with essential oils such as Roman chamomile, clary sage, geranium, lavender, neroli, sweet orange, sandalwood or ylang ylang.

To create an uplifting antidepressant blend, consider blending petitgrain oil with essential oils such as bergamot, geranium, jasmine absolute, sweet orange, neroli, rose otto, rosemary, sandalwood or ylang ylang.

To create an energising and invigorating blend, consider blending petitgrain, with essential oils such as basil, geranium, ginger, lemon, lemon myrtle, cold-pressed lime, rosemary or peppermint.

For insomnia, consider blending petitgrain with essential oils such as Roman chamomile, clary sage, fragonia, lavender, sweet marjoram, neroli or sandalwood.

Perfumery

Petitgrain is used in perfumery mainly for its refreshing, sweet-floral notes in citrus colognes and fougère style perfumes. It is often used as a replacement for the more expensive neroli oil.[2]

Mode of administration

Bath

Full body bath, foot bath

Topical

Compress, massage, ointment, skin care

Inhalation

Direct inhalation, diffuser, oil vaporiser

Safety Profile

General safety

Petitgrain oil is non-toxic, non-irritating and non-sensitising.

Contraindications

No contraindications known.

Regulatory guidelines

Petitgrain essential oil has GRAS status.

References

1. Khan I, Abourashed E. *Leung's encyclopedia of common natural ingredients used in food, drugs and cosmetics*. 3rd edn. John Wiley & Sons, New Jersey, 2010.
2. Arctander S. *Perfume and flavor materials of natural origin*. Allured Publishing, Carol Stream, 1994.
3. Weiss EA. *Essential oil crops*. CAB International, Wallingford, 1997.
4. Guenther E. *The essential oils – Vol. III*. Robert E Krieger Publishing Company, Malabar, 1949.
5. Lawrence BM. *Progress in essential oils – petitgrain or citrus leaf oils*. Perfumer & Flavorist, 2003; 28: 54-65.
6. Schmidt E, Wanner J. *Adulteration of essential oils*. In Baser KHC, Buchbauer G. eds. *Handbook of essential oils – science, technology and applications*. 2nd edn. CRC Press, Boca Raton, 2016: 707-745.
7. Lis-Balchin M. *Aromatherapy science – a guide for healthcare professionals*. Pharmaceutical Press, London, 2006.
8. Galal EE et al. *Evaluation of certain volatile oils for their antifungal properties*. Journal of Drug Research, 1973; 5(2): 235-245. Cited in Quintessential Aromatics database, 2013.
9. Davis P. *Aromatherapy: an A-Z*. 2nd edn. C.W. Daniel Company, Saffron Walden, 1999.
10. Lavabre M. *Aromatherapy workbook*. Healing Arts Press, Rochester, 1997.
11. Lawless J. *The encyclopaedia of essential oils*. Element Books, Shaftesbury, 1992.
12. Schnaubelt K. *Medical aromatherapy*. Frog, Berkeley, 1999.
13. Mailhebiau P. *Portraits in oils*. C.W. Daniel Company, Saffron Walden, 1995.
14. Worwood VA. *The fragrant mind*. Transworld Publishers, London, 1995.
15. Davis P. *Subtle aromatherapy*. C.W. Daniel Company, Saffron Walden, 1991.
16. Worwood VA. *The fragrant heavens*. Transworld Publishers, London, 1999.
17. Zeck R. *The blossoming heart – aromatherapy for healing and transformation*. Aroma Tours, East Ivanhoe, 2004.

Pine

Identification

Botanical name

Pine (Scots): *Pinus sylvestris* L.

Pine (black): *Pinus nigra* J.F.X. Arnold

Pine (dwarf): *Pinus mugo* Turra, *Pinus mugo* Turra var. *pumilio*

Pine (white): *Pinus strobus* L.

Pine (longleaf): *Pinus palustris*

Synonyms

Pine (Scots): Scotch pine, forest pine, Norway pine

Pine (dwarf): Mountain pine, dwarf mountain pine, mugo pine, pumilio pine

Pine (white): Canadian white pine needle

Pine (longleaf): Longleaf yellow pine, southern yellow pine, pitch pine

Family

Pinaceae

Botany and origins

There are many species of pine used to produce essential oil from their needles and wood, or used for the production of turpentine.[1]

P. sylvestris is a tree with leaves in two-leaved fascicles (clusters), deep fissured bark and up to 40 m high.[2]

The oil from *P. sylvestris* is considered one of the most useful and safest pine oils to use in aromatherapy.[1]

P. sylvestris is widely grown all over the Baltic states, Russia and central and southern Europe. Arctander states that the best quality *P. sylvestris* oil comes from Tryol, Austria.[3]

Dwarf pine is a prostrate shrub or pyramidal tree up to 12 m high. It is native to the mountains of central and southern Europe.[1]

Longleaf pine is a tall evergreen tree with long needles and a straight trunk. It is extensively cultivated for its timber. It exudes a natural oleoresin, which provides the largest source for the production of turpentine.[1]

Method of extraction

Pine oils are steam-distilled from the leaves and twigs of the pine trees.

A pine oil is also obtained by steam distillation of the heartwood and stump wood of *P. palustris* and other *Pinus* species. The oil is then fractionally distilled under vacuum to yield pine oil. The lighter fractions from this distillate are also known as wood turpentine. Production of this oil takes place mainly in the USA.[3]

Apart from pine essential oil being obtained from the needles and twigs of various coniferous trees of the Pinaceae family, an oil can be obtained from the oleoresin obtained from the wood. The distillate of the oleoresin is also referred to as turpentine. Turpentine oil is rich in sesquiterpene fractions such as α-muurolene (22%), longifolene (17.5%), γ-muurolene (6.0%) and δ-cadinene (5%).[4]

Characteristics

P. sylvestris oil is a clear mobile liquid with a characteristic pine, fresh top note and a distinct sweetness.[3]

P. nigra oil is a colourless to pale-yellow mobile liquid with a pleasant, balsamic pine-like, refreshing odour. The turpentine notes are very dominating and the odour has no tenacity or pleasant dryout note.[3]

P. mugo Turra var. *pumilio* oil is a clear mobile liquid with a very pleasant pine-type aroma which is described as balsamic-sweet, faintly woody and a little spicy, reminiscent of cypress and juniper berry oil.[3]

Chemical composition

Tisserand & Young state that there is considerable variation in the chemistry of *P. sylvestris* oils. They state that there are possibly two chemotypes: β-pinene and δ-3-carene.[5]

The principal compounds found in *P. sylvestris* essential oil consist mainly of 50-90% monoterpene hydrocarbons, with a small percentage of sesquiterpene hydrocarbons as well as oxygenated monoterpenes.[4]

The oils from *P. sylvestris* produced from trees in different locations in Lithuania contained over 70 constituents. The main constituents were as follows:

α-pinene (18.5-33.0%), car-3-ene (9.1-24.6%), germacrene-4-ol (13.2%), bornyl acetate (0.5-3.0%). The main sesquiterpenes were β-caryophyllene, germacrene D, bicyclogermacrene, δ and γ-cadinene, germacrene D-4-ol, cubenol (2.0-5.1%) and α-cadinol (1.9-7.7%).[4]

Analysis of the oil taken from trees in industrial and contaminated areas found that, as the level of contamination increased, the content of α-pinene, camphene and limonene increased, whereas the car-3-ene, β-pinene and terpinolene decreased.[4]

Another study confirmed that there was seasonal variation in the terpene composition of *P. sylvestris*, and that there was a variation in the chemistry of the oil from the needles compared to that of the twigs.[6]

The principal constituents found in *Pinus mugo* var. *pumilio* essential oil were as follows:

α-pinene (12.9-14.1%), δ-3-carene (6.4-12.0%), bornyl acetate (7.6%). The oil also contained sesquiterpene hydrocarbons: β-caryophyllene and germacrene D, as well as sesquiterpene alcohol germacrene D-4-ol (4.1-6.1%).[7]

Adulteration

Pine needle oils are often subject to frequent adulteration with other pine oils, camphene, pinene, isobornyl acetate and turpentine oil.[3,5,8]

Pharmacopoeias and standards

The purity, composition and physico-chemical properties of dwarf pine essential oil are defined in ISO 21093:2003 Oil of Dwarf Pine (*Pinus mugo* Turra).

History and Traditional Uses

History

Native Americans would also burn twigs and needles along with cedar and juniper for ritual smudging of the sweat lodge, in order to purify the spirit.[9]

The young macerated shoots were also added to the bath for nervous exhaustion, circulatory disorders, arthritis and skin disorders.[2]

Herbal

Pine needle oil is listed in the German Commission E Monographs for catarrhal diseases of the upper and lower respiratory tract, and for rheumatic and neuralgic ailments. However, it is contraindicated for bronchial asthma and whooping cough.[10]

Food, perfumery and flavouring

Pine needle oil is extensively used in pharmaceutical preparations for cough and cold medicines, vaporising fluids, nasal decongestants and analgesic ointments.[1] Arctander states that pine is not commonly used in perfumery, and that its use is often confined to room fresheners, disinfectants, insecticides, soaps and detergents.[3]

Other uses

Pines are amongst the most important commercial trees. Most of them have straight, unbranched, cylindrical trunks, which furnish large amounts of excellent timber.[11]

Therapeutics

Pharmacology and clinical studies

Many pharmacological studies involving pine essential oil have been published. A systemic review of these studies will not be attempted. Rather, I have chosen a selection of studies that support the traditional and clinical uses.

Acetylcholinesterase inhibitory activity

A study found that *Pinus heldreichii* subsp. *leucodermis* and *Pinus nigra* var. *calabrica* essential oils exhibited good acetylcholinesterase (AChE) and butyrylcholinesterase (BChE) inhibitory activity. This activity is relevant to the treatment of Alzheimer's disease.[12]

Anticarcinogenic activity

There is growing evidence that Pycnogenol and Flavangenol, extracts derived from the bark of *Pinus maritima*, are potential candidates for chemoprevention. Studies have confirmed that they can strongly inhibit the migration capability of human cervical cancer cells and induce apoptosis of human liver cancer cells. Pycnogenol has also been shown to exert an antileukemic effect, and protective properties against skin carcinogenesis.[13]

It was recently demonstrated that the essential oil from the needle extract of *P. sylvestris* displayed clear cytotoxic activity to breast cancer cells. It was concluded that the exact isolation and structure of the potential active compounds still needs to be conducted before pine needle extract and essential oil could serve as potential candidates for the development of novel therapeutic anticancer drugs.[13]

Antifungal activity

Lis-Bachin states that pine oil had moderate antifungal activity against 4 out of 5 fungi.[8] The results of an in vitro study confirmed that the antifungal activity of *P. sylvestris* essential oil was found to be most effective at 2.5% concentration when tested against a range of fungal organisms.[14]

Antimicrobial activity

Both dwarf pine oil and Scotch pine oil have varying degrees of antimicrobial activities. Limonene, dipentene and bornyl acetate have been reported as the main constituents responsible for the antibacterial properties.[1]

The essential oils from the needles of *Pinus halepensis, P. canariensis, P. pinaster, P. pinea* and *P. brutia* grown in Morocco were investigated for their antimicrobial activity. Only *P. pinaster* and *P. pinea* oils exhibited strong antibacterial activity.[15]

It has been reported that *P. sylvestris* can be divided into four chemotypes. The chemotype with the highest percentage of α-pinene and β-pinene had the lowest antimicrobial activity.[16]

Insecticidal activity

A study confirmed that *P. sylvestris* essential oil achieved over 85% larval mortality against mosquitoes within 24 hours. The results justify the potential use of *P. sylvestris* oil for its larvicidal activity.[17]

Wound-healing activity

The essential oils from the cones and needles of five different *Pinus* species were evaluated for their in vivo wound-healing and anti-inflammatory activities. The essential oils obtained from the cones of *Pinus pinea* and *Pinus halepensis* demonstrated the highest effect on wound-healing activity models, whereas the needle oils did not show any significant wound-healing or anti-inflammatory activities.[18]

Actions

Actions commonly cited in aromatherapy

Antimicrobial, antineuralgic, antirheumatic, antiseptic, antiviral, bactericidal, balsamic, deodorant, diuretic, expectorant, insecticidal, rubefacient, tonic[2,9,19]

Actions supported by clinical studies

Antifungal, antibacterial, antiseptic, insecticidal

Comment

The essential oil produced from the Scotch pine is the most widespread variety, and it is commonly used in aromatherapy.[2]

Schnaubelt states that the pine needle oils are used for their fresh fragrance and air-disinfectant qualities, as well as having a decongestant effect on the respiratory system. Pine oils are usually rich in monoterpene hydrocarbons, which are balanced with calming esters. *P. sylvestris* oil contains hormone-mimicking, polycyclic terpenoid compounds that are endocrine tonics which, according to Schnaubelt, help to balance the pituitary, thyroid, adrenals and ovaries.[20]

Chalchat et al. warn us against making a blanket statement that an essential oil has antimicrobial activity. Their research has identified that the antibacterial activity of *P. sylvestris* oil is dependent on the chemical composition of the oil. For example, it was found that the pine oils that had a high α-pinene and β-pinene content had the lowest antibacterial activity. They explain that to suggest that an essential oil is antimicrobial without consideration of its individual chemical composition may lead to therapeutic error.[16]

P

Aromatherapy Uses

Clinical aromatherapy

Musculoskeletal system

Pine oil has a stimulating effect on the circulation and may be used in a liniment to relieve the pain of rheumatism and arthritis, and for muscular aches from over-exertion.[21]

Psychological

Mojay states that pine oil is just as effective as rosemary and thyme for combating fatigue and nervous exhaustion.[9] It is recommended whenever we feel mental fatigue, or suffer from burnout, apathy and low self-confidence.

Respiratory system

It has excellent expectorant, balsamic and antiseptic properties, thus making it very useful for a wide variety of pulmonary complaints.[2]

Tonic

Pine oil is regarded as a tonic to the lungs, kidneys and the nervous system.[9,19] Schnaubelt considers it a tonic and adrenal stimulant, and recommends that it be used topically over the kidney area for adrenal support.[20] Pine oil is recommended during times of convalescence or following an illness that leaves one feeling weak or with severe psychological stress.[23]

Urinary system

The antiseptic properties of pine oil indicate its usefulness for conditions such as cystitis and pyelitis.[2,19]

Energetics, psyche and subtle uses

Energetics

The energetic qualities of pine oil are *warming* and *drying*. It is one of the best oils to clear *cold* phlegm and is recommended for bronchial congestion, coughing and asthmatic breathing.[9,22]

Pine oil dispels *wind, cold* and *damp* conditions, which are often associated with colds and influenza, chronic cough, excess phlegm and sinus congestion.

The oil also tonifies our *Qi*. Whenever our *Qi* is weak, we feel physically, mentally and emotionally exhausted; we suffer from apathy and have low motivation.

Pine oil strengthens the *Lungs* and balances the Metal Element. Mojay states that it has an invigorating effect on the bodily soul, the *Po*, which is seen as the source of our vital spirit.[9]

When the Metal Element is out of balance, our *Po* spirit is affected. According to TCM, whenever the *Po* is not balanced, we may experience physical pain that takes over our entire life yet seems to have no identifiable cause. We have a vague feeling that 'something isn't right' but no clear sense of why, and we may have unexpressed emotional issues. We also may refuse to accept the truth and suppress traumatic experiences that have occurred in the past.

Personality

Fischer-Rizzi beautifully describes the character of pine:

> *The tree is a symbol of an uncompromising will to live, endurance, strength, and a free spirit that refuses to conform or live in servitude … The oil awakens one's spirit and it is good for people who lack courage, perseverance, self-confidence and patience.*[23]

Pine is recommended for people who often feel responsible, not just for their own actions, but for the mistakes and suffering of others. Pine oil instils positivity and restores self-confidence, replacing undue guilt with forgiveness and self-acceptance.[9]

Worwood describes pine personalities as soft, gentle types who often go through life afraid to make a mistake. They can be self-critical and constantly apologising for everything and everyone.[24]

She explains that, like a good walk in the alpine forest, pine can help you make important decisions calmly and confidently. Pine personalities are never satisfied with themselves or their work, and always blame themselves for not having tried harder. They are often workaholics who have forgotten how to play. They can have an incredible amount of energy.[24]

According to Myers-Briggs personality types, the pine personality is likely to be an INTJ. INTJs are very responsible and dependable. They are people of very few words and tend to be private. They are punctual, precise and fastidious. They have the ability to concentrate and are difficult to distract. They are modest, unassuming and down to earth. They can be resistant to change. They can make quick critical judgements of others. They are extremely devoted in their relationships.

Subtle

Pine oil may be used to clear a meditation space, especially if the room or space cannot be devoted exclusively for this purpose.[25]

Keim Loughran & Bull explain that we live in a culture that values high energy and high performance, but tends to ignore the body's natural rhythms and its need for sleep, rest and replenishment. It is no wonder that so many people feel exhausted – physically, emotionally and spiritually. Pine will help energise the body and mind. It will align the energy of the body and focus of the will. Pine clears away feelings of being emotionally or spiritually stagnant and fills us with delight, purpose and vitality.[26]

Mojay explains that pine restores emotional positivity. It helps us to dispel any negative self-image and feelings of sorrow we may have, and replaces feelings of guilt with forgiveness and self-acceptance.[9]

Worwood states that pine teaches us that it is love and generosity of spirit that endures in the hearts of those we have loved and known, and in our children.[27]

Zeck suggests that pine oil helps us validate and strengthen our unique gifts and talents, encouraging us to believe in our self-worth.[28]

Dosage and Administration

Blending

Aromatherapy

To alleviate sinus and bronchial congestion, consider blending pine oil with essential oils such cajeput, fragonia, peppermint eucalyptus, 1,8-cineole-rich eucalypts, fragonia, manuka, myrtle, niaouli or tea tree.

For the relief of musculoskeletal pain and inflammation, consider blending pine oil with essential oils such as black pepper, cajeput, ginger, kunzea, spike lavender, peppermint or rosemary.

For combating fatigue and nervous exhaustion, consider blending pine oil with essential oils such as basil, black pepper, cardamom, ginger, lemon, peppermint or rosemary.

Perfumery

Pine oils are not commonly used in perfumery.

Mode of administration

Bath

Full body bath, foot bath

Topical

Massage, ointment

Inhalation

Direct inhalation, diffuser, oil vaporiser

P

Safety Profile

General safety

Scotch pine oil is non-toxic, non-irritating and non-sensitising.[2]

Dwarf pine oil has been reported to be a dermal irritant and dermal sensitiser to certain individuals.[1,2]

While dwarf pine is considered a dermal irritant, it is very likely that all pine oils are potential irritants if oxidised, but not when fresh.[5]

As all the pine oils contain a high percentage of monoterpene hydrocarbons, it is recommended to store them in dark airtight containers in a refrigerator to avoid oxidation. It is also advised to add an antioxidant to preparations containing pine oil.[5]

Essential oils from the Pinaceae family should only be used when the level of peroxides is kept to the lowest practical level.[5,8]

Contraindications

No contraindications known.[2]

Regulatory guidelines

P. sylvestris and *P. mugo* var. *pumilio* oils have GRAS status.

References

1. Khan I, Abourashed E. *Leung's encyclopedia of common natural ingredients used in food, drugs and cosmetics*. 3rd edn. John Wiley & Sons, New Jersey, 2010.
2. Lawless J. *The encyclopaedia of essential oils*. Element Books, Shaftesbury, 1992.
3. Arctander S. *Perfume and flavor materials of natural origin*. Allured Publishing, Carol Stream, 1994.
4. Maciag A et al. *Essential oil composition and plant-insect relations in Scots pine (Pinus sylvestris L.)*. Scientific Bulletin of the Technical University of Lodz, 2007; 71(1008): 71-95.
5. Tisserand R, Young R. *Essential oil safety*. 2nd edn. Churchill Livingstone, Edinburgh, 2014.
6. Zafra M, Garcia-Peregrin E. *Seasonal variations in the composition of Pinus halepensis and Pinus sylvestris twigs and needles essential oil*. The Journal of Agricultural Science, 1976; 86(1): 1-6. doi: 10.1017/S002185960006490X.
7. Ioannou E et al. *The genus Pinus: a comparative study on the needle essential oil composition of 46 pine species*. Phytochemistry Reviews, 2014; 13(4): 741-768. doi: 10.1007/s11101-014-9338-4.
8. Lis-Balchin M. *Aromatherapy science – a guide for healthcare professionals*. Pharmaceutical Press, London, 2006.
9. Mojay G. *Aromatherapy for healing the spirit*. Healing Arts Press, Rochester, 1999.
10. Blumenthal M et al. *The complete German commission E monographs: therapeutic guide to herbal medicine*. American Botanical Council, Austin, 1998.
11. Grieve M. *A modern herbal – Vol. II*. Dover Publications, New York, 1971.
12. Bonesi M et al. *Acetylcholinesterase and butyrylcholinesterase inhibitory activity of Pinus species essential oils and their constituents*. Journal of Enzyme Inhibition and Medicinal Chemistry, 2010; 25(5): 622-628. Cited in Quintessential Aromatics database, 2013.
13. Hoai NT et al. *Selectivity of Pinus sylvestris extract and essential oil to estrogen-insensitive breast cancer cells Pinus sylvestris against cancer cells*. Pharmacognosy Magazine, 2015; 11(Suppl 2): S290-S295. doi: 10.4103/0973-1296.166052.
14. Motiejūnaite O, Peciulyte D. *Fungicidal properties of Pinus sylvestris L. for improvement of air quality*. Medicina (Kaunas), 2004; 40(8): 787-794.
15. Hmamouchi M et al. *Chemical and antimicrobial properties of essential oils of five Moroccan Pinaceae*. Journal of Essential Oil Research, 2001; 13(4): 298-302. Cited in Quintessential Aromatics database, 2013.
16. Chalchat JC et al. *Correlation of chemical composition and antimicrobial activity – the activity of different chemotypes of Pinus sylvestris against Escherichia coli*. Plantes Medicinales et Phytotherapie, 1987; 21(1): 26-35. Cited in Quintessential Aromatics database, 2013.
17. Fayemiwo KA et al. *Larvicidal efficacies and chemical composition of essential oils of Pinus sylvestris and Syzygium aromaticum against mosquitoes*. Asian Pacific Journal of Tropical Biomedicine, 2014; 4(1): 30-34. Cited in Quintessential Aromatics database, 2013.
18. Süntar I et al. *Appraisal on the wound healing and anti-inflammatory activities of the essential oils obtained from the cones and needles of Pinus species by in vivo and in vitro experiment models*. Journal of Ethnopharmacology, 2012; 129(2): 533-540. doi: 10.1016/j.jep.2011.11.045.
19. Lavabre M. *Aromatherapy workbook*. Healing Arts Press, Rochester, 1997.
20. Schnaubelt K. *Medical aromatherapy*. Frog, Berkeley, 1999.
21. Davis P. *Aromatherapy: an A-Z*. 2nd edn. C.W. Daniel Company, Saffron Walden, 1999.
22. Holmes P. *The energetics of Western herbs – Vol. I*. Artemis Press, Boulder, 1989.
23. Fischer-Rizzi S. *Complete aromatherapy handbook*. Sterling Publishing, New York, 1990.
24. Worwood VA. *The fragrant mind*. Transworld Publishers. London, 1995.
25. Davis P. *Subtle aromatherapy*. C.W. Daniel Company, Saffron Walden, 1991.
26. Keim Loughran J, Bull R. *Aromatherapy anointing oils*. Frog, Berkeley, 2001.
27. Worwood VA. *The fragrant heavens*. Transworld Publishers, London, 1999.
28. Zeck R. *The blossoming heart – aromatherapy for healing and transformation*. Aroma Tours, East Ivanhoe, 2004.

P

Ravintsara

Identification

Botanical name

Cinnamomum camphora L.

Synonyms

Ho leaf ct. cineole. In Japanese, it is referred to as yu-sho.[1]

Family

Lauraceae

Botany and origins

C. camphora was introduced from Taiwan as an ornamental tree and now grows widely in Madagascar. The oil has often been confused with and traded as ravensara, which comes from *Ravensara aromatica*.[2]

True ravensara oil is extracted from the leaves of a common species of tree known to locals in Madagascar as *havozo* or *hazomanitra,* which means 'aromatic tree' in the Malagasy language. It has a distinctly different aroma that is very spicy and aniseed-like. The chemical profile of *Ravensara aromatica* oil is dominated by sabinene (15%), limonene (21.5%), methyl eugenol (19%) and methyl chavicol (7%).[2]

It would appear that most ravensara essential oils commercially available are, in fact, ravintsara oil from *C. camphora* tree. The similarity of the common names (ravintsara and ravensara) among English-speaking customers has perpetuated the misidentification and confusion of these oils.[2]

Juliani et al. also state that another source of confusion with *Ravensara* species is that *R. aromatica* and *Ravensara anisata* were considered different species producing different oils, whereas the plants are in fact the same. *R. aromatica* and *R. anisata* come from the same plant. For some reason it would appear that the name R. *anisata* refers to the bark oil of *R. aromatica,* while the true ravensara is extracted from the leaves.[2]

Method of extraction

Ravintsara oil is steam-distilled from the leaves of *Cinnamomum camphora.*

Characteristics

The essential oil of ravintsara is typically colourless with a fresh camphoraceous and slightly spicy aroma.[2]

Chemical composition

The chemical composition of ravintsara essential oil from Madagascar was reported as follows:

α-thujene (0.8%), α-pinene (5.0%), sabinene (12.2%), β-pinene (3.3%), myrcene (1.2%), α-terpinene (1.3%), *p*-cymene (0.1%), (*E*)-β-ocimene (0.4%), 1,8-cineole (62.6%), γ-terpinene (2.0%), terpinolene (0.3%), para menthadienol (0.3%), terpinen-4-ol (2.5%), α-terpineol (7.3%), (*E*)-caryophyllene (0.1%), α-humelene (0.4%).[2]

Adulteration

Ravintsara oil should not be confused with ravensara. There is a good chance that ravintsara may be adulterated with less expensive oils with a similar scent such as cajeput or niaouli.[3]

Pharmacopoeias and standards

At the time of writing, the purity, composition, physico-chemical properties and therapeutic use of ravintsara essential oil are not defined in any pharmacopoeia monograph or standard.

History and Traditional Uses

Traditional medicine

According to Halpern, the leaves of the tree have been used in Madagascar as a folk remedy to treat stomach aches and headaches. However, he suggests that the ravintsara tree and *C. camphora* are not the same tree. It has been stated that *C. camphora* was introduced to Madagascar in the mid-nineteenth century; however, he argues that ravintsara tree was a household medicine and has been part of Malagasy culture for centuries.[4]

Holmes provides us with a good explanation for Halpern's confusion. Holmes states that, during the mid-twentieth century, French botanists considered that the *Ravensara aromatica* tree was identical with the *C. camphora* tree. However, they were later identified to be two different species.[3] Unfortunately, all the attributed therapeutic functions and indications of *C. camphora* leaf oil reported in literature had remained with *Ravensara aromatica*.[3]

Therapeutics

Pharmacology and clinical studies

At the time of writing, no pharmacological or clinical studies for ravintsara oil could be found.

Actions

Actions commonly cited in aromatherapy

Analgesic, anti-infective, anti-inflammatory, antimicrobial, antiviral, expectorant,

R

immunostimulant, nerve restorative, vulnerary.[3]

Actions supported by clinical studies

None

Comment

While no clinical studies could be found to confirm the actions of ravintsara oil, the chemistry of ravintsara oil suggests that it has much in common with cajeput and 1,8-cineole-rich eucalyptus oils. It is high in 1,8-cineole and monoterpenes, which would make it ideal for the treatment of upper and lower respiratory tract infections.

Aromatherapy Uses

Clinical aromatherapy

Nervous system

Holmes states that ravintsara oil stimulates the mind and promotes alertness. He recommends the oil for lethargy, mental fogginess and lack of concentration.[3]

Mailhebiau states that the oil is a nerve tonic and a mental and physical stimulant, and can be used to revitalise people suffering from physical and nervous fatigue.[5]

Respiratory system

Ravintsara oil has been described as having antibacterial, immunostimulating and expectorant properties. This makes it especially useful for colds and influenza, sinusitis, rhinitis and chronic bronchitis with phlegm and cough.[3]

In *Portraits in essential oils*, Mailhebiau refers to ravensara, which I believe from his description to be ravintsara. He describes the oil as having the freshness of 1,8-cineole; however, we know that there is very little 1,8-cineole in true ravensara.[5]

Mailhebiau states that the oil has excellent antiviral properties, particularly for the flu. He recommends diluting it in a carrier oil with *Eucalyptus radiata* and using it as a massage rub. It is one of the first essential oils one should turn to as a preventative at the first signs of chills, shivers or tiredness. It is highly effective in cases of bronchitis, rhinitis and sinusitis, and for more serious pathologies such as whooping cough, especially when blended with cypress.[5]

Energetics, psyche and subtle uses

Energetics

Holmes states that ravintsara oil strengthens the *Lung Qi* and the protective *Qi*. It dispels *wind, damp* and *cold* pathogens, which are associated with colds and flu. It may, therefore, be used to prevent infection from colds and flu and to alleviate symptoms such as phlegm and coughs.[3]

It strengthens the *Shen* and raises *Yang* energy. Therefore, it may be beneficial for physical and mental fatigue, poor concentration and lethargy.[3]

According to the principles of the Five Elements, it has an affinity with the Metal Element.

Subtle

Holmes explains that ravintsara oil is as invigorating to the mind and soul as it is to the body, and suggests that the uplifting, refreshing effect will be beneficial for those individuals suffering from low self-esteem, low self-confidence, pessimism and a lack of willpower.[3]

Mailhebiau suggests blending ravintsara with *Mentha* x *piperita* and *Laurus nobilis* for people who no longer enjoy life, doubt everything and no longer know where they are through lack of aims or ideals.[5]

Dosage and Administration

Blending

Aromatherapy

To alleviate symptoms associated with respiratory infections, the common cold, bronchial congestion and coughing, consider blending ravintsara oil with essential oils such as aniseed, Atlas cedarwood, peppermint eucalyptus, 1,8-cineole-rich eucalypts, fragonia, ginger, niaouli, peppermint, pine, tea tree or thyme.

To alleviate nervous tension, stress-related conditions and anxiety, consider blending ravintsara oil with essential oils such as bergamot, clary sage, fragonia, geranium, lavender, neroli, sweet orange or sandalwood.

To alleviate fatigue and promote alertness, consider blending ravintsara oil with essential oils such as basil, clove bud, ginger, fir, lemon, pine, peppermint or rosemary.

For the relief of pain and inflammation associated with arthritis, consider blending ravintsara oil with essential oils such as black pepper, lemon-scented eucalyptus, kunzea, ginger, peppermint, pine or rosemary.

Perfumery

Ravintsara oil is not commonly used in perfumery.

Mode of administration

Bath

Full body bath, foot bath

Topical

Compress, massage, ointment, skin care

Inhalation

Direct inhalation, diffuser, oil vaporiser

Safety Profile

General safety

Holmes states that the oil is not irritating or sensitising to the skin.[3] However, Tisserand & Young state that no information is available regarding the oil's safety. They profile a Chinese ho leaf oil that contained methyl eugenol (0.1%) and safrole (0.2%), which are both known carcinogens and are restricted ingredients according to IFRA and the EU; however, Madagascan ravintsara contained no methyl eugenol or safrole.[1]

Contraindications

No contraindications known.

Regulatory guidelines

Ravintsara oil is not defined in any regulatory guideline.

References

1. Tisserand R, Young R. *Essential oil safety*. 2nd edn. Churchill Livingstone, Edinburgh, 2014.
2. Juliani H et al. *Searching for the real ravensara (Ravensara aromatica Sonn.) essential oil.* Perfumer & Flavorist, 2005; 30: 60-65.
3. Holmes P. *Aromatica: a clinical guide to essential oil therapeutics – Vol. I.* Singing Dragon, London, 2016.
4. Halpern G. *The healing trail – essential oils of Madagascar.* Basic Health Publications, North Bergen, 2003.
5. Mailhebiau P. *Portraits in oils.* C.W. Daniel Company. Saffron Walden, 1995.

Rosalina

Identification

Botanical name

Melaleuca ericifolia Smith

Synonyms

Lavender tea tree, swamp paperbark

Family

Myrtaceae

Botany and origins

An evergreen paper bark shrub that grows in low lying swamps, along creeks and behind sand dunes in northern Tasmania, southern Victoria and along the east coast of New South Wales and Queensland.[1]

It is a tall erect bushy shrub, 6-9 m high with a bushy crown and greyish, papery bark. The leaves are greyish green, narrow, 1.2 cm long, recurved and crowded. It has an erect stem, with white papery, corky bark, numerous, slender branches and a densely textured crown.[1] The distribution of this species has decreased markedly with the clearing or draining of many wetlands in which it formerly grew.[2]

Method of extraction

Rosalina essential oil is produced by steam distillation of the leaves and twigs of *M. ericifolia.*

Characteristics

Rosalina oil has a soft medicated aroma with a light floral back note. It is very similar to *M. alternifolia* except that the major constituent is linalool, not terpinen-4-ol. This makes the oil more pleasant smelling and less irritating on younger and sensitive skin.[3]

R

Chemical composition

The chemical composition of *M. ericifolia* essential oil was reported as follows:

terpinen-4-ol (0.5-3.5%), α-terpinene (1.5-4.0%), α-terpinolene (1.5-5.0%), 1,8-cineole (18-26%), *p*-cymene (1.0-4.0%), α-pinene (5.0-10.0%), α-terpineol (1.5-4.0%), aromadendrene (1.5-4.0%), limonene (1.5-5.0%), viridiflorol (0.5-3.0%), linalool (35.0-55.0 %).[3]

Webb states that some natural variation exists within this range, but it does not cause any significant variation in properties for the essential oil.[3]

Adulteration

Not reported.

Pharmacopoeias and standards

At the time of writing, the purity, composition, physico-chemical properties and therapeutic use of rosalina essential oil are not defined in any pharmacopoeia monograph or standard.

History and Traditional Uses

History

Like so many other Australian plants, *M. ericifolia*

was first identified back in the 1950s as a potential new Australian essential oil.[1]

Therapeutics

Pharmacology and clinical studies

Anticarcinogenic activity

The phenolic ether methyl eugenol, the major component of the essential oil of the leaves of *M. ericifolia*, was used as a starting scaffold to design 11 new and three known anti-tubulin agents using carbon: carbon coupling reactions. A computer-assisted approach was used to design new biaryl derivatives using colchicine-binding site of tubulin as the molecular target and colchicine as an active ligand. Several derivatives showed potent inhibitory activity against two breast cancer cell lines at the 1-4 μM dose range.[4]

Tisserand & Young state that the methyl eugenol chemotype is not commercially produced.

Antimicrobial activity

M. ericifolia essential oil has shown to possess good antibacterial, antifungal and antiviral activities.[5,6]

Actions

Actions commonly cited in aromatherapy

Antibacterial, antifungal, carminative, decongestant, immunostimulant, sedative[1,3]

R

Actions supported by clinical studies

Antibacterial, antifungal

Comment

The chemical profile of rosalina oil suggests that it would have properties similar to that of a blend of tea tree, lavender and eucalyptus essential oils. It has a higher percentage of 1,8-cineole, so it would be excellent as an expectorant for coughs and colds, while its terpinen-4-ol and linalool content suggests that it would have excellent antimicrobial properties, while at the same time being quite soothing and relaxing.

Aromatherapy Uses

Clinical aromatherapy

Antimicrobial

Webb recommends using rosalina oil for colds, influenza and sinusitis.[1] Pénoël often uses rosalina oil for children who are prone to ENT infections. He explains that rosalina oil is so mild on the skin that it can be applied two to three drops at a time along the side of the neck (on the areas of the lymph node).[7]

Insect bites

Webb states that rosalina oil is a very good anaesthetic when applied neat to insect bites.[3]

Psychological

The higher percentage of linalool means that the oil is likely to have a deeply relaxing effect. Pénoël states that linalool is soothing to the nerves, calming and to a certain degree sleep inducing:

> *Rosalina oil massaged in the back will quickly trigger a state of letting go of stress and tension and induce a deep sleep. The good thing is that this Yin action is harmonious and respects the body and the brain.*[7]

Pénoël explains that, when you wake up, you do not feel like someone who is taking pharmaceutical sleeping pills.[7]

Skin care

Rosalina oil is recommended for skin rashes, dandruff and acne.[3]

Dosage and Administration

Blending

Aromatherapy

For the relief of muscular aches and pain, consider blending rosalina oil with essential oils such as cajeput, black pepper, fragonia, kunzea, ginger, spike lavender, peppermint or rosemary.

For the relief of anxiety, stress and nervous tension, consider blending rosalina oil with essential oils such as bergamot, Atlas cedarwood, geranium, lavender, sweet orange, neroli or sandalwood.

For the relief of symptoms of colds and flu, consider blending rosalina oil with essential oils such as lemon-scented eucalyptus, 1,8-cineole-rich eucalypts, cajeput, fragonia, spike lavender, lemon, tea tree or thyme.

For acne, consider blending rosalina oil with essential oils such as bergamot, lavender or tea tree.

Perfumery

Rosalina oil is not commonly used in perfumery.

Mode of administration

Bath

Full body bath, foot bath

Topical

Compress, massage, ointment, skin care

Inhalation

Direct inhalation, diffuser, oil vaporiser

Safety Profile

General safety

No known hazards or contraindications.[8] No information on toxicity is available for rosalina, however, its chemical composition does not raise any concerns.

Contraindications

No contraindications known.[8]

Regulatory guidelines

Rosalina oil is not defined in any regulatory guideline.

References

1. Webb M. *Bush sense.* Self-published, Australia, 2000.
2. Robinson R. *Regeneration mechanisms in swamp paperbark (Melaleuca ericifolia Sm.) and their implications for wetland rehabilitation.* Victoria University, 2007.
3. Webb M. *Australian essential oil profile – rosalina.* Aromatherapy Today, 2001; 17: 32-34.
4. Abdel Bar FM et al. *Design and pharmacophore modelling of biaryl methyl eugenol analogs as breast cancer invasion inhibitors.* Bioorganic & Medicinal Chemistry, 2010; 18(2): 496-507. doi: 10.1016/j.bmc.2009.12.019
5. Barbosa LCA et al. *Chemistry and biological activities essential oils from Melaleuca L. species.* Agriculturae Conspectus Scientificus, 2013; 78(1): 11-23.
6. Williams C. *Medicinal plants in Australia – Vol. 2. Gums, resins, tannins and essential oil.* Rosenburg Publishing, Dural, 2011.
7. Pénoël D, Pénoël R. *Natural home health care using essential oils.* Osmobiose Publishing, La Drôme, 1998.
8. Tisserand R, Young R. *Essential oil safety.* 2nd edn. Churchill Livingstone, Edinburgh, 2014.

Rose

Identification

Botanical name

The two major species of rose used for essential oil production are:

- *Rosa* x *damascena* Mill.
- *Rosa* x *centifolia* L.

Synonyms

Rosa damascena is commonly known as Damask rose, Bulgarian rose, Turkish rose or otto of rose.

Rosa centifolia is commonly known as rose Maroc, cabbage rose, rose de mai, French rose, attar of rose or rose absolute.

Family

Rosaceae

Botany and origins

The Rosaceae is a large family of some 115 genera and about 3,200 species, with the genus *Rosa* L. containing approximately 150 species.[1] While there are thousands of rose varieties, there are three varieties which are typically used for rose oil production. They are:

- Damask rose from *Rosa damascena*
- Cabbage or May rose produced from *Rosa centifolia*
- *Rosa gallica*.[1]

The *Rosa* species are small prickly shrubs up to 1.2 to 2.4 m high. It is considered a native of Europe and western Asia.[2]

It has been suggested that the Mediterranean *R. gallica* is one of the species from which modern rose cultivars are derived. *R. gallica* is a vigorous spreading shrub to 1.5 m, with dense foliage and few thorns. It has fragrant, semi-double light red flowers with yellow stamens.[1]

The birthplace of the cultivated rose, *R. damascena,* was probably northern Persia or Faristan on the Gulf of Persia. It then spread across Mesopotamia, Palestine and across to Asia Minor and Greece.[3]

The European name for the Damascus rose dates from the Crusades, but it is now incorporated in its botanical name. Cultivation of *R. damascena* and production of rose oil was introduced to Bulgaria, then part of the Turkish Empire, in the fifteenth century.[1]

Commercial rose growing to produce rose oil was well established in the Kazanlik region of Bulgaria by the end of the seventeenth century. It is the Bulgarian rose oil which today is still considered the most prized of all rose oils. The Bulgarian rose industry is confined to one mountain district, having for its centre the town of Kazanlik.[3]

Under communism, Bulgaria collectivised all rose plantations and nationalised the distilling and marketing of the oil. Between 1938 and 1948, the area under rose cultivation fell from 6300 ha to 2000 ha. Since the fall of communism, the Bulgarian rose plantations have returned to private ownership.[1]

The major rose oil producing countries are France, Bulgaria, Morocco, Turkey, Italy and China.[2,4]

Method of extraction

Three main products are obtained from roses: an essential oil, a concrete and an absolute. The essential oil is obtained by steam distillation of the whole flowers, the concrete by solvent extraction of the leaves and flowers, and the absolute by further extracting the concrete.[1]

The three products vary from different cultivars or species, and also vary from the same cultivar or species grown in geographically separate areas. Weiss states that the term 'rose otto' is generally accepted to apply to the oil distilled from *Rosa damascena*, and it should be prefixed by the country of origin.[1]

Rose otto from *R. damascena* that is produced in India, China and Morocco differs from Bulgarian and Turkish otto, and should be sold as rose oil followed by the country of origin, e.g. rose oil Morocco. However, rose oil produced in Morocco and France from *R. centifolia*, in Egypt from *R. gallica* and in China from *R. rugosa* is also incorrectly often sold as rose otto. Weiss explains that experienced perfumers can readily identify them.[1]

The flowers are generally picked manually. In order to minimise loss of oil, harvesting needs to be done between 5 and 10 am as this is the period that the flowers are open and the oil content is highest.[1]

Flowers must be promptly transported to the distillery before being distilled. Weiss explains that storing bagged flowers in clean cold water retains the oil content and quality for up to three days. Temperature above 25°C during storage can decrease flower content by half, and also increase citronellol and stearoptene, but decrease the nerol and geraniol content. The oil in the petals actually increases after picking due to enzymatic activity.[1]

Rose oil is produced by a two-stage distillation process. It is a common practice to redistill the distilled water, a process known as cohobation. The yield of cohobation oil is several times higher than that from the first distillation of the flowering material. The oils from the two distillations are then blended. The phenylethyl alcohol in otto of rose is derived almost exclusively from cohobation water.[4]

According to Grieve, 4,000 kg of flowers yield 1 kg of rose oil, of which one-third comes from the first distillation, and the remaining two-thirds are a result of redistilling the waters.[3]

Rosewater is the aqueous portion of the steam distillation after rose oil has been removed.

Rose absolute is obtained by solvent extraction. Holmes refers to the solvent extraction process as 'dry-cleaning' the plant. Solvent extraction produces a more complete plant extract. However, Holmes suggests that contact with the solvent, which is usually petroleum ether, may result in minute traces of solvent in the final absolute. He suggests that, from an energetic perspective, this may devitalise the essential oil through contact with a 'dead chemical substance'.[5]

Wabner suggests that rose absolute produced by solvent extraction is superior to the distilled rose otto because rose otto actually contains synthetic constituents that are not found in nature. He proved this by doing a headspace analysis of a live rose and comparing the constituents with that of rose absolute of the same flower and rose otto of the same flower. While the chemical constituents of the rose absolute and live rose were the same, rose otto oil contained several constituents such as rose oxide and damascenone that are by-products of distillation.[6]

Characteristics

Arctander states that *R. centifolia* is excellent for the extraction of rose oil by solvent extraction. Rose absolute obtained from the concrete of *R. centifolia* flowers is also referred to as rose de mai absolute.[1]

Rose de mai absolute is an orange-yellow to brown-orange viscous liquid with a sweet, deep-rosy, very tenacious odour. The spicy notes are usually less pronounced, while the honey-like notes are similar to that of *R. damascena*.[4]

Arctander explains that Bulgarian producers had originally insisted on only producing rose otto oil; however, it is now possible to obtain a rose absolute from *R. damascena* flowers from Bulgaria. The rose absolute from *R. damascena* is an orange-yellow to brown-orange viscous liquid with a rich, warm, spicy-floral, and a very deep rose odour with a pronounced honey undertone.[1]

It is very diffusive when it is diluted or used at very low concentration of a few per cent or even less in a perfume base.[4]

Bulgarian rose otto is a pale yellow to yellowish green oil. Fresh oil is often green due to the presence of azulenes, which gradually decompose over time. When cooled to a temperature below 20°C, rose otto separates into white or colourless blades of crystals, stearoptene. Stearoptene is odourless and constitutes 15-25% of the oil. When cooled below 16°C, the oil further congeals to a translucent soft mass.[1] When it is heated with the warmth of the hands the oil will liquefy.[1]

The odour of Bulgarian rose otto is warm, deep-floral, slightly spicy and immensely rich, truly reminiscent of red roses.[4]

Rose otto obtained from *R. centifolia* is colourless to pale yellow, sometimes with a greenish tinge when fresh. It has a deep, sweet, warm, rich, but less spicy odour than Bulgarian or Turkish rose otto oils.[1]

Chemical composition

Rose is one of the most complex essential oils known. It contains more than 300 chemical compounds, of which the greater part is still unidentified. The table below identifies 86% of the rose composition. The remaining 14% of the volatile part of the oil represents about 300 substances.

A comparative chemical composition of Bulgarian rose otto and Turkish rose otto is as follows:[1]

Constituent	Bulgaria	Turkey
ethanol	1.43%	5.14%
pentanal	0.07%	0.05%
3-hexenal	0.26%	0.16%
α-pinene	0.73%	0.50%
camphene and heptanal	0.14%	0.07%
β-pinene	0.03%	0.02%
myrcene and hexanol	0.50%	0.30%
heptanol	0.02%	0.01%
hexyl acetate	0.01%	0.01%
methyl heptenone	0.04%	0.02%
octanol	0.07%	0.01%
linalool	2.18%	0.54%
cis-rose oxide and nonanal	0.43%	0.33%
trans-rose oxide	0.17%	0.18%
nonanol	0.09%	0.07%
phenylethyl alcohol, decanol and terpinen-4-ol	1.45%	1.88%
citronellol	33.40%	45.04%
nerol	5.90%	3.60%
geraniol and neral	18.47%	11.87%
geranial and carvone	0.72%	0.57%
citronellyl acetate	0.53%	0.72%
neryl acetate	0.06%	0.04%
cinnamaldehyde and C15 paraffin	0.21%	0.3%
geranyl acetate	1.60%	1.23%
eugenol and *trans*-β-damascenone	1.20%	1.19%
methyl eugenol and C16 paraffin	2.37%	3.26%
octanal	0.05%	0.02%
benzaldehyde	0.10%	0.03%

A comparative chemical composition of rose absolute from Morocco and Turkey is as follows:[1]

Constituents	Morocco	Turkey
ethanol	0.38%	ni
camphene + heptanal	0.01%	0.02%
β-pinene	0.03%	ni
linalool	0.40%	0.28%
phenylethyl alcohol + decanal + terpinen-4-ol	74.06%	72.28%
citronellol	8.77%	-
nerol	2.52%	-
citronellol + nerol	-	14.04%
geraniol + neral	5.18%	4.1%
citronellyl acetate	0.23%	0.10%
neryl acetate	0.10%	0.17%
geranyl acetate	0.38%	0.15%
eugenol+ trans-β-damascenone	0.89%	0.53%
trans-trans-farnesol	1.30%	0.20%
unidentified	5.70%	ni

ni: not identified under compound name

The oil composition varies according to the stage of flower development and rose flower parts. For example, the citronellol content in the petals from the centre of the flower is 18.9%, whereas from the outer petals it is 10.1%. The phenylethyl alcohol content is highest in the outer petals. It was also found that the chemical composition of the oil differed over the harvesting period.[1]

Adulteration

Being so expensive, rose oils are commonly adulterated. Lis-Balchin states that many rose oils sold may be completely synthetic.[7]

Rose de mai absolute is frequently adulterated with phenylethyl alcohol. Rhodinol from geranium oil, costus oil, clove bud absolute, palmarosa fractions, Peru balsam oil and synthetic laevo-citronellol are also used as an adulterant.[4]

Bulgarian rose absolute is adulterated with *R. centifolia* absolute and other adulterants such as phenylethyl alcohol, ethyl alcohol, rhodinol from geranium oil and diethyl phthalate.[4]

Rose otto is adulterated with ethyl alcohol, diethyl phthalate, rhodinol from geranium and phenylethyl alcohol.[4]

Pharmacopoeias and standards

The purity, composition and physico-chemical properties of rose oil are defined in ISO 9842:2003 Oil of Rose (*Rosa* x *damascena* Miller).

History and Traditional Uses

History

No other flower has been exalted in literature and mythology and used for so many sacred purposes as the rose. In both ancient art and literature, the rose was the predominant flower symbol. Its blossom symbolises beauty, love, youth, perfection and immortality.[8]

The word *rosa* comes from the Greek word *rodon* (red), and the rose of the ancients was a deep crimson colour, which probably suggested the Greek fable of its springing from the blood of Adonis.

Homer in his *Iliad* wrote that the body of Hector was anointed with rose before his burial. According to Islam, when Muhammad was taken up to heaven some of his sweat fell to earth from which a rose grew – who smells rose smells Muhammad.[1]

It was prized in Babylon, Assyria, China, Rome and Greece. These cultures were aware of the healing properties of rose. Pliny in his book *Natural History* discusses at great length the scent of rose: the lands and climate which produce the best scented roses, the best season, time of the day and weather for picking a rose in order to preserve its scent, the point in a rose's life when it smells strongest, the perfume of freshly gathered rose as compared to a faded rose, the use of rose perfume and so on.[9]

R

Pliny explained that the scent of roses could be improved if the bushes are pruned before March and hot water applied to induce flowering. Plutarch explained that interplanting rose plants with garlic would improve the scent of the roses.[1]

Ancient Rome had an insatiable appetite for roses and rosewater. During festivals and banquets, rose petals were strewn over the floor and along the streets. Self-indulgent Romans wore rose garlands at their feasts, as a prevention against drunkenness. To them, the rose was a sign of pleasure, the companion of mirth and wine, but it was also used at their funerals.[10]

Grieve claims that the first preparation of rosewater was by Avicenna in the tenth century. According to Grieve, rose oil was first discovered at a wedding feast of the princess Nour Djihan to the Grand Mogul Djihanguyr. A canal circling the whole garden was dug and filled with rosewater. They noticed a scum had formed on the water and, was floating on the surface. The scum turned out to be oil that the heat of the sun had caused to separate from the water.[3]

Weiss states that the history of when rose oil was first extracted is unknown; however, he cites the earliest written reference as in the ninth century when production was well established in Iran. Distillation of rose began in Persia in 1612. The production of rose oil quickly became a major industry with local cultivars finding their way east and west along the Silk Road.[1]

The term attar is derived from Farsi, *aettr*, meaning fat. In modern Turkish language, attar is known as *gulyagi* from the Farsi *gul* for rose flower.[1]

Rose and rose products were employed extensively in English medicine, notably by the well-known physician, Nicholas Culpeper, who used rose oil as an anti-inflammatory agent.[3]

An ointment of roses was used to soothe headaches, a syrup to 'comfort the heart', and rose leaves mixed with mint were applied externally as a poultice to 'quiet the over-heated spirits'.[3]

Traditional medicine

Generally, therapeutic remedies containing rose oil have a cooling and soothing influence. It is interesting to note that the fields of application of rose oil in ancient medicine are almost identical with those of modern aromatherapy.

In Chinese and Sanskrit manuscripts, rose was highly praised. Li Shih-Chin tells us of a highly fragrant rose, *R. rugosa*, which is cultivated in China:

> *Its nature is cooling, its taste is sweet with a slight bitterishness, and it acts on the spleen and liver, promoting the circulation of the blood. It is prescribed in the form of an extract for haematemesis, and the flowers are used in all diseases of the liver, to scatter abscesses, and in blood diseases generally … Essence of rose is made by distilling the flowers of* Rosa rugosa. *Its medicinal action is upon the liver, stomach, and blood. It drives away melancholy.*[11]

Herbal

The German Commission E recommends rose flower petals as a herbal tea for mild inflammations of the oral and pharyngeal mucosa.[12]

In France, rose flower buds and petals are traditionally indicated for symptomatic treatment of mild diarrhoea, topically applied for soothing and alleviating dermatological ailments, and used as a protective treatment for cracks, grazes, chapped skin and insect bites.[13]

Food, perfumery and flavouring

Nowadays, rose oil and rosewater are extensively used as fragrance components in skin care preparations, perfumes, soaps and in food flavouring.[2]

Therapeutics

Pharmacology and clinical studies

Many pharmacological studies involving rose oil have been published. A systemic review of these studies will not be attempted. Rather, I have chosen a selection of studies that support the traditional and clinical uses.

Analgesic activity

A study involving 80 patients with renal colic found that inhaling rose essential oil effectively reduced renal pain. It has been suggested that the possible mechanisms for reducing pain by inhalation is by increasing parasympathetic activity and releasing neurotransmitters such as enkephalin and endorphin, as well as reducing sympathetic activity and reducing the release of cortisol and noradrenalin.[14]

Massage with rose oil was found to reduce the severity of primary dysmenorrhoea compared to the massage therapy alone.[14]

A study investigated the effect of topically applied rose oil in a randomised, controlled clinical trial conducted on 120 women with pregnancy-related lower back pain. All participants were evaluated by Visual Analog Scale and the Roland-Morris Disability Questionnaires to assess pain intensity and its impact on daily activities before and after the intervention. A significant decrease in pain intensity was reported in the rose oil group compared to the plain carrier oil group or no intervention group. However, while rose oil also improved the functional ability of the patients in contrast with no intervention, its effect on function is not significant compared to the carrier oil group. There were also no significant adverse effects reported.[15]

Antidepresant activity

The inhalation of rose vapour was able to exert an antidepressant action in rats depressed from chronic mild stress. The increase in lipid peroxidation in the cerebral cortex associated with stress was also reduced with inhalation of rose aroma; however, there was no significant influence seen with oral ingestion. It was concluded that rose oil vapour induced protective effects on oxidative stress in depression.[16]

In a study involving 60 male patients, it was found that *R. damascena* oil improved the symptoms of depression and selective serotonin re-uptake inhibitor-induced sexual dysfunction (SSRI-ISD). In another similar study on 50 female patients suffering from depression and SSRI-ISD sexual desire, sexual orgasms and sexual satisfaction increased by rose inhalation.[14]

It has been suggested that the antidepressant activity of rose oil has an antagonistic effect on the stimulation of the post-synaptic 5-HT2 and 5-HT3 receptors, as well as an antagonistic effect on the cortico-limbic 5-HT receptors, which may also affect sexual behaviour and could be responsible for increased sexual desire.[14]

Antiepileptic activity

R. damascena essential oil was found to significantly retard the development of seizures and possessed the ability to counteract kindling acquisition in an in vivo study using male rats.[17]

Anti-inflammatory activity

The effect of rose oil and hydro-alcoholic extract of *R. damascena* on rat paw oedema induced by carrageenan was demonstrated. It was found that the essential oil had no anti-inflammatory effect, while the extract could significantly reduce oedema by inhibiting mediators of acute inflammation.[18]

Antimicrobial activity

In vitro studies have confirmed that both rose otto and absolute have wide-spectrum antimicrobial activity against *Escherichia coli, Pseudomonas aeruginosa, Bacillus subtilis, Staphylococcus aureus, Chromobacterium violaceum* and *Erwinia carotovora* strains. Rose absolute also showed antibacterial activity against both gram-negative and gram-positive bacteria.[18]

An in vivo study confirmed that Bulgarian rose oil had an inhibitory effect on *Helicobacter pylori* bacteria. It was suggested that the oil may also be anti-ulcerous; however, in vivo studies are required to confirm the concentration of rose oil required to exert an effect, and whether the oil could sufficiently penetrate the gastric mucosa to eradicate the bacteria.[19]

Antiviral activity

The antiviral effect of a combination of rose and melissa (ratio of 1:2) on herpes zoster and herpes simplex has been confirmed. According to Wabner & Wurdack, the oil is to be applied pure without dilution, two or three times a day for several days.[8]

Anxiolytic activity

The effect of rose oil inhalation on the elevated plus-maze test was investigated in adult male rats and compared with the effect of diazepam administered intraperitoneally 30 minutes before testing. Inhalation of rose oil produced an anxiolytic-like effect similar to diazepam.[20]

Another study found that 2-phenethyl alcohol and citronellol, two constituents in rose oil, produced the same anti-conflict effect in mice

R

when compared with rose oil. Further studies indicated that the effect of rose oil was not antagonised by flumazenil, a benzodiazepine antagonist. It was suggested that rose oil may have a pharmacological activity similar to non-benzodiazepine anxiolytic drugs.[21]

A clinical trial involving animals found that rose oil exhibited antianxiety effect. It was concluded that rose oil has a pharmacological activity similar to non-benzodiazepine anxiolytic drugs.[22]

Cardiovascular activity

Wabner cites a study which demonstrated that rose oil can reduce high blood pressure and arrhythmia of the heart.[8]

Hepatoprotective activity

Rose oil had considerable hepatoprotective effect against the toxic action of ethanol in an in vivo study involving rats. A histological and electron microscope investigation found that an active regeneration of the hepatocytes and rapid proliferation of Kupffer cells.[23]

Menopausal symptoms

A study investigated the effects of aromatherapy massage on menopausal symptoms in Korean climacteric women using a blend of rose, jasmine, lavender and geranium essential oils in a base of sweet almond and evening primrose oil. The aromatherapy massage was performed once a week for eight weeks. The aromatherapy group reported significantly lower menopausal symptoms; however, it could not be determined whether the benefits were from the essential oils or from the massage. It was concluded that further studies should be done.[24]

R

Neuropharmacology

An in vivo study examined the effects of *R. damascena* oil on withdrawal signs of naloxone-precipitated morphine in mice. The results of the study indicated that rose oil significantly reduced signs of withdrawal compared to the control group. It was concluded that GABAergic activity induced by flavonoids from *R. damascena* essential oil can alleviate signs of morphine withdrawal; however, further studies are required to better understand this mechanism.[25]

Damask rose oil had protective effects against aluminium-induced neurotoxicity in an in vitro study using immortalised hypothalamic neuronal cells.[26]

Sedative activity

One study investigated the effects of *Rosa damascena* on human autonomic parameters and emotional responses in healthy subjects after transdermal absorption. Five autonomic parameters were measured – blood pressure, breathing rate, blood oxygen saturation, pulse rate and skin temperature. Emotional responses were assessed by rating scales.[27]

Compared to the placebo, rose oil caused significant decreases of breathing rate, blood oxygenation saturation and systolic blood pressure, which indicated a decrease of autonomic arousal. At an emotional level, subjects in the rose oil group rated themselves as more calm, more relaxed and less alert than subjects in the control group. It was concluded that this provides some evidence for the use of rose oil in aromatherapy for the relief of depression and stress.[27]

An in vivo study found that inhalation of rose oil significantly inhibited the increase in plasma corticosterone in rats. The results suggested that chronic stress-induced disruption of the skin barrier can be limited or prevented by rose oil inhalation, possibly through its inhibitory effect on the HPA axis.[28]

A randomised controlled study investigated the effects of *R. damascena* on the sleep quality of 60 patients hospitalised in a coronary care unit. The patients in the control group received routine care, while the patients in the experimental group received routine care with rose. The sleep quality was assessed using the Pittsburgh Sleep Quality Index. It was confirmed that *R. damascena* significantly improved the sleep quality of patients hospitalised in the coronary care unit.[29]

Actions

Actions commonly cited in aromatherapy

Antidepressant, antiphlogistic, antiseptic, antispasmodic, antiviral, aphrodisiac, astringent, bactericidal, choleretic, cicatrisant, depurative, emmenagogue, haemostatic, hepatic, laxative, sedative (nervous system), stomachic, tonic (heart, liver, stomach, uterus)[30,31,32]

Actions supported by clinical studies

Antidepressant, antiseptic, anxiolytic, antiviral, bactericidal, sedative

Comment

There appears to be a growing number of studies confirming that rose oil possesses sedative and anxiolytic properties. What I found most interesting is that the evidence suggests that the most effective way to use rose oil for its sedative and anxiolytic activity is by inhalation.

Rose oil has been assigned many other diverse therapeutic properties, many of which have not yet been investigated; however, rose has, since days of antiquity, always been assigned to the heart and soul.

> *The rose, queen of flowers! Her fragrance, captured in the essential oil, is the most precious of all heavenly scents. It refreshes the soul; its fragrant poetry brings joy to the heart.*[33]

It is not surprising that many aromatherapists agree that rose oil is effective in all levels of life, for the soul, spirit and body. According to Fischer-Rizzi, rose otto heals the heart. It comforts in times of sorrow, dissolves psychological pain, refreshes a sad heart, and opens doors to love, friendship and empathy.[33]

Aromatherapy Uses

Clinical aromatherapy

Psychological

Rose oil is referred to as a gentle but potent antidepressant.[34] Rose oil may be used as a sedative for the nerves; it is useful for the treatment of palpitations, irritability and insomnia. It helps to release anger, despair and frustration.[5]

It opens the heart and soothes feelings such as anger, fear and anxiety.[33]

Reproductive system

Rose oil is valuable for the treatment of gynaecological problems. Maury comments that rose oil has an astonishing effect on the female sexual organs as a purifying and regulating agent.[35]

Rose oil is considered a tonic of the uterus.[32,34] It regulates menstruation and relieves menstrual cramps and excessive menstrual bleeding.[30,32,33,34]

Rose is recommended for functional infertility.[5] It is beneficial when it is difficult to predict ovulation dates because of an irregular cycle.[34]

Skin care

Rose oil has excellent emollient, softening and hydrating properties, which accompanied by its stimulating and antiseptic qualities, makes it ideal for all skin care, especially for mature, dry or sensitive skin.[30,31,33,34] Rose oil has a tonic and astringent effect on the capillaries and can be used for the treatment of broken capillaries, redness and inflammation of the skin.[30,34] Rosewater is also used in skin care for its soothing and mildly astringent properties.

Energetics, psyche and subtle uses

Energetics

Rose oil is classified as *cool* and *moist* in nature, and is recommended for clearing *heat* and inflammation and for alleviating anxiety and depression. It may be beneficial for hot conditions involving the *Liver* and *Gall Bladder* that result in tension, irritability, headache and constipation.[32]

According to the principles of the Five Elements, rose oil helps to balance the Fire Element and nourish the *Heart*. It helps to nourish *Yin deficiency* and calm the *Heart* and the *Shen*. Whenever we have *Yin deficiency* and the *Shen* is agitated, we may experience fatigue, insomnia, mental restlessness, nervous tension, anxiety, worry, depression, palpitations and headaches.

Personality

Worwood states that the spirit of *Rosa damascena* epitomises the gentleness of the female spirit. She suggests that rose otto is perfection personified. She explains that rose otto personalities have the wisdom to know that there are far greater things in the universe than them and that humans do make mistakes. They love cooperation and cannot understand why everyone does not operate on the same level as they do.[36]

Mailhebiau refers to rose as a miracle of nature:

> *... to simply smell it will refine our sensitivity, take us into an unknown world and disperse the shadows of our worries, anxieties and sorrows. It shows us love, not only human love which is a gift as it is – possibly the finest – from existence, but spiritual love, and we would even say divine, were this term not over-used.*[37]

According to Worwood, the character of rose absolute represents passion of the spirit with a deep, hypnotic personality – vivacious and alive. She explains that rose absolute personalities are very charming people who tend to be very emotional and expressive people. They are very creative. They are very erotic and fully aware of their sexuality – and the influence it can have on others. They prefer to work in professions that allow them free rein of their creative expression.[36]

According to Myers-Briggs personality types, the rose otto personality is likely to be an ENFP. ENFPs are outgoing, lively and spontaneous. They are very enthusiastic and their joy for life can be contagious. They have a rich imagination and active mind. Their thoughts are always wandering and their mood constantly changing. They can be inspiring and charismatic leaders. They are always involved, or in love, with someone or something new. They know how to establish instant rapport and make people feel comfortable. They love emotional intensity and enjoy expressing their feelings. They can be charming and flirtatious. They relate with warmth to many people and can appear overly enthusiastic, positive and optimistic.

According to Myers-Briggs personality types, the rose absolute personality is likely to be an ESFP.

ESFPs are friendly, witty, charming and talkative. They value and nurture their relationships, and give generously, without expecting anything in return. They are spontaneous, playful and enjoy everything they do and see. People who share their sense of fun and adventure are their favourite companions. They turn everything into a fun-filled event. They enjoy good things in life – music, dance, food, drink and entertainment. They avoid being alone. They like working in a lively and stimulating atmosphere with friendly, energetic people. They can be good at dealing with the public. They like variety and frequent change of tasks or jobs. They are enthusiastic, high-spirited and have lots of energy.

Subtle

Dziubany states that Sufis consider the red rose as the highest expression of religious experience. Dziubany cites Sufi mystic, Hazrat Inayat Khanl (1882-1927), who compares the rose with the soul:

> *The soul can be likened to the rose; as a rosebud blooms, so the soul unfolds itself, for the rosebud to bloom five conditions are required – fertile soil, bright sun, water, air and space; and the same five conditions are required for the unfoldment of the soul.*[38]

He goes on to describe the fragrance of a rose as the spiritual personality of the rose:

> *… the soul becomes like a rose, and begins to show the rose quality. Just as the rose consists of many petals held together, so the person who attains to the unfoldment of the soul begins to show many different qualities. These qualities emit fragrance in the form of a spiritual personality. The rose has a beautiful structure and the personality which proves the unfoldment of the soul has a fine structure: in manner, in dealing with others, in speech, in action.*[38]

It is no wonder that Worwood describes the personality of rose otto as one of gentleness and apparent perfection.[36]

Fischer-Rizzi also describes the rose as a symbol of completeness, stating that all parts of the rose are formed to perfection.[33]

Mojay states that the rose is the symbol of love. The compassion of rose is revealed in its ability to heal emotional wounds. Mojay says that when rejection or loss have injured one's capacity for self-love and nurturing, rose oil brings a sweet, gentle comfort, restoring the trust that makes love possible again.[32]

It is not surprising that Davis associates rose oil to the heart chakra, which is the centre of love, whether that be love for one person or universal love.[34]

It will help the heart chakra to open when grief has caused it to close down.[39] Davis also associates rose with the sacral chakra, which is the centre of creativity and sex. She describes rose as a gentle aphrodisiac, which helps to spiritualise sexual relationships.[39]

Keim Loughran & Bull state that rose is the oil that teaches us the lessons of love. They explain that the extraordinary energy of rose assists us in healing our emotional wounds so we can better give and receive love unconditionally. It is said to help us heal the pain of grief and teaches us how to forgive others when they hurt us. Rose also gently seals and protects our energy field so that we are not affected by negativity.[40]

According to Holmes, it is not surprising that rose has been a symbol for the feminine and feminine qualities, namely love, sexuality and compassion. He explains that rose supports self-esteem, sexuality and nurturing.[5]

The subtle qualities of rose otto and rose absolute are quite different. Worwood best describes the difference between the two oils. She explains that the etheric realms associate rose absolute with the desires of the human heart, while rose otto is likened to the realm of angels.[41]

Rose otto vibrates with the energy of universal love, operating in the light of unconditional love and giving. Rose otto is the quintessential fragrance of love, the love that touches every soul. It is for the love that touches our very soul. It is for the awakening of love in us that offers itself.[41]

Dosage and Administration

Blending

Aromatherapy

To alleviate anxiety, nervous tension and stress, consider blending rose absolute or rose otto with essential oils such as bergamot, Roman chamomile, clary sage, geranium, lavender, mandarin, sweet orange, patchouli, petitgrain, sandalwood, vetiver or ylang ylang.

To alleviate symptoms associated with PMS, consider blending rose absolute or rose otto with essential oils such as Roman chamomile, clary sage, geranium, lavender, sweet marjoram or ylang ylang.

To alleviate symptoms associated with menopause, consider blending rose otto with essential oils such as cypress, geranium or lavender.

To soothe sensitive skin associated with inflammation, consider blending rose otto with essential oils such as German chamomile, everlasting, lavender or sandalwood.

In skin care preparations for mature dry skin

conditions, consider blending rose absolute with essential oils such as frankincense, lavender, myrrh, patchouli or sandalwood.

Perfumery

Rose de mai absolute and rose otto are extensively used in expensive perfumes, especially in floral, chypres and oriental bases. The absolute blends very well with jasmine, neroli and other floral oils. It blends well with essential oils such as bergamot, clary sage, geranium, sandalwood, guaiacwood and patchouli.[4]

Mode of administration

Bath

Full body bath, foot bath

Topical

Compress, massage, ointment, skin care

Inhalation

Direct inhalation, diffuser, oil vaporiser

Safety Profile

General safety

Rose absolute and rose otto are non-toxic, non-irritating and non-sensitising. However, Tisserand & Young state that both rose absolute and rose otto may contain methyl eugenol, and set the maximum dermal use level at 0.6% for rose oil that contains 3.3% methyl eugenol.[42]

Contraindications

No contraindications known.

Regulatory guidelines

Both *R. damascena* and *R. centifolia* have GRAS status.

References

1. Weiss EA. *Essential oil crops*. CAB International, Wallingford, 1997.
2. Khan I, Abourashed E. *Leung's encyclopedia of common natural ingredients used in food, drugs and cosmetics*. 3rd edn. John Wiley & Sons, New Jersey, 2010.
3. Grieve M. *A modern herbal – Vol. II*. Dover Publications, New York, 1971.
4. Arctander S. *Perfume and flavor materials of natural origin*. Allured Publishing, Carol Stream, 1994.
5. Holmes P. *Rose – the water goddess*. The International Journal of Aromatherapy, 1994; 6(2): 8-11.
6. Wabner D. *A rose is a rose is a rose oil*. 2nd Australasian Aromatherapy Conference, Sydney, 1998.
7. Lis-Balchin M. *Aromatherapy science – a guide for healthcare professionals*. Pharmaceutical Press, London, 2006.
8. Wabner D, Wurdack I. *Rose oil: its use in therapy and cosmetics*. International Journal of Aromatherapy. 1989; 2(1):28-11.
9. Classen C. *Worlds of sense – exploring the senses in history and across cultures*. Routledge, London, 1993.
10. Morris E. *Fragrance – the story of perfume from Cleopatra to Chanel*. Products of Nature and Art, New York, 1984.
11. Tisserand R. *The art of aromatherapy*. C.W. Daniel Company, Saffron Walden, 1977.
12. Blumenthal M et al. *The complete German commission E monographs: therapeutic guide to herbal medicine*. American Botanical Council, Austin, 1998.
13. Committee on Herbal Medicinal Products (HMPC). *Assessment report on Rosa gallica L., Rosa centifolia L., Rosa damascene Mill., flos.* European Medicines Agency, London, 2014. Doc ref. EMA/HMPC/137298/2013.
14. Mohebitabar S et al. *Therapeutic efficacy of rose oil: a comprehensive review of clinical evidence.* Avicenna Journal of Phytomedicine, 2017; 7(3): 206-213.
15. Shirazi M et al. *The effect of topical Rosa damascena (rose) oil on pregnancy-related low back pain: a randomized controlled clinical trial.* Journal of Evidence-Based Integrative Medicine, 2017; 22(1): 120-126. doi: 10.1177/2156587216654601.
16. Naziroğlu M et al. *Rose oil (from Rosa x damascena Mill.) vapor attenuates depression-induced oxidative toxicity in rat brain.* Journal of Natural Medicine, 2013; 67(1): 152-158. doi: 10.1007/s11418-012-0666-7.
17. Ramezani R et al. *The effect of Rosa damascena essential oil on the amygdala electrical kindling seizures in rats.* Pakistan Journal of Biological Sciences, 2008; 11(5): 746-751.
18. Boskabady MH et al. *Pharmacological effects of Rosa damascena.* Iranian Journal of Basic Medical Sciences, 2011; 14(4): 295-307.
19. Boyanova L, Neshev G. *Inhibitory effect of rose oil products in Helicobacter pylori growth in vitro: preliminary report.* Journal of Medical Microbiology, 1999; 48(7): 705-706. Cited in Quintessential Aromatics database, 2013.
20. de Almeida RN et al. *Anxiolytic-like effects of rose oil inhalation on the elevated plus-maze test in rats.* Pharmacology, Biochemistry and Behavior, 2004; 77(2): 361-364.
21. Umezu T et al. *Anticonflict effects of rose oil and identification of its active constituents.* Life Sciences, 2002; 72(1): 91-102.
22. Umezu T. *Anticonflict effects of plant-derived essential oils.* Pharmacology, Biochemistry and Behavior, 1999; 64(1): 35-40. Cited in

R

the Aromatherapy Database, by Bob Harris, Essential Oil Resource Consultants, UK, 2000.
23. Kirov M et al. *Rose oil. Liptropic effect in modelled fatty dystrophy of the liver. (Morphological and enzymohistochemical study)* Medico Biologic Information, 1988; 3: 18-22. Cited in Quintessential Aromatics database, 2013.
24. Hur MH et al. *Aromatherapy massage affects menopausal symptoms in Korean climacteric women: a pilot-controlled clinical trial.* Evidence-Based Complementary and Alternative Medicine, 2008; 5(3): 325-328. Cited in Quintessential Aromatics database, 2013.
25. Maleki NA et al. *Suppressive effects of Rosa damascena essential oil on naloxone-precipitated morphine withdrawal signs in male mice.* Iranian Journal of Pharmaceutical Research, 2013; 12(3): 357-361. Cited in Quintessential Aromatics database, 2013.
26. Mizuno D et al. *An in vitro system comprising immortalized hypothalamic neuronal cells (GT1-7 cells) for evaluation of the neuroendocrine effects of essential oils.* Evidence-Based Complementary and Alternative Medicine, 2015; 2015: 343942. doi: 10.1155/2015/343942.
27. Hongratanaworakit T. *Relaxing effect of rose oil on humans.* Natural Product Communications, 2009; 4(2):291-296.
28. Fukada M et al. *Effect of 'rose essential oil' inhalation on stress-induced skin-barrier disruption in rats and humans.* Chemical Senses, 2012 37(4): 347-356. doi: 10.1093/chemse/bjr108.
29. Hajibagheri A et al. *Effect of Rosa damascene aromatherapy on sleep quality in cardiac patients: a randomized controlled trial.* Complementary Therapies in Clinical Practice, 2014; 20(3): 159-163. Cited in Quintessential Aromatics database, 2013.
30. Lawless J. *The encyclopaedia of essential oils.* Element Books, Shaftesbury, 1992.
31. Lavabre M. *Aromatherapy workbook.* Healing Arts Press, Rochester, 1997.
32. Mojay G. *Aromatherapy for healing the spirit.* Healing Arts Press, Rochester, 1999.
33. Fischer-Rizzi S. *Complete aromatherapy handbook.* Sterling Publishing, New York, 1990.
34. Davis P. *Aromatherapy: an A-Z.* 2nd edn. C.W. Daniel Company, Saffron Walden, 1999.
35. Maury M. *Marguerite Maury's guide to aromatherapy.* C.W. Daniel Company, Saffron Walden, 1964.
36. Worwood VA. *The fragrant mind.* Transworld Publishers, London, 1995.
37. Mailhebiau P. *Portraits in oils.* C.W Daniel Company, England, 1995.
38. Dziubany R. *The rose.* Retrieved Sep 17, 2017, from http://www.rahmana.de/download/the_rose.pdf
39. Davis P. *Subtle aromatherapy.* C.W. Daniel Company, Saffron Walden, 1991.
40. Keim Loughran J, Bull R. *Aromatherapy anointing oils.* Frog, Berkeley, 2001.
41. Worwood VA. *The fragrant heavens.* Transworld Publishers, London, 1999.
42. Tisserand R, Young R. *Essential oil safety.* 2nd edn. Churchill Livingstone, Edinburgh, 2014.

R

Rosemary

Identification

Botanical name

Rosmarinus officinalis L.

Synonyms

Rosmarinus coronarium

Family

Lamiaceae (Labiatae)

Botany and origins

Rosemary is a small evergreen shrub with thick, aromatic, linear leaves, which grows up to 2 m in height. It is a native to the Mediterranean region. The plant grows wild in abundance in Spain, France, Corsica, Italy, Sardinia and Tunisia. The majority of the essential oil is produced in Spain, France and Tunisia.[1]

There are three main chemotypes of *R. officinalis*:[2]

- camphor-borneol (Spain)
- 1,8-cineole (Tunisia)
- verbenone (France).

Schnaubelt explains that rosemary growing at higher altitudes will always have more camphor – as much as 20%. On the other hand, rosemary growing at sea level produces very little to no camphor.[3]

Method of extraction

Rosemary oil is steam-distilled from the leaves, flowers and twigs of *R. officinalis* and the numerous sub-varieties.

Characteristics

Rosemary oil is a pale yellow to almost colourless mobile liquid, with a strong, fresh, woody-herbaceous top note and a clean-woody-balsamic body note which fades into a dry herbaceous base note. This description is for a commercial rosemary oil from Tunisia and Spain. Arctander explains that the Tunisian oil is very uniform and of a very high quality. One reason is that the twigs are never included in the distillation.[4]

Mailhebiau describes the odour of the Spanish chemotype as strong and rather camphoraceous, the French chemotype as gentle and the Tunisian chemotype as having an odour reminiscent of eucalyptus, giving it a fresher aroma.[5]

Chemical composition

The composition of rosemary oil from 15 cultivars of rosemary grown in Sardinia varied as follows:

α-pinene (13.95-56.9%), camphene (4.5-11.8%), β-pinene (1.5-3.3%), myrcene (1.4-4.5%), limonene (4.4-7.2%), 1,8-cineole (0.7-18.7%), camphor (0.1-22.3%), α-terpineol (1.0-2.7%), borneol (0.7-15.9%), verbenone (1.3-11.5%), bornyl acetate (0.4-24.4%).[6]

The 1,8-cineole content of rosemary oil produced from plants collected in Cevoli, a region in northern Italy, was reported to be in the range of 7.3 to 8.7%, whereas the 1,8-cineole in rosemary oil from plants grown in the Lungiana region of Italy was reported to be in the range of 42.5 to 55.3%. On the other hand, the was no verbenone in the rosemary oil from the Lungiana region of Italy, whereas the rosemary oil from the Cevoli region had a verbenone content of 6.0 to 8.2%.[6]

The comparative composition of major components of Moroccan rosemary oil produced at different times of the year from the same plants was reported as follows:[7]

compound	May	November
α-pinene	5.8-6.1%	5.9-7.0%
1,8-cineole	53.6-57.3%	48.6-53.8%
camphor	9.7-13.4%	12.7-16.4%
borneol	2.4-3.2%	1.8-2.2%
verbenone	0.1-0.4%	0.5-0.7%

The oil produced in May was slightly higher in 1,8-cineole and had less camphor, whereas the November oil was slightly higher in verbenone.[7]

On the other hand, the changes in major component composition of Algerian rosemary oil produced from plants harvested at different times of the development cycle were reported as follows:[7]

compound	Full budding	Beginning of flowering	Full flowering	After flowering
α-pinene	2.5%	4.8%	16.9%	7.1%
camphene	1.7%	2.3%	trace	Trace
β -pinene	0.9%	3.4%	1.8%	3.8%
1,8-cineole	39.6%	41.7%	17.2%	16.0%
camphor	26.0%	9.3%	11.9%	11.6%
borneol	9.0%	6.7%	2.2%	2.7%
α-terpineol	4.2%	4.5%	9.3%	12.8%
bornyl acetate	2.3%	1.3%	1.7%	2.9%
β-caryophyllene	4.9%	5.4%	9.9%	13.6%

The highest 1,8-cineole content was found in oils produced from plants that had just commenced flowering.

The composition of rosemary oil from Tunisia was reported as follows:[7]

α-pinene (12.22-14.28%), camphene (4.37-4.58%), β-pinene (4.83-9.21%), myrcene (1.5-1.87%), limonene (2.35-2.85%), 1,8-cineole (44.10-49.33%), γ-terpinene (0.82-1.38%), *p*-cymene (1.12-1.44%), camphor (8.65-13.13%), linalool (0.71-0.77%), bornyl acetate (0.95-1.22%), terpinen-4-ol (0.24-0.29%), b-caryophyllene (4.49-5.11%), α-terpineol (1.24-1.4%), borneol (1.28-4.67%).

The Tunisian rosemary oil is rich in 1,8-cineole and camphor and has a lower α-pinene content. Rosemary oil from Spain typically has higher levels of α-pinene and myrcene and lower levels of 1,8-cineole. The difference in composition is mostly due to the difference in climate, soil conditions, harvesting and distillation techniques. A study in Tunisia reported, that when the pressure inside the retort is increased, the level of camphor goes up while the level of α-pinene goes drastically down.[8]

Adulteration

Rosemary oil is often adulterated with turpentine oil, fractions of turpentine oil, 1,8-cineole from eucalyptus, white camphor, synthetic camphor and fractions from the production of synthetic terpineol.[4]

The percentage of the constituents in 10 commercial samples of rosemary oil varied significantly: α-pinene (3.1 to 28.1%), 1,8-cineole (8.5 to 28.6%) and camphor (10.3 to 27.9%). It was stated that rosemary oil is often adulterated with eucalyptus oil and camphor oil. However, it was also possible that the variation was due to different chemotypes of rosemary.[9]

Schnaubelt states that rosemary is commonly adulterated and diluted. He explains that it is very important to pay close attention to the source of the oil, and that the best quality can only be provided by those producers who make the oil exclusively for the aromatherapy market.[2]

Pharmacopoeias and standards

The purity, composition and physico-chemical properties of rosemary oil are defined in several standards and monographs. The following pharmacopoeia and composition standards are available:

- ISO 1342:2012 – Essential Oil of Rosemary (*Rosmarinus officinalis* L.)
- *Community Herbal Monograph on Rosmarinus officinalis L., aetheroleum*. European Medicines Agency
- *WHO Monographs on Selected Medicinal Plants* – Vol. 4.

History and Traditional Uses

History

The generic name *Rosmarinus* is derived from the Latin *ros*, meaning dew, and *marinus*, meaning sea, referring to its habit of growing near the coast.[10]

Rosemary is probably one of the best known and most used of aromatic herbs. The ancient Egyptians favoured it, and traces of it have been found in the first dynasty tombs. To the Greeks and Romans, it was considered a sacred plant. They believed rosemary symbolised love and death.[10]

R

Rosemary has been used medicinally for centuries. Theophrastus and Dioscorides recommended it as a powerful remedy for stomach and liver problems; Hippocrates said rosemary should be cooked with vegetables to overcome liver and spleen disorders; and Galen prescribed it for jaundice.[10]

In place of more costly incense, the ancients used rosemary in their religious ceremonies. It was a custom to burn rosemary with juniper berries to purify the air and prevent infections.[10]

Rosemary was known to have a stimulating effect on the mind and be a useful aid to the memory; consequently, the herb became known as a symbol of remembrance.[10] On this account, it became the emblem of fidelity for lovers. It was used at weddings, funerals, banquets and festivals, and as incense in religious ceremonies and in magical spells. It was a custom to burn rosemary in sick chambers and in French hospitals.[11]

A sprig of rosemary was carried in the hands at funerals, being given to the mourners before they left the house to be cast on the coffin when it had been lowered into the grave.[11]

Culpeper recommended the herb for the treatment of diseases of the head and brain, the giddiness and swimmings therein, drowsiness or dullness, the dumb palsy or loss of speech, the lethargy and the falling sickness (epilepsy).[10]

It was used to prepare Hungary water, which was used to restore the vitality of paralysed limbs. Hungary water was first prepared for the Queen of Hungary and was considered very effective in the treatment of gout.[11]

Traditional medicine

Grieve stated that rosemary oil was highly regarded as a carminative and is considered an excellent stomachic and nervine, curing many cases of headaches. It was used topically as *spiritus Rosmarini* in hair lotions for its odour and effect in stimulating the hair and preventing premature baldness. The oil is used externally as a rubefacient and added to liniments as a fragrant stimulant.[11]

Herbal

Rosemary has been used since ancient times in Europe as a tonic, stimulant and carminative and in treating dyspepsia, stomach aches, headaches, head colds and nervous tension.[1]

The German Commission E recommends infusions of rosemary leaf for dyspeptic complaints. Externally it recommends the essential oil as supportive therapy for rheumatic diseases and circulatory problems.[12]

Food, perfumery and flavouring

Rosemary oil is extensively used as a fragrance component in cosmetics, soaps, detergents and perfumes.[1]

Therapeutics

Pharmacology and clinical studies

Many pharmacological studies involving rosemary essential oil have been published. A systemic review of these studies will not be attempted. Rather, I have chosen a selection of studies with an emphasis on those studies that support the traditional and clinical uses.

Alopecia areata

A random controlled study involving 84 patients with alopecia areata confirmed that a blend of *Thymus vulgaris, Lavandula angustifolia, Rosmarinus officinalis* and *Cedrus atlantica* in a base of jojoba and grapeseed oil, massaged into the scalp every night and occluded with a warm towel, showed significant statistical advantage to the treatment over the control group, with an improvement rate of 44%. A lack of response in the control group indicated a pharmacological activity of the essential oils as opposed to any effects arising from the scalp massage with carrier oils alone.[13]

A double-blind, randomised controlled study using a blend of thyme, lavender and rosemary oils confirmed that the aromatherapy group was significantly more improved than the placebo group in the treatment of localised alopecia areata.[14]

Androgenetic alopecia

A study investigated the efficacy of rosemary oil for the treatment of androgenetic alopecia and compared its effects with minoxidil 2% for a period of six months. Both groups experienced a significant increase in hair count at the end of the six months. The findings of the trial provided evidence supporting the efficacy of rosemary oil in the treatment of androgenetic alopecia.[16]

Anticolitic activity

An in vivo study investigated the effects of rosemary oil and rosemary hydroalcoholic extract on experimental colitis in rats. Rosemary oil was administered orally and intraperitoneally. Both rosemary essential oil and hydroalcoholic extract were effective in reducing colon tissue lesions.[15]

Antifungal activity

Rosemary oil is reported to have significant antifungal activity.[15] At 20 mg/mL rosemary oil exhibited good antifungal activity against *Candida albicans, Cryptococcus* and the *Mycobacterium* species.[18] Rosemary oil exhibited antifungal activity by destruction of cell walls and impairment of metabolism of *Candida albicans.*[19]

Antimicrobial activity

Rosemary oil is reported as having antimicrobial activities.[17,20] An in vitro study confirmed that rosemary oil and clove oil, when tested alone, possessed significant antimicrobial effect against a range of microorganisms. The blend of both oils was tested and reported to have a synergistic improved antimicrobial effect.[21]

Rosemary oil exhibited antimicrobial activity against drug-resistant mutants of *Mycobacterium smegmatis, Escherichia coli* and *Candida albicans.*[22]

Cognitive performance

An in vivo study on 20 healthy human volunteers showed that the improvement of cognitive tasks was significantly related to the concentration of absorbed 1,8-cineole following exposure to rosemary essential oil aroma. Furthermore, it was also found that these effects were similar for speed and accuracy performance. The relationship between 1,8-cineole levels and mood was less pronounced, but there was significant correlation between change of contentment and plasma 1,8-cineole levels. The findings of this study suggest that the compounds absorbed from rosemary essential oil affect cognition and subjective states independently through different neurochemical pathways.[23]

Drug interaction

The influence of rosemary oil on pharmacodynamics effects of diazepam and pentobarbital on experimental animals was evaluated on mice. Rosemary oil significantly reduced pentobarbital-induced sleeping time, compared to the control group. The oil also caused a significantly longer retention of mice on the rotarod, compared to the group receiving diazepam only. The results confirmed that rosemary oil had a considerable influence on diazepam and pentobarbital pharmacodynamics.[24]

Free radical scavenging activity

An in vivo study on 22 healthy humans found inhalation of rosemary enhanced the free radical scavenging activity in the body and decreased the stress hormone, cortisol, which protects the body from antioxidative stress.[25]

Hepatoprotective activity

The hepatoprotective effects of rosemary oil and the ethanolic extract were investigated in rats. Administration of rosemary ethanolic extract (0.15 g/100 g body weight) for three weeks produced the most pronounced hepatoprotective effect compared to silymarin, which was used as the reference compound.[26]

The hepatoprotective effects of rosemary have been observed in different experimental models of liver injury. Rosemary methanol extract has been effective against carbon tetrachloride (CCl_4)-induced acute liver damage in rats. The methanolic extract of rosemary could also prevent hepatotoxicity in both prevention and reversion experimental models of liver cirrhosis induced by CCl_4.[27]

The results of another study confirmed that rosemary oil mediates its hepatoprotective effects not only by scavenging of harmful free radicals, but also through activation of physiological defense mechanisms.[27]

Hyperglycaemic activity

Rosemary oil is reported to have a hyperglycaemic and insulin release inhibitory effects in a study involving rabbits.[28]

Insecticidal activity

Rosemary oil had potent insecticidal activity on lepidopteran larvae.[29]

R

Niticidal activity

An in vitro study confirmed that rosemary oil exhibited good niticidal activity on *Pediculus humanus capitis.* The alcoholic and ketonic compounds were found to be the most effective on nits.[30]

Spasmolytic activity

Rosemary oil has an inhibiting action on muscle contraction when tested on contractile electro-induced response of guinea pig ileum. The constituent borneol was found to have the greatest spasmolytic activity.[31]

Stimulating activity

Rosemary oil was also found to stimulate locomotor activity of mice when administered orally or by inhalation. 1,8-cineole, a component of rosemary oil, was used as an indicator of the level of rosemary in the blood. Dose-related increases in 1,8-cineole blood levels were found after oral and inhaled administration of rosemary oil. The component of rosemary causing the stimulating effect was not investigated.[32]

Another study was performed in 40 subjects to assess the EEG activity and the mood after three minutes of inhalation with rosemary and lavender. The lavender-treated group showed increased beta power, suggesting increased drowsiness. They also had less depressed mood and reported feeling more relaxed. The rosemary oil had decreased frontal alpha and beta power, suggesting increased alertness. It was also reported that they were faster, but not more accurate, during mathematics computations, and they had lower anxiety scores and also reported feeling more relaxed and alert.[33]

When inhaled, rosemary oil decreased blood flow and increased systolic blood pressure immediately after inhalation, resulting from stimulating sympathetic nerve activity.[34]

Another study also confirmed significantly increased blood pressure, heart rate and respiratory rate after inhalation of rosemary oil.[35]

Actions

Actions commonly cited in aromatherapy

Analgesic, antidepressant, astringent, carminative, cephalic, cholagogue, cordial, digestive, diuretic, emmenagogue, hepatic, hypertensive, nervine, rubefacient, stimulant, sudorific, tonic[36,37,38,39,40,41]

Actions supported by clinical studies

Antifungal, carminative, cephalic, digestive, hepatoprotective, nervine, tonic

Comment

The EMA assessment report on *R. officinalis* essential oil states that the pharmacological effects of the constituents found in the oil support claims for carminative and digestive ailments, such as flatulence and feelings of distension. There are also documented antibacterial and anti-inflammatory effects attributable to rosemary oil.[41]

Due to the different composition, the three principal chemotypes of rosemary oil can be applied for different purposes to achieve maximum efficiency. The camphor-borneol chemotype rosemary oil is best used as a general stimulant and is considered the most specific heart tonic of all the rosemary oils.[5] It is also suitable for muscular aches and pains.[5,37]

The cineole chemotype rosemary oil is best used for the treatment of respiratory ailments such as bronchitis, asthma and sinusitis.[5,37] It is also used to facilitate elimination from the liver and the kidneys.[37]

The verbenone chemotype rosemary oil is the most appropriate to strengthen liver and gall bladder.[5] The verbenone rosemary is considered the most gentle, non-irritant essence and is excellent for high-quality skin care preparations.[37]

Holmes states that the verbenone chemotype has the best antiviral, antibacterial and antifungal activity.[39]

However, Holmes explains that, although there are three different chemotypes of rosemary, we should not think of them as different essential oils with distinct uses. He explains:[39]

> *Each chemotype contains all three constituents (cineole, camphor and verbenone) but in different proportions. The three chemotype oils should be thought of as the extreme variants within a continuum, whose therapeutic actions and indications are essentially the same.*

Rosemary has always been well known in traditional medicine for improving mental and cognitive functions. It has also been considered a tonic and restorative action for many body functions. Holmes states that it has special emphasis on the neuroendocrine system, and that the pituitary, heart and adrenal functions are enhanced and regulated.[39]

Aromatherapy Uses

Clinical aromatherapy

Cardiovascular system

Rosemary oil is considered a tonic of the heart.[38] It is said to benefit cardiac fatigue, palpitations, low blood pressure and circulatory problems of the extremities.[42]

R

Digestive system

Holmes describes rosemary oil as a digestive and gastrointestinal stimulant. He recommends it for gastric dyspepsia with flatulence, chronic gastroenteritis and colitis.[39]

Liver tonic

Rosemary oil is recommended as a tonic for the liver and gall bladder.[38] It may be used in the treatment of gall bladder infections, biliary colic and gallstones.[36,37,42] For this purpose Fischer-Rizzi recommends warm compresses of rosemary.[42]

Mailhebiau recommends *R. officinalis* ct. bornyl acetate, verbenone for people who are very tired, with an overloaded liver, fetid breath and a grey complexion. He describes it as a 'remarkable regulator of the liver.'[5]

Musculoskeletal system

Rosemary oil makes a good analgesic and should be used for treating rheumatism, arthritis, and tired, stiff and overworked muscles.[36,37,38]

Nervous system

Rosemary oil is well known for its stimulating effect on the central nervous system. It is reputed to be a brain stimulant and is used for poor concentration and nervous debility.[36,38,42]

Holmes describes rosemary oil as a nervous and cerebral restorative, and recommends it for conditions such as mental and physical fatigue, debility, and memory or concentration loss.[39]

Mailhebiau recommends blending rosemary ct. 1,8-cineole with peppermint and lavender as an excellent treatment for alleviating headaches.[5]

Psychological

Holmes states that rosemary oil promotes motivation and self-confidence. He recommends using the oil for loss of motivation, apathy, self-neglect and feelings of pessimism.[39]

Respiratory system

Rosemary ct. 1,8-cineole oil is recommended for catarrhal conditions and respiratory ailments such as bronchitis, asthma and sinusitis.[3,37,38] Rosemary ct. verbenone oil is recommended for its mucolytic properties.[3,36,37]

Skin care

Rosemary has traditionally been used in skin and hair care.[38] It is extensively used in hair care products as it is reputed to stimulate hair growth and prevent premature baldness. It is also used for the prevention of dandruff.[11]

Energetics, psyche and subtle uses

Energetics

Holmes states that rosemary oil helps to tonify the *Qi* and strengthen the *Shen*. It is recommended for conditions associated with physical and mental fatigue, poor focus and memory, and depression. It also warms the *Lungs,* expels phlegm and dispels *wind-cold*. It is, therefore, recommended for conditions associated with chronic cough, sputum expectoration, sinus congestion, aches and pains.[39]

Mojay refers to rosemary as one of the most valuable and invigorating essential oils, describing it as an excellent tonic for the body's *Yang* energy promoting the circulation of *Qi* and *Blood*.[40]

According to the principles of TCM and the Five Elements, I would associate rosemary oil with the Wood Element.

Personality

Worwood describes the rosemary personality as a young at heart person who has found the elixir of youth. They are imaginative, happy, sensitive people with determination. They love security and aim to be in a secure position in love and life because it's within a secure environment that they can express themselves fully. Rosemary has a spirit that vibrates at an astonishing level; others often find it difficult to keep up with rosemary personalities. They have the ability to perform several tasks at once. They love a challenge and set high standards for themselves.[43]

The rosemary personality types have high ideals of themselves and consider themselves to be better than most people around them; however, not in a consciously arrogant way. They always judge with their head, rather than their heart. They are very open and trustworthy and will make good friends.[43]

Mailhebiau provides us with a character profile of each chemotype of rosemary. He describes *R. officinalis* ct. 1,8-cineole as a cheerful, youthful and sincere character, while *R. officinalis* ct. bornyl acetate, verbenone is a super human being whose stability, strength and equilibrium have no equal in love, justice and light. On the other hand, *R. officinalis* ct. camphor is an elderly man, essentially characterised by the temperament of an old moaner.[5]

According to Myers-Briggs personality types, the rosemary personality is likely to be an ESTP. ESTPs are confident, gregarious and exciting. They like being with people who share their interests and sense of fun. Adventure is pleasurable for them. They are charming and have an infectious manner. They can be assertive. They have lots of energy and are constantly on the go. They can have an intense personality and seek recognition and success. They are often not interested in dealing with interpersonal or emotional issues.

Subtle

Davis describes rosemary as a psychic protector. She recommends using the oil first thing in the morning before exposing oneself to all the external influences. Rosemary oil is associated with clear thought and is helpful wherever there is a need for clarity. It is, therefore, associated with the third eye or brow chakra.[44]

Keim Loughran & Bull explain that rosemary promotes mental clarity, allowing us to remember what we truly value. It strengthens our relationship with our spirit and strengthens our willpower so we can walk our spiritual path with purpose and intent. It also deepens our joyful, loving connection with the sustenance of faith and the tender, powerful truth that we are always with our spirit.[45]

Zeck states that the scent of rosemary stimulates the psyche while allowing us to tap into the enormous riches of the creative realm. It allows us to recharge our creative batteries and reconnect our creative fire, and allows us to tap into the next part of our cycle to emerge.[46]

R

Dosage and Administration

Blending

Aromatherapy

As a liver restorative and tonic, consider blending rosemary oil with essential oils such as lemon and everlasting.

For the relief of upper respiratory tract infections such as sinusitis and rhinitis, consider blending rosemary oil with essential oils such as cajeput, 1,8-cineole rich eucalypts, fragonia, myrtle, peppermint, pine, ravintsara or thyme.

For the relief of muscular pains, cramps, tendinitis, sprains and strains, consider blending rosemary oil with essential oils such as black pepper, cajeput, 1,8-cineole rich eucalypts, ginger, kunzea or pine.

As a mental restorative, consider blending rosemary oil with essential oils such as basil, black pepper, ginger, lemongrass, lemon, pine or peppermint.

As a hair restorative and tonic for seborrhoea, dandruff and alopecia, consider blending rosemary oil with essential oils such as Atlas cedarwood or patchouli.

Perfumery

Arctander states that rosemary oil is extensively used in perfumery for citrus colognes, fougère style perfumes, pine needle fragrances and oriental style perfumes. It blends well with cedarwood oils, citronella, labdanum, lavender, elemi, frankincense, petitgrain and thyme oils.[4]

Mode of administration

Bath

Full body bath, foot bath

Topical

Compress, massage, ointment, skin care

Inhalation

Direct inhalation, diffuser, oil vaporiser

Safety Profile

General safety

Lawless states that rosemary oil is non-toxic, non-irritating and non-sensitising.[36] However, it should not be used during pregnancy and by people suffering from epilepsy.[36,38,42]

Contraindications

A case was reported where a patient with well-controlled epilepsy experienced a seizure. It was believed that the culprit was camphor from rosemary oil, which was one of the ingredients in a commercial massage product that had been used.[47]

I agree with Tisserand & Young who explain that it is incorrect to assume that essential oils that are emmenagogues (including rosemary) are unsafe to use in pregnancy. They explain that all of the essential oils that are alleged to be emmenagogues or uterine stimulants are not powerful enough to cause miscarriage.[48]

Based on the camphor content the oil may be neurotoxic.[48] Therefore, I would prefer rosemary oil not be used during pregnancy.

Regulatory guidelines

Rosemary oil has GRAS status.

References

1. Khan I, Abourashed E. *Leung's encyclopedia of common natural ingredients used in food, drugs and cosmetics*. 3rd edn. John Wiley & Sons, New Jersey, 2010.
2. Schnaubelt K. *Advanced aromatherapy*. Healing Arts Press, Rochester, 1995.
3. Schnaubelt K. *The healing intelligence of essential oils*. Healing Arts Press, Rochester, 2011.
4. Arctander S. *Perfume and flavor materials of natural origin*. Allured Publishing, Carol

Stream, 1994.
5. Mailhebiau P. *Portraits in oils*. C.W. Daniel Company, Saffron Walden, 1995.
6. Lawrence BM. *Progress in essential oils – rosemary oil and extract*. Perfumer & Flavorist 2007; 32: 48-52.
7. Lawrence BM. *Progress in essential oils – rosemary oil*. Perfumer & Flavorist. 2001; 26: 50-63.
8. Ouahada S. *Tunisian rosemary oil*. Perfumer & Flavorist. 2000; 25: 24-25.
9. Svoboda KP, Deans SG. *A study of the variability of rosemary and sage and their volatile oils on the British market: their antioxidant properties*. Flavour and Fragrance Journal, 1990; 7(2): 81-87. Cited in Quintessential Aromatics database, 2013.
10. Le Strange R. *A history of herbal plants*. Angus and Robertson, United Kingdom, 1977.
11. Grieve M. *A modern herbal – Vol. II*. Dover Publications, New York, 1971.
12. Blumenthal M et al. *The complete German commission E monographs: therapeutic guide to herbal medicine*. American Botanical Council, Austin, 1998.
13. Hay IC et al. *Randomized trial of aromatherapy. Successful treatment of alopecia areata*. Archives of Dermatology, 1998; 134(11): 1349-1352. Cited in Quintessential Aromatics database, 2013.
14. Ozmen I et al. *Efficacy of aromatherapy in the treatment of localized alopecia areata: a double-blind placebo controlled study*. Gulhane Medical Journal, 2015; 57: 233-236. Cited in Quintessential Aromatics database, 2013.
15. Minaiyan M et al. *Effects of extract and essential oil of Rosmarinus officinalis L. on TNBS-induced colitis in rats.* Research in Pharmaceutical Sciences, 2011; 6(1): 13-21. Cited in Quintessential Aromatics database, 2013.
16. Panahi Y et al. *Rosemary oil vs minoxidil 2% for the treatment of androgenetic alopecia: a randomized comparative trial.* SKINmed, 2015; 13 (1): 15-21. Cited in Quintessential Aromatics database, 2013.
17. Bozin B et al. *Antimicrobial and antioxidant properties of rosemary and sage (Rosmarinus officinalis L. and Salvia officinalis L ., Lamiaceae) essential oils.* Journal of Agricultural and Food Chemistry, 2007; 55(19): 7879-7885. Cited in Quintessential Aromatics database, 2013.
18. Soliman FM et al. *Analysis and biological activity of the essential oil of Rosmarinus officinalis from Egypt*. Flavour and Fragrance Journal, 1994; 9(1): 29-33. Cited in the Aromatherapy Database, by Bob Harris, Essential Oil Resource Consultants, UK, 2000.
19. Steinmetz MD et al. *Transmission and scanning electronmicroscopy study of the action of sage and rosemary essential oils and eucalyptol on Candida albicans*. Mycoses, 1988; 31(1): 40-51. Cited in Quintessential Aromatics database, 2013.
20. Sienkiewicz M et al. *The potential use of basil and rosemary essential oils as effective antibacterial agents*. Molecules, 2013; 18(8): 9334-9351. doi: 10.3390/molecules18089334.
21. Fu YF et al. *Antimicrobial activity of clove and rosemary essential oils alone and in combination.* Phytotherapy Research, 2007; 21(10): 989-994. Cited in Quintessential Aromatics database, 2013.
22. Luqman S et al. *Potential of rosemary oil to be used in drug-resistant infections*. Alternative Therapies, 2007; 13(5): 54-59. Cited in Quintessential Aromatics database, 2013.
23. Moss M, Oliver L. *Plasma 1,8-cineole correlates with cognitive performance following exposure to rosemary essential oil aroma*. Therapeutic Advances in Psychopharmacology, 2012; 2(3): 103-113. doi: 10.1177/2045125312436573.
24. Milanovic I et al. *Interaction of Rosmarinus officinalis L. essential oil with diazepam and pentobarbital in experiemental animals.* Value in Health, 2014; 17(3): A15. Cited in Quintessential Aromatics database, 2013.
25. Atsumi T, Tonosaki K. *Smelling lavender and rosemary increases free radical scavenging activity and decreases level in saliva.* Psychiatry Research, 2007; 150(1): 89-96. Cited in Quintessential Aromatics database, 2013.
26. Fahim FA et al. *Allied studies on the effect of Rosmarinus officinalis L. on experimental hepatoxicity and mutagenesis.* International Journal of Food Sciences and Nutrition, 1999; 50: 413-427. Cited in Quintessential Aromatics database, 2013.
27. Rašković A et al. *Antioxidant activity of rosemary (Rosmarinus officinalis L.) essential oil and its hepatoprotective potential.* BMC Complementary and Alternative Medicine, 2014; 14: 225. doi: 10.1186/1472-6882-14-225.
28. Al-Hader AA et al. *Hyperglycaemic and insulin release inhibitory effects of Rosmarinus officinalis.* Journal of Ethnopharmacology, 1994, 43(3): 217-221. Cited in the Aromatherapy Database, by Bob Harris, Essential Oil Resource Consultants, UK, 2000.
29. Isman MB et al. *Insecticidal activities of commercial rosemary oils (Rosmarinus officinalis) against larvae of Pseudaletia unipuncta and Trichoplusia ni. in relation to their chemical composition.* Pharmaceutical Biology, 2008; 46 (1/2): 82-87.
30. Lahlou M, Berrada R. *Composition and niticidal activity of essential oils of three chemotypes of Rosmarinus officinalis L. acclimatized in Morocco.* Flavour and Fragrance Journal, 2003; 18(2): 124-127. Cited in Quintessential Aromatics database, 2013.
31. Taddei I et al. *Spasmolytic activity of peppermint, sage and rosemary essences and their major constituents.* Fitoterapia, 1988; 59(6): 463-468.

32. Kovar KA et al. *Blood levels of 1,8-cineole and locomotor activity of mice after inhalation and oral administration of rosemary oil.* Planta Medica, 1987; 53(4): 315-318. Cited in the Aromatherapy Database, by Bob Harris, Essential Oil Resource Consultants, UK, 2000.
33. Diego M et al. *Aromatherapy positively affects mood, EEG patterns of alertness and math computations.* International Journal of Neuroscience, 1998; 96(3/4): 217-224. Cited in Quintessential Aromatics Database, 2013.
34. Saeki Y, Shiohara M. *Physiological effects of inhaling fragrances.* International Journal of Aromatherapy, 2001; 11(3): 118-125. Cited in Quintessential Aromatics database, 2013.
35. Sayorwan W et al. *Effects of inhaled rosemary oil on subjective feelings and activities of the nervous system.* Scientia Pharmaceutica, 2013; 81(2): 531-542. Cited in Quintessential Aromatics Database, 2013.
36. Lawless J. *The encyclopaedia of essential oils.* Element Books, Shaftesbury, 1992.
37. Lavabre M. *Aromatherapy workbook.* Healing Arts Press, Rochester, 1997.
38. Davis P. *Aromatherapy: an A-Z.* 2nd edn. C.W. Daniel Company, Saffron Walden, 1999.
39. Holmes P. *Aromatica: a clinical guide to essential oil therapeutics – Vol. I.* Singing Dragon, London, 2016.
40. Mojay G. *Aromatherapy for healing the spirit.* Healing Arts Press, Rochester, 1999.
41. Committee on Herbal Medicinal Products (HMPC). *Assessment report on Rosmarinus officinalis L., aetheroleum and Rosmarinus officinalis L., folium.* European Medicines Agency, London, 2010. Doc ref. EMA/HMPC/13631/2009.
42. Fischer-Rizzi S. *Complete aromatherapy handbook.* Sterling Publishing, New York, 1990.
43. Worwood VA. *The fragrant mind.* Transworld Publishing, London, 1995.
44. Davis P. *Subtle aromatherapy.* C.W. Daniel Company, Saffron Walden, 1991.
45. Keim Loughran J, Bull R. *Aromatherapy anointing oils.* Frog, Berkeley, 2001.
46. Zeck R. *The blossoming heart – aromatherapy for healing and transformation.* Aroma Tours, East Ivanhoe, 2004.
47. Bozorg AM, Benbadis SR. *Essential oils as a cause of breakthrough seizure after temporal lobectomy.* Seizure, 2009; 18(8): 604-605. Cited in Quintessential Aromatics database, 2013.
48. Tisserand R, Young R. *Essential oil safety.* 2nd edn. Churchill Livingstone, Edinburgh, 2014.

Rosewood

Identification

Botanical name

Aniba rosaeodora Ducke

Synonyms

Bois de rose

Family

Lauraceae

Botany and origins

The tree is a tropical, medium-sized, slow-growing evergreen from the Amazon basin.[1]

Guenther explains that there used to be two commercial rosewood oils. One was called Cayenne oil and was produced in French Guiana. This oil is no longer commercially available. There is also the Brazilian rosewood oil produced from timber in the lower Amazon basin. It is interesting that until 1927 only the Cayenne oil was available. The two trees are closely related. However, the Guiana rosewood oil had a higher percentage of linalool (90-97%) compared to the Brazilian rosewood oil (80-90%).[2]

Sadly, the over-exploitation of rosewood has been going on since the 1920s. Guenther states that in 1929 there were almost 50 field distilleries operant in French Guiana. The demand for the wood became so great that trees were being exploited recklessly, and since no provision had ever been made for replanting, the woodcutters had to move into even more remote areas of the Amazon basin. By 1932 the trees had become so scarce that only three distilleries were able to continue operation. While the production of Cayenne rosewood oil eventually ceased, another variety of rosewood growing in the wild parts of the Amazon basin of Brazil was found to yield a similar oil. Eventually the rosewood oil from Brazil, the oil that is available nowadays, became the only commercially produced rosewood oil.[2]

In 1932, Brazil and French Guiana issued Decree No. 1455 which stipulated that only a limited quantity of rosewood oil could be produced yearly and only by those distillers who obligated themselves to replace every cut tree with a newly planted one.[2]

Then at a later date, legislation was enacted which required one new tree to be planted by the distillery for every 20 kg of rosewood oil sold. Guenther explained that the replanting had to be done under the supervision of a government inspector, who signed a receipt for every planted tree. It is obvious that the woodcutters and distilleries did not follow through with any of these initiatives taken by the Brazilian government to prevent the indiscriminate harvesting of the rosewood trees.[2]

Method of extraction

Rosewood oil is steam-distilled and occasionally water-distilled from the chipped wood of *A. rosaeodora*.[1]

Characteristics

Rosewood oil from Brazil is a colourless to pale yellow liquid of a refreshing, sweet-woody, somewhat floral-spicy odour. The top note varies considerably with the origin and quality of the oil. It is usually camphoraceous and peppery with a hint of 1,8-cineole.[1]

Chemical composition

The major constituent of rosewood oil is linalool (80-90%).[2] A commercial sample of rosewood oil had the following chemical composition:

α-pinene (0.15%), camphene (0.03%), β-pinene (0.52%), myrcene (0.04%), limonene (0.6%), *cis*-linalool oxide (1.5%), *trans*-linalool oxide (1.31%), 1,8-cineole + β-phellandrene (1.61%), linalool (85.29%), terpinen-4-ol (0.37%), caryophyllene (0.03%), α-terpineol (3.54%), geranyl acetate (0.14%).[3]

Adulteration

Rosewood is often adulterated with synthetic linalool, α-terpineol and geraniol.[4,5]

Pharmacopoeias and standards

The purity, composition and physico-chemical properties of rosewood oil are defined in ISO 3761:2005 Oil of Rosewood, Brazilian Type (*Aniba rosaeodora* Ducke or *Aniba parviflora* Meisn)

History and Traditional Uses

History

The commercial interest in rosewood oil is because of the linalool, which is an important aromatic chemical used in the fragrance industry. However, with the advent of synthetic linalool and cheaper sources of linalool from ho leaf oil from China, the production of rosewood oil has declined.[1]

In the second edition of *The Complete Guide to Aromatherapy* in 2003, I quoted Shawe, who stated that, while the *Aniba rosaeodora* species is not threatened, as a result of heavy exploitation of the trees, very few trees exceeding a 30 cm girth can be found within 20 km of riverbanks of navigable rivers. This is the only means of bulk transportation in the Amazon region.[6]

Shawe explained that the production of rosewood is not efficient. Young branch wood provides high oil yields, but is rejected on site in favour of the more readily portable trunk wood. This means that up to 60% of the wood biomass is left on site and therefore wasted. Further losses occur in sawing and chipping the wood prior to distillation, and owing to out of date equipment, oil recovery is inefficient.[6]

While substantial stands of *A. rosaeodora* still remain because they are in inaccessible parts of the Amazon, producers are now harvesting smaller trees than before, including species of *Aniba* that had previously been left untouched.[6]

Unfortunately, not much has changed – nowadays rosewood is listed in the IUCN Red List of Threatened Species as endangered.[7]

The IUCN report for rosewood states that populations of all rosewood species have seriously declined because of rosewood oil extraction. Where there has been exploitation of rosewood trees, the area has become devoid of mature trees and signs of regeneration are absent. Trees of all sizes are harvested indiscriminately with the whole tree and its roots being destroyed. Brazil is now the sole producer of the oil. Harvesting is costly and is taking place in more and more remote locations concentrated around the Amazon tributaries. Mobile distillation factories have also moved deep into the forest. The report also states that levels of exploitation have significantly declined with the increased use of synthetic oils. The good news is that substantial wild strands are believed to exist in areas which are unlikely to be exploited.[7]

In 2010, CITES (Convention on International Trade of Endangered Species of Wild Fauna and Flora) included *A. rosaeodora* in Appendix II. This refers to species that are not necessarily threatened with extinction, but in which trade must be controlled in order to avoid utilisation incompatible with their survival. This includes the trade of logs, sawn wood, veneer sheets and essential oil.[8]

According to a report cited by Cropwatch, it is not surprising to know that the over-exploitation of the tree now means that this species has become endangered, despite many of the restrictive regulations by the Brazilian government designed to help in its conservation.[9]

The same report also states that rosewood essential oil continues to be used by many leading fragrance houses even though the tree is now on the threatened list.[9]

The Brazilian National Institute for the

Environmental and Natural Resources (IBAMA) issued a set of directions to the rosewood distillers in 1998. They were as follows:

- Rosewood harvest is not permissible in certain areas.
- No trees with a diameter at breast height less than 20 cm can be felled.
- There is an annual amount of wood permitted to be distilled.
- Re-forestation must be proportionate to the tree harvest.
- A limit of 2,000 trees can be harvested annually.
- The possession of an IBAMA certificate is mandatory for oil export.[10]

Unfortunately, such directives are hopeless if they are not enforced, and despite these regulations, the species is still being exploited and is vanishing from much of its original habitat.

It was interesting to find a report on a trial conducted in French Guiana assessing the opportunity to produce essential oil from cultivated rosewood trees. The authors identified the optimum growing conditions for the trees and production of essential oil of a consistent quality. The aim of the study was to assess the influence of surrounding forest and seed provenance on tree growth and on the yield of essential oil.[11]

The results of the study support the opinion of commercial distillers in Brazil that young rosewood stems provide higher oil yields than larger mature trees. They considered harvesting is feasible at 10 years of age, whereas it had been previously reported that trees in an open-field plantation would require around 20 years of growth before being ready for felling and distillation of rosewood. The authors state that the management system they have developed would not only protect an endangered species, but also provide a sustainable source of rosewood trees for the production of essential oil.[11]

However, at the time of writing, I do not believe that this has led to production of rosewood oil from cultivated plantations of rosewood trees.

Food, perfumery and flavouring

Rosewood oil was originally produced for the fragrance and perfume industry, and the wood extensively used for furniture production.[4] Rosewood oil was extensively used as a source of natural linalool or linalyl acetate which is used in perfumery.[12]

Arctander states that ho leaf oil is a major competitor for rosewood essential oil. Ho leaf oil contains more linalool, and when the oil is rectified, its terpenes have a less harsh or penetrating aroma.[1]

R

Therapeutics

Pharmacology and clinical studies

Anticonvulsant activity

Linalool, the main constituent in rosewood, has been reported to have anticonvulsant activity in mice and rats and spasmolytic activity on isolated guinea pig ileum.[12]

A study investigated the effects of rosewood essential oil and linalool on adenylate cyclase. Both rosewood oil and linalool inhibited the cAMP accumulation stimulated by forskolin, even when the adenosine receptors were blocked with the non-selective adenosine receptor antagonist 3-isobutyl-methyl-xanthine.[13]

Antimicrobial activity

Rosewood oil is reported to have antimicrobial properties.[4,14]

Sedative activity

The sedative activity of rosewood oil was determined by measuring the potentiation of pentobarbital-induced sleeping time. The results indicated that the rosewood significantly decreased latency and increased the duration of sleep time.[15]

Actions

Actions commonly cited in aromatherapy

Antidepressant, antiseptic, bactericide, cephalic, deodorant, insecticide, stimulant[16,17]

Actions supported by clinical studies

Antispasmodic, sedative

Comment

I am disappointed that some within the aromatherapy industry continue to sell and supply rosewood oil, considering that it is listed in the IUCN Red List of Threatened Species and CITES as endangered.

I recommend that, until we can be assured of plantation-grown rosewood, which does not commercially exist at the moment, we should refrain from using rosewood essential oil in aromatherapy. There are so many other essential oils that can produce a relaxation effect without having to contribute to the destruction of the environment and endangering of a species.

Aromatherapy Uses

Clinical aromatherapy

Nervous system

Some aromatherapists have stated that rosewood's

uplifting and enlivening properties are reputed to have an overall balancing effect. It has been recommended for people who are feeling stressed, depressed and dragged down by the burdens of life.[18] The oil has also been recommended for alleviating headaches and anxiety.[16,17,18]

Skin care

Some aromatherapists have stated that rosewood oil is beneficial for treating acne, dermatitis, sensitive skin, aged skin and damaged skin.[16,17] It has been considered a very safe oil to use on the skin and its antiseptic properties makes it an excellent oil to use in a deodorant.[16,18]

Energetics, psyche and subtle uses

Subtle

Davis suggests using rosewood oil for meditation or in preparation of any spiritual healing. It has a calming effect without inducing any drowsiness. It is associated with the crown chakra.[19]

Dosage and Administration

Blending

Aromatherapy

Due to the current endangered status of rosewood, it would be irresponsible of me to provide guidelines for aromatherapy blending using rosewood oil.

Perfumery

Arctander states that rosewood oil has lost much of its importance in perfumery because of other sources of natural linalool from ho leaf and production of synthetic linalool.[1]

Mode of administration

Bath

Full body bath, foot bath

Topical

Compress, massage, ointment, skin care

Inhalation

Direct inhalation, diffuser, oil vaporiser

Safety Profile

General safety

Rosewood oil is non-toxic, non-irritating and non-sensitising.[16]

Contraindications

No contraindications known.

Regulatory guidelines

Rosewood essential oil has GRAS status.

References

1. Arctander S. *Perfume and flavor materials of natural origin.* Allured Publishing, Carol Stream, 1994.
2. Guenther E. *The essential oils – Vol. IV.* Robert E Krieger Publishing, Malabar, 1950.
3. Lawrence BM. *Essential oils 1981-1987.* Allured Publishing, Wheaton, 1989.
4. Lis-Balchin M. *Aromatherapy science – a guide for healthcare professionals.* Pharmaceutical Press, London, 2006.
5. Schmidt E, Wanner J. *Adulteration of essential oils.* In Baser KHC, Buchbauer G. eds. *Handbook of essential oils – science, technology and applications.* 2nd edn. CRC Press, Boca Raton, 2016: 707-745.
6. Shawe K. *Conservation and aromatherapy – what you need to know.* The World of Aromatherapy III Conference Proceedings, NAHA, 2000; 27-32.
7. Varty N. *Aniba rosodora.* The IUCN Red List of Threatened Species 1998: e.T33958A68966060. doi: 10.2305/IUCN.UK.1998.RLTS.T33958A68966060.en.
8. *Notification No.2010/036 concerning Annotations for Aniba rosaeodora (Brazilian rosewood), Bulnesia sarmientoi (palo santo) and Euphorbia antisyphilitica (candelilla).* CITES, Geneva, 2010.
9. *Cropwatch's Rosewood Biblio (Aniba rosaedora Ducke) together with other related & unrelated Aniba spp.* Cropwatch, 2010: 1(7). Retrieved Mar 10, 2017, from http://cropwatch.org.uk/rosewood%20Biblio%201.07.pdf
10. Lawrence BM. *Progress in essential oils – rosewood or bois-de-rose oil.* Retrieved Nov 23, 2017, from http://www.perfumerflavorist.com/fragrance/rawmaterials/natural/Progress-in-Essential-oils-420426493.html
11. Amusant N et al. *Planting rosewood for sustainable essential oil production: influence of surrounding forest and seed provenance on tree growth and essential oil yields.* Bois et Forets des Tropiques, 2015; 326 (4).
12. Khan I, Abourashed E. *Leung's encyclopedia of common natural ingredients used in food, drugs and cosmetics.* 3rd edn. John Wiley & Sons, New Jersey, 2010.
13. Sampaio LFS et al. *Linalool from rosewood (Aniba rosaeodora Ducke) oil inhibits adenylate cyclase in the retina, contributing to understanding its biological activity.* Phytotherapy Research, 2012; 26(1): 73-77. Cited in Quintessential Aromatics database, 2013.

R

14. Lobato AM et al. *Antimicrobial activity of essential oils from the Amazon.* Acta Amazonica, 1989; 19: 355-363.
15. de Almeida RN et al. *Rosewood oil induces sedation and inhibits compound action potential in rodents.* Journal of Ethnopharmacology, 2009; 124(3): 440-443. Cited in Quintessential Aromatics database, 2013.
16. Lawless J. *The encyclopaedia of essential oils.* Element Books, Shaftesbury, 1992.
17. Lavabre M. *Aromatherapy workbook.* Healing Arts Press, Rochester, 1997.
18. Davis P. *Aromatherapy: an A-Z.* 2nd edn. C.W. Daniel Company, Saffron Walden, 1999.
19. Davis P. *Subtle aromatherapy.* C.W. Daniel Company, Saffron Walden, 1991.

Sage

Identification

Botanical name

Salvia officinalis L.

Synonyms

Common sage, garden sage, Dalmatian sage

Family

Lamiaceae (Labiatae)

Botany and origins

S. officinalis is a small, evergreen, shrubby perennial with woody stems near the base and herbaceous ones above. It grows up to 0.8 m high and is native to the Mediterranean region. It is cultivated worldwide.[1]

Although there are over 900 species of sage throughout the world, only a few can be used as a raw material in herbal medicine and aromatherapy.[2]

Sage oil, usually known as Dalmatian sage oil, is produced in Bosnia. It is also produced in the USA, Bulgaria, Turkey, Malta, France and Germany. *Salvia lavandulaefolia* is closely related to *S. officinalis.* It grows wild in Spain and southwestern France.[2]

Method of extraction

Sage oil is steam-distilled from the dried leaves of *S. officinalis*.

Characteristics

Sage oil is a pale yellow, mobile liquid with a fresh, strong, warm-herbaceous and camphoraceous odour.[3]

Chemical composition

The chemical composition of sage essential oil produced from wild *S. officinalis* plants collected in Croatia in the month of June was reported as follows:

α-pinene (3.0%), camphene (1.7%), β-pinene (0.7%), myrcene (1.0%), limonene (1.0%), 1,8-cineole (13.2%), α-thujone (23.1%), β-thujone (25.0%), camphor (9.5%), linalool (0.5%), linalyl acetate (0.8%), bornyl acetate (0.9%), borneol (1.4%), α-humulene (1.2%).[4]

The chemical composition of sage essential oil produced from plants harvested in six different locations in Jordan was reported as follows:

α-thujene (0.1-1.8%), α-pinene (2.0-4.8%), camphene (0.2-3.9%), β-pinene (3.3-7.3%), myrcene (0.9-1.9%), 1,8-cineole (39.5-48.5%), *cis*-thujone (1.2-3.7%), *trans*-thujone (0.1-9.9%), camphor (8.8-25.0%), borneol (1.5-2.2%), bornyl acetate (0.2-1.3%), α-terpineol (2.6-3.1%), α-terpenyl acetate (1.4-2.9%).[5]

The composition *of S. officinalis* essential oil is highly influenced by genetics and environmental factors such as seasonality, climatic conditions and age of the plant. As a result, it does not always match the profile define by ISO 9909 described as follows:

α-thujone (18.0-43.0%), β-thujone (3.0-8.5%), camphor (4.5-24.5%), 1,8-cineole (5.5-13.0%), humulene (0-12.0%), α-pinene (1.0-6.5%), camphene (1.5-7.0%), limonene (0.5-3.0%), linalool (1% maximum) and bornyl acetate (2.5% maximum).[5]

Sage oil has been categorised into five chemotypes according to the amount of the major constituents:[5]

- camphor > α-thujone > 1,8-cineole > β-thujone
- camphor > α-thujone > β-thujone > 1,8-cineole
- β-thujone > camphor> 1,8-cineole > α-thujone
- 1,8-cineole > camphor > α-thujone > β-thujone
- α-thujone > camphor > β-thujone > 1,8-cineole.

The chemical composition of eight *S. officinalis* essential oils extracted from plants growing in different gardens in Lithuania were also examined and varied significantly:

1,8-cineole (0.7-17.6%), *cis*-thujone (4.8-9.6%), *trans*-thujone (0.8-3.2%), camphor (1.3-6.2%), borneol (3.5-8.1%), α-humulene (5.2-11.2%), viridiflorol (5.0-16.5%) and manool (7.9-15.7%).[6]

Adulteration

Sage is occasionally adulterated with other essential oils that have a similar odour profile such as cedar leaf (thuja) oil, Spanish sage, rosemary oil and various *Artemisia* oils.[3] The oil is also adulterated with β-caryophyllene, 1,8-cineole and borneol from other sources.[7] In turn, sage is also used as an adulterant in other oils.[3]

Pharmacopoeias and standards

The purity, composition and physico-chemical properties of sage oil are defined in several standards and monographs. The following pharmacopoeia and standards are available:

- ISO 9909:1997 – Oil of Dalmatian Sage
- Public Statement on *Salvia officinalis* L., aetheroleum. European Medicines Agency
- German Drug Codex.

History and Traditional Uses

History

The generic name *Salvia* is derived from the Latin *salvare*, meaning 'to save', which refers to its medicinal properties. Sage has been used by Egyptians, Greeks and Romans since ancient times.

In the Middle Ages, there was a saying, 'Why should a man die whilst sage grows in his garden?'[2]

Sixteen-century herbalist Gerard tells us that sage is good for the head and brain, and that it improves the senses and memory and restores health to those who have palsy. According to Culpeper, sage was reputed to provoke urine, bring down women's courses, stop the bleeding of wounds and cleanse foul ulcers and sores.[8]

Traditional medicine

Sage is used as a tonic, digestive, astringent and antispasmodic. It is used as a tea or infusion. It is used to reduce perspiration, to stop the flow of milk, and to treat nervous conditions, dysmenorrhoea, diarrhoea, gastritis and sore throat.[1]

Sage is mentioned in Ebers Papyrus (1500 BC) for treating itches. It was also used for labour pain, contractions, ulcers, coughing, hoarseness and perspiration.[2]

Herbal

The German Commission E recommends sage herb internally for dyspeptic symptoms and excessive perspiration. Externally it is recommended for inflammation of the mucous membranes of the nose and throat.[9]

The antioxidant properties of sage herb have been comprehensively studied and found to be related to the presence of rosmarinic acid and carnosic acid. Salvianolic acid also exhibited high antioxidant activity and is a very strong scavenger of free radicals. The aqueous extract of *S. officinalis* has been shown to have antioxidant and antiviral effects. In one study, it was observed that drinking sage tea for two weeks resulted in improved liver antioxidant status.[10]

Food, perfumery and flavouring

Dalmatian sage oil is extensively used as a flavour material. It is used in liqueurs, canned meats, spice sauces and pickles. The dried leaves are considered the most popular culinary herbs in southern Europe.[3]

Therapeutics

Pharmacology and clinical studies

Many pharmacological studies involving sage essential oil have been published. A systemic review of these studies will not be attempted. Rather, I have chosen a selection of studies that support the traditional and clinical uses.

S

Anticarcinogenic activity

An in vitro study found that *S. officinalis* oil could inhibit human head and neck squamous cell carcinoma growth.[11]

Antifungal activity

Three samples of *S. officinalis* oil exhibited broad antifungal activity against four clinical isolates of candida, dermatophytes and other filamentous fungi. The sage oils with the lower content of thujone were confirmed to be the most active.[12]

S. officinalis essential oil exhibited antifungal activity against two clinical strains of *Candida albicans,* with inhibition zones ranging from 40.5 to 19.5 mm.[13]

An in vitro study examined the antifungal and anti-inflammatory activity of *S. officinalis* oil from Jordan whose main compounds were 1,8-cineole (39.5-50.3%) and camphor (8.8-25.0%). The oil had a strong antifungal activity against dermatophyte strains, and significantly inhibited NO production stimulated by LPS in macrophages, without affecting cell viability, in concentrations up to 0.64 μL/mL.[5]

Antimicrobial activity

Sage oil is reported to have significant

antimicrobial activity on oral bacteria responsible for the development of dental disease.[14]

S. officinalis oil from Tunisia displayed strong antimicrobial vapour activity against a range of bacteria. It was suggested that the oil could be used as an eco-friendly disinfectant to manage airbourne microbes.[15]

A study compared the antimicrobial activity of *S. officinalis* oils from the same plant, but at different stages of the plant's life – young leaves and old leaves. The results indicated that the essential oils from younger leaves potentiated the inhibitory effect of antibiotics against methicillin-resistant *Staphylococcus aureus* strains.[16]

Another in vitro study also confirmed that there was a synergistic effect of *S. officinalis* oil with oxacillin against methicillin-resistant *Staphylococcus epidermis*.[17]

Antispasmodic activity

Sage oil has been reported to have antispasmodic effects. Small doses of the essential oil inhibited isolated guinea pig ileum contractions induced by electrical stimulation.[18]

Chemoprotective activity

An in vivo study involving the topical application of sage oil to mouse skin at concentrations of 5, 50 and 100% significantly inhibited chemically induced tumour growths. The observed growth inhibition was due to cytostatic and not cytotoxic effects. It was suggested that sage oil has potent suppressive activities against tumour promotion in mouse skin, and could be an effective chemopreventive against skin cancer.[19]

Cognitive performance

Many of the studies involving improvement in cognitive function involved the standardised ethanolic extracts of sage. However, one study found that the inhalation of *Salvia officinalis* essential oil could reproduce some, but not all the effects found following herbal administration. Data analysis of a study using 135 healthy volunteers found that the *S. officinalis* aroma group performed significantly better than the control group on the quality of memory and secondary memory primary outcome factors from the test battery.[20]

A systematic review of a clinical trial assessed the pharmacological properties of *Salvia* species on memory, cognitive impairment and Alzheimer's disease. It was concluded that *S. officinalis* and *S. lavandulaefolia* herbs and essential oils exert beneficial effects by enhancing cognitive performance both in healthy subjects and patients with dementia or cognitive impairment, and are safe. However, it was also stated that the beneficial effects are debased by methodological issues and believe that sage's promising effects need to be further investigated.[21]

Epileptogenic activity

A clinical trial identified that the ketone components of *Salvia officinalis* – thujone and camphor – are responsible for an increase in epileptiform seizures.[22]

Hypoglycaemic activity

An in vivo study on rats found that sage oil exhibited significant hypoglycaemic activity.[23]

Spasmolytic activity

Sage oil had a relatively weak spasmolytic effect on isolated guinea pig ileum smooth muscle in comparison to melissa or thyme essential oils. However, a water-alcohol extract of *S. officinalis* demonstrated a strong spasmolytic action on smooth-muscle contractions in isolated guinea pig ileum.[24]

Actions

Actions commonly cited in aromatherapy

Antibacterial, anti-inflammatory, antiseptic, antispasmodic, astringent, digestive, diuretic, emmenagogue, febrifuge, hypertensive, insecticidal, stimulant, stomachic, tonic, vulnerary[25,26]

Actions supported by clinical studies

Antibacterial, antifungal, antispasmodic, chemoprotective

Comment

Lawless states that *S. officinalis* oil should not be used in aromatherapy.[25] Schnaubelt explains that as an isolated constituent, thujone is undoubtedly toxic. It is a hepatotoxic and a nerve toxin; however, he explains that toxicity tests have indicated that sage oil is less toxic than it would be expected to be, based on an average thujone content of around 40%. He also explains that if the sage plant is distilled while it is still early in its life cycle when the leaves are still very small, it produces an essential oil with a very low thujone content.[27]

Aromatherapy Uses

Clinical aromatherapy

Digestive system

Sage oil strengthens and promotes digestion. It is recommended where there is a loss of appetite.[26]

Nervous system

Sage oil is recommended for general nervous debility.[28]

Reproductive system

Sage oil has a beneficial effect on the female reproductive system. It is said to imitate the hormone oestrogen, thereby regulating the menstrual cycle.[26,28,29] It is particularly beneficial for treating delayed, scanty or no menstruation with cramp, and for menopausal problems, particularly sweating.[26,28]

Skin care

Sage oil is reputed to be highly regenerative in skin care. Schnaubelt recommends a blend of sage, everlasting and rosehip oil for slow healing wounds. He suggests two applications per day for 10 days on a recent wound, or for three to six months for old scars.[29]

Lavabre states that sage is a regulator of seborrhoea and recommends using it for the treatment of acne, dermatitis, eczema, dandruff and hair loss.[26] Valnet recommends using sage for atonic wounds, sores, ulcers, insect bites and eczema.[30]

Energetics, psyche and subtle uses

Energetics

Sage oil is drying and astringent. It helps to tonify the *Qi*. It is recommended for conditions associated with physical and mental fatigue, poor focus and memory. It also warms the *Lungs*, expels phlegm and dispels *wind-cold*. It is recommended for conditions associated with chronic cough, sputum expectoration and sinus congestion. According to the principles of the Five Elements, sage oil helps to balance the Metal Element.

Personality

Mailhebiau states sage evokes the Greek goddess and huntress Artemis. Artemis is the protector of women, children, wild animals and births. He explains that the powers of life and death are contained within the archetype of sage. He describes sage as mature in age, which does not signify advance in years; however, they are wise and have authority, appealing to people's intelligence rather than their heart. The sage personality is tenacious, persistent, concise and efficient, and is a capable person who is not afraid to impose her authority and strictness.[31]

Mailhebiau states that the sage personality knows how to appear without weakness in order to reach their goals, ruthlessly combating indolence, lameness and laxity in others. However, they can easily become intolerant:

> *… she does not tolerate mistakes, either her own or those of others whom she reproached for not having her qualities as well as for their own faults.*[31]

The sage personality is described as a tireless worker, being able to achieve anything they do, and they will channel all their strength to succeed. Mailhebiau uses Queen Elizabeth I of England, Margaret Thatcher and Indira Gandhi as examples of individuals that epitomise the sage personality.[31]

According to Myers-Briggs personality types, the sage personality is likely to be an ENTJ. ENTJs are dynamic, energetic, confident and competent. They naturally move into positions where they can take charge. They enjoy confrontation and they like to engage in intellectually stimulating exchanges. They like and respect people who challenge them and have little or no respect for those that don't. They have an improvement plan for everything, including their leisure. They like to set goals and provide directions. They see obstacles as challenges. They dislike inefficiency, incompetence and indecisiveness. They are competitively driven and often considered to be workaholics. They can be very honest and direct and do not hesitate to express themselves. When stressed they can have explosive outbursts or be judgemental on themselves and others.

Subtle

Davis suggests using sage in conjunction with meditations or visualisations to develop wisdom.[32]

Worwood describes sage as a protective spirit for those who are not afraid of the spiritual forces. She states that sage encourages strength, courage and perseverance.[33]

Zeck states that sage acknowledges a deeper collective consciousness that assists us on our spiritual quest.[34]

Dosage and Administration

Blending

Aromatherapy

For the relief of musculoskeletal aches and pains, consider blending sage oil with essential oils such as cajeput, kunzea, black pepper, ginger, lavender, sweet marjoram, peppermint and rosemary.

For the relief of colds and flu, consider blending sage oil with essential oils such as bay laurel, 1,8-cineole-rich eucalypts, fragonia, fir, kunzea, lemon, manuka, myrtle, peppermint, pine, tea tree or thyme.

To promote wound healing, consider blending sage oil with essential oils such as carrot seed, everlasting, lavender or myrrh.

Perfumery

Dalmatian sage is reputed to have good tenacity. The fadeout of the odour is sweet-herbaceous and very pleasant. Arctander states that it blends well with citrus oils, lavender and rosemary. It is used to add a fresh note to fougères, chypres, colognes and aldehydic perfume bases.[3]

Mode of administration

Bath

Full body bath, foot bath

Topical

Compress, massage, ointment, skin care

Inhalation

Direct inhalation, diffuser, oil vaporiser

Safety Profile

General safety

Lawless recommends that sage oil not be used in aromatherapy.[25] The oil contains a high percentage of thujone and camphor, which have been identified as provoking epileptic seizures.

While the thujone content of sage is marginally lower than that of tansy and thuja, it is similar to that of wormwood, and therefore it has been suggested that sage oil is equally as toxic as these oils.[36] However, Schnaubelt states that sage is one of the safest of all the oils having a high thujone content, and that sage oil is less toxic than the thujone content alone would suggest.[29]

Tisserand & Young have calculated the maximum dermal use level at 0.4% based on sage oil having a maximum thujone content of 60%.[36]

Contraindications

The German Commission E states that alcoholic extracts of sage and sage essential oil are contraindicated in pregnancy and that their prolonged use may cause epileptiform convulsions.[9]

The EMA states that the benefits of sage do not outweigh the risks.[37]

Sage oil should only be used with great caution and should not be used during pregnancy, or for young children or anyone suffering from epilepsy.[25,26,29]

Tisserand & Young state that sage is a neurotoxin and should not be taken in oral doses.[36]

Davis cites cases where individuals have used only a few drops in a massage oil or bath, and the oil induced moderate to severe uterine contractions and caused excessive menstrual bleeding.[38]

Regulatory guidelines

Sage oil has GRAS status.

References

1. Khan I, Abourashed E. *Leung's encyclopedia of common natural ingredients used in food, drugs and cosmetics.* 3rd edn. John Wiley & Sons, New Jersey, 2010.
2. Altindal D, Altindal N. *Sage (Salvia officinalis) oils.* In Preedy VR. ed. *Essential oils in food preservation, flavor and safety.* Academic Press, London, 2016: 715-721.
3. Arctander S. *Perfume and flavor materials of natural origin.* Allured Publishing, Carol Stream, 1994.
4. Lawrence BM. *Progress in essential oils – sage oil part 1.* Perfumer & Flavorist, 2013; 38: 42-45.
5. Abu-Darwish MS et al. *Essential oil of common sage (Salvia officinalis L.) from Jordan: assessment of safety in mammalian cells and its antifungal and anti-inflammatory potential.* Biomedical Research International, 2013; 2013: 538940. doi: 10.1155/2013/538940.
6. Bernotiene G et al. *Essential oil composition variability in sage (Salvia officinalis L.).* Chemija, 2007; 18(4): 38-43.
7. Schmidt E, Wanner J. *Adulteration of essential oils.* In Baser KHC, Buchbauer G. eds. *Handbook of essential oils – science, technology and applications.* 2nd edn. CRC Press, Boca Raton, 2016: 707-745.
8. Grieve M. *A modern herbal – Vol. II.* Dover Publications, New York, 1971.
9. Blumenthal M et al. *The complete German Commission E monographs: therapeutic guide to herbal medicine.* American Botanical Council, Austin, 1998.
10. Hamidpour M et al. *Chemistry, pharmacology and medicinal property of sage (salvia) to prevent and cure illnesses such as obesity, diabetes, depression, dementia, lupus, autism, heart disease and cancer.* Journal of Traditional and Complementary Medicine, 2014; 4(2): 82-88. doi: 10.4103/2225-4110.130373.
11. Sertel S et al. *Anticancer activity of Salvia officinalis essential oil against HNSCC cell line (UMSCC1).* HNO, 2011; 59(12): 1203-1208. Cited in Quintessential Aromatics database, 2013.
12. Pinto E et al. *In vitro susceptibility of some species of yeasts and filamentous fungi to essential oils of Salvia officinalis.* Industrial Crops and Products, 2007; 26(2): 135-141. Cited in Quintessential Aromatics database, 2013.
13. Sookto T et al. *In vitro effects of Salvia officinalis L. essential oil on Candida albicans.* Asian Pacific Journal of Tropical Biomedicine, 2013; 3(5): 376-380. Cited in Quintessential Aromatics database, 2013.

14. Shapiro S et al. *The antimicrobial activity of essential oils and essential oil components towards oral bacteria.* Oral Microbiology & Immunology, 1994; 9(4): 202-208. Cited in the Aromatherapy Database, by Bob Harris, Essential Oil Resource Consultants, UK, 2000.
15. Bouaziz M et al. *Disinfectant properties of essential oils from Salvia officinalis L. cultivated in Tunisia.* Food and Chemical Toxicology, 2009; 47(11): 2755-2760. Cited in Quintessential Aromatics database, 2013.
16. Milenkovic M et al. *Synergistic effects of Salvia officinalis L. essential oils and antibiotics against methicillin-resistant Staphylococcus aureus.* Archives of Biological Sciences, 2015; 67(3): 949-956. Cited in Quintessential Aromatics database, 2013.
17. Chovanova R et al. *In vitro antibacterial and antibiotic resistance modifying effect of bioactive plant extracts on methicillin-resistant Staphylococcus epidermis.* International journal of Microbiology, 2013; 2013: 760969. doi: 10.1155/2013/760969.
18. Bruneton J. *Pharmacognosy.* 2nd edn. Lavoisier Publishing, Paris, 1999.
19. Gali-Muhtasib HU, Affara NI. *Chemoprotective effects of sage oil on skin papillomas in mice.* Phytomedicine, 2000; 7(2): 129-136. doi: 10.1016/S0944-7113(00)80085-9.
20. Moss L et al. *Differential effects of the aromas of Salvia species on memory and mood.* Human Psychopharmacology, 2010; 25(5): 388-396. Cited in Quintessential Aromatics database, 2013.
21. Miroddi M. *Systematic review of clinical trials assessing pharmacological properties of salvia species on memory, cognitive impairment and Alzheimer's disease.* CNS Neuroscience & Therapeutics, 2014; 20(6): 485-495. doi: 10.1111/cns.12270.
22. Steinmetz MD et al. *The activity of essential oils of sage, thuja, hyssop and certain components on the respiration of cerebral cortex slices in vitro.* Plantes Medicinales et Phytotherapie, 1985; 19(1): 35-37. Cited in the Aromatherapy Database, by Bob Harris, Essential Oil Resource Consultants, UK, 2000.
23. Essway GS et al. *The hypoglycaemic effect of volatile oil of some Egyptian oils.* Veterinary Medicine Journal, Giza, 1995; 43(2): 167-172. Cited in the Aromatherapy Database, by Bob Harris, Essential Oil Resource Consultants, UK, 2000.
24. Committee on Herbal Medicinal Products (HMPC). *Assessment report on Salvia officinalis L., folium and Salvia officinalis L., aetheroleum.* European Medicines Agency, London. Doc ref. EMA/HMPC/150801/2015.
25. Lawless J. *The encyclopaedia of essential oils.* Element Books, Shaftesbury, 1992.
26. Lavabre M. *Aromatherapy workbook.* Healing Arts Press, Rochester, 1997.
27. Schnaubelt K. *The healing intelligence of essential oils.* Healing Arts Press, Rochester, 2011.
28. Holmes P. *The energetics of Western herbs – Vol. I.* Artemis Press, Boulder, 1989.
29. Schnaubelt K. *Advanced aromatherapy.* Healing Arts Press, Rochester, 1995.
30. Valnet J. *The practice of aromatherapy.* C.W. Daniel Company, Saffron Walden, 1980.
31. Mailhebiau P. *Portraits in oils.* C.W. Daniel Company, Saffron Walden, 1995.
32. Davis P. *Subtle aromatherapy.* C.W. Daniel Company, United Kingdom, 1991.
33. Worwood VA. *The fragrant heavens.* Transworld Publishers, London, 1999.
34. Zeck R. *The blossoming heart – aromatherapy for healing and transformation.* Aroma Tours, East Ivanhoe, 2004.
35. Tisserand R, Balacs T. *Essential oil safety.* Churchill Livingstone, Edinburgh, 1995.
36. Tisserand R, Young R. *Essential oil safety.* 2nd edn. Churchill Livingstone, Edinburgh, 2014.
37. Committee on Herbal Medicinal Products (HMPC). *Public statement on Salvia officinalis L. aetheroleum.* European Medicines Agency, London, 2016. Doc ref. EMA/HMPC/41843/2009.
38. Davis P. *Aromatherapy: an A-Z.* 2nd edn. C.W. Daniel Company, Saffron Walden, 1999.

S

Sandalwood

Identification

Botanical name

This monograph will review *Santalum album* L. and *Santalum spicatum* A. DC.

Synonyms

S. album L.: White sandalwood, East Indian sandalwood, Mysore sandalwood

S. spicatum A. DC.: Australian sandalwood, Western Australian sandalwood

Family

Santalaceae

Botany and origins

There are about 16-20 species spread throughout India, Indonesia, Malaysia, Australia and the

Pacific Islands. There are six species of sandalwood that are commercially harvested in international markets:

- *S. album* (native to India and Indonesia and now cultivated in Australia)
- *S. yasi* (native to Fiji and Tonga)
- *S. austrocaledonicum* (native to New Caledonia and Vanuatu)
- *S. macgregorii* (native to Papua New Guinea and Indonesia)
- *S. spicatum* (native to Western Australia)
- *S. lanceolatum* (native to Queensland).[1]

All sandalwoods are classified as a hemiparasitic tree. In order to survive, the roots of the sandalwood tree must attach themselves to the roots of other trees to obtain their nutrients. However, the sandalwood tree will not kill its host tree.[1]

Santalum album

Santalum album is a medium-sized tree (12-15 m) that reaches maturity at 40-50 years old. The branches, bark and sapwood are odourless and the essential oil is found in the heartwood and roots. It is native to the tropical regions of Asia such as India, Sri Lanka, Malaysia and Indonesia, and cultivated in Northern Australia.[1]

S. album is indigenous to India and its distribution is limited to an area of about 9,600 km^2, mostly in the deciduous forest of the Deccan region of the Indian peninsula. The southern states of Karnataka and Tamil Nadu together account for more than 90% of the natural population of *S. album* in India.[2]

Excessive harvesting without a strategy for replanting has substantially reduced the availability of sandalwood in India. This has resulted in global shortages and soaring market prices.

Unfortunately, illegal poaching and spike disease have further contributed to the demise of sandalwood trees in India. As a result, in 1998, it was listed on the IUCN (International Union for Conservation of Nature) Red List of Threatened Species in India as a vulnerable species.[3]

S. album plantations in Australia began back in 1999. The first harvest of Indian sandalwood from plantations established in Kununurra, Western Australia, occurred in 2013.[4]

Santalum spicatum

S. spicatum, commonly referred to as Western Australian sandalwood, is typically a small evergreen tree, 3-8 m in height. It occurs in the drier inland regions of Western and South Australia. It generally grows in a wide range of soils and prefers level country, but it can be seen growing on hillsides. The tree's parasitic habit requires it to grow in association with other trees and scrubs. The two most common local hosts are *Acacia acuminata* Benth. and *A. aneura* F. Muell.[1]

Method of extraction

Sandalwood oils are obtained by steam distillation of powdered wood chips from the heartwood of the tree. The sandalwood tree must be over 30 years old before the wood is suitable for distillation. Preparing the wood for distillation is difficult as three steps are required – sawing or cleaving, chopping and grinding.[5]

The essential oil yield from old mature *S. album* trees (greater than 30 years) ranges from 6-7%. The oil content from *S. spicatum* is only 2%.[1]

Chana reported that the oil content of the heartwood of 10-year-old sandalwood trees was 0.9% compared to 30-year-old trees, which possessed 4% oil. It was also noted that the total santalols, santalyl acetate and santalenes in the oil produced from the 30-year-old heartwood were much higher.[6]

Lawrence states that 12- to 15-year-old plantations possess an oil content of between 3.5-4% and are of a similar quality of that of 30-year-old trees. It was stated that it would be economically more viable for farmers to establish sandalwood plantations if they could wait 15 years to generate a good economic return.[7]

The oil is contained primarily in the heartwood and the larger roots, therefore the rate of the heartwood formation is of utmost importance. Trees growing in favourable conditions show heartwood development at around 10 years of age. Heartwood formation accelerates rapidly from 20 years and it is at its prime in trees 30 to 60 years old. Weiss states that the proportion of heartwood to outer wood and bark is 65-85% on healthy mature trees.[1]

The sapwood and heartwood are normally sharply demarcated. The sapwood is unscented, white to whitish yellow, and the heartwood is scented and light yellowish-brown when freshly cut, changing on exposure and age to a dark reddish brown.[1]

The trees growing on dry rocky ground in India produce a harder wood with a higher oil content than trees growing on more fertile soils whose heartwood is softer with a lower oil content.[1]

When *S. spicatum* oil first became available, it was produced by a combination of solvent extraction and steam distillation; however, all *S. spicatum* oil is now extracted by steam distillation.

Characteristics

S. album oil is described as a pale yellow to yellow viscous liquid, having an extremely soft, sweet-woody and almost animal-balsamic, milky and nutty odour, presenting little or no particular top note, and remaining uniform for a considerable length of time due to its outstanding tenacity.[5]

S. spicatum oil is described as having a soft, woody, extremely tenacious and somewhat balsamic aroma. The top note is distinctly different from that of the East Indian sandalwood oil, with a rather dry-bitter, slightly resinous note similar to myrrh oil, although not as pronounced. On drying out, the odour slowly becomes very similar to the East Indian sandalwood.[5]

Weiss states that the characteristic scent of *S. album* oil is due to the various santalols and santalenes, especially *epi*-β-santalol and *trans*-β-santalol. The quality of sandalwood oil is often judged on its total alcohol content as santalol. Fresh oil often has less santalol than santalyl acetate and santalene, but this ratio often reverses with age.[1]

It is interesting that Weiss states that redistilled *S. spicatum* oil is very similar in odour to East Indian sandalwood oil. He states that the dendrolasin content is responsible for the odour difference. He also suggests that redistilled *S. spicatum* can directly replace East Indian sandalwood in perfumes, cosmetics and scented soaps.[1]

Chemical composition

The chemical composition of Indian *S. album* oil produced from the heartwood of a 25-year-old tree was reported as follows:[7]

α-santalene (0.08%), *epi*-β-santalene (0.12%), β-santelene (0.25%), curcumene (0.05%), α-santalol (43.09%), (Z)-*trans*-α-bergamotol (9.44%), *epi*-β-santalol (3.66%), β-santalol (22.53%), nuciferol (9.65%), (Z)-lanceol (0.51%).

The chemical composition of *S. album* oil produced from trees cultivated in Australia and *S. spicatum* oils produced from green wood and dead wood were reported as follows:

Constituent	S. album Australian[8]	S. spicatum green wood[9]	S. spicatum dead wood[10]
α-santalene	0.75%	1.29%	0.75%
trans-α-bergamotene	0.16%	0.46%	0.11%
epi-β-santalene	0.79%	-	0.09%
trans-β-farnesene	-	0.70%	-
β-santalene	1.21%	1.06%	0.25%
γ-curcumene	0.12%	0.15%	1.05%
ar-curcumene	0.19%	0.6%	1.41%
β-bisabolene	0.12%	0.42%	1.11%
β-curcumene	0.21%	1.15%	1.83%
nerolidol	0.21%	-	1.22%
trans-nerolidol	-	2.24%	-
dendrolasin	0.04%	2.39%	0.77%
epi-β-bisabolol	0.23%	3.86%	-
β-bisabolol	0.55%	-	0.68%
cis-α-santalol	44.49%	17.38%	1.78%
β-sinensal	1.61%	-	-
epi-α-bisabolol	0.28%	5.41%	25.01%
cis-α-*trans*-bergamotol	5.85%	3.53%	0.22%
cis-*epi*-β-santalol	3.64%	1.22%	0.18%
epi-α-santalol	0.26%	-	0.35%
cis-β-santalol	18.6%	4.81%	0.31%
cis-nuciferol, *cis*-γ-curumen-12-ol	4.18%	15.98%	13.59%
trans-farnesol	-	12.10%	0.62%
trans-β-santalol	0.36%	-	1.95%
cis-β-curumen-12-ol	1.59%	8.62%	5.95%
cis-lanceol	3.02%	2.01%	5.73%
α-sinensal	0.49%	-	1.28%
α-bisabolol acetate	-	-	0.77 %
α-bergamotol acetate	0.29%	-	0.39%

ISO 3518 for *S. album* essential oil states that the oil should have (Z)-α-santalol (41.0-55.0%) and (Z)-β-santalol (16.05-24.0%).[11]

ISO 22769 for *S. spicatum* essential oil states that the oil should have (Z)-α-santalol (15.0-25.0%) and (Z)-β-santalol (5.0–20.0%).[12]

The major constituent of the oil, α-santalol, is responsible for most biological activities of sandalwood oil. The santalols are known to add to the fine woody notes of East Indian sandalwood.[1,13]

The age at which the trees are harvested also determines the oil composition:[1]

- 10-year-old trees contain santalol (72-83%), santalyl acetate (4.5-6.5%) and santalene (3.6-7.3%).
- 30-year-old trees contain santalol (86-91%), santalyl acetate (2.6-3.4%) and santalene (1.3-2.9%).

Adulteration

Sandalwood oil is regularly adulterated. However, Guenther stated that present specifications of the various pharmacopoeias make it quite difficult to adulterate *Santalum album* oil to any considerable extent. He explains that oils of cedarwood, guaiacwood, West Indian, Western Australian and South African sandalwood oils along with oils, from copaiba balsam, and gurjun balsam have been used for this purpose.[14]

Guenther explains that the addition of cedarwood

S

oil or gurjun balsam oil increases optical rotation and decreases the specific gravity and solubility of the sandalwood oil. Copaiba balsam acts similarly except that it usually decreases the rotation slightly. *S. spicatum* oil has a lower ester number after acetylation and poorer solubility than East Indian sandalwood oil.[14]

For pharmaceutical purposes, Arctander states that sandalwood oil is usually rectified.[5]

Lawrence reports that polyethylene glycol and dioctyl phthalate have been found in commercial *S. album* oil from India.[7]

Schmidt & Wanner state that *S. album* oil is adulterated with cheaper varieties coming from Australia. However, the Australian oils are no longer considered to be 'cheap'. They state that it is easy to detect *S. spicatum* as it contains higher percentages of *cis*-nuciferol. The same can be said for *S. austrocaledonicum*, which contains higher percentages of *cis*-lanceol.[15]

Pharmacopoeias and standards

The purity, composition and physico-chemical properties of *Santalum album* are defined in ISO 3518:2002 Oil of Sandalwood (*Santalum album* L.).

The purity, composition and physico-chemical properties of *Santalum spicatum* are defined in ISO 22769:2009 Oil of Australian Sandalwood (*Santalum spicatum* (R.Br.) A.DC.).

S

History and Traditional Uses

History

Santalum album

Sandalwood's common name derives from Sanskrit *chandana*. Sandalwood is a highly prized aromatic wood that is well known for its oil, and the wood has religious and cultural significance in Asian cultures and in Buddhism.[1]

S. album is traditionally considered the most valuable variety of sandalwood and the most sought after in the industry due to its aroma and oil yield. India has been the traditional leader in sandalwood oil production for more than 5,000 years. The oil and the wood are highly esteemed by people belonging to three of the major religions of the world – Hinduism, Buddhism and Islam.[16]

The wood is recommended for worshipping Shiva. Goddess Lakshmi is believed to reside in the sandalwood tree. The Egyptians imported the wood and used it in medicine, for embalming the dead and in ritual burnings to worship the gods.[16]

It is customary in some communities among the Hindus to place a piece of sandalwood in the funeral pyre. The beige-coloured paste of sandalwood is applied to the forehead and other body parts by devotees of the god Krishna and for ritual bathing of Hindu gods.[16]

Holmes explains that, wherever Buddhism spread throughout Asia, sandalwood followed. The burning of incense sticks made from finely ground sandalwood is an example of how this precious wood has always been the aromatic foundation of Buddhist practice.[17]

The demise of S. album in India

Rashkow provides us with a detailed account of the demise of the sandalwood industry in India. He argues that, while both early nineteenth-century capitalist commodification and late nineteenth-century bureaucratic forestry department management were detrimental to the demise of the tree's population in southern India, it was not until postcolonial mismanagement by the state-run sandalwood oil industry in the 1950s-70s that the species came to the brink of extinction.[18]

Rashkow explains that precolonial conservation measures had always been in place which effectively managed sandalwood trees. He quotes Buchanan, who, in 1894, described how villages appointed a keeper of the forest. The keeper's role was to manage all the resources of the forest, including the sandalwood tree. In one area, the tradition was to harvest the sandalwood once in every 12 years.[18]

In the eighteenth century, Tipu Sultan of Mysore established the first state monopoly over all sandalwood. The British East India Company's invasion of Mysore was motivated by the need to control one of Mysore's most prized commodities – sandalwood.[18]

Rashkow states that the British monopolised the sandalwood trade in southern India and used it to balance their accounts in China. They would overexploit the species as far as the market would allow. He explains that this represented a significant departure from the precolonial period where local elites were happy to trade with outside powers, but with eyes thoroughly fixed on the domestic market.[18]

In Hawaii, the sandalwood trade collapsed by 1928, only decades after it had begun. The first shipwrecked Europeans to land on Fiji's second largest island, Vanua Levu, called it 'sandalwood island'. The sandalwood trade collapsed there within 20 years of its discovery. In the Marquesas, the British and Americans decimated sandalwood in just three years between 1814 and 1816. The same story occurred with *S. austrocaledonicum* in Vanuatu.[18]

European traders managed to decimate the sandalwood trees across the Pacific islands in a very short time span, leading to the collapse of trade in the 1830s. On the other hand, southern India's sandalwood stocks continued to provide the international market without interruption into the 1950s.[18]

Rashkow argues that one of the factors leading to the demise of sandalwood in India was the failure of 'scientific' forestry.[18]

All early attempts to cultivate sandalwood proved to be complete failures. Before the first quarter of the twentieth century, European foresters could not work out how to grow sandalwood effectively. The main reason is that sandalwood is a hemiparasite. John Scott, curator of the Royal Botanical Garden in Calcutta, discovered this back in 1871; however, it was never taken seriously. Rashkow states that, if the British plantation managers had studied how villagers cultivated sandalwood, they could have solved the problem sooner. It was also not known at the time that only the sandalwood heartwood and roots develop the essential oil, and trees only begin to develop the oil in significant quantities after about 30 years.[18]

The second major natural problem facing southern India's sandalwood was spike disease. At the end of the nineteenth century and beginning of the twentieth century, spike disease was the number one killer of trees. Even today the mystery of spike disease has not been solved and scientific investigation is ongoing to find a cure.[18]

However, an even bigger demise facing sandalwood oil came in the twentieth century. Traditionally used as an incense and pressed into attars and oils, sandalwood had always been a consumable good, but with the coming of an industrial-scale sandalwood oil factory located in the heart of sandalwood country, sandalwood production now ramped up immensely.[18]

Annual reports from Karnataka State Forest Department stated that over 480,000 sandalwood trees were harvested annually in the state each year between 1950 and 1970. In 1974, a resource report stated that there were only 350,000 trees left standing. Most alarming was that of these trees, only 4,360 had a diameter more than 30 cm. Overnight India's sandalwood industry came to a halt. Harvesting and trade in sandalwood was now banned.[18]

Rashkow states that the drive for destruction of sandalwood was because people around the world had developed a fondness for scent and natural products made with sandalwood.

> *Ironically, much of the sandalwood consumption in the West especially seems to be driven by a desire to live a 'natural' lifestyle coupled with an utter lack of awareness.*[18]

It was at this time that the illegal harvesting and smuggling of sandalwood increased. By the 1970s, the sandalwood situation was made worse by the fact that sandalwood smugglers could make more money by poaching endangered sandalwood trees than by killing elephants. Smugglers have made large fortunes from illegal poaching of sandalwood. According to one report, approximately 75% of the sandalwood leaving Karnataka is smuggled.[18]

Sandalwood in India today

A 1998 report highlighted the critical status of sandalwood in India. In all six states of India in which sandalwood is harvested, the authors expressed concern. Swaminathan explained that sandalwood is indiscriminately exploited illegally. The data on the amount of illegally harvested sandalwood is indeed alarming – representing over 30% of the total sandalwood being harvested.[2]

The report stated that no mature trees were left in the forest areas. The forests were devoid of larger girth trees. This is not only due to illegal harvesting but also to grazing and another big concern – spike disease. Spike disease has caused substantial damage and destroyed some good sandalwood bearing areas.[2]

Lawrence reports the total official auction sales of sandalwood in India dropped from 2,850 tonnes in 1993 to 1,275 tonnes in 2005. This is more than a 50% drop in such a short period. However, it has been reported that the actual annual production could be as high as 3,000-4,000 tonnes.[7] This is because of all the illegal harvesting that is now occurring. This is alarming and highlights the lack of controls in India to manage sandalwood production.

The monopoly of sandalwood trade by the governments of Karnataka, Tamil Nadu and Kerala has resulted in severe exploitation, pushing sandalwood into the vulnerable category of the IUCN Red List in 1998. The IUCN urges that it is essential to establish community and corporate sandalwood plantations in different parts of India with appropriate incentives and adequate protective measures.[16]

Unfortunately, the monopolistic control of sandalwood trees by the Indian government has not deterred the illegal and indiscriminate harvesting of sandalwood, nor has it helped to conserve the species in its natural habitat. Paradoxically, the restrictive policies of the Indian government discouraged legitimate interest in growing sandalwood trees. The landholder was responsible for the preservation of the sandalwood trees, which remain the exclusive property of the government; however very little incentive was provided to the landowner to protect the sandalwood trees.[19]

Landowners had no right to a sandalwood tree growing on their land, but were responsible for its preservation. Only the government had the right to sell or trade the wood. On extraction, the landowner was paid 75% of the net value less all the costs of extraction, transport and cleaning, which often did not amount to much. The punitive clauses in the law made landowners vulnerable to severe punishments even for minor offences related to the sandalwood trees growing on their land. In particular, the liability to preserve the trees and the fear of harassment and compensation to be paid to the government in case of theft promoted the farmers to destroy even saplings that came up naturally.[19]

Local government authorities in India have changed the Act to entitle occupants or holders of the land to be legally entitled to own the sandalwood tree on their land. However, while changes have been made to give the landowners ownership, the government still retains control over felling, sale and transport of privately owned trees. Dhanya et al. state that sandalwood laws in India should be liberalised. This will be the only way to encourage farmers to take up sandalwood cultivation.[19]

S

History of sandalwood in Australia

S. spicatum has been exported since the early days of Western Australian settlement – first to Chinese merchants in South East Asia since 1844 for use as incense, and then to other parts of Asia and mainland China. Sandalwood soon became a significant export economy, with export values being considerably more than wool prices at the time.[20]

In the period 1844 to 1929, Western Australia became a dominant exporter of sandalwood, which was purchased mainly by Chinese merchants in Singapore and Shanghai to be powdered for incense. The Australian sandalwood was considered inferior to the *S. album* from Timor and India. It was not suitable for carving given its lower oil content. However, the aromatic quality of the Western Australian sandalwood was an excellent choice for incense.[21]

By 1847 most of the wild sandalwood stands in the Avon Valley had been exhausted and cutters were venturing further and further inland.[21]

During the 1870s the Mysore sandalwood plantations in India failed to meet domestic demand and restrictions had been placed on export. This allowed the Western Australian sandalwood industry to treble in size. The peak of 9,605 tonnes exported in 1882 was, in fact, not surpassed for almost 40 years. The discovery of gold in the Pilbara region meant that Western Australia's population had increased by 46% within a very short period. While alluvial gold was easily found, there was no incentive to harvest sandalwood, but as surface gold became harder to find, sandalwood provided a welcome substitute.[21]

More than 50,000 tonnes of sandalwood was exported from the Western Australian wheat belt in the final decades of the 1800s. From the mid-nineteenth century onwards, harvesting of sandalwood continued at such a prolific rate that legislation was finally introduced in 1929 to ensure that the industry could operate sustainably and ensure the quality of the harvest continued.[20]

In 1929 the Western Australian government introduced the *Sandalwood Act 1929* to manage the harvesting of wild *S. spicatum*. This Act has been responsible for setting the quota for the number of wild trees that can be harvested. However, as the amount of *S. album* available on the international market has diminished, the pressure to harvest more *S. spicatum* from the wild increased. Nowadays the Western Australian government has acknowledged that the current rate of harvest of native sandalwood is not sustainable.[20]

Guenther states that the oil was first distilled experimentally in 1875 by Schimmel & Co in Leipzig, Germany. However, it was not until the beginning of the twentieth century that there was sporadic production of the oil by a number of small distillers in Western Australia. At the time, the oil was sold in a crude state and it had a very low santalol content.[14]

In 1921, the systemic production and scientific control of the distillation of sandalwood oil was instituted by Plaimar Ltd in Perth. At that time, the oil was of such a quality that it was considered the equivalent of the well-established and better-known East Indian sandalwood oil. According to the British Pharmacopoeia of 1932, Western Australian sandalwood was considered equally therapeutic to the Easter Indian sandalwood oil.[14]

The Western Australian sandalwood tree has had a very rough handling by scientific botanists. It was first known as *Santalum spicatum* or *S. zygnorum*. This was later changed to *Fusanus spicatus*, and then to *Eucarya spicata*. This last classification was accepted by the British Pharmacopoeia in 1932, but synonymised as *Santalum spicatum*.[14]

Guenther states that the effect of changing the botanical nomenclature upon a commercial product is far reaching. He states that for years Australian sandalwood suffered serious competition with the East Indian oil because merchants used differences in nomenclature and chemical composition for trade purposes. The change of name from the genus *Santalum* to the genus *Eucarya* created the erroneous impression that the Australian oil was an entirely different species, with a different chemical composition and therapeutic properties.[14]

Sandalwood in Australia today

New legislation was passed in 2016 to manage licensing for the harvest of sandalwood. It is now managed by the Department of Parks and Wildlife under the *Biodiversity Conservation Act 2016*. This replaces the *Wildlife Conservation Act 1950* and the *Sandalwood Act 1929*. The new legislation has set a strict quota for the amount of green wood and dead wood that can be harvested. It also enforces tougher penalties for illegal activities, as well as improving trading and processing accountability.[20]

Sandalwood harvesting on Crown land is managed by Forest Products Commission (FPC) under a contract system. The Wildlife Licensing Section of Parks and Wildlife issues a Sandalwood Act Crown land licence to the FPC with the names of all approved contractors endorsed upon it as 'authorised persons'.[22]

A government report in 2015 stated that if current levels of harvesting continued indefinitely, there would be a substantially lower frequency of larger trees within a few decades. Each year a new quota is determined for an acceptable level of harvest of wild sandalwood.[20]

FPC is responsible for the commercial harvesting, regeneration, marketing and sale of wild Western Australian sandalwood from Crown land (including land that is subject to pastoral leases). The 'sandalwood order' took effect on July 1, 2016 and set an annual quota at 2,500 tonnes – 1,250 tonnes of green wood and 1,250 tonnes of dead wood.[20]

The new legislation specifies the tree sizes that can be harvested. The current minimum circumference for living wild sandalwood trees to be harvested is 400 mm (over bark) measured at approximately 150 mm above the ground. This is equivalent to stem diameter of 126 mm.[20]

According to the 2015 government report, natural regeneration of sandalwood is being severely hampered because seedlings are grazed by feral herbivores and stock. Woylies traditionally played a critical role in the propagation and regeneration of sandalwood. The woylie is a small marsupial which feeds on sandalwood seeds, collecting and hoarding them in shallow diggings up to 80 m from the original tree, similar to the way that squirrels store acorns. Not all the seeds that the woylie buries are revisited; therefore, some of the buried seeds germinate when the winter rains come.[20]

The disappearance of the small marsupial because of feral cats and foxes has impacted on the regeneration of sandalwood in the wild. Fire, drought and climate change are additional factors that have also contributed to reduced seedling survival.[20]

FPC has commenced a regeneration program that aims to plant a minimum of 10 tonnes of seeds (around 3.5 million seeds) per year. It is estimated that this will lead to the establishment of over one million seedlings between 2016 and 2025. This figure is well in excess of the number of trees to be harvested.[22]

The establishment of *S. spicatum* plantations will take pressure off the demand to harvest wild trees. An estimated total of 20,000 ha of Western Australian sandalwood plantations has been established in Western Australia. Harvesting the *S. spicatum* plantations is anticipated to commence around 2026.[23]

Cultivation of *S. spicatum* is also being encouraged to reduce problems with salinity in many areas of wheat belt in Western Australia. Growing wheat and other grains has led to dry land salinity. These crops do not consume all of the year's rainfall, and the surplus builds up in the flat landscape, bringing salt to the surface. Plantations of sandalwood and other trees are helping to reverse this trend.[23]

S. spicatum is unique because it provides a secondary source of income for farm owners because of the seeds. The seeds are also used for planting and replanting and as 'bush food'.[23]

According to a WA government report of 2015, the illegal activities were on a very small scale; however, illegal poaching escalated around 2008 and peaked in 2013.[21]

The illegal harvesting and theft of Australian sandalwood is still a significant issue and has been addressed with the introduction of new legislation. The Act increases the penalties for the illegal harvesting of sandalwood. The maximum penalties for illegally harvested wild sandalwood are now $200,000 for individuals and $1 million for corporations.[20]

Santalum album in Australia

Experimental growing of Indian sandalwood first occurred in Kununurra in 1983 by FPC and the former Department of Conservation and Land Management. Australian Centre for International Agricultural Research (ACIAR) funded sandalwood research in Indonesia and Australia with the then WA Department of Conservation and Land Management (CALM) from 1987 to 1995. This helped develop reliable nursery techniques for mass production of high-quality seedlings, and for identifying and assessing the practicality and value of second-stage and third-stage host plants.[24]

The *S. album* in Western Australia has, over the last 20 years, become a large-scale commercial industry. One of the major companies is Tropical Forestry Services (TFS), now called Quintis. In 2017, it managed over 5.4 million trees covering 12,182 hectares of *S. album* in Western Australia, Northern Territory and Queensland.[25]

The first harvest of Indian sandalwood occurred in September 2013. The first harvest consisted of 144 hectares of sandalwood trees that were planted in 1999 and 2000.[4,26]

Cultivation of *S. album* is a challenging and laborious process. Each sandalwood tree will require at least four host trees and continuous care over a 15-year lifespan.[25]

As supplies of sandalwood oil from world sources dwindle, Australia has become the world leader in the growth and sustainable supply of *S. album.*

Traditional medicine

Sandalwood oil is traditionally used in Ayurveda, Chinese and Tibetan medical systems. It is used in the treatment of conditions such as the common cold, bronchitis, fever, dysentery, piles, scabies, infection of the urinary tract, inflammation of the mouth and pharynx, liver and gall bladder complaints, and as an expectorant, stimulant, carminative, digestive and muscle relaxant. Venous and lymphatic stasis such as varicose veins and swollen lymph nodes of the lymphatic system were also traditionally treated with sandalwood oil.[13,16]

Sandalwood was rarely mentioned in medieval European herbals. It was not until the eighteenth century when the Europeans became established in India that sandalwood became well known and highly prized in Europe.[1] It was recommended for the treatment of gonorrhoea and urinary tract infections.[27]

The German Commission E recommends 1-1.5 g of sandalwood oil for the supportive treatment of urinary tract infections.[28]

Guenther states that, during the early part of the twentieth century, a large portion of sandalwood oil produced in the world was used for medicinal purposes, particularly for the treatment of certain diseases such as gonorrhoea; however, by the 1950s the situation had entirely changed, with only 10% of the oil being used for medicinal purposes.[14]

S

Food, perfumery and flavouring

Without a doubt, sandalwood is considered one of the most precious perfumery materials from antiquity to modern times, and the popularity of sandalwood oil shows no signs of waning. The desirable attributes of sandalwood in perfumery are due to the sesquiterpene alcohols, α-santalol and β-santalol, being great fixatives.

According to Michael Edwards' research, about 47% of all perfumes created since 1790 contain sandalwood notes. In perfumery, both *S. spicatum* and *S. album* are used. Both have different aromatic profiles. Often *S. spicatum* is considered more raw, earthy and sharp.[29]

The perfume industry uses sandalwood oil extensively. It is used for its tenacious base note, which acts as a fixative, and for its ability to blend and harmonise with other essential oils.[1]

Most Indian attars use sandalwood oil as the base because of its inherent capacity to absorb most of the ethereal notes of other herbs and flowers.

Other uses

Sandalwood is considered one of the finest woods for carving, and the highest quality heartwood is often reserved for this use. It is generally used for ornamental objects and furniture. The sawdust is used in incense sticks or further powdered for use in sachets to scent stored clothes. A paste of the sandalwood powder is applied to the forehead at Hindu religious ceremonies.[1]

Therapeutics

Pharmacology and clinical studies

Many pharmacological studies involving sandalwood oils have been published. A systemic review of these studies will not be attempted. Rather, I have chosen a selection of studies that support the traditional and clinical uses.

Anti-inflammatory activity

Research involving testing the ability of sandalwood essential oil to inhibit the enzymes responsible for the inflammatory reaction at a cellular level suggests that the oil has anti-inflammatory activity.[30]

Antimicrobial activity

Beylier obtained good results with *S. spicatum* essential oil against *Staphylococcus aureus*, whereas the almost chemically identical East Indian sandalwood reported negligible activity.[31]

Australian sandalwood exhibited greater bacteriostatic activity against the yeast *Candida albicans* than tea tree. Other in vitro studies have also confirmed that Australian sandalwood is an excellent biocide against many gram-positive organisms, including *Staphyloccus aureus* and methicillin-resistant S. *aureus* (MRSA), in addition to the organism responsible for acne, thrush and tinea.[32]

S. album and *S. spicatum* essential oils exhibited antimicrobial activity against the yeast *C. albicans*, the gram-positive bacteria *S. aureus* and gram-negative bacteria *Escherichia coli, Pseudomonas aeruginosa* and *Klebsiella pneumoniae*. It was suggested that the santalols in medium or high percentage in sandalwood oils have significant influence on the antimicrobial activity of the essential oil.[33]

Antiviral activity

An in vitro study found that *S. album* oil had antiviral activity against herpes simplex virus (HSV) type 1 and 2. The authors speculated that the antiviral activity of sandalwood oil was indirectly related to the inhibition of HSV replication by glutathione.[34]

Bowles states that this means sandalwood oil could be used as a preventative for cold sores.[35]

An in vitro study demonstrated that sandalwood oil exhibited high levels of antiviral activity against acyclovir-sensitive strain KOS and acyclovir-resistant HSV-1 clinical isolates and reduced plaque formation significantly.[36]

Another in vitro study found that sandalwood demonstrated antiviral activity against HSV-2; however, it was also noted that no inhibitory effect could be observed when the essential oil was added to the cells prior to infection with HSV-2 or after the adsorption period. This indicates that sandalwood affected the HSV-2 before adsorption by interacting with the viral envelope.[37]

Chemoprotective activity

Oral doses of *S. album* increased glutathione S-transferase (GST) activity in mice studies. This suggests a possible chemoprotective activity of sandalwood oil on carcinogenesis activity.[38]

S. album oil significantly decreased papilloma in animal studies. It was suggested that the oil could be used as an effective chemoprotective agent against skin cancer.[39]

Another in vitro study involving mice concluded that sandalwood oil could be used as an effective chemoprotective against chemically induced skin cancer.[40]

Insecticidal activity

Sandalwood oil exhibited the highest adulticidal activity and maintained an efficacy of 85% over a 24-hour period. α-santalol and β-santalol proved to have the lowest LC50 values one, six and 24 hours after treatment.[41]

Sedative activity

A study investigated the effect of *S. album* oil and its component α-santalol on the autonomic nervous system and the mental and emotional wellbeing of healthy human subjects. Sandalwood oil was applied topically using a carrier oil. All subjects were supplied with breathing masks preventing any olfactory stimulation or pulmonary absorption. The sandalwood group had a significant decrease in eye-blink rate and a large decrease in systolic blood pressure. At a behavioural level, the sandalwood group also rated themselves more attentive than the control group. The authors suggested that sandalwood oil exerted its effect by interaction with hypothalamic and limbic structures that control the level of physiological and behavioural arousal. It was suggested that the activity of sandalwood oil is characterised by the concept of 'harmonisation' rather than relaxation. The authors also stated that these effects were mediated by pharmacological mechanisms.[42]

A randomised, controlled clinical trial compared the effectiveness of aromatherapy massage with 1% *S. album* oil, massage with a plain carrier oil, and sandalwood by inhalation only. The aim of this study was to evaluate the effectiveness of sandalwood in reducing anxiety in patients receiving palliative care. The researchers stated that it was difficult to make any conclusion from the results because of the small sample; however, the results supported the idea that sandalwood oil is effective in reducing anxiety.[43]

Misra & Dey suggest that because α-santalol is a strong inhibitor of both tyrosine and cholinesterase in vitro, there is potential for using sandalwood oil in the treatment of Alzheimer's.[44]

Actions

Actions commonly cited in aromatherapy

Antidepressant, anti-inflammatory, antiseptic, antispasmodic, astringent, carminative, diuretic, emollient, expectorant, sedative, tonic[45,46,47]

Actions supported by clinical studies

Anti-inflammatory, antiseptic, antiviral, chemo-protective, sedative

Comment

Sandalwood oils are among the most commonly and widely used oils in perfumery and cosmetics. The oil also has a wide range of pharmacological activities. Various studies have established the versatile pharmacological properties of sandalwood oil, ranging from antibacterial to

S

treatment of skin diseases to its chemoprotective activity.

The essential oil from *S. spicatum* contains less santalols than *S. album*; however, it also contains farnesol and nuciferols that are said to enhance the anti-inflammatory and antimicrobial properties of the oil.[48]

Aromatherapy Uses

Clinical aromatherapy

Integumentary system

Both *S. album* and *S. spicatum* essential oil are known to have an anti-inflammatory effect. The oils are effective in the treatment of psoriasis, dermatitis, eczema and various scalp irritations.[49,50]

Lymphatic system

Sandalwood is beneficial for treating venous and lymphatic stasis such as varicose veins and swollen lymph nodes. Holmes suggests that this may be due to the sesquiterpene alcohols which have an anti-inflammatory effect.[17]

Nervous system

Sandalwood oil has a relaxing effect on the nerves and may be used for hot, agitated emotional states that lead to conditions such as headache, insomnia and nervous tension.[49]

Fischer-Rizzi perfectly describes sandalwood's effects on the nervous system:

> *With sandalwood, the experience of warmth and balance fills the human heart with joy. This makes it an ideal remedy for nervous depression, fear, stress and a hectic daily tempo. When you react to others with aggression and irritation, it is time to reach for sandalwood.*[51]

Respiratory system

Sandalwood is recommended for the treatment of respiratory tract infections, especially when its soothing, demulcent effects are required.[49] It is recommended for chronic bronchitis involving a chronic dry cough.[17,46,47,49]

The anti-inflammatory and antiseptic properties of Australian sandalwood assist in the relief of symptoms of colds such as dry cough, bronchitis, sore throat, tonsillitis, earache and sinusitis.[50]

Skin care

Applied to the skin, all sandalwood oils are soothing, cooling and moisturising, and are primarily used for dry skin conditions caused by loss of moisture and skin inflammations.[49] It may be used to relieve eczema and psoriasis and for the treatment of oily skin and acne.[17,46,49]

Urinary system

Sandalwood oil has traditionally been used for the treatment of genitourinary tract infections such as cystitis and gonorrhoea.[17,46,47,49] Sandalwood is an astringent and helps to resolve mucous congestion. Sandalwood oil helps to restore the mucous membrane and minimise the risk of infection.[17]

Energetics, psyche and subtle uses

Energetics

The energetic qualities of sandalwood oil are *cooling*. It is primarily indicated for conditions of a *hot*, inflammatory and catarrhal nature – particularly where the skin, intestines, genitourinary system and *Lungs* are involved.[49]

Mojay also says that sandalwood's influence on the mind and spirit relate to its *cooling* and calming influence on the nervous system. He recommends it for *hot*, agitated, emotional states that lead to headache, insomnia and nervous exhaustion.[49]

According to the principles of the Five Elements, sandalwood is often associated with having a harmonising effect on the Earth Element; however, I would also describe the qualities of sandalwood as having a strong affinity with the Water Element. Water's spirit quality is the *Zhi*. The *Zhi* is the will to live; it represents willpower, ambition and self-actualisation. *Zhi* is the will we draw on to survive ordeals, overcome obstacles and persevere against hardships. The *Zhi* represents collectivity – our sense of being a part of a whole. Collectivity invites us to feel connected not only to each other or to God, but to country, community and the whole of creation.

Mojay states that it reduces the constant need to overthink, instilling a state in which the body, mind and spirit can realign as one. He explains that sandalwood is ideal for states of obsessive worry and worldly 'over-attachments', traits often associated with an imbalanced Earth Element.[49]

In Ayurveda, sandalwood reduces conditions associated with excess *Pitta*.

Personality

Sandalwood oil is also recommended when you react to others with aggression and irritation. The oil also helps us to make human contact and overcome isolation. Sandalwood helps us to accept others with an open heart and diminishes our egocentricity. Sandalwood fosters openness, warmth and understanding.[51]

The sandalwood personality is serene and in charge of their emotions, fully aware of their direction in life.[52]

S

They are fully aware of their direction in life, even anticipating the rocky sections ahead. She says that their inner calm is like that of an old soul.[52]

Sandalwood personalities are very intuitive. Worwood explains that it is as if they have a direct line with the universal telephone exchange and instinctively know when something is missing or not quite right. They may long for the meaning of life, appealing to the heavens to reveal a little more. They have a laidback philosophical attitude that mistakenly leads them to be accused of detachment. They are very still people who listen more than talk, and they also make wonderful healers.[52]

They are very sensual people who are not afraid of their sexuality. They will view it as one of the precious gifts we have been given to help us through this lifetime.[52]

According to Myers-Briggs personality types, the sandalwood personality is likely to be an INFP. INFPs are gentle, calm, easygoing and affirming. Integrity and commitment to what they believe in are essential. They like time alone for their many interests. They like learning and researching new things and interests. They are highly reflective, especially in understanding the mysteries and meaning of life. They have little need to impose their values on others. They prefer to gently influence and inspire. They value authenticity and depth in their relationships.

Subtle

> *Sandalwood helps humanity to have strength of conviction when standing against adversity, as it rejoins all aspects of being. It rejoices in the physical aspects of mankind, while always being aware of the spiritual self.*

Worwood beautifully describes the subtle qualities of sandalwood.[53]

Sandalwood's subtle properties are reflected in its traditional use as an aid to meditation, prayer and spiritual practice. It is reputed to quieten mental chatter that can distract a person meditating.[49,54] It is also recommended for the preparation of healing work.[54]

Sandalwood is often referred to as the fragrance of the subtle body. It is assigned to the base chakra as well as the crown chakra. Fischer-Rizzi asks – 'How can an essential oil be assigned to the base chakra and the highest chakra?' She explains that sandalwood oil has the ability to awaken the power of the kundalini, helping to connect all the chakras.[51]

Keim Loughran & Bull state that sandalwood teaches us to delight in our senses and sexuality and to appreciate the beauty of life. They also explain that it helps us make good decisions about who and what we allow in our lives.[55]

Holmes provides us with an insightful description of sandalwood that helps us understand why it has always been and always will be one of the most precious aromatic gifts to humankind. Sandalwood oil grounds us in a world of sensuous unaffected beauty, like that experienced after a deep meditation or love experience. Sandalwood helps us experience the simplicity and purity of the physical world and experience the immanence of the spirit in the physical world.[17]

Holmes explains that sandalwood helps us reflect internally, balancing the one-sided Western emphasis on the external world. It helps connect us with our soul and our intrinsic wisdom. Sandalwood naturally guides us into a meditation that integrates our body, mind and soul.[17]

Dosage and Administration

Blending

Aromatherapy

The soft, sweet, woody, balsamic aroma of sandalwood makes it one of the most beautiful oils to blend with. It does not impart a strong aroma; however, it leaves you with a very long-lasting scent and has the ability to enhance the other oils used. It imparts such a delicate, ethereal, balance, warmth and harmony to all blends.

For meditation and mindfulness practice, consider blending *S. album* or *S. spicatum* oil with essential oils such as frankincense, juniper, lavender, lemon, myrrh, patchouli, cistus, spikenard or vetiver.

To soothe sensitive skin or for the relief of eczema and dermatitis, consider blending *S. album* or *S. spicatum* oil with essential oils such as German chamomile, everlasting, lavender or neroli.

To create an uplifting, antidepressant blend, consider blending *S. album* or *S. spicatum* oil with essential oils such as bergamot, sweet orange, coriander seed, geranium, ginger, neroli, mandarin, jasmine absolute, rose absolute or ylang ylang.

Perfumery

Perfumer Roja Dove best explains the challenges of creating perfumes with sandalwood:[56]

> *It is a difficult material to balance in a creation, as it plays a trick with one's nose – at one moment it is there and then it disappears.*

The perfume industry tends to consider sandalwood as a fixative. However, the high price of sandalwood now means that perfumers use it much more carefully.

S

There are many synthetic ingredients that are reminiscent of sandalwood; however, most perfumers agree that the woody aroma chemicals that attempt to mimic the scent of sandalwood do not have the complexity, richness and depth of character of real sandalwood.

Sandalwood blends well with all aroma types; however, it is best suited to florals and other warm, woody, earthy aromas. Sandalwood complements the fresh, vibrant scent of citrus oils. At the same time, it harmonises with rich, warm resins such as frankincense, cistus or Peru balsam.

Mode of administration

Bath

Full body bath, foot bath

Topical

Compress, massage, ointment, skin care

Inhalation

Direct inhalation, diffuser, oil vaporiser

Safety Profile

General safety

Sandalwood oil is considered non-toxic, non-irritant and non-sensitising.[46] Tisserand & Young suggest that the safety profile of other sandalwood oils would be similar to East Indian sandalwood because of similar chemical profiles.[57]

Tisserand & Young reference a study which conducted a patch test on 3,542 dermatitis patients with 2% sandalwood (*S. album*) oil. Only 12 (0.345%) had a reaction. Based on this information and because of the risk of photoallergic reactions, they recommend a maximum use level of 2%.[57]

Lis-Balchin states that the RIFM recommended safety of use limit for *S. album* is 10%.[58] Another safety assessment report on *S. album* states that the oil has low acute oral and dermal toxicity in laboratory animals, and considering it has a long history of oral and topical use without any reported adverse effects, it is considered safe at present use levels.[59]

Contraindications

No contraindications known.

Regulatory guidelines

S. album oil has GRAS status.

S

References

1. Weiss EA. *Essential oil crops.* CAB International, Wallingford, 1997.
2. Radomiljac AM et al. *Sandal and its products.* Proceedings of an international seminar held on 18-19 December 1997, organised by the Institute of Wood Science and Technology (ICFRE) and Karnataka State Forest Department, Bangalore, India. ACIAR Proceedings No. 84, ACIAR, Canberra, 1998.
3. Asian Regional Workshop (Conversation & Sustainable Management of Trees, Vietnam, August 1996). *Santalum album, sandalwood.* The IUCN Red List of Threatened Species 1998: eT31852A9665066. doi: 10.2305/IUCN.UK.1998.RLTS.T31852A9665066.
4. *TFS begins Indian sandalwood harvest.* Retrieved Dec 10, 2017 from http:www.perfumerflavorist.com.networking/news/company/TFS-Corp-begins-indian-sandalwood-Harvest-222169511.html
5. Arctander S. *Perfume and flavor materials of natural origin.* Allured Publishing, Carol Stream, 1994.
6. Chana J. *Sandalwood production.* The International Journal of Aromatherapy, 1994; 6(4): 11-13.
7. Lawrence BM. *Progress in essential oils – sandalwood.* Perfumer & Flavorist, 2009; 34: 52-56.
8. Southern Cross University. *Perfect Potion Australian S. album – certificate of analysis.* 2017.
9. Southern Cross University. *Perfect Potion Australian S. spicatum greenwood – certificate of analysis.* 2017.
10. Southern Cross University. *Perfect Potion Australian S. spicatum deadwood – certificate of analysis.* 2017.
11. International Organization for Standardization. *Oil of sandalwood (Santalum album L.)* (ISO 3518:2002). 2002.
12. International Organization for Standardization. *Oil of Australian sandalwood (Santalum spicatum (R.Br.) A.DC.)* (ISO 22769:2009). 2009.
13. Khan I, Abourashed E. *Leung's encyclopedia of common natural ingredients used in food, drugs and cosmetics.* 3rd edn. John Wiley & Sons, New Jersey, 2010.
14. Guenther E. *The essential oils – Vol. V.* Robert E Krieger Publishing, Malabar, 1952.
15. Schmidt E, Wanner J. *Adulteration of essential oils.* In Baser KHC, Buchbauer G. eds. *Handbook of essential oils – science, technology and applications.* 2nd edn. CRC Press, Boca Raton, 2016: 707-745.
16. Arun Kumar AN, Joshi G, Mohan Ram HY. *Sandalwood: history, uses, present status and the future.* Current Science, 2012; 103(12): 1408-1416.
17. Holmes P. *The wisdom of being.* The International Journal of Aromatherapy, 1994; 6(4): 14-17.

18. Rashkow ED. *Perfumed the axe that laid it low: the endangerment of sandalwood in southern India.* Indian Economic & Social History Review, 2014; (51)1: 41-70. doi: 10.1177/0019464613515553.
19. Dhanya B et al. *Sandal (Santalum album L.) conservation in southern India: A review of policies and their impacts.* Journal of Tropical Agriculture, 2010; 48(1/2): 1-10.
20. O'Brien S. *Report 35 Standing committee on environment and public affairs. Inquiry into the sandalwood industry in Western Australia.* Parliament of Western Australia, Perth, 2014. Retrieved on May 15, 2017, from http://www.parliament.wa.gov.au/parliament%5Ccommit.nsf/RelatedReportsLookup/851396FFA630B66548257CD0001800EA?OpenDocument
21. Statham P. *The sandalwood industry in Australia: a history.* Proceedings of the Symposium on Sandalwood in the Pacific. Pacific Southwest Research Station, Forest Service, U.S. Department of Agriculture, Honolulu, 1990.
22. *WA sandalwood industry development plan 2008 -2020.* Australian Sandalwood Network, Forest Products Commission, Western Australia, 2008.
23. *Sandalwood.* Retrieved May 15, 2017, from http:www.fpc.wa.gov.au/sandalwood
24. Henderson W. *Sweet scent of success – sandalwood in Australia.* Retrieved on May 15, 2017, from http://aciarblog.blogspot.com.au/2014/05/sweet-scent-of-success-sandalwood-in.html
25. *Quintis Sandalwood album: our story.* Retrieved May 15, 2017, from https://quintis.com.au/our-story/
26. McConnon T. *Sandalwood company happy despite low harvest.* (Sept 20, 2013) In ABC Rural. Retrieved from http://www.abc.net.au/news/rural/2013-09-20/tfs-happy-with-sandalwood-harvest/4970344
27. Squire P. *Companion to the latest edition of the British Pharmacopoeia.* 13th edn. London, 1882.
28. Blumenthal M et al. *The complete German commission E monographs: therapeutic guide to herbal medicine.* American Botanical Council, Austin, 1998.
29. Marks-McGee A. *Indian sandalwood returns to the perfumer's palette.* Perfumer & Flavorist, 2016; 41: 40-41.
30. Baylac S, Racine P. *Inhibition of 5-lipoxygenase by essential oils and other natural fragrance extracts.* International Journal of Aromatherapy, 2003; 13(2/3): 138-142.
31. Beylier MF, Givaudan SA. *Bacteriostatic activity of some Australian essential oils.* Perfumer & Flavorist, 1979; 4(1): 23-25. Cited in Quintessential Aromatics database, 2013.
32. Lassak EV, McCarthy T. *Australian medicinal plants.* Methuen Australia, North Ryde, 1983.
33. Jirovetz L et al. *Comparative study on the antimicrobial activities of different sandalwood essential oils of various origins.* Flavour and Fragrance Journal, 2006; 21(3): 465-468. Cited in Quintessential Aromatics database, 2013.
34. Benencia F, Courreges MC. *Antiviral activity of sandalwood oil against Herpes simplex viruses -1 and -2.* Phytomedicine, 1999; 6(2): 119-123. Cited in Quintessential Aromatics database, 2013.
35. Bowles EJ. *The chemistry of aromatherapeutic oils.* 3rd edn. Allen & Unwin, Crows Nest, 2003.
36. Schnitzler P et al. *Susceptibility of drug-resistant clinical Herpes simplex virus type I strains to essential oils of ginger, thyme, hyssop and sandalwood.* Antimicrobial Agents and Chemotherapy, 2007; 51(5): 1859-1862. Cited in Quintessential Aromatics database, 2013.
37. Koch C et al. *Inhibitory effect of essential oils against herpes simplex virus type 2.* Phytomedicine, 2008; 15(1/2): 71-78. Cited in Quintessential Aromatics database, 2013.
38. Banerjee S, Ecavade A, Rao AR. *Modulatory influence of sandalwood oil on mouse hepatic glutathione S-transferase activity and acid soluble sulphydryl level.* Cancer Letters, 1993; 68(2/3): 105-109. Cited in Quintessential Aromatics database, 2013.
39. Dwivedi C, Abu-Ghazaleh A. *Chemopreventive effects of sandalwood oil on skin papillomas in mice.* European Journal of Cancer Prevention, 1997; 6(4): 399-401. Cited in Quintessential Aromatics database, 2013.
40. Dwivedi C, Zhang Y. *Sandalwood oil prevents skin tumour development in CD1 mice.* European Journal of Cancer Prevention, 1999; 8(5): 449-455. Cited in Quintessential Aromatics database, 2013.
41. Kang SH et al. *Spray adulticidal effect of plant oils against house mosquito, Culex pipiens pallens (Diptera: Culicidae).* Journal of Pesticide Science, 2009; 34(2): 100-106. Cited in Quintessential Aromatics database, 2013.
42. Hongratanaworakit T et al. *Evaluation of the effects of East Indian sandalwood oil and α-santalol on humans after transdermal absorption.* Planta Medica, 2004; 70(1): 3-7. Cited in Quintessential Aromatics database, 2013.
43. Kyle G. *Evaluating the effectiveness of aromatherapy in reducing levels of anxiety in palliative care patients: results of a pilot study.* Complementary Therapies in Clinical Practice, 2006; 12(2): 148-155. Cited in Quintessential Aromatics database, 2013.
44. Misra BB, Dey S. *TLC-bioautographic evaluation on an in vitro anti-tyrosinase and anti-cholinesterase potentials of sandalwood oil.* Natural Product Communication, 2013; 8(2): 253-256. Cited in Quintessential Aromatics database 2013.

45. Lavabre M. *Aromatherapy workbook.* Healing Arts Press, Rochester, 1997.
46. Lawless J. *The encyclopaedia of essential oils.* Element Books, Shaftesbury, 1992.
47. Davis P. *Aromatherapy: an A-Z.* 2nd edn. C.W. Daniel Company, Saffron Walden, 1999.
48. Kerr J. *Essential oil profile – Australian sandalwood.* Aromatherapy Today, 2000; 15: 8-12.
49. Mojay G. *Aromatherapy for healing the spirit.* Healing Arts Press, Rochester, 1999.
50. Webb M. *Bush sense.* Self-published, Australia, 2000.
51. Fischer-Rizzi S. *Complete aromatherapy handbook.* Sterling Publishing, New York, 1989.
52. Worwood VA. *The fragrant mind.* Transworld Publishers, London, 1995.
53. Worwood VA. *The fragrant heavens.* Transworld Publishers, London, 1999.
54. Davis P. *Subtle aromatherapy.* C.W. Daniel Company, Saffron Walden, 1991.
55. Keim Loughran J, Bull R. *Aromatherapy anointing oils.* Frog, Berkeley, 2001.
56. Dove R. *The essence of perfume – the master perfumer's definitive guide.* Black Dog, London, 2014.
57. Tisserand R, Young R. *Essential oil safety.* 2nd edn. Churchill Livingstone, Edinburgh, 2014.
58. Lis-Balchin M. *Aromatherapy science – a guide for healthcare professionals.* Pharmaceutical Press, London, 2006.
59. Burdock GA et al. *Safety assessment of sandalwood oil (Santalum album L.).* Food and Chemical Toxicology, 2008; 46(2): 421-432. Cited in Quintessential Aromatics database, 2013.

Savory

S

Identification

Botanical name

Summer savory: *Satureja hortensis* L.

Winter savory: *Satureja montana* L.

Synonyms

Summer savory: *Satureia hortensis* L., garden savory

Winter savory: *Satureia montana* L.

Family

Lamiaceae (Labiatae)

Botany and origins

Summer savory is an annual herb with oblong-linear leaves and hairy erect branches. It grows up to about 45 cm in height and is native to Europe. Winter savory is a bristly perennial subshrub with a woody base and oblong-linear leaves. It grows up to 38 cm in height.[1] There are over 200 different herbs and scrub species belonging to the *Satureja* genera.[2] In France, *S. hortensis* is cultivated and *S. montana* grows wild.[3]

Method of extraction

Summer savory oil is steam-distilled from the entire overground plant with its flowering stalks. Winter savory oil is steam-distilled from the leaves and tender stems.[1]

Characteristics

Savory oil is a pale yellow to almost colourless liquid with a fresh medicinal odour, reminiscent of sage and thyme, but with a sharpness reminiscent of cumin. The dryout has a harsh phenolic aroma.[3]

Chemical composition

The chemical composition of *S. hortensis* essential oil from Turkey was reported as follows:

carvacrol (79.17%), γ-terpinene (9.05%), *p*-cymene (3.14%), thymol acetate (2.24%), β-caryophyllene (1.48%).[4]

The chemical composition of *S. montana* essential oil was reported as follows:

carvacrol (60-75%), thymol (1.0-5.0%), *p*-cymene (10-20%), γ-terpineol (2.0-10.0%), 1,8-cineole (3.8%), borneol (12.5%), α-terpineol (2.5%).[5]

Adulteration

Lis-Balchin states that savory is often adulterated with similar oils such as high carvacrol marjoram.[6]

Pharmacopoeias and standards

At the time of writing, the purity, composition, physico-chemical properties and therapeutic use of savory essential oils are not defined in any pharmacopoeia monograph or standard.

History and Traditional Uses

History

Savory has been used as a culinary herb since antiquity in the Mediterranean countries.[3]

In ancient times, savory was supposed to belong to the Satyrs, hence the name Satureia. The Satyr was a Greek mythical creature, half-beast, half-man who roamed the woods and mountains. He was associated with pipe-playing and pursuing nymphs and vestals with vigour, making nightly visits to respectable women and prompting men to action. Satyr was a tempter who was considered dangerous and crafty.[7]

Culpeper stated that the juice dropped into the eyes removes dimness of sight if it proceeded from thin humours distilled from the brain. He also suggested heating the juice with oil of roses and dropping into the ears to remove noise and singing and deafness. He also explained that summer savory expels tough phlegm from the chest and lungs, quickens the dull spirits in the lethargy and eases sciatica when applied outwardly.[7]

S. hortensis was a popular seasoning herb in the Ancient Roman and Greek civilisations. The English name of the plant savory refers to its pleasant and spicy taste. It is also one of the herbs used in the ingredients of *herbes de Provence* – rosemary, thyme, oregano, marjoram along with savory and some other herbs. It is added to bouquets garnis, and in some cases is used as a replacement for parsley.[8]

Traditional medicine

Savory has been used as a medicinal herb in folk medicine for the digestive system. Traditionally it has been used for healing and to relieve pain from bone and muscle, as well as treating nausea, diarrhoea and cramps.[8]

Valnet states that in the old days a decoction of savory in wine was used to treat mouth and throat ulcers. Toothache was relieved by rubbing the essential oil directly onto the decayed tooth.[9]

Herbal

Both summer savory and winter savory are used as a tea for the carminative, expectorant and tonic properties. Both varieties of savory can be used for treating stomach and intestinal disorders such as cramps, nausea and indigestion. Summer savory oil is reported to have excellent antimicrobial properties.[1]

Food, perfumery and flavouring

The oil is mainly used for flavouring sauces, seasonings, canned meats, pickles and vinegars.[3] Savory is included in many digestive liqueurs.[9]

Therapeutics

Pharmacology and clinical studies

Many pharmacological studies involving savory essential oils have been published. A systemic review of these studies will not be attempted. Rather, I have chosen a selection of studies that support the traditional and clinical uses.

Acetylcholinesterase (AChE) inhibitory activity

AChE is the main enzyme involved in Alzheimer's disease. *S. montana* oil had strong inhibitory activity on AChE.[10]

Antifungal activity

An in vitro study confirmed that *S. montana* oil had strong antifungal activity against *Trichophyton violaceum, Trichophyton rubrum, Trichophyton tonsurans, Trichophyton mentagrophytes* and *Pyricularia oryzae*.[2]

A randomised, controlled clinical trial study was conducted on 80 patients (mean age 62.91 ± 7.34) in two groups treated either with *S. hortensis* oil at 1% gel or placebo, applied two times daily for denture stomatitis. Denture stomatitis is an inflammatory process of the oral mucosa associated with the presence of *Candida albicans* or other microorganisms which are the most common causative agent of oral candidiasis. The study concluded that *S. hortensis* oil in the gel base significantly reduced the candida colony count.[11]

S. hortensis oil had strong antifungal activity on the planktonic, biofilm formation and mature biofilms of *C. albicans* isolates from buccal lesions of HIV (+) individuals.[12]

Antimicrobial activity

A review of the many *Satureja* species indicates that the high presence of carvacrol is the main indicator of the antimicrobial activity of savory essential oil.[10]

Antinociceptive activity

A study found that the hydroalcoholic extract of *S. hortensis* was much more effective than the essential oil in reducing pain responses in an in vivo study using mice.[10]

Antispasmodic activity

S. hortensis essential oil has been reported to have antispasmodic activity on isolated rat ileum contractions induced by potassium chloride and acetylcholine.[13]

Antiviral activity

The aqueous extract of *S. montana* has been found to have exerted strong antiviral activity on human immunodeficiency virus-1 (HIV-1).[2,10]

Insecticidal activity

A review of many *Satureja* species indicates that the oils have proven insecticidal and larvicidal activity against a range of insect species such as *Ephestia kuehniella, Culex quinquefasciatus* and *Culex pipiens*.[10]

Actions

Actions commonly cited in aromatherapy

Anticatarrhal, antispasmodic, aphrodisiac, astringent, bactericidal, carminative, cicatrisant, emmenagogue, expectorant, fungicidal, stimulant, vermifuge[14,15]

Actions supported by clinical studies

Antifungal, antimicrobial, antinociceptive, insecticidal

Comment

Mailhebiau states that *S. montana* oil is preferable to *S. hortensis* oil.[16] Lawless states that savory essential oil should not be used in aromatherapy because it is a dermal toxin and irritant.[14]

Schnaubelt states that the preferred method of use is internally. Taken internally, it counteracts enteritis, enterocolitis and nervous exhaustion.[17]

Considering the risk of dermal irritation or sensitisation, I would recommend that savory essential oil only be used by professionally trained aromatherapists.

Aromatherapy Uses

Clinical aromatherapy

Antimicrobial

Mailhebiau states that *S. montana* oil has immunostimulating properties and that it is ideal to use for genitourinary and gastrointestinal infections. However, he warns that essential oils with high phenols should not be used on children.[16]

Digestive system

Mailhebiau states that *S. montana* oil regularises intestinal peristalsis and is indicated in cases of diarrhoea, flatulence and constipation, especially when used with cinnamon, clove bud and rosemary ct. verbenone.[16]

Musculoskeletal system

Mailhebiau suggests blending savory with lavender and adding it to *Hypericum perforatum*-infused oil to make an analgesic blend for rheumatism.[16]

Nervous system

Savory oil is also recommended for physical debility and fatigue; however, Mailhebiau explains that it should not be used excessively. He recommends blending it with lemon to give to people who are physically rundown and have metabolic disturbance.[16]

Energetics, psyche and subtle uses

Energetics

The energetic qualities of savory oil are similar to thyme oil. Savory oil is a *hot* and invigorating essential oil. It increases *Qi*, stimulates and warms the *Lungs* and dispels *wind cold*. It is therefore indicated for the onset of infections with stiff muscles, aches and pains, chills and fatigue.

Savory oil can be used to dispel any *cold* condition involving weakness, congestion or infection of the *Lungs*. It is particularly beneficial for chronic fatigue, shallow breathing, catarrhal coughs and bronchitis. Savory oil is associated with the Metal and Water Elements.

Subtle

Keim Loughran & Bull state that winter savory helps us to appreciate, connect and understand the wisdom and spirituality of nature.[18]

Dosage and Administration

Blending

Aromatherapy

To prevent colds and flu, consider blending savory oil with essential oils such as bay laurel, clove bud, cinnamon bark, 1,8-cineole-rich eucalyptus oils, fragonia, lemon, ravintsara, tea tree or thyme.

For the relief of rheumatic aches and pains, consider blending savory oil with essential oils such as cajeput, kunzea, spike lavender, sweet marjoram, pine or rosemary ct. camphor.

To alleviate mental and physical fatigue, consider blending savory oil with essential oils such as lemon, peppermint or rosemary.

Perfumery

Savory is occasionally used in perfumery to impart an interesting fresh, herbaceous and medicinal aroma to perfumes. It is used to create forest-type, chypre and fougère style perfumes. It blends well with citrus oil, oakmoss absolute, lavender, pine needle oils and rosemary.[3]

Mode of administration

Bath

It is not recommended for use in a bath.

Topical

Consider using it in a massage or balm; however, the percentage must not exceed 1% and it must not be used on people with sensitive skin or diseased or damaged skin.

Inhalation

Direct inhalation, diffuser, oil vaporiser

Safety Profile

General safety

Summer and winter savory essential oils are dermal irritants and mucous membrane irritants.[14,19]

Lawless states that they should not be used in aromatherapy.[14] Tisserand & Young state that people with sensitive, diseased or damaged skin and children under the age of two should not use the oils.[20] Tested at 6% in petrolatum on human volunteers, summer savory oil was not irritating or sensitising.[21]

Contraindications

Lawless states that it should be avoided during pregnancy.[14]

Toxicity

Essential oils such as savory that are rich in phenols generally have strong antibacterial activity and tend to be corrosive to tissues. However, Tisserand & Young also state that the carvacrol present in savory does not appear to present a high risk as an irritant. They state that the maximum dermal use level should be 1.5% for summer savory and 1.2% for winter savory. They also state that the oil may contain methyl eugenol, and this may inhibit blood clotting. People on diabetic medication, anticoagulant medication, or having major surgery, peptic ulcers, haemophilia and other bleeding disorders should use with caution.[20]

Regulatory guidelines

Savory oil has GRAS status.

References

1. Khan I, Abourashed E. *Leung's encyclopedia of common natural ingredients used in food, drugs and cosmetics*. 3rd edn. John Wiley & Sons, New Jersey, 2010.
2. Jafari F et al. *A critical overview on the pharmacological and critical aspects of popular Satureja species*. Journal of Acupuncture and Meridan Studies, 2016; 9(3): 118-127. doi: 10.1016/j.jams.2016.04.003.
3. Arctander S. *Perfume and flavor materials of natural origin*. Allured Publishing, Carol Stream, 1994.
4. Gormez A et al. *Chemical composition and antibacterial activity of essential oils of two species of Lamiaceae against phytopathogenic bacteria*. Polish Journal of Microbiology, 2015; 64(2): 121-127.
5. Lawrence BM. *Essential oils 1981-1987*. Allured Publishing, Wheaton, 1989.
6. Lis-Balchin M. *Aromatherapy science – a guide for healthcare professionals*. Pharmaceutical Press, London, 2006.
7. Grieve M. *A modern herbal – Vol. II*. Dover Publications, New York, 1971.
8. Hassanzadeh MK et al. *Summer savory (Satureja hortensis L.) oils*. In Preedy VR. ed. *Essential oils in food preservation, flavor and safety*. Academic Press, London, 2016: 757-764.
9. Valnet J. *The practice of aromatherapy*. C.W Daniel Company, Saffron Walden, 1980.
10. Tepe B, Cilkiz M. *A pharmacological and phytochemical overview on Satureja*. Pharmaceutical Biology, 2016; 54(3): 375-412. doi: 10.3109/13880209.2015.1043560.
11. Sabzghabaee AM et al. *Clinical evaluation of essential oil of 'Satureja hortensis' for the treatment of denture stomatitis*. Dental Research Journal, 2012; 9(2): 198-202.
12. Sharifzadeh A et al. *Chemical composition and antifungal activity of Satureja hortensis L. essential oil against planktonic and biofilm growth of Candida albicans isolates from buccal lesions of HIV (+) individuals*. Microbial Pathogenesis, 2016; 96: 1-9. doi: 10.1016/j.micpath.2016.04.014.
13. Hajhashemi V et al. *Antispasmodic and anti-diarrhoeal effect of Satureja hortensis L. essential oil*. Journal of Ethnopharmacology, 2000; 71(1/2): 187-192. doi: 10.1016/S0378-8741(99)00209-3.
14. Lawless J. *The encyclopaedia of essential oils*. Element Books, Shaftesbury, 1992.
15. Lavabre M. *Aromatherapy workbook*. Healing Arts Press, Rochester, 1997.
16. Mailhebiau P. *Portraits in oils*. C.W Daniel Company, Saffron Walden, 1995.
17. Schnaubelt K. *Medical aromatherapy*. Frog, Berkeley, 1999.
18. Keim Loughran J, Bull R. *Aromatherapy and subtle energy techniques*. Frog, Berkeley, 2000.
19. Tisserand R, Balacs T. *Essential oil safety*. Churchill Livingstone, Edinburgh, 1995.
20. Tisserand R, Young R. *Essential oil safety*. 2nd edn. Churchill Livingstone, Edinburgh, 2014.
21. Opdyke DLJ. *Monographs on fragrance raw materials*. Pergamon Press, Oxford, 1979.

Spearmint

Identification

Botanical name

Mentha spicata L.

Synonyms

Mentha viridis, common spearmint

Family

Lamiaceae (Labiatae)

Botany and origins

Spearmint is a hardy, branched perennial herb with bright green, lance-shaped leaves with finely toothed edges and a smooth surface.[1]

Although it is native to Europe, it is now very common in North America and western Asia. The USA is the major producer of spearmint. Smaller quantities of spearmint oil are produced in Europe.[2]

In some countries the use of mint as a culinary herb and herbal tea does not differentiate between spearmint and *Mentha viridis*, known as 'garden mint'.[2]

Native spearmint was introduced to the USA as a garden plant by the British, who settled in New England. By the seventeenth century spearmint had been established as an important crop in Massachusetts. Over the next 100 years, spearmint cultivation moved to the midwest sates of Ohio, Michigan, Indiana and Wisconsin. Spearmint was first introduced into India during the British occupation.[3]

S

Method of extraction

Spearmint oil is produced by steam-distillation of the fresh flowering tops of *M. spicata*.

Characteristics

Spearmint oil is a pale olive or pale yellow mobile liquid with a warm, slightly green, herbaceous, penetrating aroma reminiscent of the odour of the crushed herb.[2]

Chemical composition

The chemical composition of North American Scotch spearmint essential oil from the Midwest was reported as follows:

carvone (65.8-71.6%), 1,8-cineole (1.4-1.6%), limonene (13.7-17.3%), myrcene (0.8-1.1%), 3-octyl acetate (0.1-0.2%), *trans*-sabinene hydrate (1.0-1.4%), β-bourbonene (0.9-1.2%), *trans*-carveol (0.3-0.5%), *cis*-carveol (0.3-0.5%).[4]

The ISO standard for spearmint oil states that it should contain 55% or more carvone.[5]

Adulteration

Spearmint is commonly adulterated with synthetic laevo-carvone.[6]

Pharmacopoeias and standards

The purity, composition and physico-chemical properties of spearmint essential oil are defined in ISO 3033-1:2005 Oil of Spearmint – Part 1: Native Type (*Mentha spicata* L.).

Spearmint oil is listed in the British and French pharmacopoeias.

History and Traditional Uses

History

The use of spearmint dates back to the ancient Greeks who used it in their bath water. The Romans introduced spearmint into Britain, where it was used to stop milk from curdling. Grieve explains that the ancients used mint to scent their bath water and as a restorative, as we use smelling salts today. In medieval times, it became a feature in oral hygiene and was used to heal sore gums and for whitening teeth.[1]

It is thought that the first record of spearmint cultivation was a garden plant of large European convents and monasteries in the ninth century. It became popular in England in the eighteenth century as an ingredient of mint sauce, a traditional sauce served with lamb or mutton.[3]

Herbal

Spearmint herb has been used in both Western and Eastern cultures as an aromatic, stomachic, stimulant, antiseptic, local anaesthetic and antispasmodic in treating indigestion.[7]

Food, perfumery and flavouring

Spearmint oil is primarily used as a flavouring in toothpastes, chewing gum, candy and mouthwashes.[2,7]

Therapeutics

Pharmacology and clinical studies

Antiemetic activity

A randomised, double-blind clinical trial examined the efficacy of spearmint and peppermint oils in preventing chemotherapy-induced nausea and vomiting. It was found that there was a significant reduction in the intensity and number of emetic events in the first 24 hours with spearmint and peppermint, when compared with the control group. No adverse effects were reported and the cost of the treatment was also reduced when the essential oils were used.[8]

Antifungal activity

An in vitro study reported that spearmint oil exhibited significant antifungal activity. It was found to be more effective than the synthetic antifungal drugs miconazole and ketoconazole.[9]

Another in vitro study also reported that spearmint oil had more potent antifungal activity than commercial fungicide, bifonazole. The researchers suggested that spearmint oil could be used as a natural preservative and fungicide in food preservation.[10]

Anti-inflammatory activity

An in vitro study found that spearmint oil at a 0.1% concentration suppressed TNF-α-induced neutrophil adherence. This suggests that low concentration of spearmint oil has anti-inflammatory activity.[11]

Antimicrobial activity

Spearmint oil is reported to have antimicrobial properties.[12,13]

An in vitro study confirmed that spearmint oil inhibits and reduces *Vibrio* spp. biofilm. It was suggested that further investigation should explore the use of natural products such as spearmint oil in antibiofilm adhesion, and use in the food industry as a preservative against vibrio contamination.[14]

Antispasmodic activity

A study investigating the antispasmodic effect of spearmint on guinea pig ileum was investigated. It was found that the (-)-carvone found in spearmint oil reduced the contraction induced by high K^+ and was almost 100 times more potent than verapamil. The researchers stated that (-)-carvone had a potent calcium channel blocker-like action.[15]

Actions

Actions commonly cited in aromatherapy

Antidepressant, antiseptic, antispasmodic, carminative, cephalic, cholagogue, hepatic, insecticide, restorative, stimulant[16,17,18]

Actions supported by clinical studies

Antiemetic, antifungal, antimicrobial, antispasmodic

Comment

Grieve states that the properties of spearmint oil resemble those of peppermint, being a stimulant, carminative and antispasmodic; however, she states its effects are less powerful and it is better adapted for children's maladies.[1]

Lis-Balchin states that she cannot understand why spearmint is compared to peppermint, as the chemical composition of spearmint is totally different to that of the other mint oils such as peppermint. She also explains that spearmint oil was not ever commonly used in herbal medicine. Traditionally, it has been used as a flavour ingredient, so she is surprised that many aromatherapy books offer many uses for spearmint oil and compare it to peppermint.[5]

Holmes states that spearmint is an underrated oil in the therapeutic arena. Unfortunately, this is because the aroma of spearmint is synonymous with toothpaste, mouthwashes and chewing gum.[18]

Aromatherapy Uses

Clinical aromatherapy

Digestive system

Grieve states that spearmint is an excellent choice for children with digestive problems such as nausea, flatulence, constipation and diarrhoea.[1] Spearmint oil is recommended for indigestion and hepatobiliary disorders, and it relieves flatulence, hiccups and nausea.[16,17,18]

Nervous system

Spearmint oil has an uplifting effect, reducing mental strain and fatigue, stress and depression.[16,17,18]

Psychological

Holmes states that spearmint oil promotes emotional stability and renewal. He recommends it for irritability, negative feelings, emotional and mental confusion and lethargy, especially in the morning. He explains that it is mildly stimulating and promotes alertness.[18]

Holmes suggests that spearmint may be beneficial for those who are unable to let go of distressing feelings and negative emotions.[18]

Respiratory system

Used as an inhalation, it can be used to decongest sinus problems, catarrhal conditions and asthma.[16,17,18]

Holmes suggests that spearmint is a very effective oil for acute respiratory infection associated with thick, purulent mucus. He explains the oil is rich in ketones which act as a mucolytic expectorant.[18]

Skin care

Spearmint oil is recommended for the treatment of acne, dermatitis and congested skin.[16]

Energetics, psyche and subtle uses

Energetics

Holmes explains that spearmint oil is *cooling* and it helps to regulate the *Liver Qi* and harmonise the *Shen*. When the *Liver Qi* is constrained and there is *Shen* disharmony, we may experience irritability, mood swings and feelings of frustration.[18]

According to the principles of the Five Elements, spearmint oil strengthens the Wood Element and balances the Earth Element.

Dosage and Administration

Blending

Aromatherapy

For the relief of indigestion, bloating and nausea, consider blending spearmint with essential oils such as black pepper, cardamom, sweet fennel, ginger, mandarin or peppermint.

To help clear and expel excess mucus and phlegm, consider blending spearmint with essential oils such as aniseed, cajeput, 1,8-cineole-rich eucalypts, myrtle, niaouli, pine or tea tree.

To alleviate anxiety, nervous tension, stress and irritability, consider blending spearmint oil with essential oils such as bergamot, lavender, cold-pressed lime, mandarin, neroli or sweet orange.

Perfumery

Arctander states that spearmint is used in perfumery for its peculiar herbaceous-green effect in lavender fougère or jasmine compositions. He states that carvone, the principal constituent of spearmint, blends well with certain notes of the jasmine complex.[2]

Mode of administration

Bath

Full body bath, foot bath

Topical

Compress, massage, ointment, skin care

Inhalation

Direct inhalation, diffuser, oil vaporiser

Safety Profile

General safety

Spearmint oil is non-toxic, non-irritating and non-sensitising.[16] (-)-carvone has been identified as a skin sensitiser. The IFRA standard recommends a maximum of 1.2% for either isomer of carvone in a leave-on product. Tisserand & Young, therefore, recommend a dermal maximum of 1.7% based on 71.6% (-)-carvone content in spearmint oil.[19]

Contraindications

No contraindications known.

Regulatory guidelines

Spearmint has been granted GRAS status.

References

1. Grieve M. *A modern herbal – Vol. II.* Dover Publications, New York, 1971.
2. Arctander S. *Perfume and flavor materials of natural origin.* Allured Publishing, Carol Stream, 1994.
3. Morris M. *Commercial mint species grown in the United States.* In Lawrence BM. ed. *Mint: the genus Mentha.* Taylor & Francis Group, London, 2007: 421-495. (Medical and Aromatic Plants – Industrial Profiles; 44).
4. Lawrence BM. *Progress in essential oils – spearmint oil.* Perfumer & Flavorist, 2004; 29: 85-88.
5. Lis-Balchin M. *Aromatherapy science – a guide for healthcare professionals.* Pharmaceutical Press, London, 2006.
6. Schmidt E, Wanner J. *Adulteration of essential oils.* In Baser KHC, Buchbauer G. eds. *Handbook of essential oils – science, technology and applications.* 2nd edn. CRC Press, Boca Raton, 2016: 707-745.
7. Khan I, Abourashed E. *Leung's encyclopedia of common natural ingredients used in food, drugs and cosmetics*. 3rd edn. John Wiley & Sons, New Jersey, 2010.
8. Tayarani-Najaran Z et al. *Antiemetic activity of volatile oil from Mentha spicata and Mentha x piperita in chemotherapy-induced nauseas and vomiting*. Ecancermedicalscience, 2013; 7: 290. doi: 10.3332/ecancer.2013.290.
9. Pandey KP et al. *Antifungal efficacy of Taxodium and Menthe oils against human pathogenic fungi.* Flavour and Fragrance Journal, 2002; 17(6): 443-444. Cited in Quintessential Aromatics database, 2013.
10. Soković MD et al. *Chemical composition of essential oils of Thymus and Mentha species and their antifungal activities*. Molecules, 2009; 14(1): 238-249. Cited in Quintessential Aromatics database, 2013.
11. Abe S et al. *Suppression of tumor necrosis factor-α-induced neutrophil adherence responses by essential oils.* Mediators of Inflammation, 2003; 12(6): 323-328. Cited in Quintessential Aromatics database, 2013.
12. Montes MA. *Antibacterial activity of essential oils from aromatic plants growing in Chile.* Fitoterapia, 1998; 69(2): 170-172. Cited in the Aromatherapy Database, by Bob Harris, Essential Oil Resource Consultants, UK, 2000.
13. Mkaddem M et al. *Chemical composition and antimicrobial and antioxidant activities of mentha (longifolia L. and viridis) essential oils.* Journal

of Food Science, 2009; 74(7): M358-M363. Cited in Quintessential Aromatics database, 2013.
14. Snoussi M et al. *Mentha spicata essential oil: chemical composition, antioxidant and antibacterial activities against planktonic and biofilm cultures of Vibrio spp. strains.* Molecules, 2015; 20(8): 14402-14424. Cited in Quintessential Aromatics database, 2013.
15. Souza F et al. *(-)-carvone: antispasmodic effect and mode of action.* Fitoterapia, 2013; 85: 20-24. Cited in Quintessential Aromatics database, 2013.
16. Lawless J. *The encyclopaedia of essential oils.* Element Books, Shaftesbury 1992.
17. Lavabre M. *Aromatherapy workbook.* Healing Arts Press, Rochester, 1997.
18. Holmes P. *Aromatica: a clinical guide to essential oil therapeutics – Vol. I.* Singing Dragon, London, 2016.
19. Tisserand R, Young R. *Essential oil safety.* 2nd edn. Churchill Livingstone, Edinburgh, 2014.

Spikenard

Identification

Botanical name

Nardostachys jatamansi DC

Synonyms

Nard, Indian nard

Family

Valerianaceae

Botany and origins

Spikenard is also known as 'false' Indian valerian root. It is tender aromatic herb with a pungent rhizome root.[1]

Spikenard oil, sometimes known as nard oil, is obtained from the roots of two species of *Nardostachys* which are erect perennial members of the Valerianaceae family. The first of these is *Nardostachys jatamansi* which can be found in the Himalayan region of India.[1] It usually grows at an elevation of 3000 to 5000 m from the Punjab to Sikkim and Bhutan.[2]

Another species of which very little is known is *Nardostachys chinensis*. It is an ancient Chinese medicinal plant from which a Chinese spikenard oil is obtained. This latter oil is of very little interest because very little is available commercially.[1]

Nepal has banned the export of unprocessed spikenard and encouraged cultivation in order to minimise the harvesting of wild plants.[3] *N. jatamansi* is now listed as 'Critically Endangered' according to the IUCN Red List of Threatened Species.[4]

It is considered an important medicinal plant in India, and also grows in Nepal, Bhutan, Myanmar and southwest China. It has been targeted by medicinal plant collectors. It is threatened by overgrazing, loss of habitats and forest degradation. The species is collected from its wild habitat in an indiscriminate way, causing the natural population of the species to rapidly decline.[4]

Method of extraction

Spikenard oil is steam-distilled from the dried and crushed roots and rhizomes.

Characteristics

Spikenard oil is a pale yellow to amber coloured liquid with a heavy, sweet-woody, spicy-animal odour reminiscent of valerian, ginger, cardamom and Atlas cedarwood.[1]

Chemical composition

The chemical composition of spikenard oil was reported as follows:

β-maaliene (5.98%), aristolene (3.04%), β-gurjunene (20.60%), seychellene (3.32%), α-patchoulene (1.27%), α-gurjunene (5.4%), β-selinene (1.24%), valencene (1.43%), γ-gurjunene (0.79%), 7-*epi*-α-selinene (1.54%), maaliol (8.21%), patchouli alcohol (5.92%), 9-aristolen-12-ol (5.97%), valeranone (8.05%), valerenal (3.09%).[5]

Adulteration

There are a number of *Nardostachys* species and other plants which yield roots that are sold commercially as 'Indian valerian root'. That is why there is so much variation in the odour of spikenard oil. Spikenard is frequently adulterated with borneol, patchouli oil, isobornyl, valerianate, terpinyl valerianate, terpineol and eugenol.[1]

Pharmacopoeias and standards

At the time of writing, the purity, composition, physico-chemical properties and therapeutic use of spikenard essential oil are not defined in any pharmacopoeia monograph or standard.

History and Traditional Uses

History

Spikenard is regularly mentioned in the Bible. During biblical times, spikenard would have come from India. Spikenard was then used in incense and expensive perfumes. It was, therefore, not surprising that when Mary Magdalene used spikenard to perfume the feet of Christ, she was rebuked by those around her, but not by Christ:

> *Then took Mary a pound of ointment of spikenard, very costly, and anointed the feet of Jesus, and wiped his feet with her hair: and the house was filled with the odour of the ointment.*[6]
>
> John 12:3 (King James Version)

The scent of spikenard was also associated with royalty:

> *While my king sitteth at his table, my spikenard sendeth forth the smell thereof.*[6]
>
> Song of Solomon 1:12 (King James Version)

Traditional medicine

Traditional therapeutic uses include tonic, cooling, antipyretic and laxative properties. It was used for the treatment of skin diseases, throat troubles, ulcers, leprosy and diseases of the blood. Dioscorides suggests that the herb is 'warming and drying', good for nausea, flatulent indigestion, menstrual problems, inflammations and conjunctivitis.[7]

S

Spikenard has a very long history of use as a medicinal herb in Ayurveda. The roots and rhizomes of *N. jatamansi* have been used to treat epilepsy, hysteria and mental weakness. It also has cardioprotective activity and is used in the treatment of neural diseases.[8]

In India, it is reputed to have a protective effect in Parkinson's disease, epilepsy and cerebral ischemia, and has free radical scavenging activity. It is reputed to lower norepinephrine, as well as serotonin in the brain.[9]

In Ayurveda, spikenard is attributed with the following qualities: *Medhya* (brain tonic), *Rasayana* (rejuvenation to the mind), *Nidhrajnana* (promotes sleep), *Manasrogaghna* (alleviates mental diseases), *Pachana* (digestive), *Kasawasahara* (alleviates cough and breathing difficulties), *Dahaprasha-mana* (stops burning sensations) and *Roma sanjanana* (promotes hair growth).[10]

Therapeutics

Pharmacology and clinical studies

Antifungal activity

Spikenard had potent inhibitory activity against filamentous formation of *Candida albicans*. However, the inhibition against the growth of the yeast form was weak.[11]

Anti-inflammatory activity

The results of a study confirmed that ethanolic extracts of *Nardostachys jatamansi* rhizome demonstrated strong anti-inflammatory potential in experimental animals against acute, subacute and chronic model induced inflammation.[9]

Sedative activity

The vapour inhalation of a hexane extract of spikenard had a sedative effect on mice.[12]

Inhalation of valerena-4,7(11)-diene isolated from spikenard oil had a profound sedative effect on mice. The strongest sedative activity was observed at a dose of 0.06%. The continuous sleep time of pentobarbital-treated mice was prolonged by about 2.7 times with valerena-4,7(11)-diene, an effect similar to that of chlorpromazine administered orally.[13]

Actions

Actions commonly cited in aromatherapy

Anti-inflammatory, bactericidal, deodorant, fungicidal, laxative, sedative, tonic[7]

Actions supported by clinical studies

Sedative

Comment

Some clinical and pharmacological studies have examined the therapeutic properties of spikenard herb in Ayurvedic medicine. Spikenard has been described as one of the most important psychotropic herbs in Ayurveda.[8]

The essential oil of spikenard is very rich in sesquiterpene compounds. Jatamansone, one of the main sesquiterpene compounds present in the oil, is reported to have anticonvulsant and sedative activities. Studies have also found that jatamansone reduced aggression and restlessness in hyperkinetic children. Some believe that *N. jatamansi* could provide us with cures for degenerative diseases such as Alzheimers's disease and Parkinson's disease.[8]

Unfortunately, this precious plant is on the verge of extinction. Conservation strategies must be implemented to ensure the long-term future of spikenard.[8]

Aromatherapy Uses

Clinical aromatherapy

Nervous system

It has been suggested that spikenard may have

similar sedative properties to that of valerian.[14]

Schnaubelt states that spikenard is probably the most powerful sedative in aromatherapy.[15] Lawless recommends using it to alleviate insomnia, nervous indigestion, migraines and stress.[7] Mojay explains that spikenard has a calming effect on the mind and it helps to soothe the deepest forms of anxiety.[16]

Skin care

Gumbel suggests that, in skin care, spikenard is balancing, soothing and rejuvenating.[14] Schnaubelt states that it helps to restore balance to all skin types and can be used to treat psoriasis. He recommends blending it with lavender oil.[15]

Energetics, psyche and subtle uses

Energetics

Mojay explains that spikenard helps to calm the *Heart*, balancing the *Shen* and settling emotions. He compares it to valerian and recommends it for nervous tension, anxiety and insomnia. He states that it helps regulate the flow of *Liver Qi*.[16]

Subtle

Gumbel describes spikenard as the ultimate essential oil to find inner balance in the emotional, spiritual and physical interplay of energies.[14] Schnaubelt recommends rubbing spikenard over the heart or the solar plexus to provide a sedative effect.[15]

Worwood states that the fragrance of spikenard carries with it the bonds of human existence: the chains that bind us to the emotions which we may be fearful of releasing. She says that its purpose is to release the past from the shackles of our own making, those which relentlessly bind us to repeating actions which affect the freedom of the spirit.[17]

Keim Loughran & Bull state that spikenard embodies wholeness, promotes a sense of hope and helps comfort and balance the heart, especially for people who take on the cares of the world. They explain that to be willing to open our hearts, and truly feel and empathise with others, is an act of courage. However, there is a tendency to cut ourselves off from feelings in response to the suffering around the world. We often do this by perceiving those who suffer to be 'different' from us, or by assuming that they are to blame for their predicament. Spikenard will teach us to be truly compassionate – feeling for others in their time of suffering – without becoming depleted. It will help us to keep our hearts open to those around us, ever ready to offer compassion in times of need.[18]

Spikenard is recommended for the type of individual who is searching for spiritual certainty. It nourishes both the heart and the soul, and through its serenity and earthly humility, it gives us the strength to be devoted to our chosen path.[7]

Dosage and Administration

Blending

Aromatherapy

To alleviate stress, anxiety and nervous tension, consider blending spikenard oil with essential oils such as German chamomile, clary sage, lavender, frankincense, geranium, myrrh, neroli, patchouli, sandalwood or vetiver.

To alleviate insomnia, consider blending spikenard oil with essential oils such as Roman chamomile, lavender, sweet marjoram, neroli or sandalwood.

For sensitive skin, consider blending spikenard oil with essential oils such as German chamomile, everlasting, lavender, patchouli or sandalwood.

In subtle aromatherapy to comfort the heart, consider blending spikenard oil with essential oils such as bergamot, lavender, neroli, rose otto or sandalwood.

Perfumery

Spikenard oil is used in perfumery in oriental style perfumes, heavy florals, fougère style perfumes, woody bases and animal-amber style perfumes.[1]

The complex, spicy, earthy aroma of spikenard blends well with warm spicy oils such as cardamom, ginger and black pepper. It also blends well with the sweet, warm resin oils such as opopanax, cistus and benzoin. It creates depth and tenacity when it is blended with rich florals such as rose absolute and jasmine. Together with oakmoss absolute, galbanum, or pine needle oil, it creates a lush, green, earthy natural aroma.

Mode of administration

Bath

Full body bath, foot bath

Topical

Compress, massage, ointment, skin care

Inhalation

Direct inhalation, diffuser, oil vaporiser

Safety Profile

General safety

Spikenard is non-toxic, non-irritating and non-sensitising.[7]

Contraindications

No contraindications known.

Regulatory guidelines

Spikenard essential oil is not defined in any regulatory guideline.

References

1. Arctander S. *Perfume and flavor materials of natural origin*. Allured Publishing, Carol Stream, 1994.
2. Lawrence BM. *Essential oils 1981-1987*. Allured Publishing, Wheaton, 1989.
3. Tisserand R, Young R. *Essential oil safety*. 2nd edn. Churchill Livingstone, Edinburgh, 2014.
4. Ved D et al. *Nardostachys jatamansi*, The IUCN Red List of Threatened Species. 2015: eT50126627A50131395. doi: 10.2305/IUCN.UK.2015-2.RLTS.T50126627A50131395.en.
5. Lawrence BM. *Progress in essential oils – spikenard oil*. Perfumer & Flavorist, 2010;35: 55-56.
6. *King James Bible online*. https://www.kingjamesbibleonline.org
7. Lawless J. *The encyclopaedia of essential oils*. Element Books, Shaftesbury, 1992.
8. Disket J et al. *A review on spikenard (Nardostachys jatamansi DC.) – an 'endangered' essential herb of India*. International Journal of Pharmaceutical Chemistry, 2012; 2(3): 52-60.
9. Singh RK et al. *Evaluation of anti-inflammatory potential of Nardostachys jatamansi rhizome in experimental rodents*. Journal of Coastal Life Medicine, 2014; 2(1): 38-43.
10. Purnima MB, Kothiyal P. *A review article on phytochemistry and pharmacological profiles of Nardostachys jatamansi DC – medicinal herb*. Journal of Pharmacognosy and Phytochemistry, 2015; 3(5): 102-106.
11. Inouye S et al. *Composition, antifungal and radical scavenging activities of 15 rare oils*. International Journal of Essential Oil Therapeutics, 2010; 4(1/2): 1-10. Cited in Quintessential Aromatics database, 2013
12. Takemoto H et al. *Sedative effects of vapor inhalation of agarwood oil and spikenard extract and identification of their active compounds*. Journal of Natural Medicine, 2008; 62(1): 41-46. Cited in Quintessential Aromatics database, 2013.
13. Takemoto H et al. *Evaluation of volatile components from spikenard: valerena-4,7(11)-diene is a highly active sedative compound*. Journal of Natural Medicines, 2009; 63(4): 380-385. Cited in Quintessential Aromatics database, 2013.
14. Gumbel D. *Principles of holistic skin therapy with herbal essences*. Karl F Haug Publishers, Heidelberg, 1986.
15. Schnaubelt K. *Medical aromatherapy*. Frog, Berkeley, 1999.
16. Mojay G. *Aromatherapy for healing the spirit*. Healing Arts Press, Rochester, 1999.
17. Worwood VA. *The fragrant heavens*. Transworld Publishers, London, 1999.
18. Keim Loughran J, Bull R. *Aromatherapy and subtle energy techniques*. Frog, Berkeley, 2000.

S

Spruce

Identification

Botanical name

Norway spruce: *Picea abies* L.

Hemlock spruce: *Tsuga canadensis* L.

Black spruce: *Picea mariana* (Mill.) Britton

White spruce: *Picea glauca* (Moench) Voss

Synonyms

Norway spruce: Common spruce, European spruce

Hemlock spruce: Eastern hemlock, hemlock

Black spruce: Canadian black pine

White spruce: Canadian spruce

Family

Pinaceae

Botany and origins

Spruce is a large evergreen tree up to 50 m tall, also known as hemlock spruce. Spruce is native to the east coast of the USA. Arctander states that the oil is usually derived from several different botanical sources.[1]

Tudge states that several of the hemlocks epitomise the image of what a conifer tree should look like – tall, dark, with needle-leaved like spruces, but the *T. canadensis* of the eastern United States are smaller, slower growing and often cut into hedges.[2]

The word spruce originates from *spruse* which literally means 'from Prussia'.[3]

Method of extraction

Spruce essential oil is steam-distilled from the needles and twigs from several different botanical sources of spruce trees.

Characteristics

Spruce oil is a pale yellow to colourless oil with a very pleasant, balsamic-fresh odour and a slightly fruity undertone. The odour characteristics can vary according to the origin of the oil and the botanical species used.[1]

Chemical composition

The chemical composition of *T. canadensis* essential oil was reported as follows:

tricyclene (1.3%), α-pinene (12.1%), camphene (13.4%), β-pinene (16.0%), limonene (12.0%), β-phellandrene (4.9%), *p*-cymene (0.1%), terpinolene (3.7%), *p*-cymenene (0.2%), bornyl acetate (37.6%), terpinen-4-ol (0.1%), β-caryophyllene (0.9%), citronellyl acetate (0.1%), α-terpineol (0.6%), borneol (0.1%), α-terpinyl acetate (0.1%), piperitone (0.6%), geranyl acetate (0.2%).[4]

The chemical composition of *Picea mariana* essential oil was reported as follows:

α-pinene (13.7%), camphene (8.1%), limonene (5.2%), bornyl acetate (36.8%), β-pinene (14.2%), camphor (4.9%), δ-3-carene (3.4%), β-myrcene (2.8%), β-phellandrene (2.1%), borneol (1.4%).[5]

Adulteration

No information is available on possible adulteration of spruce oil. While adulteration may not occur, I can imagine that there may be challenges in obtaining spruce oil that is species pure. This is confirmed by Guenther, who states that spruce oil is not usually derived from one single well-defined species of spruce, but from mixed branches and leaves of four different species of spruce. As no distinction is made in the collection of the distillation material, the physico-chemical properties of commercial spruce oil may vary significantly.[6]

Pharmacopoeias and standards

At the time of writing, the purity, composition, physico-chemical properties and therapeutic use of spruce essential oil are not defined in any pharmacopoeia monograph or standard.

History and Traditional Uses

Herbal

The British Herbal Pharmacopoeia recommends an infusion or decoction of hemlock bark for the treatment of diarrhoea, cystitis, leucorrhoea, stomatitis and gingivitis.[7]

In the nineteenth century, the North American colonists made spruce beer, which was the tops of spruce infused in beer. Spruce beer was used as an antiscorbutic. The British Navel Surgeon James Lind in 1753 had high praise for spruce beer:

> *The Newfoundland spruce beer, made of the black spruce, either fresh or dried, or from its essence, is an excellent medicine. The beer must be drunk daily, and parts affected with the eruption bathed with it night and day.*[8]

Captain James Cook used it to preserve the health of his crew and prevent scurvy.[8]

A 1905 book, *Curative foods from the cook: in place of drugs from the chemist*, noted that spruce beer made with the Norway spruce fir is an agreeable and wholesome beverage, very useful against scurvy and for chronic rheumatism.[8]

Food, perfumery and flavouring

Spruce oil is extensively used in room fresheners, perfumes, bath products and household cleaning products.[1]

Other uses

Spruce is one of the species most commonly used as a 'Christmas tree'.[5] Spruce is extensively used for its timber as a building material. In North America, it is commonly referred to by several different names such as North American timber and SPF lumber (a combination of spruces, pines and firs). All species yield a high-grade timber with relatively small tight knots. It is generally recommended for indoor construction purposes only.[9]

Therapeutics

Pharmacology and clinical studies

Antimicrobial activity

The essential oil extracted from *P. abies* was found to have antimicrobial activity against a range of gram-positive bacteria and fungi.[10]

Nootropic activity

An in vivo study found that treatment with black spruce oil enhanced memory function in rats, and that the underlying mechanism of its action may be attributed to its acetylcholinesterase (AChE) inhibition activity.[11]

Actions

Actions commonly cited in aromatherapy

Antimicrobial, antiseptic, antitussive, astringent, diaphoretic, diuretic, expectorant, nervine, rubefacient, tonic[12,13]

Actions supported by clinical studies

Antimicrobial

S

Comment

Spruce essential oil is not listed in any pharmacopeia. There is a lack of clinical data for the therapeutic uses of spruce oil in aromatherapy; however, I am very interested in Schnaubelt's comment regarding the chemical profile of many of the pine needle essential oils. He explains that they have a balance of stimulating monoterpene and calming esters. He states that they contain hormone-mimicking, polycyclic terpenoid compounds that are endocrine tonics, re-establishing hormonal balance in the pituitary, thyroid, adrenals and ovaries.[14]

Holmes states that, while white spruce and black spruce have similar functions, only black spruce has the restorative action on the neuroendocrine-immune functions. White spruce has a higher monoterpene content that would make it more useful as a stimulating oil and an analgesic for aches and pains. He explains that white spruce acts as a stimulating expectorant with mucolytic action.[15]

It would be exciting to see research conducted to confirm the use of spruce oil as a tonic of the neuroendocrine-immune system.

Aromatherapy Uses

Clinical aromatherapy

Musculoskeletal system

Spruce oil is recommended for the relief of muscular aches and pains, poor circulation and rheumatism.[12]

Psychological

Holmes recommends black spruce for mental fatigue and burnout. He suggests using it whenever one feels low motivation, low stamina and vitality, and depression.[15]

Zeck beautifully describes the tonifying effect of spruce on our psyche:

> *When suffering lingers too long and defeat and exhaustion pervade all areas of your life, refreshing aromatic spruce descends deep into the unlimited energy reserves that lie dormant within your being.*
>
> *Like the warmth of a radiant sun upon your face, spruce activates the release of a healthy energy flow from the adrenal glands to refresh and bring strength to each new day.*[16]

Respiratory system

Spruce oil is very effective for the treatment of asthma, bronchitis, colds and flu, coughs and respiratory weakness.[12]

Tonic

Schnaubelt notes that a number of pine needle oils have a balance of stimulating monoterpene and calming esters. They are endocrine tonics, re-establishing hormonal balance in the pituitary, thyroid, adrenals and ovaries.[14]

Energetics, psyche and subtle uses

Energetics

According to the principles of TCM, spruce oil tonifies the *Qi* and *Yang* and strengthens the *Shen*.[15] Whenever our *Qi* and *Shen* are weak, we may experience fatigue and recurring infections, have low motivation and may suffer from depression.

Black spruce also tonifies the *protective Qi* which helps protect us from colds, influenza and recurring infections.[15]

Black spruce tonifies the *Lungs* and *Kidney Yang Qi*. Whenever we experience *Lung* and *Kidney Yang deficiency*, we may experience chronic cough, wheezing, chest pain, low stamina, mental and physical fatigue, backache and fearfulness.[15]

Subtle

Spruce promotes communication of inner feelings. It is said to bring objectivity and clarity to the intuitive mind. Spruce teaches us to walk our spiritual path with 'practical feet', moving forward and making choices with grounded wisdom and intuitive understanding. Spruce supports intuition and teaches us about compassion – for ourselves and others. It will allow us to feel compassion despite our mistakes and fears.[17]

Lavabre states that spruce oil is excellent for balancing energy and recommends it for any type of psychic work because of its opening and elevating quality.[13]

Holmes states that inhaling black spruce oil evokes strength and endurance at the level of the soul. He describes the aroma as centring, strengthening and energising. It helps us find the inner strength whenever we need to face challenging situations. The oil will help us draw energy from the deeper wellspring of connected, deep inner strength and hope. It connects us to our collective past, our ancestral wisdom, becoming a source of deep and enduring strength for the future.[15]

Dosage and Administration

Blending

Aromatherapy

For the relief of musculoskeletal conditions such as inflammation, tension and pain, consider blending spruce with essential oils such as black pepper, ginger, kunzea, spike lavender, pine or rosemary.

For the relief of coughs and respiratory congestion, consider blending with essential oils such as aniseed, cajeput, cypress, 1,8-cineole-rich eucalypts, fragonia, niaouli, pine and thyme.

To alleviate fatigue, lack of stamina, adrenal burnout and stress, consider blending spruce with essential oils such as bergamot, black pepper, ginger, lemon, galbanum, grapefruit, cold-pressed lime, pine, rosemary or vetiver.

Holmes recommends a blend of black spruce and scotch pine as a neuroendocrine-immune restorative tonic.

Perfumery

Spruce is excellent in 'fresh' perfume types. It blends well with all other pine oils and with oils that have a rich green note such as oakmoss absolute and galbanum. Spruce also blends well with herbaceous scents such as lavandin and rosemary.[1]

Mode of administration

Bath

Full body bath, foot bath

Topical

Compress, massage, ointment, skin care

Inhalation

Direct inhalation, diffuser, oil vaporiser

Safety Profile

General safety

The overall composition of spruce oil means that it is a safe and non-toxic essential oil. However, skin sensitisation may occur if the oil is oxidised, therefore, old or oxidised oil should not be used.[5]

Contraindications

No contraindications known.

Regulatory guidelines

Spruce essential oil has GRAS status.

References

1. Arctander S. *Perfume and flavor materials of natural origins*. Allured Publishing, Carol Stream, 1994.
2. Tudge C. *The secret life of trees*. Allan Lane, London, 2005.
3. *Spruce*. In *Online etymology dictionary*. Retrieved Sep 15, 2017, from http://etymonline.com/index.php?allowed_in_frame=0&search=Spruce
4. Lawrence BM. *Progress in essential oils – Canadian hemlock oil*. Perfumer & Flavorist, 2009; 34: 59.
5. Tisserand R, Young R. *Essential oil safety*. 2nd edn. Churchill Livingstone, Edinburgh, 2014.
6. Guenther E. *The essential oil– Vol. VI*. Robert E Krieger Publishing, Malabar, 1952.
7. *British herbal pharmacopoeia*. British Herbal Medicine Association, Bournemouth, 1983.
8. Crellin KK. *A social history of medicines in the twentieth century: to be taken three times a day*. Pharmaceutical Products Press, New York, 2004.
9. Canada Wood Group. *SPF products*. Retrieved November 11, 2017, from http://canadawood.org/products/spf/
10. Radulescu V et al. *Chemical composition and antimicrobial activity of essential oil from shoots spruce (Picea abies L)*. Revista de Chimie, 2011; 62: 69-74.
11. Kharade P. *Screening of black spruce for nootropic activity in rats*. Retrieved Sep 15, 2017 from http://hdl.handle.net/123456789/2130
12. Lawless J. *The encyclopaedia of essential oils*. Element Books, Shaftesbury, 1992.
13. Lavabre M. *Aromatherapy workbook*. Healing Arts Press, Rochester, 1997.
14. Schnaubelt K. *Advanced aromatherapy*. Healing Arts Press, Rochester, 1995.
15. Holmes P. *Aromatica: a clinical guide to essential oil therapeutics – Vol. I*. Singing Dragon, London, 2016.
16. Zeck R. *The blossoming heart – aromatherapy for healing and transformation*. Aroma Tours, East Ivanhoe, 2004.
17. Keim Loughran J, Bull R. *Aromatherapy and subtle energy techniques*. Frog, Berkeley, 2000.

Tagetes

Identification

Botanical name

Tagetes minuta L., *Tagetes patula* L. and *Tagetes erecta* L.

Synonyms

Taget, African marigold, French marigold, *Tagetes glandulifera* Schrank

Family

Asteraceae (Compositae)

Botany and origins

Tagetes is a strongly scented herb about 0.3 to 1 m high with bright orange, daisy-like flowers and soft green oval leaves.[1]

Tagetes is native to South America and Mexico. It grows wild in South Africa, Europe, Asia and North America. The oil is produced in South Africa, France, Argentina and Egypt.[2]

It grows semi-wild and is cultivated on a comparatively large scale in the western parts of India. *T. patula* flowers are occasionally used for the adulteration of saffron since the dried petals of tagetes have an appearance similar to that of true saffron.[2]

T

Tagetes is also known as 'French marigold'. This often leads to confusion with *Calendula officinalis*, the common marigold. Most commercial tagetes oil is distilled from *T. minuta*, but oils from *T. patula* are occasionally available.[3]

Method of extraction

Tagetes essential oil is produced from the steam distillation from the fresh flowering herb. An absolute is obtained by solvent extraction from the fresh flowering herbs.[2]

Characteristics

The essential oil of tagetes is a dark yellow to orange-yellow coloured mobile liquid that solidifies on exposure to air, daylight and moisture. The odour is intensely herbaceous-green, with a sweet-fruity undertone and a somewhat bitter herbaceous dryout.[2]

The oil oxidises and resinifies quickly and becomes very viscous when exposed to air and moisture. Old tagetes oil is viscous, dark amber brown and lacks the typical fruity top note.[2]

Chemical composition

Lawrence compared the major chemical constituents of seven commercial samples of tagetes oil. The major constituents were found to vary as follows:

limonene (5.0-7.0%), (*Z*)-β-ocimene (27.9-54.5%), dihydrotagetone (5.1-28.0%), (*E*)-tagetenone (0.5-3.2%), (*Z*)-tagetone (2.4-9.3%), (*Z*)-tagetenone (0.3-7.6%).[4]

The main constituent, tagetone, is an unstable ketone. It is responsible for the peculiar aroma and for the resinification and instability of the oil.[2]

Adulteration

Not reported.

Pharmacopoeias and standards

At the time of writing, the purity, composition, physico-chemical properties and therapeutic use of tagetes essential oil are not defined in any pharmacopoeia monograph or standard.

History and Traditional Uses

History

Tagetes has a long history of use as a food, medicine, ornamental, and in rituals and sociocultural ethnopractices. In Chile and Argentina, the plant is used in stews and is considered a highly prized flavouring agent. In other parts of the world, it is used to make hot or cold beverages as well as a herbal tea.[5]

In certain regions of South America, it is referred by the Incan name, *huacatay*. A paste is used to make a popular potato dish called *ocopa*. In Nepal, marigold garlands are used in almost every household during the Tihar festival. The flowers are also used in religious festivals in India, Portugal and Mexico. The flowers are used to decorate the Hindu temples in India.[5]

Traditional medicine

The flower heads and foliage of *T. erecta* are used as anthelmintic and emmenagogue, and in treating colic.[1]

In China, the flower heads of *T. erecta* are used in decoctions for the treatment of whooping cough, colds, colic, mumps, sore eyes and mastitis. In India, the juice from the leaves of *T. erecta* is used as a treatment for eczema. In Peru, the aerial parts of *T. minuta* are used in a decoction as a digestive, vermifuge, cholagogue and a sedative in gastric pain.[1]

Herbal

The herb of *T. minuta* is used as a stomachic, carminative, diuretic and diaphoretic.[1]

Food, perfumery and flavouring

Tagetes oil is used as a flavour component in many food products, including alcoholic and non-alcoholic beverages. The highest average maximum use level reported is 0.003% in condiments and relishes.[1]

Other uses

Tagetes oil finds limited use in perfumery, but is often used for flavouring tobacco and in many other food substances. Tagetes extract is approved for use in chicken feed to give the characteristic yellow colour to egg yolks and the yellow colour of chicken's skin. *T. erecta* flowers are used as a mosquito repellent.[1]

T. minuta has excellent antinematicidal activity. It is often grown alongside other crops such as tomato, eggplant and potato to keep the nematode population in the soil under control and to protect the plants from nematode damage.[5]

In Kenya, an infusion of *T. minuta* is used for the treatment of snake bites in the Luo and Kamba communities. In parts of Kenya, the plant is used for protection against mosquito bites and it is also used to protect livestock from ticks.[5]

Therapeutics

Pharmacology and clinical studies

Antidepressant activity

A study found that tagetes oil had a negative modulation on GABAergic function – meaning that the oil may have antidepressant-like properties. GABAergic neurotransmission is important in anxiety and stress responses. The in vivo effects of the oil were investigated on rat behaviour. However, it must be noted that the oil was administered subcutaneously at a dose of 0.3 mL/kg.[9]

Antifungal activity

The essential oil of *T. patula* has antifungal activity.[1,6]

Antimicrobial activity

The essential oil from the flowering heads of *T. minuta* was tested in vitro against a range of microorganisms. The oil demonstrated antimicrobial activity against all the tested microorganisms such as *Bacillus subtilis, Escherichia coli, Salmonella typhi, Staphylococcus aureus* and *Aspergillus niger*, but not *Microsporum gypseum*.[7]

Antioxidant activity

The oil of *T. minuta* significantly reduced NADH oxidase, inducible nitric oxide synthase and TNF-α mRNA expression in cells. This means that tagetes oil can modulate and diminish immune responses. The essential oil was found to have radical scavenging and anti-inflammatory activities, and could be used as a safe effective source of natural antioxidants in treatments against oxidative damage and stress associated with some inflammatory conditions.[8]

Larvicidal activity

α-terthienyl found in *T. erecta* is reported to be a nematocide and larvicide. The essential oil of *T. patula* also demonstrated larvicidal effect against three species of mosquito.[1]

Plantar lesions

The essential oil, paste and tincture of *T. erecta* was used in a double-blind, placebo-controlled trial to assess its efficacy in the treatment of hyperkeratotic plantar lesions. The treatment was effective for the reduction of corn and callus width, length and pain levels.[10]

Actions

Actions commonly cited in aromatherapy

Anti-inflammatory, antispasmodic, bactericidal, bronchodilator, carminative, diaphoretic, emmenagogue, fungicidal, hypotensive, stomachic[1,11]

Actions supported by clinical studies

Antimicrobial, antioxidant, insecticidal, larvicidal

Comment

There appears to be extensive ethnobotanical usage to support the role of tagetes extracts and essential oil for their insecticidal activity and in traditional agricultural practices.

There is a lack of clinical studies to support many of the properties attributed to tagetes essential oil. Some studies indicate that tagetes oil may have antioxidant activity and is useful as a treatment for hyperkeratotic plantar lesions. It is also well known that the essential oil is relatively unstable, so care should be taken to ensure you are using fresh essential oil.

Aromatherapy Uses

Clinical aromatherapy

Integumentary system

Tagetes is recommended for the treatment of bunions, calluses, corns and fungal infections.[10,11]

Dosage and Administration

Blending

Aromatherapy

For the treatment of fungal foot infections,

consider blending tagetes oil with essential oils such as myrrh, patchouli or tea tree.

Perfumery

Tagetes oil is used in creating herbaceous fragrances, and occasionally used for floral based fragrances with oils such as jasmine and gardenia. Modern aldehydic style perfumes also benefit from trace amounts of tagetes oil.[1]

Mode of administration

Topical

I would not recommend tagetes oil for massage purposes. It would be best used for topical applications for the treatment of bunions, calluses, corns and fungal infections. Use a 0.01% dilution of the appropriate blend of essential oils to the chosen carrier oil.

Safety Profile

General safety

Tagetes oil should be used with caution on the skin as it is possible that it may cause dermal sensitisation.[11]

IFRA recommends that tagetes oil and tagetes absolute be limited to a maximum 0.01% except for wash-off products. Tisserand & Young state that there appears to be a high risk of phototoxicity, even though the oil's psoralen content is very low. It is possible that another phototoxic compound found in the oil, α-terthienyl, is responsible.[3]

T

Contraindications

No contraindications known.

Toxicity

Davis and Lawless state that tagetone, one of the main constituents found in tagetes oil, may be a harmful or toxic component.[11,12] However, I could not find any clinical or research data to support this claim.

Regulatory guidelines

Tagetes has been approved for food use.[1]

References

1. Khan I, Abourashed EA. *Encyclopedia of common natural ingredients used in food, drugs and cosmetics*. 3rd edn. John Wiley and Sons, New Jersey, 2010.
2. Arctander S. *Perfume and flavor materials of natural origin*. Allured Publishing, Carol Stream, 1994.
3. Tisserand R, Young R. *Essential oil safety*. 2nd edn. Churchill Livingstone, Edinburgh, 2014.
4. Lawrence BM. *Essential oils 1992-1994*. Allured Publishing, Carol Stream, 1995.
5. Cornelius WW, Wycliffe W. *Tagetes (Tagetes minuta) oils*. In Preedy VR. ed. *Essential oils in food preservation, flavor and safety*. Academic Press, London, 2016: 791-802.
6. Garg SC, Dengre SI. *Antifungal efficacy of some essential oils*. Pharmazie. 1988; 43(2): 141-142. Cited in Quintessential Aromatics database, 2013.
7. Razdan TK et al. *Chemical composition and antimicrobial activity of the oil of Tagetes minuta Linn*. Parfumerie und Kosmetik, 1986; 67(1): 52-54. Cited in Quintessential Aromatics database, 2013.
8. Karimian P, Kavoosi G, Amirghofran Z. *Anti-oxidative and anti-inflammatory effects of Tagetes minuta essential oil in activated macrophages*. Asian Pacific Journal of Tropical Biomedicine, 2014; 4(3): 219-227. Cited in Quintessential Aromatics database, 2013.
9. Martijena ID et al. *Anxiogenic-like and antidepressant–like effects of the essential oil from Tagetes minuta*. Fitoterapia, 1998; 69(2): 155-160. Cited in Quintessential Aromatics database, 2013.
10. Khan MT et al. *Podiatric treatment of hyperkeratotic plantar lesions with marigold Tagetes erecta*. Phytotherapy Research, 1996; 10(3): 211-214. Cited in Quintessential Aromatics database, 2013.
11. Lawless J. *The encyclopaedia of essential oils*. Element Books, Shaftesbury, 1992.
12. Davis P. *Aromatherapy: an A-Z*. 2nd edn. C.W. Daniel Company, Saffron Walden, 1999.

Tangerine

Identification

Botanical name

Citrus reticulata Blanco var. 'tangerine'

Synonyms

Citrus nobilis var. *deliciosa*

Family

Rutaceae

Botany and origins

The botanical origin of tangerine and mandarin are similar. They are both considered to be varieties of the same species. Weiss treats mandarin and tangerine as one species. He states that the name tangerine is used in English-speaking countries but mandarin elsewhere.[1]

The tangerine fruit is much larger than the mandarin, almost globoid, and its peel is usually yellow or pale yellow to reddish. The tangerine represents a lower stage of horticultural development of the mandarin, which with intensive cultivation and after a sufficient period of time evolved into a mandarin.[2]

Method of extraction

Tangerine oil is cold-pressed from the peel of the ripe fruit of *C. reticulata*.

Characteristics

The oil is orange-coloured, mobile and with a fresh, sweet odour, reminiscent of bitter orange and Valencia orange oil, rather than mandarin. It completely lacks the characteristic dryness and note of mandarin oil, and it also has a much 'thinner' body.[3]

Chemical composition

The chemical composition of tangerine oil was reported as follows:

α-pinene (1.00%), myrcene (2.03%), limonene (91.23%), γ-terpinene (3.09%), and trace amounts of citronellal, linalool, neral, neryl acetate, geranyl acetate, geraniol, thymol and carvone.[4]

Reeve et al. compare the chemical composition of a typical Sicilian red mandarin and Chinese tangerine. They explain that the typical level of limonene present in the Chinese tangerine is around 90%, whereas the level of limonene in Sicilian red mandarin oil is approximately 73%. The γ-terpinene is typically present at 4% in the Chinese tangerine oil and around 17% in Sicilian red mandarin oil. The methyl-*N*-methyl anthranilate, which is characteristic of the Sicilian red mandarin, is often not found in the Chinese tangerine oil.[5]

Adulteration

Tangerine oil is often adulterated with synthetic dimethyl anthranilate.[6]

Pharmacopoeias and standards

At the time of writing, the purity, composition, physico-chemical properties and therapeutic use of tangerine essential oil are not defined in any pharmacopoeia monograph or standard.

History and Traditional Uses

History

There is very little history of tangerine. The word tangerine was originally used to describe fruit coming from Tangier, Morocco, from where the first shipment of tangerines was allegedly sent to mainland Europe in the mid-1840s. It was originally known as a tangerine orange.[5]

Traditional medicine

The peel of tangerine has long been used in traditional herbal medicines. The dried external part of the peel has stomachic and tonic properties and it is also used to relieve toothache and earache. Evidence suggests an association between citrus peel consumption and protection against coronary heart disease and stroke.[7]

Food, perfumery and flavouring

Apart from its use in aromatherapy, tangerine oil is extensively used in flavours, from where it gives interesting modifications with sweet and bitter orange, grapefruit and lime oils. It is used in flavour compositions for soft drinks, candy and liqueurs.[3]

Therapeutics

Pharmacology and clinical studies

Antibacterial activity

The essential oil from immature tangerine fruit exhibited the highest antibacterial activity against *Escherichia coli*. In the case of *Staphylococcus aureus*, the oil was mostly active at the mature stages of fruits.[7]

Other studies have confirmed that the fresh tangerine peel essential oil was bioactive against a range of bacteria. The antibacterial activity of tangerine essential oil has been reported to be associated with the monoterpene hydrocarbons, which diffuse into and damage bacterial cell membrane.[7]

Antifungal activity

The antifungal activity of tangerine essential oil has been reported against some common foodborne and phytopathogenic fungi. The essential oil displayed concentration-dependent inhibitory activity against *Aspergillus nidulans, A. niger* and *Fusarium oxysporum*.[7]

Actions

Actions commonly cited in aromatherapy

Antispasmodic, digestive, lymphatic, sedative[8,9]

Actions supported by clinical studies

Antibacterial, antifungal

Comment

Therapeutically, tangerine oil has similar properties to mandarin and orange oils.

Aromatherapy Uses

Clinical aromatherapy

Digestive system

Tangerine oil has a tonic effect on the digestive system, and it may be used for calming the intestines and relieving flatulence.[9,10]

Nervous system

Lavabre states that tangerine oil is soothing and sedating, and recommends it to alleviate insomnia, nervousness, emotional shock and grief.[10]

Pregnancy

It is often recommended for use during pregnancy in a massage oil to prevent stretch marks.[8,9]

Skin care

Tangerine oil is recommended for acne, congested and oily skin.[8]

Dosage and Administration

Blending

Aromatherapy

For the relief of anxiety, nervous tension and stress-related conditions, consider blending tangerine oil with essential oils such as bergamot, geranium, lavender, neroli, petitgrain, sandalwood or ylang ylang.

To alleviate depression, consider blending tangerine oil with essential oils such as bergamot, geranium, jasmine absolute, lavender, neroli, sweet orange, patchouli, rose absolute, sandalwood or ylang ylang.

To alleviate fatigue, consider blending tangerine oil with essential oils such as black pepper, coriander seed, ginger, grapefruit, lemon, petitgrain or rosemary.

To alleviate indigestion, consider blending tangerine oil with essential oils such as black pepper, coriander seed, ginger, sweet fennel, peppermint or spearmint.

To help prevent and reduce stretch marks during pregnancy, consider blending tangerine oil with essential oils such as lavender and neroli in a vegetable oil base of apricot kernel, avocado, rosehip or wheatgerm.

Perfumery

Arctander states that tangerine essential oil does not have a sufficiently characteristic aroma to be of interest in perfumery. It is used as a modifier in colognes and a top note in aldehydic perfumes.[3]

Mode of administration

Bath

Full body bath, foot bath

Topical

Compress, massage, skin care

Inhalation

Direct inhalation, diffuser, oil vaporiser

Safety Profile

General safety

Tangerine oil is non-toxic, non-irritating and non-sensitising. Old or oxidised tangerine oil should not be used as it may cause skin sensitisation.[6]

Contraindications

No contraindications known.

Regulatory guidelines

Tangerine oil has GRAS status.

References

1. Weiss EA. *Essential oil crops.* CAB International, Wallingford, 1997.
2. Guenther E. *The essential oils – Vol. III.* Robert E Krieger Publishing, Malabar, 1950.
3. Arctander S. *Perfume and flavor materials of natural origin.* Allured Publishing, Carol Stream, 1994.
4. Lawrence BM. *Tangerine oil.* Perfumer and Flavorist, 1980; 5(6): 27.
5. Reeve D et al. *Riding the citrus trail: when is a mandarin a tangerine?* Perfumer & Flavorist, 2002; 27: 20-23.
6. Tisserand R, Young R. *Essential oil safety.* 2nd edn. Churchill Livingstone, Edinburgh, 2014.
7. Mandal S, Mandal M. *Tangerine (Citrus reticulata L. var.) oils.* In Preedy VR. ed. *Essential oils in food preservation, flavor and safety.* Academic Press, London, 2016: 803-811.
8. Lawless J. *The encyclopaedia of essential oils.* Element Books, Shaftesbury, 1992.
9. Davis P. *Aromatherapy: an A-Z.* 2nd edn. C.W. Daniel Company, Saffron Walden, 1999.
10. Lavabre M. *Aromatherapy workbook.* Healing Arts Press, Rochester, 1997.

T

Tarragon

Identification

Botanical name

Artemisia dracunculus L.

Synonyms

Estragon

Family

Asteraceae (Compositae)

Botany and origins

Tarragon is a perennial herb with an erect, branched stem, up to 1.2 m in height. It is a native of southern Russia and western Asia. It is cultivated in Europe, USA, Argentina and many other countries.[1]

There are two varieties traded:

- *A. dracunculus* cv. 'Sativa': French tarragon
- *A. dracunculus:* Russian tarragon.

The Russian tarragon does not have the same fine flavour or aroma as the French tarragon. The major oil producers of tarragon are France and the United States.[1]

Method of extraction

Tarragon oil is steam-distilled from the whole above-ground part of the herb.

Characteristics

Tarragon oil is a colourless to very pale-yellow liquid with a sweet-anisic, green-spicy and slightly celery-like aroma. With age, tarragon oil tends to resinify, becoming dark yellow, sticky, and viscous and losing its fresh green note and pleasant aroma.[2]

Chemical composition

The comparative chemical composition of French and Russian tarragon essential oil is reported as follows:[3]

Constituent	French oil	Russian oil
α-pinene	0.51%	0.28%
sabinene	0.06%	41.34%
myrcene	0.13%	2.69%
limonene	2.26%	-
β-ocimene	10.0%	12.65%
γ-terpinene	8.89%	7.52%
linalool	10.04%	0.15%
terpinen-4-ol	-	1.32%
citronellyl formate	-	2.25%
methyl chavicol	74.46%	-
geranyl acetate	-	1.47%
methyl eugenol	0.79%	6.27%
eugenol	0.28%	-
elemicin	0.28%	17.16%

The chemical composition of a sample of tarragon essential oil from plants growing in the Himalaya region of India was reported as follows:

α-pinene (1.05%), myrcene (1.93%), 1,8-cineole (7.75%), (Z)-β-ocimene (15.79%), (Z)-β-ocimene (3.7%), α-terpinolene (10.1%), *trans*-anethole (28.1%), α-copaene (2.78%), elemicin (10.08%).[4]

This oil had no methyl chavicol and methyl eugenol, which are found in most tarragon oils. It was stated that this tarragon oil was different due to its chemotype variability, and it could be considered as an alternative source of tarragon oil.[4]

Adulteration

Arctander states that adulteration with estragole (synthetic or derived from pine oil) is a big problem for tarragon oil.[2] Tarragon oil is also commonly adulterated with synthetic anethole, eugenol from cinnamon leaf oil, synthetic estragole, and *cis*- and *trans*-ocimene from other sources.[5]

Pharmacopoeias and standards

The purity, composition and physico-chemical properties of tarragon essential oil are defined in ISO 10115:2013 Essential Oil of Tarragon (*Artemisia dracunculus* L.)

History and Traditional Uses

History

Hemphill states that there is very little recorded history of tarragon before the thirteenth century, when Ibn Baitar, an Arab physician living in Spain, described the virtues of *tarkhum*, Arabic for dragon. It was not until the sixteenth century that it became commonly used as a condiment and was cultivated by the French, who referred to it as estragon, meaning little dragon. The dragon reference is believed to come from the appearance of its coiled serpent-like root system, or the belief that tarragon was an antidote to the venom of snakes.[6]

Traditional medicine

The dried aerial parts of *A. dracunculus* are used orally to treat epilepsy in Iranian traditional medicine.[4]

T

Herbal

In herbal medicine, tarragon is used as a stomachic, diuretic, hypnotic, and emmenagogue, and in treating toothache.[1] Alcohol herbal extracts of tarragon were reported to have antidiabetic activity.[4]

Valnet recommends tarragon for anorexia, dyspepsia, hiccup, dysmenorrhoea, intestinal parasites and rheumatic conditions. He recommends using an herbal infusion of the herb, to use the herb in foods, and also suggests 2 drops of the essence in honey water.[7]

Food, perfumery and flavouring

The herb tarragon is commonly used as a domestic cuisine herb. The oil is extensively used as a flavouring component in numerous food products, including non-alcoholic beverages, candy, meat and meat products, condiments and relishes.[1]

Tarragon oil is also used as a fragrance component in soaps, detergents and perfumes.[1]

Hemphill states that French tarragon herb is worshipped by cooks for its characteristic licorice-anise aroma and tart, lingering, appetite-appealing flavour.[6]

Therapeutics

Pharmacology and clinical studies

Acetylcholinesterase inhibitory activity

A range of essential oils including *A. dracunculus* L were tested for their acetylcholinesterase (AChE) inhibitory activity. The results indicated that all the oils exhibited AChE inhibitory activity, except for *A. dracunculus* from Hungary, while tarragon oil from France showed the most potent inhibitory activity. Eugenol was found to be a potent AChE inhibitor.[8]

Anticonvulsant activity

Tarragon oil exerted dose- and time-dependent anti-seizure activity in both maximal electroshock and pentylenetetrazole models of experimental seizures.[9]

Antimicrobial activity

Tarragon oil was reported to have strong antimicrobial activity. The methyl chavicol content was not responsible for the antimicrobial activity.[1]

An in vitro study using essential oil from French tarragon grown in Scotland was found to inhibit a range of bacteria including *Escherichia coli, Pseudomonas aeruginosa, Streptococcus faecalis* and *Yersinia enterocolitica*.[10]

Tarragon oil extracted from plants growing in Iran had strong antibacterial activity on two important pathogen bacteria (*Staphylococcus aureus* and *E. coli*). The MIC for *E. coli* was 2500 μg/mL and for *S. aureus* it was 1250 μg/mL.[11]

Antinociceptive activity

The results of nociceptive tests in rats and mice confirmed that tarragon oil administered intraperitoneally at doses of 10, 30, 100 and 300 mg/kg showed significant analgesic activity. It was noted that the antinociceptive effect of the oil appears to be due to mechanisms independent of activation of opioid receptors, since naloxone, an opioid antagonist, failed to antagonise the antinociceptive effect of the essential oil. The researchers state that this finding supports the use of tarragon in traditional medicine for the treatment of painful disorders.[12]

Actions

Actions commonly cited in aromatherapy

Antiseptic, antispasmodic, carminative, digestive, diuretic, emmenagogue, stimulant, stomachic, vermifuge[13,14]

Actions supported by clinical studies

Analgesic, antimicrobial

Comment

Schnaubelt states that tarragon oil is one of aromatherapy's strongest antispasmodics.[14]

I would like to see more studies examine the antispasmodic and antinociceptive activities of the essential oil. However, the methyl chavicol and methyl eugenol content concerns me. Tisserand & Young recommend the dermal maximum of 0.1% tarragon based on 87.3% methyl chavicol content and 1.5% methyl eugenol.[15]

If you do use tarragon oil, it should only be for a short term and definitely not for oral doses. There can be so much variability in the chemical composition of the oil, so it is imperative that you know the country of origin and the chemical profile of the oil you are about to use.

Aromatherapy Uses

Clinical aromatherapy

Digestive system

Tarragon oil is recommended for dyspepsia, flatulence, hiccups, intestinal spasm, nervous indigestion and sluggish digestion.[13]

Reproductive system

Tarragon oil is recommended for amenorrhoea, dysmenorrhoea and PMS.[13]

Dosage and Administration

Blending

Aromatherapy

For the relief of dyspepsia, intestinal spasm and nervous indigestion, consider blending tarragon oil with essential oils such as sweet fennel, ginger, cardamom or peppermint.

For the relief of amenorrhoea and dysmenorrhoea, consider blending tarragon oil with essential oils such as Roman chamomile, clary sage, lavender or sweet marjoram.

Perfumery

It is used in very small amounts in perfumery in chypre, fougères and green floral bases. It blends well with galbanum, lavender and oakmoss absolute.

Mode of administration

Bath

I prefer not to use tarragon oil in a bath.

Topical

Compress, massage, ointment

Inhalation

Direct inhalation, diffuser, oil vaporiser

Safety Profile

General safety

Lawless states that tarragon is moderately toxic and should be used in moderation, and recommends avoiding tarragon oil during pregnancy.[13]

Contraindications

Avoid use during pregnancy.[13]

Toxicity

Tisserand & Young recommend that tarragon essential oil not be taken in oral doses. They state that it is a potential carcinogenic based on the high levels of estragole and methyl eugenol.[15]

The genotoxicity of Italian *A. dracunculus* oil with a methyl chavicol content of 60.46% was determined by the Zimmermann test. The essential oil of tarragon was found to be genotoxic.[3]

Regulatory guidelines

Tarragon essential oil has GRAS status.

References

1. Khan I, Abourashed E. *Leung's encyclopedia of common natural ingredients used in food, drugs and cosmetics.* 3rd edn. John Wiley & Sons, New Jersey, 2010.
2. Arctander S. *Perfume and flavor materials of natural origin.* Allured Publishing, Carol Stream, 1994.
3. Lawrence BM. *Progress in essential oils – tarragon oil.* Perfumer & Flavorist, 2002; 27: 51-56.
4. Tak IR et al. *Phytochemical studies on the extract and essential oils of Artemisia dracunculus L. (tarragon).* African Journal of Plant Science, 2014; 8(1): 72-75. doi: 10.5897/AJPS2013.1145.
5. Schmidt E, Wanner J. *Adulteration of essential oils.* In Baser KHC, Buchbauer G. eds. *Handbook of essential oils – science, technology and applications.* 2nd edn. CRC Press, Boca Raton, 2016: 707-745.
6. Hemphill I. *Spice notes.* Pan Macmillan Australia, Sydney, 2000.
7. Valnet J. *The practice of aromatherapy.* C.W. Daniel Company, Saffron Walden, 1980.
8. Dohi S et al. *Acetylcholinesterase inhibitory activity and chemical composition of commercial essential oils.* Journal of Agricultural and Food Chemistry, 2009; 57(10): 4313-4318. Cited in Quintessential Aromatics database, 2013.
9. Sayyah M et al. *Anticonvulsant activity and chemical composition of Artemisia dracunculus L. essential oil.* Journal of Ethnopharmacology, 2004; 94(2/3): 283-287. Cited in Quintessential Aromatics database, 2013.
10. Dean SG, Svoboda KP. *Antibacterial of French tarragon (Artemisia dracunculus L.) essential oil and its constituents during ontology.* Journal of Horticultural Science. 1988; 63(3): 503-508. Cited in Quintessential Aromatics database, 2013.
11. Raeisi M et al. *Essential oil of tarragon (Artemisia dracunculus) antibacterial activity on Staphylococcus aureus and Escherichia coli in culture media and Iranian white cheese.* Iranian Journal of Microbiology, 2012; 4(1): 30-34.
12. Maham M et al. *Antinociceptive effect of the essential oil of tarragon (Artemisia dracunculus).* Pharmaceutical Biology, 2014; 52(2): 208-212. doi: 10.3109/13880209.2013.824007.
13. Lawless J. *The encyclopaedia of essential oils.* Element Books, Shaftesbury, 1992.
14. Schnaubelt K. *Advanced aromatherapy.* Healing Arts Press, Rochester, 1995.
15. Tisserand R, Young R. *Essential oil safety.* 2nd edn. Churchill Livingstone, Edinburgh, 2014.

Tea tree

Identification

Botanical name

Melaleuca alternifolia Cheel

Synonyms

Ti-tree, narrow-leaved paperbark

Family

Myrtaceae

Botany and origins

M. alternifolia is a shrub or small tree which grows up to 5-7 m, usually with a single trunk but multiple stems may originate from a common rootstock. The trees coppice quickly and vigorously. *M. alternifolia* is confined to the warmer, wetter, east coast of Australia. It naturally prefers swampy areas, drainage lines and riverbanks. Most of the oil available nowadays is from commercial plantations.[1]

The name *Melaleuca* is derived from the Greek word *melos* (dark, black) and *leukon* (white). This name was apparently given to the first species described, *M. leucadendron*, which had white papery bark on the higher stems and branches and a black lower trunk. The common name of paperbark refers to the paper-like bark, which can often be peeled from the larger trees in broad strips.[1]

T

Method of extraction

Tea tree oil is water- or steam-distilled from *M. alternifolia*.

Characteristics

Tea tree oil is a pale yellowish green to almost clear mobile liquid, with a warm, spicy, aromatic odour reminiscent of nutmeg, cardamom and sweet marjoram, but with a strong emphasis on the terpinene and terpineol notes.[2]

Chemical composition

The chemical composition of tea tree was reported as follows:

α-pinene (2.1%), β-pinene (0.4%), sabinene (0.2%), myrcene (0.4%), α-phellandrene (0.8%), α-terpinene (7.1%), limonene (1.4%), 1,8-cineole (3.0%), γ-terpinene (15.7%), *p*-cymene (6.2%), terpinolene (3.4%), linalool (0.2%), terpinen-4-ol (45.4%), α-terpineol (5.3%).[1]

There has been much research done on the microbiological activity of the essential oil with regards to the terpinen-4-ol to cineole ratio.[1] The Australian Standard for tea tree oil (AS 2782 – 1985) requires that the 1,8-cineole content shall not exceed 15% and the terpinen-4-ol content shall be at least 30%.[3] Maintaining quality control when harvesting from the bush has been a problem because physically identified trees of *M. alternifolia* may produce oil with 1,8-cineole content ranging from 0 to 65%.[1]

There has been no evidence to support the fact that tea tree oil with lower levels of 1,8-cineole is considered superior to tea tree oil with higher levels of 1,8-cineole (5-15%). Southwell says that the antifungal and anthelmintic activities may actually be enhanced by 1,8-cineole. It was also identified that the antimicrobial properties of tea tree oil did not vary when the terpinen-4-ol content was maintained constant and the 1,8-cineole content varied from 20% to 1.5%.[4]

However, another study tested the major components of tea tree oil, including 1,8-cineole, terpinen-4-ol, *p*-cymene, linalool, α-terpinene, γ-terpinene, α-terpineol and terpinolene. The constituents were tested against a range of microorganisms and only terpinen-4-ol inhibited all of the microorganisms. In a previous study, the whole oil failed to inhibit pseudomonas – one of the test organisms.[5]

Adulteration

Tea tree oil is often adulterated by the addition of α-pinene and β-pinene from different sources, and γ-terpinene from terpenes resulting from citrus oil production. Synthetic terpinen-4-ol is also used.[6] Lis-Balchin states blending occurs to a large extent using tea tree oils from different species and localities.[7]

Arctander states that tea tree oil has been used as an adulterant for nutmeg oil and sweet marjoram oil.[2]

Pharmacopoeias and standards

The purity, composition and physico-chemical properties of tea tree are defined in several standards and monographs.

- ISO 4730:2017 Essential oil of Melaleuca, Terpinene-4-ol Type (Tea Tree Oil)
- AS 2782-2009 Oil of Melaleuca, Terpinene-4-ol Type (Tea Tree Oil)
- WHO Monographs on Selected Medicinal Plants – Vol. 2
- Assessment Report on *Melaleuca alternifolia* (Maiden and Betch) Cheel, *M. linariifolia* Smith, *M. dissitiflora* F. Mueller and/or other species of *Melaleuca*, aetheroleum. European Medicines Agency.

History and Traditional Uses

History

The Australian Aborigines have long recognised the virtues of tea tree. The leaves were simply crushed in the hand and the volatile oil inhaled to relieve colds and headaches. The name tea tree was first used by Captain Cook in 1777, when the leaves of melaleuca or leptospermum were brewed to make a tea to prevent scurvy. The common name of tea tree applies to a number of species of *Leptospermum* and *Melaleuca*.[1]

Tea tree oil was first distilled in Australia in the 1920s. Williams cites Professor McKern's 1960 review of the natural plant products industry of Australia:

> *The term tea tree is applied in Australia to a large group of shrubs and trees belonging to such genera as Melaleuca, Leptospermum, Kunzea etc. Nearly all produce an oil in greater or lesser amounts, but the commercial term 'tea tree oil' is reserved for the product distilled from the foliage of Melaleuca alternifolia (family Myrtaceae), one of the paper-barked tea trees of the north Coast of New South Wales.*[8]

McKern goes on to explain the therapeutic qualities of tea tree:

> *Extensive investigation has shown the oil to possess valuable bactericidal properties, and at the present time overseas demand for this oil for medicinal and dental use is very strong. The advantage that the oil possesses over other germicides is its ability to penetrate deeply into infected animal tissue and pus, and at the same time it has a very low level of toxicity to the host. It is also of value in dealing with obstinate fungal infections.*[8]

Williams explains that tea tree oil has travelled a very rocky road to success. The commercial production of tea tree oil was very tedious and laborious. The remote locations where the tree is found around Bungawalbyn Creek in New South Wales is a swampy habitat characterised by soggy environmental obstacles to the collection of the raw material.[8]

The development of a reliable source of supply was the only way to overcome these challenges. In the late 1970s, cultivation of the tree was undertaken by Thursday Plantation. This subsequent development of sophisticated oil extraction processes and reliable chemotypes of the plant were essential to developing a successful industry. Tea tree oil has progressively gained a remarkable level of support from good pharmacological and clinical research. This was the stimulus that eventually led to its outstanding success in the local and international marketplace.[8]

Traditional medicine

In 1930, Humphery described the medicinal properties of tea tree:

> *An essential oil extracted from a variety of tea tree growing in profusion on the North coast of New South Wales was brought to my notice about twelve months ago. Analysis by Mr. W.R. Penfold, Curator and Economic Chemist of the Sydney Technological Museum, showed that it was non-toxic, non-irritating and eleven to thirteen times stronger than carbolic as a germicide (Rideal-Walker coefficient).*
>
> *Dirty wounds, such as the result of street accidents, may be washed or syringed out with a 10% watery lotion, the solvent properties will loosen and bring away the dirt which is usually ground in, and the tissues will remain fresh and retain their natural colour. Dressings dipped in a 2.5% solution may then be applied, changed every twenty four hours and healing will readily take place.*
>
> *The pus solvent properties led me to try the lotion for perionychia which is usually so disheartening and so frequently results in the loss of the nail or deformity. Here the results were excellent. Infections which resisted treatment of various kinds for months, were cured in less than a week. The fingers were dressed with lint soaked in 10% solution and changed every twenty four hours.*
>
> *Twenty drops in a tumbler of warm water used as a gargle quickly clear up a sore throat in the early stages; it should be an excellent prophylactic for many infective conditions which gain entrance to the body through the naso-pharynx.*[9]

An article in the *Sydney Technological Museum Bulletin* of 1946 mentions an interesting use for tea tree oil:

> *An interesting application of the oil, the germicidal and healing properties have reduced to a minimum infection of skin injuries, especially abrasions to the hands by metal filings and turnings. Large quantities of Melaleuca alternifolia oil were used for this purpose in the various ammunition annexes during world war II.*[8]

The British Pharmaceutical Codex of 1949 reports that tea tree oil has germicidal properties and is used topically for the treatment of furunculosis, tinea, paronychia, impetigo, thrush and stomatitis, and as an inhalant in coryza.[10]

Food, perfumery and flavouring

Tea tree oil is used in soaps, toothpastes, deodorants, disinfectants and mouth gargles. It has some limited use in perfumery.

Therapeutics

Pharmacology and clinical studies

Many pharmacological studies involving tea tree oil have been published. A systemic review of these studies will not be attempted. Rather, I have chosen a selection of studies with an emphasis on those studies that support the traditional and clinical uses.

Acne

A clinical trial involving 124 teenage patients evaluated the effectiveness of 5% tea tree oil in a gel for treating mild to moderate acne when compared with 5% benzoyl peroxide lotion. The results confirmed that both 5% tea tree gel and the 5% benzoyl peroxide lotion had a significant result on reducing the patient's acne by reducing the number of inflamed and non-inflamed lesions.[11]

Anticarcinogenic activity

Tea tree oil and terpinen-4-ol were able to impair the growth of human M14 melanoma cells. It was more effective on the resistant variants, which express high levels of P-glycoprotein in the plasma membrane, overcoming resistance to caspase-dependent apoptosis exerted by P-glycoprotein-positive tumour cells.[12]

Terpinen-4-ol induced a significant growth inhibition of colorectal, pancreatic, prostate and gastric cancer cells in a dose-dependent manner. Terpinen-4-ol and various anticancer agents (oxaliplatin and fluorouracil) demonstrated a synergistic inhibitory effect on cancer cell proliferation.[13]

Antifungal activity

An in vitro study confirmed the antifungal activity of tea tree oil against *Candida albicans* and non-*albicans Candida* species. The minimum concentration required for killing the organisms was 0.25% and 0.5% for *C. albicans* and non-*albicans Candida* species, respectively.[14]

Onychomycosis is a common cause of nail disease that is caused by *Trichophyton rubrum* and *Candida* species. A double blind trial compared 1% clotrimazole and 100% tea tree oil by applying them directly to the toenails twice daily for six months. The results showed similar improvement in clinical assessment, nail appearance and symptomatology. Both preparations were comparable in efficacy and cost.[15]

A review article by Carson et al. reported the antifungal activity of tea tree oil against a range of fungal species, which had been published in more than 15 papers. The minimum inhibitory concentrations (MICs) were in the range between 0.03 and 0.5% and fungicidal concentrations from 0.12 to 25%. The exception was *Aspergillus niger* with a minimum fungicidal concentration (MFC) value up to 8%. However, it was noted that these essays were conducted with a fungal conidia that are known to be relatively impervious to chemical agents. Subsequent assays showed that the germinated conidia are significantly more susceptible to tea tree oil than non-germinated conidia. It was also noted that tea tree oil vapours have been demonstrated to inhibit fungal growth and affect sporulation.[16]

A study found that terpinen-4-ol was more active than tea tree oil and strongly enhanced fluconazole activity against fluconazole-resistant *C. albicans* strains. The results of the study demonstrated that combining tea tree oil with conventional drugs such as fluconazole may help treat difficult yeast infections.[17]

Anti-inflammatory activity

A number of studies have examined tea tree oil's ability to reduce inflammation. In one study, the application of 100% tea tree oil significantly reduced skin inflammation in a group of volunteers injected with histamine. Another type of inflammation reaction tested was 'contact' hypersensitivity to nickel, often found in jewellery. The study found that applying 100% tea tree oil significantly reduced skin inflammation in some, but not all patients.[11]

Antimicrobial activity

The antimicrobial properties of tea tree oil are well documented through clinical studies.[14,15,18,19]

The antibacterial activity of tea tree oil was demonstrated against methicillin-susceptible (MSSA) and methicillin-resistant (MRSA) *Staphylococcus aureus*.[18]

MICs have been determined for many organisms including coagulase-negative *Staphylococci* (0.06-3% v/v), *Staphylococcus aureus* (including MRSA) (0.12-0.5%), *Streptococcus* spp. (0.03-0.12%), vancomycin-resistant *Enterococci* (VRE) (0.5-1%), *Acinetobacter baumannii* (0.06-1%), *Escherichia coli* (0.12-0.25%), *Klebsiella pneumoniae* (0.12-0.5%), *Candida albicans* (0.12-0.25%), other *Candida* species (0.12-0.5%) and *Malassezia furfur* (0.12-0.25%). It was also stated that many organisms that colonise the skin transiently have been shown to be more susceptible to tea tree oil than commensal organisms.[19]

A study examining the mode of antimicrobial action of tea tree oil reported that the oil inhibited respiration and increased the permeability of bactericidal cytoplasmic and yeast plasma membranes. In the case of *E. coli* and *S. aureus*, tea tree oil also caused potassium ion leakage. It was concluded that the ability of tea tree oil to disrupt the permeability barrier of cell membrane structures and the accompanying loss of chemiosmotic control is the most likely source of its lethal action at minimum inhibitory levels.[20]

The EMA assessment report for tea tree states that, while tea tree oil exhibited a broad-spectrum antimicrobial activity in vitro, its efficacy in vivo remains unsubstantiated.[10]

Antiviral activity

Until 2005 there was little research on the antiviral activity of tea tree oil. However, a study by Carson and her colleagues at the University of Western Australia was the first to show that tea tree oil has significant antiviral activity against the *Herpes simplex* virus which causes cold sores. The in vitro study clearly demonstrated that tea tree oil and several of its components can inactivate the herpes virus.[11]

Tea tree oil had an inhibitory effect on influenza virus replication at doses below the cytotoxic dose. Terpinen-4-ol, terpinolene and α-terpineol were the main active components. The results also revealed that viral replication was significantly inhibited if tea tree oil was added within two hours of infection, indicating an interference with an early step of the viral replicative cycle of influenza virus.[21]

A study investigated the antiviral activity of tea tree oil and eucalyptus oil aerosols in a range of concentrations against influenza A virus and *E. coli* phage M13. The study found that both essential oil aerosols possessed strong antiviral action and were capable of inactivating model viruses with efficacy of more than 95% within 5-15 minutes of exposure.[22]

Insecticidal activity

Tea tree oil has demonstrated promising acaricidal activity against scabies mites in vitro, and has been successfully used as an adjuvant topical medication for the treatment of crusted scabies, including cases that did not respond to standard treatments.

A study confirmed that house dust mites showed 100% mortality in vitro after exposure to a 10% tea tree oil formulation. Preclinical investigations have demonstrated that tea tree oil does have superior scabicidal activities when compared with commonly used scabicidal agents such as permethrin cream and ivermectin. The authors suggested that tea tree oil could be a cost-effective, simple-to-use topical treatment that could be implemented in remote communities as a traditional medicine for the long-term management of scabies and pyoderma in children.[23]

Tea tree oil was more effective than nerolidol against head lice, with a 100% mortality at 30 minutes at 1% concentration. On the contrary, nerolidol expressed a more pronounced ovicidal activity, inducing the failure of 50% of the eggs to hatch at 1% concentration after 4 days. The same effect was achieved by using 2% concentration of tea tree oil. The authors of the study suggested combining tea tree oil with nerolidol to ensure effective treatment for head lice in 30 minutes and the abortive effect on louse eggs after 5 days.[24]

Oral health

A study examined the role of tea tree oil on a range of oral bacteria. The study confirmed that all 162 different bacteria were inhibited or completely killed by using concentrations of 2% tea tree oil. Two bacteria often associated with dental caries – *Streptococcus mutans* and *Lactobacillus rhamnosus* – were rapidly killed by 0.5% tea tree oil.[11]

Carson et al. cite a study comparing the effects of mouthwashes containing either 0.34% tea tree oil, 0.1% chlorhexidine or placebo on plaque formation on eight volunteers. The volunteers had their teeth professionally cleaned, and for the next four days they rinsed twice daily with one of the treatments and did not clean their teeth in any other manner. The teeth were clinically evaluated daily for the four days. The plaque index from the tea tree mouthwash treatment did not differ from the placebo mouthwash, whereas the chlorhexidine mouthwash differed significantly on all days. In this study, it was concluded that tea tree oil treatment was considered ineffective at reducing plaque regrowth or the vitality of plaque organisms.[25]

In another study, the effect of 0.2% tea tree oil mouthwash was evaluated on oral flora. It was confirmed that the tea tree oil could reduce the number of *Mutans streptococci* and the total number of oral bacteria, and that residual activity maintained these reduced levels for two subsequent weeks.[25]

A study evaluated the antibacterial and anti-inflammatory efficacy of a mouth rinse containing tea tree oil and comparing it with two mouthwashes containing chlorhexidine and a placebo. The results of the study confirmed that tea tree oil and chlorhexidine are effective treatments. Tea tree oil provided a better improvement in Gingival Index and Full Mouth Bleeding Score; however, it was least effective in the control of bacterial plaque. It was concluded that further studies are needed and that tea tree oil could be a valuable non-toxic adjunct in the management of gingivitis.[26]

Actions

Actions commonly cited in aromatherapy

Antibacterial, antifungal, anti-inflammatory, antiseptic, bactericide, cicatrisant, expectorant, immunostimulant, insecticide, vulnerary[27,28,29]

Actions supported by clinical studies

Antibacterial, antifungal, anti-inflammatory, antiseptic, antiviral, bactericide, insecticide

Comment

A body of evidence supporting the use of tea tree oil has grown dramatically over the last 10 years. Carson, Hammer & Riley have compiled the most extensive document that reviews all published and unpublished tea tree oil literature up to 2006. The literature was compiled into a database. More than 500 tea tree oil publications were found including research articles, reviews, conference abstracts or presentations, books and theses. They state that, while a wealth of information now supports the long-held beliefs that tea tree oil has antimicrobial and anti-inflammatory properties, larger randomised clinical evidence is now required to cement a place for tea tree oil as a topical medicinal agent.[25]

Aromatherapy Uses

Clinical aromatherapy

Genitourinary system

Tea tree oil has been recommended for the treatment of thrush, vaginitis, cystitis and pruritis.[10,27,28,29,30]

Immune system

Davis states that tea tree oil is a very powerful immune-stimulant, so when the body is threatened with any infection, tea tree increases its ability to respond. She recommends tea tree oil for debilitating illnesses such as glandular fever, and for people who repeatedly succumb to infections or who are very slow to recover from any illness.[31]

Psychological

Holmes recommends tea tree oil for chronic mental and physical fatigue, and states that the oil is indicated for minor depression.[32]

Respiratory system

Tea tree oil is recommended for the treatment of asthma, bronchitis, catarrh, coughs, sinusitis and whooping cough.[10,27,28,29]

Restorative

Holmes states that the chemistry of tea tree oil, with about 50% monoterpene alcohols with monoterpene hydrocarbons and 1,8-cineole, indicates that the oil is likely to be a restorative rather than a stimulant or relaxant. He recommends using tea tree oil for treating weakness of the nervous and immune systems, and of the brain and heart.[32]

Skin care

Tea tree is recommended for the treatment of acne, athlete's foot, blisters, burns, cold sores, dandruff, herpes, insect bites, oily skin, rashes, verrucae, warts and wounds.[27,28,30]

To treat athlete's foot, it is advised to dilute pure tea tree oil with equal amounts of water or vegetable oil before applying to the affected area three times a day with a cotton ball.[10]

Davis recommends placing a single drop of neat tea tree oil on the centre of the wart every day and covering it with plaster.[31]

Energetics, psyche and subtle uses

Energetics

Holmes recommends tea tree for dispersing *wind cold* conditions. *Wind cold* is characterised as the onset of respiratory tract infections with aches and pains, chills and a dislike for cold.[33]

Tea tree oil tonifies the *Qi* and strengthens the *Shen*. Whenever we experience *Qi* deficiency and our *Shen* is weak, we experience fatigue, lethargy, poor focus and depression. Tea tree oil also clears *heat* and dispels toxins. It is therefore recommended for treating boils, swollen glands, inflammation, abscesses and ulcers.[32]

Holmes states that, unlike cajeput and niaouli, which are considered to be more *warming*, tea tree oil is more *cooling*, and is recommended for *hot* conditions associated with weakness. He suggests that tea tree oil will excel in patients with chronic inflammation or low-grade fever as part of their overall weak condition.[32]

According to Mojay, tea tree oil strengthens the defensive *Qi*. It can be used to eradicate harmful pathogens and prevent the recurrence of infections. Tea tree oil helps to strengthen the Metal Element. It strengthens the bodily soul, the *Po*, which supports a positive outlook and the healing instinct.[29]

Personality

Mojay states that the strong, bittersweet spiciness of tea tree essential oil invigorates the heart and mind, uplifting the spirit and building confidence.[29]

According to Myers-Briggs personality types, the tea tree personality is likely to be an INTP. INTPs are quiet, reserved and highly independent. They like to be precise. They have a natural curiosity to understand the universe and to examine its universal truths and principles. They may be good at developing complex systems and conceptual models, but prefer to leave the implementation to others. They have high standards of intellectual and professional competence. They can have difficulty explaining their deep thoughts so that others can understand. They dislike supervising others or resolving conflict. They appear to be concerned with their thoughts, interests and work, and can neglect their relationships. They prefer calm, conflict-free atmosphere. They can appear to be formal and distant with strangers and acquaintances, but are generally open-minded and accepting of people once they know them.

Subtle

Tea tree oil is recommended for physically delicate individuals who struggle not only with their bodies, but with the feelings of victimisation and doom that often accompany chronic ill-health.[29]

Zeck suggests that tea tree oil will promote patience and understanding and help us to be more tolerant when dealing with challenging situations.[34]

Dosage and Administration

Blending

Aromatherapy

To treat fungal infections such as athlete's foot or nail fungus, consider blending tea tree oil with essential oils such as palmarosa and thyme ct. linalool.

To prevent colds or flu, consider blending tea tree oil with essential oils such as fragonia, lemon, manuka, niaouli, ravintsara, oregano or thyme.

For the treatment of herpes and cold sores, consider blending tea tree oil with essential oils such as melissa or ravintsara.

To treat scabies and headlice infestation, consider blending tea tree oil with essential oils such as clove bud and kunzea.

For the treatment of acne, consider blending tea tree oil with essential oils such as bergamot, geranium, lavender, neroli, palmarosa, rosalina or sandalwood.

For the relief of weepy eczema, consider blending tea tree oil with essential oils such as German chamomile, lavender, myrrh or cistus.

To alleviate fatigue and neurasthenia, consider blending tea tree oil with basil, bergamot, black pepper, lemon, lime, geranium, peppermint, petitgrain, palmarosa or rosemary.

As a natural insect repellent, consider blending tea tree oil with essential oils such as Buddha wood, cedarwood, citronella, kunzea, lemon-scented tea tree, 1,8-cineole-rich eucalypts, peppermint eucalyptus, spike lavender, niaouli, palmarosa or peppermint.

Perfumery

Arctander states that in perfumery tea tree oil is often used for its warm-spicy, aromatic and fresh character in spicy colognes and aftershaves. The oil blends well with clove, nutmeg, rosemary and oakmoss absolute.[2]

Mode of administration

Bath

Full body bath, foot bath, sitz bath

Topical

Compress, massage, ointment, skin care

Tea tree is extensively used in gels, creams, ointments, oral rinses, soaps and shampoos. Braun & Cohen recommend the following dosages:[35]

- *onychomycosis* – 100% essential oil applied twice daily
- *tinea pedis* – 10% essential oil in a cream base applied twice daily
- *contact dermatitis* – 20 to 50% tea tree oil preparation
- *acne* – 5% essential oil in cream or gel base applied daily
- *dermatitis in dogs* – 10% preparation applied twice daily for four weeks
- *dandruff* – 5% essential oil in shampoo daily for at least four weeks
- *gingivitis* – 2.5% oral gel, brush teeth with preparation twice daily for five days
- *MRSA* – 2 to 4% nasal ointment and 5% tea tree oil body wash used for five days.

Some of the above percentages recommended are very high and I would not consider them for commercial products, only under professional practitioner supervision.

An Australian government document recommends the following typical concentration in cosmetic formulations – moisturisers (1.25%), body lotions (1.25%), shampoos and conditioners (0.2%), mouthwashes (0.2%), face cleansing washes (0.7%), hand washes (0.7%), soaps (2%), foot sprays (2%), foot powders (1%), shaving products (2%), post-waxing treatments (1.25%) and deodorants (2%).[11]

Inhalation

Direct inhalation, diffuser, oil vaporiser

Safety Profile

General safety

Tea tree oil is non-toxic and non-irritant, but possibly sensitising to some individuals.[27]

Researchers found that tea tree oil that had been stored in clear glass bottles changed significantly. The most interesting thing was a rapid increase in the levels of *p*-cymene, one of the minor components of tea tree oil. The *p*-cymene content has increased from 3% to over 30% in the light-exposed oil in clear glass bottles. Terpinen-4-ol, the primary antimicrobial fraction of the oil, was oxidised to 1,2,4-trihydroxymenthane. This dramatic oxidation effect was barely apparent in the oil protected by amber glass bottles, which maintained a composition nearly identical with the control throughout the trial.[36]

p-cymene has been identified as a potent skin irritant which causes painful episodes of erythema and oedema of the skin. Oxidised tea tree oil with high *p*-cymene content caused slow-healing and extensive chemical burns when applied to the skin.[36]

There have been some reported cases of sensitisation to tea tree after repeated exposure. This has typically manifested as a skin inflammation or rash. 10 separate human patch test studies involving almost 9,400 people examined the sensitisation potential of tea tree oil. In the patch test studies, an average of 1.6% of people displayed some allergic reaction to tea tree. However, it was also reported that in several patch tests degraded tea tree oil was used. The incident of sensitisation in the patch test studies may, therefore, be an overestimate due to the peroxides and their degradation products in the oils tested.[11]

Tea tree oil has to be stored in airtight containers, and protected from light and heat, in order to avoid oxidation, which will have greater potential for skin sensitisation. An Australian government report states that, while 100% tea tree oil is a weak skin sensitiser in susceptible individuals, oxidised tea tree oil has a greater risk to cause skin sensitisation.[11]

The Australian Tea Tree Oil Industry Association has developed a code of practice and guidelines to ensure the quality of tea tree oil supplied to the market. The guideline recommends that consumers discard opened bottles of tea tree oil that are more than 12 months old.[11]

Contraindications

No contraindications known.

Regulatory guidelines

Tea tree oil does not have GRAS status; however, it has been granted temporary acceptability in foods.[7]

In Australia, the Medicines Evaluation Committee approved undiluted tea tree oil as a 'mild antiseptic for minor cuts, abrasions, bites and stings and minor burns.' [10]

References

1. Weiss EA. *Essential oil crops*. CAB International, Wallingford, 1997.
2. Arctander S. *Perfume and flavor materials of natural origin*. Allured Publishing, Carol Stream, 1994.
3. Standards Australia. *Essential oils – oil of melaleuca, terpinen-4-ol type*. (AS 2782-1985). 1985.
4. Southwell IA et al. *Is cineole detrimental to tea tree oil?* Perfumer and Flavorist, 1996; 21:7-10.
5. Carson CF, Riley TV. *Antimicrobial activity of the major components of the essential oil of Melaleuca alternifolia*. Journal of Applied Bacteriology, 1995; 78(3): 264-269.
6. Schmidt E, Wanner J. *Adulteration of essential oils*. In Baser KHC, Buchbauer G. eds. *Handbook of essential oils – science, technology and applications*. 2nd edn. CRC Press, Boca Raton, 2016: 707-745.
7. Lis-Balchin M. *Aromatherapy science – a guide for healthcare professionals*. Pharmaceutical Press, London, 2006.
8. Williams C. *Medicinal plants in Australia – Vol. 2. Gums, resins, tannins and essential oil*. Rosenburg Publishing, Dural, 2011.
9. Humphery EM. *A new Australian germicide*. Medical Journal of Australia, 1930; 1: 417-418.
10. Committee on Herbal Medicinal Products (HMPC). *Assessment report on Melaleuca alternifolia (Maiden and Betch) Cheel, M. linariifolia Smith, M. dissitiflora F. Mueller and/or other species of Melaleuca, aetheroleum*. European Medicines Agency, London, 2014. Doc ref. EMA/HMPC/320932/2012.
11. *The effectiveness and safety of Australian tea tree oil*. Rural Industries Research and Development Corporation, Barton, 2007. RIRDC Publication No. 07/143. Retrieved Oct 3, 2017, from https://rirdc.infoservices.com.au/items/07-143
12. Calcabrini A et al. *Terpinen-4-ol, the main component of Melaleuca alternifolia (tea tree) oil inhibits the in vitro growth of human melanoma cells*. The Journal of Investigative Dermatology, 2004; 122(2): 349-360.
13. Shapira S et al. *Terpinen-4-ol: a novel and promising therapeutic agent for human gastrointestinal cancers*. PLoS One, 2016; 11(6): e0156540. doi: 10.1371/journal.pone.0156540.

T

14. Hammer KA et al. *In vitro activity of essential oils, in particular Melaleuca alternifolia (tea tree) oil and tea tree oil products, against Candida ssp.* Journal of Antimicrobial Chemotherapy, 1998; 42(5): 591-595.
15. Buck DS et al. *Comparison of two topical preparations for the treatment of onychomycosis: Melaleuca alternifolia (tea tree) oil and clotrimazole.* Journal of Family Practice, 1994; 38(6): 601-605.
16. Carson CF, Hammer KA, Riley TV. *Melaleuca alternifolia (tea tree) oil: a review of antimicrobial and other medicinal properties.* Clinical Microbiological Reviews, 2006; 19(1): 50-62. doi: 10.1128/CMR.19.1.50-62.2006.
17. Mertas A et al. *The influence of tea tree oil (Melaleuca alternifolia) on Fluconazole activity against fluconazole-resistant Candida albicans.* BioMed Research International, 2015; 2015: 590470. doi: 10.1155/2015/590470.
18. Carson CF et al. *In-vitro activity of the essential oil of Melaleuca alternifolia against Streptococcus spp.* Journal of Antimicrobial Chemotherapy, 1996; 37(6): 1177-1181.
19. Carson CF, Riley TV, Cookson BD. *Efficacy and safety of tea tree oil as a topical antimicrobial agent.* Journal of Hospital Infection, 1998; 40: 175- 178.
20. Cox SD et al. *The mode of antimicrobial action of the essential oil of Melaleuca alternifolia (tea tree oil).* Journal of Applied Microbiology, 2000; 88(1): 170-175.
21. Garozzo A et al. *Activity of Melaleuca alternifolia (tea tree) oil on influenza virus A/PR/8: study on the mechanism of action.* Antiviral Research, 2011; 89(1): 83-88. doi: 10.1016/j.antiviral.2010.11.010.
22. Usachev E et al. *Antiviral activity of tea tree and eucalyptus oil aerosol and vapour.* Journal of Aerosol Science, 2013; 59: 22-30. doi: 10.1016/j.jaerosci.2013.01.004.
23. Thomas J et al. *Therapeutic potential of tea tree oil for scabies.* American Journal of Tropical Medicine and Hygiene, 2016; 94(2): 258-266. doi: 10.4269/ajtmh.14-0515.
24. Di Campli E et al. *Activity of tea tree and nerolidol alone or in combination against Pediculus capitis (head lice) and its eggs.* Parasitology Research, 2012; 111(5): 1985-1992. doi: 10.1007/s00436-012-3045-0.
25. Carson CF, Hammer KA, Riley TV. *Compilation and review of published and unpublished tea tree oil literature.* Rural Industries Research and Development Corporation, Barton, 2005. RIRDC Publication No 05/151.
26. Salvatori C et al. *A comparative study of antibacterial and anti-inflammatory effects of mouthrinse containing tea tree oil.* Oral & Implantology, 2017; 10(1): 59-70. doi: 10.11138/orl/2017.10.1.059.
27. Lawless J. *The encyclopaedia of essential oils.* Element Books, Shaftesbury, 1992.
28. Lavabre M. *Aromatherapy workbook.* Healing Arts Press, Rochester, 1997.
29. Mojay G. *Aromatherapy for healing the spirit.* Healing Arts Press, Rochester, 1999.
30. Schnaubelt K. *Advanced aromatherapy.* Healing Arts Press, Rochester, 1995.
31. Davis P. *Aromatherapy: an A-Z.* 2nd edn. C.W. Daniel Company, Saffron Walden, 1999.
32. Holmes P. *Aromatica: a clinical guide to essential oil therapeutics – Vol. I.* Singing Dragon, London, 2016.
33. Holmes P. *The energetics of Western herbs – Vol I.* Artemis Press, Boulder, 1986.
34. Zeck R. *The blossoming heart – aromatherapy for healing and transformation.* Aroma Tours, East Ivanhoe, 2004.
35. Braun L, Cohen M. *Herbs & natural supplements: an evidence-based guide – Vol. 2.* 4th edn. Elsevier, Chatswood, 2015.
36. Dean C. *Australian tea tree oil.* Australasian Aromatherapy Conference, Sydney, 1998.

T

Tea tree, lemon-scented

Identification

Botanical name

Leptospermum petersonii F.M. Bailey

Synonyms

Leptospermum citratum (J.F. Bailey & C.T. White) Challinor, Cheel & A.R. Penfold, citratum

Family

Myrtaceae

Botany and origins

It is an evergreen shrub native to southern Queensland and northern New South Wales, which grows to a height of 8 m (frequently less) with a single main trunk to 8 cm. If it is cut or damaged, multiple stems arise from the stump. The tree is often planted as an ornamental or kept clipped as a hedge.[1]

It has broad, flat, light green leaves that are about 3.5 cm long with a strong aromatic lemon scent.[2]

A report from the Queensland Forest Service Bulletin in 1928 mentioned that it was a rare species found only in the coastal regions. It also stated at the time that:

> *... it does not exist naturally in any commercial availability, but may be cultivated readily. The seed is scarce, but the Queensland Forest Service has planted several plots of it for the purposes of seed supply.*[3]

The origins of the botanical name are from Greek words, (*leptos*) meaning slender and (*sperma*) meaning seeds. It is named after W.J. Peterson, the original collector in 1905.[2]

Method of extraction

The oil is produced by the steam distillation of the leaves and terminal branchlets of *L. petersonii*.

Characteristics

Lemon-scented tea tree oil is a colourless to pale yellow or greenish coloured liquid with a powerful fresh, citrus-like odour.[2] Guba compares it to other essential oils rich in citral such as lemon verbena, may chang, lemongrass or melissa.[4]

Chemical composition

Studies by Penfold in 1942 established that there were three chemotypes. They are the citral chemotype, the citronellal chemotype and the geranyl acetate/geraniol chemotype.[3]

The geranyl acetate type is characterised by a fragrant rose aroma, while the citral type is the lemon-scented type.[2]

The chemical composition of *L. petersonii* essential oil obtained from five different regions in Australia was reported as follows:

α-pinene (0.1-12.3%), myrcene (0.1-0.3%), limonene (trace-0.1%), citronellal (6.8-46.2%), linalool (1.2-1.8%), isopulegol (0.5-1.3%), pinocarvone (1.3-2.7%), neral (13.5-31.3%), geranial (22.8-45.4%), citronellol (0.7-1.9%), geraniol (2.4-2.7%), spathulenol (0.05-1.0%), citronellic acid (0.6-1.3%).[5]

Adulteration

Weiss states that *L. petersonii* oil is subject to adulteration with essential oils such as lemon-scented eucalyptus, lemongrass and citronella.[1]

Pharmacopoeias and standards

At the time of writing, the purity, composition, physico-chemical properties and therapeutic use of lemon-scented tea tree oil are not defined in any pharmacopoeia monograph or standard.

T

History and Traditional Uses

History

The oil was first described in 1918 by Richard Challinor, Edwin Cheel and Arthur Penfold. It gained some popularity in the essential oil industry as a fragrance where it was incorporated into personal care and perfumery products. However, in 1950, the only commercial plantations were located in Kenya, which was part of the British Empire.[3] Weiss states that no lemon-scented tea tree plantations existed in Australia.[1]

Food, perfumery and flavouring

The oil is rich in citral and citronellal, making it ideal for use in flavourings and fragrances, as well as providing excellent insect repellent properties.[1]

Therapeutics

Pharmacology and clinical studies

Antifungal activity

Lemon-scented tea tree oil has been reported to display potent antifungal activity against *Candida albicans* and *Aspergillus fumigatus*. It was reported to have displayed more potent antifungal activity than *Backhousia citriodora* (lemon myrtle) oil and *Cymbopogon citratus* (lemongrass) oil.

It was suggested that the oil's mode of action is through direct disturbance of the fungal cell membrane.[6]

Antioxidant activity

An in vitro study confirmed that lemon-scented tea tree oil had very high antioxidant activity. It has been suggested that the antioxidant effect of essential oils is of special interest in disease with an inflammatory response.[7]

Insecticidal activity

A study evaluated the repellency of 11 Australian native plants in 55 formations against *Aedes aegypti*, *Culex quinquefasciatus* and *Culex annulirostris* under laboratory conditions. All the oils, including *L. petersonii*, provided some protection against the three mosquito species. A blend of the best performing oils – *L. petersonii*, *Prostanthera melissifolia* and *M. alternifolia* – was also tested. It was concluded that these oils from Australian native plants offer limited protection against mosquitos, and have commercial potential as a short-term insect repellent.[8]

Lemon-scented tea tree oil has an antifeedant effect and also inhibits larval growth and oviposition against the diamondback moth, *Plutella xylostella*, under laboratory conditions. It was concluded that lemon-scented tea tree oil has modest potential for development as a botanical insecticide.[9]

Actions

Actions commonly cited in aromatherapy

Antibacterial, antifungal, antitiviral, expectorant, insecticidal[2,4]

Actions supported by clinical studies

Antibacterial, antifungal, insecticidal

Comment

Essential oils rich in aldehydes are considered very effective for the treatment of fungal infections and are very effective insect repellents; however, dermal sensitisation is likely due to the high citral content.

Aromatherapy uses

Clinical aromatherapy

Antiseptic

Guba states that lemon-scented tea tree oil is an excellent air antiseptic, destroying airborne moulds and bacteria when diffused.[4]

Colds and flu

Its excellent antimicrobial indicates that it will provide good protection against colds and flu. When it is diffused into the atmosphere, it will relieve sinusitis and head colds. It can be a wonderful air purifier and antiseptic.[2]

Webb recommends using it as a throat gargle to protect against throat infection.[2] I would only add one drop to a glass of warm water.

Musculoskeletal system

Guba states that lemon-scented tea tree oil is effective for treating joint inflammation such as rheumatoid arthritis, nerve inflammations such as viral neuritis, and to alleviate muscular soreness.[4]

Psychological

The fresh citrus aroma of lemon-scented tea tree oil means it can also be used to aid concentration and space clearing.[2]

Skin care

Lemon-scented tea tree oil is often recommended for oily skin and acne; however, there is a high risk of skin sensitisation, so I would prefer that the oil not be used topically on individuals with sensitive skin.

Dosage and Administration

Blending

Aromatherapy

For the relief of colds and flu, consider blending lemon-scented tea tree oil with essential oils such as peppermint eucalyptus, 1,8-cineole-rich eucalypts, fragonia, kunzea or tea tree.

To create a natural insect repellent, consider blending lemon-scented tea tree oil with essential oils such as citronella, 1,8-cineole-rich eucalypts, niaouli, spike lavender, peppermint or tea tree.

Guba states that the effect of lemon-scented tea tree oil is dose-dependent. It is more cooling and sedative when it is used in low dosages (<1%), while it is more tonifying and energising when it is used at higher percentages.[4]

Perfumery

Weiss states that the main use of lemon-scented tea tree oil is in perfumery because it has a very diffusive quality that allows it to be used in very small quantities to impart a very distinctive note.[1]

Mode of administration

Bath

Due to the high level of citral, I would not recommend using lemon-scented tea tree oil in a bath.

Topical

Massage, ointment

Inhalation

Direct inhalation, diffuser, oil vaporiser

Safety Profile

General safety

The oil is rich in aldehydes such as citral and citronellal, which may cause sensitisation reaction if used undiluted.

Tisserand & Young state that it should not be used if your skin is hypersensitive, diseased or damaged, and it should not be used on children under two years of age. They further advise that the maximum dilution should not be more than 0.8% to avoid skin sensitisation.[10]

Contraindications

No contraindications known.

Regulatory guidelines

Lemon-scented tea tree oil is not defined in any regulatory guideline.

References

1. Weiss EA. *Essential oil crops.* CAB International, Wallingford, 1997.
2. Webb M. *Australian essential oil profile – lemon tea tree.* Aromatherapy Today, 2001; 20: 32-34.
3. Williams C. *Medicinal plants in Australia – Vol. 2. Gums, resins, tannins and essential oil.* Rosenburg Publishing, Dural, 2011.
4. Guba R. *Lemon tea tree.* Essential News, Vol. 2, 2000.
5. Lawrence BM. *Progress in essential oils – lemon-scented tea tree oil.* Perfumer & Flavorist, 2009; 34: 52-53.
6. Hood JR et al. *The effect of Leptospermum petersonii essential oil on Candida albicans and Aspergillus fumigatus.* Medical Mycology, 2010; 48(7): 922-931.doi: 10.3109/13693781003774697.
7. Zhao Q, Bowles EJ, Zhang HY. *Antioxidant activities of eleven Australian essential oils.* Natural Product Communications, 2008; 3(5): 837-842. Cited in Quintessential Aromatics database, 2013.
8. Maguranyi SK et al. *Are commercially available essential oils from Australian native plants repellents to mosquitoes?* Journal of the American Mosquito Control Association, 2009; 25(3): 292-300. doi: 10.2987/09-0016.1.
9. Purwatiningsih et al. *Efficacy of Leptopsermum petersonii oil, on Plutella xylostella, and its parasitoid, Trichogramma pretiosum.* Journal of Economic Entomology, 2012; 105(4): 1379-1384. doi: 1603/EC11382.
10. Tisserand R, Young R. *Essential oil safety.* 2nd edn. Churchill Livingstone, Edinburgh, 2014.

Thyme

T

Identification

Botanical name

Thymus vulgaris L.

Synonyms

Red thyme, garden thyme, common thyme

Family

Lamiaceae (Labiatae)

Botany and origins

There are more than 300 different varieties of thyme. The most common species is *Thymus vulgaris,* known as garden or common thyme. Other species include *Thymus serpyllum,* known as wild thyme, creeping thyme or mother thyme, *Thymus zygis,* known as Spanish thyme, and *Thymus citriodorus,* known as lemon thyme.[1]

Mailhebiau states that there are six different chemotypes of *T. vulgaris*. The two most common ones are located close to the Mediterranean Sea at a low altitude: the thymol type and the carvacrol type.[2] *T. vulgaris* ct. linalool prefers the sun and south-exposed slopes.[3]

The geraniol chemotype is rare and mixed with the linalool type. It is mainly located in high altitudes, on well-exposed slopes at an altitude of 1000-1200 m. The 4-thujanol chemotype is very rare and located between the thymol-carvacrol one and that of linalool. The composition of the 4-thujanol chemotype is very similar to that of *Origanum marjorana* (sweet marjoram). The last chemotype is mainly found in the eastern Mediterranean area and is the α-terpinyl acetate one.[3]

A cluster analysis based on 85 *T. vulgaris* essential oils revealed as many as 20 chemotypes. The most common chemotype was the thymol chemotype. Other chemotypes included the linalool chemotype, the geranial chemotype, the carvacrol chemotype, the borneol chemotype and the sabinene hydrate/terpinen-4-ol chemotype.[4]

Lavabre suggests that the geographic location or growing conditions do not seem to make so much difference to the chemotype:

> *As seductive as this theory might be, the reality is slightly different. There is in the wild, a predominance of the thymol and carvacrol chemotypes in the dryer and warmer areas, while the milder chemotypes are more abundant under milder conditions. But more than seven years of wild harvesting of thyme have shown me that different chemotypes can be found everywhere. Furthermore, most of the commercial production of chemotyped thyme comes from the same area in southern France and several farmers grow all chemotypes on their farm.*[5]

On the other hand, Schnaubelt states that the growers have been very skilled in cloning thyme plants whose attractive fragrance will potentially provide an essential oil with a desirable composition such as a higher percentage of linalool.[6]

He also explains that the elevation does influence the biosynthesis of the components found in thyme oil. *p*-cymene is the compound immediately preceding thymol in its biosynthesis, and the biosynthesis process goes through to the last step in plants that grow at lower altitudes – this means that *p*-cymene adds on a hydroxyl group which converts it into thymol or carvcrol.[6]

Method of extraction

Thyme oil is produced by water and steam distillation of the dried or partially dried leaves and flowering tops of thyme.[7] Grieve states that the fresh herb should be collected on a dry day when it is just coming into flower. The lower portions of the stem, together with the yellow and brown leaves, should be rejected and the herb taken to the distillery as soon as possible.[8]

Characteristics

Red thyme oil is a brownish-red, orange-red coloured liquid with an intense warm herbaceous odour that is somewhat spicy and distinctly aromatic.[9]

Wild thyme, distilled from *T. serpyllum,* is a pale yellow mobile liquid with a fresh, somewhat sharp-terpene, woody-herbaceous odour and a spicy-phenolic undertone.[9]

Chemical composition

The chemical composition of *T. vulgaris* and *T. serpyllum* was reported as follows:[3]

Constituent	*T. vulgaris*			*T. serpyllum*
	Thymol chemotype	Carvacrol chemotype	Linalool chemotype	
α-thujone	4.6%	4.9%	0.26%	1.53%
α-pinene	0.75%	4.3%	0.3%	0.7%
camphene	0.3%	0.8%	0.27%	0.2%
β-pinene	0.34%	0.35%	-	0.17%
p-cymene	26.0%	33.9%	2.0%	25.0%
α-terpinene	24.0%	44.85%	0.28%	4.85%
linalool	4.2%	4.2%	77.5%	3.4%
borneol	0.65%	0.8%	0.2%	-
β-caryophyllene	3.55%	2.5%	2.8%	2.5%
thymol	34.0%	5.5%	2.2%	8.3%
carvacrol	4.7%	24.5%	trace	14.2%
geraniol	-	-	-	9.0%

A selection of oils from *T. vulgaris* collected from different locations in the Languedoc region (France) were found to have the following range of major constituents:[10]

1,8-cineole (0-3.8%), *p*-cymene (0-29.0%), γ-terpinene (0-23.5%), linalool (0.1-13.4%), sabinene hydrate (0-3.3%), terpinene-4-ol (0.1-5.0%), α-terpineol (0-6.1%), myrcen-8-ol (0-1.7%), geraniol (0-8.9%), thymol (21.4-72.9%), carvacrol (0.8-26.8%), β-caryophyllene (0.2-7.8%).

Please note that sabinene hydrate is also referred to as 4-thujanol, thuyan-4-ol, thuyanol or thujanol.

Adulteration

Arctander states that thyme oil is frequently adulterated or contaminated with origanum oil and fractions of various Spanish essential oils. He also states that origanum oil may often end up being sold as thyme oil merely because of the lack of knowledge from the broker's side.[9]

Synthetic thymol and carvacrol are often used to adulterate thyme oil. White thyme is mostly blended and synthetic.[11] Lis-Balchin states that ajowan is often added or substituted. White thyme is often a compounded blend of pine oil fractions, terpineol, rosemary, eucalyptus and red thyme fractions.[12]

Schnaubelt suggests that, as the *T. vulgaris* ct. thujanol is only available from dedicated suppliers to the aromatherapy industry, the quality of the essential oil is likely to be good.[13]

Pharmacopoeias and standards

The purity, composition and physico-chemical properties of *Thymus zygis* oil are defined in ISO 14715:2010 – Oil of Thyme Containing Thymol, Spanish Type [*Thymus zygis* (Loefl.)L.]

There is no ISO standard available at the time of writing for *Thymus vulgaris*.

History and Traditional Uses

History

The name thyme originates from the Greek word *thymon*, meaning 'to fumigate'. Others derive the name from the Greek word *thumus*, meaning courage – as the plant was associated with bravery.[8]

Grieve states that the antiseptic properties of thyme were well known in classic times.[8]

Pliny explained that when burnt, it helped repel all venomous creatures. The Greeks believed that thyme denoted graceful elegance. In the days of chivalry, it was customary for ladies to embroider a bee hovering over a sprig of thyme on scarves they presented to knights. In France, wild thyme was a symbol of extreme Republicanism. Tufts of thyme would be sent out with the summons to a Republican meeting.[8]

The Roman soldiers bathed in a bath infused with the herb before entering battle, and in the Middle Ages sprigs of thyme were woven into the scarves of knights departing for the Crusades. St Hildegarde prescribed thyme for plague and paralysis, leprosy and body lice. Thyme was a strewing herb in Britain and was included in the posies carried by judges and kings to protect them from disease in public.[8]

In 1887, Chamberland demonstrated the

bactericidal action of thyme oil. Cadéac & Meunier examined the antimicrobial activity on typhus and glanders bacillus in 1889. Morel & Rochaix in 1921-22 studied its effect on meningococcus, Eberth's bacillus and diphtheria bacillus, and staphylococcus.[14]

Thymol is the principal active constituent of thyme oil. It is a powerful antiseptic for both internal and external uses; it was extensively used to medicate gauze and wool for surgical dressings. It resembles carbolic acid in its action, but it is less irritating to wounds and its germicidal action is greater.[8]

Traditional medicine

The seventeenth century herbalist Nicholas Culpeper stated that thyme strengthens the lungs, helps expel phlegm, and is an excellent remedy for shortness of breath. He recommended it for the treatment of whooping cough.[5]

Culpeper recommended infusion of wild thyme in cases of drunkenness, and to take just before going to bed to prevent troublesome nightmares.[8] Grieve states that the oil of thyme is also employed as a rubefacient and counterirritant for the treatment of rheumatism.[8]

Thyme was used along with clove, lemon and chamomile essential oils as a disinfectant and antiseptic in hospitals until World War I. As it could kill yellow fever organisms, and was seven times stronger than carbolic acid, it was sprayed onto the clothes of soldiers during the Crimean War to protect against disease and lice.[8]

T

Herbal

Valnet describes thyme as one of the herbs that is blessed with a large number of therapeutic properties.[14] The German Commission E recommends thyme herb for the relief of symptoms of bronchitis and whooping cough, and for catarrh of the upper respiratory tract.[15]

The WHO monograph for thyme herb reports that it is used in traditional and folk medicine for the treatment of dyspepsia and other gastrointestinal disturbances, coughs due to cold, bronchitis and whooping cough, and laryngitis and tonsillitis. Topical applications of thyme have been used in the treatment of minor wounds, the common cold and disorders of the oral cavity.[16]

Food, perfumery and flavouring

Thyme oil is used in toothpastes, soaps, detergents, creams, lotions and perfumes with a maximum level of use at 0.8%. Lemon thyme is extensively used in spice blends and for culinary purposes. Thyme is widely used as a herb and flavouring ingredient in baked goods, meat products, condiments and relishes, processed vegetables and soups.[7]

The antioxidant property of thyme oil can be utilised to prevent a number of pathological disorders such as atherosclerosis, cancer, inflammation and rheumatoid arthritis. It is also used to prevent rancidity and preserve foods.[7]

Therapeutics

Pharmacology and clinical studies

Many pharmacological studies involving thyme essential oil have been published. A systemic review of these studies will not be attempted. Rather, I have chosen a selection of studies that support the traditional and clinical uses.

Acetylcholinesterase inhibitory activity

Bone & Mills cite a study in which thyme essential oil and its constituents carvacrol and thymol displayed inhibitory activity on acetylcholinesterase activity in an in vitro study, with carvacrol being 10-fold more potent than thymol, but two orders of magnitude less potent than the plant alkaloid galantamine used for the treatment of Alzheimer's disease.[17]

Antifungal activity

An in vitro study confirmed that thyme oil completely inhibited the growth of different fungal isolates at concentrations of 0.25, 0.5 and 1%.[18] In one study, the sabinene hydrate chemotype, the linalool chemotype and the geraniol chemotype displayed the lowest antifungal activity, whereas the thymol chemotype showed the strongest antifungal activity.[4]

Anti-inflammatory activity

An in vitro study found that carvacrol in thyme oil was the major component responsible for suppression of COX-2 expression and an activator of PPARα and γ. PPARγ-dependent suppression of COX-2 promotor activity was observed in response to carvacrol. The results of this study provide us with an important understanding of the role of carvacrol for management of inflammatory and lifestyle diseases.[19]

A study identified that thyme essential oil has anti-inflammatory effects in vivo; however, the isolated compounds thymol and carvacrol displayed antagonist effects. Thymol has an irritant effect that involves histamine, prostaglandins and inflammatory mediators. It was concluded that carvacrol may be the compound responsible for the anti-inflammatory effects of thyme oil. It was also suggested that the inhibitory effect of carvacrol on leukocyte migration contributes to its anti-inflammatory action, in addition to the irritant effect of thymol.[20]

Antimicrobial activity

It is not surprising that Lis-Balchin states that hundreds of research papers have investigated thyme oil and its extremely effective antimicrobial activity in vitro.[12]

The results of an in vitro study confirm that *T. vulgaris* oil exhibited extremely strong antibacterial activity against all of the clinical strains of *Acinetobacter*. The oil also demonstrated very good efficacy against multidrug-resistant strains of tested bacteria. The bacteria were sensitive to thyme oil at concentrations of 0.25, 0.5. 0.75 and 1 μl/mL. It was stated that these are relatively low concentrations compared to the high concentration of antibiotics usually required.[21]

The high antimicrobial activity is due to the presence of phenols such as carvacrol and thymol. It has been suggested that these compounds are responsible for inactivation of enzymes in charge of energy production and structure synthesis.[22] Studies have concluded that thymol possesses the largest activity spectrum.[22,23]

An in vitro study confirmed that *T. vulgaris* oil exhibited strong antibacterial activity against *Salmonella enteritidis, Salmonella thyphimurium, Staphylococcus aureus*, methicillin-resistant *S. aureus* (MRSA), *Escherichia coli* and *Bacillus cereus*.[23]

Antioxidant activity

Thyme oil and thymol exhibit significant antioxidant activity according to in vitro and in vivo studies.[24] Lis-Balchin states that high antioxidant activity has been reported in all the thyme essential oils.[12]

Antitussive activity

The antitussive activity of thyme oil is attributed to the phenolic constituents – thymol and carvacrol.[16]

Antiviral activity

Thyme oil demonstrated antiviral activity against herpes simplex virus (HSV)-1, HSV-2 and an acyclovir-resistant strain of the virus. It has been suggested that thyme essential oil interferes with the viral envelope.[24]

Expectorant activity

Experimental evidence suggests that thyme oil has secretomotoric activity. Increase in mucous secretion of the bronchi after treatment with thyme extracts has been observed.[16]

Hepatoprotective activity

The hepatoprotective activity of thyme oil was investigated against acetaminophen-induced hepatic damage in mice. The results of the study confirmed that pre-treatment with thyme oil protected the functional integrity of hepatocytes and cellular membrane from damage by toxic reactive metabolites, produced by acetaminophen biotransformation.[25]

Insecticidal activity

Thyme oil has been reported to be lethal to mosquito larvae. Its major monoterpenes were also found to effectively repel mosquitoes. α-terpinene was active at 2%.[7]

Four chemotypes of *T. vulgaris* oil were tested for their insecticidal activity. The thymol chemotype was also found to be the most larvicidal against *Culex quinquefasciatus* larvae. In the control sample, the adult emergence from the larvae was 77%, whereas in the thyme oils there was only 5.3% to 16% emergence.[26]

Actions

Actions commonly cited in aromatherapy

Analgesic, antifungal, antioxidant, antirheumatic, antiseptic, antispasmodic, antitussive, bactericide, cardiac, carminative, cicatrisant, emmenagogue, expectorant, hypertensive, insecticide, nervine, rubefacient, stimulant, sudorific, tonic, vermifuge[1,5,2]

Actions supported by clinical studies

Analgesic, antibacterial, antifungal, antioxidant, antirheumatic, antiviral, expectorant, rubefacient

Comment

Thyme oil has strong antimicrobial activity and is often used for the treatment of common infections such as bronchitis and upper respiratory tract infections.

Lavabre states that thyme is one of the most important oils in aromatherapy. He states that the *Thymus* genus shows amazing adaptability and offers us broad-spectrum healing qualities.[5]

When using thyme oil in aromatherapy, it is imperative that you are aware of the chemotype you are using. Very often the chemotype is not specified and the commercial grade thyme oil, which is usually very high in thymol, is used. The risk of irritation and sensitisation can be very high.

Schnaubelt states that the *T. vulgaris* ct. thuyanol is non-toxic and non-irritating. He states that this oil has outstanding antiviral and antibacterial qualities. He explains that the thuyanol chemotype combines the mild qualities of the higher altitude linalool and geraniol chemotypes with the more aggressive antimicrobial thyme oils of lower altitude.[6]

Holmes states that thyme ct. geraniol and thyme ct. thuyanol are very similar to the thyme ct. linalool; however, he makes the following clinical differentiations:[28]

- Thyme ct. geraniol is recommended as a cardiac restorative and for heart weakness.
- Thyme ct. thuyanol is an arterial circulatory stimulant with warming as well as tonifying actions. It is especially useful for viral and bacterial infections of the respiratory system and the urogenital system.

Aromatherapy Uses

Clinical aromatherapy

Antimicrobial

Thyme oil has strong, broad-spectrum, antimicrobial activity and is recommended for the treatment of a wide range of infections, especially respiratory, gastrointestinal, urinary and genital. Holmes recommends using the linalool chemotype for:[28]

- fungal infections associated with *Candida* spp. such as intestinal dysbiosis, candidiasis, fungal stomatitis, chronic sinusitis, cystitis and vaginitis.
- bacterial infections associated with *S. aureus* and *Streptococcus pneumoniae* such as sinusitis, bronchitis, whooping cough, pneumonia, colitis, microbial intestinal toxicosis, intestinal dysbiosis, urinary infections, dermatitis or psoriasis.
- viral infections associated with immune or intestinal microflora deficiency, viral enteritis, pharyngitis, bronchitis or pleurisy.

Schnaubelt states that thyme ct. thuyanol oil is a strong antiseptic oil that is well suited to external and internal use. He explains that in French style aromatherapy it is used in mild genital washes for chlamydia, cervicitis, vaginitis and salpingitis.[13]

Digestive system

Thyme oil is a digestive stimulant and a carminative. It promotes appetite, eases abdominal distention and relieves flatulence.[1,27] Mojay states that the strong antimicrobial properties of thyme can help to counteract intestinal putrefaction, gastroenteritis and candidiasis.[27]

Immune system

Thyme oil is recommended for all infections. It stimulates the production of white blood corpuscles, so it strengthens the body's immune system.[29] Mailhebiau says that *T. vulgaris* ct. thymol is an excellent immunostimulant, particularly where there have been repeated infectious pathologies.[2]

Musculoskeletal system

Thyme oil is used to ease gout, rheumatic pain and arthritis, and sporting injuries. It is recommended for fixed pain of a contracted or cramping nature.[1]

Nervous system

It is considered a nerve tonic and an intellectual and mental stimulant, which is beneficial in cases of nervous depression and mental fatigue. It is also recommended for headaches and stress-related complaints.[1,5]

Psychological

Holmes states that *T. vulgaris* ct. linalool oil promotes emotional stability and renewal. He recommends using it to alleviate emotional confusion, mood swings, feeling disconnected, and general feelings of distress and stuck emotions stuck, and to help us let go of negative feelings.[28]

Mailhebiau states that the linalool chemotype is helpful for children suffering psychological problems due to parental lack of understanding and conflicts, and who are unbalanced by family disharmony, due to its strong antidepressive and stimulating effect on the psyche.[29]

Respiratory system

As a respiratory tonic, antiseptic and expectorant, thyme may be used for any cold condition involving weakness, congestion or infection of the lungs. It will benefit chronic fatigue, shallow breathing, catarrhal coughs and bronchitis, especially when there is copious, clear or white catarrh.[1,30]

T. vulgaris ct. linalool has excellent infection-fighting properties. It has a higher percentage of monoterpene alcohols and is considered gentle and safe to use with children. When blended with myrtle, it helps calm spasmodic coughing fits.[2]

T. vulgaris ct. thymol has excellent bronchopulmonary and immunostimulant properties, and is ideal for treating colds, coughs, sore throats, bronchitis, whooping cough and asthma.[2]

According to Valnet, an aqueous solution of 5% thyme oil kills *Typhus bacillus* in 2 minutes. It can kill colon bacillus in 2-8 minutes, staphylococcus in 4-8 minutes and streptococcus and *Diphtheria bacillus* in 4 minutes.[14]

Skin care

Schnaubelt recommends using *T. vulgaris* ct. linalool for skin infections, as it is non-irritating.[13]

Tonic

Thyme oil is particularly effective for people who are fatigued, depressed or lethargic.[28] It is very useful during convalescence, and it stimulates the appetite. It helps to revive and strengthen both the body and mind, and is reputed to stimulate the brain and improve memory. It stimulates the circulation and may be used to raise low blood pressure.[1,14,30]

Energetics, psyche and subtle uses

Energetics

Mojay refers to thyme oil as one of the most energetically *hot* and invigorating essential oils.[27]

Thyme increases *Qi*, stimulates and warms the *Lungs* and dispels *wind cold*. It is indicated for the onset of infections with stiff muscles, aches and pains, chills and fatigue.[31]

Thyme will dispel any *cold* condition involving weakness, congestion or infection of the *Lungs*. It is particularly beneficial for chronic fatigue, shallow breathing, catarrhal coughs and bronchitis. It also tonifies the *Yang Qi* of the *Heart*, strengthening the heartbeat and improving circulation.[27]

Thyme is associated with the Metal and Water Elements. Mojay explains that thyme has always been a traditional remedy to dispel melancholy; hence, it helps revive the bodily soul, the *Po*, which is associated with the Metal Element. When the *Po* is weak, we have feelings of pessimism and self-doubt and are withdrawn.[27]

Thyme has always been associated with instilling courage and strength associated with willpower. According to the principles of TCM, these are qualities associated with the Water Element and spirit, *Zhi*. When the *Zhi* is strong, we have self-confidence and have no fear.

According to Holmes, thyme oil tonifies the *Qi* and strengthens the *Shen*. Whenever the *Qi* and *Shen* are weak, we experience physical and mental fatigue, debility and depression. Holmes also states that thyme oil helps to strengthen the *Lung Qi*. Whenever the *Lung Qi* is weak, we experience shallow breathing, chronic weak cough and are susceptible to respiratory tract infections.[28]

Personality

According to Mailhebiau, *T. vulgaris* ct. thymol corresponds to a strong and stocky man, living close to nature, who is a very physical person whose mind is healthy and clear. He works hard and never gets lost in sterile intellectualism. He lives simply in a world he does not understand well, while relying on simple and sure values.[29]

On the other hand, he describes *T. vulgaris* ct. linalool as an introverted young man, with a difficult temper, who may look outwardly as fragile as he is strong in his deep self.[29]

Subtle

Mojay describes the subtle effects of thyme as energising and dispelling despondency. He suggests that the oil will restore morale at the deepest level. Thyme seeks to imbue both spiritual fortitude and bodily vigour.[27]

Worwood exquisitely describes the subtle qualities of *T. vulgaris* oil:

> *There is fire within the soul of thyme, the fire to summon the most mighty angels to our assistance – the force of compassion, the forgiveness in might, the enlightenment of the mind and spirit, the revealing of truth. In the power and might of the heavens, where pretense does not exist, we cannot hide – least of all from ourselves.*[32]

Zeck states that the strong and fiery scent of thyme oil activates our vital force to encourage our willpower, and strengthens our resolve in breaking negative patterns or bad habits. She explains that thyme oil provides us with a dynamic quality of energy that strengthens our physical body and willpower. It will also harness our healing powers.[33]

Keim Loughran & Bull state that thyme oil relieves fear and apathy and helps to clear energy blockages. It strengthens the solar plexus chakra by promoting self-confidence and courage. At the same time, it also helps to balance the third eye chakra by reactivating the left brain after a subtle energy session. It also promotes focus and concentration. It also strengthens the crown chakra by restoring spiritual fortitude.[34]

Cunningham states that thyme has the effect of closing down the psychic mind in favour of the conscious intellectual mind. This may be particularly beneficial for people who tend to be dreamy, detached or immersed in their spiritual life to the detriment of their physical wellbeing.[35]

Dosage and Administration

Blending

Aromatherapy

For the relief of muscular aches and pains and arthritis, consider blending thyme oil with essential oils such as black pepper, cajeput, kunzea, ginger, spike lavender, sweet marjoram, peppermint, pine or rosemary.

For the relief of respiratory tract congestion and coughs, consider blending thyme oil with essential oils such as cajeput, cypress, 1,8-cineole-rich eucalypts, fragonia, kunzea, rosalina, myrtle, peppermint, pine, spruce or tea tree.

As an immune stimulant to help prevent infections, consider blending thyme oil with essential oils such as cinnamon bark, clove bud, fragonia, 1,8-cineole-rich eucalypts, lemon, rosalina, rosemary or tea tree.

For the relief of anxiety, nervous tension and stress-related conditions, consider blending thyme ct. linalool oil with essential oils such as bergamot, fragonia, geranium, lavender, palmarosa, neroli, sweet orange or sandalwood.

Perfumery

Thyme oil is generally not used in perfumery; however, Arctander states that it does find some use in soap perfumes where its power and freshness can introduce a hint of medicinal notes. He states that very small amounts of thyme oil may lend body and a sweet freshness to lavender, fougère, citrus and spicy style colognes. However, Arctander explains that the high phenol content in thyme also makes it unstable and can cause discoloration.[9]

Mode of administration

Bath

Thyme ct. thymol is sensitising, therefore, it is not recommended for use in a bath.

Valnet recommends 500 g of thyme herb boiled in 4 L of water and then added to the bath water for the relief of arthritis, gout, rheumatism and debility.[14]

Topical

Thyme ct. thymol – massage, ointment; Thyme ct. linalool – massage, ointment, skin care

Inhalation

Direct inhalation, diffuser, oil vaporiser

Ingestion

Schnaubelt suggests that ingesting up to 5 drops of thyme ct. thujanol oil 3 or 4 times per day to prevent oncoming infection has been done without any undesirable side effects.[6]

Safety Profile

General safety

Thyme ct. linalool and thyme ct. thujanol oils are reported to have no known hazards and no contraindications.[36]

Lawless states that thyme oil is non-toxic and non-irritating, but is a sensitiser for some individuals.[1]

Lavabre states that thyme ct. thymol oil should never be applied externally.[5]

Contraindications

Tisserand & Young caution oral use of thyme ct. thymol oil, thyme ct. carvacrol oil and thyme ct. thymol/carvacrol oil for people on anticoagulant medication, or with major surgery, peptic ulcers, haemophilia and other bleeding disorders. They explain that thymol and carvacrol both inhibit platelet aggregation. These oils also have moderate risk as a mucous membrane irritant. They suggest that the maximum dermal use level is 1.3%.[36]

Braun & Cohen state that thyme oil can cause nausea and vomiting, headache, dizziness, convulsions, and cardiac or respiratory arrest if taken internally.[24]

Regulatory guidelines

Thyme essential oil has GRAS status.

References

1. Lawless J. *The encyclopaedia of essential oils.* Element Books, Shaftesbury, 1992.
2. Mailhebiau P. *Portraits in oils.* C.W. Daniel Company, Saffron Walden, 1995.
3. Soulier J. *Thyme folder.* Aromatherapie Records 1995; 1: 38–49.
4. Satyal P et al. *Essential oil characterization of Thymus vulgaris from various geographic locations.* Foods, 2016; 5(4): 70. doi: 10.3390/foods5040070.
5. Lavabre M. *Aromatherapy workbook.* Healing Arts Press, Rochester, 1997.
6. Schnaubelt K. *The healing intelligence of essential oils.* Healing Arts Press, Rochester, 2011.
7. Khan I, Abourashed E. *Leung's encyclopedia of common natural ingredients used in food, drugs and cosmetics.* 3rd edn. John Wiley & Sons, New Jersey, 2010.
8. Grieve M. *A modern herbal – Vol II.* Dover Publications, New York, 1971.
9. Arctander S. *Perfume and flavor materials of natural origin.* Allured Publishing, Carol Stream, 1994.
10. Lawrence BM. *Progress in essential oils: thymol-rich thymus vulgaris oils – part 1.* Retrieved on Jan 19, 2018 from http://www.perfumerflavorist.com/flavor/trends/progress-in-Essential-Oils-Thymol-rich-Thymus-vulgaris-oils-part1-4519121133.html
11. Schmidt E, Wanner J. *Adulteration of essential oils.* In Baser KHC, Buchbauer G. eds. *Handbook of essential oils – science, technology and applications.* 2nd edn. CRC Press, Boca Raton, 2016: 707-745.
12. Lis-Balchin M. *Aromatherapy science – a guide for healthcare professionals.* Pharmaceutical Press, London, 2006.
13. Schnaubelt K. *Medical aromatherapy.* Frog, Berkeley, 1999.
14. Valnet J. *The practice of aromatherapy.* C.W. Daniel Company, Saffron Walden, 1980.
15. Blumenthal M et al. *The complete German commission E monographs: therapeutic guide to herbal medicine.* American Botanical Council, Austin, 1998.

T

16. *WHO monographs on selected medicinal plants – Vol. 2*. World Health Organization, Geneva, 2004.
17. Bone K, Mills S. *Principles and practice of phytotherapy*. 2nd edn. Elsevier, Edinburgh, 2013.
18. Radwan IA et al. *Effect of thyme, clove and cinnamon essential oils of Candida albicans and moulds isolated from different sources*. American Journal of Animal and Veterinary Sciences, 2014; 9(4): 303-314. doi: 10.3844/ajavssp.2014.303.314.
19. Hotta M et al. *Carvacrol, a component of thyme oil, activates PPARalpha and gamma and suppresses COX-2 expression*. Journal of Lipid Research, 2010; 51(1): 132-139. doi: 10.1194/jlr.M900255-JLR200.
20. Fachini-Queiroz FC et al. *Effects of thymol and carvacrol, constituents of Thymus vulgaris L. essential oil, on the inflammatory response*. Evidence-Based Complementary and Alternative Medicine, 2012: 657026. doi: 10.1155/2012/657026.
21. Lysakowska M et al. *The activity of thyme essential oil against Acinetobacter spp*. Central European Journal of Biology, 2011; 6(3): 405-413. doi: 10.2478/s11535-011-0008-x.
22. Chemat S et al. *Composition and antimicrobial activity of thyme (Thymus algeriensis genuinus) essential oil*. The Journal of Essential Oil Research, 2012; 24(1): 5-11. doi: 10.1080/10412905.2012.645303.
23. Boskovic M. *Antimicrobial activity of thyme (Tymus vulgaris) and oregano (Origanum vulgare) essential oils against some food-borne microorganisms*. Procedia Food Science, 2015; 5: 18-21.
24. Braun L, Cohen M. *Herbs & natural supplements: an evidence-based guide – Vol. 2*. 4th edn. Elsevier, Chatswood, 2015.
25. Grespan R et al. *Hepatoprotective effect of pretreatment with Thymus vulgaris essential oil in experimental model of acetaminophen-induced injury*. Evidence-Based Complementary and Alternative Medicine, 2014; 2014: 954136. doi: 10.1155/2014/954136.
26. Pavela R et al. *Mosquitocidal activities of thyme oils (Thymus vulgaris L.) against Culex quinquefasciatus (Diptera: Culicidae)*. Parasitology Research, 2009; 105(5): 1365-1370. doi: 10.1007/s00436-009-1571-1.
27. Mojay G. *Aromatherapy for healing the spirit*. Healing Arts Press, Rochester, 1999.
28. Holmes P. *Aromatica: a clinical guide to essential oil therapeutics – Vol. I*. Singing Dragon, London, 2016.
29. Mailhebiau P. *Approach to the characterology of thymes*. Aromatherapy Records, 1995; 1: 57-60.
30. Davis P. *Aromatherapy: an A-Z*. 2nd edn. C.W. Daniel Company, Saffron Walden, 1999.
31. Holmes P. *The energetics of Western herbs – Vol. I*. Artemis Press, Boulder, 1986.
32. Worwood VA. *The fragrant heavens*. Transworld Publishers, London, 1999.
33. Zeck R. *The blossoming heart – aromatherapy for healing and transformation*. Aroma Tours, East Ivanhoe, 2004.
34. Keim Loughran J, Bull R. *Aromatherapy & subtle energy techniques*. Frog, Berkeley, 2000.
35. Cunningham S. *Magical aromatherapy*. Llewellyn Publications, St Paul, 1989.
36. Tisserand R, Young R. *Essential oil safety*. 2nd edn. Churchill Livingstone, Edinburgh, 2014.

Tuberose absolute

Identification

Botanical name

Polianthes tuberosa L.

Family

Agavaceae

Botany and origins

Tuberose is a tender, tall, slim perennial that grows up to 50 cm high, with long, slender leaves, a tuberous root and large, fragrant, white, lily-like flowers. It is a native of Central America and is cultivated in France, India, Morocco, Egypt and on the Comoro Islands.[1]

The plant is related to narcissus and jonquil. The tuberose flower is one of the few flowers which continues to produce a scent long after it has been removed from the plant.[1]

It takes 1,200 kg of tuberose buds to produce 200 g of the absolute. Master Perfumer Roja Dove states that, unfortunately, nearly all the tuberose used in perfumery is synthetically replicated. The synthetic version tends to have an almost sickly quality, far removed from the natural oil which is rich, sensual and narcotic.[2]

Method of extraction

The concrete or absolute is prepared from the hand-picked flowers by solvent extraction.[1]

Characteristics

Tuberose absolute is a dark orange to brown coloured viscous liquid with a very heavy floral,

T

almost nauseatingly sweet, heavy spicy aroma reminiscent of honeysuckle, Peru balsam, orange flower absolute and ylang ylang residue fractions.[1]

Chemical composition

The major constituents of tuberose absolute were reported as follows:

methyl palmitate (14.5%), methyl benzoate (12.2%), benzyl benzoate (10.4%), ethyl oleate (5.3%), α-terpineol (4.0%), 1,8-cineole (3.8%), methyl salicylate (3.6%), farnesol (3.5%), methyl anthranilate (2.4%), methyl eugenol (2.2%), benzyl salicylate (2.1%), palmitic acid (1.4%), oleic acid (1.3%), δ-decalactone (0.1-1.0%), jasminlactone (0.1-1.0%).[3]

Adulteration

Tuberose absolute is considered one of the most expensive natural aromatic compounds. It is subject to extensive adulteration. Absolutes of longoza, narcissus, ylang ylang, Peru balsam, helichrysum, methyl benzoate, methyl anthranilate, methyl *p*-toluate, methyl salicylate and many other natural and synthetic aromatic materials have been used to adulterate tuberose.[1]

Pharmacopoeias and standards

At the time of writing, the purity, composition, physico-chemical properties and therapeutic use of tuberose absolute are not defined in any pharmacopoeia monograph or standard.

T

History and Traditional Uses

History

Simon de Tovar, a physician of Seville, received the plant in 1594, and from Spain it was taken to France and Italy. For centuries, it was grown in Grasse; however, nowadays the production in France is a fraction of what it was at the turn of the twentieth century. Morocco and India have now become the leading producers of tuberose.[4]

Food, perfumery and flavouring

Tuberose absolute is used extensively in fine floral fragrances.[1]

Therapeutics

Pharmacology and clinical studies

There has been very little research into the pharmacological or clinical uses of tuberose.

One study stated that the essential oil distilled from the flowers of tuberose showed more antibacterial activity at lower concentration on gram-negative than gram-positive bacteria.[5]

Actions

Actions commonly cited in aromatherapy

Narcotic[6]

Actions supported by clinical studies

None.

Comment

Tuberose absolute is not commonly used in aromatherapy; however, essential oils with a rich floral aroma often promote emotional healing and stability. They are used whenever we feel anxiety, or suffer from frustration, acute depression, irritability and emotional confusion.

Aromatherapy Uses

Clinical aromatherapy

Tuberose absolute is not commonly used in aromatherapy.

Energetics, psyche and subtle uses

Energetics

Tuberose absolute regulates the *Qi* of the *Heart* and harmonises the *Shen*. Whenever we experience disharmony of the *Shen*, we may experience feelings of moodiness, anxiety, irritability, restlessness and insomnia. We lack inspiration and insight and there is no 'heart and soul' to life.

According to the principles of the Five Elements, tuberose strengthens and balances the Fire Element. According to the principles of Ayurveda, tuberose strengthens the *Pitta* dosha, reduces excess *Kapha* dosha and balances the *Vata* dosha.

Personality

Worwood describes the personality profile of tuberose as daring, attractive, hypnotic, charming, extroverted and spontaneous. Tuberose should be used to promote enthusiasm, sensuality, expressiveness, sensitivity and motivation.[7]

Worwood explains that the tuberose personality loves danger and will take big risks just for the sake of some fun. They have an obsessive nature and they will use their skills of seduction to get exactly what they want. Their physical appearance is very important to them. They will always be nicely dressed. They love power of any kind – sexual, economic and political. Tuberose personalities' biggest challenge in life is to learn to love genuinely and to forget superficialities and appreciate people for their good qualities.[7]

According to Myers-Briggs personality types, the tuberose personality is likely to be an ESFP. ESFPs are friendly, witty, charming and talkative. They value and nurture their relationships, give generously, without expecting anything in return. They are spontaneous and playful, and enjoy everything they do and see. People who share their sense of fun and adventure are their favourite companions. They turn everything into a fun-filled event. They enjoy good things in life – music, dance, food, drink and entertainment. They avoid being alone. They like working in a lively and stimulating atmosphere with friendly, energetic people. They can be good at dealing with the public. They like variety and frequent change of tasks or jobs. They are enthusiastic, high-spirited and have lots of energy.

Subtle

Keim Loughran & Bull state that tuberose calms and soothes strong emotions, promotes motivation and enthusiasm, and invites love into our life.[8]

Worwood explains tuberose embodies forgiveness and rediscovering of self-love when the self is lost and the spirit low. She also explains that this is the essential oil for reaching the true self in a world in which it is easy to be without hope. When all seems lost, it brings the ego into the spirit to bring balance and harmony.[9]

Dosage and Administration

Blending

Aromatherapy

To alleviate irritability, anger and frustration, consider blending tuberose absolute with essential oils such as bergamot, geranium, lavender, jasmine absolute, mandarin, sweet orange, patchouli, rose absolute, sandalwood or ylang ylang.

To alleviate depression, despair and low self-esteem, consider blending tuberose absolute with essential oils such as benzoin, bergamot, geranium, lavender, jasmine absolute, Peru balsam, sweet orange, rose absolute or ylang ylang.

Perfumery

Tuberose absolute is often used to create extravagant heavy sweet floral and tenacious perfumes. It blends well with other rich floral oils such as jasmine, rose and ylang ylang. It complements heavy resins such as Peru balsam, and opopanax to create rich oriental and fantasy type perfumes.

Mode of administration

Bath

Full body bath, foot bath

Topical

Compress, massage, ointment, skin care

Inhalation

Direct inhalation, diffuser, oil vaporiser

Safety Profile

General safety

Tisserand & Young state that, since tuberose absolute may contain methyl eugenol, it may be a skin sensitiser. It should therefore not be used topically for people with hypersensitive, diseased or damaged skin, and on children under two years of age.[10]

IFRA recommends that tuberose absolute should not be used at levels over 0.02%; however, Tisserand & Young recommend a dermal maximum of 1.2% based on 1.7% methyl eugenol content.[10]

Contraindications

No contraindications known.

Regulatory guidelines

Tuberose absolute has GRAS status.

References

1. Arctander S. *Perfume and flavor materials of natural origin*. Allured Publishing, Carol Stream, 1994.
2. Dove R. *The essence of perfume – the master perfumer's definitive guide*. Black Dog, London, 2014.
3. Lawrence BM. *Progress in essential oils – tuberose absolute*. Perfumer & Flavorist, 2004; 29: 57-58.
4. Morris E. *Fragrance – the story of perfume from Cleopatra to Chanel*. Products of Nature and Art, New York, 1984.
5. Lodhia MH et al. *Antibacterial activity of essential oils from palmarosa, evening primrose, lavender and tuberose*. Indian Journal of Pharmaceutical Sciences, 2009; 71(2): 134-136. doi: 10.4103/0250-474X.54278.
6. Lawless J. *The encyclopaedia of essential oils*. Element Books, Shaftesbury, 1992
7. Worwood VA. *The fragrant mind*. Transworld, London, 1995.
8. Keim Loughran J, Bull R. *Aromatherapy and subtle energy techniques*. Frog, Berkeley, 2000.
9. Worwood VA. *The fragrant heavens*. Transworld, London, 1999.
10. Tisserand R, Young R. *Essential oil safety*. 2nd edn. Churchill Livingstone, Edinburgh, 2014.

T

Turmeric

Identification

Botanical name

Curcuma longa L.

Synonyms

Curcuma, Indian saffron

Family

Zingiberaceae

Botany and origins

Turmeric, also known as curcuma, is a perennial tropical herb that belongs to the ginger family. It grows up to 1 m high with a thick rhizome root.[1]

It is a native of South Asia where it has been known and used for thousands of years as a spice and common medicinal plant. It is cultivated extensively in India, China, Indonesia and other tropical countries, and it no longer grows wild.[1]

As many as 133 species of curcuma have been identified worldwide. Most of them have common local names and are used medicinally. India produces almost all the world's turmeric and consumes 80% of it. Erode, a city in the south Indian state of Tamil Nadu, is the world's largest producer of turmeric and the most important trading centre for turmeric.[2]

T

Method of extraction

The essential oil is produced by steam distillation from the dried rhizome. An essential oil is also available from the fresh and dried leaves.

Characteristics

Turmeric rhizome oil is a yellow to dark orange liquid with a fresh, spicy odour reminiscent of ginger and galangal.[3] The yellow colour of turmeric is due to curcuminoids, (0.3-5.4%) the main one being curcumin.[4]

Chemical composition

The major volatile principles found in turmeric oil from the rhizomes are sesquiterpene compounds: α- and β-turmerone and *ar*-turmerone. The chemical composition of the oil from ground turmeric rhizome was reported as follows:

eugenol (8%), (*E*)-caryophyllene (2%), *ar*-curcumene (1.8%), α-zingiberene (2.8%), β-sesquiphellandrene (2.8%), *ar*-turmerone (22.7%), turmerone (26%), curlone (16.8%).[5]

Adulteration

Not reported.

Pharmacopoeias and standards

At the time of writing, the purity, composition, physico-chemical properties and therapeutic use of turmeric essential oil are not defined in any pharmacopoeia monograph or standard.

Turmeric rhizome is officially listed in many herbal pharmacopoeias.

History and Traditional Uses

History

Turmeric is a plant with a very long history of medicinal use, dating back 4,000 years to the Vedic culture in India. In South East Asia, turmeric is not only used as a spice but as an ingredient in many religious ceremonies. Because of its bright yellow colour, it is often referred to as Indian saffron.[2]

The word turmeric derives from the Latin word *terra merita* (meritorious earth), referring to the colour of ground turmeric, which resembles a mineral pigment.[2]

Traditional medicine

In Ayurveda, turmeric has been attributed with many medicinal properties including strengthening the overall energy of the body, relieving gas, dispelling worms, improving digestion, regulating menstruation, dissolving gallstones and relieving arthritis. In Pakistan and Afghanistan, turmeric is used to cleanse wounds and stimulate their recovery by applying on a piece of burnt cloth that is placed over the wound.[2]

Turmeric paste is used by women in some parts of India to remove superfluous hair. In some parts of India, the paste is applied to the skin of the bride and groom before a wedding ceremony. Turmeric is used to expel excess *Kapha* or phlegm, as well as to open blood vessels in order to improve blood circulation.[2]

As a spice, it is used in food, including rice dishes, to improve digestion and reduce gas and bloating. It is considered a cholagogue and stimulates bile production in the liver, which is said to improve the body's ability to digest fats.[2]

Herbal

The German Commission E recommends turmeric rhizome for the treatment of dyspeptic conditions.[6]

Turmeric is extensively used in TCM. It is officially listed in the Pharmacopoeia of the People's Republic of China as well as in the Japanese Herbal Medicines Codex, and is used in these countries and Korea for a range of conditions including abdominal distention, kidney pain and amenorrhoea.[7]

In India turmeric is extensively used in Ayurveda and is officially listed in the Ayurvedic Pharmacopoeia of India. In Ayurvedic medicine turmeric has a long history of use as an anti-inflammatory drug for arthritis. A turmeric paste is used topically to treat ulcers and scabies.[7]

Bone & Mills state that indications for the use of turmeric and curcumin that are supported by clinical trials include conditions such as rheumatoid arthritis, postoperative inflammation, osteoarthritis, precancerous conditions, tropical pancreatitis, inflammatory bowel disease and chronic uveitis.[8]

Food, perfumery and flavouring

The ground roots of turmeric are extensively used as a spice and for making curry powder. Turmeric is also used as an antioxidant in capsules and tablets.[1]

Therapeutics

Pharmacology and clinical studies

Many pharmacological studies involving turmeric rhizome and its essential oil have been published. However, almost all of the studies involve curcumin, which is not found in the essential oil.

Antidiabetic activity

The antidiabetic activity of turmeric oil was investigated in its ability to inhibit glucosidase enzymes. It was found to inhibit the glucosidase enzymes more effectively than the reference standard drug acarbose. *ar*-turmerone, the major volatile component in turmeric rhizome, also displayed potent α-glucosidase and α-amylase inhibition.[9]

Antifungal activity

Turmeric oil is reported to possess fungicidal activity comparable with standard antifungal drugs.[10]

The antifungal activity of turmeric oil and curcumin was examined against 15 isolates of dermatophytes, four isolates of pathogenic moulds and six isolates of yeasts. The results confirmed that turmeric oil inhibited all 15 isolates of dermatophytes at dilutions of 1:40 to 1:320. None of the isolates were inhibited by curcumin.[11]

Anti-inflammatory activity

An in vivo study examined the anti-inflammatory activity of oral administration of turmeric oil on mice. The results demonstrated that turmeric oil had significant anti-inflammatory activity. In one study, turmeric essential oil displayed dose-dependent inhibition of second phase carrageenan-induced paw oedema. This suggested the inhibition of inflammatory mediators and scavenging of free radicals.[12]

Turmerone and *ar*-turmerone are reported to be some of the constituents responsible for turmeric's anti-inflammatory activity.[5]

Another study compared the anti-inflammatory activity of turmeric oil and standard curcumin against dextran sodium sulfate-induced colitis. The study found that a combination of the essential oil and standard curcumin provide more effective anti-inflammatory activity.[13]

Antimicrobial activity

Turmeric oil displayed slightly better antimicrobial activity against gram-negative bacteria, *Proteus vulgaris* and *Klebsiella pneumoniae,* than cephalosporin antibiotic Cefalexin. It is also reported that the oil has the best antimicrobial activity on *Candida albicans.*[5]

Antinociceptive activity

An in vivo study examined the antinociceptive activity of oral administration of turmeric essential oil on mice. The results demonstrated that turmeric oil had significant antinociceptive activity.[12]

Gastroprotective activity

The gastroprotective activity of turmeric and ginger essential oils was evaluated in an in vivo study using rats. Oral doses of turmeric essential oil were found to inhibit ulcer by 84.7%. Histopathological examination showed that ethanol-induced lesions such as necrosis and hemorrhage of the stomach wall were significantly reduced after oral administration of the essential oil.[14]

Hepatoprotective activity

Extracts of both turmeric and curcumin have been found to prevent and reduce carbon tetrachloride-induced liver damage. Curcumin appears to be responsible for turmeric's hepatoprotective activity.[15]

Actions

Actions commonly cited in aromatherapy

Analgesic, antiarthritic, anti-inflammatory, antioxidant, bactericidal, cholagogue, digestive, diuretic, hypotensive, rubefacient, stimulant[1,16]

Actions supported by clinical studies

Antiarthritic, antifungal, anti-inflammatory, digestive, gastroprotective

Comment

Most of the studies involving turmeric have focused on the curcuminoids that are only found in the herbal extracts, not the essential oil. Turmeric oil does possess some of the activities attributed to the turmeric rhizome as a herb; however, I would prefer to use the fresh rhizome or dried powdered turmeric to obtain the full therapeutic benefits of turmeric.

This can be done by taking 1.5-3 g/day of powdered turmeric in water or a smoothie, or using it in cooking. Tablet formulas are readily available with other anti-inflammatory herbs, where the curcuminoids are formulated with phospholipid to increase relative absorption.

Aromatherapy Uses

Clinical aromatherapy

Digestive system

Turmeric oil is recommended for the treatment of digestive problems and liver congestion.[16]

Musculoskeletal system

Turmeric oil is recommended for the treatment of arthritis and rheumatism.[16]

Energetics, psyche and subtle uses

Energetics

Bone & Mills describe turmeric rhizomes as being *Blood* and *Qi* tonics with analgesic qualities.[8]

According to the principles of TCM, the properties of turmeric are described as *warming*. It helps dispel *cold* conditions associated with the digestive system, respiratory system and reproductive system.

According to the principles of Ayurveda, turmeric has a stimulating effect on the *Pitta* dosha. Turmeric is ideally suited to reduce excess *Kapha*.

Dosage and Administration

Blending

Aromatherapy

For the relief of indigestion, consider blending turmeric oil with essential oils such as black pepper, sweet fennel, ginger, sweet orange or rosemary.

For the relief of inflammation associated with osteoarthritis and joint pain, consider blending turmeric oil with essential oils such as black pepper, cajeput, ginger, kunzea, nutmeg, spike lavender or rosemary.

Perfumery

Arctander states that turmeric oil is used in perfumery to create a warm-woody, dry powdery note in oriental and fantasy style perfumes.[3]

Turmeric oil blends well with other spice oils such as galangal, ginger, black pepper, with sweet citrus oils such as mandarin or sweet orange, with sweet florals such as ylang ylang or jasmine absolute, and resins such as benzoin or cistus.

Mode of administration

Bath

Full body bath, foot bath

Topical

Compress, massage, ointment, skin care

Inhalation

Direct inhalation, diffuser, oil vaporiser

Safety Profile

General safety

Turmeric oil is non-toxic, non-irritant and non-sensitising.[16]

Contraindications

No contraindications known.

Regulatory guidelines

Turmeric essential oil has GRAS status.

References

1. Khan I, Abourashed E. *Leung's encyclopedia of common natural ingredients used in food, drugs and cosmetics*. 3rd edn. John Wiley & Sons, New Jersey, 2010.
2. Prasad S, Aggarwal BB. *Turmeric, the golden spice*. In Benzie IFF, Wachtel-Galor S. eds. *Herbal medicine: biomolecular and clinical aspects*. 2nd edn. CRC Press, Boca Raton, 2011: 263-288.
3. Arctander S. *Perfume and flavor materials of natural origin*. Allured Publishing, Carol Stream, 1994.
4. Balacs T. *Turmeric oil*. The International Journal of Aromatherapy, 1994; 6(1): 12-15.
5. Stanojevic J et al. *Chemical composition, antioxidant and antimicrobial activity of turmeric essential oil. (Curcuma longa L.)* Advanced Technologies, 2015; 4(2): 19-25. doi: 10.5937/savteh1502019S.
6. Blumenthal M et al. *The complete German commission E monographs: therapeutic guide to herbal medicine*. American Botanical Council, Austin, 1998.
7. Committee on Herbal Medicinal Products (HMPC). *Assessment report on Curcuma longa L. rhizoma*. European Medicines Agency, London, 2010. Doc ref. EMEA/HMPC/456848/2008.

8. Bone K, Mills S. *Principles and practices of phytotherapy*. 2nd edn. Churchill Livingstone, Edinburgh, 2013.
9. Lekshmi PC et al. *Turmeric (Curcuma longa L.) volatile oil inhibits key enzymes linked to type 2 diabetes.* International Journal of Food Sciences and Nutrition, 2012; 63(7): 832-834. Cited in Quintessential Aromatics database, 2013.
10. Sarker SD, Nahar L. *Bioactivity of turmeric.* In Ravindran PN, Nirmal Babu K, Sivaraman K. eds. *Turmeric: the genus Curcuma*. CRC Press, Boca Raton, 2007: 257-295. (Medical and Aromatic Plants – Industrial Profiles; 45).
11. Apisariyakul A et al. *Antifungal activity of turmeric extracted from Curcuma longa (Zingiberaceae).* Journal of Ethnopharmacology, 1995; 49(3): 163-169. Cited in Quintessential Aromatics database, 2013.
12. Liju VB et al. *An evaluation of antioxidant, anti-inflammatory and antinociceptive activities of essential oil from Curcuma longa. L.* Indian Journal of Pharmacology, 2011; 43(5): 526-531. doi: 10.4103/0253-7613.84961.
13. Toden S et al. *Essential turmeric oils enhance anti-inflammatory efficacy of curcumin in dextran sulfate sodium-induced colitis*. Scientific Reports, 2017; 7: 814. doi: 10.1038/s41598-017-00812-6.
14. Liju VB, Jeena K, Kuttan R. *Gastroprotective activity of essential oils from turmeric and ginger.* Journal of Basic and Clinical Physiology and Pharmacology, 2015; 26(1): 95-103. doi: 10.1515/jbcpp-2013-0165.
15. Braun L, Cohen M. *Herbs & natural supplements: an evidence-based guide – Vol. 2.* 4th edn. Elsevier, Chatswood, 2015.
16. Lawless J. *The encyclopaedia of essential oils.* Element Books, Shaftesbury, 1992.

Valerian

Identification

Botanical name

European valerian: *Valeriana officinalis* L.

Indian valerian: *Valeriana jatamansi* Jones

Synonyms

European valerian: common valerian, garden valerian, *Valeriana fauriei* Briq.

Indian valerian: *Valeriana wallichii* DC.

Family

Valerianaceae

Botany and origins

Valeriana officinalis is a perennial herb with deeply dissected leaves, which grows up to 1.5 m high. It is a native of Asia, and it grows in most parts of Asia and Europe. The plant is cultivated in Russia, the Baltic states, Belgium, Germany and France.[1]

An essential oil is also produced from *Valeriana wallichii or Valeriana jatamansi*, commonly known as Indian valerian. This plant grows wild and is cultivated in the northern mountainous regions of India. It is generally considered to have a poorer odour to the European valerian oil.[1]

Another valerian oil is obtained from kesso root, the rhizomes of the Japanese variety of *V. officinalis*. The aroma of kesso root oil is much drier and more woody than the European valerian root oil. As the Japanese oil is much less expensive, it is often used to adulterate the European valerian oil.[1]

Tisserand & Young explain that the chemical composition of valerian oil can vary significantly depending on the country of origin. Factors such as cultivar, plant age and harvest time may all play a role in contributing to such chemical variability. They also warn us that in some parts of the world valerian has become a threatened species and it has been prohibited from harvesting in the wild. It is imperative that plants be cultivated.[2]

Because of over-exploitation, Bulgaria has prohibited the collection of wild growing *V. officinalis* for commercial purposes.[2]

Method of extraction

Valerian essential oil is steam-distilled from the rhizomes of *V. officinalis*.

Characteristics

Valerian oil is an olive-green to olive-brown coloured liquid and a warm woody, balsamic-earthy odour with a distinct musk-like character of great tenacity. Arctander states that a fresh-green, slightly camphoraceous top note is typical in the odour of a good oil. Upon aging or poor storage conditions, the oil turns darker, becomes more viscous and acquires an unpleasant odour of isovaleric acid.[1]

Indian valerian oil is a pale brown or amber-yellow coloured oil with a balsamic-woody, slightly spicy-earthy aroma and a distinct note of

V

valerian acid. The musk-like and patchouli-like camphoraceous notes are quite distinctive.[1]

Generally, Indian valerian oil is considered to have an inferior odour to the European valerian oil.[1]

Chemical composition

A total of 84 compounds, representing more than 93% of the total essential oil, were identified in *V. officinalis* root oil samples obtained from Estonia. The main components were isovaleric acid (0-2.1%), α-pinene (0.4-3.6%), α-fenchene (0.6-5.8%), camphene (0.6-5.9%), bornyl acetate (8.8-33.7%), myrtenyl acetate (2.0-7.2%), *allo*-aromadendrene (0.3-7.6%), myrtenyl isovalerate (1.1-2.5%), spathulenol (0.7-4.1%), sesquiterpene alcohol (0.8-6.6%), valerianol (0.3-16.7%), valeranone (0.5-9.4%), valerenal (trace-14.7%) and valereneic acid (0-0.9%).[3]

One study found that the essential oil extracted from the dried roots varied significantly from oil from the fresh roots. The essential oil from the dried root contained a higher amount of free isovaleric acid (13.0%) in comparison to fresh roots (0.2%). It was suggested that this may be due to enzymatic hydrolysis of isovaleric esters upon drying. Higher contents of borneol and sesquiterpene hydrocarbons were also found in the dried root oil.[4]

Twenty-one compounds were identified in the oil of *V. jatamansi* distilled from the roots of plants collected India. The oil was predominated by oxygenated sesquiterpenes (33.2-84.7%), followed by sesquiterpene hydrocarbons (13.5-61.6%), whereas monoterpene hydrocarbons and oxygenated monoterpenes were less than 2%. The major compounds identified were patchouli alcohol (0.4-63.7%), maaliol (2.9-53.8%), seychellene (4.1-27.4%), calarene/β-gurjunene (3.0-20.8%) and α-santalene (0.6-12.0%). Other compounds were bornyl acetate (0.6-1.5%), α-guaiene (0.7-2.3%), α-bulnesene/δ-guaiene (0.7-6.3%), 7-*epi*-α-selinene (0.4-1.4%), kessane (2.1-3.3%), spathulenol (0.7-3.4%), viridiflorol (0.9-7.1%), α-patchoulene (0.8-6.6%) and β-patchoulene (0.4-0.8%).[5]

Two chemotypes have been identified: chemotype one is characterised by the prevalence of patchouli alcohol and chemotype two by the prevalence of maaliol.[5]

Adulteration

Valerian oil is often adulterated with synthetic bornyl isovalerate; however, Arctander states that the characteristic sweetness and musky undertone is only obtainable from the true unadulterated oil.[1]

Pharmacopoeias and standards

At the time of writing, the purity, composition, physico-chemical properties and therapeutic use of valerian root essential oil are not defined in any pharmacopoeia monograph or standard.

History and Traditional Uses

History

Dioscorides and Galen extolled the use of valerian as an aromatic and diuretic. It was also used for certain kinds of epilepsy. In the Middle Ages, it was called 'all heal', a name which still applies in some parts of the world.[6]

It is said to have been named after Valerius, who first used it in medicine. Others say it derives its name from the Latin word *valere* (to be in health). Grieve states that we first see the use of the word *Valeriana* in the ninth or tenth century. Valerian was first used for epilepsy by Fabius Calumna in 1592, having cured himself of the disease with it.[6]

Culpeper recommended the use of the herb and root for its many comforting virtues. Gerard tells us that herbalists of his time thought it was excellent for those burdened and for such as be troubled with croup and other like convulsions, and also for those that are bruised with falls.[6]

In the Middle Ages, the roots were not only used as a medicine, but also as a spice and a perfume. Grieve explains that *V. jatamansi*, the nard of the ancients, believed to be the spikenard, has a much more pleasant odour than the European valerian.[6]

Traditional medicine

In traditional medicine, valerian root is used as an antispasmodic, carminative, stomachic and sedative. It is often recommended for the treatment of migraines, insomnia, hysteria, neurasthenia, fatigue, stomach cramps and other nervous conditions – usually as a tea or an infusion.[7]

In Ayurveda, the roots of *Valeriana jatamansi* are used for the treatment of ulcers, convulsions, jaundice, cardiac debility, dry cough, asthma, seminal weakness, skin diseases, leprosy, general debility and improving sleep.[5]

Herbal

Many studies have been performed in animals and in humans to investigate the sleep-inducing activity of valerian root. A double-blind study using aqueous extract of common valerian root confirmed that valerian root decreased sleep latency in eight human subjects who had difficulties falling asleep.[7]

Many other clinical trials have been conducted using preparations of valerian and the overall results support its sleep-enhancing effects.[8]

The German Commission E recommends an infusion or a tincture of valerian for restlessness and sleeping disorders of a nervous nature.[9]

Food, perfumery and flavouring

Valerian root oil is used in perfumery for its musky-woody aroma. It is sometimes used for tobacco flavouring. It is also used as a flavour component in many major food products, including alcoholic liqueurs.[7]

Therapeutics

Pharmacology and clinical studies

Many pharmacological studies involving valerian essential oil have been published. A systemic review of these studies will not be attempted. Rather, I have chosen a selection of studies that support the traditional and clinical uses.

Anti-inflammatory activity

Valerian oil exhibited significant topical anti-inflammatory activity in mice.[10]

Autonomic nervous system activity

In depressed subjects, hand massage with valerian oil had a prolonged stimulatory effect on parasympathetic activity compared to the group with just hand massage. Hand massage with valerian oil enhanced sympathetic activity in normal healthy subjects, but not in depressed patients. In depressed patients, valerian oil enhanced parasympathetic nerve activity after hand massage.[11]

Lis-Balchin cites studies in which valerian oil reduced stress and systolic blood pressure in humans.[12]

Sedative activity

Schnaubelt explains that many of the individual constituents in valerian oil contribute to the neurophysiological activity of valerian root. Therefore, he suggests that most scientists investigating valerian favour the opinion that not one single constituent is responsible for the efficacy of valerian, but a synergy of many constituents.[13]

Valeranone, valerenal and valerenic acid found in valerian oil were found to possess central depressive properties. In vivo studies found that valerenic acid had similar central nervous depressant properties to that of pentobarbital. Other compounds in valerian oil did not have similar effect when administered at the same dose. The results indicated that valerenic acid may contribute to the calming effect of valerian.[14]

Valerian oil and some of its major constituents such as borneol, isoborneol, bornyl acetate and isobornyl acetate all had sedative effects after inhalation on mice.[15]

Pizzorno & Murray state that pharmacological studies confirm that both valepotriates and valerenic acid are capable of binding to GABA receptors, much like the benzodiazepines. However, they state that valerian does not have the side effects such as impaired mental function or morning hangover. They also explain that there are other compounds that do not bind to GABA receptors that have been shown to have sedative effect, therefore, they conclude that other mechanisms may be more important, including valerenic acids modulating GABA receptors or promoting the release of GABA.[16]

Pizzorno & Murray explain that another mechanism of action of valerian constituents is acting as an agonist to adenosine receptors. They explain that adenosine is not a typical hormone or neurotransmitter, but is an important neuromodulator in the central and peripheral nervous systems. A neuromodulator is a compound that has a modulatory effect on neuronal activity – increasing or decreasing the rate at which nerve cells fire. They state that valerian has been shown to act as an adenosine agonist.[16]

Sleep-inducing activity

Valerenic acid found in valerian oil has been shown to significantly decrease the motility of mice and increase pentobarbital-induced sleeping time. The study also found that valeranone possessed similar sedative activity to the other sesquiterpenes found in valerian oil. It was noted that the valerenic acid was partly responsible for the sleep-inducing effects of valerian, whilst the sedative effects could be attributed to the essential oil and the valepotriates found only in the herbal extract.[17]

A randomised clinical trial was conducted in an adult intensive care unit, with 41 subjects in the experimental group and 44 subjects in the control group. Experimental groups received valerian essential oil acupressure on the Shenmen, Neiguan and Yongquan acupuncture points. The results indicated that, after receiving valerian acupressure, patients' sleeping hours increased, wake frequency reduced and Stanford Sleepiness Scale measures on the next morning declined.[18]

Another study tested the pharmacological properties of valerian oil and its major components. The study found that all the components tested and valerian oil had a sedative or muscle relaxant activity. The study found that valerenic acid and valerenal were most sedative at low doses. The researchers stated that the sedative activity was found mostly in the oxygenated fractions of the essential oil.[19]

Inhalation of valerian oil significantly prolonged the pentobarbital-inducing sleep time, whereas lemon oil inhalation significantly shortened it. Many studies have reported that valerian oil exerted a good effect for sleep when used internally; however, this study suggested that the inhalation of valerian may enhance sleep.[20]

Actions

Actions commonly cited in aromatherapy

Antispasmodic, anxiolytic, bactericidal, carminative, hypnotic, sedative, spasmolytic[21,22]

Actions supported by clinical studies

Anxiolytic, sedative, spasmolytic

Comment

Review of traditional uses and clinical data supports valerian root extract and essential oil as having CNS-depressant and sleep-enhancing activities.

Aromatherapy Uses

Clinical aromatherapy

Nervous system

Valerian oil is recommended for insomnia, nervous indigestion, migraine and nervous tension.[21]

Energetics, psyche and subtle uses

Energetics

Valerian oil is beneficial for *Yin deficiency* conditions and calms the *Shen*. Symptoms associated with *Yin deficiency* include restlessness, irritability, night sweats and insomnia. When the *Shen* is agitated, we may experience restlessness, irritability, insomnia, tinnitus, dizziness and palpitations. According to the principles of TCM and the Five Elements, valerian oil helps cool excess *heat* associated with the Fire Element and helps to balance the Earth Element.

According to the principles of Ayurveda, valerian oil helps to balance the *Kapha* dosha, cools *Pitta* and reduces excess *Vata*.

Subtle

Keim Loughran & Bull state that valerian oil will comfort the heart.[23]

Dosage and Administration

Blending

Aromatherapy

For anxiety, restlessness, nervous tension and insomnia, consider blending valerian root oil with essential oils such as Roman chamomile, Atlas cedarwood, clary sage, lavender, patchouli, sandalwood or vetiver.

Perfumery

Arctander states that valerian root is used in perfumery for its musky-woody balsamic notes, which give an interesting effect when blended with essential oils such as patchouli, costus or oakmoss. He states that it is used to create modern chypre style perfumes and also blends well with pine oils, the cedarwood oils and lavender.[1]

Mode of administration

Bath

Full body bath, foot bath

Topical

Massage

Inhalation

Direct inhalation, diffuser, oil vaporiser

Safety Profile

General safety

Valerian oil is non-toxic, non-irritating and no adverse skin reactions reported.[21]

Contraindications

No contraindications known.[2,21]

Pizzorno & Murray state that there is some concern that valerian may prolong thiopental- and pentobarbital-induced sleep. This indicates the need to avoid concurrent use of valerian and barbiturates.[16]

Regulatory guidelines

Valerian root oil has GRAS status.

References

1. Arctander S. *Perfume and flavor materials of natural origin.* Allured Publishing, Carol Stream, 1994.
2. Tisserand R, Young R. *Essential oil safety.* 2nd edn. Churchill Livingstone, Edinburgh, 2014.
3. Raal A et al. *Variation in the composition of the essential oil of Valeriana officinalis L. roots.* Proceedings of the Estonian Academy of Sciences. Chemistry, 2007; 56(2): 67-74.
4. Lopes D, Strobl H, Kolodriejczyk P. *Influence of drying and distilling procedures on the chemical composition of valerian oil (Valeriana officinalis L.).* Journal of Essential Oil Bearing Plants, 2005; 8(2): 134-139. doi: 10.1080/0972060X.2005.10643433.
5. Raina AP, Negi KS. *Essential oil composition of Valeriana jatamansi Jones from Himalayan*

regions of India. Indian Journal of Pharmaceutical Sciences, 2015; 77(2): 218-222.
6. Grieve M. *A modern herbal – Vol. II.* Dover Publications, New York, 1971.
7. Khan I, Abourashed E. *Leung's encyclopedia of common natural ingredients used in food, drugs and cosmetics.* 3rd edn. John Wiley & Sons, New Jersey, 2010.
8. Krystal AD, Ressler I. *The use of valerian in neuropsychiatry.* Empirical Evaluations of Selected Herbal Remedies, 2001; 6(10): 841-847. doi: 10.1017/S1092852900001668.
9. Blumenthal M et al. *The complete German commission E monographs: therapeutic guide to herbal medicine.* American Botanical Council, Austin, 1998.
10. Agnihotri S et al. *Chemical composition, antimicrobial and topical anti-inflammatory activity of Valeriana jatamansi Jones.* Journal of Essential Oil Bearing Plants, 2011; 14(4): 417-422. Cited in Quintessential Aromatics database, 2013.
11. Komori T. *Effect of hand massage with lemon or valerian oil on autonomic nerve activity in depressed and healthy subjects.* International Journal of Essential oil Therapeutics, 2010; 4(3/4): 95-100. Cited in Quintessential Aromatics database, 2013.
12. Lis-Balchin M. *Aromatherapy science – a guide for healthcare professionals.* Pharmaceutical Press, London, 2006.
13. Schnaubelt K. *Essential oil and receptor science.* 2nd International Scientific Aromatherapy Symposium, Grasse, 1999.
14. Hendriks H et al. *Central nervous depressant activity of valerenic acid in the mouse.* Planta Medica, 1985; 51(1): 28-31. Cited in Quintessential Aromatics database, 2013.
15. Buchbauer G et al. *Effect of valerian root, borneol, isoborneol, bornyl acetate and isobornyl acetate on the motility of laboratory animals (mice) after inhalation.* Pharmazie, 1992; 47(8): 620-622. Cited in Quintessential Aromatics database, 2013.
16. Pizzorno JE, Murray MT. *Textbook of natural medicine.* 4th edn. Churchill Livingstone, St Louis, 2013.
17. Houghton PJ. *The scientific basis for the reputed activity of valerian.* Journal of Pharmacy and Pharmacology, 1999; 51(5): 505-512. Cited in Quintessential Aromatics database, 2013.
18. Chen JH et al. *The effectiveness of valerian acupressure on the sleep of ICU patients: A randomized clinical trial.* International Journal of Nursing Studies, 2012; 49(8): 913-920. Cited in Quintessential Aromatics database, 2013.
19. Hendriks H et al. *Pharmacological screening of valerenal and some other components of essential oil of Valeriana officinalis.* Planta Medica, 1981; 42(1): 62-67. Cited in Quintessential Aromatics database, 2013.
20. Komori T et al. *The sleep-enhancing effect of valerian inhalation and sleep-shortening effect of lemon inhalation.* Chemical Senses, 2006; 31(8): 731-737. Cited in Quintessential Aromatics database, 2013.
21. Lawless J. *The encyclopaedia of essential oils.* Element Books, Shaftesbury, 1992.
22. Bone K, Mills S. *Principles and practices of phytotherapy.* 2nd edn. Churchill Livingstone, Edinburgh, 2013.
23. Keim Loughran J, Bull R. *Aromatherapy anointing oils.* Frog, Berkeley, 2001.

V

Verbena

Identification

Botanical name

Aloysia triphylla (L'Her) Britton

Synonyms

Lippia citriodora, Aloysia citriodora Palau, lemon verbena

Family

Verbenaceae

Botany and origins

The plant grows up to 2 m high, with light green lancet-shaped leaves and small white blossoms at the tips of the branches. Originally from Chile and Argentina, lemon verbena is nowadays cultivated in southern France, Algeria, Morocco, Tunisia and Italy.[1]

Method of extraction

The essential oil is produced by steam distillation of the leaves of verbena.

Characteristics

Verbena oil is a pale yellow to yellow or olive-greenish coloured liquid with an intensely fresh, lemony fruity-floral fragrance.[1]

Chemical composition

Lemon verbena oil distilled from the fresh leaves of lemon verbena growing in Greece was found to possess the following composition:

α-pinene (0.4%), sabinene (0.7%), (*Z*)-β-ocimene (1.3%), myrcene (0.6%), geranial (38.7%), neral (24.5%), geraniol (6.0%), limonene (5.8%), β-caryophyllene (1.8%), germacrene D + *ar*-curcumene (3.1%), spathulenol (0.9%), zingiberene (0.6%), bicyclogermacrene (2.4%), (*E*)-nerolidol (0.9%), nerol (0.9%).[2]

Three chemotypes of lemon verbena have been identified. The most commonly encountered chemotype is the neral/geranial-rich lemon verbena oil. The major constituents of the second chemotype are sabinene (11.2%), limonene (40.3%), and citronellal (21.6%), while the third chemotype contained β-thujone (73.4%) as the only major constituent.[2]

Adulteration

True verbena oil is expensive and it is subject to extensive adulteration with oils such as Spanish verbena, lemongrass, lemon and citronella.[3]

Arctander states that true verbena is non-existent.[1]

Pharmacopoeias and standards

At the time of writing, the purity, composition, physico-chemical properties and therapeutic use of verbena essential oil are not defined in any pharmacopoeia monograph or standard.

V

History and Traditional Uses

Traditional medicine

Fischer-Rizzi states that in the past, midwives gave a woman in the last phases of childbirth a strong tea of lemon verbena to stimulate contractions of the uterus.[4]

Herbal

Grieve states that the use of verbena herb is similar to that of mint, orange flowers or melissa as a stomachic and antispasmodic in dyspepsia, indigestion and flatulence, stimulating skin and stomach.[5]

Verbena has been traditionally used in herbal medicine for nervous conditions that manifest as digestive complaints. An infusion of lemon verbena makes a refreshing and cooling summertime drink. It has also been recommended for all kinds of digestive upsets and for congestion of the liver.[4]

Food, perfumery and flavouring

Verbena oil is commonly used in perfumery and citrus colognes.[1,3]

Therapeutics

Pharmacology and clinical studies

Antimicrobial activity

An in vitro and in vivo study confirmed that lemon verbena possesses strong bactericidal effects on the growth of *H. pylori* even under acidic conditions, and may have potential as a new therapeutic agent for helicobacter infections.[6]

Antiviral activity

An in vitro study examined the inhibitory effect of lemon verbena on dengue virus. The study found that the inhibitory effect of lemon verbena seemed to cause direct virus inactivation before adsorption on host cell.[7] Another in vitro study examined the antiviral activity of citral, limonene and lemon verbena essential oil. Citral and lemon verbena were found to possess antiviral activity.[8]

Actions

Actions commonly cited in aromatherapy

Antiseptic, antispasmodic, carminative, detoxifying, digestive, febrifuge, sedative, stomachic[3]

Actions supported by clinical studies

Antimicrobial, antiseptic

Comment

Lemon verbena possesses a unique aroma, which Fischer-Rizzi describes like the morning when everything seems fresh, new and promising.[4]

Apart from the antimicrobial activity, very few studies have investigated the properties of lemon verbena oil. This may be because the chance of adulteration is high and the genuine oil is very costly.

Aromatherapy Uses

Clinical aromatherapy

Nervous system

Verbena oil is recommended for the relief of anxiety, insomnia, nervous tension and stress-related conditions.[3] The oil may be used to relieve tiredness and overcome apathy, listlessness and disinterest.[5]

Energetics, psyche and subtle uses

Subtle

Fischer-Rizzi suggests that verbena oil is ideal for people who continue to live in the past or who miss opportunities and the beauty of the present moment.[4]

Keim Loughran & Bull state that verbena oil clears and cleanses the room and dispels negativity. They also recommend using it to promote creativity.[9]

Dosage and Administration

Blending

Aromatherapy

To create an uplifting and refreshing blend to dispel negativity, consider blending verbena oil with essential oils such as bergamot, lemon, neroli, sweet orange or rosemary.

To alleviate anxiety, nervous tension and stress-related conditions, consider blending verbena oil with essential oils such as bergamot, geranium, lavender, lemon or sandalwood.

To create an effective antimicrobial blend for use in a diffuser, consider blending lemon verbena oil with essential oils such as bergamot, clove bud, cinnamon bark, lemon-scented eucalyptus, 1,8-cineole-rich eucalypts, fragonia, manuka or rosemary.

Perfumery

Arctander states that verbena oil can be found in the 'old-fashioned' citrus colognes where it imparts a delightful freshness and clean top note, which is superior to the effects that can be obtained with lemon oil. He recommends blending it with citrus oils, neroli, palmarosa, spice oils, olibanum or elemi.[1]

Mode of administration

Bath

Due to the risk of dermal sensitisation I would not recommend using verbena oil in a bath.

Topical

Massage, ointment

Inhalation

Direct inhalation, diffuser, oil vaporiser

Safety Profile

General safety

Verbena oil is non-toxic; however, it is a potential dermal irritant and dermal sensitiser. It is reported to be photosensitising.[3,10]

Tisserand & Young recommend that the maximum percentage for dermal application be 0.9%. Lemon verbena oil should be avoided by people with hypersensitive, diseased or damaged skin, and on children under two years of age.[10]

Contraindications

No contraindications known.

Regulatory guidelines

IFRA states that lemon verbena should not be used as a fragrance ingredient because it is sensitising. The oil is also prohibited as a fragrance ingredient in the EU.[10]

References

1. Arctander S. *Perfume and flavor materials of natural origin*. Allured Publishing, Carol Stream, 1994.
2. Lawrence BM. *Progress in essential oils – lemon verbena*. Perfumer and Flavorist 2011; 36: 55-58.
3. Lawless J. *The encyclopaedia of essential oils*. Element Books, Shaftesbury, 1992.
4. Fischer-Rizzi S. *Complete aromatherapy handbook*. Sterling Publishing, New York, 1990.
5. Grieve M. *A modern herbal – Vol. II*. Dover Publications, New York, 1971.
6. Ohno T et al. *Antimicrobial activity of essential oils against Helicobacter pylori*. Helicobacter, 2003; 8(3): 207-215. Cited in Quintessential Aromatics database, 2013.
7. Ocazionez RE et al. *Virucidal activity of Colombian Lippia essential oils on dengue virus replication in vitro*. Memorias do Instituto Oswaldo Cruz, 2010; 105(3): 304-309. Cited in Quintessential Aromatics database, 2013.
8. Gómez LA et al. *Comparative study on in vitro activities of citral, limonene and essential oils from Lippia citriodora and L. alba on yellow fever virus*. Natural Product Communications, 2013; 8(2): 249-252. Cited in Quintessential Aromatics database, 2013.
9. Keim Loughran J, Bull R. *Aromatherapy and subtle energy techniques*. Frog, Berkeley, 2000.
10. Tisserand R, Young R. *Essential oil safety*. 2nd edn. Churchill Livingstone, Edinburgh, 2014.

Vetiver

Identification

Botanical name

Vetiveria zizanioides (L.) Nash

Synonyms

Khus, khus-khus, *Andropogon muricatus*, vetivert

Family

Poaceae (Gramineae)

Botany and origins

Vetiveria zizanioides is a tall, densely tufted perennial grass, which is native to the tropical regions of northern India. The main rootstock is a stout, branching rhizome developing an extensive but not deeply penetrating fibrous mat of aromatic roots.[1]

In most areas, vetiver will not bloom, and even the flowers produce sterile seeds. Vetiver does not send out lateral stems underground. It must use the ramet method to propagate. This explains why vetiver does not spread and become a weed. It has a very fast-growing potential, and the ramet roots can grow 60 cm deep within 10 weeks after planting. The plant is fast growing and it can grow into a grass hedge within 3-4 months.[2]

In addition to the essential oil, the roots contain fructose, sucrose, glucose and, interestingly, free glycerol, not usually found in plants. The mature roots have a pleasant aroma and the highest essential oil content.[1]

Vetiver is endemic to India but was transported around the world more than a century ago.[3] The original use of vetiver was to prevent soil erosion, since its abundant lacework or rootlets will prevent the loss of soil on mountainous slopes against excessive erosion which occurs during the wet season.[4]

Java was the major exporter of vetiver prior to the Second World War. Although commonly planted in the Philippines, it is not cultivated to produce an essential oil.[1]

Vetiver was introduced to Réunion Island with other essential oil crops in the mid-1950s. The finest quality vetiver is referred to as Bourbon vetiver and originates from Réunion.[1]

Vetiver is grown commercially for oil in Java, the Seychelles, Réunion, Brazil, Haiti and Japan.[1] In India, oils produced from vetiver collected in the wild and from cultivated vetiver are differentiated by calling the former khus oil and the latter vetiver oil.[4]

According to Lawrence, there are two main chemotypes of vetiver oil. He explains that vetiver (khus) oil produced in India originates from a fertile form, and the one grown outside of India is a non-seeding, sterile form. Khus oil is primarily made for the Indian domestic market, while the rest of the world uses the oil produced from the sterile form.[3]

Method of extraction

Vetiver oil is steam-distilled from cleaned and washed rootlets which are dried, cut and chopped, then soaked in water before distillation.

Characteristics

Vetiver oil is an amber to brownish coloured viscous oil whose odour is sweet and heavy-woody, earthy, reminiscent of the roots and wet soil, with a rich undertone of 'precious wood'. The oil produced from rootlets that are too young tends to display some 'green' potato-peel-like or asparagus-like top notes.[4]

Chemical composition

Lawrence states that vetiver oil is one of, if not the most, complex essential oils produced.[3]

The chemical composition of Bourbon vetiver comprised sesquiterpene hydrocarbons (42 compounds, 25%), sesquiterpene alcohols (24 compounds, 45%), sesquiterpene ketones (10 compounds, 12%) and some acids that were not identified.[5]

The chemical composition of the major oxygenated components of vetiver oil from Réunion was reported as follows:

khusimol (21.5%), β-vetivone (3.2%), α-vetivone (5.8%), unknown ketone (10.5%), elemol (0.7%), 10-*epi*-γ-eudesmol (1.2%), β-eudesmol (5.5%), vetiverenol + cyclocopacamphenol (6.8%), vetiselinenol (11.1%), unknown alcohol (3.7%).[5]

Lawrence cites a study that confirmed that endophytic bacteria found inside the vetiver roots were capable of sesquiterpenoid biotransormations.[3]

The unique earthy odour of vetiver is due to two sesquiterpene ketones: α-vetivone and β-vetivone.[6]

Adulteration

Vetiver oil is occasionally adulterated with oils from roots of other grasses or it may be cut with fractions from the isolation of vetiverol. It is also adulterated with caryophyllene, cedarwood derivatives and amyris oil.[4]

Pharmacopoeias and standards

The purity, composition and physico-chemical properties of vetiver oil are defined in ISO 4716:2013 Essential Oil of Vetiver [*Chrysopogon zizanioides* (L.) Roberty, syn. *Vetiveria zizanioides* (L.) Nash].

History and Traditional Uses

History

Vetiver has long been valued in India for its aromatic properties. In Sri Lanka, it is known as 'oil of tranquillity.'[1] Vetiver is also known as *khus khus* in India, 'miracle grass' in Thailand and *xiang-gen-cao* or *yan-lan-cao* in China and Taiwan.[4]

In India, the dried thin, wiry roots are woven into fans, screens and mats to scent the houses. As the hot, dry breeze enters through the verandas, the vetiver screens which are wet then refresh, cool and scent the house.[1]

Traditional medicine

A drink is made from the fresh rhizomes and is taken as a stimulant and tonic.[1] In Ayurvedic medicine, vetiver is used to alleviate thirst, heatstroke, fever and headaches. The oil is applied as part of a liniment to relieve inflammatory disorders of the joints and skin, and it has been used for rheumatoid arthritis.[7]

In Ayurvedic medicine, a decoction of the roots is used for dissolving kidney stones.[1]

Food, perfumery and flavouring

Vetiver oil is extensively used in perfumery.[4]

Other uses

Vetiver's massive, deep, strong fibrous roots and thick thatch of stiff leaves has led to its extensive use in other areas such as:[8]

- *Soil erosion control* – vetiver's root structures have been known to grow as many as 3-4 m in one year. The deep root structures and rigid grass above ground make vetiver an effective plant for soil erosion control.
- *Decontamination treatment of soil and water* – it is commonly used in waste water treatment and has been shown to remove nitrates, phosphates and heavy metal contaminants from soil and water.
- *Animal feed* – the young vetiver leaves can be ground to feed fish and livestock, but mature leaves cannot be used because their nutritive value is lower than other grasses.
- *Botanical pesticide management* – it has been observed that the vetiver plant grown in close proximity to other plants could inhibit to a substantial degree the attack upon that plant by certain insects.
- *A biofuel* – vetiver leaves are high in cellulose. Dry biomass yields exceed 370 t/ha per year. It can be harvested three to four times a year. The leaves can also be used as a substrate for ethanol production through alkali pretreatment followed by enzyme hydrolysis and yeast fermentation.

Another novel but very practical use of vetiver is the vetiver latrine. This is a very simple concept where vetiver is planted around a small concrete slab above the pit. Instead of bricks and mortar, the long roots of the grass stabilise the pit and are also able to remove environmental contaminants. Above the ground, the blades of the grass provide a tall, thick privacy screen that is also storm proof. Once the latrine is filled, the slab and seedlings can be transferred to a new pit. This concept has been tested in 2012 in remote villages in Haiti and was considered very successful.[9]

Therapeutics

Pharmacology and clinical studies

Many pharmacological studies involving vetiver essential oil have been published. A systemic review of these studies will not be attempted. Rather, I have chosen a selection of studies that support the traditional and clinical uses.

Anticonvulsant activity

Vetiver oil demonstrated significant anticonvulsant activity in an animal study.[10]

Anti-inflammatory activity

A study stated that vetiver oil may suppress inflammatory responses by regulating the expression of inflammation-related enzymes heme oxygenase-1, inducible nitric oxide synthase and cyclooxygenase-2, and the inflammatory cytokines tumour necrosis factor-α, interleukin-1β and interferon-β.[11]

Antimicrobial activity

Vetiver oil was found to have very effective antimicrobial activity against cultures of *Trichomonas vaginalis* in an in vitro study.[12] Another in vitro study found vetiver at up to 1:1000 dilution in dimethyl sulphoxide was very effective against *Staphylococcus aureus*.[13]

Antioxidative activity

Vetiver oil exhibited potent lipid peroxidation inhibitory activity to moderate the bleaching of β-carotene and to maintain the cellular glutathione (GSH) levels. Vetiver oil markedly decreased melanin production and tyrosine activity in α-melanin-stimulating-hormone (α-MSH-) stimulated B16 cells. These results demonstrated

V

that the activity of vetiver oil on melanogenesis might be a result of its potent antioxidative ability, which is reflected in the decreased cellular oxidant and malondialdehyde (MDA) levels and the recovered activities of superoxide dismutase (SOD), glutathione peroxidase (GPX) and catalase (CAT) in α-MSH-stimulated B16 cells. It has been suggested that vetiver essential oil has the potential to become an ingredient in future hypopigmentation drugs, foods and cosmetics.[14]

Anxiolytic activity

An in vivo study using rats confirmed that the inhalation of vetiver oil exhibited anxiolytic-like activity. It was found that vetiver oil significantly increased c-fos expression in the amygdala, known to be involved in anxiety.[15]

It has been suggested that the anxiolytic or sedative effect of vetiver was through GABAergic activity.[10]

Autonomic nervous system activity

Vetiver oil inhalation significantly increased total waking and reduced slow-wave sleep time in animal studies. The results of the EEG study suggest that the aroma of vetiver oil increases brain activity and alertness.[10]

Human subjects who inhaled vetiver essential oil showed faster reaction times and stimulation of sympathetic nerve activity. It was suggested that the oil may help subjects to improve performance and alertness during a visual determination task. It was also concluded that the stimulating effects of vetiver oil may be beneficial for learning and memory processes.[16]

Dementia

A blend of lavender, sweet marjoram, patchouli and vetiver essential oils was blended into an aqueous cream and 5 g was gently massaged five times a day onto the bodies and limbs of 56 aged care facility residents (age range 70-92 years) with moderate to severe dementia. Participants were divided into two groups, and following a baseline period in which there was no massage at all, followed by massage with cream only, the groups received four weeks of massage with cream and essential oils or four weeks of massage with only cream, and then received the other treatment for four weeks.[17]

During the period of oil application, both groups showed a significant decrease in the average frequency and severity of dementia-related behaviours occurring at times other than during nursing care, compared with the baseline and the 'no oil' periods. However, it was noted that resistance to nursing care procedures increased, which may reflect increased mental alertness and awareness caused by the oils.[17]

Insecticidal activity

Sixty-one essential oils were screened for their insecticidal activity against *Aedes aegypti* (mosquito) larvae. Vetiver essential oil was found to be the most toxic, causing over 50% mortality at a 50 mg/L concentration.[18]

Actions

Actions commonly cited in aromatherapy

Antiseptic, antispasmodic, mild rubefacient, sedative, tonic, vermifuge[19]

Actions supported by clinical studies

Anti-inflammatory, anxiolytic, insecticidal, sedative, tonic

Comment

Holmes states that vetiver possesses therapeutic potential that is still largely unexplored yet very rich in possibilities. He states that very few remedies exert the same depth of restorative action as vetiver oil. He explains that it influences the body's four core systems – the nervous, endocrine, gastrointestinal and immune systems.[20]

Schnaubelt states that vetiver oil is almost exclusively composed of sesquiterpenoid constituents. Due to the complexity of these compounds, there are many unknown interactions between them and the various transmitter-receptor systems, which may have surprising implications for their pharmacological properties.[21]

Aromatherapy Uses

Clinical aromatherapy

Musculoskeletal system

Vetiver oil is a mild rubefacient and may be used for arthritis, rheumatism and muscular pain.[19,22,23]

Psychological

Vetiver oil is relaxing and is beneficial for anyone experiencing stress, anxiety, insomnia or depression.[19,20,22]

Vetiver oil is recommended for physical, mental and emotional burnout which results from total exhaustion.[7] Holmes states that vetiver oil promotes cognitive flexibility and emotional security. Vetiver helps to dispel worry, obsessions, compulsions, repetitive and excessive thinking, the inability to let go, and feelings of insecurity and vulnerability.[20]

Reproductive system

Vetiver is reputed to regulate hormonal secretions

V

of oestrogen and progesterone.[7,24,25] This makes vetiver an ideal oil to use during menopause, where both the hormones need supplementing and its grounding and cooling effects will help to reduce the symptoms of hot flushes.[7]

Holmes suggests that vetiver is useful for PMS because of endocrine and emotional reasons. Vetiver is recommended for PMS caused by oestrogen deficiency that often displays weepiness and depression, and PMS associated with progesterone deficiency that typically presents feelings of unworthiness.[7]

Skin care

Vetiver oil assists in strengthening the body's connective tissue. It is beneficial for weak, loose or simply fatigued skin.[26] Holmes suggests using it during and after childbirth to minimise stretch marks.[7]

Gumbel states that vetiver oil mainly influences the subcutis. Its application is especially recommended where the skin has become atrophic and slack and where there is too little adipose tissue built up. The resorptive power of the skin is stimulated, so that tissue development will be strengthened and vitalised.[26]

Tonic

Holmes refers to vetiver as a neuroendocrine restorative, recommending the oil for hypotonic conditions involving chronic neurohormonal deficiencies with fatigue, debility, burnout, neurasthenia, nervous breakdown, depression associated with chronic stress, overwork or disease. He also recommends vetiver oil as a gastrointestinal restorative for conditions such as malabsorption syndrome with fatigue, weight loss, gut hyperpermeability, gluten sensitivity, peptic ulcer, ulcerative colitis and anaemia.[20]

Energetics, psyche and subtle uses

Energetics

Vetiver is *cool* and *moist*. It clears *heat*, nourishes, calms and uplifts.[20,25] Mojay describes vetiver's ability to reconnect us to mother earth:

> *Whether mentally exhausted from overwork, or out of touch with our body and its needs, vetiver sedates and yet restores us – centres and reconnects us – closing the gap between spirit and matter.*[25]

It nourishes and supports *Yin Qi*, which is the body's restorative and metabolic functions. It is for this reason that Mojay recommends using vetiver for poor appetite, weight loss, anaemia and malabsorption.[25]

Holmes states that vetiver oil nourishes the blood and *Yin*, clears *heat* and calms the *Shen*. Vetiver will be beneficial for *Yin deficiency* conditions. Symptoms associated with *Yin deficiency* include hot spells, fever, restlessness, irritability, night sweats and insomnia.[20]

When the *Shen* is agitated, we may experience restlessness, irritability, insomnia, tinnitus, dizziness and palpitations. According to the principles of TCM, vetiver essential oil helps cool excess *heat* associated with the Fire Element and helps to balance the Earth Element.

According to the principles of Ayurveda, vetiver oil helps to balance the *Kapha* dosha, cools *Pitta* and reduces excess *Vata*.

Personality

Vetiver personalities are often strong and intellectual and are aware of their surroundings. They are very interested in the esoteric side of life, particularly the journeys of the shamans and voyages to uncover the earth's mysteries.[27]

Worwood explains that there is nothing delicate about the vetiver personality – it's very much of the here and now. While they can often be gentle and wise in spirit, friends will turn to vetiver for advice, which will be blunt and straight. She states that vetiver personalities revel in the sensuality of life. They are the person who needs to hold and feel something in order to fully appreciate all aspects of an object.[27]

According to Myers-Briggs personality types, the vetiver personality is likely to be an ISTP. ISTPs are quiet and they prefer to stand back and observe. They can be difficult to understand and remain a mystery to many people. They are independent and do not like to behave to the rules of society. They appear cool, dispassionate and analytical. They can be very disorganised in things where they have no interest. They dislike supervising or being supervised. They tend to ignore rules, policies and regulations when they can get in the way of results. They tend to remain calm in a crisis. They have little need for talking or socialising. They often have poor interpersonal skills and seem detached or uncaring to those who are not close to them.

Subtle

Vetiver is beneficial for anyone who needs to be brought into close contact with the earth, to ground and centre their energies.[22]

Fischer-Rizzi beautifully describes the grounding qualities of vetiver:

> *This essential oil connects us to earth's energies. It is a source of vital energy and regeneration. The earthy fragrance of the oil supports all of those who have lost touch with the earth and their roots. Vetiver nourishes people who have cold feet*

or have their heads in the clouds. When we lose contact with the ground beneath us, with reality, we pay the price of a weakened immune system. When in touch with the earth, we breathe fresh air, enjoy the magic of an open fire, and feel the wind blow through our hair.[24]

Keim Loughran & Bull state that vetiver balances and grounds us so that we can be receptive to spiritual energy. They recommend using vetiver oil whenever we feel ungrounded or confused, whenever we feel unsafe in the world and when our personal boundaries are vulnerable and weak.[28]

The oil is recommended as protection against oversensitivity and may be applied to the solar plexus to prevent becoming a 'psychic sponge'. To do this, apply one drop of vetiver oil on the fingertips and gently massage it to the solar plexus in an anticlockwise direction.[29] Vetiver oil helps to balance our base or root chakra.[23,29]

Zeck recommends using vetiver if we are feeling threatened by the demands of our own soul for change. The earthy quality of vetiver will embrace, sustain and re-establish a balanced relationship between heart, body and mind.[30]

Worwood states that vetiver oil will stop the turmoil of unanswerable questions swirling in our mind. She explains that vetiver oil will help us remain calm when unsettling events affect our spiritual self and when we face adversity.[31]

V

Holmes beautifully describes vetiver as mother earth's gift to humankind. He states that vetiver represents the nurture and self-empowerment given to us by our earth mother:

As she shows us her deepest mysteries, we can become more open to her beauty, feel the deep connection of all of life and come to realise on an instinctive level that her density and ours are really one.[20]

Dosage and Administration

Blending

Aromatherapy

For the temporary relief of arthritis and rheumatic pain, consider blending vetiver oil with essential oils such as black pepper, German chamomile, cajeput, kunzea, spike lavender or rosemary.

For the relief of anxiety, nervous tension and stress-related conditions, consider blending vetiver oil with essential oils such as bergamot, lavender, cold-pressed lime, jasmine absolute, neroli, patchouli, sandalwood and ylang ylang.

For the relief of chronic neurasthenia with exhaustion, consider blending vetiver oil with essential oils such as clary sage, geranium, lemon, cold-pressed lime, pine or rosemary ct. verbenone.

Perfumery

Vetiver oil is extensively used in perfumery, not only as a fixative, but also as an odour contributor in fougère, chypre, modern woody-aldehydic or amber-aldehydic, oriental, moss and wood style bases. It blends well with essential oils such as opopanax, patchouli, sandalwood, oakmoss absolute, lavender and clary sage.[4]

Jouhar states that vetiver essential oil is an excellent fixative for rose and opopanax perfumes.[32]

Mode of administration

Bath

Full body bath, foot bath

Topical

Massage, ointment, skin care

Inhalation

Direct inhalation, diffuser, oil vaporiser

Safety Profile

General safety

Vetiver oil is non-toxic, non-irritating and non-sensitising.[19]

Contraindications

No contraindications known.

Regulatory guidelines

Vetiver oil is approved by the FDA for food use.[33]

References

1. Weiss EA. *Essential oil crops.* CAB International, Wallingford, 1997.
2. Chou ST, Shih Y, Lin CC. *Vetiver grass (Vetiveria zizanioides) oils.* In Preedy VR. ed. *Essential oils in food preservation, flavor and safety.* Academic Press, London, 2016: 843-848.
3. Lawrence BM. *Progress in essential oils – vetiver oil and extract.* Perfumer & Flavorist, 2016; 41: 54. Retrieved July 1, 2017, from http://www.perfumerflavorist.com
4. Arctander S. *Perfume and flavor materials of natural origin.* Allured Publishing, Carol Stream, 1994.
5. Lawrence BM. *Progress in essential oils – vetiver oil.* 2008; 33: 56-61.
6. Anonis DP. *Woody notes in perfumery – vetiver and derivatives. Part I.* Perfumer & Flavorists, 2004; 29: 30-36.
7. Holmes P. *Vetiver oil.* The International Journal of Aromatherapy, 1993; 5(3): 13-15.

8. Balasankar D et al. *Traditional and medicinal uses of vetiver.* Journal of Medicinal Plants Studies, 2013; 1(3): 191-200.
9. *The vetiver latrine.* Retrieved on Nov 23, 2017, from http://www.vetiver.org/LAICV2F/2%20Environmental%20Protection/E5Lee_TE.pdf
10. Cheaha D et al. *Modification of sleep-waking and electroencephalogram induced by vetiver essential oil inhalation.* Journal of Intercultural ethnopharmacology. 2016;5(1):72-78. doi: 10.5455/jice.20160208050736.
11. Chou ST et al. *Study of the chemical composition, antioxidant activity and anti-inflammatory activity of essential oil from Vetiveria zizanioides.* Food Chemistry, 2012; 134(1): 262-268. Cited in Quintessential Aromatics database, 2013.
12. Viollon C et al. *Antagonistic activities, in vitro, of some essential oils and natural volatile compounds in relation to the growth of Trichomonas vaginalis.* Fitoterapia, 1996: 67(3): 279-281. Cited in Quintessential Aromatics database, 2013.
13. Gangrade SK et al. *Evaluation of some essential oils for antibacterial properties.* Indian Perfumer, 1990; 34(3): 204-208. Cited in Quintessential Aromatics database, 2013.
14. Peng HY et al. *Effect of Vetiveria zizanioides essential oil on melanogenesis in melanoma cells: downregulation of tyrosinase expression and suppression of oxidative stress.* The Scientific World Journal, 2014; 2014: 213013. doi: 10.1155/2014/213013.
15. Saiyudthong S et al. *Anxiety-like behaviour and c-fos expression in rats that inhaled vetiver essential oil.* Natural Product Research, 2015; 29(22): 2141-2144. Cited in Quintessential Aromatics database, 2013.
16. Matsubara E et al. *Volatiles emitted from the roots of Vetiveria zizanioides suppress the decline in attention during a visual display terminal task.* Biomedical Research, 2012; 33(5): 299-308.
17. Bowles EJ et al. *Effects of essential oils and touch on resistance to nursing care procedures and other dementia-related behaviours in a residential care facility.* International Journal of Aromatherapy. 2002;12(1):22-29. Cited in Quintessential Aromatics database, 2013.
18. Chantraine JM et al. *Insecticidal activity of essential oils on Aedes aegypti larvae.* Phytotherapy Research, 1998; 12(5): 350-354. Cited in Quintessential Aromatics database, 2013.
19. Lawless J. *The encyclopaedia of essential oils.* Element Books, Shaftesbury, 1992.
20. Holmes P. *Aromatica: a clinical guide to essential oil therapeutics – Vol. I.* Singing Dragon, London, 2016.
21. Schnaubelt K. *Medical aromatherapy.* Frog, Berkeley, 1999.
22. Davis P. *Aromatherapy: an A-Z.* 2nd edn. C.W. Daniel Company, Saffron Walden, 1999.
23. Lavabre M. *Aromatherapy workbook.* Healing Arts Press, Rochester, 1997.
24. Fischer-Rizzi S. *Complete aromatherapy handbook.* Sterling Publishing, New York, 1990.
25. Mojay G. *Aromatherapy for healing the spirit.* Healing Arts Press, Rochester, 1999.
26. Gumbel D. *Principles of holistic skin therapy with herbal essences.* Karl F Haug, Heidelberg, 1986.
27. Worwood VA. *The fragrant mind.* Transworld Publishers, London, 1995.
28. Keim Loughran J, Bull R. *Aromatherapy anointing oils.* Frog, Berkeley, 2001.
29. Davis P. *Subtle aromatherapy.* C.W. Daniel Company, Saffron Walden, 1991.
30. Zeck R. *The blossoming heart – aromatherapy for healing and transformation.* Aroma Tours, East Ivanhoe, 2004.
31. Worwood VA. *The fragrant heavens.* Transworld Publishers, London, 1999.
32. Jouhar AJ. *Poucher's perfumes, cosmetics and soaps – Vol. 1: The raw materials of perfumery.* 9th edn. Springer-Science+Business Media, Dordrecht, 1991.
33. Opdyke DLJ. *Monographs on fragrance raw materials.* Pergamon Press, Oxford, 1979.

V

Violet leaf absolute

Identification

Botanical name

Viola odorata L.

Synonyms

Sweet violet

Family

Violaceae

Botany and origins

A small, tender, perennial plant with dark green, heart-shaped leaves and fragrant violet-blue flowers. The plants are cultivated mainly in Italy and France.[1]

Method of extraction

The concrete is obtained by solvent extraction of the leaves and an absolute by further extraction of the concrete.[1]

Characteristics

The leaf absolute is an intense dark green viscous liquid with a strong green-leaf odour and delicate floral undernote.[1]

Chemical composition

The chemical composition of violet leaf absolute was reported as follows:

2-*trans*-6-*cis*-nonadien-1-al, *n*-hexanol, n-octen-2-ol-1, benzyl alcohol, tertiary octenol, heptenol, octenal and traces of eugenol.[2]

Adulteration

Violet leaf absolute is subject to adulteration with synthetic 2,6-nonadien-1-al (one of the constituents responsible for the absolute's distinctive odour), chlorophyll extracts and other synthetic aromatics not found in the true absolute.[1]

Pharmacopoeias and standards

At the time of writing, the purity, composition, physico-chemical properties and therapeutic use of violet leaf absolute are not defined in any pharmacopoeia monograph or standard.

History and Traditional Uses

Herbal

Both the leaf and flowers have been used in traditional herbal medicine for congestive pulmonary conditions and sensitive skin conditions such as weak capillaries.[3] The British Herbal Pharmacopeia lists the dried flowers and leaf as a specific for eczema and skin eruptions with serious exudate, particularly associated with rheumatic conditions.[4]

Food, perfumery and flavouring

Violet leaf absolute is used in expensive perfumery to bring about a green violet note.[1]

Therapeutics

Pharmacology and clinical studies

At the time of writing there are no clinical or pharmacological studies to confirm any of the therapeutic properties of violet leaf absolute.

Actions

Actions commonly cited in aromatherapy

Analgesic (mild), anti-inflammatory, antiseptic, decongestant, diuretic, expectorant[3]

Actions supported by clinical studies

None of the actions commonly cited in aromatherapy can be supported by clinical studies.

Comment

Violet leaf is typically used in perfumery for its intense natural green aroma. A review of traditional uses and clinical data could not confirm any clinical applications for violet leaf oil in aromatherapy.

The pleasant fresh green note of violet leaf absolute may be beneficial for improving mood and reducing the symptoms of stress-induced disorders such as anxiety and depression.

Aromatherapy Uses

Clinical aromatherapy

Lymphatic system

Arcier recommends violet leaf absolute for the treatment of fluid retention.[5]

Nervous system

Violet leaf absolute has also been suggested for dizziness, headaches, insomnia and nervous exhaustion.[3]

Respiratory system

Arcier recommends violet leaf absolute as an effective expectorant of the respiratory tract.[5]

Skin care

Violet leaf absolute is used for the treatment of skin problems such as acne, eczema, thread veins and wounds.[3] Davis states that violet leaf is antiseptic and has healing properties that are beneficial for treating acne, oily skin and large pores. It may also be useful for thread viens.[6]

Energetics, psyche and subtle uses

Subtle

Worwood recommends violet leaf absolute for those who are shy and timid. It gives them the courage to speak and be heard. She explains that violet leaf offers understanding and empathy and a way into the great open void of love.[7]

Dosage and Administration

Blending

Aromatherapy

For use in subtle aromatherapy, consider blending violet leaf absolute with essential oils such as bergamot, geranium, lavender or sandalwood.

Perfumery

Violet leaf absolute is extensively used in perfumery. It gives a blend incredible diffusion and a delicate naturalness at very low concentrations.

It is ideal to use when creating high-class chypre or aldehydic-woody fragrances.[1]

It blends well with rich florals such as boronia absolute, tuberose absolute and narcissus absolute. It also compliments fresh citrus oils such as lemon, cold-pressed lime and grapefruit.

Mode of administration

Bath

Full body bath, foot bath

Topical

Compress, massage, ointment, skin care

Inhalation

Direct inhalation, diffuser, oil vaporiser

Safety Profile

General safety

Violet leaf absolute is non-toxic and non-irritant. It had previously been reported as being sensitising to some individuals; however, Tisserand & Young state that there is no evidence to support this claim. They believe that it may have been caused by an adulterated oil.[8]

Contraindications

No contraindications known.

Regulatory guidelines

Violet leaf absolute has GRAS status.

References

1. Arctander S. *Perfume and flavor materials of natural origin*. Allured Publishing, Carol Stream, 1994.
2. Lawrence BM. *Essential oils 1976-1978*. Allured Publishing, Wheaton, 1979.
3. Lawless J. *The encyclopaedia of essential oils*. Element Books, Shaftesbury, 1992.
4. British Herbal Medicine Association Scientific Committee. *British Herbal Pharmacopoeia*. BHMA, Bournemouth, 1983.
5. Arcier M. *Aromatherapy*. The Hamlyn Publishing Group, London, 1990.
6. Davis P. *Aromatherapy: an A-Z*. 2nd edn. C.W. Daniel Company, Saffron Walden, 1999.
7. Worwood VA. *The fragrant heavens*. Transworld Publishing, London, 1999.
8. Tisserand R, Young R. *Essential oil safety*. 2nd edn. Churchill Livingstone, Edinburgh, 2014.

Wintergreen

W

Identification

Botanical name

Gaultheria procumbens L.

Synonyms

Gaultheria

Family

Ericaceae

Botany and origins

Wintergreen is a native of eastern North America and grows wild in the eastern states, from the southern part of Canada to Georgia in the southeast of the USA.[1]

It is a small evergreen herb up to 15 cm high, with slender creeping stems, erect twigs, leathery serrated leaves and drooping white flowers.[2]

Method of extraction

Wintergreen oil is derived by water distillation of the leaves of *G. procumbens*. Prior to distillation, the leaves are exposed to enzymatic action in warm water. During this process, methyl salicylate is formed as a decomposition product from a glycoside in the plant material.[1]

Characteristics

The oil is a pale yellow to yellow-pink coloured liquid with an intense sweet-aromatic odour.[1]

The odour is distinctively different from synthetic methyl salicylate. Wintergreen essential oil is slightly laevorotatory, while sweet birch and synthetic methyl salicylate are optically inactive.[3,4]

Chemical composition

The main constituent found in wintergreen oil is methyl salicylate (98%). Most commercial wintergreen oils are in fact synthetic methyl salicylate.[4]

Adulteration

Wintergreen oil is used interchangeably with sweet birch oil or methyl salicylate. It is, therefore, very difficult to obtain genuine essential oil from the leaves of *G. procumbens*.[4]

Pharmacopoeias and standards

The purity, composition and physico-chemical

properties of wintergreen oil are defined in ISO 21390:2005 Oil of Wintergreen, China (*Gaultheria yunnanensis* (Franch.) Rehd.), Redistilled.

History and Traditional Uses

Traditional medicine

Wintergreen oil is recommended for external application as a liniment because of its anti-inflammatory and antirheumatic properties. It is a specific for rheumatoid arthritis.[5,6]

Herbal

The leaves have been used as a tea for colds, headaches, stomachaches, fevers and kidney ailments. Externally it is used for rheumatism, sore muscles and lumbago.[4]

Food, perfumery and flavouring

The oil is used extensively in the USA as a flavouring for toothpaste, chewing gum and soft drinks.[2,4] Wintergreen oil is used for similar flavouring purposes as sweet birch oil, though its use level is lower than that of birch oil.[4]

Therapeutics

Pharmacology and clinical studies

Analgesic activity

The topical application of rubefacients containing salicylates may be efficacious in the treatment of acute pain. Salicylates have the ability to suppress the synthesis of prostaglandins, which have an integral role in the management of pain and inflammation.[7]

The anti-inflammatory activity in mice was comparable with aspirin, but had the advantage of not having gastric ulcerogenic effect.[4] However, other trials of musculoskeletal and arthritic pain suggest moderate or poor efficacy. A report concluded that efficacy estimates for rubefacients are unreliable owing to a lack of good clinical trials.[8]

Antibacterial activity

An in vitro study confirmed that wintergreen oil had strong antibacterial activity. It was found to be more effective against MRSA and MSSA growth than vancomycin.[9]

Miticidal activity

Eight two essential oils were tested for their miticidal activity on mites such as *Dermatophagoides pteronyssinus, Dermatophagoides farinae* and *Tyrophagus putrescentiae*. Wintergreen oil was found to have a very powerful miticidal activity.[10]

Actions

Actions commonly cited in aromatherapy

Analgesic, anti-inflammatory, antirheumatic, antitussive, astringent, carminative, diuretic, emmenagogue, stimulant[2]

Actions supported by clinical studies

Analgesic, anti-inflammatory, antirheumatic

Comment

Many aromatherapists do not recommend the use of wintergreen oil in aromatherapy. The oil was traditionally used and still is used in many over-the-counter products for its anti-inflammatory and analgesic activity. I believe that the essential oil has an important use in aromatherapy products for treating arthritis and rheumatic pain. Schnaubelt states that it is highly irritant if used in too high a concentration, therefore, it should always be blended with other essential oils.[11]

Aromatherapy Uses

Clinical aromatherapy

Musculoskeletal system

Many aromatherapists state that wintergreen oil is toxic and should not be used in aromatherapy; however, the British Herbal Pharmacopoeia recommends using wintergreen externally as a liniment.[5]

Considering that methyl salicylate is extensively used in many commercial analgesic and antiarthritic ointments and balms, I believe that wintergreen oil may be useful in aromatherapy for topical applications for the relief of short-term acute musculoskeletal pain.

A combination of wintergreen oil and peppermint oil is commonly used because it is believed to give far better pain relief than either wintergreen oil or peppermint oil alone.[12]

Dosage and Administration

Blending

Aromatherapy

For the temporary relief of the pain of rheumatism and arthritis, consider blending wintergreen oil with essential oils such as black pepper, cajeput, clove bud, 1,8-cineole-rich eucalypts, ginger, kunzea, lemon-scented eucalyptus, rosemary or peppermint.

Perfumery

Wintergreen is commonly used for flavouring; however, it does find some limited use in perfumery. It may be used to create fougères and forest notes.[1]

Mode of administration

Bath

Not recommended for use in bath.

Topical

Massage, ointment. For massage, use a 1.0% dilution of the appropriate blend of essential oils to the chosen carrier oil. This equates to 2 drops of essential oil to 10 mL of carrier oil.

Inhalation

Not commonly used by inhalation.

Safety Profile

General safety

Many aromatherapists state that wintergreen should not be used in aromatherapy. Tisserand & Young state that the maximum dermal use level is 2.4% and the maximum adult daily oral dose is 175 mg.[13]

Although prolonged skin contact with methyl salicylate may cause dermatitis, it is generally safe in topical formulations.[14]

Contraindications

Methyl salicylate applied topically or orally can inhibit platelet aggregation and potentiate the action of warfarin, therefore, wintergreen essential oil is contraindicated with anticoagulant medication, after major surgery, and for people with haemophilia and other bleeding disorders. It should not be used during pregnancy and breastfeeding. It should not be used or given to children. It should not be given to people with salicylate sensitivity.[13]

Oral administration of wintergreen oil and other oils with a high methyl salicylate content is contraindicated for people with gastroesophageal reflux disease, and should be avoided altogether in children due to the risk of developing Reye's syndrome.[13]

Toxicity

Numerous cases of methyl salicylate poisoning have been reported. Signs of methyl salicylate poisoning included CNS excitation, rapid breathing, fever, high blood pressure, convulsions and coma.[13] Studies indicate that compounds containing salicylates such as wintergreen potentiate blood-thinning drugs such as warfarin.[7,13]

Approximately 5 mL of pure wintergreen is equivalent to approximately 7000 mg of salicylate or 21.7 adult aspirin tablets. Ingestion of as little as 4 mL in a child can be fatal. Prevention of accidental ingestion of methyl salicylate-containing products must be achieved by keeping the products out of reach of children, using child-resistant bottles and restricting the size of the openings of the bottles, and appropriate labels.[15]

Dermal exposure to methyl salicylate was associated with LD_{50} of 2 g/kg. The lowest lethal oral dose of methyl salicylate was reported in women at 355 mg/kg, in men at 101 mg/kg and in children at 228 mg/kg.[14]

The oral administration of methyl salicylate (up to 0.5 mL) in rats during organogenesis increased the rate of abnormalities, particularly of the central nervous system. This does represent 5 times the lethal human dose. It has been reported that pregnant hamsters treated orally or topically with 175 mg/100 g of methyl salicylate exhibited central nervous system teratogenicity. However, another study found that the topical application of methyl salicylate did not cause congenital defects when used at doses up to 6000 mg/kg/day. It has been noted that the doses in many of these studies is significantly higher than the adult lethal dose on mg/kg basis.[14]

Regulatory guidelines

Wintergreen essential oil has GRAS status. Health Canada has set a maximum for methyl salicylate of 1% for topical products.[13]

Several regulatory agencies have established recommended toxicity levels for oral exposure to methyl salicylate. The United States Environmental Protection Agency's Biopesticide and Pollution Prevention Division, Norwegian Food Safety Authority, European Food Safety Authority and the Joint FAO/WHO Expert Committee on Food Additives (JECFA 2002) all recommend an acceptable daily intake for methyl salicylate of 0.5 mg/kg per day.[16]

A critical review of the available literature for the oral exposure to methyl salicylate analysed the quality of the studies available and the current mode of action. Following the review of all the available literature, Green et al. recommended that the acceptable daily intake (ADI) for methyl salicylate is 11 mg/kg/day, which is 22 times higher than the current ADI recommended by most regulatory authorities of 0.5 mg/kg body weight.[16]

References

1. Arctander S. *Perfume and flavor materials of natural origin.* Allured Publishing, Carol Stream, 1994.

2. Lawless J. *The encyclopaedia of essential oils.* Element Books, Shaftesbury, 1992.
3. Lis-Balchin M. *Aromatherapy science – a guide for healthcare professionals.* Pharmaceutical Press, London, 2006.
4. Khan I, Abourashed E. *Leung's encyclopedia of common natural ingredients used in food, drugs and cosmetics.* 3rd edn. John Wiley & Sons, New Jersey, 2010.
5. British Herbal Medicine Association Scientific Committee. *British herbal pharmacopoeia.* BHMA, Bournemouth, 1983.
6. Hoffman D. *A new holistic herbal.* Element Books, Shaftesbury, 1996.
7. McGuffin M et al. eds. *American herbal products association's botanical safety handbook.* CRC Press, Boca Raton, 1997.
8. Mason L et al. *Systemic review of efficacy of topical rubefacients containing salicylates for the treatment of acute and chronic pain.* BMJ, 2004; 328(7446): 995. doi: 10.1136/bmj.38040.607141.EE.
9. Sharma PR et al. *Ten highly effective essential oils inhibit growth of methicillin resistant Staphylococcus aureus (MRSA) and methicillin sensitive Staphylococcus aureus (MSSA).* International Journal of Pharmacy and Pharmaceutical Sciences, 2013; 5(1): 52-54. Cited in Quintessential Aromatics database, 2013.
10. Watanabe F et al. *Killing activities of the volatiles emitted from essential oils for Dermatophagoides pteronyssinus, Dermatophagoides farinae and Tyrophagus putrescentiae.* Shyoyakugaku Zasshi, 1989; 43(2): 163-168. Cited in Quintessential Aromatic database, 2013.
11. Schnaubelt K. *Advanced aromatherapy.* Healing Arts Press, Rochester, 1995.
12. Herbert PR, Barice EJ, Hennekens CH. *Treatment of low back pain: the potential clinical and public health benefits of topical herbal remedies.* The Journal of Alternative and Complementary Medicine, 2014; 20(4): 219-220. doi: 10.1089/acm.2013.0313.
13. Tisserand R, Young R. *Essential oil safety.* 2nd edn. Churchill Livingstone, Edinburgh, 2014.
14. Alsaad A et al. *Toxicology and teratology of the active ingredients of professional therapy MuscleCare products during pregnancy and lactation: a system review.* BMC Complementary and Alternative Medicine, 2015; 15:14. doi: 10.1186/s12906-015-0585-8.
15. Botma M et al. *Laryngeal oedema caused by accidental ingestion of oil of wintergreen.* International Journal of Pediatric Otorhinolaryngology, 2001; 58(3): 229-232. doi: 10.1016/S0165-5876(01)00453-0.
16. Green T et al. *A critical review of the literature to conduct a toxicity assessment for oral exposure to methyl salicylate.* Critical Reviews in Toxicology, 2017; 47(2): 98-120. doi: 10.1080/10408444.2016.1236071.

Yarrow

Identification

Botanical name

Achillea millefolium L.

Synonyms

Milfoil, common yarrow

Family

Asteraceae (Compositae)

Botany and origins

Yarrow is a perennial creeping herb, growing to a height of 10 to 60 cm, with erect stems, lace-like leaves divided into feathery leaflets, and a composite head of numerous tiny, daisy-like flowers, white or pink in colour. It grows wild all over Europe, western Asia and the United States. It is mostly cultivated in Germany, Belgium, Hungary and Yugoslavia.[1]

Method of extraction

Yarrow oil is steam-distilled from leaves and flowering tops of *A. millefolium*.

Characteristics

Yarrow oil is a dark-blue or greenish-blue to dark-olive-coloured oil, with a sharp, somewhat camphoraceous odour, drying out in a sweeter, faint and pleasant note. The bluish colour is due to the presence of azulenes.[1]

Chemical composition

High biodiversity within the yarrow species is responsible for the wide range of chemical constituents.[2] Yarrow oil is generally considered to be of value because of its richness in chamazulene; however, Lawrence states that a survey of literature reveals that the chamazulene-rich yarrow oils are not as common as the other chemotypes.[3]

The chemical composition of yarrow oil produced in Egypt was reported as follows:

β-pinene (2.7%), α-phellandrene (0.9%), limonene (9.7%), terpinene (2.5%), β-phellandrene (59.7%), terpinolene (2.9%), linalool (2.3%), camphor (2.4%), linalyl acetate (6.3%), cadinene (3.3%), neral (1.5%), geranial (0.2%), geranyl acetate (0.4%).[3]

On the other hand, yarrow oil produced from plants harvested from nine different regions in Lithuania was categorised into three groups:

- Group 1: β-pinene/1,8-cineole group
- Group 2: chamazulene group
- Group 3: nerolidol group.[3]

Constituent	Group 1	Group 2	Group 3
α-pinene	3.0-7.4%	3.4-5.3%	2.1-7.1%
camphene	trace-2.7%	0-1.4%	0.6-2.8%
sabinene	3.3-14.0%	3.4-5.2%	2.0-8.5%
β-pinene	11.8-31.1%	9.7-30.2%	5.5-21.3%
myrcene	0.2-2.1%	0.9-2.2%	0.5-1.1%
α-terpinene	trace-1.2%	0-0.7%	0.5-1.4%
p-cymene	0-1.6%	trace-1.9%	0.7-1.3%
1,8-cineole	8.1-17.0%	5.3-16.0%	4.4-9.0%
γ-terpinene	0.3-3.4%	0.2-1.7%	1.1-3.8%
camphor	trace-3.4%	0.3-1.8%	1.5-4.9%
cis-chrysanthenol	0-0.2%	0-1.5%	0.2-0.4%
borneol	trace-4.1%	0.4-3.8%	3.1-6.5%
terpinen-4-ol	0.9-3.4%	1.2-2.1%	1.2-5.5%
α-terpineol	0.2-3.0%	0.6-2.8%	trace-1.3%
cis-chrysanthenyl acetate	-	0-1.7%	0-3.8%
bornyl acetate	0.2-4.0%	0-1.2%	0.3-4.9%
β-caryophyllene	3.5-5.9%	4.5-8.7%	3.4-5.0%
α-humulene	trace-1.5%	0.3-1.4%	0-0.9%
germacrene D	1.1-4.2%	1.9-4.9%	1.4-3.8%
δ-cadinene	0.6-2.4%	0.6-2.4%	0.7-2.5%
(*E*)-nerolidol	0.5-7.8%	0-5.8%	8.2-13.5%
spathulenol	0.5-2.4%	0.5-1.5%	0.3-1.8%
caryophyllene oxide	1.4-8.0%	1.1-5.4%	2.5-5.3%
viridiflorol	0-5.1%	0-6.5%	0.9-3.1%
10-*epi*-γ-eudesmol	0.3-11.0%	0-1.6%	1.2-8.3%
1-*epi*-cubenol	0.3-1.9%	0-2.2%	0.6-2.1%
himachalol	0-1.9%	0-3.5%	0-1.5%
selin-11-en-4α-ol	0.5-3.9%	0-2.2%	1.2-7.0%
α-bisabolone oxide A	0-2.2%	0-0.03%	0.3-3.1%
(*E*,*E*)-farnesol	0-1.7%	0-0.5%	0-2.8%
chamazulene	0-6.8%	9.8-23.2%	0-0.1%

The major chemical components of yarrow essential oil extracted from plants growing at an altitude of 2300 m in Iran were 1,8-cineole (18.6%), camphor (13.9%), borneol (9.4%), terpinolene (8.6%), γ-terpinolene (6.8%), thujone (4.3%), farnesol (2.3%) and chamazulene (2.3%), whereas essential oil extracted from plants grown at 700 m were terpinolene (81%), borneol (4.2%), β-pinene (3.5%) and chamazulene (2.9%).[4]

Adulteration

Lis-Balchin states that yarrow is often used to adulterate German chamomile oil.[5] Arctander states that it could be possible that German chamomile is co-distilled with yarrow; however, he claims that the resulting product would hardly fool anyone familiar with real German chamomile.[1]

Yarrow oil is often adulterated with thuja oil, Siberian fir and synthetic constituents such as isobornyl acetate and camphene.[1]

Pharmacopoeias and standards

At the time of writing, the purity, composition, physico-chemical properties and therapeutic use of yarrow essential oil are not defined in any pharmacopoeia monograph or standard.

History and Traditional Uses

History

The common name for the plant, 'yarrow', is a corruption of its Anglo-Saxon name, *gearwe*, while its specific name, *millefolium*, refers to its finely divided, feathery leaves.[6]

Yarrow was esteemed as a vulnerary, and its old names of Soldier's Wound Wort and Knight's Milfoil testify to this. The term *Achillea* originates from Achilles, the legendary Greek warrior who apparently made an ointment from the leaves, using it to treat his warriors wounded in the siege of Troy.[6]

By the 1450s, yarrow was extensively used for its therapeutic properties. Herbalist Gerard recommended the herb for headaches and toothache, and to stop nosebleed. Culpeper informed us that yarrow is 'drying and binding'. He recommended a poultice for treating piles and an ointment of the leaves to cure wounds.[6]

The herb is still prescribed for its diaphoretic, stimulant and tonic effects, mainly in warm infusions as a way of opening the pores to induce perspiration in the treatment of colds and influenza.[6]

Traditional medicine

The *Achillea* genus is widespread all over the world, and its species have been used by local people in folk and traditional herbal medicines.

In New Mexico and southern Colorado, *A. millefolium* is called *plumajillo*, or 'little feather', because of the shape of the leaves. Native Americans and early settlers used yarrow for its astringent qualities that made it effective in wound healing and to stop bleeding.[7]

Herbal

The herb is recommended for lack of appetite, stomach cramps, flatulence, gastritis, enteritis, internal or external bleeding of all kinds, wounds, sores and skin rashes.[8,9]

The fresh herb is used as a poultice for the treatment of sores and wounds, while the dried herb is recommended for internal bleeding, especially menstrual and haemorrhoidal.[8]

The German Commission E recommends yarrow herb internally for loss of appetite and dyspeptic ailments. As a sitz bath, yarrow is recommended for painful, cramp-like conditions of psychosomatic origins.[10]

In Western herbalism, yarrow is also recommended for treatment of fever, the common cold, essential hypertension, thrombotic conditions and amenorrhoea.[11]

Most of the pharmacological research confirming the therapeutic actions of yarrow involves the use of the aqueous alcoholic extract of yarrow.[11]

Food, perfumery and flavouring

Yarrow oil is not commonly used in perfumery. Yarrow oil is used in bitters and vermouths.[8]

Therapeutics

Pharmacology and clinical studies

Anti-inflammatory activity

The sesquiterpene compounds found in yarrow contribute to the oil's anti-inflammatory activity.[7]

Antimicrobial activity

An in vitro study confirmed the antimicrobial activity of yarrow essential oil against methicillin-resistant *Staphylococcus aureus* (MRSA), *S. aureus*, *Pseudomonas aeruginosa*, *Escherichia coli* and *Bacillus cereus*.[12]

Yarrow oil from France confirmed the antimicrobial activity against common bacteria and fungi.[13]

Actions

Actions commonly cited in aromatherapy

Anti-inflammatory, antirheumatic, antiseptic, antispasmodic, astringent, carminative, cicatrisant, diaphoretic, digestive, emmenagogue, expectorant, haemostatic, stomachic, tonic, wound healing[14,15]

Actions supported by clinical studies

Anti-inflammatory, antimicrobial

Comment

Yarrow essential oil is very complex as it contains monoterpene hydrocarbons, monoterpene alcohols, esters, sesquiterpenes, lactones, oxides and ketones. It is likely that the chemistry of the oil contributes to the many properties traditionally attributed to the oil.

Many studies have confirmed the diverse therapeutic actions of the herbal extract of yarrow; however, very few studies have confirmed the bioactivities of yarrow essential oil. There is a chance that many of the properties that we have assigned to yarrow oil have been appropriated from the herbal extract of yarrow.

Tisserand & Young state that yarrow is a very polymorphic species.[16] This is confirmed by the chemical variability that exists in yarrow oil. This may significantly impact on the pharmacological activity of the oil.

Aromatherapy Uses

Clinical aromatherapy

Circulatory system

Yarrow oil is beneficial for treating varicose veins and haemorrhoids. For this purpose, it should be blended with cypress oil and used as a compress or liniment.[17]

Digestive system

Yarrow oil may be used to alleviate stomach cramps and gall bladder pain.[14,18]

Integumentary system

Yarrow oil is highly valued for its treatment of wounds. Its antiseptic, astringent, styptic and anti-inflammatory properties contribute to its excellent affinity with skin problems, and it may be used to soothe irritated skin and to help heal infections. Used in compresses, it may also be excellent for eczema and allergic skin reactions.[14,15,17,18,19]

Reproductive system

For infections of the pelvic region, yarrow oil is recommended in a sitz bath or compress. For vaginal infections and irritations, a douche is recommended.[18] It is also recommended to help alleviate menstrual pain because it is an emmenagogue.[18,19]

Yarrow oil is recommended as a balancing remedy during menopause. During hormonal system changes, the oil helps keep psychological equilibrium intact and supports reorganisation of shifting energies.[18]

Energetics, psyche and subtle uses

Energetics

According to the principles of TCM, yarrow oil is *cooling* and *drying*. It is recommended for inflammatory conditions. Yarrow also stimulates the *Liver* and regulates the flow of *Qi*, making it beneficial for indigestion, intestinal colic and releasing stagnant *Qi* and the blocked emotions that go with it.[19]

Subtle

Fischer-Rizzi states that yarrow helps to balance *Yin* and *Yang* energies. She explains that the scent of yarrow makes possible the meeting of heaven and earth. The oil balances the highs and lows, internal and external, so that our thoughts may be in heaven while our feet remain solidly on the ground.[18]

Mojay compares yarrow to everlasting oil, which is ideal for deeply repressed anger and bitterness. Yarrow is considered most appropriate for people whose feelings of anger and rage are subconsciously linked to vulnerability and emotional wounds. It is, therefore, beneficial to help such people release the bitterness of hidden rage and relinquish their tears.[19]

Fischer-Rizzi says that yarrow helps us reconcile opposing forces. This makes the oil a perfect companion in times of major life changes such as mid-life crisis, menopause or other times of transition.[18]

Worwood states that yarrow is the fragrance for dreaming and visionary experiences. It helps us tap into our intuition.[20]

Zeck states that yarrow will bring balance and stability to our life whenever we need emotional stability or at times of major life changes.[21]

Dosage and Administration

Blending

Aromatherapy

For the treatment of wounds, consider blending yarrow oil with essential oils such as everlasting, frankincense, lavender or myrrh.

For alleviating menstrual pain, consider blending yarrow oil with essential oils such as clary sage, Roman chamomile, lavender or sweet marjoram.

To give us courage and strength in times of major life changes, consider blending yarrow oil with essential oils such as cypress, fragonia, everlasting or neroli.

Perfumery

The oil is not commonly used in perfumery; however, it could be used for its unique fresh-herbaceous note.

Mode of administration

Bath

Full body bath, foot bath, sitz bath

Topical

Compress, massage, ointment, skin care

Inhalation

Direct inhalation, diffuser, oil vaporiser

Safety Profile

General safety

Yarrow oil has been reported to be non-toxic and non-irritating.[14] The sesquiterpene lactones found in yarrow are frequently responsible for dermatitis of an allergic origin.[9]

Contraindications

No contraindications known.

Toxicity

Yarrow oil contains several ketones – camphor, thujone and isoartemisia ketone. Whitton states that, while some ketones are gentle and safe to use on the skin and often have mucolytic properties, they can be neurotoxic in large and prolonged doses. Whitton explains that yarrow should not be used continuously or too frequently, and recommends never using it on babies, children or pregnant women.[22]

However, Tisserand & Young cite a study in which yarrow oil inhibited convulsions induced by cardazol, a GABA antagonist, suggesting that the presence of thujone (a potentiator of GABA-mediated responses) in the oil may not present a risk.[16]

My concern is that there is too much chemical variability in yarrow oil, so it is important to know the exact chemical composition of the yarrow oil you are using.

Regulatory guidelines

Yarrow oil does not have GRAS status; it has been approved for use in alcoholic beverages only.[8]

References

1. Arctander S. *Perfume and flavor materials of natural origin.* Allured Publishing, Carol Stream, 1994.
2. Judzentiene A. *Atypical chemical profiles of wild yarrow (Achillea millefolium L.) essential oils.* Records of Natural Products, 2016; 10(2): 262-268.

Y

3. Lawrence BM. *Progress in essential oils – yarrow oil.* Perfumer and Flavorist, 2003; 28: 63-74.
4. Mazandarani M et al. *Essential oil composition and antibacterial activity of Achillea millefolium L. from different regions in North east of Iran.* Journal of Medicinal Plant Research, 2013; 7(16): 1063-1069. doi: 10.5897/JMPR12.961.
5. Lis-Balchin M. *Aromatherapy science – a guide for healthcare professionals.* Pharmaceutical Press, London, 2006.
6. Le Strange R. *A history of herbal plants.* Angus and Robertson, United Kingdom, 1977.
7. Saeidnia S et al. *A review on phytochemistry and medicinal properties of the genus Achillea.* DARU, 2011; 19(3): 173-186.
8. Khan I, Abourashed E. *Leung's encyclopedia of common natural ingredients used in food, drugs and cosmetics.* 3rd edn. John Wiley & Sons, New Jersey, 2010.
9. Bruneton J. *Pharmacognosy.* 2nd edn. Lavoisier Publishing, Paris, 1999.
10. Blumenthal M et al. *The complete German commission E monographs: therapeutic guide to herbal medicine.* American Botanical Council, Austin, 1998.
11. Bone K. *A clinical guide to blending liquid herbs.* Churchill Livingstone, Edinburgh, 2003.
12. Sevindik E et al. *Determination of the chemical composition and antimicrobial activity of the essential oils of Teucrium polium and Achillea millefolium grown under North Anatolian ecological conditions.* Biotechnology & Biotechnological Equipment, 2016; 30(2): 375-380. doi: 10.1080/13102818.2015.1131626.
13. El-Kalamouni C et al. *Antioxidant and antimicrobial activities of the essential oil of Achillea millefolium L. grown in France.* Medicines, 2017; 4(2): 30. doi: 10.3390/medicines4020030.
14. Lawless J. *The encyclopaedia of essential oils.* Element Books, Shaftesbury, 1992.
15. Lavabre M. *Aromatherapy workbook.* Healing Arts Press, Rochester, 1997.
16. Tisserand R, Young R. *Essential oil safety.* 2nd edn. Churchill Livingstone, Edinburgh, 2014.
17. Schnaubelt K. *Advanced aromatherapy.* Healing Arts Press, Rochester, 1995.
18. Fischer-Rizzi S. *Complete aromatherapy handbook.* Sterling Publishing, New York, 1990.
19. Mojay G. *Aromatherapy for healing the spirit.* Healing Arts Press, Rochester, 1999.
20. Worwood VA. *The fragrant heavens.* Transworld Publishers, London, 1999.
21. Zeck R. *The blossoming heart – aromatherapy for healing and transformation.* Aroma Tours, East Ivanhoe, 2004.
22. Whitton S. *Yarrow.* Aromatherapy Quarterly, 1994; 40: 14-17.

Ylang ylang

Identification

Botanical name

Cananga odorata (Lam.) Hook.f. & Thomson

Synonyms

Cananga

Family

Annonaceae

Botany and origins

Ylang ylang originates from South East Asia, although it is now native in Burma, Malaysia, Papua New Guinea and other Pacific Islands. It was introduced to the tropical countries of Africa, Asia, the Caribbean and the French colonies of the Indian Ocean.[1]

Ylang ylang essential oil is primarily produced in Indonesia and Madagascar, with smaller amounts from Réunion, Comoro Island and the Philippines.[1]

Cananga is a fast growing, tall, evergreen tree which grows up to 35 m; however, under cultivation it is pruned to about 3 m. The tree bears numerous large, yellow-green, strongly scented flowers. It flowers all year-round; however, the main flower harvests are in the early dry season.[1]

Two types of oil are produced from the flowers of *C. odorata*: cananga oil from forma *macrophylla* and ylang ylang oil from forma *genuina*. Cananga oil has a higher sesquiterpene content but is low in alcohols and esters; conversely, ylang ylang contains a proportion of alcohols and esters.[1]

Method of extraction

Ylang ylang essential oil is produced by steam and water distillation of the freshly picked flowers from *C. odorata.* Distillation is carried out in small stills since the flowers would suffer considerably by the weight and pressure of a heavy charge of flowers.[2]

Modern Madagascan distilleries produce four and often five fractions or grades of ylang ylang:

extra, first, second and third. The quality and price decreases in the same order.[1]

The fractions are usually separated by controlling the specific gravity of the distillate. By controlling the specific gravity, producers make the interruptions at the moment when they feel that the oil can be classified within one of these groups.[1]

However, Arctander states that there are no standards for the physico-chemical properties of ylang ylang extra or any of the other grades. He claims it is usually left to the distillers' discretion to make the correct fractionation during the distillation.[2]

The extra is usually considered the most desirable grade and is accordingly the most expensive, even though it does usually amount to almost half the yield of the oil.[2]

Arctander states that most people are simply after a good 'extra' oil and a good 'third' oil and that there is no interest in the first- or second-grade oils.[2]

The four or five grades of ylang ylang are fractionated according to the following approximate distillation times and specific gravity:[3]

- Ylang ylang extra superior comes from the first half hour of distillation. Its specific gravity is > 0.965.
- Ylang ylang extra comes during the next hour of distillation. Its specific gravity is 0.955-0.965.
- Ylang ylang 1st grade is obtained during the third hour of distillation. Its specific gravity is 0.945-0.955.
- Ylang ylang 2nd grade is obtained between the fourth and sixth hour of distillation. Its specific gravity is 0.932-0.940.
- Ylang ylang 3rd grade is collected after the sixth hour of distillation and will often continue for up to 16 hours. This is why it often has a burnt note. The specific gravity should be 0.905-0.910.

A ylang ylang complete oil is often available. The name suggests that the oil should be the natural distillate from the uninterrupted water and steam distillation of the *C. odorata* flowers; however, the complete is made by blending ylang ylang extra, grade 1 and grade 2 fractions.[2]

Characteristics

Ylang ylang extra is a pale yellow oil with a powerful floral and intensely sweet odour. The base note becomes more pleasant, softer and sweet.[2]

Ylang ylang complete is usually a yellowish, somewhat oily liquid with a powerful and intensely sweet, but soft balsamic floral odour with a floral woody undertone.[2]

Ylang ylang third grade is a yellowish oily liquid with a sweet-floral odour and balsamic-woody base note, and a tenacious and very sweet-balsamic undertone.[2]

Chemical composition

The chemical composition of the various grades of ylang ylang was reported as follows:[1]

Constituent	Extra	1st grade	2nd grade	3rd grade
α-pinene	0.3%	0.1%	0.1%	0.1%
p-cresyl methyl ether	8.4%	3.1%	1.0%	0.4%
benzyl alcohol	0.5%	0.2%	-	-
p-cresol	0.1%	0.1%	-	-
methyl benzoate	4.0%	1.0%	0.3%	0.1%
linalool	10.3%	5.5%	3.2%	2.0%
benzyl acetate	12.6%	4.2%	1.2%	0.5%
α-terpineol	0.1%	-	-	-
methyl salicylate	0.1%	0.1%	-	-
geraniol	0.2%	0.2%	0.2%	-
linalyl acetate	0.2%	0.2%	0.2%	-
safrole	0.3%	0.1%	0.1%	-
methyl anthranilate	0.1%	-	-	-
eugenol	0.2%	0.2%	0.4%	0.3%
geranyl acetate	4.0%	3.0%	2.2%	2.0%
isoeugenol	0.2%	0.4%	-	-
β-caryophyllene	6.8%	11.5%	12.8%	16.3%
α-caryophyllene	3.1%	4.2%	4.1%	8.8%
farnesene	18.0%	16.8%	17.0%	21.0%
δ-cadinene	8.9%	15.1%	20.4%	16.3%
γ-cadinene	2.0%	5.3%	7.0%	7.5%
nerolidol	0.5%	0.8%	0.5%	1.8%
(*Z*),(*E*)-farnesol	0.9%	1.7%	1.7%	1.4%
benzyl benzoate	4.3%	8.5%	9.7%	1.7%
benzyl salicylate	1.9%	1.2%	2.7%	1.7%

Adulteration

Adulteration of ylang ylang essential oil occurs frequently. The various fractions – extra, first, second or third – are often blended together. The blending of the fractions fortunately will not affect the purity of the oil as all are from the same botanical source. However, *Cananga odorata* (Lam.) Hook. F. Thomson forma *macrophylla*, commonly known as cananga oil, is also used for adulteration. Blending is also done with linalyl acetate, benzyl acetate, synthetic geraniol from various sources, methyl benzoate, benzyl alcohol, methyl salicylate, bay leaf oil, cedarwood terpenes, lavandin residues and traces of synthetic ethyl vanillin.[4]

Arctander also states that it is not uncommon in

Indonesia and the Philippines for the ylang ylang flowers to be contaminated with the flowers of *Artabotrys suaveolens*.[2]

The specific gravity was usually considered the most effective way to verify the grade of the ylang ylang. However, recently it was found that heating ylang ylang 3rd grade would increase its specific gravity from the low 0.900 to the mid 0.950 – essentially turning ylang ylang 3rd grade into ylang ylang extra. Hellivan states that this type of adulteration of heating ylang ylang 3rd grade and blending it with ylang ylang extra has created a crisis and damaged the integrity of the ylang ylang industry.[3]

Pharmacopoeias and standards

The purity, composition and physico-chemical properties of ylang ylang essential oil are defined in ISO 3063: 2004 Oil of Ylang Ylang (*Cananga odorata* (Lam.) Hook. f. et Thomson forma *genuina*).

History and Traditional Uses

History

The history of ylang ylang oil is very recent. Weiss states that the first distillation of ylang ylang occurred in the middle of the nineteenth century in the Philippines. The introduction of ylang ylang to Réunion is credited to a French expedition under a Captain d'Etchevery in 1770, although the oil was not produced for another 100 years. By the end of the nineteenth century, commercial plantations with about 200,000 trees were established. Large volumes of high-quality ylang ylang oil were produced between 1918 and 1928, but the world depression of the 1930s and competition from Madagascar caused a major decline in the Réunion ylang ylang plantations.[1]

The cananga trees were introduced to Madagascar on the small island of Nossi-Be. The ylang ylang industry in Madagascar is credited to Rev Raimbault. By 1950, eight large and many smaller distilleries were in operation. Cananga was introduced to the Comoros at the beginning of the twentieth century. By the early 1980s there were reported to be nearly a million trees.[1]

Traditional medicine

In Java and Vietnam, the dried flowers of *C. odorata* are used to treat malaria-like symptoms. The fresh flowers are pound into a paste and used for treating asthma. Traditional healers from Northern Mariana Islands use the flowers and bark to treat pneumonia and stomach ache.[5]

Mojay explains that the medicinal properties of ylang ylang were first identified at the beginning of the twentieth century by French chemists Garnier and Rechler. They discovered that the oil was effective against malaria, typhus and infections of the intestinal tract.[6]

Food, perfumery and flavouring

Ylang ylang has long been considered one of the most important essential oils in perfumery. The higher grades are generally used in perfumes, while the lower grades are used for soaps and detergents.[7]

Therapeutics

Pharmacology and clinical studies

Many pharmacological studies involving ylang ylang essential oil have been published. A systemic review of these studies will not be attempted. Rather, I have chosen a selection of studies that support the traditional and clinical uses.

Antiepileptic activity

Ylang ylang oil was found to be one of the most popular choices from a range of essential oils used in a clinical trial to examine the effectiveness of essential oils to control epileptic seizures.

Three methods of using the essential oils were employed:

- hypnosis, where the patients were taught autohypnosis and once in the hypnotic state, were invited to smell their chosen oil
- inhaling the essential oil from a pillow three times a week on going to bed, accompanied with six, twice weekly full body massages with the same essential oil
- a combination of the first two but without the bedtime inhalation of method two.

In all three methods, the patients were encouraged to smell the oil if a seizure was threatening or likely. The results of the study indicated that one-third of the patients that used aromatherapy massage and hypnosis were seizure-free after one year; many were seizure-free after two years, although there were relapses, particularly in the aromatherapy massage-only group. The hypnosis-only group was the least successful. The most successful group was the combination of aromatherapy massage and hypnosis. While this trial was not a properly controlled study, it does provide the basis for more studies to examine the potential role of aromatherapy for the management of epileptic seizures.[8]

Antimicrobial activity

Ylang ylang oil demonstrated relatively low antibacterial activity against *E. coli*. The oil also did not show any antimicrobial activity against *Malassezia furfur*, which is a fungal pathogen associated with seborrhoeic dermatitis. On the

Y

other hand, another study demonstrated that *C. odorata* oil with germacrene D (20%) and β-caryophyllene (17%) exhibited slight fungicidal activity against *Trichophyton mentagrophytes* using agar diffusion assay.[5]

Anxiolytic activity

A pilot study with 34 professionals from a nursing group participated in a study to examine the effect of ylang ylang oil applied by cutaneous application or inhalation on anxiety, self-esteem perception, and physiological parameters such as blood pressure and body temperature. The study verified that ylang ylang oil significantly altered the self-esteem perception in the three groups; however, the study also concluded that there was no difference in the analysis between groups for anxiety or for physiological parameters.[9]

An in vivo study examined the anxiolytic activity of ylang ylang oil by inhalation on mice. The study confirmed that ylang ylang essential oil had an anxiolytic effect. It was suggested that the major constituent benzyl benzoate might act on the 5-HTnergic and DAnergic pathways.[10]

Hypotensive activity

Fifty-two human subjects were divided into three groups: an essential oil group, a placebo group and a control group to examine the effects of aromatherapy on blood pressure and stress responses. A blend of lavender, ylang ylang and bergamot was used by inhalation method once a day for four weeks. To evaluate the effects, blood pressure and pulse, serum cortisol levels, catecholamine levels, subjective stress and state anxiety were measured before and after the treatment in the three groups.[11]

The blood pressure, pulse, subjective stress, state anxiety and serum cortisol levels were significantly statistically different. The results suggest that inhalation of essential oils can be considered an effective nursing intervention that reduces stress responses and serum cortisol, as well as the blood pressure of clients with essential hypertension.[11]

Another study using 44 human participants divided into an experimental group and a control group also found that aromatherapy was effective in lowering systolic blood pressure and sympathetic nervous system activity. This time a blend of lemon, lavender and ylang ylang oils was prepared in a ratio of 2:2:1 and the blend was administered by inhalation.[12]

Another study investigated the effects of essential oil inhalation on the 24-hour ambulatory blood pressure and salivary cortisol level in 83 prehypertensive and hypertensive subjects. The experimental group was asked to inhale a blend of lavender, ylang ylang, sweet marjoram and neroli essential oils (20:15:10:2), whereas the placebo group inhaled an artificial fragrance. The daytime diastolic blood pressure of the experimental group presented with significant decreases in comparison with the measurements of the placebo and control group. There was no significant difference in night-time diastolic blood pressures.[13]

The daytime systolic blood pressures during the 24-hour ambulatory blood pressure measurement of the experimental group also presented with significant decreases in comparison to the placebo and control groups. The experimental group also displayed significant decreases in the concentration of salivary cortisol in comparison to the two other groups. It was suggested that essential oils have an immediate and continuous effect on the reduction of blood pressure and stress reduction.[13]

A study examined the effects of ylang ylang oil on blood pressure by inhalation on 29 healthy men who were randomly divided into two groups – ylang ylang group and control group. The results demonstrated that ylang ylang significantly decreased the systolic and diastolic blood pressure and reduced the heart rate. This study confirmed that ylang ylang oil inhibited the sympathetic nervous system, whereas it activated the parasympathetic nervous system.[14]

Sedative activity

The inhalation of ylang ylang oil significantly decreased both systolic and diastolic blood pressure and pulse rate, indicating that the inhalation of ylang ylang oil can decrease autonomic nervous system (ANS) arousal. The same study also demonstrated that the subjects felt more attentive and alert after inhaling ylang ylang. It was suggested that the effect of inhaling ylang ylang oil is characterised as 'harmonisation', which resulted in the uncoupling of physiological (reduced ANS arousal) and behavioural arousal processes (increased behavioural activation).[15]

A study investigated the effects of ylang ylang oil on human physiological parameters and self-evaluation after transdermal absorption. 40 healthy human volunteers participated in the study. Ylang ylang oil caused a significant decrease in blood pressure and a significant increase in skin temperature. At a behavioural level, the subjects in the ylang ylang oil group rated themselves more calm and relaxed than the people in the control group.[16]

A study revealed that ylang ylang oil aroma acted significantly differently on the cognitive performance of a healthy group of human volunteers as compared to the control group and the peppermint group. The ylang ylang group experienced reduced alertness and increased calmness, but no enhancement of cognitive performance and a longer processing speed.[17]

Actions

Actions commonly cited in aromatherapy

Antidepressant, antiseptic, aphrodisiac, hypotensive, nervine, sedative, tonic[18,19]

Actions supported by clinical studies

Anxiolytic, hypotensive, sedative

Comment

Many studies have shown that ylang ylang essential oil has sedative, relaxing and harmonisation effects. This explains why ylang ylang oil is commonly used in aromatherapy to reduce blood pressure and stress.

Holmes explains that ylang ylang has both a relaxing and a regulating action. He refers to it as a 'deep systemic relaxant' for treating tense conditions in their acute phase such as nervous tension, anxiety, spasms, while also calming brain functions and enhancing parasympathetic activity.[20]

I agree with Holmes when he describes ylang ylang as a remedy for the soul as much as for the body, and that it deserves more exploration than it has received thus far.

Y

Aromatherapy Uses

Clinical aromatherapy

Circulatory system

Ylang ylang is recommended for treating palpitations and reducing high blood pressure.[6,18,19,21]

Nervous system

Ylang ylang is known for its ability to slow down over-rapid breathing and over-rapid heartbeat. These symptoms are usually associated with shock, anxiety and anger.[18,19,22]

Holmes states that ylang ylang promotes emotional stability and can be used to reduce irritability, moodiness, frustration, anger and emotional instability. It is also recommended for acute depression, with anxiety or agitation and feelings of despair and self-destructiveness.[20]

The oil is renowned as an antidepressant and is particularly beneficial for treating nervous depression, and feelings of anger, rage and frustration.[21] Ylang ylang is commonly classified as an aphrodisiac. This is undoubtedly due to ylang ylang's ability to reduce stress and anxiety, often associated with sexual inadequacy.[6,19,22]

Reproductive system

Ylang ylang has proven beneficial for treating PMS, especially associated with extreme mood swings that occur just before the onset of menstruation. For this purpose, Fischer-Rizzi recommends blending ylang ylang with clary sage and neroli. This blend should be used in a bath, massage oil or vaporiser.[21]

Skin care

Added to a skin care preparations, ylang ylang oil is beneficial in softening and balancing the moisture in the skin. It is recommended in hair care to treat split ends.[21] It can be used in a shampoo base, or massaged into the tips of the hair after shampooing with a base oil such as apricot kernel or jojoba.

Ylang ylang is recommended for both dry and oily skin and is reputed to have a balancing action on sebum production.[18,19,22]

Energetics, psyche and subtle uses

Energetics

Ylang ylang is *cooling*, clearing *heat* from the *Heart*, when severe nervous tension leads to palpitations, hypertension and tachycardia.[6]

According to the principles of TCM, ylang ylang regulates the *Qi* and harmonises the *Shen*. It also helps to spread the *Liver Qi*. Whenever the *Liver Qi* is constrained and we experience disharmony of the *Shen*, we may experience feelings of moodiness, anxiety, irritability, restlessness and insomnia.[20]

Ylang ylang has an affinity with the Wood and Fire Elements.

Personality

Fischer-Rizzi best describes the ylang ylang personality:

> *The spirit of ylang ylang usually fits the person naturally drawn to it. Upon inhaling ylang ylang with its heavy seductive, sweet aroma one can imagine a fiery, temperamental, passionate and erotic person with an awesome radiance and confidence never losing her balance. She would also dress in bright and colourful clothing and loves to wear jewellery.*[21]

Therefore, ylang ylang is recommended for the woman who does not allow herself to live, who hides her femininity, dresses drably, and does not care what she looks like. She lacks self-confidence, may be extremely frustrated, and appears nervous, depressed and tense.[21]

Fischer-Rizzi recommends using ylang ylang for men to become less harsh towards themselves and others. It allows them to get in touch with their feminine side and nurtures their understanding and intuition. Many men may find the rich floral scent of ylang ylang overwhelming. If this is the case, ylang ylang should be blended with sweet orange, bergamot or sandalwood.[21]

The ylang ylang person is extremely passionate and feminine, charismatic, erotic and sensual. Neither male or female ylang ylang personalities are happy alone, flourishing best when they have an audience to applaud their achievements. They are described as having a fiery, passionate nature and would sacrifice everything for love. However, they fall in and out of love easily.[23]

Worwood states that ylang ylang personalities prefer jobs that allow them to express the aesthetic side of life, or any profession that involves exciting physical pursuits. She also explains that they can easily make a mountain out of a molehill. If they do not have their own way, they will get upset and unleash their anger.[23]

According to Myers-Briggs personality types, the ylang ylang personality is likely to be an ESFP. ESFPs are friendly, witty, charming and talkative. They value and nurture their relationships, give generously, without expecting anything in return. They are spontaneous and playful, and enjoy everything they do and see. People who share their sense of fun and adventure are their favourite companions. They turn everything into a fun-filled event. They enjoy good things in life – music, dance, food, drink and entertainment. They avoid being alone. They like working in a lively and stimulating atmosphere with friendly, energetic people. They can be good at dealing with the public. They like variety and frequent change of tasks or jobs. They are enthusiastic, high-spirited and have lots of energy.

Subtle

Ylang ylang helps to create a feeling of peace and dispels anger, which is often a hindrance to meditation, healing and all spiritual activities.[24]

Keim Loughran & Bull explain that ylang ylang helps us to confidently deal with our fears and to recognise whether or not they are appropriate or useful.[25]

Zeck explains that ylang ylang will allow you to transform your anger and become mindful of how you are affecting others. It promotes the capacity for growth and deepening of relationships.[26]

Ylang ylang oil helps strengthen the sacral chakra by promoting our sexuality and creativity. It also supports the solar plexus chakra by promoting self-confidence, and nurtures the heart chakra by promoting love.

Dosage and Administration

Blending

Aromatherapy

To alleviate the symptoms of depression, consider blending ylang ylang oil with essential oils such as bergamot, frankincense, geranium, lavender, jasmine absolute, mandarin, neroli, rose absolute, sweet orange, patchouli or sandalwood.

For the relief of anxiety, frustration, irritability, nervous tension and stress, consider blending ylang ylang oil with essential oils such as bergamot, Atlas cedarwood, fragonia, frankincense, geranium, lemon, lavender, palmarosa, petitgrain, neroli, sweet orange, patchouli, rose absolute, rosemary or sandalwood.

As a cardiovascular relaxant or for reducing hypertension, consider blending ylang ylang oil with essential oils such as lavender, may chang, sweet marjoram or neroli.

Perfumery

Ylang ylang extra is mainly used in high-class perfumes of a floral and heavy oriental type. Arctander states that there would not be any floral type perfume where ylang ylang was not used.[2]

Ylang ylang blends well with bergamot, resin oils such as benzoin, Peru balsam and opopanax, and spice oils such as cinnamon and clove, and certainly complements other strong florals such as gardenia absolute, tuberose absolute and jasmine absolute. It also complements sweet citrus oils such as sweet orange and mandarin, and blends perfectly with sandalwood oil.

Mode of administration

Bath

Full body bath, foot bath

Topical

Compress, massage, ointment, skin care

Inhalation

Direct inhalation, diffuser, oil vaporiser

Safety Profile

General safety

Ylang ylang oil is non-toxic, non-irritating and non-sensitising. Excessive use may cause nausea or headaches.[18,22]

Tisserand & Young state that there is a moderate risk of skin sensitisation, and caution should be exercised on people with hypersensitive, diseased or damaged skin, and children, under two years of age.[27]

According to IFRA guidelines, the maximum dermal use level for ylang ylang is 0.8%. Tisserand & Young confirm that there is no clear consensus on which constituent is responsible for the risk of skin reactions. They suspect isoeugenol.[27]

Opdyke states that when ylang ylang oil was tested at 10% dilution on 25 human volunteers, it was not irritating.[28]

Contraindications

No contraindications known.

Regulatory guidelines

Ylang ylang oil has GRAS status.

References

1. Weiss EA. *Essential oil crops.* CAB International, Wallingford, 1997.
2. Arctander S. *Perfume and flavor materials of natural origin.* Allured Publishing, Carol Stream, 1994.
3. Hellivan PJ. *Natural stories: ylang ylang.* Perfumer & Flavorist, 2008; 33: 47-51.
4. Schmidt E, Wanner J. *Adulteration of essential oils.* In Baser KHC, Buchbauer G. eds. *Handbook of essential oils – science, technology and applications.* 2nd edn. CRC Press, Boca Raton, 2016: 707-745.
5. Tan LTH et al. *Traditional uses, phytochemistry and bioactivities of cananga odorata (ylang-ylang).* Evidence-Based Complementary and Alternative Medicine, 2015; 2015: 896314. doi: 10.1155/2015/896314.
6. Mojay G. *Aromatherapy for healing the spirit.* Healing Arts Press, Rochester, 1999.
7. Khan I, Abourashed E. *Leung's encyclopedia of common natural ingredients used in food, drugs and cosmetics.* 3rd edn. John Wiley & Sons, New Jersey, 2010.
8. Betts T. *Use of aromatherapy (with or without hypnosis) in the treatment of intractable epilepsy – a two-year follow-up study.* Seizure, 2003; 12(8): 534-538. Cited in Quintessential Aromatics database, 2013.
9. Gnatta JR et al. *Aromatherapy with ylang ylang for anxiety and self-esteem: a pilot study.* Revista da Escola de Enfermagem da USP, 2014; 48(3): 492-499. doi: 10.1590/S0080-623420140000300015.
10. Zhang N et al. *The anxiolytic effect of essential oil of Cananga odorata exposure on mice and determination of its major active constituents.* Phytomedicine, 2016; 23(14): 1727-1734. doi: 10.1016/j.phymed.2016.10.017.
11. Hwang JH. *The effects of the inhalation method using essential oils on blood pressure and stress responses of clients with essential hypertension.* Journal of Korean Academy of Nursing, 2006; 36(7): 1123-1134. Cited in Quintessential Aromatics database, 2013.
12. Cha JH et al. *Effects of aromatherapy on changes in the autonomic nervous system, aortic pulse wave velocity and aortic augmentation index in patients with essential hypertension.* Journal of Korean Academy of Nursing, 2010; 40(4): 705-713. Cited in Quintessential Aromatics database, 2013.
13. Kim IH et al. *Essential oil inhalation on blood pressure and salivary cortisol levels in prehypertensive and hypertensive subjects.* Evidence-Based Complementary and Alternative Medicine, 2012; 2012: 984203. doi: 10.1155/2012/984203.
14. Jung DJ et al. *Effects of Ylang-ylang aroma on blood pressure and heart rate in healthy men.* Journal of Exercise Rehabilitation, 2013; 9(2): 250-255. doi: 10.12965/jer.130007.
15. Hongratanaworakit T, Buchbauer G. *Evaluation of the harmonising effect of ylang ylang oil on humans after inhalation.* Planta Medica, 2004; 70(7): 632-636. Cited in Quintessential Aromatics database, 2013.
16. Hongratanaworakit T, Buchbauer G. *Relaxing effect of ylang ylang on humans after transdermal absorption.* Phytotherapy Research, 2006; 20(9): 758-763. doi:10.1002/ptr.1950.
17. Moss M et al. *Modulation of cognitive performance and mood by aromas of peppermint and ylang-ylang.* International Journal of Neuroscience, 2008; 118(1): 59-77. Cited in Quintessential Aromatics database, 2013
18. Lawless J. *The encyclopaedia of essential oils.* Element Books, Shaftesbury, 1992.
19. Lavabre M. *Aromatherapy workbook.* Healing Arts Press, Rochester, 1997.
20. Holmes P. *Aromatica: a clinical guide to essential oil therapeutics – Vol. I.* Singing Dragon, London, 2016.
21. Fischer-Rizzi S. *Complete aromatherapy handbook.* Sterling Publishing, New York, 1990.
22. Davis P. *Aromatherapy: an A-Z.* 2nd edn. C.W. Daniel Company, Saffron Walden, 1999.
23. Worwood VA. *The fragrant mind.* Transworld Publishers, London, 1995.
24. Davis P. *Subtle aromatherapy.* C.W. Daniel Company, Saffron Walden, 1991.
25. Keim Loughran J, Bull R. *Aromatherapy anointing oils.* Frog, Berkeley, 2001.
26. Zeck R. *The blossoming heart – aromatherapy for healing and transformation.* Aroma Tours, East Ivanhoe, 2004.
27. Tisserand R, Young R. *Essential oil safety.* 2nd edn. Churchill Livingstone, Edinburgh, 2014.
28. Opdyke DLJ. *Monographs on fragrance raw materials.* Pergamon Press, Oxford, 1979.

Y

Appendices

Appendix 1 • Glossary

Appendix 2 • Properties

Appendix 3 • Essential oils

Appendix 4 • A typical material safety data sheet

Appendix 5 • Summary of cautions and contraindications

Appendix 6 • Useful addresses

Appendix 1 • Glossary

Absolute
Products obtained from a concrete, a pomade or a resinoid by extraction with ethanol at room temperature. The resulting ethanol solution is generally cooled and filtered to eliminate the waxes. The ethanol is then eliminated by distillation.

AchE
Acetylcholinesterase is an enzyme that catalyzes the breakdown of acetylcholine and some other choline esters that function as neurotransmitters.

ACOS
Australian Certified Organic Standard.

Adulteration
Any material added to a whole, genuine essential oil which alters its original composition or odour.

Albedo
The pith or inner rind of a citrus fruit.

Alcohol
An organic compound containing one or more hydroxyl groups attached directly to carbon atoms.

Aldehyde
An organic compound containing a carbonyl group of atoms and a hydrogen atom bonded to the carbon atom of the carbonyl group.

Allelopathy
The adverse effect which one plant has on another, caused by the exudation of chemicals into the soil which supresses the growth of nearby plants.

Allergen
A substance which causes an allergic reaction.

Allergy
Tendency to react unfavourably to a certain substance that is normally harmless to most people.

Anaerobic
A type of organic respiration which does not require oxygen. Many bacteria are anaerobic.

Angiogenesis
The induction of blood-vessel growth, often associated with a particular organ or tissue, or with a tumour.

Anticholinergic
An agent that blocks the neurotransmitter acetylcholine in the central and the peripheral nervous system.

Aromacology
The study of the psychological effects of odours, particularly those of essential oils used in aromatherapy.

Aromatic chemicals
Any chemical with an aroma or flavour, which is usually synthetic.

Aromatic water
Aqueous distillates remaining from water or steam distillation after the essential oil has been separated.

Artefact
A compound produced during distillation and other processes, or storage of an essential oil.

Atom
The smallest particle of an element which can take part in a chemical change.

Atomic number
The number of protons in the nucleus of an atom, which is equal to the number of electrons that the atom contains.

Balsam
A natural exudate from a plant.

Benzene ring
The molecular structure of the cyclic, unsaturated, aromatic hydrocarbon benzene C6H6.

Biocide
A chemical agent that destroys life by poisoning, especially a pesticide, herbicide or fungicide.

Biofilm
A complex structure adhering to surfaces that are regularly in contact with water, consisting of colonies of bacteria that secrete a mucilaginous protective coating in which they are encased.

Boiling point
The temperature at which a liquid boils.

CAM
Complementary and alternative medicine.

Carbonyl group
The divalent group of atoms consisting of a carbon atom joined to an oxygen atom by a double bond.

Carboxylic acid
Organic compounds containing one or more carboxyl groups.

Carcinogen
Cancer-causing substance.

Carcinogenesis
Refers to the inception or production and growth of cancer.

Carrier oil
A fixed oil of vegetable origin.

CDC
Centers for Disease Control.

Chassis
The arrangement of glass plates and the surrounding wooden frame used in the enfleurage process.

Chemotype
Variation in the chemical composition of an essential oil produced from two or more plants of the same species.

Chronic
Referring to a disease that develops slowly, persists over a long time, or is recurring.

Chypre
In perfumery, a chypre-style perfume is based on oakmoss and sandalwood.

CITES
Convention on International Trade in Endangered Species of Wild Fauna and Flora.

Clonic
A word applied to short spasmodic movements.

CNS
Central nervous system.

Cohobation
A process of redistillation of the distillation water in order to recover dissolved essential oil.

Concrete
Extracts obtained with non-aqueous solvents from fresh, natural raw materials. A concrete consists mainly of waxy components of plant materials. Mainly prepared for the production of absolutes.

Constituent
Specific component of an essential oil accurately defined.

Coppiced
The regrowth of a tree in the form of thin stems after felling to leave a stump.

Covalent bond
A bond between two atoms consisting of a shared pair of electrons.

COX-2
Cyclooxygenase-2, an enzyme that acts to speed up the production prostaglandins that play a key role in promoting inflammation.

Cultivar
A plant variety produced from a naturally occurring species that has been developed and maintained by cultivation.

Cutaneous
Belonging to the skin.

Cytochrome P450
A collective name for a group of metabolic enzymes found in many tissues, especially the liver. They are responsible for the phase I detoxification of foreign molecules.

Cytotoxicity
The degree to which an agent has specific destructive action on certain cells.

Decarboxylate
A chemical reaction that removes a carboxyl group and replacement with a hydrogen atom.

Diastole
Relaxation phase of the cardiac cycle.

Digestion
Process of breaking down food into absorbable particles.

Distillation
The process of vaporising a substance in a distillation vessel and collecting the product of cooling the vapour in a separate vessel.

EEG
Electroencephalograph – instrument used to study electrical activity of the brain.

Efferent
Carrying away from a given point, such as a motor neuron that carries nerve impulses away from the central nervous system.

Element
A substance composed of atoms. The nuclei of all the atoms contain the same number of protons.

EMA
European Medicines Agency

Endophytes
An organism, especially a fungus or microorganism, that lives inside a plant, in a parasitic or mutualistic relationship.

Enfleurage
The process of extracting essential oil from flowers. The flowers are placed on trays of fat which absorb the oil. The oil is then solvent extracted.

ENFJ
Myers Briggs personality type – extraverting, intuiting, feeling, judging.

ENFP
Myers Briggs personality type – extraverting, intuiting, feeling, perceiving.

ENTJ
Myers Briggs personality type – extraverting, intuiting, thinking, judging.

ENTP
Myers Briggs personality type – extraverting, intuiting, thinking, perceiving.

EPA
Environmental Protection Agency

ESFJ
Myers Briggs personality type – extraverting, sensing, feeling, judging.

ESFP
Myers Briggs personality type – extraverting, sensing, feeling, perceiving.

Essential oil
A product obtained from natural distillation or expression.

Ester
Organic compound formed by the union of an acid and an alcohol with the elimination of water.

ESTJ
Myers Briggs personality type – extraverting, sensing, thinking, judging.

ESTP
Myers Briggs personality type – extraverting, sensing, thinking, perceiving.

Ether
An organic compound which is characterised by the presence of an oxygen atom bonded to two hydrocarbon chains, ring systems or other hydrocarbon molecular structures.

EU
European Union.

Evaporation
The change of a liquid or solid to a gas or vapour phase.

Expression
The physical change of a liquid or solid to the vapour state.

FDA
Food and Drug Administration

Fixative
A material that is capable of prolonging the effects of the main fragrance theme of a perfume.

Fixed oil
Non-volatile, fatty, generally vegetable oil.

Flash point
The temperature, under standardised conditions, at which a liquid begins to evolve flammable vapours.

Flavedo
The coloured part of the rind of a citrus fruit.

Floral water
Also known as hydrosol. The water collected when plants are distilled to extract essential oils.

Fougére
Fougére style perfumes are based on coumarin in combination with oakmoss and lavender.

Fractional distillation
A distillation process in which portions of the distillate have different boiling points, or ranges of boiling point, and are collected in separate receivers.

Functional group
The smallest part of an organic molecule consisting of a single atom or group of atoms that substitutes for a hydrogen atom and has a profound effect upon the properties of the molecule as a whole.

Furanocoumarins
Derivatives of coumarins.

Gas liquid chromatography
An analytical technique for separating the constituents of a minute sample of a mixture of volatiles and recording the results of the analysis. The results of the analysis are recorded as a series of peaks, each one corresponding, with respect to its position, to a constituent of the sample.

GDV
Gas discharge visualisation. A biometric tool using Kilian photography, that can be used to capture the physiological and psychoemotional status of a person through electrophotonic emissions from the fingertips.

Genotoxic
An agent that damages cellular DNA, resulting in mutations or cancer.

GLC
see Gas liquid chromatography.

GMP
Good manufacturing practice.

GRAS
Generally recognized as safe.

GST
Glutathione S-transferase are a group of detoxification enzymes which use glutathione.

Gynaecomastia
Abnormal overdevelopment of the breasts in a male.

Headspace
The space bounded by the walls of a container, the closure and the surface of its contents.

Headspace analysis
Analysis done by GLC, of the gas or vapour present in a headspace.

Heartwood

The internal, non-living part of a woody stem, branch or trunk.

Hemiparasite

A parasitic plant that needs some or all of its nutritional requirements from another living plant.

Hepatotoxicity

Having a harmful of toxic effect on the liver.

Homeostasis

State of balance within the body; maintenance of body conditions within set limits.

Hormone

Secretion of an endocrine gland; chemical messenger that has specific regulatory effects on certain other cells.

Hydrocarbon

A compound composed of molecules consisting of atoms of carbon and hydrogen only.

Hydrolysis

The decomposition of a compound by water.

Hydrosol

Also known as floral water. The water that is recovered from the distillation process. Considered beneficial in skin care.

Hydroxyl group

The functional group –OH, present in water molecules and molecules of alcohols, and distinguished from the hydroxide ion by its electronic configuration and lack of negative charge.

Hypersensitivity

Exaggerated reaction of the immune system to a substance that is normally harmless to most people; allergy.

IARC

International agency for research on cancer.

IFOAM

International Federation of Organic Agriculture Movements.

IFRA

International Fragrance Research Association. A voluntary body, based in Switzerland, which advises the perfume industry on the safety of fragrance ingredients.

Inflammation

The production of redness, swelling, heat and pain in a tissue in response to chemical or physical injury, or an infection.

Infra-red spectroscopy

A spectroscopic instrumental technique measuring the absorption of infra-red radiation over a range of frequencies by molecules of a substance.

INFJ

Myers Briggs personality type – introverting, intuition, feeling, judging.

INFP

Myers Briggs personality type – introverting, intuition, feeling, perceiving.

Infused oil

Produced by the immersion of plant material in a vegetable oil, often gently heated to release aromatic constituents from the plant into the oil.

INTJ

Myers Briggs personality type – introverting, intuition, thinking, judging.

INTP

Myers Briggs personality type – introverting, intuition, thinking, perceiving.

In vitro

In an artificial environment, such as a test tube; not inside a living organism.

In vivo

Relates to biological processes or study occurring or conducted in the living organism.

ISFJ

Myers Briggs personality type – introverting, sensing, feeling, judging.

ISFP

Myers Briggs personality type – introverting, sensing, feeling, perceiving.

ISO

The International Organization for Standardisation.

Isomers

Compounds that have the same molecular formula but different structures and hence different properties.

Isoprene

The basic building unit of a group of chemicals called terpenes (2-methylbuta-1,3-diene), molecular formula C5H8.

ISTJ

Myers Briggs personality type – introverting, sensing, thinking, judging.

ISTP

Myers Briggs personality type – introverting, sensing, thinking, perceiving.

IUCN

International Union for Conservation of Nature.

Ketone

An organic compound characterised by the presence in its molecules of a carbonyl functional group bonded to two hydrocarbon radicals.

Lactone
An organic compound characterised by the presence in its molecules of an ester functional group as part of a ring system.

LD_{50}
Lethal dose 50%. It is a traditionally accepted method of determining toxicity. The value is the dosage required to kill 50% of the group of animals used in the test (usually rats or mice). LD_{50} values are usually expressed in grams of the toxic substance per kilogram of body weight.

Maceration
The process of allowing a definite weight of extractable matter to soak in a closed vessel for several days, in a definite weight of alcohol of given strength to produce a tincture.

MBC
Minimum bactericidal concentration.

Menopause
Time at which menstruation ceases.

MFC
Minimum fungicidal concentration.

MIC
Minimum inhibitory concentration.

Molecular formula
The formula expressing the true number of atoms of the different elements present in a molecule of a compound.

Monoterpene
A terpene of molecular formula C10H16.

MRSA
Methicillin-resistant Staphylococcus aureus.

MSSA
Methicillin-sensitive Staphylococcus aureus.

MSDS
Material safety data sheet

Narcotic
Substance that induces stupor and eventually unconsciousness. Can be used in the relief of severe pain.

Nature identical
Designates a synthetic organic compound of the same composition and molecular structure as the same compound as it occurs in nature.

Neurotoxic
Having a harmful or toxic effect on the nervous system.

Neurotransmitter
Chemical released from the ending of an axon that enables a nerve impulse to cross a synapse.

NO
Nitric oxide

Nucleus
In chemistry it refers to the positively, central body of an atom. In biology it is the dense, organised proteinaceous body found in the protoplasm of a plant or animal cell, containing hereditary material and controlling the metabolic activities of the cell.

Occlusions
The covering of the skin with an impermeable material which prevents evaporation of a volatile substance from the skin.

Odorant
A substance having an odour.

Odour
There is no accurate description of this term. It explains what an individual perceives via their nose as the scent of any material.

Odour threshold
The least concentration, or highest dilution, at which the odour of an odorant can be detected under standardised conditions.

Olfactory
Pertaining to the sense of smell.

Optical rotation
Angle through which the plane of polarisation of light is rotated when polarised light passes through a layer of liquid. Unless otherwise specified, the measurement is by sodium light in a 1 mm layer at 20°C. Essential oils may be dextrorotatory (+) or laevorotatory (-) according to whether the plane of polarisation is rotated to the left or right.

Organic chemistry
The study of the chemical behaviour of compounds of carbon, other than carbon containing ionic compounds such as carbonates and similar molecular compounds such as carbon dioxide.

Oxidation
The addition of oxygen to, or the removal of hydrogen or electrons from a molecule or atom. Also used as a general term indicating the changes in essential oil composition when exposed to air.

Oxide
A compound of oxygen with another element. The most commonly occurring oxide in essential oils is 1,8-cineole.

Pathogenic
Disease producing.

Percutaneous
By diffusion through the skin.

Peristalsis
Wavelike movements in the walls of an organ or duct that propel its contents forward.

pH
A measure of the acidity or alkalinity of an aqueous solution, expressed as a numerical value on a scale from 0 (extremely acidic) to 14.0 (extremely alkaline). A pH value of 7.0 expresses neutrality.

Phenols
The organic benzenoid compound C6H5OH or any other compound of which the molecules each have one or more hydroxy groups bonded directly to a benzene ring.

Phenyl propane derivatives
The name given to compounds of phenol that have a three-carbon-atom chain attached.

Pheromone
A chemical messenger used as a signal between individuals.

Photosynthesis
The manufacture of the sugar glucose in the leaves of a green plant from carbon dioxide and water in the presence of chlorophyll, using sunlight as a source of energy and with the evolution of oxygen.

PMS
Premenstrual syndrome.

Polar
A term used to describe a molecule which has a partial positive and negative charge. Polar molecules are generally water-soluble.

Polarised light
Light with a specific plane of polarisation.

Polarimeter
An instrument for measuring the optical rotation.

Polymorphism
The occurrence of more than one form of individual in a single species within an interbreeding population.

Pomade
Perfumed fat obtained as a result of enfleurage.

Positional isomer
An isomer that differs in respect of the position of the functional group in their molecules.

Prostaglandins
Group of hormones.

Proton
A positively charged particle of unit atomic mass, which occurs in the nuclei of all atoms.

QMS
Quality management system

Qi
A term used in traditional Chinese medicine and holistic therapies, referring to the life force.

Quorum sensing
Biofilm formation, virulence factors production, and resistance to antimicrobials are regulated by the quorum sensing process, a bacterial communication system.

Ramet
Sprouted from the single parent plant.

Rectification
The process in which an essential oil is distilled a second time to remove unwanted constituents (also known as redistillation).

Refractive index
Ratio of the velocity of light in a vacuum to its velocity in a substance. It varies with the wavelength of light used.

Refractometer
An instrument for measuring the refractive index.

Resinoid
An extract obtained from dried, natural, raw materials by use of non-aqueous solvents.

RIFM
Research Institute for Fragrance Materials. A voluntary organisation, based in the USA, for testing the safety of perfume ingredients.

Scarification
A process of scraping as used in the expression of citrus oils from the peel of the fruit.

Sesquiterpene
A terpene with the molecular formula $C_{15}H_{24}$. These constituents are based on 1½ terpene units.

Specific gravity
The ratio of the weight of a substance to the weight of an equal volume of water measured at a stated temperature.

Solvent
Hexane, petroleum ether, acetone or methanol, often used to extract essential oils from plant materials or their extracts.

Solvent extraction
Extraction by solvents.

Still
Any form of distillation equipment.

Still note
An unpleasant, vegetable-like note commonly found in freshly distilled essential oils, caused by the presence of organic sulphides. Still notes can be eliminated by brief aeration of the essential oils.

Synergy
The increased effect achieved by two or more substances working together. The effect of the whole is greater than the sum of its separate parts.

Taxonomy
The science of defining and naming groups or biological organisms on the basis of shared characteristics.

TCM
Traditional Chinese medicine.

Teratogenic effect

Leading to the production of foetal abnormalities.

Terpeneless oil
Essential oils from which the monoterpene hydrocarbons have been removed.

Terpenes
Naturally occurring unsaturated hydrocarbon compounds. They constitute a large number of compounds present in plants and essential oils.

Terpenoid
Essential oil constituents based on the isoprene skeleton, but containing a functional group.

TGA
Therapeutic Goods Administration

TNF
Tumour necrosis factor is a proinflammatory cytokine that is produced by white blood cells. It has an antineoplastic effect but causes inflammation.

Volatile oil
See essential oil.

WHO
World Health Organization

Appendix 2 • Properties

Abortifacient
An agent capable of inducing abortion.

Acaricidal
An agent that kills mites and ticks.

Alterative
An agent that cleanses the blood and corrects impure blood conditions.

Analgesic
An agent that relieves or diminishes pain.

Anaphrodisiac
An agent that reduces sexual desire.

Anthelmintic
An agent that destroys or expels intestinal worms.

Anti-allergenic
An agent that reduces the symptoms of allergies.

Antiangiogenic
An agent that can destroy or interfere with the fine network of blood vessels needed by tumours to grow and metastasize.

Anti-arthritic
An agent that combats arthritis.

Antibacterial
An agent that is capable of destroying or inhibiting the growth of bacteria.

Anticarcinogenic
An agent that neutralises the effects of a cancer-causing substance and can prevent or delay tumour formation.

Anticatarrhal
An agent that reduces the production of mucous.

Anticoagulant
An agent that can slow or prevent the clotting of blood.

Anticolitic
An agent that can reduce inflammation of the colon.

Anticonvulsive
An agent that arrests or controls convulsions.

Antidepressant
An agent that is uplifting and counteracts melancholy.

Antidiabetic
An agent that aids in blood glucose management or improves management of diabetes.

Anti-emetic
An agent that reduces the incidence and severity of vomiting.

Antiepileptic
An agent that is used to treat epileptic seizures, an anticonvulsant.

Antifungal
An agent capable of destroying or inhibiting the growth of fungi.

Antiglycation
An agent that prevents damage to proteins caused by sugar molecules. Glycation is a normal process of everyday metabolism; however, the rate of glycation determines the speed of the aging process.

Anti-inflammatory
An agent that alleviates inflammation.

Antimicrobial
An agent that resists or destroys pathogens.

Antinociceptive
An agent that reduces sensitivity to a painful stimulus.

Antioxidant
An agent that inhibits oxidation.

Antiphlogistic
An agent that reduces inflammation.

Antipruritic
An agent that relieves sensations of itching or prevents its occurrence.

Antirheumatic
An agent that helps to relieve rheumatism.

Antiseptic
An agent that destroys or controls pathogenic bacteria.

Antispasmodic
An agent that prevents and eases spasms and relieves cramps.

Antisudorific
An agent that reduces sweating.

Antitussive
An agent that relieves coughing.

Antiulcerogenic
An agent that prevents or reduces ulcers.

Antiviral
An agent that can destroy or inhibit the growth and reproduction of viruses.

Anxiolytic
An agent that is capable of reducing anxiety.

Aphrodisiac
An agent that provokes sexual interest and excitement.

Astringent
An agent that contracts, tightens and binds tissues.

Bactericide
An agent that destroy bacteria.

Balsamic
Usually applies to a resin – a soothing and healing agent.

Cardiac
An agent having a stimulating effect on the heart.

Cardioprotective
An agent that protects the heart from damage by toxins or ischaemia.

Carminative
An agent that settles the digestive system and the expulsion of gas from the intestines.

Cephalic
An agent that is stimulating and clears the mind.

Chemoprotective
An agent that reduces the incidence of cancer.

Cholagogue
An agent that increases the secretion and flow of bile production into the duodenum.

Choleretic
An agent that aids the excretion of bile by the liver, so that there is a greater flow of bile.

Cholinergic
An agent that mimics the action of acetylcholine or of the parasympathetic nervous system.

Cicatrisant
An agent that promotes the formation of scar tissue.

Convulsant
An agent that causes convulsions.

Cordial
An agent that is invigorating and stimulating.

Cytophylactic
An agent that encourages growth of skin cells.

Decongestant
An agent that relieves or reduces congestion.

Demulcent
An agent that soothes, softens and allays irritation of mucous membranes.

Deodorant
An agent that destroys or inhibits odours.

Depurative
An agent that helps to purify the body, particularly the blood.

Diaphoretic
An agent that promotes perspiration.

Digestive
An agent that aids the digestion of food.

Disinfectant
An agent that prevents and combats the spread of disease.

Diuretic
An agent that increases the secretion and expulsion of urine.

Emetic
An agent that induces vomiting.

Emmenagogue
An agent that promotes and regulates menstrual flow.

Emollient
An agent used externally to soothe and soften the skin.

Epileptogenic
An agent with the capacity to induce epilepsy.

Expectorant
An agent that expels mucus in the respiratory system.

Febrifuge
An agent that cools and reduces high body temperature.

Fungicide
An agent that destroys fungal infections.

Galactagogue
An agent that increases the secretion of milk.

Gastroprotective
An agent that protects the gastric mucosa from aggressive or irritating agents.

Germicidal
An agent that destroys germs or microorganisms.

Haemostatic
An agent that arrests bleeding and haemorrhage.

Hepatic
An agent that stimulates and aids function of the liver.

Hepatoprotective
An agent that is able to prevent damage to the liver.

Hypertensive
An agent that increases blood pressure.

Hypoglycaemic
An agent that lowers blood sugar levels.

Hypolipidaemic
An agent that can lower high levels of fats (lipids), such as cholesterol in the blood.

Hypnotic
An agent that produces sleep.

Hypotensive
An agent that lowers blood pressure.

Immunostimulant
An agent that stimulates the immune system.

Insecticide
An agent that kills insects.

Larvicide
An agent that kills larvae.

Laxative
An agent that aids bowel evacuation.

Miticide
An agent that kills mites.

Molluscicide
An agent that kills mollusks.

Mucolytic
An agent that dissolves or breaks down mucus.

Nervine
An agent that strengthens or tonifies the nerves and nervous system.

Neuroprotective
An agent that protects against neurotoxicity.

Nootropic
An agent that enhances or improves cognitive function.

Oestrogenic
An agent that stimulates the action of oestrogen.

Parasiticide
An agent that kills parasites.

Parturient
An agent that promotes labour and the delivery in childbirth.

Pediculicide
An agent that kills lice.

Prophylactic
An agent that prevents disease.

Refrigerant
An agent that lowers abnormal body heat.

Relaxant
An agent that causes relaxation of the mind or the body.

Rubefacient
An agent that is warming and increases blood flow.

Sedative
An agent that reduces nervousness, distress or agitation.

Soporific
An agent that induces sleep.

Spasmogenic
An agent that causes spasms.

Spasmolytic
An agent that reduces spasms or cramps.

Splenic
An agent that is a tonic to the spleen.

Stimulant
An agent that stimulates the physiological functions of the body.

Stomachic
An agent that is a digestive aid and tones the stomach.

Styptic
An agent that is astringent, especially preventing external bleeding.

Sudorific
An agent that promotes or increases perspiration.

Teratogenic
An agent that injures the fetus.

Tonic
An agent that strengthens and improves bodily performance.

Uterine
An agent that is a tonic to the uterus.

Vasoconstrictor
An agent that causes contraction of blood vessel walls.

Vasodilator
An agent that causes dilation of blood vessels.

Vermifuge
An agent that causes expulsion of worms.

Vulnerary
An agent that prevents tissue degeneration and promotes healing of wounds.

Appendix 3 • Essential oils

Common and botanical names, including plant family, part of plant used, origin of raw material and trade quantities of the essential oil.[1]

HQ – high quantities (> 1,000 t/a); MQ – medium quantities (100-1,000 t/a); LQ – low quantities (<100 t/a)

Common name	Botanical name	Plant family	Part of plant	Wild or cultivated	Trade quantities
Amyris	*Amyris balsamifera* L.	Rutaceae	Wood	Wild	LQ
Angelica root	*Angelica archangelica* L.	Apiaceae	Root	Cult	LQ
Aniseed	*Pimpinella anisum* L.	Apiaceae	Fruit	Cult/wild	LQ
Basil	*Ocimum basilicum* L.	Lamiaceae	Herb	Cult	LQ
Bay laurel	*Laurus nobilis* L.	Lauraceae	Leaf	Cult/wild	LQ
Bay, West Indian	*Pimenta racemosa* (Mill.) J.W. Moore	Myrtaceae	Leaf	Cult	LQ
Bergamot	*Citrus surantium* Risso et Poit	Rutaceae	Fruit peel	Cult	MQ
Black pepper	*Piper nigrum* L.	Piperaceae	Fruit	Cult	LQ
Buchu	*Agathosma betulina* (P.J Bergius) *Pillans; A. crenulata* (L.) Pillans	Rutaceae	Leaf	Wild	LQ
Cade	*Juniperus oxycedrus* L.	Cupressaceae	Wood	Wild	LQ
Cajeput	*Melaleuca cajuputi* Powell	Myrtaceae	Leaf	Wild	LQ
Camphor	*Cinnamomum camphora* L.	Lauraceae	Wood	Cult	LQ
Caraway	*Carum carvi* L.	Apiaceae	Seed	Cult	LQ
Cardamom	*Elettaria cardamomum* (L.) Maton	Zingiberaceae	Seed	Cult	LQ
Carrot seed	*Daucus carota* L.	Apiaceae	Fruit	Cult	LQ
Cedarwood, Atlas	*Cedrus atlantica* (Endl.) Manetti ex Carriere	Pinaceae	Wood	Wild	MQ
Cedarwood, Himalayan	*Cedrus deodara* (Roxb. Ex D.Don) G.Don	Pinaceae	Wood	Wild	MQ
Cedarwood, Texas	*Juniperus Mexicana* Schiede	Cupressaceae	Wood	Wild	MQ
Cedarwood, Virginian	*Juniperus virginiana* L.	Cupressaceae	Wood	Wild	MQ
Celery seed	*Apium graveolens* L.	Lamiaceae	Seed	Cult	LQ
Chamomile, German	*Matricaria recutita* L.	Asteraceae	Flower	Cult	LQ
Chamomile, Roman	*Anthemis nobilis* (L.) All.	Asteraceae	Flower	Cult	LQ
Cinnamon bark	*Cinnamomum verum J.Presl*	Lauraceae	Bark	Cult	LQ
Cinnamon leaf	*Cinnamomum verum J.Presl*	Lauraceae	Leaf	Cult	LQ
Citronella, Sri Lanka	*Cymbopogon nardus* L.	Poaceae	Leaf	Cult	HQ
Citronella, Java	*Cymbopogon winterianus* Jowitt.	Poaceae	Leaf	Cult	HQ
Clary sage	*Salvia sclarea* L.	Lamiaceae	Flowering herb	Cult	MQ
Clove bud	*Syzygium aromaticum* (L.) Mer. & L.M. Perry	Myrtaceae	Bud	Cult	LQ
Clove leaf	*Syzygium aromaticum* (L.) Mer. et L.M. Perry	Myrtaceae	Leaf	Cult	HQ
Coriander seed	*Coriandrum sativum* L.	Apiaceae	Fruit	Cult	LQ
Cornmint	*Mentha arvensis* L.	Lamiaceae	Leaf	Cult	HQ
Cumin	*Cuminum cyminum* L.	Apiaceae	Fruit	Cult	LQ
Cypress	*Cupressus sempervirens* L.	Cupressaceae	Leaf/twigs	Wild	LQ
Dill	*Anethum graveolens* L.	Apiaceae	Herb/fruit	Cult	LQ
Dill, India	*Anethum sowa* Roxb.	Apiaceae	Fruit	Cult	LQ
Elemi	*Canarium luzonicum* (Blume) A.Gray.	Burseraceae	Resin	Wild	LQ

Common name	Botanical name	Plant family	Part of plant	Wild or cultivated	Trade quantities
Eucalyptus, blue mallee	*Eucalyptus polybractea* R.T. Baker	Myrtaceae	Leaf	Cult/wild	HQ
Eucalyptus, lemon-scented	*Corymbia citriodora* Hook	Myrtaceae	Leaf	Cult/wild	HQ
Eucalyptus, peppermint	*Eucalyptus dives* Schauer	Myrtaceae	Leaf	Cult/wild	MQ
Everlasting	*Helichrysum angustifolium* (L.) DC.	Asteraceae	Flower	Cult/wild	LQ
Fennel, sweet	*Foeniculum vulgare* Mill.	Apiaceae	Fruit	Cult	LQ
Fir needle, Canadian	*Abies balsamea* (L.) Mill.	Pinaceae	Leaf/twig	Wild	LQ
Fir needle, Siberian	*Abies sibirica* Ledeb.	Pinaceae	Leaf/twig	Wild	LQ
Fragonia	*Agonis fragrans* J.R.Wheeler & N.G.Marchant	Myrtaceae	Leaf	Cult	LQ
Frankincense	*Boswellia spp.*	Burseraceae	Resin	Wild	MQ
Galbanum	*Ferula galbaniflua* Boiss.& Buhse	Apiaceae	Resin	Wild	LQ
Geranium	*Pelargonium* spp.	Geraniaceae	Leaf	Cult	MQ
Ginger	*Zingiber officinale* Roscoe	Zingiberaceae	Rhizome	Cult	LQ
Grapefruit	*Citrus x paradisa* Macf.	Rutaceae	Fruit peel	Cult	LQ
Guaiacwood	*Bulnesia sarmienti* Lorentz ex Griseb.	Zygophyllaceae	Wood	Wild	MQ
Hyssop	*Hyssopus officinalis* L.	Lamiaceae	Leaf	Cult	LQ
Jasmine absolute	*Jasminum grandiflorum* L.	Olreaceae	Flower	Cult	LQ
Juniper berry	*Juniperus communis* L.	Cupressaceae	Fruit	Wild	LQ
Kanuka	*Kunsea ericoides* (A.Rich.) Joy Thomps.	Myrtaceae	Leaf	Wild	LQ
Kunzea	*Kunsea ambigua* (Sm.) Druce	Myrtaceae	Leaf	Wild	LQ
Lavandin	*Lavendula angustifolia* Mill. x *L. latifolia* Medik.	Lamiaceae	Flowering tops	Cult	HQ
Lavender	*Lavendula angustifolia* Mill.	Lamiaceae	Flowering tops	Cult	MQ
Lavender, spike	*Lavendula latifolia* Medik.	Lamiaceae	Flowering tops	Cult	LQ
Lemon	Citrus limon (L.) Osbeck	Rutaceae	Fruit peel	Cult	HQ
Lemongrass, East Indian	*Cymbopogon flexuosus* (Nees ex Steud.) H.Wats.	Poaceae	Leaf	Cult	LQ
Lemongrass, West Indian	*Cymbopogon citratus* (DC.) Stapf	Poaceae	Leaf	Cult	LQ
Lemon myrtle	*Backhousia citriodora* F.Muell.	Myrtaceae	Leaf	Cult	LQ
Lime	*Citrus aurantifolia* (Christm.) Swingle	Rutaceae	Fruit peel	Cult	MQ
Mandarin	*Citrus reticulata* Blanco	Rutaceae	Fruit peel	Cult	MQ
Manuka	*Leptosperum scoparium* J.R. Forster & G. Forster	Myrtaceae	Leaf	Wild	LQ
Marjoram, sweet	*Origanum majorana* L.	Lamiaceae	Herb	Cult	LQ
May chang	*Litsea cubeba* (Lour.) Pers.	Lauraceae	Fruit/leaf	Cult	MQ
Melissa	*Melissa officinalis* L.	Lamiaceae	Leaf	Cult	LQ
Myrrh	*Commiphora myrrha* (Nees) Engl.	Burseraceae	Resin	Wild	LQ
Myrtle	*Myrtus communis* L.	Myrtaceae	Leaf	Cult/wild	LQ
Neroli	*Citrus x aurantium* L.	Rutaceae	Flower	Cult	LQ
Niaouli	*Melaleuca quinquenervia* (Cav.) S.T. Blake	Myrtaceae	Leaf	Cult/wild	LQ
Nutmeg	*Myristica fragrans* Houtt.	Myristicaceae	Seed	Cult	LQ
Oakmoss absolute	*Evernia prunastri* L.	Usneaceae	Lichen	Wild	LQ
Opopanax	*Commiphora guidottii* Chiov.	Burseraceae	Resin	Wild	LQ
Orange, sweet	*Citrus sinensis* (L.) Osbeck	Rutaceae	Fruit peel	Cult	HQ
Oregano	*Origanum* ssp.	Lamiaceae	Herb	Cult/wild	LQ

Common name	Botanical name	Plant family	Part of plant	Wild or cultivated	Trade quantities
Palmarosa	*Cymbopogon martini* (Roxb.) W Watson	Poaceae	Leaf	Cult	LQ
Parsley seed	*Petroselinum crispum* (Mill.) Fuss	Apiaceae	Fruit	Cult	LQ
Patchouli	*Pogostemon cablin* (Blanco) Benth.	Lamiaceae	Leaf	Cult	HQ
Pennyroyal	*Mentha pulegium* L.	Lamiaceae	Leaf	Cult	LQ
Peppermint	*Mentha x piperita* L.	Lamiaceae	Leaf	Cult	HQ
Petitgrain	*Citrus* x *aurantium* L.	Rutaceae	Leaf	Cult	LQ
Pine needle	*Pinus silvestris* L.	Pinaceae	Leaf/twig	Wild	LQ
Ravinstara	*Cinnamomum camphora* L.	Lauraceae	Flower	Cult/Wild	LQ
Rosalina	*Melaleuca ericifolia* Smith	Myrtaceae	Leaf	Cult/Wild	LQ
Rose	*Rosa* x *damascena* Miller	Rosaceae	Flower	Cult	LQ
Rosemary	*Rosmarinus officinalis* L.	Lamiaceae	Herb	Cult/wild	LQ
Rosewood	*Aniba rosaeodora* Ducke	Lauraceae	Wood	Wild	LQ
Sage, Dalmation	*Salvia officinalis* L.	Lamiaceae	Herb	Cult/wild	LQ
Sage, Spanish	*Salvia lavandulifolia* L.	Lamiaceae	Herb	Cult/wild	LQ
Sandalwood	*Santalum album* L.	Santalaceae	Wood	Cult/wild	LQ
Sandalwood, Australian	*Santalum spicatum* A. DC.	Santalaceae	Wood	Wild	LQ
Sandalwood, New Caledonian	*Santalum austrocaledonicum Viell.*	Santalaceae	Wood	Wild	LQ
Savory	*Satureja hortensis* L.; *Satureja montana* L.	Lamiaceae	Leaf	Cult/wild	LQ
Spearmint	*Mentha spicata* L.	Lamiaceae	Leaf	Cult	MQ
Spikenard	*Nardostachys jatamansi* DC	Valerianaceae	Root	Wild	LQ
Spruce, black	*Picea mariana* (Mill.) *Britton*	Pinaceae	Needles	Cult/wild	LQ
Tagetes	*Tagetes patula* L; *Tagetes erecta* L.	Asteraceae	Herb	Cult	LQ
Tangerine	*Citrus reticulata* Blanco var. tangerine	Rutaceae	Fruit peel	Cult	MQ
Tarragon	*Artemisia dracunculus* L.	Asteraceae	Herb	Cult	LQ
Tea tree	*Melaleuca alternifolia* Cheel	Myrtaceae	Leaf	Cult	LQ
Tea tree, lemon scented	*Leptospermum petersonii* F.M. Bailey	Myrtaceae	Leaf	Cult	LQ
Thyme	*Thymus vulgaris* L.	Lamiaceae	Herb	Cult	LQ
Tuberose absolute	*Polianthese tuberosa* L.	Agavaceae	Flower	Cult	LQ
Turmeric	*Curcuma longa* L.	Zingiberaceae	Rhizome	Cult	LQ
Valerian	*Valeriana officinalis* L.	Valerianaceae	Root	Cult	LQ
Verbena	*Aloysia triphylla* (L'Her) Britton	Verbenaceae	Herb	Cult	LQ
Vetiver	*Vetiveria zizanoides* L. Nash	Poaceae	Root	Cult	MQ
Wintergreen	*Gaultheria procumbens* L.	Ericaceae	Leaf	Wild	LQ
Ylang ylang	*Cananga odorata* Hook. F.et Thoms.	Annonaceae	Flower	Cult	MQ

Reference

1. Franz C, Novak J. *Sources of essential oils,* from *Handbook of essential oils – science, technology and applications.* 2nd edn, Baser KHC, Buchauer G. eds, CRC Press, Boca Raton, 2016. Pages 43-86.

Appendix 4 • A typical material safety data sheet

MSDS:
Date of Issue: 25/01/2018

1. IDENTIFICATION

Product Name: **Juniperberry Essential Oil**

Manufacturer's Product Code:

Company:
Address:
Telephone Number:

Emergency Telephone Number: In Australia: 13 1126 (Poisons Information Centre)

2. HAZARDS IDENTIFICATION

This material is classified as: **HAZARDOUS, DANGEROUS GOOD**.

3. COMPOSITION/INFORMATION ON INGREDIENTS

Dangerous Goods Class and Subsidiary Risk:	Class 3
UN Number:	1993
Hazchem Code:	3[Y]E
Poisons Schedule Number:	Not applicable
Packing Group:	II

Chemical Name	**CAS Number**
Juniperberry Essential Oil	8002-68-4

4. FIRST AIDS MEASURES

Health Effects:

Acute:	None under normal conditions of use.
Swallowed:	Capable of causing irritation.
Eye:	Capable of causing irritation.
Skin:	Undiluted oil is capable of causing irritation.
Inhaled:	None under normal conditions of use.

First Aid:

Swallowed:	Immediately remove from the mouth, rinse and give water to effectively dilute the product. Contact a doctor, or the Poisons Information Centre in your capital city for further advice (in Australia phone 13 1126).
Eye:	Irrigate with copious amounts of water for at least 15 minutes and seek medical attention if effects persist.
Skin:	Remove contaminated clothing. Wash affected areas.
Inhaled:	Not applicable.
Advice to Doctor:	Treat symptomatically.

5. FIRE FIGHTING MEASURES

Flash Point:	41°C
Extinguishing Media:	CO_2, dry powder, foam
Special Measures:	Use standard fire fighting procedures
Extinguishing Procedures:	When heated to decomposition, produces acrid smoke and fumes.
Packing Group:	II

6. ACCIDENTAL RELEASE MEASURES

Personal Precautions:	Avoid inhalation and direct contact with skin and eyes. Use individual protective equipment in case of major spillages.
Environmental Precautions:	Keep away from drains, soils, surface and ground water.
Cleaning Up Method:	Remove all potential ignition sources. Contain spilled material. Cover.
For Spillage:	Wipe small spills with cloth. Absorb larger spills with sand, sawdust or similar porous material. Sweep up and transfer to an approved disposal container.

7. HANDLING AND STORAGE

Storage and Transport:	Store in a cool, dry place away from sunlight, strong oxidising agents, naked flames and points of ignition. Transport as per local government regulations.
Precautions in Handling:	Apply good manufacturing practice, ensuring good ventilation. Observe good personal hygiene and do not eat, drink or smoke whilst handling.
Fire Protection:	Keep away from ignition sources and naked flame.

8. EXPOSURE CONTROL/PERSONAL PROTECTION

Respiratory Protection:	Avoid breathing product vapour. Apply local ventilation where possible.
Ventilation:	Ensure good ventilation of work area.
Hand Protection:	Avoid all skin contact. Use chemically resistant gloves if required.
Eye Protection:	Use safety glasses.
Work/Hygiene Practices:	Wash hands with soap and water after handling.

9. PHYSICAL AND CHEMICAL PROPERTIES

Physical Description:	Clear, colourless to pale yellow mobile liquid with a fresh, warm, rich balsamic, woody-sweet, pine-needle like odour.
Flash Point:	41°C

10. STABILITY AND REACTIVITY

Reactivity:	No significant reactivity hazards by itself or in contact with water. Avoid contact with strong acids, alkali, or oxidising agents.
Decomposition:	Liable to cause smoke and acrid fumes during decomposition.

11. TOXICOLOGICAL INFORMATION

No information available.

12. ECOLOGICAL INFORMATION

Biodegradability:	Not available
Precautions:	Prevent surface contamination of soil, ground and surface water.

13. DISPOSAL CONSIDERATION

Avoid disposing to drainage system and into the environment. Seek expert advice.

14. TRANSPORT INFORMATION

Road (ADR/RID):	Class 3 Packing Group II
Air (IATA):	Class 3 Packing Group II
Sea (IMDG):	Class 3 Packing Group II

15. REGULATORY INFORMATION

Hazards:	Harmful, irritant, dangerous to the environment
Symbols:	Xn, Xi, N
Risk Phrases:	R10 Flammable liquid
	R20/22 Harmful by inhalation and if swallowed.
	R36/37/38 Irritating to eyes, respiratory system and skin.
	R41 Risk of serious damage to eyes.
	R43 May cause sensitisation by skin contact.
	R50/53 Very toxic to aquatic organisms; cause long term adverse effects in the aquatic environment.
	R65 Harmful: May cause lung damage if swallowed.
Safety Phrases:	S2 Keep out of reach of children.
	S16 Keep away from sources of ignition - no smoking.
	S23 Do not breathe vapours.
	S24/25 Avoid contact with skin and eyes.
	S26 In case of contact with eyes, rinse immediately with plenty of water and seek medical advice.
	S27 Take all contaminated clothes off immediately.
	S28 After contact with skin, wash immediately with plenty of soap and water.
	S37/39 Wear suitable gloves and eye/face protection.
	S46 If swallowed, seek medical advice immediately and show this container or label.
	S51 Use in well ventilated areas only.
	S61 Avoid release into the environment.
	S62 If swallowed, do not induce vomiting, seek medical advice immediately and show the container or label.

16. OTHER INFORMATION

Disclaimer: The information contained in this Material Safety Data Sheet has been compiled from data considered to be accurate. The data is believed to be reliable, however it must be noted that due to the nature of the product, values for certain properties can vary depending upon the source of the material.

Perfect Potion disclaims any liability for any injury or loss arising from the use of this information or the materials described. It is the responsibility of the user to determine the appropriate precautions for safe handling based on their application.

Appendix 5 • Summary of cautions and contraindications

Contraindications in aromatherapy are likely to create debate. The following list should be used as a guide for the safe use of essential oils. Essential oils that are not commonly available have not been listed in this appendix.

Never to use - essential oils that may be toxic to use in aromatherapy

Dweck states that the following essential oils are considered dangerous in aromatherapy:[1]

> almond (bitter, unrectified) contains hydrocyanic acid; boldo leaf contains ascaridole; calamus contains β-asarone; camphor brown & camphor yellow contain safrole; fig leaf absolute; horseradish contains allyl isocyanate; lanyana contains thujones; *Melaleuca bracteata* contains very high methyl eugenol; mustard contains allyl isocyanate; parsley herb contains apiole; pennyroyal contains pulegone; perilla contains perrilla ketone; savin contains sabinyl acetate; sassafras contains safrole; tansy contains thujone; white wormwood and wormwood contain thujones; wormseed contains ascaridole.

Tisserand & Young state that there are no essential oils that are considered extremely toxic or very toxic. They list the following essential oils as being moderate oral toxins:[2]

> almond (bitter, unrectified), boldo, calamus (tetraploid form), Himalayan cedarwood, pennyroyal, thuja, white wormwood, wormseed.

Tisserand & Young state that the following essential oils are considered moderate dermal toxins:[2]

> boldo, cassia, cinnamon bark, savory, oregano and rose absolute.

The only reason that rose absolute is listed is because of its possible methyl eugenol content. The IFRA states that the maximum dermal use of rose absolute should be 0.012%.[2] Please note that not all rose absolutes contain methyl eugenol.

Essential oils that are dermal irritants

Essential oils that are considered to have a high risk of dermal irritation at a range of 0 to 0.1% include:[2]

> horseradish, mustard, massoia.

I recommend that these oils not be used in aromatherapy.

Essential oils that are considered to have a moderate risk of dermal irritation at a range of 0.2 to 1.0% include:[2]

> immortelle absolute, wild mountain sage, garlic.

I recommend that these oils be used with extreme care in aromatherapy.

Essential oils that are considered to have a low risk of dermal irritation at a range of 1.1 to 20% include:[2]

> ajowan, oregano, wild marjoram, Mexican oregano, winter savory, thyme ct. carvacrol, thyme ct. thymol, summer savory, thyme ct. limonene, thyme ct. borneol, Siberian fir, dwarf pine.

I recommend that these oils be used with care in aromatherapy.

Essential oils that are dermal sensitisers

Essential oils that are considered high-risk dermal sensitisers at a range of 0 to 0.1% include:[2]

> costus, elecampane, fig leaf absolute, massoia, saffron absolute, lavandin or lavender absolute, cassia, cinnamon bark, oakmoss absolute, tree moss absolute.

I recommend that these oils not be used in aromatherapy.

Essential oils that are considered moderate-risk dermal sensitisers at a range of 0.2 to 1.0% include:[2]

> tea leaf absolute, lemon verbena absolute, clary sage absolute, ginger lily absolute, Peru balsam, clove bud, cinnamon leaf, clove leaf, clove stem, opopanax, styrax, jasmine absolute, lemon myrtle, lemongrass, wild mountain sage, exotic basil, may chang, narcissus, lemon scented tea tree, ylang ylang, cananga, melissa and lemon verbena.

I recommend that these oils be used with extreme care on people with sensitive, diseased or damaged skin.

Essential oils that are considered low-risk dermal sensitisers at a range of 1.1 to 20.0% include:[2]

> lemon leaf, lemon basil, spearmint, benzoin resinoid, tolu balsam resinoid, basil ct. linalool, lemon thyme, jasmine sambac absolute, palmarosa, tea tree, geranium, citronella, catnip and perilla.

I recommend that these oils be used with care on people with sensitive, diseased or damaged skin.

Essential oils not to use with anticoagulant medication

Sweet birch and wintergreen oils should not be taken in any form by individuals on warfarin (an anticoagulant).[2]

Tisserand & Young state that the following oils should not be taken in oral doses by individuals taking aspirin, heparin or warfarin:[2]

> ajowan, aniseed, aniseed myrtle, anise (star), basil ct. estragole, basil (holy), bay (West Indian), betel, birch (sweet), cassia, cinnamon bark, cinnamon leaf, clove bud, clove leaf, clove stem, cornmint, fennel (bitter), fennel (sweet), garlic, lavandin, leek, marjoram (wild), onion, oregano, oregano (Mexican), patchouli, pimento berry, pimento leaf, ravensara bark, savory, tarragon, thyme ct. borneol, thyme (thymol & carvacrol ct.), wintergreen.

Epilepsy

Based on data presented by Tisserand & Young the following oils are potential convulsants when used dermally or orally:[2]

> western red cedar, all wormwood oils, buchu, calamint, hyssop ct. pinocamphone; sage (Dalmatian), pennyroyal, thuja.

There is no safe oral dose for these oils. I would recommend that people with epilepsy do not use these oils.

The following oils are considered to be potential convulsants at a very low dermal limit (2.5% or less):[2]

> birch (sweet), boldo, tansy, all mugwort oils, ho leaf ct. camphor, tansy, wintergreen.

I recommend that people with epilepsy do not use these oils.

The following oils all contain camphor as a constituent and are considered to be potential convulsant essential oils:[2]

> rosemary ct. camphor, rosemary ct. verbenone, yarrow ct. chamazulene, Spanish lavender, Spanish sage, spike lavender.

These essential oils may stimulate an epileptic seizure in people who have epilepsy, therefore I would recommend that people with epilepsy exercise caution when using these essential oils.

High blood pressure

Davis recommends that the following essential oils should not be used by anyone suffering from high blood pressure:[3]

> hyssop, rosemary (no chemotype specified), sage (Dalmatian).

However, Tisserand & Young state that some essential oils may be a risk for some classes of hypertension, and it may be prudent to exercise some caution in certain cases of hypertension. They state that until we know more about the risks, these should be no case for contraindication of any essential oils.[2]

I would exercise caution using any of the above essential oils for people suffering from hypertension or people taking medications for hypertension.

Photosensitisation

The following essential oils are known to be phototoxic:[1,2]

> angelica root, bergamot, cumin, fig leaf absolute, grapefruit, lemon (expressed), lime (expressed), opopanax, orange (bitter, expressed), rue, tagetes.

If the above oils have been used topically, do not expose the skin to sunlight or sunbed rays for 12 hours.

Pregnancy

The following essential oils should be avoided by any route throughout pregnancy and lactation:[1,2]

> aniseed, star anise, aniseed myrtle, sweet birch, buchu ct. diosphenol, buchu ct. pulegone, carrot seed, cassia, cinnamon bark, costus, blue cypress, Indian dill seed, sweet fennel, bitter fennel, ho leaf ct. camphor, hyssop ct. pinocamphone, Spanish lavender, mugwort, myrrh, oregano, parsley leaf, parsley seed, pennyroyal, rue, Dalmatian sage, Spanish sage, savin, tansy, thuja, Western red cedar, wintergreen, wormwood.

Davis recommends that the following essential oils should not be during pregnancy:[1]

> basil, birch, atlas cedarwood, clary sage, cypress, hyssop, jasmine, juniper berry, sweet marjoram, myrrh, peppermint, rosemary, tarragon, thyme.

References

1. Dweck AC. *Toxicology of essential oils reviewed*. Personal Care, 2009; 65-77.
2. Tisserand R, Young R. *Essential oil safety*. 2nd edn, Churchill Livingstone, Edinburgh, 2014.
3. Davis P. *Aromatherapy: A-Z*. 2nd ed. C.W. Daniel Company, Saffron Walden, 1999.

Appendix 6 • Useful addresses

The following details are correct at the time of publication.

Aromatherapy associations

Australia

IAAMA – International Aromatherapy and Aromatic Medicine Association
https://wwwiaama.org.au

Canada

CCFA – Canadian Federation of Aromatherapy
www.cfacanada.com

BCAPA – British Columbia Association of Practicing Aromatherapists
https:/www.bcapa.org

Japan

The Aroma Environment Association of Japan
English website – http://www.aromakankyo.or.jp/english/aeaj.html
Japanese website – http://www.aromakankyo.or.jp/

Japanese Society of Aromatherapy
English website – http://aroma-jsa.jp/english/index.html
Japanese website – http://aroma-jsa.jp/index.html

Korea

KAEAS – The Korean Association of Essential Oils, Aroma and Spa
www.kaeas.com

New Zealand

NZROHA – New Zealand Register of Holistic Aromatherapists
www.aromatherapy.org.nz

South Africa

AromaSA – The Aromatherapy Association of South Africa
http://aromasa.org.za

United Kingdom

IFA – The International Federation of Aromatherapists
www.ifaroma.org

IFPA – International Federation of Professional Aromatherapists
https://ifpaaroma.org

USA

AIA – Alliance of International Aromatherapists
http://www.alliance-aromatherapists.org

NAHA – National Association of Holistic Aromatherapy
https://naha.org

Essential oil suppliers

To ensure you are buying the best quality essential oils available, choose a supplier that is able to meet the criteria outline for quality assurance and quality control specified in this book. Please refer to Chapter 5.

Essential oil research database

An extensive aromatherapy research database has been developed by Bob Harris of Quintessential Aromatics. Once you have subscribed you are able to search two databases. The first is the bioactivity database which allows you to search by essential oil, by year, by author or title of the research paper. The second is the component database which allows you to search on essential oil constituents.

http://www.quintessential.uk.com/

Aromatherapy journals

Aromatherapy Today

Aromatherapy Today is an international aromatherapy journal published in Australia for those who are passionate about aromatherapy. It is a progressive journal that keeps you informed with the latest information and research being undertaken within aromatherapy.

For more details go to
http://www.aromatherapytoday.com/

The International Journal of Clinical Aromatherapy

The *International Journal of Clinical Aromatherapy* (IJCA) is dedicated to practitioners working with essential oils in healthcare and related professions. Th IJCA is dedicated to those healthcare professionals who require a source of evidence-based information in a professional format. Two issues are published per year (June and December), and since 2014 the IJCA is only available in e-format. It is edited by Rhiannon Lewis and Gabriel Mojay.

For more details go to https//ijca.net/

Botanical Index

General Index